AF324161

CURRENT THERAPY IN GENITOURINARY SURGERY

SURGICAL TITLES IN THE CURRENT THERAPY SERIES

CURRENT THERAPY IN GENITOURINARY SURGERY

SECOND EDITION

MARTIN I. RESNICK, M.D.

Lester Persky Professor and Chief
Division of Urology
Case Western Reserve University
School of Medicine
Cleveland, Ohio

ELROY D. KURSH, M.D.

Associate Professor
Division of Urology
Case Western Reserve University
School of Medicine
Cleveland, Ohio

B.C. Decker
An Imprint of Mosby–Year Book

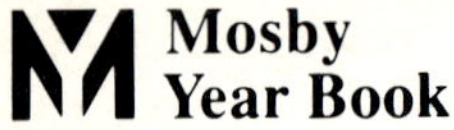

Mosby
Year Book

Dedicated to Publishing Excellence

Publisher: George Stamathis
Senior Managing Editor: Lynne Gery
Project Supervisor: Arofan Gregory

SECOND EDITION

Copyright © 1992 by Mosby–Year Book, Inc.
A B.C. Decker imprint of Mosby–Year Book, Inc.

All rights reserved. No part of this publication may be reproduced,
stored in a retrieval system, or transmitted, in any form or by any
means, electronic, mechanical, photocopying, recording, or otherwise,
without prior written permission from the publisher.

Previous edition copyrighted 1987

Printed in the United States of America

Mosby–Year Book, Inc.
11830 Westline Industrial Drive
St. Louis, MO 63146

Permission to photocopy or reproduce solely for internal or personal use is
permitted for libraries or other users registered with the Copyright Clearance
Center, provided that the base fee of $4.00 per chapter plus $.10 per page is
paid directly to the Copyright Clearance Center, 27 Congress Street, Salem, MA
01970. This consent does not extend to other kinds of copying, such as copying for
general distribution, for advertising or promotional purposes, for creating new collected
works, or for resale.

Current therapy in genitourinary surgery/[edited by] Martin
  I. Resnick, Elroy D. Kursh—2nd ed.
      p. cm. — (Current therapy series)
  Includes bibliographical references and index.
  ISBN 1-55664-350-0
  1. Genitourinary organs—Surgery. I. Resnick, Martin I.
II. Kursh, Elroy D. III. Series.
  [DNLM: 1. Urogenital Neoplasms—surgery. 2. Urogenital System—
surgery. WJ 168 C9765]
  RD571.C88 1992
  6174´6059—dc20
  DNLM/DLC   91-28435
  for Library of Congress   CIP

92 93 94 95 96 GW/MY/MY 9 8 7 6 5 4 3 2 1

CONTRIBUTORS

JØRN AAGAARD, M.D.

Former Fellow, Division of Urology, University of Wisconsin School of Medicine, Madison, Wisconsin

MARK C. ADAMS, M.D.

Assistant Professor of Urology, Indiana University School of Medicine, Indianapolis, Indiana

PAUL E. ANDREWS, M.D.

Fellow in Urology, Mayo Graduate School of Medicine, Rochester, Minnesota

GERALD L. ANDRIOLE, M.D.

Associate Professor of Urologic Surgery, Washington University School of Medicine, St. Louis, Missouri

ARMEN G. APRIKIAN, M.D.

Fellow, Urologic Surgery, Memorial Sloan-Kettering Cancer Center, New York, New York

DEAN G. ASSIMOS, M.D.

Associate Professor of Surgery (Urology), Bowman Gray School of Medicine of Wake Forest University, Winston-Salem, North Carolina

R. BREWER AULD, M.D., M.B., FRCSC

Associate Professor, Department of Urology, Dalhousie University Faculty of Medicine; Staffman, Department of Urology, Camp Hill Medical Centre, Halifax, Nova Scotia, Canada

SAID A. AWAD, M.B., FRCSC

Professor and Head, Department of Urology, Dalhousie University; Head, Department of Urology, Active Staff, Victoria General Hospital, Halifax, Nova Scotia, Canada

R. JOSEPH BABAIAN, M.D.

Professor of Urology, The University of Texas M. D. Anderson Cancer Center, Houston, Texas

RICHARD K. BABAYAN, M.D.

Professor of Urology, Boston University School of Medicine, Boston, Massachusetts

ROBERT A. BADALAMENT, M.D.

Assistant Professor, Division of Urology, The Ohio State University College of Medicine, Columbus, Ohio

NEIL H. BANDER, M.D.

Associate Professor of Surgery/Urology, New York Hospital-Cornell Medical Center; Department of Surgery (Urology) and Department of Medicine (Clinical Immunology), Memorial Sloan-Kettering Cancer Center, New York, New York

LILLY BARBA, M.D.

Transplant Physician, Department of Nephrology, Harbor-UCLA Medical Center, Torrance, California

JOSEPH G. BARONE, M.D.

Resident in Urology, Robert Wood Johnson Medical School, University of Medicine and Dentistry of New Jersey, New Brunswick, New Jersey

DAVID M. BARRETT, M.D.

Professor and Chair, Department of Urology, Mayo Medical School, Rochester, Minnesota

GEORG BARTSCH, M.D.

Professor, Department of Urology, University of Innsbruck, Innsbruck, Austria

STUART B. BAUER, M.D.

Associate Professor of Surgery (Urology), Harvard Medical School; Associate in Surgery (Urology), The Children's Hospital, Boston, Massachusetts

JOHN A. BELIS, M.D.

Professor of Urology, The Pensylvania State University College of Medicine, Hershey, Pennsylvania

ARNOLD M. BELKER, M.D.

Clinical Professor, Division of Urology, Department of Surgery, University of Louisville School of Medicine, Louisville, Kentucky

MARK F. BELLINGER, M.D.

Associate Professor of Urologic Surgery, University of Pittsburgh School of Medicine; Chief, Pediatric Urology, The Childrens Hospital of Pittsburgh, Pittsburgh, Pennsylvania

A. BARRY BELMAN, M.D., M.S. (Urology)

Professor of Urology and Pediatrics, George Washington University School of Medicine; Chairman; Department of Urology, Childrens Hospital, Washington, D.C.

ALAN H. BENNETT, M.D.

Professor of Surgery (Urology), Albany Medical College; Head, Division of Urological Surgery, Albany Medical Center, Albany, New York

MITCHELL C. BENSON, M.D.

Herbert Irving Assistant Professor of Urology, Columbia University College of Physicians and Surgeons; Director, Urologic Oncology, J. Bentley Squier Urological Clinic, Columbia-Presbyterian Medical Center, New York, New York

JERRY G. BLAIVAS, M.D.

Professor and Vice-Chairman, Department of Urology, Columbia University College of Physicians and Surgeons, New York, New York

DAVID A. BLOOM, M.D.

Associate Professor of Surgery, University of Michigan Medical School, Ann Arbor, Michigan

DONALD R. BODNER, M.D.

Assistant Professor of Surgery (Urology), Case Western Reserve University School of Medicine, Cleveland, Ohio

STUART D. BOYD, M.D.

Associate Professor of Urology, University of Southern California School of Medicine, Los Angeles, California

R. BRUCE BRACKEN, M.D.

Professor and Director, Division of Urology, University of Cincinnati Medical Center, Cincinnati, Ohio

MICHAEL K. BRAWER, M.D.

Associate Professor, Department of Urology, University of Washington School of Medicine; Chief, Section of Urology, Seattle Veterans Affairs Medical Center, Seattle, Washington

CHARLES B. BRENDLER, M.D.

Associate Professor of Urology, The Johns Hopkins University School of Medicine, Baltimore, Maryland

PETER N. BRETAN, Jr., M.D.

Assistant Professor in Residence, Department of Surgery, Division of Urology, University of California Los Angeles School of Medicine, Los Angeles; Director of Surgical Transplantation and Assistant Chief of Urology, Harbor-UCLA Medical Center, Torrance, and Director of Surgical Transplantation, Saint Mary Medical Center, Long Beach, California

WILLIAM A. BROCK, M.D., F.A.C.S., F.A.A.P.

Professor of Urology, Albert Einstein College of Medicine; Chief, Division of Pediatric Urology, Schneider Children's Hospital, Long Island Jewish Medical Center, New York, New York

STANLEY A. BROSMAN, M.D.

Clinical Professor of Surgery (Urology), University of California Los Angeles School of Medicine, Los Angeles, California

REGINALD BRUSKEWITZ, M.D.

Associate Professor of Surgery, Division of Urology, University of Wisconsin School of Medicine, Madison, Wisconsin

ANTON J. BUESCHEN, M.D.

Professor and Director, Department of Surgery, Division of Urology, University of Alabama School of Medicine, Birmingham, Alabama

JOHN R. BURNS, M.D.

Professor of Urology, University of Alabama School of Medicine; Attending Physician, Veterans Administration Medical Center, Birmingham, Alabama

ANTHONY A. CALDAMONE, M.D., F.A.C.S., F.A.A.P.

Associate Professor of Surgery (Urology), Brown University Program in Medicine; Chief of Pediatric Urology Rhode Island Hospital, Providence, Rhode Island

EDWARD W. CAMPBELL, Jr., M.D.

Associate Professor of Urology, University of Maryland School of Medicine; Consulting Urologist, Loch Raven Veterans Hospital, Baltimore, Maryland

CULLEY C. CARSON, M.D.

Professor of Urology, Duke University Medical Center, Durham, North Carolina

H. BALLENTINE CARTER, M.D.

Assistant Professor, Department of Urology, The Johns Hopkins University School of Medicine, Baltimore, Maryland

MICHAEL F. CARTER, M.D.

Chief of Staff, Northwestern Memorial Hospital, Chicago, Illinois

PATRICK C. CARTWRIGHT, M.D.

Assistant Professor of Surgery and Pediatrics, University of Utah School of Medicine; Staff, Primary Children's Medical Center, Salt Lake City, Utah

ALEXANDER S. CASS, M.B.B.S., F.R.C.S.

Associate Professor, University of Minnesota Medical School; Staff Urologist, Hennepin County Medical Center, Minneapolis, Minnesota

J. ROBERT CASSADY, M.D.

Professor and Head, Department of Radiation Oncology, University of Arizona Health Sciences Center, Tucson, Arizona

PARAMJIT S. CHANDHOKE, M.D.

Dornier/American Foundation for Urologic Disease Scholar and Instructor, Division of Urologic Surgery, Washington University School of Medicine, St. Louis, Missouri

BERNARD M. CHURCHILL, M.D., FRCSC

Professor of Urology, University of Toronto Faculty of Medicine; Chief, Division of Urology, Hospital for Sick Children, Toronto, Ontario, Canada

RALPH V. CLAYMAN, M.D.

Professor of Urologic Surgery and Radiology, Washington University School of Medicine, St. Louis, Missouri

MARC S. COHEN, M.D.

Associate Professor of Surgery (Urology), University of Florida College of Medicine; Attending Urologist, University of Florida Associated Hospitals and Shands Teaching Hospital, and Staff Physician, Gainesville Veterans Administration Hospital, Gainesville, Florida

E. DAVID CRAWFORD, M.D.

Professor and Chairman, Division of Urology, University of Colorado School of Medicine, Denver, Colorado

KENNETH B. CUMMINGS, M.D., F.A.C.S.

Professor of Surgery and Chief, Division of Urology, Robert Wood Johnson Medical School, University of Medicine and Dentistry of New Jersey, New Brunswick, New Jersey

CHARLES J. DEVINE, Jr., M.D.

Professor of Urology, Eastern Virginia Medical School, Norfolk, Virginia

CHRISTOPHER M. DIXON, M.D.

Assistant Professor of Urology, Medical College of Wisconsin, Milwaukee, Wisconsin

JOHN P. DONOHUE, M.D.

Distinguished Professor and Chairman of Urology, Indiana University School of Medicine, Indianapolis, Indiana

JOSEPH R. DRAGO, M.D.

Chief, Division of Urology, Louis Levy Professor of Cancer, Director of Urologic Oncology, and Professor, Department of Surgery, The Ohio State University College of Medicine, Columbus, Ohio

MICHAEL J. DROLLER, M.D.

Professor and Chairman, Department of Urology, Mount Sinai School of Medicine of the City University of New York; Attending Physician, Department of Urology, Mount Sinai Medical Center, New York, New York

JOHN W. DUCKETT, M.D.

Professor of Urology and Surgery, University of Pennsylvania School of Medicine; Chief of Urology, Children's Hospital of Philadelphia, Philadelphia, Pennsylvania

JACK S. ELDER, M.D.

Associate Professor of Urology and Pediatrics, Case Western Reserve University School of Medicine; Director of Pediatric Urology, Rainbow Babies and Children's Hospital, Cleveland, Ohio

OTMAR ENNEMOSER, M.D.

Department of Urology, University of Innsbruck, Innsbruck, Austria

DEBORAH R. ERICKSON, M.D.

Fellow in Urology, Center for Health Sciences, University of California Los Angeles School of Medicine, Los Angeles, California

MARC S. ERNSTOFF, M.D.

Associate Professor of Medicine, Dartmouth Medical School; Associate Professor of Medicine, Dartmouth-Hitchcock Medical Center, Hanover, New Hampshire

MAJID ESHGHI, M.D., F.A.C.S.

Associate Professor of Urology, New York Medical College; Chief, Section of Endo-Urology, Westchester County Medical Center, Valhalla, New York

WILLIAM R. FAIR, M.D.

Professor of Surgery (Urology), Cornell University Medical College; Chief, Urologic Surgery Service, and Vice Chairman, Academic Affairs, Memorial Sloan-Kettering Cancer Center, New York, New York

JEFF FEGAN, M.D.

Fellow in Mineral Metabolism, University of Texas Southwestern Medical Center at Dallas, Dallas, Texas

CASIMIR F. FIRLIT, M.D., Ph.D.

Professor of Urology, Northwestern University School of Medicine; Chairman, Division of Urology, and Head of Renal Transplantation, Children's Memorial Hospital, Chicago, Illinois

HUGH A. G. FISHER, M.D., F.A.C.S.

Associate Professor of Surgery (Urology), Albany Medical College; Attending Urologist, Albany Medical Center Hospital, Albany, New York

JOHN M. FITZPATRICK, M.Ch., F.R.C.S.I.

Professor of Surgery, University College, Dublin; Consultant Urologist, Mater Misericordiae Hospital, Dublin, Ireland

ROBERT C. FLANIGAN, M.D., F.A.C.S.

Professor and Chairman, Department of Urology, Loyola University Medical Center, Maywood, Illinois

JONATHAN FLEISCHMANN, M.D., M.M.S., F.A.C.S.

Assistant Professor of Surgery (Urology), Case Western Reserve University School of Medicine, Cleveland, Ohio

L. SUZANNE FLOM, M.D.

Attending Pediatric Urologist, Children's Memorial Hospital, Chicago, Illinois

RICHARD S. FOSTER, M.D.

Assistant Professor of Urology, Indiana University School of Medicine, Indianapolis, Indiana

JACKSON E. FOWLER, Jr., M.D.

Professor and Chairman, Division of Urology, University of Mississippi School of Medicine; Professor and Chairman, Division of Urology, University of Mississippi Medical Center and Veterans Administration Medical Center, Jackson, Mississippi

FLOYD A. FRIED, M.D.

John S. Rhodes Professor of Surgery and Chief of Urology, University of North Carolina at Chapel Hill School of Medicine, Chapel Hill, North Carolina

EUGENE F. FUCHS, M.D.

Professor of Surgery (Urology), Oregon Health Sciences University, Portland, Oregon

JERZY B. GAJEWSKI, M.D., FRCSC

Assistant Professor, Department of Urology, Dalhousie University Faculty of Medicine; Staffman, Department of Urology, Camp Hill Medical Centre, Halifax, Nova Scotia

GLEN S. GERBER, M.D.

Resident in Urology, University of Chicago Medical School, Chicago, Illinois

ROBERT P. GIBBONS, M.D., F.A.C.S.

Clinical Professor of Urology, University of Washington School of Medicine; Head, Section of Urology and Renal Transplantation, Virginia Mason Clinic, Seattle, Washington

MARTIN E. GLEAVE, M.D., FRCSC

Fellow, Department of Urology, The University of Texas M. D. Anderson Cancer Center, Houston, Texas

JAMES F. GLENN, M.D., F.A.C.S., F.R.C.S. (HON.)

Professor of Surgery, University of Kentucky College of Medicine; Attending Surgeon, University of Kentucky Medical Center, Lexington, Kentucky

DAVID A. GOLDFARB, M.D.

AFUD-Bard Scholar and Clinical Associate, Department of Urology, Cleveland Clinic Foundation, Cleveland, Ohio

MARC GOLDSTEIN, M.D.

Associate Professor of Surgery, Cornell University School of Medicine, New York, New York

SAM D. GRAHAM, Jr., M.D.

Associate Professor of Surgery (Urology), Emory University School of Medicine; Chief, Division of Urology, Emory Clinic, Atlanta, Georgia

JOHN T. GRAYHACK, M.D.

Herman L. Kretschmer Professor of Urology,
Northwestern University Medical School; Chief
of Urology, Northwestern Memorial Hospital,
Chicago, Illinois

H. BARTON GROSSMAN, M.D.

Professor, Department of Surgery, Section of Urology,
University of Michigan Medical School; Director of
Urologic Oncology Program, Cancer Center, University
of Michigan Medical Center, Ann Arbor, Michigan

W. GRAHAM GUERRIERO, M.D.

Professor of Urology, Baylor College of Medicine;
Director of Abdominal Organ Transplantation and
Director of Urodynamics Laboratory, The Methodist
Hospital, Houston, Texas

GABRIEL P. HAAS, M.D.

Assistant Professor, Department of Urology, Wayne
State University School of Medicine, Detroit, Michigan

THOMAS HAKALA, M.D.

Professor and Chief, Urologic Surgery and Renal
Transplantation, Department of Surgery, University of
Pittsburgh School of Medicine, Pittsburgh, Pennsylvania

NEHEMIA HAMPEL, M.D., F.A.C.S.

Associate Professor of Urology, Case Western Reserve
University School of Medicine; Chief, Section of Urology, Veterans Affairs Medical Center, Cleveland, Ohio

PHILIP M. HANNO, M.D.

Professor and Chairman, Department of Urology,
Temple University School of Medicine, Philadelphia,
Pennsylvania

LLOYD H. HARRISON, M.D.

Professor of Surgical Sciences (Urology), Bowman Gray
School of Medicine of Wake Forest University; Staff,
North Carolina Baptist Hospital and Forsyth Memorial
Hospital, Winston-Salem, North Carolina

CHARLES L. HEATON, M.D.

Professor of Dermatology, University of Cincinnati
College of Medicine, Cincinnati, Ohio

TERRY W. HENSLE, M.D.

Director of Pediatric Urology, Babies' Hospital,
Columbia-Presbyterian Medical Center, New York,
New York

FRANK HINMAN, Jr., M.D.

Clinical Professor of Urology, University of California
San Francisco School of Medicine, San Francisco,
California

ANNE-MARIE HOULE, M.D., FRCSC

Assistant Professor, McGill University Faculty of
Medicine; Staff, Division of Urology, Montreal
Children's Hospital, Montreal, Quebec, Canada

JEFFRY L. HUFFMAN, M.D.

Associate Professor of Urology, University of Southern
California School of Medicine, Los Angeles, California

WILLIAM C. HULBERT, Jr., M.D., F.A.A.P.

Assistant Professor of Urologic Surgery and Pediatrics,
University of Rochester School of Medicine, Rochester,
New York

JOHN J. HUTTER, Jr., M.D.

Chief, Section of Pediatric Hematology/Oncology, and
Director, Clinical Pediatric Oncology, University of
Arizona Health Sciences Center, Tucson, Arizona

JEFFREY M. IGNATOFF, M.D., F.A.C.S.

Associate Professor of Clinical Urology, Northwestern
University Medical School; Senior Attending Physician
and Head, Urologic Oncology, Evanston Hospital,
Evanston, Illinois

KENDALL A. ITOKU, M.D.

Chief Resident, Department of Surgery (Urology),
Brown University Program in Medicine, Providence,
Rhode Island

STEPHEN C. JACOBS, M.D.

Professor and Chairman, Division of Urology University
of Maryland School of Medicine; Chief of Urology,
University of Maryland Medical Systems, Baltimore,
Maryland

GÜNTER JANETSCHEK, M.D.

Assistant Professor, Department of Urology, University
of Innsbruck, Innsbruck, Austria

JONATHAN P. JAROW, M.D.

Assistant Professor of Urology, Bowman Gray School
of Medicine of Wake Forest University, Winston-Salem,
North Carolina

GERALD H. JORDAN, M.D.

Associate Professor of Urology, Eastern Virginia
Medical School, Norfolk, Virginia

DAVID B. JOSEPH, M.D.

Assistant Professor of Surgery (Urology), University of
Alabama at Birmingham School of Medicine; Chief of
Pediatric Urology, The Children's Hospital of Alabama,
Birmingham, Alabama

LAURENCE B. KANDEL, M.D.

Assistant Professor of Urology, State University of New York at Stony Brook School of Medicine; Director, Long Island Kidney Stone Unit, Stony Brook, New York

GEORGE W. KAPLAN, M.D., M.S.

Clinical Professor of Surgery and Pediatrics and Chief of Pediatric Urology, University of California at San Diego School of Medicine; Chief of Urology, Children's Hospital, San Diego, California

WILLIAM E. KAPLAN, M.D.

Associate Professor of Urology, Northwestern University School of Medicine; Director of Neurologic Urology, Northwestern Memorial Medical Center and Children's Memorial Hospital, and Attending in Pediatric Urology, Children's Memorial Hospital, Chicago, Illinois

ROBERT KAY, M.D.

Head, Section of Pediatric Urology, Cleveland Clinic Foundation, Cleveland, Ohio

MITCHELL C. KAYE, M.D.

Resident, Department of Urology, Cleveland Clinic Foundation, Cleveland, Ohio

RAJA B. KHAULI, M.D.

Director, Transplantation Services; Associate Professor of Surgery (Urology) and Physiology, University of Massachusetts Medical Center, Worcester, Massachusetts

ANTOINE E. KHOURY, M.D., FRCSC

Assistant Professor, University of Toronto Faculty of Medicine; Staff, Division of Urology, Hospital for Sick Children, Toronto, Ontario, Canada

LOWELL R. KING, M.D.

Professor of Urology and Associate Professor of Pediatrics, Duke University School of Medicine; Head, Section on Pediatric Oncology, Duke University Medical Center, Durham, North Carolina

ERIC A. KLEIN, M.D.

Staff, Department of Urology, Cleveland Clinic Foundation, Cleveland, Ohio

BARRY A. KOGAN, M.D.

Associate Professor of Urology and Pediatrics, and Chief, Pediatric Urology Service, University of California San Francisco School of Medicine, San Francisco, California

MARTIN A. KOYLE, M.D., F.A.A.P., F.A.C.S.

Associate Professor of Surgery (Urology), University of Colorado Health Sciences Center; Chief of Pediatric Urology, The Children's Hospital, Denver, Colorado

R. LAWRENCE KROOVAND, M.D.

Professor of Surgery (Pediatric Urology) and Pediatrics, and Head, Section on Pediatric, Adolescent, and Reconstructive Urology, Bowman Gray School of Medicine of Wake Forest University, Winston-Salem, North Carolina

KENNETH A. KROPP, M.D.

Professor of Surgery and Pediatrics, and Chairman, Division of Urology, Medical College of Ohio, Toledo, Ohio

SANJAYA KUMAR, M.D.

Resident, Division of Urology, University of Massachusetts Medical Center, Worcester, Massachusetts

ELROY D. KURSH, M.D.

Associate Professor of Surgery (Urology), Case Western Reserve University School of Medicine, Cleveland, Ohio

DONALD L. LAMM, M.D., F.A.C.S.

Professor and Chairman, Department of Urology, West Virginia University School of Medicine, Morgantown, West Virginia

PAUL H. LANGE, M.D.

Professor and Chairman, University of Washington School of Medicine, Seattle, Washington

MICHAEL J. LEMMERS, M.D.

Chief Resident in Urology, Oregon Health Sciences University, Portland, Oregon

HERBERT LEPOR, M.D.

Professor, Department of Urology, Medical College of Wisconsin, Milwaukee, Wisconsin

STEPHEN B. LEVINE, M.D.

Professor of Psychiatry, Case Western Reserve University School of Medicine; Medical Director, Center for Human Sexuality, University Hospitals of Cleveland, Cleveland, Ohio

GARY LIESKOVSKY, M.D.

Associate Professor of Urology, University of Southern California School of Medicine, Los Angeles, California

W. MARSTON LINEHAN, M.D.

Associate Professor of Surgery, Uniformed Services University of the Health Sciences; Head, Urologic Oncology Section, Surgery Branch, Division of Cancer Therapy, National Cancer Institute, National Institutes of Health, Bethesda, Maryland

LARRY I. LIPSHULTZ, M.D.

Professor of Urology, Scott Department of Urology, Baylor College of Medicine, Houston, Texas

STEFAN A. LOENING, M.D., F.A.C.S.

Professor of Urology, University of Iowa School of Medicine, Iowa City, Iowa

TOM F. LUE, M.D.

Associate Professor, Department of Urology, University of California San Francisco School of Medicine; Attending Physician, University of California Hospitals, San Francisco, California

BERNARD LYTTON, M.B., F.R.C.S.

Donald Guthrie Professor of Surgery and Professor of Surgery (Urology), Yale University School of Medicine; Attending Physician, Yale-New Haven Hospital, New Haven, Connecticut

REZA S. MALEK, M.D., M.S., FRCSC, F.A.C.S.

Professor of Urology, Mayo Medical School; Consultant, Department of Urology, Mayo Clinic and Mayo Foundation, Rochester, Minnesota

JAMES MANDELL, M.D.

Associate Professor of Surgery (Urology), Harvard Medical School; Associate in Surgery, Children's Hospital, Boston, Massachusetts

MICHAEL MARBERGER, M.D.

Professor of Urology and Chief, Department of Urology, Krankenstalt Rudolfstiftung, Vienna, Austria

JACK W. McANINCH, M.D.

Professor of Urology, University of California San Francisco School of Medicine; Chief of Urology, San Francisco General Hospital, San Francisco, California

JAMES G. McCOY, M.D.

Resident, Department of Urology, University of Iowa Hospitals and Clinics, Iowa City, Iowa

DAVID L. McCULLOUGH, M.D.

Professor and Chairman, Department of Urology, Bowman Gray School of Medicine of Wake Forest University, Winston-Salem, North Carolina

EDWARD J. McGUIRE, M.D.

Professor and Section Head, Section of Urology, and Associate Chairman, Department of Surgery, University of Michigan Medical School, Ann Arbor, Michigan

GORDON A. McLORIE, M.D., FRCSC

Assistant Professor, University of Toronto Faculty of Medicine; Staff, Division of Urology, Hospital for Sick Children, Toronto, Ontario, Canada

KEVIN T. McVARY, M.D.

Assistant Professor of Urology, Northwestern University Medical School; Attending Urologist, Northwestern Memorial Hospital, Chicago, Illinois

WINSTON K. MEBUST, M.D.

Professor of Surgery (Urology) and Chairman, Section of Urology, University of Kansas Medical Center, Kansas City, Kansas

MANI MENON, M.D.

Chairman, Division of Urologic and Transplantation Surgery, and Professor of Surgery and Physiology, University of Massachusetts Medical Center, Worcester, Massachusetts

EDWARD M. MESSING, M.D.

Associate Professor of Surgery and Human Oncology, and Chief of Urologic Oncology, University of Wisconsin Medical School, Madison, Wisconsin

ELI K. MICHAELS, M.D.

Assistant Professor, Division of Urology, University of Illinois College of Medicine at Chicago, Chicago, Illinois

GREGOR MIKUZ, M.D.

Professor and Chairman, Department of Pathology, University of Innsbruck, Innsbruck, Austria

D. FRANKLIN MILAM, M.D.

Emeritus Professor of Urology, West Virginia School of Medicine, Morgantown, West Virginia

JAMES L. MOHLER, M.D.

Assistant Professor of Surgery (Urology), and Director of Urologic Oncology, University of North Carolina at Chapel Hill School of Medicine, Chapel Hill, North Carolina

DROGO K. MONTAGUE, M.D.

Head, Section of Prosthetic Surgery, Department of Urology, and Director, Center for Sexual Function, Cleveland Clinic Foundation, Cleveland, Ohio

JAMES E. MONTIE, M.D.

Chairman, Department of Urology, Cleveland Clinic Florida, Ft. Lauderdale, Florida

PHILLIP F. NASRALLAH, M.D.

Associate Professor of Urology, Northeastern Ohio Universities College of Medicine; Chief, Division of Urology, Children's Hospital Medical Center, Akron, Ohio

PETER T. NIEH, M.D.

Senior Staff Urologist, Lahey Clinic Medical Center, Burlington, Massachusetts

JOHN C. NORBECK, M.D.

Fellow, Pediatric and Reconstructive Urology, Taubman Medical Center, Ann Arbor, Michigan

ANDREW C. NOVICK, M.D.

Chairman, Department of Urology, Cleveland Clinic Foundation, Cleveland, Ohio

ROBERT D. OATES, M.D.

Assistant Professor of Urology, Boston University School of Medicine, Boston, Massachusetts

CARL A. OLSSON, M.D.

Professor and Chairman, Department of Urology, Columbia University College of Physicians and Surgeons, New York, New York

CHARLES Y. C. PAK, M.D.

Distinguished Chair in Mineral Metabolism, University of Texas Southwestern Medical Center at Dallas, Dallas, Texas

ANGELO S. PAOLA, M.D.

Resident in Urology, Department of Urology, West Virginia University School of Medicine, Morgantown, West Virginia

PAUL C. PETERS, M.D.

Professor and E. E. and Greer Garson Fogelson Distinguished Chair in Urology, University of Texas Southwestern Medical Center at Dallas, Dallas, Texas

STEVEN P. PETROU, M.D.

Senior Associate Consultant, Mayo Clinic Jacksonville, Jacksonville, Florida

RONALD R. PFISTER, M.D., F.A.A.P., F.A.C.S.

Professor of Surgery and Pediatrc Urology, University of Colorado School of Medicine, Denver, Colorado

J. EDSON PONTES, M.D.

Professor and Chairman, Department of Urology, Wayne State University School of Medicine, Detroit, Michigan

KEVIN PRANIKOFF, M.D.

Associate Professor of Urology, State University of New York at Buffalo School of Medicine; Clinical Director of Urology, Erie County Medical Center, Buffalo, New York

GLENN M. PREMINGER, M.D.

Associate Professor of Urology, Radiology, and Internal Medicine, University of Texas Southwestern Medical Center at Dallas, Dallas, Texas

RONALD RABINOWITZ, M.D., F.A.A.P., F.A.C.S.

Professor of Urologic Surgery and Pediatrics, University of Rochester School of Medicine; Chief of Pediatric Urology, Strong Memorial Hospital, Chief of Urology, Rochester General Hospital, and Attending Pediatric Urologist, University of Rochester Children's Disability Center, Rochester, New York

LESLIE M. RAINWATER, M.D.

Chief Resident Associate in Urology, Mayo Graduate School of Medicine, Rochester, Minnesota

SHLOMO RAZ, M.D.

Professor of Surgery (Urology), University of California Los Angeles School of Medicine, Los Angeles, California

MARTIN I. RESNICK, M.D.

Lester Persky Professor and Chief, Division of Urology, Case Western Reserve University School of Medicine, Cleveland, Ohio

ALAN B. RETIK, M.D.

Professor of Surgery (Urology), Harvard Medical School; Chief, Division of Urology, Children's Hospital, Boston, Massachusetts

THOMAS J. ROHNER, Jr., M.D.

Professor of Surgery (Urology), The Pennsylvania State University College of Medicine; Chief, Division of Urology, Milton S. Hershey Medical Center, Hershey, Pennsylvania

NICHOLAS A. ROMAS, M.D.

Professor of Clinical Urology, Columbia University College of Physicians and Surgeons; Director of Urology, St. Luke's-Roosevelt Hospital Center, New York, New York

STEVEN A. ROSENBERG, M.D., Ph.D.

Staff, Surgery Branch, National Cancer Institute, National Institutes of Health, Bethesda, Maryland

GILBERT ROSS, Jr., M.D.

Professor of Surgery (Urology), University of Missouri-Columbia School of Medicine, Columbia, Missouri

JONATHAN ROSS, M.D.

Fellow in Pediatric Urology, Children's Hospital of Michigan, Detroit, Michigan

JONATHAN H. ROSS, M.D.

Chief Resident, Department of Urology, Cleveland Clinic Foundation, Cleveland, Ohio

A. M. SASSINE, M.D.

Resident in Urology, University Clinics of Brussels, Brussels, Belgium

IHOR S. SAWCZUK, M.D.

Assistant Professor of Urology, Columbia University College of Physicians and Surgeons; Assistant Attending, Columbia-Presbyterian Medical Center, New York, New York

PETER N. SCHLEGEL, M.D.

Assistant Professor of Urology, Cornell University Medical College, and Staff Scientist, Center for Biomedical Research, The Population Council; Assistant Attending Surgeon, The New York Hospital, New York, New York

CLAUDE C. SCHULMAN, M.D., Ph.D.

Professor of Urology, University of Brussels; Chief, Department of Urology, Erasme University Hospital, and Department of Pediatric Urology, Children's University Hospital, Brussels, Belgium

DAVID M. SCHWALB, M.D.

Urology Fellow, Memorial Sloan-Kettering Cancer Center, New York, New York

STEVEN H. SELMAN, M.D., F.A.C.S.

Professor of Surgery (Urology), and Director of Urologic Research, Medical College of Ohio, Toledo, Ohio

ELLEN SHAPIRO, M.D.

Associate Professor of Urology and Pediatrics, Medical College of Wisconsin; Pediatric Urologist, Children's Hospital of Wisconsin, Milwaukee, Wisconsin

JOEL SHEINFELD, M.D.

Assistant Attending Surgeon, Urology Service, Memorial Sloan-Kettering Cancer Center, New York, New York

STEVEN W. SIEGEL, M.D.

Head, Section of Female Urology and Urodynamics, Department of Urology, Cleveland Clinic Foundation, Cleveland, Ohio

DONALD G. SKINNER, M.D.

Professor and Chief, Department of Urology, University of Southern California School of Medicine, Los Angeles, California

EILA C. SKINNER, M.D.

Assistant Professor of Urology, University of Southern California School of Medicine, Los Angeles, California

ARTHUR D. SMITH, M.D.

Professor of Urology, Albert Einstein College of Medicine of Yeshiva University, Bronx; Chairman, Department of Urology, Long Island Jewish Medical Center, New Hyde Park, New York

ROBERT B. SMITH, M.D.

Professor of Surgery (Urology), University of California Los Angeles School of Medicine; Chief of Urology, Wadsworth Veterans Affairs Medical Center, Los Angeles, California

OLOF E. SOHLBERG, M.D.

Resident, University of Washington School of Medicine, Seattle, Washington

R. ERNEST SOSA, M.D.

Assistant Professor of Surgery (Urology), The New York Hospital-Cornell University Medical Center, New York, New York

J. PATRICK SPIRNAK, M.D.

Associate Professor, Division of Urology, Case Western Reserve University School of Medicine; Director of Urology, MetroHealth Medical Center, Cleveland, Ohio

THOMAS H. STANISIC, M.D.

Professor of Surgery (Urology), University of Arizona Health Sciences Center, Tucson, Arizona

BARRY S. STEIN, M.D., F.A.C.S.

Chairman and Professor, Division of Urology, Brown University Program in Medicine; Surgeon-in-Chief, Department of Urology, Rhode Island Hospital, Providence, Rhode Island

RALPH A. STRAFFON, M.D.

Associate Clinical Professor of Surgery
(Urology), Case Western Reserve University School of
Medicine; Chief of Staff, Cleveland Clinic Foundation,
Cleveland, Ohio

STEVAN B. STREEM, M.D.

Staff, Department of Urology, Cleveland Clinic
Foundation, Cleveland, Ohio

RAY E. STUTZMAN, M.D.

Associate Professor of Urology, The Johns Hopkins
University School of Medicine; Chief, Division of
Urology, The Francis Scott Key Medical Center,
Baltimore, Maryland

ERNEST M. SUSSMAN, M.D.

Fellow in Urology, Center for Health Sciences,
University of California Los Angeles School of
Medicine, Los Angeles, California

EMIL A. TANAGHO, M.D.

Professor and Chairman, Department of Urology,
University of California San Francisco School of
Medicine, San Francisco, California

EDWARD S. TANK, M.D.

Professor of Surgery and Pediatrics, Oregon Health
Sciences University, Portland, Oregon

RODNEY J. TAYLOR, M.D., F.A.C.S.

Associate Professor of Surgery and Chief, Section of
Urologic Surgery, University of Nebraska Medical
Center, Omaha, Nebraska

ANTHONY J. THOMAS, Jr., M.D.

Head, Section on Male Infertility, Department of
Urology, Cleveland Clinic Foundation, Cleveland, Ohio

J. BRANTLEY THRASHER, M.D.

Chief Resident in Urology, Fitzsimons Army Medical
Center, Aurora, Colorado

RALPH J. TORRENCE, M.D.

Clinical Instructor, Division of Urology, Department of
Surgery, Washington University School of Medicine,
St. Louis, Missouri

E. DARRACOTT VAUGHAN, Jr., M.D.

James J. Colt Professor of Urology, The New York
Hospital-Cornell University Medical Center,
New York, New York

ANDREW C. von ESCHENBACH, M.D.

Professor and Chairman, Department of Urology, The
University of Texas M. D. Anderson Cancer Center,
Houston, Texas

R. DIXON WALKER, M.D.

Professor of Surgery and Pediatrics, University of
Florida College of Medicine; Chief of Pediatric
Urology, Shands Hospital, Gainesville, Florida

PATRICK C. WALSH, M.D.

David Hall McConnell Professor and Director,
Department of Urology, The Johns Hopkins University
School of Medicine, Baltimore, Maryland

McCLELLAN M. WALTHER, M.D.

Senior Investigator, Urologic Oncology Section,
National Institutes of Health, Bethesda, Maryland

GARY R. WALTON, M.D.

Resident in Urology, Columbia University College of
Physicians and Surgeons and J. Bentley Squire
Urological Clinic, Columbia-Presbyterian Medical
Center, New York, New York

W. BEDFORD WATERS, M.D.

Associate Professor of Urology, Loyola University of
Chicago Stritch School of Medicine, Maywood, Illinois

ALAN J. WEIN, M.D.

Professor and Chairman, Division of Urology,
University of Pennsylvania School of Medicine; Chief of
Urology, Hospital of the University of Pennsylvania,
Philadelphia, Pennsylvania

JEFFREY N. WEISS, M.D.

Chief Resident, Department of Urology, Long Island
Jewish Medical Center, New Hyde Park, New York

EARL F. WENDEL, M.D.

Associate Professor of Clinical Urology, Northwestern
University Medical School; Attending Physician,
Northwestern Memorial Hospital, Chicago, Illinois

IHN SEONG WHANG, M.D.

Resident in Urology, Columbia University College of
Physicians and Surgeons and J. Bentley Squire
Urological Clinic, Columbia-Presbyterian Medical
Center, New York, New York

RICHARD D. WILLIAMS, M.D.

Professor and Head, Department of Urology, University
of Iowa College of Medicine, Iowa City, Iowa

TIMOTHY G. WILSON, M.D.

Instructor in Urology, University of Southern California School of Medicine, Los Angeles; Surgeon, Department of Urology and Urologic Oncology, City of Hope National Medical Center, Duarte, California

CHI-REI YANG, M.D.

Chief, Division of Urology, Department of Surgery, Taichung General Hospital, Taichung City, Taiwan, Republic of China

MICHAEL J. YOUNG, M.D.

Chief Resident, Department of Urology, Loyola University Medical Center, Maywood, Illinois

AUGUST ZABBO, M.D.

Assistant Professor, Division of Urology and Division of Biology and Medicine, Brown University Program in Medicine; Chief of Urology, Providence Veterans Affairs Hospital, Providence, Rhode Island

HORST ZINCKE, M.D.

Professor of Urology, Mayo Medical School; Consultant, Departments of Urology and Surgery, Mayo Clinic and Foundation, Rochester, Minnesota

ADRIAN W. ZORGNIOTTI, M.D.

Professor of Clinical Urology, New York University School of Medicine, New York, New York

Vicki, Andy, and Jeff

Dee, Matt, and Francie

All would agree that urologic practice is changing rapidly. Associated with these changes is the increasing availability of options for both diagnosing and treating specific disorders. In many instances, controversy tends to be the norm and "standard practice" is becoming increasingly gray. Obviously, when one is faced with a clinical problem, a single decision must be made regarding a particular approach. It was with this thought in mind that *Current Therapy in Genitourinary Surgery* was conceived.

The monograph is a compilation of opinions, thoughts, and practices of many experts in the field. Each contributor was asked to address a specific topic and to explain his or her particular approach. Justification is often provided but is not necessary. References are purposely omitted because it is the intent of the editors to have the authors express their opinion based solely on their own experience. With this basic information it is anticipated that the reader will be able to follow the recommendations of the author or, if disagreement exists, use this recommendation to decide on other approaches.

This second edition of *Current Therapy in Genitourinary Surgery* is essentially a new book. Though many authors of the first edition have also contributed to this one, their assignments were different and repetition of chapters by the same author is at a minimum. Authors have given their assigned topics much thought and consideration and have described their own treatment preferences. Many are recognized experts in the treatment of the specific clinical problems they were asked to discuss and have devoted much of their professional careers to these particular areas. We are greatly indebted to them for their efforts.

Our thanks and appreciation go to B.C. Decker, Mosby–Year Book, and particularly to our editor, Mr. William Lamsback, who has worked so closely with us. We also extend our thanks to Mrs. Barbara Goldberg, who has been so helpful in collating all manuscripts and maintaining a friendly dialogue with our many authors and with our publisher.

Martin I. Resnick, M.D.
Elroy D. Kursh, M.D.

CONTENTS

CURRENT THERAPY IN
GENITOURINARY SURGERY

BENIGN AND MALIGNANT TUMORS OF THE GENITOURINARY TRACT

ADRENAL GLANDS

CUSHING'S SYNDROME AND CUSHING'S DISEASE

RALPH A. STRAFFON, M.D.

In 1932, Harvey Cushing described a syndrome characterized by weakness, central obesity, cutaneous striae, plethora, diabetes mellitus, hypertension, and osteoporosis. He believed it represented a disorder of the pituitary gland that he called "pituitary basophilism." The findings were later established as secondary to excessive production of cortisol by the adrenal cortex.

Three basic problems may cause Cushing's syndrome:

1. Excess production of adrenocorticotropic hormone (ACTH) by the pituitary gland. This may be caused by increased production of cortisol-releasing factor (CRF) by the hypothalamus, by ACTH-secreting microadenomas of the pituitary gland, and in rare cases, by an obvious basophilic or chromophobe adenoma of the pituitary gland. Approximately 70 percent of patients with Cushing's syndrome have Cushing's disease.
2. An extra-adrenal ACTH-producing tumor, the most common being oat cell carcinomas of the lung, thymic tumors, and islet cell tumors of the pancreas. These extra-adrenal ACTH-producing tumors account for 5 to 10 percent of cases of Cushing's syndrome.
3. Primary tumors of the adrenal cortex, either benign adenomas or malignant adenocarcinomas, which account for 20 to 25 percent of cases of Cushing's syndrome.

DIFFERENTIAL DIAGNOSIS

The differential diagnosis in Cushing's syndrome is made by a series of laboratory studies. All patients with Cushing's syndrome have a high serum cortisol level with loss of normal circadian rhythm of cortisol secretion (Table 1). Low doses of dexamethasone (0.5 mg orally 4 times daily for 2 days) will suppress serum cortisol levels

Table 1 Differential Diagnosis of Cushing's Syndrome

All patients with a high serum cortisol level should undergo the dexamethasone suppression test (low dose and high dose)
Cortisol output suppressed
Cushing's disease producing bilateral adrenal hyperplasia
Cortisol output not suppressed, then measure ACTH level
High ACTH level—extra-adrenal ACTH-producing tumor
Low ACTH level—primary adrenal cortical tumor

in healthy subjects, but will not suppress cortisol levels to normal in patients with Cushing's syndrome. If a low dose of dexamethasone is not effective, a high dose of dexamethasone (2 mg orally 4 times daily for 2 days) should be administered, which will suppress serum cortisol levels to normal in patients with bilateral adrenal hyperplasia due to Cushing's disease. Those patients in whom a high dose of dexamethasone does not suppress serum cortisol levels usually have a primary adrenal tumor or an extra-adrenal ACTH-producing tumor.

The ACTH level should then be measured. If it is low, ACTH production is being suppressed by the cortisol produced by an adrenal tumor. If it is high, ACTH production is being produced by an extra-adrenal source. Unusually high levels of cortisol are frequently seen in patients with malignant tumors of the adrenal cortex. The free cortisol level in urine is usually elevated, as are the metabolites of cortisol (e.g., 17 hydroxycorticosteroid). In patients exhibiting virilism, the 17-ketosteroids are usually elevated.

THERAPEUTIC ALTERNATIVES

Once the diagnosis of Cushing's syndrome is made, treatment should ensue, since the 5-year survival rate of patients with untreated Cushing's syndrome is about 50 percent. The plan of treatment obviously depends on an accurate, differential diagnosis of the cause of Cushing's syndrome.

Treatment of Patients with Cushing's Disease

If a pituitary tumor is identified, either by x-ray studies of the sella turcica or by high-resolution computed tomography (CT) scanning of the pituitary gland, the initial treatment of choice in most centers is hypophysectomy. Large pituitary tumors, such as a chromophobe adenoma, producing visual field defects and other neurologic signs should be removed surgically. Open hypophysectomy, usually requiring the transfrontal approach, is used for these larger tumors. Transsphenoidal hypophysectomy is the treatment of choice for patients with normal pituitary glands or those containing microadenomas. This procedure is successful in correcting the hypercortisolism in 85 percent of patients with microadenomas of the pituitary gland.

In some centers, pituitary irradiation is the treatment of choice for patients with Cushing's disease. The remission rate achieved with radiation is about 50 percent, and a long interval is common between the completion of treatment and the remission of the symptoms and signs of Cushing's disease.

If pituitary ablation fails to relieve the symptoms of Cushing's disease, bilateral total adrenalectomy is the treatment of choice. In addition, bilateral adrenalectomy may be the procedure of choice in selected patients with advanced Cushing's disease and no obvious pituitary tumor on radiologic examination.

Postoperatively, patients treated by hypophysectomy require exogenous cortisol as well as thyroid and gonadal replacement therapy.

Extra-Adrenal ACTH-Producing Tumors

The most satisfactory treatment for this cause of Cushing's syndrome is surgical removal of the tumor producing ACTH. Although occasionally an isolated tumor identified by CT scanning can be removed, most of these tumors are malignant and complete removal is impossible. Aminoglutethimide, metyrapone, or mitotane can be administered to control the excess secretion of cortisol and some of the symptoms of Cushing's syndrome.

Primary Adrenal Corticol Tumors

Localizing the Adrenal Tumor

The surgeon must localize an adrenal tumor causing Cushing's syndrome. Intravenous pyelograms, even with laminograms, are seldom helpful in localizing an adrenal tumor unless it is very large. CT has been quite accurate in localizing adrenal tumors if they are larger than 1 cm. Sector CT scans of the adrenal area are even more sensitive and are sometimes of great value.

Adrenal venograms may be useful, particularly in studying patients with small adrenal tumors. This procedure can be combined with measuring cortisol levels in the adrenal venous blood. Adrenal angiograms are helpful in patients with large adrenal tumors in identifying blood supply to the tumor. This information may facilitate surgical removal.

Nonfunctioning Adrenal Tumors

The widespread use of CT of the upper abdomen identifies many patients with incidental adrenal masses.

The differential diagnosis of an incidentally discovered adrenal mass should include a functioning adrenal tumor, an adrenal cyst, a nonfunctioning adrenal adenoma or carcinoma, and metastatic carcinoma involving the adrenal gland. Nonfunctioning adrenal masses present a difficult decision, since 20 percent of adrenal carcinomas are nonfunctioning. The size of the mass may be helpful in the physician's decision whether to remove the mass or simply follow the patient with periodic CT of the adrenal area. If the mass is nonfunctioning, smaller than 3 cm, and not enhanced by contrast material, it may be followed by periodic CT. Any change in the size of the lesion is an indication for surgical removal.

Surgical Approach to the Adrenal Gland

Flank Approach. This approach, through a standard flank incision, is seldom used because it exposes the adrenal gland poorly. Some surgeons, however, still employ it.

Posterior Approach. This is an excellent approach to the adrenal gland for either bilateral or unilateral lesions that are not too large. It is particularly useful for bilateral adrenalectomies in patients with bilateral adrenal hyperplasia when pituitary ablation has failed to relieve the symptoms of Cushing's syndrome.

Place the patient in the prone position and approach the adrenal gland through the bed of the twelfth rib on the left side and the eleventh rib on the right side. On the right side, retract the kidney downward and free the apex of the adrenal gland and lateral margins from surrounding tissue, using Liga clips for hemostasis. Identify the inferior vena cava and doubly ligate and divide the short adrenal vein. The gland can then be easily removed.

Retract the kidney on the left side downward, exposing the left adrenal gland. Again, mobilize the apex and lateral margins of the adrenal gland, using Liga clips to secure hemostasis. The left adrenal vein, draining into the left renal vein, is doubly ligated and divided. The adrenal gland is then quite easy to remove.

Thoracoabdominal Approach. This is an excellent approach for large adrenal tumors, particularly on the right side. Make the incision in the eighth or ninth intercostal space, crossing the upper abdomen, and reaching the linea alba midway between the xiphoid and the umbilicus. Divide the diaphragm in a circumferential manner, which allows the liver to be pushed upward into the chest cavity.

Transabdominal Approach. The anterior, subcostal approach is used most commonly for pheochromocytomas, but can also be used for removing moderate-sized cortical tumors of the adrenal gland. Expose the right adrenal gland by mobilizing the duodenum (Kocher's maneuver) and hepatic flexure medially. Retract the kidney downward and the liver and gallbladder gently upward. On the left side, mobilize the splenic flexure medially, taking care to avoid injuring the spleen. The left renal vein is easily identified, and the left adrenal vein can be doubly ligated and divided. The adrenal gland can be mobilized and removed.

A "radical" adrenalectomy is indicated in most cases of primary adrenal tumor, since it may be difficult to be sure if the tumor is malignant or benign. In selected patients with large adrenal tumors, a kidney may be removed en bloc with the adrenal tumor, since it is sometimes involved with the adrenal tumor.

Preparing the Patient for Operation

The patient with Cushing's syndrome who requires removal of an adrenal tumor or a bilateral adrenalectomy should undergo surgery in the best medical condition possible. Patients with advanced Cushing's syndrome are sometimes given aminoglutethimide (1 g per day) and/or metyrapone (2 to 3 g per day) to reduce the level of cortisol production and reverse some of the signs and symptoms of Cushing's syndrome. Supplemental use of dexamethasone may be necessary to prevent adrenal insufficiency.

The patient must receive steroid replacement therapy (Table 2). Water-soluble preparations of cortisol given intravenously are particularly useful both intraoperatively and immediately postoperatively.

Postoperative Course

Bilateral adrenalectomy for bilateral adrenal hyperplasia in patients in whom hypophysectomy failed or who are not candidates for this treatment require continuous steroid maintenance therapy. Patients must be alerted to the signs and symptoms of adrenal insufficiency, which may develop when they are exposed to any stressful situation, such as severe infection or trauma. Increase the dose of steroid replacement therapy at these times.

Adrenalectomy for benign adenoma is initially managed as in a patient who has had a bilateral adrenalectomy, since the remaining adrenal gland has usually atrophied because of the high cortisol levels produced by the adrenal adenoma. The remaining gland will recover and begin to produce endogenous cortisol so that replacement therapy can be eventually discontinued. This may take from 1 to several months.

After bilateral adrenalectomy or removal of an adrenal adenoma, the signs and symptoms of Cushing's syndrome gradually regress. Hypertension usually subsides, although it may persist in some patients in whom it has been present for a long time. Diabetes mellitus, if present, may not disappear completely, but insulin requirements are usually reduced. Osteoporosis does not progress but usually is slow to heal, particularly in adults. The patient's mental state and general appearance generally change toward normal over 3 to 6 months.

Adrenalectomy for Adrenal Carcinoma

An adrenalectomy for adrenal carcinoma producing Cushing's syndrome is less apt to be curative because

Table 2 Steroid Replacement Therapy During and After Adrenalectomy for Cushing's Syndrome

Cortisone acetate (Cortone) 100–200 mg IM the evening before surgery and the morning of surgery

Cortisone acetate 100 mg IM postoperatively (in the recovery room)

Water-soluble cortisol (Solu-Cortef) may be given IV during and after surgery at about 10 mg/hr

Cortisone acetate 75 mg IM every 8 hr for the first 2 postoperative days

Cortisone acetate 75 mg IM every 12 hrs for the third and fourth postoperative days

Maintenance doses of cortisone acetate 25 mg orally twice daily, in combination with fludrocortisone 0.1 mg/day; continue this for at least 1 mo or longer after surgery

Further maintenance therapy depends on each clinical situation

frequently metastases have occurred before the primary tumor is removed. Since most of these tumors are resistant to radiotherapy and are not dramatically responsive to chemotherapy, complete surgical excision offers the only real hope for cure.

If residual or metastatic tumor is present, treat the patient with mitotane postoperatively (2 to 6 g per day in divided doses). Increase the dose until cortisol levels are normal or until toxicity produced by the drug prevents any larger doses. Drug reactions usually involve the gastrointestinal tract, neuromuscular system, and skin. Bone marrow depression and liver damage have not been reported. Follow the patient's response to therapy with periodic serum cortisol determinations. Although this is not proved, the use of prophylactic mitotane may be justified in patients with "surgically cured" adenocarcinoma because of the poor prognosis currently being achieved through surgical treatment.

The results of treating patients with Cushing's syndrome are excellent unless one is dealing with an adrenocortical carcinoma. In my experience, if an adrenal carcinoma is completely excised, the 5-year survival rate will vary between 58 and 66 percent depending on tumor size. With malignant lymph nodes, residual carcinoma, or evidence of metastases, survival rates are markedly reduced.

Nelson's Syndrome

Before transsphenoidal hypophysectomy was introduced, Cushing's disease, when not due to an obvious pituitary tumor, was treated by bilateral adrenalectomy. Approximately 10 percent of these patients with a normal-appearing sella turcica on radiographic examination, before bilateral adrenalectomy, develop a pituitary tumor that is nearly always a chromophobe adenoma. This tumor may develop in months or up to 10 to 15 years after the bilateral adrenalectomy. Treatment of patients with this tumor, called Nelson's syndrome, consists of hypophysectomy.

PHEOCHROMOCYTOMA

GARY R. WALTON, M.D.
IHN SEONG WHANG, M.D.
MITCHELL C. BENSON, M.D.

Pheochromocytomas are rare tumors arising from chromaffin cells. Chromaffin cells are so named because of their unique histologic appearance. They contain catecholamine-filled granules that stain brown when treated with chromates. It is the unregulated secretion of catecholamines that is responsible for the clinical syndrome that accompanies this tumor.

Patients with an unsuspected pheochromocytoma may experience significant morbidity secondary to extreme hypertension, and a hypertensive crisis triggered by surgery or trauma is potentially lethal. Pheochromocytomas may also be malignant.

DIAGNOSIS

Presentation, Signs, and Symptoms

The highest incidence of pheochromocytomas occurs during the fourth and fifth decades of life. There is no strong predisposition to the condition on the basis of gender. Approximately 90 percent of patients with a pheochromocytoma experience hypertension. However, only 0.1 percent of all hypertensive patients have a pheochromocytoma. Of patients with hypertension secondary to pheochromocytoma, 50 percent demonstrate a sustained elevation in blood pressure while the remainder experience paroxysmal hypertension. Half of the patients with sustained hypertension have superimposed paroxysmal episodes. In some instances it may be difficult to differentiate essential hypertension from hypertension secondary to pheochromocytoma. However, hypertension secondary to pheochromocytoma is often more severe. These patients may present with diastolic pressures as high as 140 mm Hg.

Episodes of paroxysmal hypertension can be precipitated by physical, emotional, or pharmacologic stimuli, such as bending over, being frightened, or smoking. Typical paroxysmal attacks are characterized by various combinations of headache, diaphoresis, palpitations, weakness, and agitation. Patients may present with psychiatric instability or abdominal pain. The triad of headache, diaphoresis, and palpitations is present in more than 90 percent of patients. If none of these three symptoms is present, the likelihood of a hypertensive patient harboring a pheochromocytoma is extremely low. The frequency of attacks can vary from several times per year to several times per day. The duration of a given episode ranges from minutes to hours. In general, a paroxysm will last less than 1 hour. Patients with sustained hypertension are often hypermetabolic and may present with weight loss and demonstrate glycosuria, hyperglycemia, leukocytosis, and pyrexia.

The chronically increased catecholamine levels in patients with pheochromocytoma result in persistent vasoconstriction, and patients tend to be hypovolemic. Paradoxically, this elevated catecholamine level may lead to postural hypotension as well as secondary polycythemia. Even in patients who do not demonstrate signs of hypermetabolism, the elevated catecholamines may suppress insulin secretion, leading to fasting hyperglycemia in 50 percent of patients.

Ten percent of pheochromocytomas are associated with a variety of familial conditions. These include von Hippel-Lindau disease (hemangioblastoma of the cerebellum, pancreatic and renal cysts, hepatoblastoma, retinal angiomata, and renal cell cancers), von Recklinghausen's disease (café au lait spots and neurofibromas), and multiple endocrine neoplasia syndrome (MEN) IIA and IIB. The MEN IIA syndrome is the most common of the familial causes of pheochromocytoma and is characterized by hyperparathyroidism secondary to hyperplasia or adenomas, medullary carcinoma of the thyroid, and pheochromocytoma. MEN IIB is more rare and is characterized by pheochromocytoma, medullary cancer of the thyroid, corneal nerve thickenings, gastrointestinal tract ganglioneuromatosis, and marfanoid body habitus. The evaluation of patients with pheochromocytoma should include an investigation for signs and manifestations of these disorders.

Differential Diagnosis

The differential diagnosis of pheochromocytoma includes hyperthyroidism, carcinoid syndrome, porphyria, adverse reactions to medications (theophylline toxicity or clonidine withdrawal), diencephalic epilepsy (a seizure disorder with paroxysmal hypertension), all causes of headaches, and other causes of hypertension. The latter includes hyperaldosteronism, Cushing's disease and Cushing's syndrome, renovascular disease, renal parenchyma disorders, and coarctation of the aorta. Pheochromocytomas most commonly present with accelerated hypertension or paroxysmal episodes as previously described. A high index of suspicion is necessary to lead to appropriate biochemical testing and a definitive diagnosis.

Biochemical Diagnosis

Biochemical tests for pheochromocytoma are based on measuring urine or blood levels of catecholamines (dopamine, norepinephrine, and epinephrine) or their degradation products: homovanillic acid (HVA), vanillylmandelic acid (VMA), dihydoxyphenylglycol (DHPG) and the metanephrines, normetanephrine and metanephrine (Fig. 1). Under normal conditions, the adrenal medulla predominantly synthesizes epinephrine. The enzyme responsible for conversion of norepinephrine to epinephrine, phenylethanolamine-*N*-methyltransferase, is found only in the adrenal, and the overproduction of

$$\text{Tyrosine} \xrightarrow{1} \text{Levadopa} \xrightarrow{2} \text{Dopamine} \xrightarrow{3} \text{Norepinephrine} \xrightarrow{4} \text{Epinephrine}$$

	HVA	DHPG	Metanephrine
		Normetanephrine	VMA
		VMA	

Figure 1 Synthetic and degradative pathways. 1 = tyrosine hydroxylase; 2 = aromatic L-amino acid decarboxylase; 3 = dopamine *B*-hydroxylase; 4 = phenylethanolamine-*N*-methyltransferase.

epinephrine is highly correlated with an adrenal medullary tumor. Under usual circumstances, extra-adrenal tumors produce only norepinephrine.

Twenty-four hour urine samples are the preferred means of detection because of their excellent sensitivity. The intermittent excretion of catecholamines makes spot urine samples less accurate. Blood samples must be collected in accordance with rigorously standardized procedures to prevent stress-induced elevations in catecholamine levels. The patient should be fasting and resting in the supine position for 30 minutes before venipuncture. Many suggest waiting 20 minutes after venous access is achieved before obtaining a blood sample for analysis. In either urine or serum, free or unconjugated catecholamines should be measured to prevent interference from dietary conjugated catecholamines such as those found in bananas. The clinician should be aware that methyldopa (Aldomet) can significantly decrease catecholamine levels and should be discontinued 1 week before testing.

Typically, a 24-hour urine sample for the measurement of free catecholamines and either VMA or metanephrines is our initial screening test, as this diagnoses more than 95 percent of cases of pheochromocytomas. Because recent consumption of bananas, vanilla, or coffee can affect VMA determinations, the patient should be advised to avoid these food products for 72 hours before testing. Duncan et al demonstrated measuring 24-hour urinary free norepinephrine via a combined gas chromatography–mass spectrometry technique to have a 100 percent sensitivity and 98 percent specificity. Specificity improved to 99 percent when a 24-hour urinary DHPG measurement was included. If the first results are equivocal or if it is clinically indicated, a second 24-hour urine sample for the measurement of catecholamines and DHPG is sent.

In the rare instance that all tests prove equivocal, a provocative test can be considered. These tests can be quite dangerous and should be performed in a hospital setting with appropriate monitoring and informed consent. The safest of all the provocative tests is probably the clonidine suppression test. The test is performed by measuring plasma norepinephrine levels before and 3 hours after the oral administration of 0.3 mg of clonidine. Plasma norepinephrine levels decrease with essential hypertension while they remain elevated with a pheochromocytoma.

Localization

Pheochromocytomas can occur anywhere chromaffin cells arise from their neuroectodermal origins. The adrenal medulla contains the largest collection of these cells, and accordingly, 90 percent of pheochromocytomas occur in the adrenal medulla (Table 1). The "rule of tens" is still largely true for pheochromocytomas: 10 percent are extra-adrenal, 10 percent are bilateral, and 10 percent are malignant. Ninety percent of extra-adrenal neoplasms are below the diaphragm, and the majority of these are located in the upper periaortic region at the level of the renal vessels. The remainder occur anterior to the aortic bifurcation at the organ of Zuckerkandl or in the lumbar sympathetic chains.

There are three major imaging studies used to localize a pheochromocytoma: computed tomography (CT), magnetic resonance imaging (MRI), and meta-iodobenzlyguanidine (MIBG) scanning. CT is currently the initial localizing procedure of choice and is 97 percent accurate for neoplasms larger than 1 cm at adrenal sites. Most pheochromocytomas are larger than 2 cm in diameter when diagnosed. To image the adrenals accurately, thin sectioning beginning 2 cm above and extending to 2 cm below each adrenal gland should be routinely performed. MRI is equivalent to CT for localizing adrenal masses greater than 2 cm in size but is believed by some to be less sensitive than CT for the detection of lesions smaller than 2 cm. MRI has the advantage of being able to identify different tissue characteristics, and pheochromocytomas tend to be hyperintense on T2-weighted images compared with the liver and other possible adrenal neoplasms. Thus MRI may be useful in the preoperative evaluation of adrenal lesions of unknown origin. MIBG is a radionuclide scan employing an I-131–tagged guanethidine analog. MIBG is similar to norepinephrine, and like norepinephrine, is taken up by chromaffin cells and packaged in adrenergic granules. At the dosage employed for clinical localization, MIBG has no known pharmacologic effects on normal adrenal medulla or pheochromocytomas. There are no reports of MIBG-induced hypertensive crises. MIBG is most valuable in detecting ectopic tumors. Its sensitivity is 90 percent. False-positive MIBG scans can occur with neuroblastomas, carcinoids, and medullary thyroid carcinomas. Because of the I-131 label, patients should be pretreated with an iodine solution (Lugol's Solution) to prevent thyroid uptake. Treatment should begin 48 hours before the test and continue for 72 hours afterwards.

Venous sampling and arteriography are rarely needed for localization. However, for the infrequent patient with positive biochemical tests in whom radiologic imaging studies fail to detect the tumor, venous sampling may be the only means of localizing the pheochromocytoma. A patient should never undergo

Table 1 Location of Pheochromocytomas

Location	Percentage
Adrenal	90
Extra-adrenal	10
Below the diaphragm	90
Perirenal vessels	50
Near the organ of Zuckerkandl	25
Other sites including bladder and the lumbar sympathetic chains	25
Above the diaphragm	10
Usually in the posterior mediastinum	

arteriography without prior adrenergic blockade, as arteriography can induce a hypertensive crisis.

PHEOCHROMOCYTOMA OF THE BLADDER

Since pheochromocytoma of the bladder was first reported in 1953 by Zimmerman, approximately 100 cases have been cited. It accounts for only 0.06 percent of all bladder tumors. The presenting symptoms can be similar to those of bladder tumors and include gross or microscopic hematuria that is sometimes associated with pain. However, specific for pheochromocytoma of the bladder are symptoms of syncope, palpitations, headaches, or sweating either associated with or following voiding.

These tumors grow slowly and may occur anywhere in the bladder, but are found most often at the dome. Measurements of urinary catecholamine levels are helpful in making the diagnosis, but no more so than in other pheochromocytomas. The diagnosis is made by cystoscopy, imaging, and biopsy. As with all pheochromocytomas, alpha-adrenergic blockade should be instituted before the procedure is begun if the diagnosis is suspected. Partial cystectomy is recommended for treatment. There is a 10 to 20 percent recurrence rate and a 5 percent incidence of metastatic disease. Whether or not the high incidence of recurrence is secondary to multifocality is not known.

PHEOCHROMOCYTOMA DURING PREGNANCY

Pheochromocytoma during pregnancy is rare and only about 150 cases have been reported. It produces symptoms similar to those found in nonpregnant patients. These symptoms may be overlooked, however, because of the rarity of the tumor and its mimicry of eclampsia and preeclampsia. Potentially fatal hypertensive crisis may be precipitated by anesthesia, vaginal delivery, mechanical effects of the gravid uterus, uterine contractions, and even vigorous fetal movements.

Special care must be taken when one is employing imaging modalities in pregnancy. Ultrasonography, CT, and MRI may all be capable of localizing the tumors. Ultrasonography is safe but may not be sufficiently sensitive, especially if an extra-adrenal tumor is present. CT remains sensitive but results in high fetal radiation exposure and should be used only if MRI is not able to localize the tumor. MRI gives good images without ionizing radiation but is less sensitive than CT in diagnosing tumors less than 2 cm. MRI has been employed in the localization of an ectopic pheochromocytoma in a pregnant patient.

Management of pheochromocytomas discovered during pregnancy presents the clinician with unique challenges. The key to maternal survival is early diagnosis. If the diagnosis is made prior to the 24th week of gestation, early exploration after adequate alpha-adrenergic blockade is recommended. If the diagnosis is made after the 24th week of gestation, the patient should have her hypertension controlled by medical management until a cesarean section is feasible. Cesarean section should be followed by the immediate exploration and removal of the tumor. Medical management can include phenoxybenzamine, prazosin, and labetalol (Normodyne). These medications have not been reported to have adverse effects on the fetus, especially when given during the second half of pregnancy. In laboratory animals, however, mutagenesis has been reported to occur with the use of phenoxybenzamine. As with any medications believed to be indicated during pregnancy, the mother should be warned about possible effects upon the fetus.

A recent review of pheochromocytoma during pregnancy by Harper et al reveals that there has been improvement in management and maternal survival. Prior to 1969, the maternal mortality rate was reported to be 48 percent. This decreased to 26 percent from 1969 to 1979 and further improved to 17 percent during the period of 1980 to 1987. When the diagnosis was made antepartum, the maternal mortality was only 11 percent, emphasizing the importance of early diagnosis and early therapy. First trimester surgery was associated with the highest rate of fetal loss (90 percent), while fetal loss during the second trimester was 67 percent. The overall fetal mortality from a maternal pheochromocytoma was 50 percent. A diagnosis of pheochromocytoma should be considered in pregnant women with severe, intermittent, or paroxysmal hypertension presenting during the first half of pregnancy.

PHEOCHROMOCYTOMA IN CHILDREN

Pheochromocytoma occurring in a child was first reported in 1904 by Marchetti. Only 20 percent of pheochromocytomas occur in children. Unlike adults, where multiplicity of tumors occurs in only 10 percent of patients, children have synchronous multiple tumors in more than one-third of cases. The presenting symptoms are headaches, visual blurring, hypertension, and diaphoresis. In children, the hypertension tends to be sustained rather than paroxysmal. The differential diagnosis in children includes that of the adult plus neuroblastoma, Wilms' tumor, ganglioneuroma, and Riley-Day syndrome (dysautonomia).

Due to the higher incidence of tumor multiplicity in children, total body imaging studies are necessary for complete localization. As in adults, CT is the most sensitive modality. MIBG can be used for detection of pheochromocytomas in children. The thyroid gland should be blocked with Lugol's Solution to prevent inadvertent I-131 uptake. The dosage in children is one drop per day starting 24 hours before the study and continuing for 7 days afterwards. Since CT and MRI have fewer potential adverse effects, MIBG scanning is not often utilized. MRI is currently the initial imaging modality of choice in older children, since it avoids radiation exposure and is capable of tissue typing. Younger children may be too fearful of MRI to tolerate the procedure. Although angiography is rarely necessary, if it is performed, prior adrenergic blockade should be initiated and arterial blood pressure monitoring is indicated. Drugs used to treat severe hypertension and hypotension as well as cardiac arrhythmias must be available in the angiography suite. Venous sampling is sometimes necessary to localize residual tumors not imaged preoperatively.

Although according to the *Physicians' Desk Reference,* its safety and efficacy has not been "proven" in children, phenoxybenzamine is the alpha-adrenergic blocking agent of choice. The recommended starting oral dosage is 1 to 2 mg per kilogram per day divided in four doses. The dose is increased until normal blood pressure is achieved. The side effects of phenoxybenzamine include nasal congestion and orthostatic hypotension.

In children, an anterior transperitoneal or thoracoabdominal surgical approach is suggested. Either of these approaches allows for exploration of both adrenals, the para-aortic ganglia, and the retroperitoneal space. The incidence of multiple tumors (i.e., one-third of patients) mandates that thorough palpation be performed even in the absence of a preoperative suggestion of tumor multiplicity.

Prognosis in children depends on the benign or malignant nature of the tumor. A lifetime follow-up with initially semiannual and thereafter annual measurement of urinary catecholamine levels is recommended.

FAMILIAL PHEOCHROMOCYTOMA

Familial pheochromocytoma occurs secondary to an autosomal dominant inheritance with a high degree of penetrance. The incidence of multiple tumors is approximately 50 percent, and most are bilateral adrenal tumors. Although familial pheochromocytoma can occur as an isolated tumor, most familial pheochromocytomas are associated with other syndromes. These include neurofibromatosis, von Hippel-Lindau disease, and MEN types IIa and IIb. Of these, MEN IIa is the most common.

MEN IIa is a syndrome that also has an autosomal dominant inheritance. It is characterized by synchronous or metachronous occurrence of medullary thyroid carcinoma, pheochromocytomas, and hyperparathyroidism secondary to parathyroid hyperplasia or adenoma. Almost all patients with MEN IIa develop medullary thyroid carcinoma, but only 50 percent develop clinical evidence of pheochromocytoma or parathyroid hyperplasia. The pheochromocytomas are usually bilateral and frequently multiple. It has been reported that hyperplasia of the adrenal medulla precedes the development of pheochromocytoma. Some surgeons have advocated that if a pheochromocytoma develops, bilateral adrenalectomy should be performed to prevent contralateral occurrence and to diminish the risk of metastatic disease from delayed diagnosis. Since there is a high likelihood that a patient with MEN IIa will develop a contralateral adrenal pheochromocytoma, we agree with prophylactic contralateral adrenalectomy. In fact, many patients undergoing prophylactic adrenalectomy will demonstrate microscopic evidence of subclinical pheochromocytoma. Patients presenting with medullary thyroid carcinoma should be screened for parathyroid hyperplasia and pheochromocytoma. Relatives of patients with MEN IIa should be evaluated for the associated endocrinopathies even if they are asymptomatic.

MALIGNANT PHEOCHROMOCYTOMA

Approximately 10 percent of pheochromocytomas are malignant. The 5-year survival with malignant pheochromocytoma has been reported to be 44 percent. The malignant tumors are often functional and, like their benign counterparts, produce catecholamines. However, unlike benign tumors, they can also secrete large quantities of earlier precursor substances such as levodopa and dopamine (see Fig. 1). This occurs secondary to the mutational loss of the capability to complete the metabolic pathway.

The rarity of malignant pheochromocytoma makes the study of its natural history difficult. Some authors have noted the existence of two subsets of patients that have distinct outcomes. About one-half of the patients have a relatively rapid demise and die within 4 to 5 years. The other half appear to have a more indolent course and may live for 20 years or more without definitive cytotoxic therapy.

In general, the experience with chemotherapy and radiation therapy has been poor. Radiation therapy is often useful only for palliation of bone pain. Recently, there have been encouraging reports using combination chemotherapy and using MIBG at a therapeutic as opposed to a diagnostic dosage. In one report, the use of cyclophosphamide, vincristine sulfate, and dacarbazine (CVD) has had an overall objective response rate of 57 percent, with a mean duration of 21 months. A group in France, using MIBG at doses of 850 to 9,700 rad, has shown a clinical response in seven of 12 patients. However, there were no complete remissions. According to one study of a group at the University of Michigan, four of ten patients responded when MIBG at doses of up to 18,000 rad were used. These results are encouraging; however, further research is warranted. It is important to note that these patients treated with therapeutic doses of I-131–labeled MIBG should receive Lugol's Solution, six drops per day starting the first day before therapy. Lugol's Solution should be continued for 4 weeks.

Cytotoxic chemotherapy can induce hypertensive crisis, and adrenergic blockade is necessary before any therapy can be initiated. In addition to alpha-adrenergic blockers, beta-blockers and alpha-methyl *L*-tyrosine (Metyrosine) can be used. Metyrosine inhibits tyrosine hydroxylase, the rate-limiting enzyme in catecholamine synthesis. It has proven useful in patients not responsive to other medications and in those with heavy tumor burdens. It should not be considered a first-line therapy because of frequent side effects, including sedation, diarrhea, extrapyramidal reactions, and crystalluria.

TREATMENT

Surgery

The treatment of pheochromocytoma is surgical excision unless there is a contraindication to surgery or if metastatic disease from a malignant pheochromocytoma is present. Before one proceeds with surgery, it is imperative that appropriate pharmacologic management be initiated.

Preoperative Adrenergic Blockade

Alpha-adrenergic blockade along with a high-sodium diet helps expand the contracted plasma volume. This prevents or diminishes the hypotension associated with tumor removal. The adrenergic blockade also moderates fluctuations in blood pressure encountered during the induction of anesthesia and the surgical procedure itself. In spite of adequate adrenergic blockade, the hypertensive response to intraoperative tumor palpation, which in some instances can be useful at exploration, is usually not totally eliminated. Prophylactic preoperative blood transfusions have not been used at our institution, although they are recommended by some authors.

The long-acting, oral alpha-blocking agent phenoxybenzamine (Dibenzyline) is the most widely used primary agent. The patient begins with a dose of 10 mg twice per day, and the dose is increased by 10-mg increments every 3 days until the blood pressure is under adequate control. Doses as high as 40 to 100 mg per day may be needed. Side effects of phenoxybenzamine and all alpha-blocking agents include postural hypotension, compensatory tachycardia, and nasal congestion. If intolerable side effects preclude adequate adrenergic blockage, blood pressure can be further controlled with an angiotensin-converting enzyme (ACE) inhibitor such as captopril (Capoten). Prazosin has also been employed

as a primary alpha-adrenergic–blocking agent. It is shorter acting than phenoxybenzamine, however, and has been reported to result in less adequate intraoperative blood pressure control.

Beta-blockers can be added for treatment of heart rates greater than 110 beats per minute or tachyarrhythmias but should never be started prior to alpha-blockade. The use of beta-blockers without prior alpha-adrenergic blockade can lead to unopposed vasoconstriction, hypertensive crisis, and possible myocardial infarction or cerebral vascular accident. The patient can be started on propranolol, 10 mg three times per day, which can be increased as needed. Selective beta-blockers should be considered in the patient with asthma.

Intraoperative Monitoring and Anesthetic Technique

The surgeon should consult with the anesthesiologist before surgery to ensure the use of proper monitoring and the availability of appropriate pharmacologic agents. Since removal of a pheochromocytoma is one of the most demanding operative procedures from an anesthetic standpoint, several points should be stressed. Direct monitoring of intra-arterial pressure is mandatory for following the rapid changes in blood pressure. To ensure adequate intravascular volume following tumor excision, central venous monitoring is used. A Swan-Ganz catheter may prove useful in some clinical situations. We recommend the placement of a Foley catheter to monitor urine output.

Enflurane (Ethrane) has been a good choice for general anesthesia. Certain drugs should be avoided. Halothane (Fluothane) lowers the threshold for catecholamine-induced arrhythmias. Morphine releases histamine and could lead to a hypertensive crisis. Sodium nitroprusside (Nipride) is an excellent choice for treating intraoperative hypertension since it is short-acting and can be easily titrated. Arrhythmias should be treated first by controlling blood pressure and then with more specific agents — usually propranolol for supraventricular arrhythmias and lidocaine for ventricular arrhythmias.

After the tumor is isolated from the systemic circulation, there is typically a rapid decrease in blood pressure. Although preoperative adrenergic blockade will blunt this response, it can be quite pronounced. The treatment is volume replacement, and central venous pressure monitoring facilitates the safe and rapid administration of fluid. Low-dose pressors may be needed in this clinical situation.

Surgical Approaches

The surgical approach depends on whether solitary, multiple, or extra-adrenal tumors are present. The majority of patients have a solitary, unilateral adrenal lesion. As mentioned earlier, CT is 97 percent accurate in locating adrenal lesions larger than 1 cm. Patients not in a high-risk group for tumor multiplicity who are found to have a solitary adrenal lesion on complete abdominal imaging have a low probability of ectopic tumors. Unless the tumor is large, this category of patients is approached via a flank incision. If the tumor is greater than 6 cm, a transdiaphragmatic thoracoabdominal incision is employed to minimize tumor manipulation during the dissection.

If there are multiple or ectopic tumors, the patient must be explored through a transabdominal or thoracoabdominal incision to allow full exposure of all abdominal structures. Patients at high risk for multiple ectopic pheochromocytomas must be approached via such an incision. These include all patients with extra-adrenal tumors, all with MEN syndromes, and all patients younger than 18 years of age. At our institution, a thoracoabdominal incision is usually employed, although both the chevron and extended midline incisions are adequate.

The main venous drainage of the adrenal gland is through a solitary vein that drains in a consistent fashion into the renal vein on the left side and directly into the vena cava on the right side. On the right side, the vein is quite short and care must be taken not to avulse it from the vena cava. Unlike nephrectomy, in which procedure ligation of the renal vein prior to arterial ligation leads to renal engorgement and more difficult dissection, early ligation of the adrenal vein prior to ligation of the adrenal artery helps diminish fluctuations in blood pressure. Surgical excision of the adrenal begins laterally, where the blood supply is sparse and continues around the medial aspect of the gland. The inferior attachments are the last to be taken, so that downward traction on the kidney can be used to displace the adrenal gland without direct manipulation. To ensure adequacy of resection, a margin of periadrenal fat is taken with the specimen when possible.

Postoperative Care

Postoperatively, the patient should be monitored in an intensive care setting with arterial and central venous lines and a Foley catheter in place. After tumor excision, volume replacement is the primary treatment of hypotension, although direct-acting pressor agents such as phenylephrine or norepinephrine may be needed for brief periods. This is especially true if hypotension is resulting in an inadequate renal perfusion (low urine output). Sudden repositioning should be avoided, as orthostatic hypotension will continue until the preoper-

atively administered adrenergic-blocking agents are no longer active (i.e., within 2 to 4 days).

After pheochromocytoma removal, catecholamine suppression of insulin decreases. With increased insulin secretion, patients may become hypoglycemic and the patient's blood glucose should be followed closely for the first 48 hours. Intravenous fluids should contain glucose.

Rarely, the patient remains hypertensive for several days after surgery. This may be secondary to fluid shifts, autonomic instability, or elevated catecholamine stores within adrenergic neurons. In fact, urinary VMA often continues to be elevated for several days after excision of the pheochromocytoma. Persistent hypertension may also be caused by irreversible renal damage or underlying essential hypertension. The question of residual or metastatic pheochromocytoma should be raised if hypertension continues. Repeat urinary catecholamines should be measured not less than 2 weeks postoperatively since false elevations may occur from tissue stores.

LONG-TERM CARE

Patients should have their blood pressure checked every 3 months for the first year. Urine samples for catecholamines should be sent every 6 months for the first 2 years and then annually for the next 3 years to ensure that no residual tumor is present. As mentioned previously, children should be monitored for life since they are at significantly greater risk for recurrence. Patients developing recurrent symptoms should be evaluated promptly.

SUGGESTED READING

Chatal JF, Carbonnel B. Comparison of iodobenzylguanidine imaging with computerized tomography in locating pheochromocytoma. J Clin Endocrinol Metab 1985; 61:769–772.

Duncan MW, Compton P, Lazarus L, Smythe GA. Measurement of norepinephrine and 3,4-dihydroxyphenylglycol in urine and plasma for the diagnosis of pheochromocytoma. N Engl J Med 1988; 319:136–142.

Greene JP, Guay AT. New perspectives in pheochromocytoma. Urol Clin N Am 1989; 16:487–503.

Harper MA, Murnaghan GA, Kennedy L, et al. Phaeochromocytoma in pregnancy. Five cases and a review of the literature. Br J Obstet Gynecol 1989; 96:594–606.

McEwan AJ, Duncan A. Radioiodinated iodobezylguanidines for diagnosis and therapy. Appl Radiat Isot 1986; 37:765–775.

NEUROBLASTOMA

L. SUZANNE FLOM, M.D.
WILLIAM E. KAPLAN, M.D.

Neuroblastoma, the most common extracranial solid tumor in infancy and childhood, accounts for approximately 50 percent of all neonatal malignancies. The presence of the tumor in utero has been documented by cases in which the tumor has invaded the placenta and caused maternal flushing and hypertension from catecholamine secretion. Ninety percent of cases of neuroblastoma present within the first 8 years of life and more than half of the patients are younger than 2 years of age at presentation. Most patients have metastatic disease at the time of diagnosis. In contrast to the advances made in the treatment of most childhood cancers, the prognosis for children with neuroblastoma remains poor.

Among newborns dying of other causes, neuroblastoma in situ can be detected in the adrenal medulla in one of 250 patients. However, the clinical attack rate is approximately one in 10,000 children. This would suggest that most of these tumors must either disappear, mature, or convert to other forms with increasing age of the child.

Neuroblastomas arise from embryonal cells of the neural crest that eventually form the sympathetic ganglia and adrenal medulla. In 75 percent of patients, the primary tumor is retroperitoneal: 50 percent arise in the adrenal medulla and 25 percent arise in the paraspinal sympathetic ganglia. Approximately 20 percent of tumors arise in the posterior mediastinum and less than 5 percent arise in the neck and pelvis.

DIAGNOSIS

The presenting symptoms are variable and may include fatigue, anorexia, weight loss, bone pain, abdominal pain, emesis, diarrhea, and paralysis. Most abdominal tumors tend to remain asymptomatic until metastatic disease brings the child to medical attention. Large tumors may become evident because of symptoms caused by the mass itself (e.g., early satiety, change in bowel habits, urinary frequency).

A mass may be discovered by the parents or on routine physical examination. Ultrasonography is usually the initial imaging modality for a child with a palpable abdominal mass. It will help define the precise origin of the mass, its morphology, and its relation to other structures. Neuroblastoma can usually be distinguished from Wilms's tumor by its extrarenal location. However, ultrasonography has limited value in detecting metastatic disease to retroperitoneal and retrocrural lymph nodes. Similarly, extradural extension of tumor into the vertebral canal cannot be detected. Despite these limitations, ultrasonography remains the modality of choice for the initial screening of a neonatal abdominal mass.

In 50 percent of patients, a plain film of the abdomen will reveal microcalcifications, which are usually located in the prevertebral or paravertebral space. This can be demonstrated approximately 80 percent of the time on computed tomography (CT).

CT is superior to ultrasonography and conventional radiography for detection and delineation of primary and metastatic neuroblastoma, as well as recurrent tumor. It can determine the extension of tumor to retroperitoneal lymph nodes, to liver, around central vessels, and into the vertebral canal. Thus, it has improved on other imaging techniques for indicating tumor operability. Serial CT scanning provides a method for monitoring the response of therapy in inoperable cases and in assisting the surgeon in evaluating the feasibility of delayed excision after radiation or chemotherapy. Recent experience with magnetic resonance imaging (MRI) suggests that it is especially valuable in detecting extradural extension of tumor. It is also capable of documenting bone marrow involvement and major vessel encroachment by tumor.

Presurgical and pretreatment quantification of biochemical markers associated with neuroblastoma is essential in patients with suspected disease. Despite the fact that there are no clinical manifestations of elevated serum catecholamine levels, approximately 90 percent of patients will have elevated urinary catecholamines—vanillylmandelic acid (VMA) or homovanillic acid (HVA) or both. A ratio of VMA:HVA greater than 1.5 is associated with an improved prognosis. Levels of these catecholamines can also be used to monitor disease status once treatment begins.

Serum ferritin and neuron-specific enolase (NSE) have also been shown to have prognostic value. Increased serum ferritin levels are associated with a significantly worse prognosis than normal levels. This correlation appears independent of the stage or patient's age at the time of diagnosis. The duration of survival is indirectly related to the height of the ferritin elevation. Similarly, normal NSE levels suggest improved survival in patients of any age. However, in infants younger than 1 year of age, high NSE levels are associated with a particularly poor prognosis.

Bone marrow aspirations and biopsies are indicated in all patients suspected of having neuroblastoma. Detection of characteristic syncytial clumps is enhanced by sampling multiple sites. Screening with monoclonal antibodies improves the yield. Fifty to 70 percent of aspirates will be positive for tumor.

Operative tumor specimens can be studied for the presence of the n-*myc* oncogene and DNA—flow cytometry (evaluating for chromosomal ploidy). Regardless of age or stage, n-*myc* amplification portends refractory disease. Chromosomal ploidy appears to have prognostic significance; hyperdiploid tumors behave less virulently.

Radiologic evidence of bony metastases is seen in approximately half of the patients at the time of diagnosis. Radiographic skeletal surveys and radionuclide bone scans are used to indicate the presence of bone metastases. Radiolabeled metaiodobenzylguanidine (MIBG) allows imaging of nonosseous as well as osseous sites. MIBG structurally resembles catecholamine precursors. It is specifically taken up by adrenergic tissue. The sensitivity for primary neuroblastoma is more than 90 percent, and for neuroblastoma with a high level of catecholamine excretion, more than 95 percent. Sensitivity to tumor relapse and all localizations of metastases and bone marrow infiltration in the follow-up phase is 70 percent. MIBG has also been used for therapeutic purposes. In addition, monoclonal antibodies may be employed to detect primary as well as metastatic neuroblastoma.

STAGING AND PROGNOSIS

The patient's age, site of tumor, and stage of disease at the time of initial diagnosis are the main determinants of prognosis. Even when the stage of their disease is similar, infants younger than 1 year of age have a much better prognosis than children older than 1 year.

Tumors arising in the chest or neck have a better prognosis than those arising in the abdomen. Thoracic neuroblastomas are associated with an overall survival rate of 61 percent, compared with the 20 percent survival rate of patients with abdominal tumors. Adrenal tumors result in the highest mortality rate.

Stage appears to be the most important prognostic factor. Proposed in 1971, the Evans's system is the one used most commonly. Stage I is confined to the organ or structure of origin. Stage II includes tumor extending in continuity beyond the organ of origin but not crossing the midline. Ipsilateral lymph nodes may be positive. The prognosis for Stages I and II is excellent, with survival exceeding 80 percent. Stage III tumors extend across the midline. Regional lymph node involvement may be noted. Encasement of the great vessels may preclude complete surgical excision. Slightly more than one-third of the patients will survive. Stage IV is disseminated disease, with survival being dismal at 5 to 7 percent regardless of therapy. Little impact has been made on Stage IV survival data in more than 20 years. Stage IV-S comprises a unique group of patients in whom the primary tumor would otherwise be Stage I or Stage II but who also have distant metastases confined to liver, skin, and/or bone marrow (with a negative skeletal survey). Most commonly seen in infancy, Stage IV-S usually regresses spontaneously. Without treatment, more than 80 percent of patients will survive.

TREATMENT

The treatment of choice for Evans's Stage I or II tumors is complete surgical resection. The guidelines for surgery depend on the site of the primary. The basic principle is to resect the primary tumor completely, if this can be accomplished without removal of or perma-

nent damage to any vital structures. Most neuroblastomas arise within the abdomen. Whether or not the tumor can be safely excised is usually decided at the time of laparotomy. Complete excision is usually impossible in large upper retroperitoneal tumors that arise in the celiac axis and wrap around the great vessels. Because these tumors are vascular and fragile, attempted removal can lead to uncontrolled operative hemorrhage. Surgical cytoreduction is generally not attempted. In these cases, a biopsy of the most accessible site from which the diagnosis can be established should be performed and the then operation terminated.

Excision of tumor in the adrenal gland usually requires a concomitant nephrectomy in order to remove all gross tumor. Patients should undergo bowel preparation preoperatively, as occasionally a segment of bowel adheres to the tumor and requires resection in order for all gross tumor to be removed. Because of the high incidence of nodal metastases and the important prognostic role they play, regional lymph nodes should be sampled. If the primary site is in the pelvis, then periaortic lymph nodes from the aortic bifurcation up to the renal vessels should be sent to pathology. A liver biopsy is generally advocated in order to assess the liver histologically. Whenever possible, the spleen should be salvaged. Pneumovax should be administered if splenectomy becomes necessary.

In the 10 to 15 percent of neuroblastoma patients who at the time of diagnosis have resectable disease without lymph node involvement, survival rates of 80 to 100 percent have been achieved with surgery alone. Improved staging techniques, alluded to previously, allow a more confident assignment of patients to this group. These results hold both when the tumor is entirely excised as well as when microscopic residual disease confined to the tumor bed remains.

Five to ten percent of patients with neuroblastoma have Stage IV-S disease. Because in these patients, survival is excellent at close to 90 percent, even without treatment, management is somewhat controversial. Infants who succumb due to Stage IV-S lesions often die as a result of a rapidly enlarging liver causing compression of vital organs or respiratory compromise, sepsis as a result of malnutrition, and immunosuppression or coagulopathies. Therapeutic approaches have included low-dose chemotherapy, low-to-moderate doses of radiation to reverse hepatomegaly, and marsupialization with silastic patches to relieve intra-abdominal pressure.

If tumor cells are recovered on bone marrow aspirate, if the serum ferritin and/or NSE levels are high, or if there is n-*myc* amplification, the use of intensive systemic chemotherapy is favored. The absence of both dangerous organomegaly and these biologic markers seems to identify the infants with Stage IV-S disease who would do well without any treatment.

Chemotherapy has been used in patients with Stage II tumors with residual disease, especially in those older than 1 year of age, with positive lymph nodes, and/or with unfavorable histology. Some centers use radiation therapy.

In unresectable Stage III tumors and in metastatic (Stage IV) disease, intensive multimodal chemotherapy, including cyclophosphamide (Cytoxan), *CIS*-platinum, VP-16, and doxorubicin hydrochloride (Adriamycin), has been utilized. Delayed primary or "second look" laparotomy is then undertaken for complete resection, or at least reduction, of residual disease. A recent approach to the patient with previously treated metastatic neuroblastoma has been the use of supralethal chemotherapy with or without irradiation and allogenic or autologous bone marrow reconstitution. Some centers purge the autologous marrow with monoclonal antibodies directed against neuroblastoma. Recent data suggest that disease-free survivors are in the group of children who are transplanted before the development of progressive disease.

Monoclonal antibodies are currently used in three types of treatment trials: (1) the in vivo administration of antibody used as a carrier of cytotoxic materials; (2) the use of the antibody for the ex vivo purging of bone marrow in conjunction with bone marrow transplant; and (3) the ex vivo use of antibody to deplete T cells from allogenic marrow and thus reduce the incidence of graft versus host disease.

Other therapeutic modalities currently under investigation include the administration of drugs that have a direct effect on the catecholamine biosynthetic pathway and the administration of maturing agents to the tumor, causing it to differentiate to a non-life–threatening form.

SUGGESTED READING

Evans AE, et al. Advances in neuroblastoma research. New York: Alan R. Liss, 1987.

Seeger RC, Broden GM, Sathes H, et al. Association of multiple copies of the n-*myc* oncogene with rapid progression of neuroblastomas. N Engl J Med 1985; 303:1111–1116.

Shimada H, Chatten J, Newton WA, et al. Histopathologic prognostic factors in neuroblastic tumors; definitions of subtypes of ganglioneuroblastomas. Journal of the National Cancer Institute 1984; 73:405–413.

ADRENOCORTICAL CARCINOMA

MARTIN E. GLEAVE, M.D., FRCSC
R. JOSEPH BABAIAN, M.D.

Adrenocortical carcinoma (ACC) is an uncommon malignancy with an incidence of approximately one in 1.7 million. It accounts for less than 0.02 percent of all cancers and 0.2 percent of all deaths due to cancer. It most frequently presents between the third and fifth decades of life, with approximately 40 percent of these neoplasms having clinically evident endocrine function. The paucity of patients with ACC seen by any one investigator or groups and its relative resistance to current multimodal therapy has prevented unanimity of opinion as to what, other than surgery, constitutes optimum treatment.

CLINICAL PRESENTATION AND DIAGNOSIS

Patients with ACC can present with various clinical syndromes depending on the functional status of the neoplasm and the age and sex of the patient. Masculinization or precocious puberty resulting from the production of androstenedione and dehydroepiandrosterone sulfate (DHEAS) and their conversion to testosterone can occur in up to 80 percent of females and prepubescent boys. Feminization resulting from the conversion of excessive DHEA to estrogen can occur in men and may cause impotency, loss of libido, or gynecomastia. Cushing's syndrome occurs secondary to excess glucocorticoid production, and Conn's syndrome, although rare, results from mineralocorticoid excess.

Diagnosis of this malignancy is often delayed because the adrenal glands are anatomically inaccessible to physical examination and because they grow quite large before causing symptoms, some of which are nonspecific. In contrast to females and prepubescent boys, the majority of men and older patients (fifth to seventh decades of life) with ACC tend to present with clinically nonfunctioning neoplasms. Consequently, this latter group may present following a long history of vague upper abdominal or flank discomfort, weight loss, fatigue, or palpable abdominal mass, and are more apt to have advanced disease.

Computed tomography (CT) is the preferred imaging modality for assessing an incidentally found retroperitoneal mass and is frequently the clinical investigative study employed to define a presumed abdominal mass (Fig. 1). CT scanning provides valuable information regarding nodal status, invasion into adjacent structures or organs (including the ipsilateral kidney), venous or caval extension (Fig. 2), and the status of the contralateral kidney. Excretory urography may reveal a suprarenal mass with either inferior or lateral displacement of the ipsilateral kidney. As with CT imaging, the nephrotomograms of the urogram may reveal speckled calcifications secondary to hemorrhage. The ultrasonogram can confirm the solid nature of a lesion as well as determine tumor extension into the inferior vena cava.

Arteriography is of limited value in either the diagnosis or clinical staging of ACC, although it may help determine whether a large neoplasm is of renal or

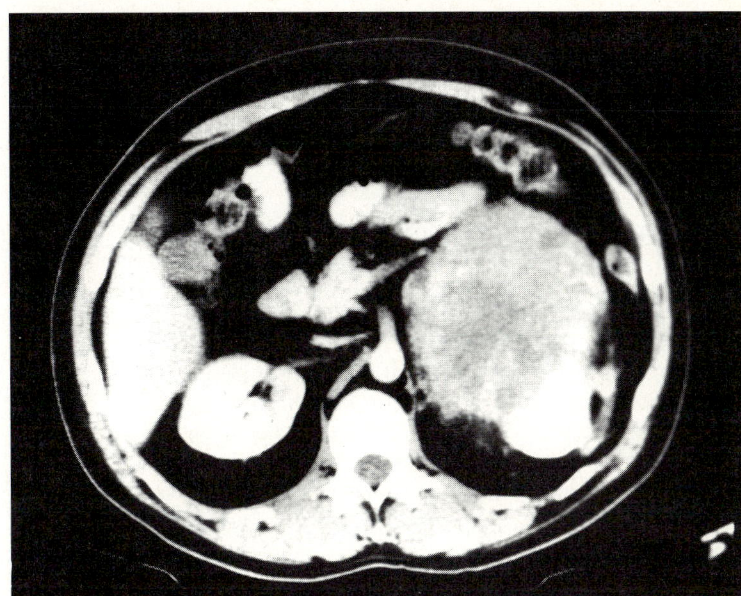

Figure 1 CT scan demonstrating a large, inhomogeneous left adrenal mass. No obvious nodal or venous extension is seen.

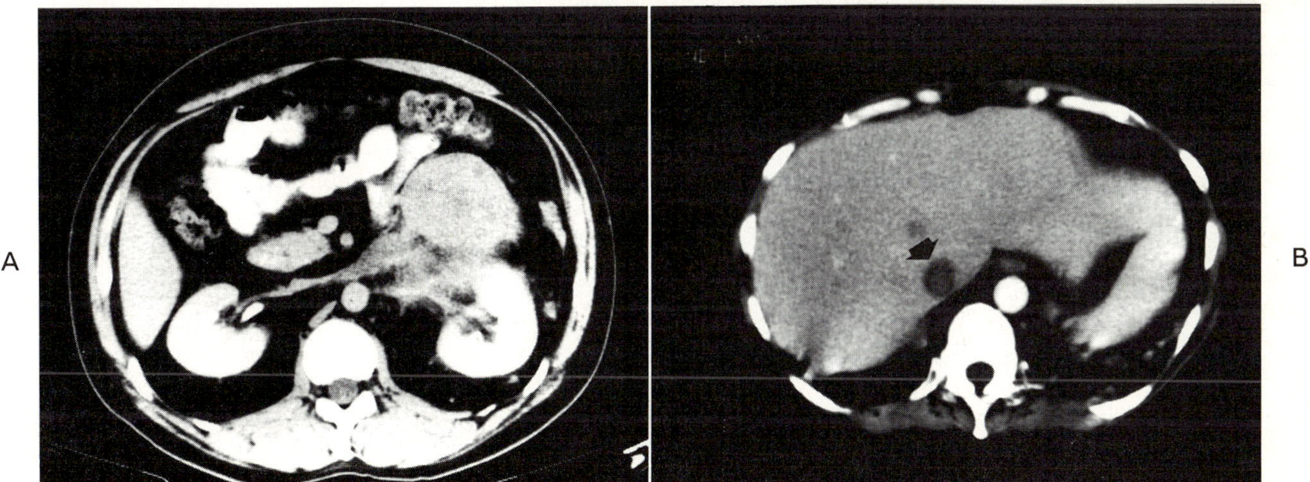

A

B

Figure 2 CT scan demonstrating (*A*) extension of a left adrenal cortical carcinoma into the left renal vein, and (*B*) large intrahepatic caval thrombus (*arrow*) from a right adrenal carcinoma.

adrenal origin and may help map out the tumor's blood supply. Venocavography may be useful to assess possible caval extension associated with large tumors or to define the extent of involvement (Fig. 3). Fine-needle aspiration (FNA) does not distinguish between an adrenal adenoma and carcinoma because their cytologic features are indistinguishable. Indeed, the only reliable indicator of malignancy for an adrenal neoplasm is the presence of metastasis. However, FNA may help to differentiate metastatic lesions from primary adrenal neoplasms.

Recently, magnetic resonance imaging (MRI) has emerged as a possible method for characterization of adrenal masses. The normal adrenal gland is isointense or hypointense to the liver on T1- and T2-weighted images. Proponents suggest that ACC can be differentiated from adenomas on the basis of the former's increased signal intensity ratio (adrenal/liver or adrenal/ fat) on T1- and T2-weighted images (Fig. 4); increased lipid content ($>7\%$); or longer T2 relaxation time. Further clinical experience is needed to determine the role and limitations of MRI in ACC characterization and staging.

Hormonal studies to ascertain the functional status of an adrenal tumor and to differentiate a carcinoma from a pheochromocytoma with its biochemical implications are recommended (Table 1). In addition, any hormonal abnormalities can serve as useful markers to monitor the response to therapy. These clinical investigations are combined with a metastatic evaluation consisting of a serum chemistry profile (including liver function tests), chest x-ray examination, and bone scan. The most common sites of metastasis, in decreasing order of frequency, are lung, liver, retroperitoneal lymph nodes, and bone.

There is no universally accepted staging system, but one of the utilized systems is the surveillance, epidemiology, and end results classification (SEER) (Table 2 and Fig. 5).

Treatment

Surgery remains the mainstay of treatment of ACC. Surgical extirpation of the primary tumor is performed with a regional lymphadenectomy in all suitable operative candidates who do not present with distant metastasis. Patients with regionally advanced disease (i.e., nodal or contiguous organ involvement) would not necessarily be excluded from undergoing surgery. Neither chemotherapy nor radiotherapy has been effective in curing this malignancy, and the rarity of this neoplasm precludes the development of meaningful therapeutic trials using these modalities. Because of its adrenolytic activity, mitotane (Ortho-para DDD) has palliative efficacy in the treatment of metastatic disease.

Because of the high retroperitoneal location and the large size of most adrenal carcinomas, we prefer the thoracoabdominal incision. We believe this incision enhances exposure and facilitates complete extirpation of the mass upon which cure is predicated.

Surgery

Anatomy

Weighing between 3 and 6 g, each adrenal gland is within Gerota's fascia on the superiomedial aspect of the kidney and receives 6 to 7 ml per gram per minute of blood (approximately twice the renal blood flow). The arterial vascular supply is multiple and variable, being derived from the aorta and branches of the inferior phrenic and renal arteries (Fig. 6). In contrast to the arterial supply, the venous drainage is relatively constant, beginning as capillary networks in the cortex, which coalesce to form a central vein that enters directly into the inferior vena cava (IVC) on the right and into the superior border of the midrenal vein on the left.

Because of its rich vascular supply, friability, and high retroperitoneal location, the adrenal gland can bleed excessively during surgery. On the right side, the central vein is short and friable and can be easily torn or avulsed with excessive lateral retraction on the mass or with medial retraction on the IVC. Compared with the right adrenal gland, the left adrenal gland is more elongated and situated lower on the superiomedial aspect of the kidney, which means the superior blood supply is lower than its counterpart. This, along with the overlying liver, makes dissection of the right upper adrenal border more difficult than that of the left. On the left, care must be taken anterior to the adrenal gland where the tail of the pancreas and splenic artery are situated. Additionally, because the left adrenal gland

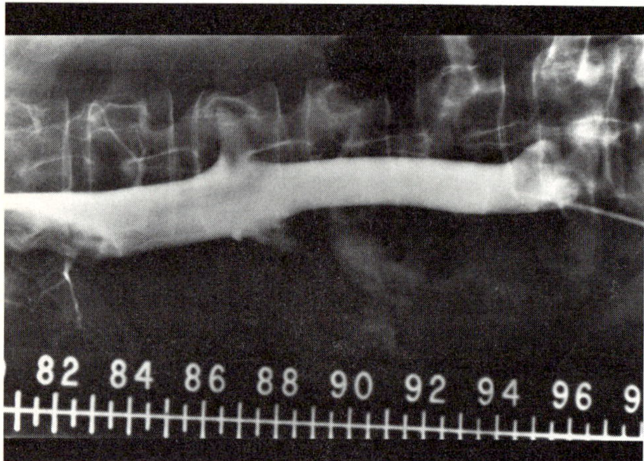

Figure 3 Venocavagram of the patient with right adrenal carcinoma in Fig. 2B demonstrating caval thrombus cephalad to renal veins and extending into the intrahepatic vena cava.

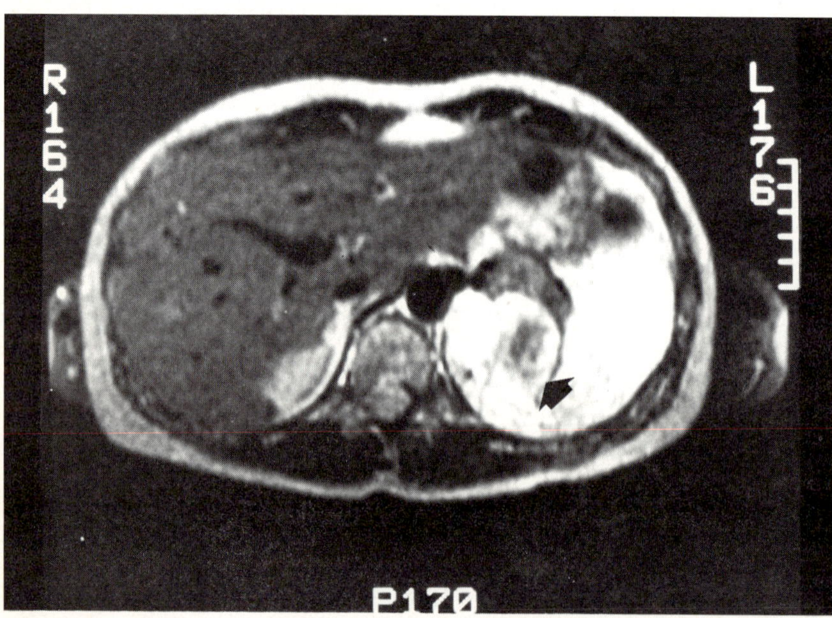

Figure 4 T2 weighted MRI demonstrating increased signal intensity ratio (adrenal/liver) of a local recurrence of left adrenal cortical carcinoma (*arrow*) 1 year after left adrenalectomy.

Table 1 Clinical Features of Adrenal Cortical Carcinoma

Presentation	Laboratory Investigation	Imaging Studies
Local		CT
Abdominal discomfort or mass		Optional:
Distant		Ultrasonography
Fatigue	Abnormal liver function tests,	Angiography
Weight loss	anemia	MRI
Bone pain		
Endocrine function status		
Masculinization	↑ Serum and urinary 17-KS,	
Feminization	17-OHCS, serum testosterone	
Precocious puberty	(female), estrogen (male)	
	and DHEA	
Cushing's syndrome	↑ Cortisol, ↓ ACTH, failure	
	of high-dose dexamethasone	
	to suppress cortisol	
Conn's syndrome	↑ aldosterone, ↓ plasma renin	
	activity; ↓ K^+	
Rule out pheochromocytoma	Normal serum and urinary	
	catecholamines and metanephrines	

Table 2 Staging of Adrenal Cortical Carcinoma

SEER	Size of Primary Tumor	Nodes	Invasion of Adjacent Organs	Metastasis	TNM
I	< 5 cm	−	−	−	T1,N0,M0
(Local)	> 5 cm	−	−	−	T2,N0,M0
II	Any size	−	+	−	T3,N0,M0
(Regional)	Any size	+	−	−	T1–2,N1,M0
III	Any size	−/+	−/+	+	T1–3,N0–1,M1
(Metastatic)	Any size				

SEER = Surveillance, epidemiology, and end results classifications.

overlies the left renal hilum, this region must be dissected with care to avoid injury to the renal vessels.

Preoperative Management

Specific considerations when patients who have functional ACCs are prepared for surgery include perioperative steroid replacement because of both pituitary and contralateral adrenal gland suppression. Patients with nonfunctioning neoplasms do not require steroid replacement. However, one must keep in mind the possibility of an absent adrenal gland in patients who have had a contralateral nephrectomy. Patients with Cushing's syndrome require optimization of nutritional status, electrolytes, and glucose, which is best achieved with a 1- to 2-week preoperative course of metyrapone. Perioperative histamine (H_2) receptor blockade should be considered for stress ulcer prophylaxis in patients with Cushing's syndrome. The rare patient with an aldosterone-secreting ACC should have his or her hypertension and hypokalemia corrected with spirono-lactone before surgery.

The patient should be informed that a chest tube will be used postoperatively and of the possible removal of contiguous organs, particularly with large lesions. Bowel preparation with polyethylene glycol and antibiotics as well as a knowledge of contralateral renal function are necessary if a bowel resection or ipsilateral nephrectomy is anticipated.

Technique

We prefer and recommend the thoracoabdominal approach in patients suspected of having ACC, although other incisions such as the Chevron can be utilized. Because of the lack of curative adjuvant therapy, complete removal of the malignancy, regional lymphadenectomy, and an en bloc removal of surrounding involved organs afford the best chance for cure.

After induction of general anesthesia and secure positioning of the endotracheal tube, the patient is placed in an exaggerated torque position with sand bags placed under the ipsilateral flank and hemithorax. Careful positioning is especially important in patients with Cushing's syndrome who may have advanced osteoporosis and friable skin. The patient is positioned so the kidney rest is between the twelfth rib and the iliac crest. To provide easy and comfortable access for the surgeon, the patient's flank should be close to the edge of the table. Because venous return and ventilation

STAGING OF ADRENOCORTICAL CARCINOMA

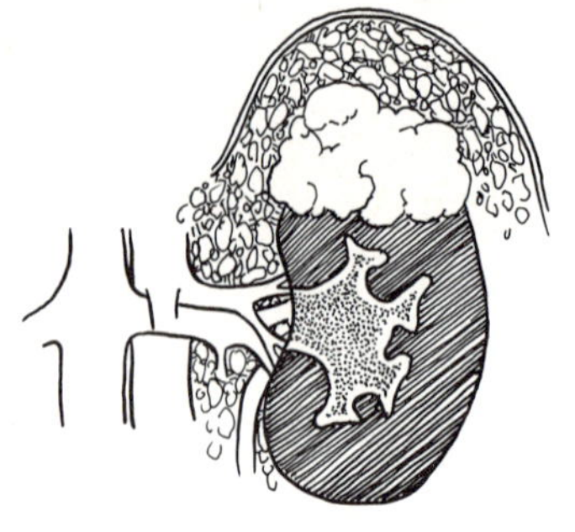

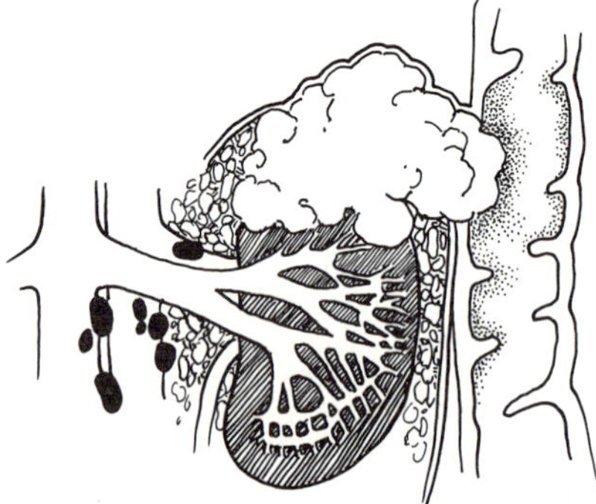

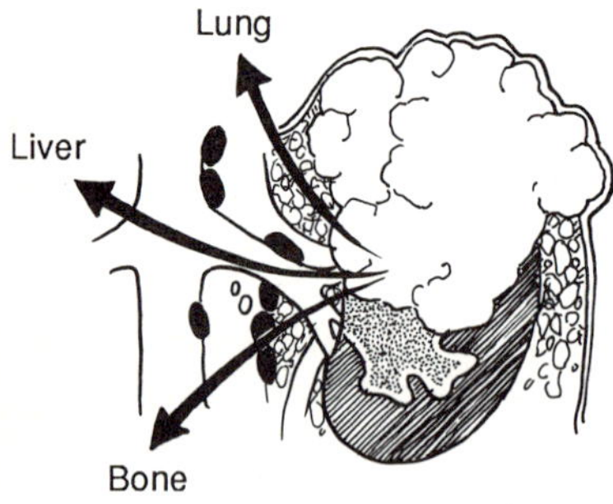

Figure 5 Staging of adrenocortical carcinoma according to the surveillance, epidemiology, and end results (SEER) classification.

pressures can be affected, the table is flexed slowly with attention paid to the patient's blood pressure and heart rate. The patient is secured to the table with adhesive tape across the hips and shoulders, with the bottom leg flexed to 90 degrees and the top leg straight, separated by a pillow. The lower contralateral arm is extended and secured on an arm board, while the upper ipsilateral arm is well supported on an elevated adjustable padded arm support, ensuring no pressure points on the axilla or elbow.

The size of the tumor dictates the level of incision, although for most lesions, a ninth intercostal incision is adequate. With smaller lesions, a supra-11 extrapleural, extraperitoneal approach or subcostal incision can be considered. The thoracoabdominal incision starts at the posterior axillary line, extends anteromedially along the ninth interspace, across the costal margin, and crosses gradually inferomedially toward the umbilicus just across the midline. The external, internal, and innermost intercostals are incised on the superior edge of the tenth rib to avoid injuring the ninth neurovascular bundle, and the latissimus dorsi and serratus posterior inferior muscles are incised at the posterior aspect of the incision. The costal margin is divided, and the external and internal obliques along with the transversus abdominal and rectus muscles are divided in the line of the incision just beyond the linea alba. A finger placed posteriorly on the superior aspect of the tenth rib can be used to push off the costovertebral ligament and thus "unhinge" the lower rib and allow for wider exposure. The diaphragm is incised in the direction of its fibers, the peritoneal cavity is opened, and the retroperitoneal space is developed bluntly. Retraction is provided posteriorly with a Finochietto and anteriorly with a Balfour retractor. The lungs, liver, and bowel are protected from injury with moistened towels. The liver

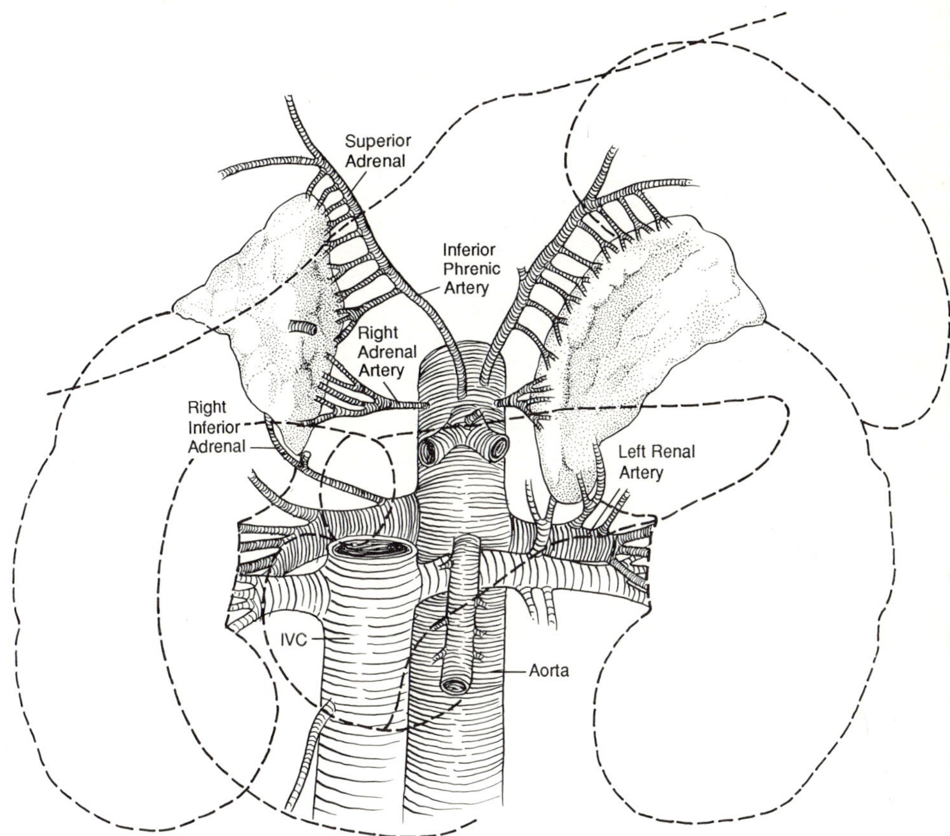

Figure 6 The adrenal glands receive their arterial supply through branches from the inferior phrenic, aorta, and renal arteries.

and retroperitoneum can now be examined for metastases, and the IVC is palpated for the presence of a tumor thrombus. Biopsy of suspicious lesions is performed as necessary. A solitary pulmonary or hepatic metastasis, if resectable, is removed at the time of adrenalectomy, if possible.

For right-sided lesions, the hepatic flexure is mobilized medially by incising the white line of Toldt. If necessary, the right triangular and coronary ligaments are divided sharply to allow the liver to be swung superomedially. The IVC is exposed by Kockerizing the duodenum, and the single adrenal vein is identified by dissecting along the lateral border of the IVC with gentle retraction on the mass and IVC (Fig. 7). The vein is isolated and tied off in continuity with 2–0 silk ties. On the left, the splenic flexure is mobilized medially similar to the hepatic flexure, and care is taken to pack away the spleen to avoid retractor injuries. The anterior surface of Gerota's fascia is now incised and the perirenal space entered and developed bluntly. The tumor's mobility and adherence to the adjacent organs is assessed. Mobilization of the mass begins at any opportune point. The subdiaphragmatic fatty tissue adhering to the superior aspect of the adrenal gland contains multiple arterial branches, which are divided after the application of hemiclips or 2–0 silk ties (Fig. 8). Similarly, arterial branches from the renal artery and aorta are divided. The left adrenal vein is identified as it enters the renal vein by dissecting distally along the superior surface of

the renal vein with gentle cephalad retraction on the mass and downward traction on the renal vein.

If the tumor cannot be dissected off the kidney with complete assurance of negative margins, an en bloc nephrectomy is performed. Similarly, invasion into adjacent organs may necessitate splenectomy, partial pancreatectomy, colectomy, or partial hepatectomy. Once the mass is excised and hemostasis secured, a regional retroperitoneal lymph node dissection is carried out with removal of perihilar, subcrural, and adjacent fatty lymphatic tissue around the great vessels.

Prior to closure, a 28-French chest tube is directed posteriorly in the pleural cavity and exteriorized through a stab wound two intercostal spaces above the incision along the anterior axillary line, secured in position with skin sutures, and connected to suction. The diaphragm is closed with running 2–0 Vicryl and the abdominal wall musculature is closed in layers with running 0 Vicryl. Posteriorly, the ribs are reapproximated with interrupted No. 1 Vicryl sutures above the ninth and below the tenth ribs, with care taken to avoid injury to the neurovascular bundle. The latissimus dorsi and external oblique are closed with running Vicryl. No abdominal drains are necessary.

Rarely, a tumor thrombus can involve the IVC in a fashion similar to renal cell carcinoma. For right-sided lesions with thrombus below the level of the hepatic veins, the IVC is isolated superiorly and inferiorly, along with the ipsilateral and contralateral renal vessels, with

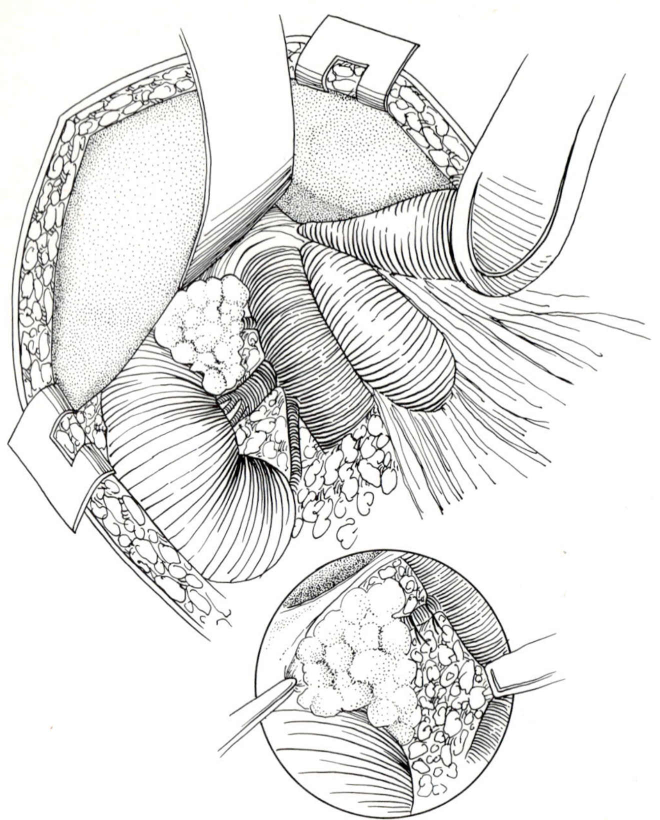

Figure 7 Exposure of a right adrenal tumor via a thoracoabdominal incision. The duodenum has been Kockerized to expose the single right adrenal vein which is ligated and divided in continuity (*inset*).

Rumel clamps. Cephalad control of a subdiaphragmatic thrombus can be obtained by passing a Rumel clamp between the right atrium and diaphragm and performing a Pringle maneuver just prior to cavotomy. The cavotomy is closed with running 4–0 Prolene, using a Scitinsky to reapproximate the opposing caval walls. Atrial extension requires cardiac bypass procedures. We consider suprahepatic IVC invasion by the tumor thrombus inoperable, while IVC resection with right nephrectomy is the procedure of choice for a subhepatic IVC thrombus with invasion. IVC thrombus extension from a left ACC is much less common, but when a diagnosis is confirmed preoperatively, an effective approach is an anterior transabdominal approach using a Chevron or midline incision with a median sternotomy if supradiaphragmatic control is necessary. Alternatively, a right thoracoabdominal incision with the patient in a modified right torque position with transverse extension across the upper abdomen provides good access to the IVC and left adrenal mass.

Surgical Complications

Intraoperative hemorrhage may develop from avulsion of the right adrenal vein and can be controlled with local pressure and suture ligature with 5–0 Prolene. Bleeding may also result from failure to ligate the multiple small superior adrenal vessels before division or before injury to lumbar or posterior vertebral veins.

The large size and high retroperitoneal location of adrenocortical carcinoma makes it possible to injure adjacent organs through either overzealous retraction or dissection. On the left side, a splenic laceration may necessitate splenectomy, although bleeding from smaller lesions may be controlled with the application of Gelfoam or Avitene and gentle pressure. An unrecognized pancreatic injury will have serious postoperative consequences such as pancreatitis and pseudocyst formation. A superficial laceration can be closed by tacking with several fine chromic sutures, while deeper injuries usually require partial pancreatectomy and formal closure of the main pancreatic duct with Prolene sutures and drainage with a closed suction system. Postoperative follow-up requires sequential serum amylase determination and abdominal ultrasonography to detect any fluid collections. On the right side, liver lacerations from retractor injuries or tumor invasion can be controlled with suture ligature of visible vessels. Unrecognized duodenal injuries, like pancreatic injuries, can be serious. If there is injury, two-layer closure with interrupted 2–0 Vicryl, with care taken not to narrow the lumen of the bowel, is performed with insertion of a nasogastric tube. When bowel function returns postoperatively, an upper gastrointestinal series is done to ensure that no leakage occurs before removal. Injuries to the ascending or descending colon may also occur, but with adequate preoperative bowel preparation, a two-layer closure of any laceration is appropriate in the absence of gross contamination. When one is performing

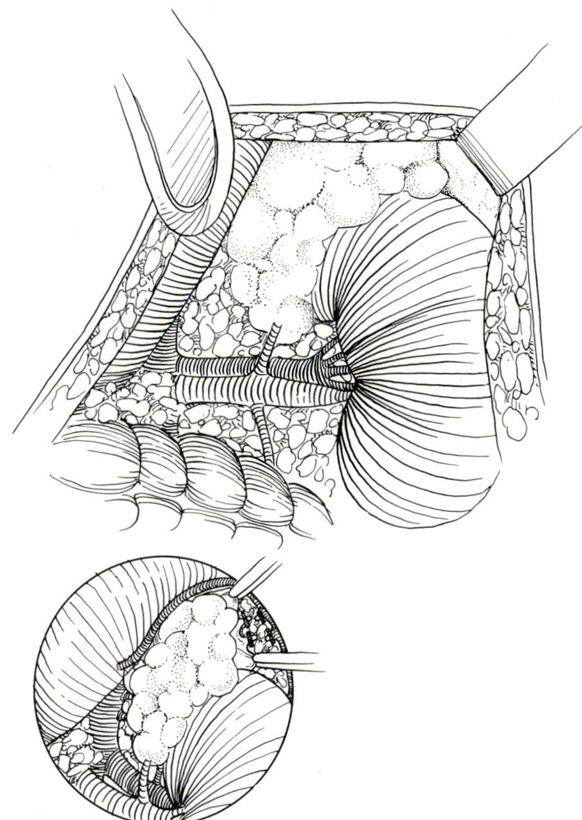

Figure 8 Exposure of a left adrenal tumor via a thoracoabdominal incision. The spleen has been packed away superiorly and Gerota's fascia opened. The superior adrenal arterial branches in subdiaphragmatic tissue are clamped, divided, and tied (*inset*).

a cavotomy for an IVC thrombus, a fatal air embolism may occur if all the intracaval air is not removed before removal of the cephalad clamp.

Adrenal insufficiency may result in patients with functional lesions or in patients with nonfunctioning lesions and an absent contralateral adrenal gland. Perioperative steroid coverage with gradual postoperative weaning prevents this problem. As with any major intra-abdominal procedure, atelectasis, ileus, and postoperative hemorrhage may also occur. Because of the catabolic and anti-inflammatory effects of elevated corticosteroids, patients with Cushing's syndrome may be at risk for increased wound complications secondary to problems with wound healing and infection.

RADIOTHERAPY

Although ACC is considered a radioresistant tumor, radiotherapy has been reported to have favorable palliative effects. Radiotherapy is indicated for (1) painful bony metastases; (2) unresectable local recurrences; and (3) incomplete resection, encompassing the adrenal bed postoperatively. The roles of intraoperative radiotherapy and interstitial implantation are undefined.

CHEMOTHERAPY

Ortho-para DDD (OPDDD), or mitotane, was introduced in 1960 for the treatment of ACC after earlier investigation of the agent as an insecticide revealed adrenolytic activity in dogs. OPDDD blocks steroid 11-hydroxylation and is specifically adrenolytic, possibly by affecting mitochondrial function at doses between 0.5 and 3 g per day.

OPDDD is indicated in inoperable, recurrent, and metastatic ACC, starting at doses of 1 to 2 g per day and increasing gradually to 8 to 10 g per day or until intolerable side effects result. Its role in adjuvant therapy continues to be evaluated; we currently advocate its use postoperatively. Daily steroid, and occasionally mineralocorticoid, maintenance is necessary during its administration. Monitoring serum drug levels to maintain concentrations between 14 and 25 µg per milliliter may optimize therapeutic efficacy, although disappointing response rates of approximately 30 percent have been reported. The functional status of the tumor does not affect the response rate to this drug. Side effects are largely dose-dependent, occurring at doses greater than 4 to 6 g per day; these include nausea, vomiting, diarrhea, drowsiness, weakness, visual disturbances, depression, ataxia, and skin rashes.

Attempts to improve the variable response rates to mitotane with various chemotherapeutic regimens have also been unsuccessful. Close to half of 110 patients seen at the University of Texas M. D. Anderson Cancer Center over a 40-year period received chemotherapy, either alone or in combination with OPDDD. Adriamycin and cyclophosphamide were probably the most effective drugs, but overall the results were dismal. Responses have also been noted with cisplatin-based therapy, suramin, and combinations of OPDDD with streptozocin.

Significant palliation against the adverse effects of excessive steroids from metastatic functioning ACC can be achieved with agents that block steroidogenesis. Metyrapone, which blocks cortisol production, is well tolerated at doses of 1 to 2 g per day. Ketoconazole, an antifungal imidazole derivative, and aminoglutethimide, which blocks the conversion of cholesterol to pregnenolone, are two alternative drugs.

PROGNOSIS

ACC is a highly malignant tumor and has a poor prognosis. Cure is possible only with total surgical excision of local or limited regional disease. The average survival rate of untreated patients is less than 3 months from the time of presentation. In a recent series of 110 patients managed at M. D. Anderson Cancer Center, 5- and 10-year survival rates of 23 and 10 percent, respectively, were reported. Fifty percent of patients were dead within 2 years of diagnosis. There was no difference in survival rate between men and women or between functioning and nonfunctioning tumors. Improved survival may be seen through stage migration because of increased discovery of incidentalomas, but clearly, new therapeutic modalities are needed.

ADRENAL INCIDENTALOMAS

With the wider application of CT and ultrasonographic scans for investigation of vague abdominal symptomatology, more adrenal masses are being discovered incidentally. As the incidence of benign lesions is much higher than that of malignant ones, management decisions must be based on the statistical chance of a particular lesion being malignant to avoid unnecessary surgery. Our approach to an incidentaloma is based on the size and biochemical activity of the lesion. The possibility that a lesion may represent a metastatic deposit, with primaries from the lung, breast, and thyroid being the most common, must be considered. Adrenal pseudotumors, such as gastric, pancreatic, or other retroperitoneal masses, may masquerade as adrenal tumors radiographically. With any incidentaloma, a biochemical evaluation should be performed consisting of serum cortisol, DHEAS, adrenocorticotropic hormone (ACTH), catecholamines, and if indicated clinically, aldosterone, estrogens, and testosterone. If serum cortisol is elevated, a high-dose dexamethasone suppression test is performed. A 24-hour urine sample is collected for 17-KS, 17-OHCS, cortisol, catecholamines, and metanephrines.

Although MRI holds promise in distinguishing adrenal adenomas from carcinomas, no reliable imaging or biochemical method is available. However, fine-needle aspiration can be used to confirm a metastatic deposit.

Any biochemically functioning mass, regardless of size, is excised because of the potential symptoms that can result and because of the increased risk of malignancy. Any solid mass that is 5 cm or larger, regardless of functional activity, is also excised because according to autopsy studies, only one in 12,000 adenomas ever reach this size. Cystic 6-cm masses are aspirated under CT guidance and followed conservatively only if negative cytologically. Nonfunctioning lesions less than 5 cm in size are 1,000 times more likely to be benign than malignant and therefore are followed. The incidence of adenomas of this size in autopsy series ranges from 2 to 9 percent. We repeat CT scans at 3-month intervals during the first year, and if the lesion continues to grow, we recommend surgery.

SUGGESTED READING

Barzilay JI, Pazianos AG. Adrenocortical carcinoma. Urol Clin North Am 1989; 16:457–468.
Bretan PN, Lorig R. Adrenal imaging: computed tomographic scanning and magnetic resonance imaging. Urol Clin North Am 1989; 16:505–514.
Copeland PM. The incidentally discovered adrenal mass. Ann Intern Med 1983; 98:940–945.
Didolkar MS, Bescher RA, Elias EG, Moore RH. Natural history of adrenal cortical carcinoma: a clinicopathologic study of 42 patients. Cancer 1981; 47:2153–2161.
Venkatesh S, Hickey RC, Sellin RV, et al. Adrenal cortical carcinoma. Cancer 1989; 64:765–769.

PRIMARY ALDOSTERONISM

JAMES F. GLENN, M.D., F.A.C.S., F.R.C.S. (HON.)

Primary aldosteronism is one of the surgically curable forms of vascular hypertension. Of course, renovascular arterial disease is far more prevalent as a surgically curable entity, followed by pheochromocytoma, which accounts for perhaps 2 percent of the hypertensive population. Aldosteronism is probably the underlying etiology in one of every 100 hypertensives.

One of the most interesting advances in modern endocrinology was the identification of aldosteronism by Jerome Conn in 1955 when he observed that many hypertensive patients coming to autopsy had so-called "nonfunctioning" adenomas of the adrenal, while normotensive patients exhibited a much lower incidence of such adenomas at postmortem examination. On this basis, Conn postulated that perhaps as many as 20 percent of hypertensive patients had hyperaldosteronism, although this was of course an overestimation.

Hyperaldosteronism may be either primary or secondary. The secondary form may be observed in conjunction with renovascular hypertension and with malignant hypertension. It may also result from antihypertensive therapy. Renin-secreting tumors of the kidney and ectopic hyper-reninism may also cause hyperaldosteronism. Alcohol abuse has been incriminated as a cause of secondary hyperaldosteronism, and the secondary type has also been noted in conjunction with pheochromocytoma and Cushing's syndrome. Clearly, some of these entities causing secondary hyperaldosteronism require surgical intervention; however, this is beyond the scope of this chapter.

It is primary hyperaldosteronism with which we are concerned here, and we can now identify four or more subtypes of the primary disease. The most common form of primary aldosteronism is that caused by a unilateral aldosterone-producing adenoma (APA) or aldosteronoma, amenable to surgical cure. The second-most common form is idiopathic hyperaldosteronism (IHA), which is caused by bilateral adrenal hyperplasia, an entity which does not respond well to surgical intervention, with the patient becoming steroid-dependent after undergoing bilateral adrenalectomy and often continuing to exhibit hypertension. There is a subgroup of IHA in which diffuse or focal hyperplasia may be found in only one adrenal, but this is relatively rare. Primary aldosteronism may also be of the glucocorticoid-suppressible type, secondary to an aldosterone-producing renin-responsive adenoma, or it may be associated with an aldosterone-producing carcinoma of the adrenal. The latter tumors are generally very large and commonly produce a variety of steroids in addition to aldosterone.

It is critical to differentiate between hyperaldosteronism caused by unilateral aldosteronoma as opposed to that caused by bilateral adrenal hyperplasia, since surgery is almost always totally curative of hypertension and the associated clinical components of aldosteronism with solitary adenoma. Patients with bilateral hyperplasia generally exhibit persistent hypertension, and consequently medical management is the treatment of choice. On the other hand, in those unusual instances of unilateral hyperplasia, removal of the affected adrenal may result in lowering of blood pressure, sometimes to normal levels. Clearly, such patients are potential candidates for surgery, since removal of the one adrenal does not cause hypoadrenalism.

CLINICAL PRESENTATION

The clinical manifestations of primary aldosteronism may be variable, but the classical symptoms are those of muscle weakness, polyuria, paresthesias, and intermittent paralysis, headache, and even tetany. Hypertension and hypokalemia with hyperkaluria are the hallmarks of aldosteronism, but the symptoms and signs may be highly variable.

A presentation of hypertension and serum potassium levels of less than 3.5 mEq per liter strongly suggests the diagnosis of aldosteronism. If the presenting serum potassium level is less than 3 mEq per liter, there is almost certainly an adenoma present. If the serum potassium level is borderline or equivocal, hypokalemia can be accentuated by small doses of diuretics. However, the level of serum potassium alone is not a satisfactory differentiating feature, since hypertension and hypokalemia have other causes as well, such as overingestion of licorice, use of chewing tobacco, Liddle's syndrome, and hyperdeoxycorticosteronism.

DIAGNOSIS

Demonstration of excessive aldosterone secretion with markedly elevated plasma or urinary aldosterone values confirms the diagnosis. Serial tests may be necessary since aldosterone production and excretion may be episodic. A relatively simple and very useful method of confirming the diagnosis of aldosteronism is the sodium loading test, in which a high-sodium diet of 2 to 3 g of sodium cloride taken three times daily for 5 days is used, or in which intravenous salt loading with 2 L of normal saline daily for 3 days is employed. Normal subjects or patients with essential hypertension exhibit suppressed aldosterone excretion (<14 μg per 24 hours), while patients with aldosteronism have urinary aldosterone values in excess of 14 μg per day. Patients with aldosteronism have persistently high potassium levels, whereas normal individuals and essential hypertensives exhibit high levels of sodium excretion and an inversely low level of urinary potassium.

In differentiating aldosteronism secondary to adenoma from that due to bilateral hyperplasia, postural stimulation is a useful test. Resting levels of plasma renin, cortisol, and aldosterone are determined after at least 2 hours of recumbency, preferably early in the morning. Repeat determinations are accomplished after 4 hours of ambulation and moderate activity. The patients with adenomas exhibit suppressed plasma renin activity and low levels of aldosterone, while in patients with hyperplasia, plasma renin levels are generally not suppressed and the aldosterone level remains elevated. This test is not totally reliable and has a specificity of only about 80 percent.

Measurement of 18-hydroxycorticosterone (18-OHB) is also useful in differentiating adenoma from hyperplasia, although there is some overlap in the levels of 18-OHB in patients with APA as opposed to those with IHA. Generally, patients with APA exhibit plasma 18-OHB levels greater than 100 ng per deciliter, while patients with IHA have levels less than 100 ng per deciliter.

Finally, it must be emphasized that patients presenting with hypertension and a serum potassium of 3 mEq per liter almost certainly have a solitary aldosteronoma, and one may then proceed directly to localization studies.

LOCALIZATION

Large adrenal tumors may be appreciated on a plain radiograph of the abdomen, although additional studies are almost always necessary in primary aldosteronism. An intravenous pyelogram may reveal displacement of the kidney if an adenoma is of sufficient size. Computed tomography (CT) will localize up to 90 percent of adenomas, although tumors less than 1 cm in diameter may be very difficult to appreciate. Since adrenal hyperplasia cannot be detected, a normal CT scan does not differentiate between hyperplasia and a small adenoma. Ultrasonography is not sensitive enough to be used as a screening or localization procedure for most adrenal tumors, including aldosteronomas.

Experience with magnetic resonance imaging (MRI) is limited, but the technique has definite advantages. The adrenals are seen as homogeneous low-intensity structures, distinct from surrounding fat, while adenomas may have increased signal intensity as compared with normal adrenal tissue. Currently, MRI is probably no more definitive than CT scanning, but further evaluation is warranted.

Adrenal scintigraphy using 131 I-19-iodocholesterol or the new scanning agent, 6-beta-131 I-iodomethyl-19-norcholesterol (NP-59), offers approximately 75 percent accuracy in localizing aldosteronomas. The patients are pretreated with dexamethasone, 1 mg four times daily for 3 days, in conjunction with Lugol's solution, to prevent thyroid uptake. NP-59 scanning will then disclose definitive uptake by APA, whereas IHA patients will exhibit only mild bilateral, symmetrical adrenal uptake. Scintigraphy is used only when other studies are ambiguous.

Adrenal venous sampling for measurement of aldosterone offers considerable technical difficulty, including difficulty in catheterizing the right adrenal vein or veins. Measurement of cortisol gives confidence in the reliability of sample capture. If APA is present, the ratio of the concentration of aldosterone from the involved adrenal to the contralateral normal gland is usually 10:1 or greater.

SURGERY

The decision for surgical intervention in a patient with primary aldosteronism is a collaborative one between the surgeon and the endocrinologist. Clearly, patients with overt aldosteronism secondary to an identifiable adenoma should have the benefit of surgical treatment, since cure of hypertension, hypokalemia, and the other manifestations of aldosteronism can be predicted with confidence. Furthermore, since aldosteronomas are almost invariably solitary and unilateral, preservation of the contralateral adrenal results in no endocrinologic disability for the patient. Surgery for unilateral adrenal hyperplasia, aldosterone-producing carcinoma, or other subtypes of primary aldosteronism is more difficult. A trial of medical management might be undertaken before surgery in any of these patients, although suspected carcinoma may impel prompt intervention.

The surgical approach to the adrenals is dictated by the diagnosis, the localization studies, the anatomy of the particular patient, and the preference and experience of the surgeon. The classical flank approach, transabdominal exploration, thoracoabdominal exposure, or some variation of the posterior approach to the adrenals all may be employed successfully.

The flank approach, subcostally or through the bed of the eleventh or twelfth rib, is infrequently employed since it offers no particular advantages and is more debilitating due to extensive dissection and division of musculature, as well as increased postoperative pain and prolonged convalescence.

The transabdominal approach to the adrenals may be desirable if there is a very large adenoma or if both adrenal glands must be explored. Mobilization of the hepatic and splenic flexures of the colon permits access to the retroperitoneal space. A midline incision may be employed, but a generous subcostal Chevron incision is usually more desirable.

A thoracolumbar or thoracoabdominal incision may be preferred for very large tumors since they offer maximal exposure. Such an approach is preferred if malignancy is suspected. Concomitant node dissection is most readily accomplished with the thoracoabdominal or thoracolumbar exposure. The disadvantages of these incisions include the time-consuming nature of opening and closing the wound, the relatively traumatic nature of the incision, and the attendant postoperative discomfort and disability.

In my experience and that of others dealing with patients with adrenal disorders, the posterior approach to the adrenal is ideally suited to patients with solitary aldosteronomas or unilateral hyperplasia. The posterior approach may be accomplished through a hockey stick incision, resecting the twelfth rib; through the bed of the eleventh or even the tenth rib, resecting the rib itself; or through a supracostal incision just above the eleventh rib, which is cut and reflected inferiorly. My own preference is for resection of the eleventh rib, entering the retroperitoneal space through the periosteum, which provides good substance for the subsequent closure.

The patient is placed prone on the operating table, which is flexed to approximately 35 degrees. The lower portion of the rib cage anteriorly should be over the kidney bar, which can then be elevated to further accentuate the flexion. An oblique incision is made over the eleventh rib, carrying this down through subcutaneous fat and the scanty musculature which covers the rib. The periosteum is incised and elevated from the underlying rib. The rib is then freed from the underlying periosteum in the usual fashion.

A point of technique relates to incision of the rib bed. This should be initiated laterally to avoid injury to the diaphragm and pleura. After the initial lateral incision is made, blunt dissection is carried medially and upward, sweeping the fibers of the diaphragm superiorly. In this way, entry into the pleural cavity is avoided, and of course, the abdominal cavity will not be entered.

A self-retaining retractor, preferably the Finochietto with the small blades, is then introduced and Gerota's fascia is exposed. An incision is made in Gerota's and the perinephric fat is dissected to expose the upper pole of the kidney. Minimal mobilization of the kidney is required, and a padded Deaver retractor can be introduced to displace the kidney inferiorly. This maneuver almost invariably brings the adrenal gland into view.

Fat is dissected from around the adrenal before any attempt is made to control the vasculature. Once the adrenal is exposed, the primary objective is control of venous drainage. On the left, there is usually a solitary inferior adrenal vein emptying into the renal vein, easily identified and controlled by either hemoclips or silk ligature. On the right, there may be one or more adrenal veins emptying into the vena cava or, in some instances, into the right renal vein. Arterial supply of the adrenals is highly variable, usually consisting of multiple small arteries of minimal caliber. Metal clips are advantageous for arterial control.

Dissection of the left adrenal is made relatively simple by the pulsatile aorta which is readily palpable and visable.

Dissection of the right gland is a bit more tedious, since it tends to wrap around the vena cava. However, in the case of aldosteronoma or unilateral hyperplasia, there are clear cleavage planes, and no difficulty with dissection should be encountered.

After the adrenal is removed, the bed of the gland is almost always dry. If hemostasis is incomplete with persistent capillary oozing, a Gelfoam sponge may be employed. Drains of any sort should not be necessary. Returning the kidney to its normal position further aids in hemostasis.

Closure of the incision is facilitated by lowering the kidney bar and decreasing the flex in the operating table. Nonabsorbable sutures of 2–0 or 3–0 silk or similar material are employed for multiple interrupted sutures in the periosteal bed. Overlying musculature and sub- cutaneous tissues are approximated with interrupted absorbable sutures. The skin may be closed according to the preference of the surgeon, but I have found that vertical mattress sutures of 4–0 silk are most satisfactory.

Unilateral adrenalectomy for adenoma or hyper- plasia requires no supplemental steroid management. In the case of aldosteronoma, electrolyte balance is achieved spontaneously. However, serum values of so- dium and potassium should be monitored. Although blood loss in adrenalectomy under these circumstances is generally negligible, volume adjustment will occur and it is imperative to accomplish appropriate fluid replace- ment based upon urinary output. Hypertensive patients with primary aldosteronism secondary to solitary ade- noma usually become normotensive within a few hours after surgery.

SUGGESTED READINGS

Bravo EL. Primary aldosteronism. Urol Clin North Am 1989; 16:481–486.

Conn JW. Primary aldosteronism: a new clinical syndrome. J Lab Clin Med 1955; 45:3–10.

Donohue JP, Weinberger MH, Hollifield JW, et al. Primary aldosteronism: diagnosis, localization and treatment. Intern J Nephrol Urol Androl 1980; 1:141–150.

Glenn JF. Adrenal surgery. In: Glenn JF, ed. Urologic surgery 4th ed. Philadelphia: JB Lippincott, 1990:1–25.

Noth RH, Biglieri EG. Primary aldosteronism. Med Clin North Am 1988; 72:1117–1131.

Young WF Jr, Klee GG. Primary aldosteronism: diagnostic evaluation. Metabol Clin North Am 1988; 17:367–395.

LOCALIZED RENAL CELL CARCINOMA

JAMES E. MONTIE, M.D.

Localized renal cell carcinoma (RCC) is a cancer that can be treated. Treatment options are primarily surgical without appreciable controversy: patients tolerate the surgery well with minimal negative functional impact, and the results are generally good. Compared with prostatic cancer, the treatment options are not nearly as controversial nor are the results so conflicting. Compared with bladder cancer, the morbidity of the treatment is much less. Unless RCC patients present with metastatic disease or an extremely large tumor, urologists can feel confident that they are doing "the right thing" that will help the patient most of the time.

DIAGNOSIS

The presentation of RCC has fundamentally changed in the last 10 to 15 years. Long recognized as a disease called the "great imitator" that could mimic other diseases, RCC was frequently a diagnostic problem. RCC now rarely fills that role. Improved imaging studies easily identify a mass in the kidney, often without the clinician looking for it. Abdominal computed tomography (CT) is readily obtained for a variety of nonspecific abdominal or systemic complaints; the clinician has no need to specifically search for RCC to make the diagnosis. As a consequence of this improved imaging capability, more cases of RCC are identified incidentally prior to any symptoms; an asymptomatic RCC also is often smaller in size. In 1932, approximately 70 percent of RCCs were greater than 10 cm; in 1950 to 1960, 30 to 40 percent were greater than 10 cm; today, only 10 to 15 percent are of this large size, and the average size is 6 to 7 cm.

The "incidental" renal mass is an entity that will confront all urologists and may well be one of the most common circumstances in which RCC is diagnosed. At the University of Michigan from 1961 to 1973, 13 percent of RCCs treated were found incidentally, compared with 48 percent from 1980 to 1985. There is evidence to support the observation that this incidental tumor will be smaller and less aggressive than the symptomatic lesion.

PREOPERATIVE IMAGING STUDIES

Once a solid or indeterminate mass has been identified in the kidney, value judgments must be made on the use of multiple imaging studies. Intravenous urography, ultrasonography, CT, magnetic resonance imaging (MRI), angiography, and inferior venacavography all can provide valuable information. However, it is not necessary to obtain all studies in all patients. The incremental benefit afforded by additional studies may be small. Ultrasonography, CT, and MRI often provide similar information on the nature of the mass; MRI offers the advantage of excellent delineation of the extension of RCC into the renal vein (RV) or inferior vena cava (IVC), but cost and logistic considerations dictate its use only in specific situations. Angiography is obtained less frequently and does not add a great deal to staging. When the cancer is large, angiography can provide helpful information to the surgeon, such as the demonstration of multiple renal arteries, which occur in 25 percent of individuals. A summary of the local staging of RCC is presented in Figure 1.

Two specific areas of caution need to be emphasized. First, the functional and anatomic status of the contralateral kidney needs to be ascertained before nephrectomy. Approximately 3 percent of RCCs are bilateral. Second, the status of the RV must also be certain before surgery. If an RV thrombus is present, one must be sure that it does not extend into the IVC; if it does, the precise level of involvement must be known. This information is critical for planning the surgical approach, and there should be no surprises in the operating room. The status of the RV can often be known from either CT or ultrasonography, but occasionally MRI and inferior venacavography are necessary. It is prudent to obtain enough information from a variety of studies to be sure of the extent of the vascular involvement of a RCC.

DIFFERENTIAL DIAGNOSIS

All solid renal parenchymal masses are not RCCs; benign and malignant lesions can be difficult to distin-

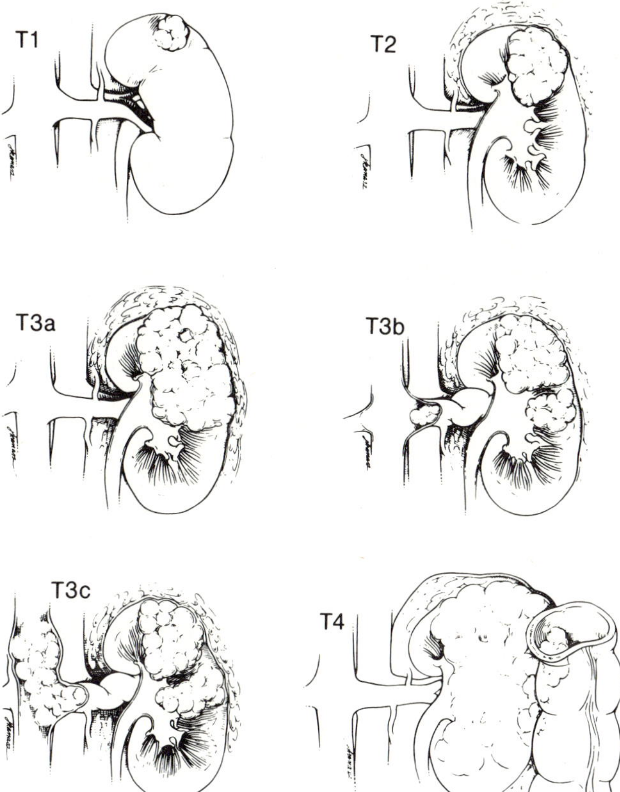

Figure 1 TNM staging of renal cell carcinoma based on the 1983 and 1988 American Joint Commission on Cancer Manual for Staging of Cancer. T1: tumor 2.5 cm or less, limited to the kidney. T2: tumor more than 2.5 cm, limited to the kidney. T3a: tumor invades the adrenal gland or perinephric tissues but not beyond Gerota's fascia. T3b: tumor grossly extends into the renal vein. T3c: tumor grossly extends into the inferior vena cava. T4: tumor invades beyond Gerota's fascia. (Republished with permission by Montie JE, Pontes JE, Bukowski RM. Clinical management of renal cell carcinoma. Chicago: Year Book, 1990.)

guish before removal of the mass (Table 1). Occasionally, removal of the kidney is justified, even though the mass ultimately is not a confirmed RCC. However, small lesions that may be benign (such as an oncocytoma, an angiomyolipoma, or a complex cyst) can be removed entirely by a partial nephrectomy in carefully selected patients. Some inflammatory lesions may resolve with antibiotics. Rare malignant lesions, such as an adult Wilms' tumor or a renal lymphoma, may be best treated with initial chemotherapy. Although these lesions are much less common than RCC, there are often characteristic aspects of the clinical presentation or of imaging studies that point to the unusual lesion.

PREOPERATIVE PREPARATION

Preoperative preparation for nephrectomy generally requires no unusual intervention. If the patient has

Table 1 Differential Diagnosis of Small, Solid Renal Masses

Renal cell carcinoma
Oncocytoma
Complex cyst
Angiomyolipoma
Adenoma
Other

undergone one or several imaging studies using intravenous contrast medium, care must be taken that there is no temporary renal dysfunction. This is particularly important in patients with compromised renal function, atherosclerosis, or diabetes. Hydration prior to imaging studies and surgery maintains an adequate intravascular volume. For a transabdominal or thoracoabdominal nephrectomy, a mechanical bowel preparation is helpful; if the tumor is large and could directly involve either the bowel or the colonic mesentery, a mechanical and antibiotic bowel preparation should be given.

Anemia is very common in patients with symptomatic RCC, especially larger cancers. Weight loss is also common, although usually not severe; perioperative total parenteral nutrition is seldom necessary. Preoperative staging for metastases usually includes a chest x-ray and CT or ultrasonography of the liver; an elevated alkaline phosphatase level or symptoms of bone pain justify a bone scan, and neurologic symptoms warrant a head CT scan.

PREOPERATIVE ANGIOINFARCTION

During the late 1970s there was considerable interest in preoperative angioinfarction of the kidney. A value was claimed for angioinfarction combined with nephrectomy in patients with pre-existing metastases; however, a randomized Southwest Oncology Group trial has identified no significant benefit, and this rationale has been abandoned. Some have claimed that the operation was easier after angioinfarction, but minimal data support this observation. The negative aspects of the postinfarction syndrome of pain, nausea and vomiting, and fever and the actual risk of the angioinfarction are noteworthy. There may be a role for angioinfarction of the kidney in patients with an IVC thrombus that is well vascularized; angioinfarction often leads to shrinkage of the thrombus and thus may provide some benefit. Appropriate patient selection, timing of surgery after the infarction, and the potential adverse effect of making the thrombus more adherent to the IVC wall need to be studied.

SURGICAL APPROACH FOR TOTAL NEPHRECTOMY

Most RCCs require a total nephrectomy. Surgical anatomy of the kidney allows the nephrectomy to be performed either inside or outside Gerota's fascia. The logic supporting a radical nephrectomy (outside Gerota's fascia) is compelling. Renal cancers commonly invade perinephric fat (60 to 70 percent) but rarely penetrate through Gerota's fascia. Dissection outside Gerota's fascia avoids many of the friable, dilated veins on the surface of the tumor and makes the operation easier. For a small cancer, an extrafascial nephrectomy may not be absolutely necessary, but use of a radical nephrectomy is a good general principle to follow.

Radical nephrectomy can be performed through a variety of surgical approaches, each with specific advantages. The most common approach is an anterior, transperitoneal exposure through a bilateral transverse incision. The hardest part of the radical nephrectomy is control of the main renal artery (RA) and main RV. Since these structures are close to the midline, it is wise to divide both rectus muscles to allow best exposure. The transperitoneal approach allows the surgeon to mobilize the colon and small bowel medially off the kidney, exposing the RA, RV, and great vessels without manipulation of the kidney. The "no touch" technique is firmly ingrained in surgical teaching, although it is supported more by the advantage of minimizing bleeding from collateral vessels than by the theoretical but unsubstantiated decrease in the number of circulating tumor cells.

A thoracoabdominal approach gives excellent exposure but is reserved for larger upper pole lesions, because it takes longer to open and close and puts the patient at some additional risk associated with a thoracotomy. For some tumors with an intrahepatic IVC thrombus, a large thoracoabdominal incision through the eighth or ninth intercostal space is the preferred approach.

The flank approach can be used for a radical nephrectomy; the kidney is of necessity manipulated more before exposure and isolation of the RA and RV. However, the flank approach is particularly valuable in obese patients, allowing the large panniculus to fall anteriorly. Either the 11th or 12th rib incision can be used, depending on the body habitus, location of the kidney, and site of the cancer.

Patients with a larger IVC thrombus present unique problems. Most commonly, a transverse upper abdominal incision is combined with a median sternotomy. This affords good exposure for both kidneys, the intraabdominal great vessels, and the heart if bypass is necessary.

RADICAL NEPHRECTOMY

As with most operations, the ease of performing nephrectomy is very dependent on adequate exposure. Two approaches can be used to expose the great vessels and renal hilum. The right colon and duodenum or left colon and jejunum are reflected medially for right- and left-sided cancers, respectively. The white line of Toldt is incised, and sharp dissection reflects the colon medially. Care must be taken not to dissect into the colonic mesentery. As medial retraction continues, either the duodenum or jejunum is exposed. On the right the hepatic flexure of the colon must be mobilized and the peritoneum incised medially to the porta hepatis. This exposes the anterior surface of the IVC. On the left side, the splenocolic ligaments must be divided, with care taken to avoid direct traction on the splenic attachments (Fig. 2). Failure to release the splenic flexure of the colon adequately is a common cause of traction injuries to the spleen. Mobilization of the jejunum medially exposes the anterior surface of the aorta, with cephalad exposure limited by the origin of the superior mesenteric artery.

An alternative approach is to incise the retroperitoneum medial to the inferior mesenteric vein. This is commonly used for retroperitoneal node dissections for testicular cancer, but also clearly can be used for a nephrectomy.

A self-retaining ring retractor has proved immensely valuable for renal surgery. A self-retaining retractor does not *provide* exposure but does *maintain* it superbly after the dissection affords the exposure; both surgeon and first assistant have both hands free to dissect, while a second assistant uses the suction, etc. Proper use of packs prevents injury to the liver, spleen, and bowel. The value of proper exposure that allows both the surgeon and the assistant to participate in the dissection cannot be overemphasized.

The initial step in the nephrectomy is ligation of the RA. On the right, the RA courses behind the IVC and RV. There are usually no branches from the right RV before branching into the hilum. The RV is mobilized with clips, cautery, or ligature to control lymphatics and small collateral vessels. A large medial cancer can abut

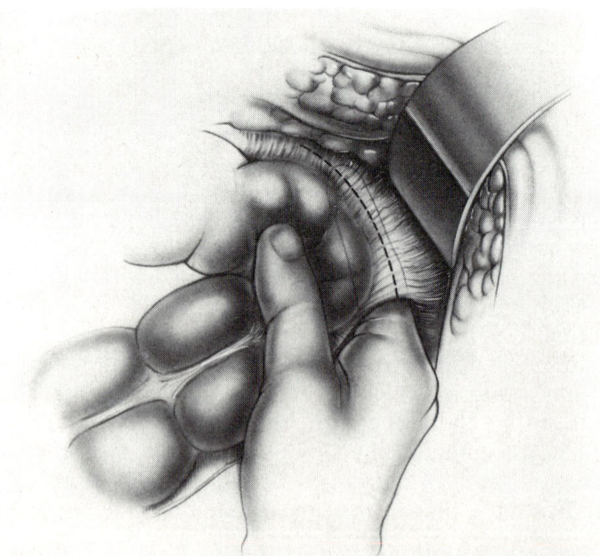

Figure 2 It is necessary to sharply divide the splenocolic ligament to avoid traction on the spleen during medial mobilization of the colon. Inadequate division of this ligament can lead to traction injuries on the splenic capsule.

or even displace the IVC or aorta, making exposure of the RV difficult. A large cancer may also have many dilated, thin-walled collaterals from the arteriovenous shunting within the tumor. If mobilization of the RV is difficult, the right RA can be approached *between* the aorta and IVC, avoiding the collateral vessels. The origin of the right RA is reliably just below the entrance of the

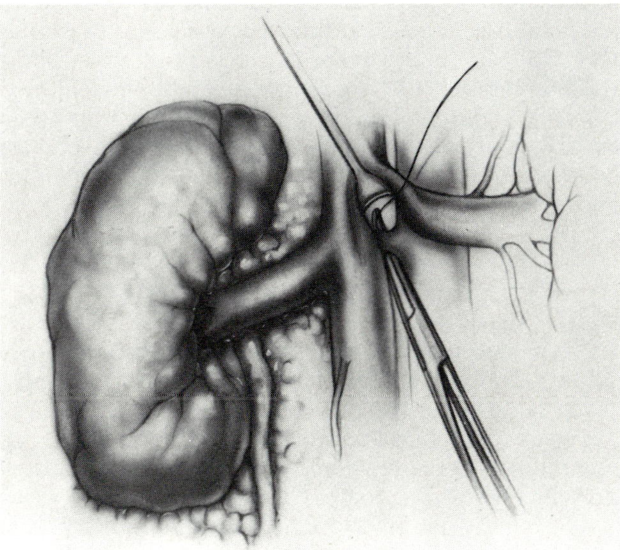

Figure 3 Ligation of the right renal artery close to the aorta, between the aorta and vena cava. The junction of the left renal vein and inferior vena cava is retracted superiorly.

left RV into the IVC (Fig. 3). Ligation of the RA early in the procedure avoids an increase in venous pressure and the engorgement of venous collaterals in the kidney that is seen with initial ligation of the RV.

If exposure of the RA is difficult, a single tie can be placed on the RA to stop blood flow into the kidney, and attention is then turned to further mobilization and division of the RV. Both the RA and RV are triply ligated with two ties close to the IVC or aorta.

After the RA and RV have been divided, the dissection proceeds inferiorly by identifying the plane between the psoas muscle and Gerota's fascia, clipping and dividing lymphatics and collateral vessels. Bleeding can be encountered from friable collaterals or lumbar veins. The right spermatic or ovarian vein is divided close to the entrance to the IVC, and the ureter is ligated separately. The dissection continues around the lower pole and then up the lateral aspect of the kidney. Access to the superior pole is provided by incising the peritoneum under the liver. RCC rarely invades the liver directly, but care must be taken to avoid blunt dissection into the parenchyma of the liver with larger upper pole tumors. The adrenal is usually removed with the kidney, especially with upper pole cancers. However, the adrenal is infrequently involved and can be left undisturbed if desired because of previous contralateral surgery or bilateral disease. The right adrenal vein enters the IVC several centimeters above the RV, usually at approximately the same level as or higher than the superior margin of the kidney. The adrenal vein is very short, entering the posterolateral side of the IVC, and needs to be specifically identified and ligated.

On the left side, problem areas include adequate mobilization of the jejunum and pancreas off the kidney

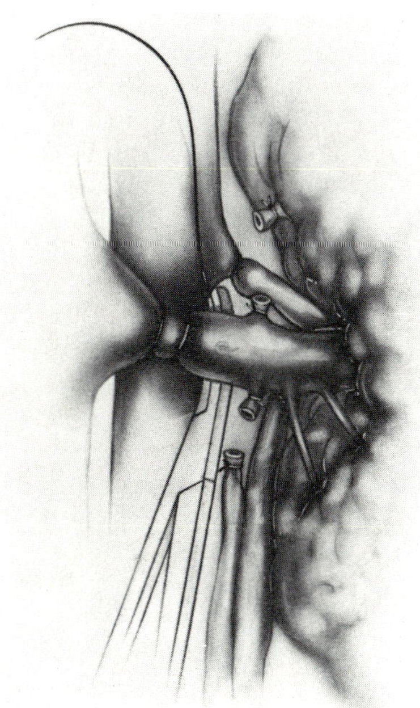

Figure 4 Mobilization of the left renal vein requires division of the adrenal vein, gonadal vein, and posterior lumbar vein. Injury to one of these branches can cause considerable bleeding, and ligation early in the dissection is a valuable approach.

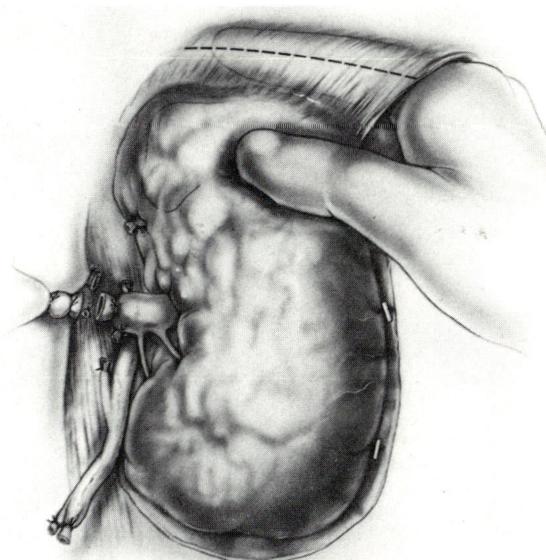

Figure 5 Dissection of the upper pole must stay behind the peritoneum to avoid injury to the spleen. Maintenance of the appropriate plane can occasionally be difficult with large upper pole tumors.

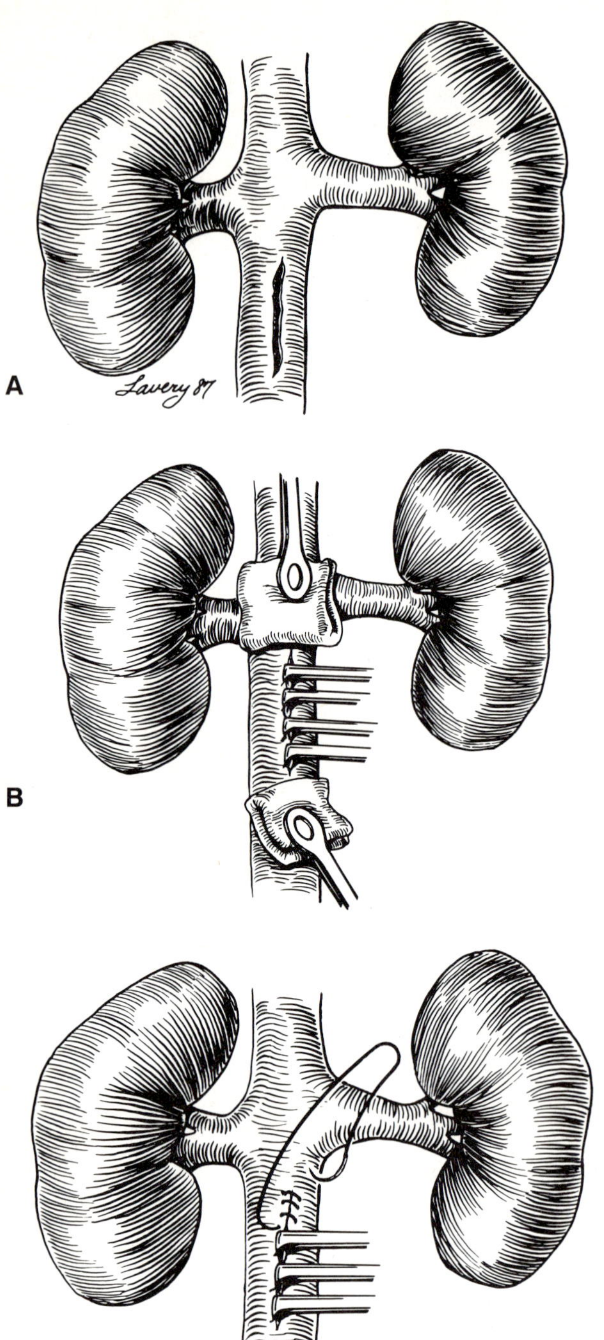

Figure 6 *A,* Laceration in the inferior vena cava. *B,* Proximal and distal control of the cava are obtained by compressing the cava with sponge sticks. Allis clamps are then sequentially applied to the tear, ultimately providing control. *C,* The tear is closed with a running vascular suture, sequentially removing the Allis clamps as the laceration is closed. This allows the tear to be closed under direct vision and minimizes the potential for compromise of the vena cava lumen. (Republished with permission by Surgery of inferior vena cava tumor thrombus. Novick AC, Montie JE. Stewart's operative urology. Baltimore: Williams & Wilkins, 1989.)

and avoidance of any splenic injury. The left adrenal vein, gonadal vein, and posterior lumbar vein must be divided to allow mobilization of the RV and subsequent exposure of the RA (Fig. 4). The left adrenal is lower than on the right, lying just above the hilum. Splenic injuries are avoided by staying behind the peritoneum as the upper pole is dissected (Fig. 5).

Troublesome venous bleeding can be seen from the stump of the left lumbar vein entering the paraspinous musculature; suture ligatures may be needed to control this. If a major injury to the IVC occurs, one must resist the temptation to use large suture ligatures immediately. Control of the IVC injury with compression and then Allis clamps allows control of bleeding and enough exposure to close the injury precisely without compromising the IVC lumen (Fig. 6).

PARTIAL NEPHRECTOMY

A partial nephrectomy may be used more commonly for a unilateral RCC when there is an identifiable potential for future compromise of total renal function. Diabetes, hypertension, stone disease, atherosclerotic renal disease, or azotemia of any cause can justify preservation of renal parenchyma.

Specific issues in the operative technique of a partial nephrectomy are covered in more detail in other chapters. Both angiography (now, commonly digital subtraction angiography) and CT or MRI provide valuable information. An angiogram gives a "road map" of renal vessels supplying the cancer, and CT delineates the location in the kidney. During the operation, mobilization and inspection of the entire kidney surface, temporary occlusion of the main RA, achievement of surface hypothermia with a saline slush solution, and resection of a 1- to 2-cm margin of normal renal parenchyma are important technical considerations. Removal of a central lesion is facilitated by extensive dissection of the RA and RV branches in the hilum after the kidney has been cooled and softened. Precise hemostasis with 4-0 absorbable sutures, closure of the collecting system in the tumor bed in the kidney, and reapproximation of the kidney on itself are important for proper healing.

Enucleation appears to offer little advantage over partial nephrectomy and exposes the patient to a potential unnecessary risk of residual cancer in the tumor fossa. Thus, enucleation is reserved for situations in which there is no alternative.

INCIDENTAL RENAL MASS

The widespread use of abdominal CT and ultrasonography identifies asymptomatic solid or complex renal masses of uncertain histology or behavior. The most common diagnosis is RCC, and although preoperative confirmation is difficult, the standard approach has been through a radical nephrectomy. Other diagnoses noted include an oncocytoma, a complex cyst, a true adenoma, or an angiomyolipoma. A subset of the incidental mass, i.e., the very small (2- to 3-cm) lesion, may be either benign or suitable for a resection that does not sacrifice a large amount of normal kidney. The value of avoiding a total nephrectomy is uncertain, since experience with renal transplant donors has not definitely identified subsequent hypertension or clinical deterioration of renal function. Animal studies suggest that glomerulosclerosis, proteinuria, and hypertension can be a consequence of extreme loss of functioning nephrons on the basis of the hyperfiltration theory. Clinical observations confirming a significant risk associated with a total nephrectomy for cancer when there is a normal contralateral kidney have not been identified. Nevertheless, removal of an entire kidney for a benign lesion of 2 to 3 cm is undesirable. Percutaneous biopsy of the mass is useful only if it is unequivocally positive for cancer, because a negative biopsy is unreliable in absolutely excluding cancer. Sampling variability within the mass, RCCs that can have an "oncocytic" appearance, and pleomorphic areas in benign tumors such as angiomyolipomas are all areas of uncertainty. In addition, the local and systemic recurrence rate for unifocal, unilateral, small RCCs will probably be less than 5 percent. However, until this reasoning is validated by clinical experience, evidence supports a total nephrectomy if the mass is thought to be malignant.

IVC THROMBECTOMY

Tumor propagation into the RV and IVC complicates removal of the kidney. Preoperative definition of the extent of the thrombus is mandatory. The classification system of IVC involvement into four levels is valuable and is based on modifications needed in the surgical technique (Fig. 7).

Collaboration with other surgical colleagues may be needed in resection of an IVC thrombus. For a urologist not comfortable with vascular techniques, assistance from a vascular surgeon is appropriate; a large thrombus may require a cardiopulmonary bypass and cardiac surgical help is needed. In some cases, a cardiac team may need to be aware of the case and be available for back-up. This suggests that the procedure should be performed in an operating room suitable for cardiopulmonary bypass, with a perfusion machine immediately available. To perform it in a standard urology room invites chaos if the cardiac team is needed in the event of an emergency during extraction of the thrombus.

A large thrombus obstructing the IVC complicates the operation from the onset. Venous collaterals in the abdominal wall and retroperitoneum may bleed profusely; mobilization of the bowel, normally done easily with blunt dissection, can be tedious. Precise hemostasis is essential, especially if bypass with anticoagulation is anticipated.

The method of extraction of the IVC thrombus depends on the extent of involvement (Table 2). A level

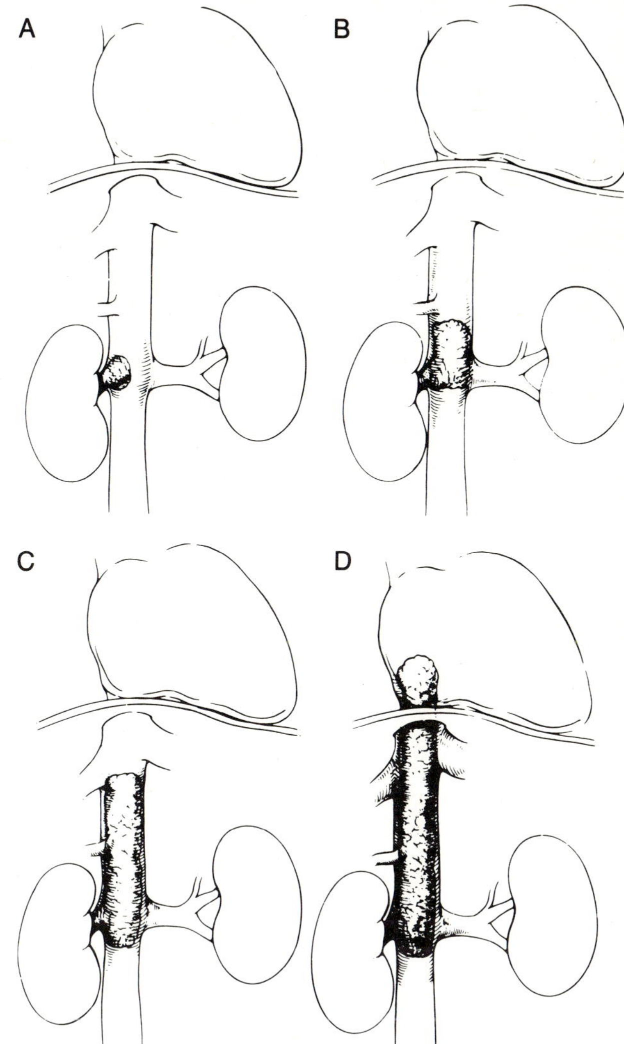

Figure 7 *A*, Level I thrombus, which extends into the vena cava but is more than 2 cm away from the renal ostia. *B*, Level II thrombus extends more than 2 cm from the renal ostia but does not go above the main hepatic veins. *C*, Level III intrahepatic thrombus, which extends up into the major portion of the intrahepatic vena cava so that control cannot be obtained above the thrombus but below the hepatic veins. *D*, Level IV thrombus with extension to the level of the diaphragm or intracardiac area.

I lesion means that the thrombus can be removed after placing a Satinsky clamp on the IVC, since only the RV ostial area of the IVC is involved. The opening in the IVC is closed with a running vascular suture. A level II lesion suggests that the thrombus is larger but still below the hepatic veins. The IVC will need to be completely controlled above and below the thrombus; the contralateral renal vein is occluded and individual lumbar veins must be ligated. However, since the thrombus is below the hepatic veins, a clamp can be placed above the thrombus without interfering with hepatic circulation. A level III thrombus is more complicated. The intrahepatic extension to the thrombus includes the hepatic veins,

Table 2 Level of IVC Involvement

Level of Thrombus	Operative Technique
I: Renal: <2 cm from renal ostia	Satinksy clamp on IVC
II: Infrahepatic: >2 cm from renal ostia but below main hepatic veins	Control of IVC above thrombus but below hepatic veins, contralateral renal vein, IVC below tumor thrombus, lumbar veins
III: Intrahepatic: intrahepatic IVC, below diaphragm	Control of IVC at diaphragm, porta hepatis, superior mesenteric artery, inferior mesenteric artery, renal vein, IVC below tumor thrombus, lumbar veins, or cardiac bypass with or without circulatory arrest
IV: Supradiaphragmatic or atrial	Cardiac bypass with or without circulatory arrest

and two approaches are possible, each with its own advantages.

Probably the simpler approach requires control of all tributaries in and out of the subdiaphragmatic IVC; the proximal IVC below the thrombus, the distal IVC at the diaphragm, the contralateral renal vein, the porta hepatis, and the superior and inferior mesenteric arteries need to be controlled and occluded. A thoracoabdominal incision is used for this technique, reflecting the liver medially to expose the retrohepatic IVC; anticoagulation is not necessary. This approach works well for the thrombus that can be extracted easily, since the ischemia time for the liver is approximately 30 minutes. If the IVC is occluded at the diaphragm without control of the hepatic arterial and portal circulation, the liver becomes engorged and enlarged; pressure in the intrahepatic IVC increases dramatically.

An alternative approach for a large intrahepatic IVC thrombus consists of cardiopulmonary bypass, with or without circulatory arrest. Bypass offers the advantage of complete control over the patient during extraction of the thrombus, without the risk of sudden hypotension; more time is available to remove small fragments of the thrombus and reconstruct the IVC. Circulatory arrest is an adjunct to cardiopulmonary bypass that relies on profound hypothermia (18° to 20° C) to protect metabolic functions. With hypothermic cardioplegia, 95 percent of the patient's blood volume is drained into the bypass machine and there is no flow to any organ. Unsurpassed exposure of the interior of the IVC allows extraction of the thrombus, previously the most difficult portion of the procedure, to be done easily under a controlled circumstance. A very long cavotomy, 15 cm or more, can be closed easily. The disadvantages are the increased complexity of the procedure, the risk of cardiopulmonary bypass (very low in individuals without significant coronary artery disease), the risk of profound hypothermia, and the need for temporary anticoagulation. Profound hypothermia has been tolerated well, with few identified neurologic, hepatic, or renal adverse consequences. A coagulopathy has been noted in a small percentage of patients and is corrected with blood-product replacement. This technique is suitable for procedures that markedly enlarge and occlude the IVC or approach the diaphragm.

A level IV thrombus extends into the heart. Cardiac bypass is appropriate, again with or without circulatory arrest, using the same techniques as described above.

An intraoperative tumor embolization to the lung is a catastrophic event with few survivors. The risk may be higher with a smaller thrombus that is more friable and less adherent to the wall of the IVC. Prevention is paramount.

LYMPHADENECTOMY

Controversy exists over the value of a retroperitoneal lymphadenectomy in association with a radical nephrectomy. Variability in patterns of initial lymphatic drainage from the kidney has caused some to question the feasibility of resection of first-echelon lymph nodes. Although instances of aberrant drainage bypassing paracaval, interaortocaval, and para-aortic lymph nodes are documented, this type of spread is unusual. More data support a consistent drainage from the right kidney to the para-, pre-, retro-, and interaortocaval lymph nodes and from the left kidney to the pre- and periaortic lymph nodes. Proponents of an extended lymphadenectomy recommend removal of all these nodes on each side respectively from the diaphragm to the bifurcation of the great vessels. Recent data, although uncontrolled and potentially biased, support this extensive resection; Giuliani and colleagues reported a 5-year survival rate of 52 percent in 20 patients with nodal involvement without venous extension. This figure is appreciably better than those in other series and may be partially a consequence of more precise pathologic staging of the nodes. My practice in the past has been to perform a very limited node dissection just around the hilum, based on the assumption that early nodal involvement would be seen in this area, and that the only patients helped by node dissection are the ones with earliest involvement. This reasoning may not be entirely accurate, and the recent data supporting a more aggressive lymphadenectomy are certainly provocative. Further dissection around the great vessels can be difficult because of enlargement of collateral vessels from the kidney. A prospective evaluation of the lymphadenectomy issue would be welcome.

SUGGESTED READING

Giuliani L, Giberti C, Martorana G, Rovida S. Radical extensive surgery for renal cell carcinoma: long-term results and prognostic factors. J Urol 1990; 143:468–474.

Konnak JW, Grossman HB. Renal cell carcinoma as an incidental finding. J Urol 1985; 134:1094–1096.

Marshall FF, Dietrick DD, Baumgartner WA, Reitz BA. Surgical management of renal cell carcinoma with intracaval neoplastic extension above the hepatic veins. J Urol 1988; 139:1166–1172.

Montie JE, Pontes JE, Bukowski RM. In: Clinical management of renal cell cancer. Chicago: Year Book, 1990.

Novick AC, Kaye MC, Cosgrove DM, et al. Experience with cardiopulmonary bypass and deep hypothermic circulatory arrest in the management of retroperitoneal tumors with large vena caval thrombi. Ann Surg 1990; 212:472–477.

Novick AC, Streem SB, Montie JE, et al. Conservative surgery for renal cell carcinoma: a single-center experience with 100 patients. J Urol 1989; 141:835–839.

Skinner DG, Pritchett TR, Lieskovsky G, et al. Vena caval involvement by renal cell carcinoma: surgical resection provides meaningful long-term survival. Ann Surg 1989; 210:387–393.

Steckler RE, Riehl RA Jr, Vaughan EO Jr. Hyperfiltration-induced renal injury in normal man: myth or reality. J Urol 1990; 144: 1323–1327.

METASTATIC RENAL CELL CARCINOMA

W. MARSTON LINEHAN, M.D.
McCLELLAN M. WALTHER, M.D.
STEVEN A. ROSENBERG, M.D., Ph.D.

It is estimated that more than 20,000 people per year will develop renal cell carcinoma in the United States and that more than 10,000 will eventually die of this disease. Although the 5-year survival rate for patients with localized renal cell carcinoma is greater than 90 percent, only 10 to 15 percent of patients in whom metastatic disease develops will survive for 24 months. Currently there is no effective standard form of therapy available for patients with advanced renal cell carcinoma.

ADJUVANT NEPHRECTOMY AND ANGIOINFARCTION

Adjuvant nephrectomy is often recommended for patients with metastatic renal cell carcinoma who have signs or symptoms such as hypercalcemia, pain, hemorrhage, or hypertension. Although there have been anecdotal reports of regression of metastatic foci after nephrectomy, the reported incidence of spontaneous regression after nephrectomy in patients with metastatic renal cell carcinoma is low—less than 1 percent. Nephrectomy and resection of metastases are often performed when a patient has a solitary, isolated focus of metastatic disease. Nephrectomy combined with either resection or treatment with radiation therapy to a single metastatic focus has been reported to be associated with a 5-year survival rate of 20 to 40 percent.

Some clinicians perform angioinfarction of the kidney by embolization of the renal artery with alcohol, autologous blood clot, or inert substances such as steel coils in patients with metastatic renal cell carcinoma. This procedure, which is associated with neither an increased incidence of regression of metastatic foci or prolonged survival is primarily employed when there is a very large or vascular tumor or when the surgeon believes that preoperative embolization will enable the performance of a more safe procedure. Angioinfarction is used occasionally in patients who are not surgical candidates who have significant pain, bleeding, or other symptoms from the tumor.

RADIATION THERAPY

The most frequent sites of hematogenous spread of renal cell carcinoma are the lung, bones, and brain. Palliative radiation therapy of painful osseous metastases often induces significant relief of symptoms. Although spinal vertebral body metastases from renal cell carcinoma often produces painful lesions, a tumor at this location can progress insidiously and result in paraplegia with little or no warning. If tumor involvement at this site is suspected, a magnetic resonance imaging (MRI) scan can be a highly sensitive test for detection of the lesion and characterization of the extent of its destruction. An MRI scan may sometimes detect a lesion that was not detectable on either computed tomography (CT) or bone scan. Radiation therapy to the spine in patients with osseous metastases can help prevent the local progression of disease and may prevent or retard the development of more significant sequelae.

The development of a CNS metastasis from renal cell carcinoma requires prompt attention. Depending on the location of the metastatic lesion and the condition of the patient, neurosurgical removal may be considered. If it is not possible or if it is inappropriate to consider surgical removal of a CNS metastasis, radiation therapy can induce significant palliative results in the majority of patients.

CHEMOTHERAPY AND HORMONAL THERAPY

A very large number of chemotherapeutic agents have been evaluated in the treatment of patients with metastatic renal cell carcinoma, with disappointing results. One of the most commonly used agents has been vinblastine sulfate. The objective response rate in patients with advanced renal cell carcinoma is approximately 15 percent. The use of the combination chemotherapeutic regimens, which is associated with increased toxicity compared with single-agent therapy, has achieved slightly higher response rates. In patients with metastatic kidney cancer, however, few durable long-term remissions have been reported with chemotherapy. There have been some recent encouraging results associated with the use of continuous infusion of floxuridine (FUDR) by means of programmable automated pumps. Further studies with larger numbers of patients are necessary to determine the role of this form of therapy in patients with metastatic renal cell carcinoma.

Several animal studies were performed during the 1960s and 1970s that suggested that hormonal therapy might be an effective strategy for kidney cancer. These studies led to the use of various forms of hormonal therapy in patients with metastatic renal cell carcinoma. Although these forms of therapy are associated with little morbidity, however, the objective response rates to such agents as medroxyprogesterone acetate are very low, less than 10 percent. Currently, hormonal therapy is most often used in patients who are not candidates for treatment with other forms of therapy.

IMMUNOTHERAPY

Since 1984, patients with advanced renal cell carcinoma have been treated with a new form of therapy developed in the Surgery Branch of the National Cancer Institute: adoptive immunotherapy. Adoptive immunotherapy involves the transfer of immunologic agents with antitumor activity to the tumor-bearing host. The initial forms of adoptive immunotherapy in the Surgery Branch involved the use of a lymphokine, interleukin-2 (IL-2), which was administered either alone or in combination with lymphokine-activated killer (LAK) cells. Interleukin-2, previously called T cell growth factor, is a naturally occurring substance which has been shown to induce proliferation of lymphocytes. LAK is defined as the incubation of lymphocytes in IL-2 which results in the generation of cells capable of lysing fresh tumor cells in short-term chromium-51 release assays. In experimental animals, the administration of recombinant IL-2 either alone or with LAK cells has been shown to be capable of inducing the regression of established tumors at several sites. In these preclinical studies there was greater antitumor effect in the animals treated with higher doses of IL-2 and in those treated with the combination of IL-2 plus adoptively transferred cells (LAK).

Patients who are treated with immunotherapy in the Surgery Branch have metastatic measurable disease and good performance status. No patient is eligible for therapy who has been treated with any form of therapy for 1 month before the initiation of immunotherapy. Patients who have a history of other types of cancer

(except for basal carcinoma of the skin) are also not eligible for therapy. Patients are excluded from study who have major illnesses of the cardiovascular, pulmonary, or gastrointestinal systems. Patients who have CNS metastasis are not eligible for this form of therapy. All patients undergo a complete radiographic evaluation, including a chest tomography and/or chest CT, abdominal CT, head CT, or MRI and bone scan. Patients older than 50 years of age undergo a stress thallium or stress mugga examination and pulmonary function testing. Patients with significant abnormalities of the cardiovascular or pulmonary systems are not eligible for immunotherapy.

The patient's renal function and serum calcium are also evaluated before they are considered for therapy. It is essential that the patient have normal renal function before the initiation of therapy. Patients with renal insufficiency will not tolerate high-dose IL-2–based immunotherapy. If a patient has hypercalcemia and the primary kidney tumor has not been removed, nephrectomy may help return the serum calcium to a normal level. If hypercalcemia persists, the patient is not considered an appropriate candidate for high-dose IL-2–based therapy. Hypercalcemia can be associated with renal insufficiency and altered sensorium. Patients who have significant hypercalcemia are not considered appropriate candidates for immunotherapy.

Patients with metastatic renal cell carcinoma have been treated in the Surgery Branch of the National Cancer Institute with a number of immunotherapeutic regimens, including IL-2, IL-2 plus LAK, IL-2 plus alpha-interferon, interleukin-4 (IL-4), IL-2 plus IL-4, and cyclophosphamide plus IL-2 and tumor-infiltrating lymphocytes (TIL). Patients have been treated both after cytoreductive nephrectomy and with their primary kidney tumor in place.

Patients who undergo cytoreductive nephrectomy before being considered for immunotherapy have had their kidney tumors removed by either a thoracoabdominal, transabdominal, or flank approach. Unless the tumor is an unusually large upper pole tumor or involves the spleen or liver directly, an attempt is made to remove it via a transabdominal, subcostal, or flank approach. A thoracoabdominal incision is often associated with more morbidity than a transabdominal approach and its use could potentially be associated with a delay in entering therapy. When the primary kidney tumor is removed, an attempt is made to remove all disease in the retroperitoneum that can be resected safely. The patient is then seen in follow up approximately 6 weeks after surgery. At this time, restaging radiographic studies are performed, and if the patient has recovered from surgery and has a normal postnephrectomy creatinine, he or she is considered for immunotherapy.

Because relatively few responses have been observed in the primary kidney tumor of patients treated with IL-2–based therapies in the Surgery Branch, most patients have undergone cytoreductive nephrectomy before therapy. However, the role of cytoreductive nephrectomy in patients with advanced renal cell carcinoma treated with IL-2–based immunotherapy has not been determined. We have demonstrated that therapy with IL-2 or IL-2 plus LAK therapy can be safely administered shortly after therapy in carefully selected patients with metastatic renal cell carcinoma. Nevertheless, in our experience, approximately one-third of patients were not able to enter therapy after cytoreductive nephrectomy, because of either disease- or surgery-related issues that developed between the time of surgery and the time at which therapy was initiated. A randomized trial is required to determine the role of surgery in the treatment of patients with metastatic renal cell carcinoma undergoing immunotherapy. A potential advantage of pretherapy nephrectomy is that there will be less bulk of disease to treat after surgery. Thus far, we have not seen significant responses in the primary tumors in many patients treated with the kidney in place. However, disadvantages of pretherapy nephrectomy are that it could potentially delay the initiation of immunotherapy and that, in our experience, only approximately two-thirds of patients have been able to enter therapy after surgery.

Either complete or partial response has been seen in approximately 35 percent of patients treated with IL-2 plus LAK and in 20 percent of patients treated with IL-2 alone. There was a complete response in approximately 10 percent of patients. These regressions can be durable; of the patients achieving a complete or partial response, some have not developed recurrence past 30 months.

Patients with metastatic renal cell carcinoma have also responded to treatment with the combination of IL-2 plus alpha-interferon. In 46 patients treated with this combination in the Surgery Branch of the National Cancer Institute, a complete response was noted in four patients and a partial response in 11. From this study it appeared that response rates may be related to the dose used and that the highest dose might produce the best response. Although the response rates in patients treated with the highest doses of IL-2 plus alpha-interferon were high (>35 percent), it has not been demonstrated in a randomized trial that this regimen is better than the use of either agent alone or superior to therapy with IL-2 plus LAK (Table 1).

The use of high-dose IL-2–containing regimens is associated with significant side effects. The primary side effect associated with the use of IL-2 is related to a capillary leak syndrome induced by this agent. In patients undergoing IL-2–based therapy, hypotension, renal insufficiency, weight gain, pulmonary insufficiency, neuropsychiatric effects, hepatic insufficiency, malaise, hematopoietic suppression, and other effects can develop. The side effects of this agent are transient and reverse after IL-2 therapy has been discontinued. Deaths have been associated with treatment-related causes in 1.5 percent of patients in the Surgery Branch treated with IL-2–based therapies.

In an effort to develop a more potent cell for adoptive transfer, preclinical studies have been performed with lymphocytes derived from the tumor itself, tumor-infiltrating lymphocytes (TILs). In a number of murine studies, TIL was found to be a more potent cell that often had specific antitumor reactivity. These and other preclinical studies led to the conduct of a pilot trial demonstrating that the treatment of patients with the combination of cyclophosphamide, IL-2, and TIL is a practical and feasible strategy. In patients with metastatic renal cell carcinoma who are candidates for TIL therapy, the primary kidney tumor or an accessible metastatic lesion is removed and TILs from the tumor are activated and expanded in the presence of IL-2. The TILs are then transferred back to the patient, along with IL-2 or IL-2 plus alpha-interferon. Although response has been observed in those patients with advanced kidney cancer who are undergoing this form of therapy, several modifications and changes are being made in attempt to make this a more effective and less toxic form of therapy.

Although in several patients, adoptive immunotherapy has been associated with significant regression of disease for a prolonged duration, this form of therapy is still in the early stages of development. Efforts evaluating the use of the combination of lymphokines as well as new modifications of adoptively transferred cells, such as TIL, are ongoing and it is hoped will lead to the development of an effective and less toxic form of therapy for patients with advanced renal cell carcinoma.

Table 1 Results of Immunotherapy for the Treatment of Renal Cell Carcinoma at the Surgery Branch of the National Cancer Institute

	IL-2 + LAK		IL-2 Alone	
	Total No. of Patients (72)	*Duration (Months)*	*Total No. of Patients (52)*	*Duration (Months)*
CR	8	(30+, 27+, 23+, 15, 13, 11, 9, 6)	4	(34+, 28+, 27+, 25+)
PR	17	(36+, 21+, 19, 13, 11, 11, 9, 7, 7, 6, 6, 6, 6, 3, 2, 1, 1)	8	(27+, 27+, 25+, 21+, 21+, 19+, 15+, 3+)
CR + PR	23 (35%)		12 (22%)	

CR = complete response; PR = partial response.
Adapted from Rosenberg SA, Lotze MT, Yang JC, et al. Experience with the use of high-dose interleukin-2 in the treatment of 652 patients with cancer. Ann Surg 1989; 210:474–485.

SUGGESTED READING

Linehan WM, Shipley W, Longo D. Cancer of the kidney and ureter. In DeVita VT, Hellman S, Rosenberg SA, eds. Principles and practices of oncology. Philadelphia: JB Lippincott, 1989: 979.

Robertson CN, Linehan WM, Pass HI, et al. Preparative cytoreductive surgery in patients with metastatic renal cell carcinoma treated with adoptive immunotherapy with interleukin-2 or interleukin-2 plus LAK cells. J Urol 1990; 144:614–618.

Rosenberg SA, Lotze MT, Muul LM, et al. A progress report on the treatment of 157 patients with advanced cancer using lymphokine activated killer cells and interleukin-2 or high-dose interleukin-2 alone. New Engl J Med 1987; 316:889–897.

Rosenberg SA, Lotze MT, Yang JC, et al. Experience with the use of high-dose interleukin-2 in the treatment of 652 patients with cancer. Ann Surg 1989; 210:474–485.

Rosenberg SA, Lotze MT, Yang JC, et al. Combination therapy with interleukin-2 and alpha-interferon for the treatment of patients with advanced cancer. J Clin Oncol 1989; 7:1863–1874.

Topalian SL, Solomon D, Avis FP, et al. Immunotherapy of patients with advanced cancer using tumor-infiltrating lymphocytes and recombinant interleukin-2: a pilot study. J Clin Oncol 1988; 6:839–853.

RENAL CELL CARCINOMA IN THE SOLITARY KIDNEY

JAMES E. MONTIE, M.D.

It has been over 30 years since Vermooten first suggested the use of a partial nephrectomy in the treatment of patients with renal cell carcinoma. The large experience obtained with renal preservation during kidney transplantation or renovascular procedures has been translated into expertise that can be applied to a partial nephrectomy. This improved understanding of the ability of the kidney to tolerate ischemia has been the main factor opening the possibility for partial nephrectomy as a reliable procedure for renal cell carcinoma. This chapter will outline considerations of patient selection, surgical technique and complications, and results obtained at the Cleveland Clinic Foundation in the treatment of patients with renal cell carcinoma in the solitary kidney.

PATIENT SELECTION

Patients should be considered for a partial nephrectomy if it is necessary to preserve functioning renal parenchyma. An anatomic solitary kidney, because of either congenital absence or surgical removal of the contralateral kidney for a benign or malignant process, is the strongest indication for a partial nephrectomy. Functional impairment of total renal function because of a systemic disease or a local abnormality in either kidney also justifies considering a partial nephrectomy. We are now considering a partial nephrectomy in patients who have adequate renal function at present, but who may be at a higher risk for developing renal failure in the future. An example of this might be a patient with severe diabetes or hypertension or one with contralateral renal artery disease. In a patient with bilateral renal parenchymal disease, preserving a portion of one kidney may not necessarily prevent renal failure, but may delay its onset. Currently, I do not feel it appropriate to do a partial nephrectomy for renal cancer when there is a normal contralateral kidney in an otherwise healthy individual.

Any patient with a carcinoma in a solitary functioning kidney should be evaluated for the possibility of a partial nephrectomy. A careful search for any metastases should include a bone scan, chest computed tomography (CT), and head CT scan (studies not normally performed in all patients with renal cell carcinoma).

If the patient has identifiable metastases, systemic treatment for renal cell carcinoma is so poor that cure is very unlikely. In this circumstance, surgical treatment of the primary tumor in the solitary kidney may be ill advised because it exposes the patient to the risks of the surgery, including renal failure, without the potential benefit of a long-term cure. It is rare that a lesion amenable to a partial nephrectomy causes symptoms that cannot be controlled by nonoperative techniques such as an angioinfarction.

Patients with a solitary functional kidney have varying degrees of compromise of total renal function. The operative risk to kidney function varies greatly with the size and location of the cancer. A 6-cm cancer on the lower pole can be removed with very little risk to total kidney function. A 6-cm lesion located directly in the hilum may be much more difficult to remove. In general, the risk to the kidney is less when an in situ partial nephrectomy is performed than when an ex vivo bench excision with autotransplantation is necessary. These are important considerations when discussing the options of partial nephrectomy, total nephrectomy and later dialysis, or nonoperative treatment with the patient.

Certainly occasional patients have widespread involvement of the kidney, and a partial nephrectomy is not feasible. One must then consider either a total nephrectomy with dialysis or subsequent transplantation or nonoperative treatment. Results with kidney transplantation have improved in the last 10 years because of safer immunosuppression. Thus, in a relatively young patient who had no evidence of metastatic disease, I would not hesitate to offer this alternative. Twelve months of dialysis is advised to select patients who are destined to relapse early.

On the other hand, keep in mind that the natural history of renal cell carcinoma can be quite indolent (especially a primary tumor). The patient must be aware that any procedure done on a solitary kidney can cause renal failure. Although the risk may be low in peripheral tumors, the patient must be appraised of this possibility. Frequently it is worthwhile to have the patient counseled preoperatively by the medical-renal service, which is familiar with home peritoneal dialysis, hemodialysis, and renal transplantation. It is often necessary to have assistance from the social work department on the availability of dialysis treatment. All these topics must be thoroughly discussed with patients before the procedure so that they understand the risks involved.

SURGICAL TECHNIQUE AND COMPLICATIONS

Both renal arteriography and abdominal CT scans are valuable in planning a partial nephrectomy. The arteriogram defines the blood supply to the tumor and the remaining normal kidney; CT is probably more precise in delineating the extent of the tumor, especially with lesions in the hilum.

Debate exists on the efficacy of enucleation of a small tumor compared with a partial nephrectomy that includes a margin of normal parenchyma. Enucleation was proposed because of the presence of a well-defined pseudocapsule apparent around some renal cell carcinomas. Several studies have now documented that although this pseudocapsule may exist around small tumors, larger cancers may not have this feature and may directly invade the surrounding parenchyma. In my opinion, the cancers suited for enucleation are very tiny lesions (1 to 2 cm). An incision at the junction of the cortex with the cancer allows an easy, blunt dissection of the tumor away from the parenchyma. The tumor "shells" out easily with minimal bleeding in the bed and with a grossly intact lesion. However, even in this circumstance the margin can be involved, with malignant cells on pathologic examination. At this point, I am not aware of local recurrences resulting specifically from this observation, but follow-up is short and caution must be maintained in advising enucleation. A patient with multiple tumors in a kidney, as in von Hippel–Lindau syndrome, is the one who may need enucleation of the tumors. In usual circumstances, normal tissue is wise.

I generally perform a partial nephrectomy in situ through the flank so that the kidney can be cooled without exposing the abdomen to the slush solution. Exposure is usually very good with this approach, even for complicated reconstructions. If a limited partial nephrectomy is being done for a surface lesion, cooling of the kidney is often not necessary. Isolate the renal artery in case unanticipated bleeding is encountered. Mobilize the entire kidney, including the renal artery and vein.

Mannitol is started at the beginning of the operation; if the renal artery is to be clamped, 20 to 40 mg of furosemide (Lasix) is also given. As with a donor nephrectomy for a kidney transplant, ensure a brisk diuresis from the kidney before clamping the renal artery.

If using surface hypothermia, place a rubber dam around the kidney, occlude the renal artery with a bulldog clamp, and pack the kidney in the saline slush solution. The renal vein is not occluded. Allow 5 to 10 minutes for the core temperature of the kidney to drop.

Start the partial nephrectomy by incising the cortex with a scalpel and then using the back handle of the scalpel to separate the parenchyma. Use sharp dissection as necessary; manual compression of the kidney can minimize venous back-bleeding. Larger vessels are suture ligated with absorbable suture. Avoid repeated clamping and unclamping of the renal artery because this may increase the ischemic injury.

With superficial tumors of the cortex, it is possible to remove the tumor without entering the collecting system, and the risk of urinary extravasation or leakage is low. The collecting system, which is opened during the resection of a larger lesion, should be closed under direct vision. I often place a double-J ureteral stent from the renal pelvis to the bladder to provide optimal drainage of the kidney. A nephrostomy tube is usually not left in place during an in situ partial nephrectomy.

Closure of the kidney on itself minimizes the potential for urinary leakage. I certainly prefer this to leaving an exposed, raw surface of parenchyma that is packed with perinephric fat. Even if the tumor has been excised in a longitudinal dimension, the parenchyma can be reapproximated in either a transverse or longitudinal direction depending on how it comes together with the least tension. The cooled kidney can be manipulated in many directions. Close the kidney with interrupted 2-0 chromic mattress sutures and then remove the clamp from the renal artery. Rarely, it may be necessary to reopen the closure of the kidney if a significant arterial bleeder has been missed.

A closed drain or a Penrose drain is placed and brought out through a separate stab wound. Because ischemia may be present in the area where the kidney was reapproximated, delayed extravasation from the collecting system is possible; thus the drain is usually left for 7 to 10 days. It may take several weeks for a fistula such as this to heal.

The risk of renal artery thrombosis is low. Although there have been reported cases of damage to the intima of the renal artery purely from clamping of the artery, this is a rare complication. Adequate venous drainage can be a problem after a large or complicated partial nephrectomy, especially if there has been venous invasion by the tumor. Renal vein thrombosis and subsequent renal failure have occurred in two patients at Cleveland Clinic Foundation.

The technique of ex vivo partial nephrectomy is not markedly different from in situ partial nephrectomy. Perform a radical nephrectomy, ensuring a brisk diuresis before dividing the pedicle. Flush the kidney through the main renal artery with Sack's or Collins' solution until the venous effluent is clear. Remove the perinephric fat from the kidney and excise the tumor, taking care to

Table 1   Renal Cell Cancer in the Solitary Kidney

Enucleation	Partial Nephrectomy In Situ	Partial Nephrectomy Ex Vivo
Technically easiest	Done with renal artery occlusion and surface hypothermia	Used for larger lesions, especially in hilum
Least risk to kidney		
? Incomplete excision in some cases	Applicable in most cases	Technically most difficult
Best suited for multiple small lesions as in von Hippel–Lindau syndrome	Moderate risk to kidney	Greatest risk to patient and to kidney
		? Best "cancer" procedure

maintain the proper orientation of the kidney to avoid injuring the main renal vessels or ureter. Several arterial branches can be identified by perfusing the kidney through the artery, and venous branches can be identified by perfusing through the renal vein. Suture the collecting system to provide a watertight closure. The kidney is reapproximated on itself and then autotransplanted into the iliac fossa in the pelvis. Often a nephrostomy tube and internal stent are used.

In my early experience with a partial nephrectomy for renal cell carcinoma, there was a greater tendency to perform an ex vivo excision than there is today. Quite large tumors can be successfully treated by an in situ partial nephrectomy. Nevertheless, the decision to perform an in situ or an ex vivo procedure can be difficult. In the former case, tumor spillage or incomplete resection is more likely; in the latter, the risk of the operation is higher. I have erred in both directions.

During a partial nephrectomy for a tumor of the hilum or lower pole, take care to preserve the blood supply to the ureter and renal pelvis. The danger is higher during an ex vivo excision and autotransplantation because collateral blood supply from the lower ureter is divided. Occasionally an ex vivo repair can be made by perfusing the kidney on the abdominal wall without dividing the ureter. In this setting, place a noncrushing clamp across the ureter during the period of renal ischemia to prevent perfusion and warming of the kidney from the ureteral blood supply.

Any procedure in a solitary kidney potentially exposes the patient to a complication that was once thought to be rare but that is being recognized more often. Injury to the adrenal gland can be minimal and yet acute adrenal insufficiency can develop in the postoperative period; this can be a difficult diagnosis to establish. Fever, hypotension, and abdominal pain can suggest a picture of sepsis or an acute abdomen, and a high index of suspicion must be maintained.

RESULTS

When the literature is searched to evaluate the results of partial nephrectomy, 5-year survival rates in the range of 60 to 80 percent are found. These results have often been compared with the overall survival rates of 50 to 60 percent seen in all patients with resectable renal cell carcinoma. Clearly this favorable survival rate for partial nephrectomy is secondary to patient selection. The survival rate of similarly staged patients treated by either partial or total nephrectomy is the figure that should be evaluated. Most patients treated by a partial nephrectomy have stage 1 cancers and usually have small tumors. The comparable survival rate of patients with stage 1 cancers treated by total nephrectomy is 70 to 80 percent. Thus, firm evidence exists that a partial nephrectomy does not lower overall survival by a great deal. Articles that have suggested worse results have ignored the role of the cancer in the contralateral kidney as possibly being the more important determinant of survival.

A partial nephrectomy does introduce the added risk of a local recurrence or a new tumor in the kidney. The local recurrence rate can be considered a specific evaluation of the efficacy of a partial nephrectomy. The literature provides a local recurrence rate of 9 to 17 percent; in my own institution, the figure was 13 percent. Some of these patients can be salvaged with a second operation, which is usually a total nephrectomy. In my opinion, there is an undeniable risk of a local recurrence after a partial nephrectomy that is not present after a total nephrectomy. In a patient with a solitary functioning kidney, this increased risk may be entirely justifiable. However, in a patient with a normal contralateral kidney, I do not believe this a justifiable risk.

Interestingly, the local recurrence rate has been higher for in situ partial nephrectomy than for ex vivo partial nephrectomy. This is noteworthy when one considers that the larger tumors are chosen for an ex vivo approach (Table 1).

In summary, partial nephrectomy for renal cell carcinoma should be considered in all patients in whom there is good reason to preserve renal parenchyma.

BILATERAL RENAL CELL CARCINOMA

ANDREW C. von ESCHENBACH, M.D.

The only available therapy that has curative potential in renal cell carcinoma is surgery. Unfortunately, early in its course, renal cell carcinoma typically produces no symptoms so that, at diagnosis, the disease may be beyond surgical cure. Indeed, there is clinical evidence of metastasis in around 25 to 50 percent of cases at presentation. Half of all patients treated surgically for localized cancer eventually develop metastases. Nevertheless, the failure of all other forms of therapy, including irradiation, chemotherapy, and immunotherapy, to improve survival has fostered an aggressive surgical approach to the disease.

The approximately 2 percent of cases in which renal involvement is bilateral are not excluded from aggressive surgery. In these patients, currently accepted management alternatives run the gamut from bilateral radical nephrectomy (which involves chronic dialysis or renal transplantation) to noninterventional supportive management. Options between these two poles are total tumor excision with nephron salvage and palliative management, which entails segmental renal angioinfarction. Total tumor excision is usually accomplished by radical nephrectomy of the most involved renal unit and contralateral partial nephrectomy. Other surgical methods that are employed to remove all tumor while at the same time preserving renal parenchyma are tumor excision or enucleation (if the tumors are on the renal surface), and ex vivo bench surgery to remove central lesions with renal reconstruction and autotransplantation.

The surgeon who must choose among these options is confronted with a variety of complex questions that must be answered when evaluating and planning therapy for the patient with bilateral disease. Is the disease a manifestation of multifocality or is the involvement of the contralateral kidney an expression of extensive metastasis? Is the tumor burden amenable to surgical extirpation that, nevertheless, preserves sufficient renal function for dialysis-free survival? What is the optimal surgical approach to maximize tumor ablation while minimizing morbidity? Thus the management of bilateral renal cell carcinoma must be highly individualized according to the nature and extent of the tumor at presentation and the clinical status of the patient.

At The University of Texas M. D. Anderson Cancer Center at Houston, we consider surgical therapy to be appropriate only when the preoperative assessment indicates that in situ surgery can render the patient tumor free without need for total renal ablation and dependence on chronic dialysis. Our cancer center does not provide facilities for chronic dialysis, and it is my philosophy and that of my co-workers that renal tumor surgery likely to entail bench surgery, transplantation, or chronic dialysis should be done at a center that provides full support. If such an extensive surgical procedure is demanded, a patient at our center is offered referral to another institution.

We are philosophically opposed to surgical procedures that render the patient anephric because of the consequences of long-term chronic dialysis, and the fact that, when tumors are so extensive as to demand bilateral nephrectomies, the disease is usually already beyond surgical cure. By avoiding surgery these patients are spared pointless morbidity, and in our experience some may survive productively for long periods. At M. D. Anderson, we have had two patients survive 3 years and one 14 years without nephrectomy. The surgical management I most often employ is radical nephrectomy of the most involved kidney and partial nephrectomy to remove the tumor in the contralateral kidney.

TOTAL TUMOR EXCISION WITH RENAL PARENCHYMAL PRESERVATION

At M. D. Anderson, total tumor excision in bilateral renal cell carcinoma requires rigid adherence to the guidelines for the selection of patients and a careful preoperative assessment for therapy planning. In most circumstances a radical nephrectomy is performed on the side of major tumor involvement, and a partial nephrectomy or tumorectomy is done on the contralateral side. In every instance the intent is to preserve sufficient renal parenchyma for dialysis-free survival. Since the goal of therapy is surgical cure, it is imperative that an extensive and meticulous evaluation exclude the presence of metastases before undertaking the surgery.

Selection and Preoperative Evaluation

Patients should be free of concurrent serious medical problems and have an average life expectancy for their age. They should be able to withstand the required extensive surgical procedure. There should be no contraindications to renal dialysis, which may become necessary postoperatively, if there is a transient period of renal insufficiency. Lungs, liver, bones, and retroperitoneal lymph nodes must be clinically free of metastases. The routine preoperative assessment thus comprises a complete blood count; biochemical profile (SMA-12), including measurements of sodium, potassium, chlorine, and carbon dioxide levels; urinalysis, urine culture, and coagulation profile; assessment of renal function by serum creatinine and blood urea nitrogen levels and by creatinine clearance with (as indicated) differential renal scan and renal function studies; electrocardiography; computed tomography (CT) of the abdomen and pelvis, with and without contrast material; and bilateral renal arteriography (anteroposterior and oblique views) and a celiac-axis arteriogram. Venacavography and bone scanning or bone radiography are also performed as indicated.

Although renal arteriography is no longer a routine part of the preoperative evaluation in unilateral renal tumors, I consider it essential in bilateral disease. An examination of the architecture of the renal vasculature aids in planning the surgical approach. Should segmental resection be the option chosen, the arteriogram can be used as a guide to microdissection of the tumor and reconstruction of the kidney.

Preoperative Preparation

As time and the patient's condition permit, 2 to 3 U of autologous blood can be harvested and stored prior to surgery. If the patient is not hemodynamically stable or if the hemoglobin level is below 11 g per deciliter, the surgeon must rely on heterologous transfusions.

The patient is admitted to the hospital 24 hours before surgery, and preoperative studies are re-evaluated. A central venous catheter is placed in a subclavian vein, and a chest film is obtained to make certain that the catheter tip is in the proper position in the superior vena cava, that no pneumothorax or hemothorax has occurred, and that the heart and lungs are normal. A mechanical bowel cleansing is performed to facilitate surgery and in anticipation of postoperative ileus.

Surgical Procedure

The surgical procedure begins with a retroperitoneal lymph node dissection, with analysis of the nodes by frozen section. Renal surgery is not performed unless the lymph nodes are microscopically free of disease. Radical nephrectomy is performed on the side where the kidney is most involved by tumor. On the contralateral side a partial nephrectomy is performed by first completely mobilizing the entire kidney along with its surrounding perinephric fat. The perihilar region is dissected to expose the renal vessels, pelvis, and ureters. At this juncture of the procedure the surgical approach is predicated on the size, location, and number of tumors present in this kidney.

If the tumor is a solitary lesion and is located at one of the poles of the kidney, a guillotine partial nephrectomy is performed without occlusion of the renal vessels. The perinephric fat is removed from the uninvolved portion of the kidney, but is left intact over the tumor-bearing portion of the kidney. The kidney, having been completely mobilized, is grasped with one hand and is compressed between the thumb (on its anterior surface) and the index finger (on its posterior surface). A sharp transverse incision is made through the kidney at a point that leaves a 1.0-cm margin of normal kidney beyond the tumor. While the index finger and thumb maintain hemostasis by compression of the kidney, vessels are ligated with figure-of-eight 3-0 chromic sutures, and then the renal collecting system is closed with interrupted 3-0 chromic sutures.

When the tumor is on the surface of the midportion of the kidney, the procedure is somewhat similar, except that a wedge resection of the tumor rather than guillotine amputation is performed. For multiple tumors

that are encapsulated and on the surface, enucleation can be performed; however, in order to reduce the likelihood of local tumor recurrence, I prefer to excise an adequate margin of normal renal parenchyma. A 1-cm margin is recommended whenever possible, but it is often difficult to achieve a uniform margin around the entire tumor mass, and at some points the margins may have to be less generous. After the tumor-bearing portion of the kidney is removed, a careful inspection of the specimen should be made to evaluate the margins; if they are inadequate, more of the kidney is removed.

Although I do not believe that there is any significant advantage to using the 10,600-nm carbon dioxide laser as a scalpel in renal surgery, the 1,060-nm neodymium-yttrium aluminum garnet (Nd:YAG) laser can be used to coagulate the cut surface of the kidney after tumor resection. This can provide additional hemostasis and, most important, produces a zone of coagulation 3 to 5 mm deep with thermal destruction of any microscopic tumor extension. This may conceivably reduce the risk of local recurrence, although the incidences of the potential problems of delayed bleeding or infection associated with producing a deep zone of necrotic residual renal tissue remain to be defined.

Although the adrenal gland can be a site of tumor involvement, either by metastasis or by direct extension, an attempt should be made to preserve at least one of the adrenal glands. Preservation should be considered particularly in the adrenal gland least likely to be at risk for tumors.

Before, during, and after the procedure the patient should be adequately hydrated and a brisk diuresis maintained by the judicious use of diuretics, if necessary. Occlusion of the renal vessels and renal cooling are not routinely employed in order to avoid inadvertent injury to the renal artery and renal ischemia. The vessels are completely exposed, however, and can be quickly secured in a bleeding emergency. At times, preoperative assessment of the renal arteriogram may indicate that the tumor-bearing portion of the kidney is supplied by a discrete and accessible artery. Such a vessel can be carefully dissected free in the hilum and injected with indigo carmine dye to delineate the zone of the kidney that it supplies; if surgically appropriate, the vessel can be ligated and the tumor-bearing portion of the kidney amputated.

After adequate hemostasis is achieved and it has been determined that there is satisfactory closure of the collecting system, the remnant kidney is returned to its normal anatomic location. Because leakage of urine occurs in the early postoperative period, drains are placed in the perinephric space and brought out in the flank. The bowel is returned to its normal anatomic position, and the abdomen is closed.

Postoperative Problems

There may be a brief period of renal insufficiency during the postoperative course, especially if the kidney has been extensively manipulated. Other than renal insufficiency, the major postoperative problems that can occur are bleeding, infection, and prolonged urinary leakage. Meticulous attention to hemostasis and to closure of the urinary collecting system may curtail leaking and bleeding, and the use of prophylactic systemic antibiotics may prevent complications of infection.

DISCUSSION

Bilateral renal cell carcinomas, whether they present synchronously or asynchronously, offer a perplexing and difficult problem to urologic surgeons. Since surgery has been the only effective method of disease eradication, many surgeons have been extremely aggressive and even heroic in their efforts to remove all tumor. However, this approach must be tempered by certain realities. No surgical therapy for the primary lesion results in improved survival when metastases are present, and therefore surgery should be considered only after a meticulous search has failed to demonstrate evidence of metastatic disease.

Recently compiled evidence suggests that the outlook for patients with bilateral renal tumors is related to the stage of the tumor and the adequacy of the surgical extirpation. In selected patients, 5-year survival after surgery is approximately 70 percent, with local recurrences approaching 10 percent. As tumors become more extensive (stage II; >6 cm in size), the likelihood of metastases increases, and treatment success, regardless of the therapy employed for the primary, is less likely.

Comparisons of in vivo excision and bench surgery in bilateral renal cell carcinoma do not reveal any differences in survival. Although there are certain theoretical advantages to ex vivo surgery, mainly that careful tumorectomy in a bloodless field lessens the risk of tumor recurrence, we have not advocated it as a routine procedure. Such surgery requires not only facilities for proper handling of the kidney, but also extraordinary expertise in microvascular techniques. The risk of damage to the residual renal parenchyma on account of the ischemia that is inherent in the ex vivo perfusion, and the surgical risks associated with the vascular anastomosis and autotransplantation of the kidney into the pelvis, make this a formidable undertaking.

When one considers the stated objective of rendering the patient tumor free while preserving sufficient renal parenchyma for dialysis-free survival, it is apparent that the realization of such an objective becomes less probable when the tumor burden demands heroic surgery. Simply stated, those patients whose tumor stage is low and in whom the size and number of lesions are limited, so that the surgical intervention is straightforward and readily performed with minimal risks, are the ones who are destined to do well after bilateral tumor surgery. On the other hand, extensive tumors involving the central portion of the kidneys and requiring extensive surgery are not likely to be amenable to any attempt at cure by excision.

My philosophy has been to avoid total bilateral nephrectomy because of the morbidity associated with chronic dialysis. As with bench surgery, when this approach is the only possible method of tumor extirpation, the disease is usually beyond surgical cure.

When cure is not a possibility, my management, with the patient's consent, is supportive. Renal function is maintained without dialysis; when it seems advisable, local symptoms may be controlled by selective embolization of the branches of the renal artery that supply the tumor mass. It has been my experience that patients with bilateral tumors can survive for prolonged periods if there is relatively indolent local disease. When disease progresses and becomes life threatening, we have offered patients the opportunity for systemic chemotherapy and/or biologic response modifiers.

Until proven, effective therapy for systemic disease becomes available, surgery should be performed only in bilateral renal cell carcinoma when cure may be expected. Surgery is indeed the treatment of choice, but with the admonition of "Physician, do no harm."

WILMS' TUMOR

JONATHAN H. ROSS, M.D.
ROBERT KAY, M.D.

Wilms' tumor is the most common genitourinary malignancy of childhood. Over the past century, its successful treatment has been a challenge to surgeons and oncologists alike. When it was characterized by Wilms in 1899, the prognosis for children with cancer of the kidney was dismal. As a result of persistent research, patient survival now approaches 90 percent. However, that success is tempered by the failure to treat effectively some patients with advanced disease and by the significant toxicity from treatment suffered by some who do survive. Although great progress has been made, new frontiers in the evaluation and treatment of Wilms' tumor persist.

HISTOPATHOLOGY

Grossly, Wilms' tumors are roughly spherical masses with a variegated surface on cross section. Soft, myxomatous areas alternate with gray, cartilaginous tissue. Areas of hemorrhagic necrosis are common.

Histologically, classical Wilms' tumor is a triphasic tumor consisting of renal blastema, "stromal" elements, and regions of epithelial differentiation. The National Wilms' Tumor Study (NWTS) has defined favorable and unfavorable histologic subtypes. Favorable histology refers to a tumor consisting of the classic triphasic elements. Tumors containing anaplastic elements are considered of unfavorable histology because they are generally associated with a poorer prognosis. In addition to anaplasia, the first NWTS identified sarcomatous tissue subtypes that also carried a poor prognosis and were considered unfavorable histologic variants. These sarcomatous subtypes were of the clear-cell sarcoma pattern, the rhabdomyosarcomatoid pattern, and the hyalinizing pattern. Further study of these tumors has led to the reclassification of the sarcomatous Wilms' tumors as separate nonWilms' entities. They are now referred to as clear-cell sarcoma of the kidney (CCSK) and malignant rhabdoid tumor of the kidney (MRTK), accounting for approximately 4 percent and 2 percent of childhood renal tumors, respectively. Therefore, only Wilms' tumors with anaplastic elements (approximately 5 percent of all Wilms' tumors) are considered of unfavorable histology.

EPIDEMIOLOGY AND GENETICS

Wilms' tumor is the most common genitourinary malignancy of childhood, affecting approximately one in 10,000 children. Wilms' tumor is bilateral in approximately 5 percent of cases, and 12 percent of unilateral cases are multifocal. A bimodal age distribution exists, with unilateral Wilms' tumors occurring at a median age of 40 months and with bilateral tumors occurring at a median age of 28 months. Wilms' tumor occurs equally in males and females and is extremely rare in adults and neonates.

Many congenital anomalies have been found in association with this tumor. Among the most common are genitourinary anomalies and hemihypertrophy, both of which occur in 3 percent of patients with Wilms' tumor. The most common genitourinary anomalies are hypospadias and cryptorchidism. Aniridia is another important association. While slightly less than 1 percent of Wilms' tumor patients have aniridia, one-third of patients with sporadic aniridia will develop Wilms' tumor. Most patients with aniridia and Wilms' tumor have been found to have a deletion on the short arm of chromosome 11, where loci for genes related to genitourinary anomalies, mental retardation, and various growth factors have also been identified.

Several syndromes associated with Wilms' tumor have been described. The most common is the Beckwith-Wiedemann syndrome which consists of exomphalos, macroglossia, high birth weight, and gigantism. These patients are at an increased risk for the development of Wilms' tumor as well as other intra-abdominal malignancies, such as adrenocortical carcinoma and hepatoblastoma.

Only 1 percent of patients with Wilms' tumor have a positive family history for Wilms' tumor. However, the association of this tumor with various congenital anomalies, and the finding that patients with bilateral disease present at an earlier age suggests the existence of a subpopulation of Wilms' tumor patients with a genetic predisposition for the formation of the tumor. Cases of familial Wilms' tumor, usually in siblings or cousins, have been reported, but only recently have a significant number of patients survived to child-bearing age. Studies of their offspring suggest that the risk of Wilms' tumor developing in the offspring of patients with a history of sporadic unilateral disease is at most 2 percent, although the risk is probably higher for the offspring of patients with multifocal disease or a positive family history.

PRESENTATION AND EVALUATION

Unlike children with other malignancies, patients with Wilms' tumor often appear quite healthy. Indeed, the most common presentation for Wilms' tumor is an abdominal mass noted by a parent or physician. A palpable abdominal mass is present in as many as 95 percent of patients. Other signs and symptoms that are often present include abdominal pain, vomiting, fever, hypertension, and occasionally, hematuria.

In high-risk patients, such as those with aniridia, hemihypertrophy, or nephroblastomatosis, surveillance protocols should be put into effect to detect the occurrence of a Wilms' tumor as early as possible. They should undergo a physical examination and ultrasonography every 3 months until they are approximately 7 years of age, after which the intervals may become more prolonged. In this way, a certain number of Wilms' tumors will present as asymptomatic lesions discovered during routine surveillance.

Since most children with Wilms' tumor present with an abdominal mass, the initial evaluation usually involves radiographic studies to characterize the mass and identify its origin. An intravenous urogram (IVU) was the traditional first study when Wilms' tumor was suspected. It may still be used and can be diagnostic in 95 percent of patients, with neuroblastoma being the most common misdiagnosis. Ultrasonography began to replace IVU because of its ease of use and noninvasiveness. In addition to its excellent imaging of the kidney and its tumor, ultrasonography is able to detect caval tumor thrombus (which is present in approximately 4 percent of patients) and, in some cases, nephroblastomatosis.

Recently, computed tomography (CT) has begun to replace ultrasonography as the initial study for a young child presenting with an abdominal mass suspicious for a neoplasm. At the same time, a CT scan of the chest may be obtained to identify possible pulmonary metastases. It is even possible that as more experience is gained, the use of CT may eventually preclude the need for contralateral exploration in patients with Wilms' tumor. Magnetic resonance imaging (MRI) appears to be comparable to CT in localizing and characterizing Wilms' tumors. MRI is highly accurate in distinguishing Wilms' tumors from neuroblastomas, and it is better than CT in identifying caval involvement. On the other hand, MRI has the disadvantages of expense and limited availability, and, as with CT, sedation is often required.

Once the diagnosis of Wilms' tumor is made, the evaluation is completed with a chest radiograph or chest CT to rule out pulmonary metastases. A routine urinalysis, blood chemistries including measurement of serum creatinine, and a complete blood count should be obtained. A measurement of serum creatinine is important for ruling out associated renal insufficiency that might have an impact on operative approach. Elevated liver function tests or alkaline phosphatase might spur further evaluation for metastatic disease.

After the initial evaluation, further studies may be indicated. The vena cava should be evaluated initially with ultrasonography. In the patient with caval tumor thrombus, cavography or MRI should be performed to delineate clearly the extent of the thrombus. Approximately 20 percent of patients with caval thrombus have intra-atrial extension. Therefore, if inferior vena cavography fails to demonstrate the superior extent of the thrombus, superior vena cavography or echocardiography is indicated.

Angiography is rarely indicated in unilateral cases. In cases of bilateral Wilms' tumor, angiography is sometimes warranted as an aid in planning appropriate renal-sparing operations.

STAGING

Staging of Wilms' tumor as designated by the NWTS is of prognostic significance, and careful staging is essential for the selection of appropriate therapy (Table 1). It should be noted that in the absence of distant metastases or bilateral involvement, an appropriate stage can be assigned only after surgical exploration. Stage I tumors do not extend beyond the kidney and are completely excised. Stage II tumors are those which extend beyond the kidney (including microscopic capsular penetration) but are completely excised. The presence of tumor thrombus also indicates a stage II

Table 1 Staging of Wilms' Tumor

Stage	Description
I	Limited to kidney, completely excised
II	Extrarenal extension (completely excised), biopsied or local tumor spillage
III	Residual nonhematogenous intra-abdominal disease or gross tumor spillage
IV	Hematogenous metastases
V	Bilateral tumors

tumor. Furthermore, any time that a tumor is biopsied or there is local tumor spillage intraoperatively, the tumor is classified as a stage II tumor. Any tumor with residual disease limited to the abdomen is classified as stage III. This includes cases with positive lymph nodes, peritoneal implants, or gross tumor spillage at the time of surgery. A positive surgical margin also warrants a stage III classification. Any tumor with hematogenous metastases is classified a stage IV tumor. The most common sites of metastatic spread are the lung, liver, bones, and brain. Bilateral Wilms' tumors are designated stage V. This should not be construed to imply a poor prognosis; bilateral disease is a special case and is discussed in a separate section.

NEPHROBLASTOMATOSIS

Nephroblastomatosis is defined as the persistence of metanephric blastema beyond 36 weeks of gestational age. This embryonic tissue is normally present during the development of the kidney. As the ureteric bud encounters the metanephric blastema, the latter is induced to develop into mature renal tissue. Nephroblastomatosis represents an aberration in this developmental process, characterized by the presence of "rests" of this blastemal tissue.

Since nephroblastomatosis was first described by Hou and Holman in 1961, the association between nephroblastomatosis and Wilms' tumor has become increasingly evident. It has been estimated that nearly 50 percent of kidneys with Wilms' tumor contain areas of nephroblastomatosis. As many as 100 percent of patients with bilateral Wilms' tumor may have areas of nephroblastomatosis.

The natural history of nephroblastomatosis is ill-defined. Circumstantial evidence suggests an etiologic relationship between nephroblastomatosis and Wilms' tumor. There is a strong association between nephroblastomatosis and bilateral and multifocal Wilms' tumor, and Wilms' tumor has been known to develop in patients previously diagnosed with nephroblastomatosis. There are also histologic, ultrastructural, and chromosomal findings that suggest a close histogenetic relationship.

However, it is apparent that not all nephroblastomatoses develop into Wilms' tumors. The autopsy incidence of perinatal nephroblastomatosis is as high as 1 percent, much higher than the incidence of Wilms' tumor. Therefore, the vast majority of nephroblastomatoses must either regress or evolve into clinically insignificant benign entities.

Because of epidemiologic evidence that nephroblastomatosis progresses to Wilms' tumor in only a small number of cases, treatment of nephroblastomatosis should be conservative. When it is discovered incidentally, no treatment is indicated, although close follow-up may be warranted. A brief course of chemotherapy may be considered for patients with very large lesions.

Patients with multifocal nephroblastomatosis in a kidney removed for Wilms' tumor are at an increased risk for contralateral disease and should undergo ultrasonographic examination every 3 months.

Contralateral nephroblastomatosis in a patient with Wilms' tumor represents a special case. The majority of these lesions respond to the modalities used to treat the initial tumor. When contralateral lesions are discovered, they should be removed only if this can be accomplished with good preservation of functional parenchyma. In cases of extensive nephroblastomatosis, a renal-sparing procedure on the side with the Wilms' tumor may be appropriate. Clearly these patients are at increased risk for clinically significant disease, and careful surveillance is essential postoperatively. These patients should be re-explored when a growing lesion is detected.

TREATMENT

Except in special circumstances, radical nephrectomy is the first step in the treatment of Wilms' tumor. A transperitoneal approach is used so that the contralateral kidney may be explored. Thorough evaluation of the contralateral kidney by complete mobilization and visual inspection of all surfaces is essential. The discovery of bilateral disease or contralateral nephroblastomatosis significantly changes the treatment of the disease, and historically, as many as one-third of bilateral tumors are discovered only at laparotomy. If the findings of contralateral exploration are negative, an ipsilateral nephrectomy is performed. Lymph nodes should be sampled, but extensive lymphadenectomy is not indicated. Tumor extending beyond the kidney should be excised if this can be easily accomplished. Excision of involved normal organs should be avoided. Residual tumor should be marked with surgical clips to aid in planning of postoperative therapy.

All patients with Wilms' tumor receive postoperative adjunctive therapy. The two most important prognostic indicators are stage and histology (Table 2). Postoperative therapy therefore is stratified based on tumor stage and histology. With the discovery of the efficacy of adjunctive radiation—and later of the chemotherapeutic agents actinomycin D and vincristine sulfate—survival for patients with Wilms' tumor has improved dramatically during the past century.

In the United States, most patients are treated according to the NWTS protocol. The protocol for NWTS-4 is shown in Figure 1. Stage I and II patients are treated with actinomycin D and vincristine sulfate. Radiation and doxorubicin are added for stage III and IV tumors (patients with stage IV tumors should receive flank irradiation only if the primary tumor is locally advanced). Patients with tumors of unfavorable histology that are staged greater than stage I receive irradiation, actinomycin D, vincristine sulfate, and doxorubicin. These patients are then randomized to a "cyclophosphamide" or "no cyclophosphamide" arm.

Although not part of an official protocol, preoperative chemotherapy may be appropriate in special circumstances. A brief preoperative course of chemotherapy may be effective in decreasing the size of the tumor, which may reduce the risk of intraoperative tumor spillage.

Table 2 4-Year Relapse-Free Survival in NWTS-3

Stage/Histology	Survival
I/Favorable	90%
II/Favorable	88%
III/Favorable	79%
IV/Favorable	75%
I-IV/Unfavorable	63%

However, major changes in tumor histology can occur in a significant number of patients, leading to potential errors in assignment of postoperative treatment regimens. There is also some concern that patients might be artificially "downstaged" by preoperative therapy. These patients might receive less aggressive therapy postoperatively than the true biologic nature of their tumor warrants. Finally, 5 percent of patients diagnosed preoperatively with Wilms' tumor are found to have some other lesion at the time of surgery. Thus there is a risk of treating a small percentage of patients inappropriately with preoperative chemotherapy. Because of these concerns, preoperative chemotherapy should not be used routinely. However, it can be helpful in patients with large tumors that are considered inoperable or hazardous to remove. It is also reasonable to consider this treatment in patients with large tumors who are at high risk for intraoperative tumor rupture. In cases in which preoperative chemotherapy is being considered, a tissue diagnosis by needle aspiration or open biopsy should be obtained.

While radical nephrectomy is the standard operation for Wilms' tumor, a role for renal-sparing procedures in selected patients is evolving. This approach is already standard in treatment of bilateral Wilms' tumors, and its adoption has not adversely affected survival in this group. Furthermore, pathologic study of Wilms' tumor kidneys has made it clear that the Wilms' tumor/nephroblastomatosis complex is often a diffuse disease involving both kidneys. It could be argued that conservative operations would allow surgical treatment of metachronous contralateral disease without rendering the patient anephric.

In patients treated with current chemotherapy regimens, however, there is a very low incidence of metachronous bilateral Wilms' tumor (e.g., fewer than 1 percent of the patients enrolled in NWTS-3). Also, a significant number of patients with *unilateral* multifocal disease would benefit from unilateral nephrectomy. It must be remembered that current regimens that include unilateral nephrectomy are extremely effective. Given the rarity of metachronous bilateral disease and our ability to detect this disease early with ultrasonography, radical nephrectomy remains the standard treatment.

The experience with parenchyma-sparing procedures in selected cases does suggest that it is a reasonable alternative in patients at high risk for

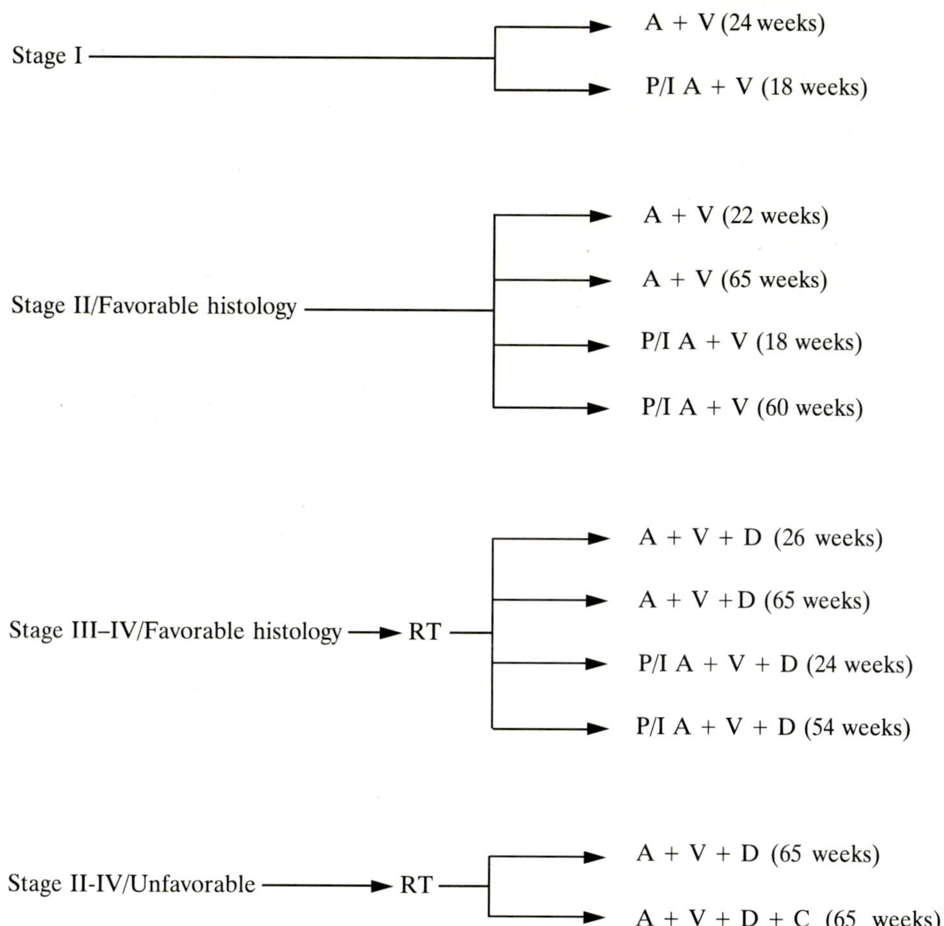

Figure 1 Postoperative treatment protocol for NWTS-4. A = actinomycin D; V = vincristine sulfate; D = Doxorubicin; C = cyclophosphamide; P/I = pulsed, intensive therapy; RT = radiation therapy.

significant renal loss. This would include patients with solitary kidneys and renal insufficiency and perhaps those with congenital anomalies or a family history of Wilms' tumor. These last patients are at increased risk for multifocal disease and a significant number may indeed be discovered with small tumors while surveillance protocols are in effect.

Adults and neonates with Wilms' tumor also warrant special consideration. The prognosis for adult Wilms' tumor is poorer than for childhood disease. This is due in part to a higher percentage of stage III and IV disease in adults. But even stage-for-stage survival is worse for adults than for children. Adults should therefore undergo radical nephrectomy followed by aggressive chemotherapy. Flank irradiation, which is standard for locally advanced disease, should also be considered for adults with stage II tumors and possibly for those with stage I tumors. Because true Wilms' tumor is extremely rare in neonates, experience in its treatment is limited. However, reduced doses of chemotherapy are appropriate, and some patients may be cured with nephrectomy alone.

FOLLOW-UP

Patients with Wilms' tumor must be followed for the development of recurrent or metastatic disease as well as for the development of acute or long-term complications of treatment. The vast majority of recurrences occur within 2 years of nephrectomy. The most common sites of relapse are the lungs, followed by intra-abdominal relapses and those occurring at the bone and brain. Periodic chest radiographs are obtained to rule out pulmonary metastases. Urinalyses and periodic renal ultrasonography are performed to monitor the contralateral kidney and intra-abdominal sites. Ultrasonography has been effective in identifying small tumors in high-risk patients. In patients with nephroblastomatosis or bilateral Wilms' tumor, more intense monitoring may be indicated. In patients at high risk for local recurrence in the flank, periodic CT scans should be obtained.

Recurrences must be treated aggressively, with surgical resection of tumor in the abdomen or chest, followed by chemotherapy and/or radiotherapy. In this way, a significant number of patients can be salvaged.

Patients who suffer early relapses that occur while they are receiving chemotherapy do poorly.

Toxicity is significant following multimodal therapy. Bone marrow suppression is the most common acute toxicity encountered. Long-term complications of radiation include skeletal changes such as scoliosis and kyphosis, and ovarian failure. Increased perinatal mortality and low birth weights among the children of women who have received radiation therapy for Wilms' tumor have also been reported. Focal segmental glomerulosclerosis has developed in the contralateral nonirradiated kidneys of some patients, resulting in hypertension and proteinuria.

With the dramatic increase in the long-term survival of patients with Wilms' tumor, there has been increasing concern regarding the eventual development of secondary malignancies in these patients. This risk approaches 20 percent 30 years after treatment and probably results from a combination of mutagenic therapy and a predisposition to the development of malignancies in these patients. Therefore, efforts to decrease the exposure of low-risk patients to mutagenic therapy is important in reducing the number of deaths due to secondary malignancies.

BILATERAL WILMS' TUMOR

Bilateral Wilms' tumor—occurring in 5 percent of patients—offers a unique challenge to the physician. Total excision of all tumor at the time of the initial laparotomy without compromising renal function can be difficult, as most cases of bilateral Wilms' tumor are characterized by diffuse or multifocal involvement of at least one of the kidneys. When patients with Wilms' tumor have undergone bilateral nephrectomy and transplant, the outcome has been poor, with the majority of deaths occurring from sepsis related to the combined effects of chemotherapy and immunosuppression. A conservative approach should therefore be undertaken in patients with bilateral Wilms' tumors.

Patients are biopsied to confirm the histologic diagnosis. Initially this was done as an open procedure. More recently, needle biopsy has been sufficient. When needle biopsy is used, one must realize that focal areas of unfavorable histology may be missed. Furthermore, one must rely on radiologic staging that is not always accurate.

Once the diagnosis is confirmed, treatment is given according to the NWTS protocol. Patients are followed radiographically during treatment and explored after a stable response to treatment has occurred (roughly 3 months). Exploration may be necessary sooner if the tumors are not responding, or it may be delayed if a response is continuing. At exploration, small residual tumors are excised and appropriate postoperative adjuvant treatment is administered. If large tumors are present, patients may require additional chemotherapy or irradiation followed by another exploration before residual tumor can be excised. Operations that may lead to eventual loss of renal function such as bilateral nephrectomy or large excisions with autotransplantation should be performed only after repeated trials of chemotherapy and irradiation have failed to make more conservative measures possible. Because of radiation's potential deleterious effect on residual renal function in these patients, it should be reserved for those cases unresponsive to chemotherapy or in which the tumor is locally advanced. Obviously patients with bilateral tumors require close long-term surveillance after treatment.

The outlook for synchronous bilateral Wilms' tumor is improving, with 3-year survivals reported of approximately 75 percent. Stage for stage (based on the most advanced lesion), survivals have been comparable for patients with bilateral tumors and those with unilateral tumors. However, the combination of unfavorable histology, advanced stage, and bilateral disease is virtually lethal. These are patients in whom more aggressive management, including early aggressive excision, may be indicated.

SUGGESTED READING

Blute ML, Kelalis PP, Offord KP, et al. Bilateral Wilms' tumor. J Urol 1987; 138:968–973.

D'Angio GJ, Breslow N, Beckwith JB, et al. Treatment of Wilms' tumor: results of the third National Wilms' Tumor Study. Cancer 1989; 64:349–360.

Knudson AG Jr, Strong LC. Mutation and cancer: a model for Wilms' tumor of the kidney. J Nat Cancer Inst 1972; 48:313–324.

Lemerle J, Voute PA, Tournade MF, et al. Effectiveness of preoperative chemotherapy in Wilms' tumor: results of an International Society of Paediatric Oncology (SIOP) clinical trial. J Clin Oncol 1983; 1:604–609.

Machin GA. Persistent renal blastema (nephroblastomatosis) as a frequent precursor of Wilms' tumor: a pathological and clinical review (parts 1–3). Am J Pediatr Hematol Oncol 1980; 2:165–171, 253–261, and 353–362.

CONGENITAL MESOBLASTIC NEPHROMA

JAMES MANDELL, M.D.

Congenital mesoblastic nephroma is a highly interesting neoplasm, the etiology, pathology, and clinical course of which, although well recognized, are still incompletely understood. Although it is generally considered benign, documented cases of recurrence and/or metastases have been published. The varied clinical and pathologic presentation make this an important lesion with which to be familiar.

The overall incidence of this lesion in childhood is relatively small, representing approximately 3 percent of renal tumors submitted to the National Wilms' Study Group. It is, however, the *most common solid renal neoplasm seen in the neonate.* The term "congenital" denotes its very early postnatal presentation as well as the well-documented association with polyhydramnios. There is a distinct male predominance.

The most common mode of presentation is the finding of a unilateral, palpable renal mass in a term newborn or very young infant with no antecedent abnormal maternal or gestational history. The mean age at presentation is approximately 3 months. Possible associated signs or symptoms include hypertension, hypercalcemia, or hematuria. At least one case with elevated plasma renins has been documented.

The diagnosis is usually suspected on the basis of clinical history as well as the radiologic findings of a solitary, solid renal mass by ultrasonography, intravenous urography, or another imaging modality. Calcifications have also been described in association with this lesion. The description of contrast uptake or "function" by this lesion is probably related to the interspersed entrapped nephrons remaining with the tumor.

The pathologic findings are generally fairly consistent. Ingrowth of connective tissue into the previously normal kidney, composed of sheets of spindle-shaped cells (Fig. 1), is seen. Ultrastructurally, these cells are thought to be fibroblasts or myofibroblasts. The pattern appears to be an infiltrative one. The outcome of patients with this histology is almost uniformly good. Those patients who have had incomplete resection tend to have recurrences locally and usually do well with completed removal. Rarely, a case of recurrence or metastasis is reported, usually in the older infant.

A more cellular variant of congenital mesoblastic nephroma exists, with a presentation and outcome that are distinct. As opposed to the "typical" lesion, these tend to present slightly later in infancy. In addition to increased cellularity, there is a higher mitotic index. Many recurrences have been reported, with several deaths cited. The only significant variable appears to be positive margins at the initial surgical resection. This tumor appears more closely related both pathologically and clinically to the clear-cell sarcoma than to the more benign congenital mesoblastic nephroma.

The link between congenital mesoblastic nephroma, the more cellular variant, and Wilms' tumor remains to be elucidated. At least one case of congenital mesoblastic nephroma in a patient with Beckwith-Wiedemann syndrome has been reported, supporting the concept of an early common cellular origin among these lesions.

What then is the recommended treatment and follow-up for patients with congenital mesoblastic nephroma. In the "typical" cases with a neonatal presentation, after appropriate diagnostic evaluation, complete nephrectomy is indicated. It is recommended by several authors, and I tend to agree, that a transperitoneal approach is best. This permits the most surgical options, and makes complete resection more feasible. My opinion

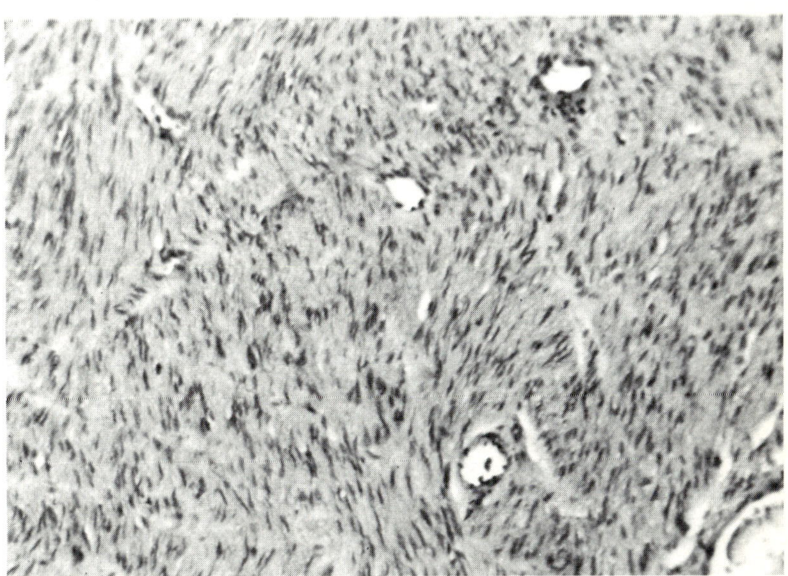

Figure 1. Photomicrograph of congenital mesoblastic nephroma showing the swirling pattern of spindle shaped cells.

differs, however, with regard to the concept of "radical nephrectomy" in these cases, since the ipsilateral adrenal gland can be spared. No adjunctive therapy is needed if the classical histologic findings are seen, with an adequate margin of resection. Follow-up surveillance with ultrasonography should be continued.

If the histology is that of the cellular variant, I believe the most judicious course is to provide treatment adjunctively with a chemotherapy regimen used for the clear-cell sarcoma protocol. If the tumor margin is compromised, especially in this cell type, then re-resection should be performed.

SUGGESTED READING

Gormley TS, Skoog SJ, Jones RV, Maybee D. Cellular congenital mesoblastic nephroma: what are the options? J Urol 1989; 142: 479–483.

Howell CG, Othersen HB, Kiviat NE, et al. Therapy and outcome in 51 children with mesoblastic nephroma: a report of the National Wilms' Tumor Study. J Pediatr Surg 1982; 17:826–831.

Snyder HM 3d, Lack EE, Chetty-Baktavizian A, et al. Congenital mesoblastic nephroma: relationship to other renal tumors of infancy. J Urol 1981; 126:513–516.

Hartman DS, Lesar MS, Madewell JE, et al. Mesoblastic nephroma: radiologic-pathologic correlation of 20 cases. Am J Roentgenol 1981; 136:69–74.

RENAL ANGIOMYOLIPOMA

GERALD L. ANDRIOLE, M.D.

Renal angiomyolipoma is an unusual benign tumor of the kidney that accounts for less than 1 percent of all renal tumors in adults. Most of the patients (60 to 80 percent) with renal angiomyolipoma have a history of tuberous sclerosis, a congenital syndrome associated with epilepsy, mental retardation, and skin lesions. Patients with tuberous sclerosis may have multiple bilateral angiomyolipomas, and renal angiomyolipoma may coexist with renal cell carcinoma in up to 30 percent of these patients. Renal angiomyolipomas unassociated with tuberous sclerosis usually present as a single lesion within one kidney. These patients are often asymptomatic (40 to 60 percent) but may present with signs and symptoms of life-threatening hemorrhage (5 to 15 percent), flank pain (30 to 40 percent), or hematuria (20 to 30 percent). The propensity of these tumors to hemorrhage is thought to be due to the absence of normal elastic tissue within the walls of the blood vessels.

Histologically, these benign tumors consist of varying proportions of mature (or occasionally immature) adipose tissue, atypical blood vessels, and smooth muscle cells. Occasionally, angiomyolipomas may exhibit certain features compatible with malignancy such as capsular penetration, local recurrence, or invasion of the renal vein or inferior vena cava. These features are thought to be more often secondary to tumor multifocality or incomplete ablation of the tumors than to metastasis per se.

Most angiomyolipomas can be accurately diagnosed by radiography. Computed tomographic (CT) scanning (Fig. 1) often provides unequivocal evidence of renal angiomyolipoma because of the presence of fat with Hounsfield units less than -20 within the lesion. However, some patients whose tumors are predominantly myomatous, or in whom the fatty component consists of immature fat, or in whom blood has infiltrated the fatty portion of the lesion may have indeterminate CT scans. In these patients, additional radiographic studies are necessary to support the diagnosis of angiomyolipoma. Ultrasonography and magnetic resonance imaging (MRI) usually provide significant additional diagnostic information. Angiomyolipomas are typically hyperechoic with respect to the normal adjacent renal parenchyma on ultrasonography (Fig. 2). This pattern is due to the fatty component of the tumor and may be absent if only a small amount of fat is contained within the lesion. MRI may also be employed to detect fat within these lesions. This is usually best seen on T1-weighted images in which adipose tissue imparts a characteristic high signal intensity (Fig. 3). Renal arteriography is ordinarily not very helpful in distinguishing angiomyolipoma from renal cell carcinoma, but can be of considerable value to the surgeon in guiding partial nephrectomy, if this therapy is employed.

In spite of these diagnostic tools, a certain proportion of renal angiomyolipomas (up to 30 percent) may not be completely distinguished from renal cell carcinoma by radiographic studies. In this situation, the renal mass must be considered a potential renal cell carcinoma and treated accordingly.

The critical features that determine the management of patients with suspected renal angiomyolipoma are (1) the presence and severity of symptoms, (2) the size of the lesion, and (3) the degree of certainty of the radiographic diagnosis. Since these lesions are benign,

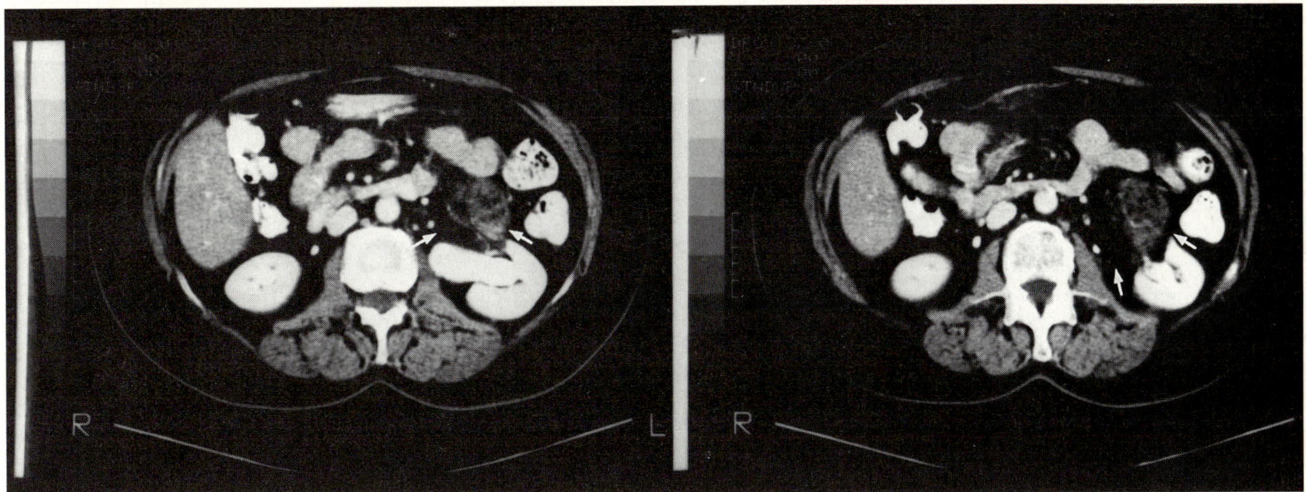

Figure 1   Computed tomography scans demonstrating a 4-cm angiomyolipoma on the anterior surface of the right kidney. Note the fatty density within the lesion, even after administration of intravenous contrast material.

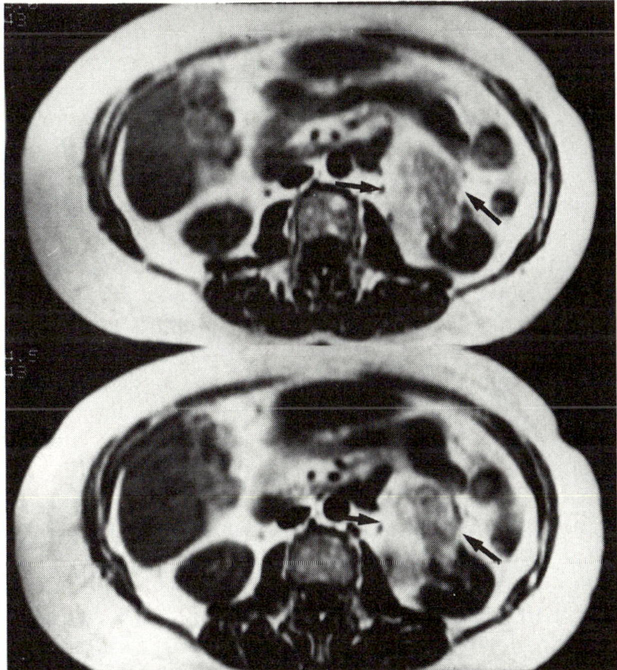

Figure 2   T1-weighted MR scans of the patient in Figure 1 demonstrating an angiomyolipoma of the lower pole of the kidney. Fat in the lesion and the subcutaneous space imparts a characteristic high signal intensity.

patients who have small lesions that meet the radiographic criteria of angiomyolipoma and who are asymptomatic may need no therapy other than observation and interval follow-up. On the other hand, severely symptomatic patients and those with indeterminate radiographic studies should undergo excision of the lesion regardless of tumor size. Since the risk of potentially life-threatening hemorrhage from renal angiomyolipoma increases directly with the size of the lesion, this factor alone can also be an important determinant of management.

The management of patients with suspected angiomyolipoma is shown in schematic form in Figure 4. The rationale for each branch of the decision tree and the preferred techniques are discussed more completely below.

PREFERRED APPROACH TO PATIENTS WITH SUSPECTED ANGIOMYOLIPOMA

The treatment of renal angiomyolipoma should be individualized depending on the certainty of the radiographic diagnosis, the size of the lesion, and the presence and severity of symptoms. From a conceptual point of view, patients should be initially stratified into two groups: those in whom the radiographic diagnosis is unequivocal, and those in whom the radiographic diagnosis is suspicious for angiomyolipoma but in whom renal cell carcinoma cannot be entirely ruled out. This distinction is critical and depends to a large extent on the quality of the radiographic studies. For example, the attenuation value of fat within an angiomyolipoma may be spuriously high if significant "volume averaging" occurs as a consequence of improper placement of the cursor box, because of motion artifact, or if thick slices of 1 cm or more (rather than the ideal narrow collimation of 2 to 5 mm) are employed. When the radiographic (especially CT) findings are indeterminate, the urologist should carefully scrutinize the studies to be certain that these factors have not contributed to the uncertainty. As discussed above, up to 30 percent of renal angiomyolipomas may be radiographically indeterminate, even when the ideal radiographic studies are performed.

Patients presenting with severe or life-threatening urinary or retroperitoneal hemorrhage should be taken for immediate surgical exploration if a renal mass lesion is

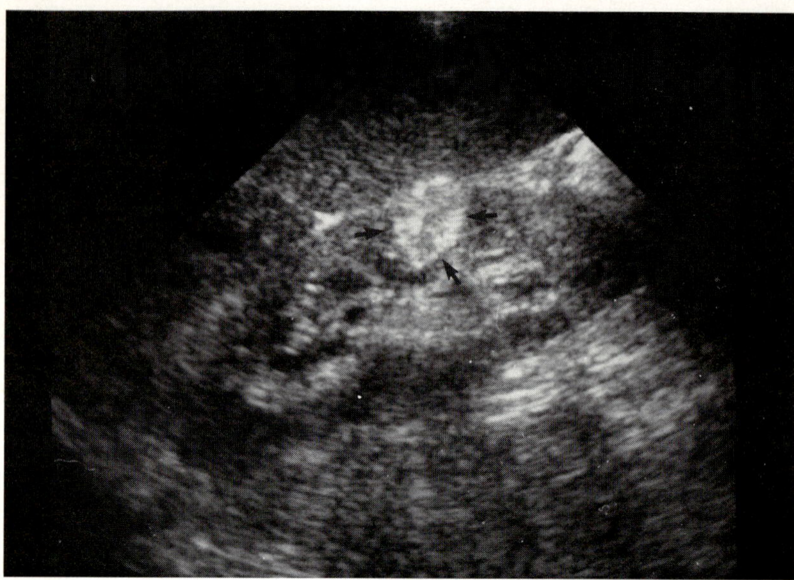

Figure 3 A renal ultrasound scan demonstrating the typical hyperechoic appearance of a renal angiomyolipoma. (Courtesy of Dr. William B. Middleton, Mallinckrodt Institute of Radiology.)

identified. A radical nephrectomy will ordinarily be performed if the contralateral kidney functions normally. If the clinical condition of the patient allows, an expeditious partial nephrectomy may be attempted. However, this is neither always possible nor desirable, because the risk of intraoperative and postoperative complications is increased if partial nephrectomy rather than total nephrectomy is performed. The technique of exploration and radical nephrectomy in cases of severe hemorrhage from renal masses should embrace the same principles advocated in cases of trauma (i.e., early control of the renal vessels via an anterior transperitoneal approach). The technique of partial nephrectomy, if chosen, is described below.

Patients with symptomatic (e.g., occasional flank pain or hematuria) and radiographically indeterminate renal masses should undergo elective open-flank exploration with a view to performing a "radical" partial nephrectomy. Frozen section of the excised lesion should be performed during surgery. If renal cell carcinoma is found, a complete radical nephrectomy should be performed. On the other hand, if the frozen section confirms the diagnosis of renal angiomyolipoma, no further renal excision is necessary. Patients with angiomyolipoma treated by partial nephrectomy should initially be followed on a semiannual basis with renal ultrasonography or CT to detect possible recurrence of the lesion within the kidney, the renal fossa, or rarely, the regional lymph nodes. The preference for either CT or ultrasonography depends on the body habitus of the patient and the ability of the radiologist to image confidently the pertinent structures.

The technique of "radical" partial nephrectomy for radiographically indeterminate renal mass lesions begins with a flank incision, complete mobilization of the entire envelope of Gerota's fascia, and isolation of the ureter, renal artery, and vein. Helpful information about the number and location of renal arteries may be obtained by preoperative angiography, but this is not essential. Before the renal vasculature is occluded, Gerota's fascia is opened at a site remote from the tumor and the perinephric fat and fascia is dissected off the normal renal parenchyma toward the lesion. This dissection is performed to within 1 cm of the lesion. At this point, a Lahey bag is placed around the pedicle of the specimen, iced slush is packed within the bag, around the kidney, and the renal artery and vein are sequentially occluded with bulldog clamps. The patient may be "insulated" from the iced slush by placing abdominal pads outside the Lahey bag along with a sump-a-sucker to aspirate any melted saline. Intravenous mannitol is given a few minutes before occlusion of the renal vasculature. The renal capsule is then scored with electrocautery and the renal parenchyma is divided bluntly, often with the back of a scalpel. The lesion is amputated with a 1- to 2-cm rim of normal renal parenchyma surrounding it and with the perinephric fat and Gerota's fascia covering it. Transected vessels in the parenchyma of the kidney are suture ligated with fine chromic sutures (4-0), and the collecting system, if entered, is closed with running chromic suture (3-0). The integrity of the collecting system should be assessed by instilling dilute indigo carmine into the renal pelvis with a 21-gauge needle. If extravasation is noted, placement of a nephrostomy tube should be considered. Interrupted horizontal mattress sutures of 2-0 chromic incorporating the renal capsule and a 5- to 7-mm edge of the renal cortex are placed along the length of the nephrotomy. A tongue of perinephric fat may be placed beneath the row of mattress sutures before they are tied for further tamponade and compression. These sutures are tied snugly but not overzealously, care being taken not to pull them through the renal capsule or parenchyma. The occlusion of the renal vein and artery are sequentially removed and the kidney is inspected for viability and hemostasis. Care is taken to replace the kidney within the renal fossa so

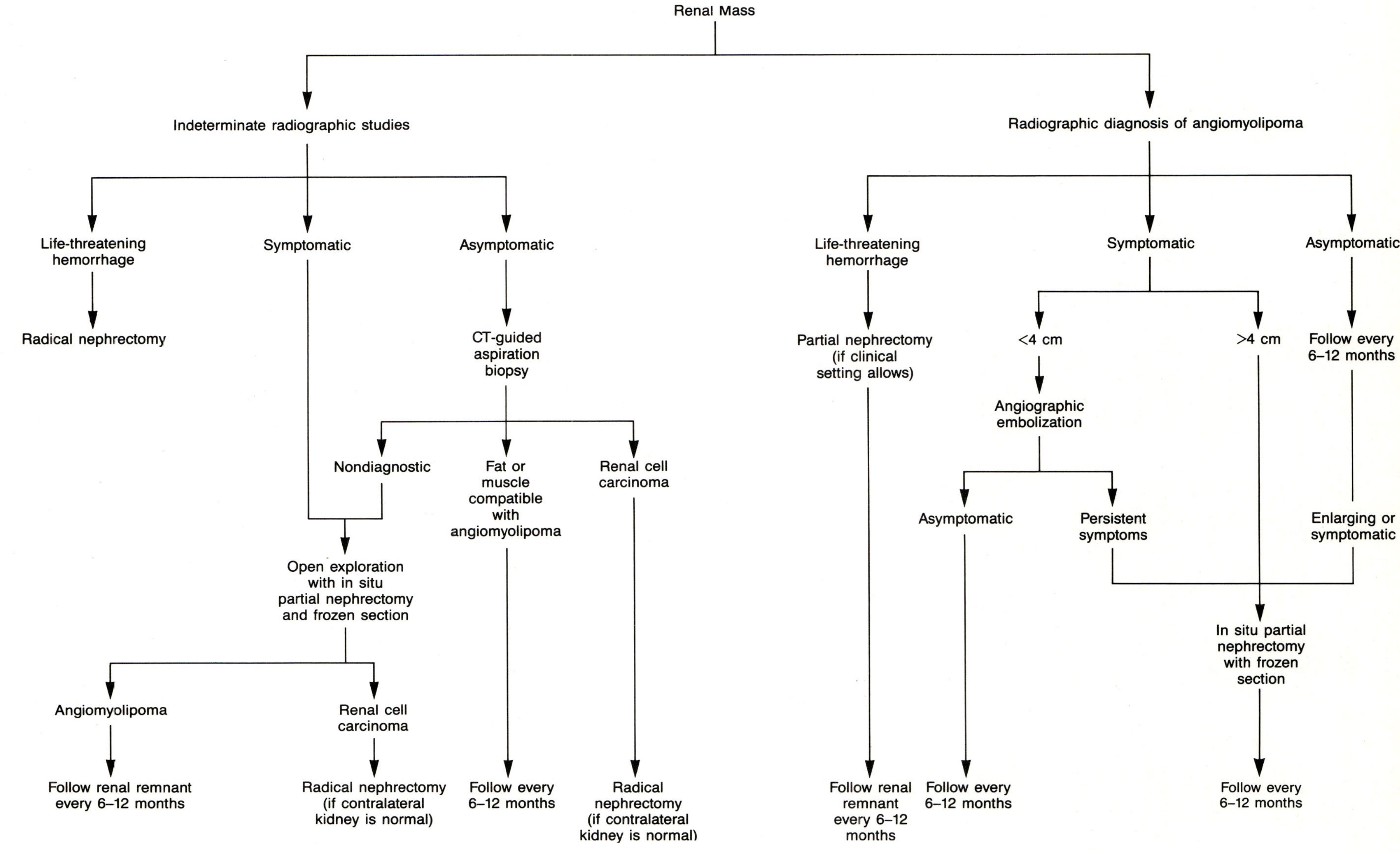

Figure 4 Proposed algorithm for management of patients with suspected renal angiomyolipoma.

that the ureter does not kink or adhere to the raw nephrotomy site.

If the diagnosis of angiomyolipoma is confirmed by frozen section, a drain is placed in proximity to the kidney. On the other hand, if renal cell carcinoma is noted, the radical nephrectomy is completed, provided that the contralateral kidney is normal.

Patients who have indeterminate renal mass lesions and are asymptomatic can be managed with open exploration as described above, or may be advised to undergo CT-guided needle biopsy (or aspiration cytology) of the suspicious lesion. Ordinarily, an 18- to 22-gauge needle may be employed to biopsy or aspirate the lesion. Automatic firing mechanisms facilitate harvesting of core specimens for histologic views. If cytology is preferred, multiple passes through the lesion in different directions should be performed during maximal aspiration with a 10-ml syringe. When material enters the syringe, the suction is relieved and the needle withdrawn. If the biopsy shows renal cell carcinoma, radical nephrectomy is indicated. However, renal angiomyolipoma may be diagnosed by the finding of fat or muscle cells histologically or cytologically compatible with the diagnosis of angiomyolipoma. In this event, patients may be followed conservatively with semiannual CT scans or renal ultrasonography. If the biopsy or aspirate is clearly diagnostic of either renal cell carcinoma or angiomyolipoma, this procedure may spare the patient the need for an operation. However, as not uncommonly occurs (in 20 to 60 percent, depending on the collective skills of the radiologists, pathologists, and cytologists), the CT-guided needle biopsy (or aspiration) may not be clearly diagnostic of either renal cell carcinoma or angiomyolipoma. In this case, open surgical exploration with in situ partial nephrectomy as described above is necessary.

Patients in whom the radiographic diagnosis of angiomyolipoma is unequivocal (usually on the basis of a CT scan) are treated differently. In these patients, both the presence of symptoms and the size of the lesion are important determinants of management.

Patients presenting with very severe symptoms of pain or with life-threatening hemorrhage from renal angiomyolipoma should undergo urgent partial or total nephrectomy, depending on the severity of the clinical situation. Although every effort should be made to preserve as much renal parenchyma as possible, in some cases total nephrectomy is unavoidable.

Patients with renal angiomyolipomas that are only moderately or intermittently symptomatic should be treated according to the size of the lesion (either above or below 4 cm in diameter). Patients with moderately symptomatic renal angiomyolipomas that are less than 4 cm in size can be followed if the symptoms are very mild, but usually should undergo radiographic embolization of the lesion with alcohol. This generally can be performed with less loss of renal parenchyma than that caused by partial nephrectomy. Ordinarily, a subselective arterial injection of absolute alcohol is well tolerated and easily diffuses throughout the entire tumor, producing complete infarction. Balloon occlusion proximal to the injection site will prevent reflux of alcohol into other arteries and tissues. Usually, 15 to 25 ml of alcohol is instilled into the lesion for 5 to 7 minutes, after which the alcohol is aspirated. Alcohol embolization, however, may not be appropriate for larger tumors, those with arteriovenous fistulas, or those with large aneurysmal dilations, because these factors may be associated with vessel rupture or significant systemic uptake of alcohol. If the radiographic embolization is unsuccessful because of technical difficulties, or if the patient has persistent symptoms after embolization, partial nephrectomy as described above should be performed.

Patients who have relatively large renal angiomyolipomas (over 4 cm in diameter) and are moderately symptomatic are ideal candidates for nephron-sparing partial nephrectomy. In all cases, intraoperative frozen section should be performed to substantiate the preoperative diagnosis of angiomyolipoma.

Patients with an unequivocal radiographic diagnosis of renal angiomyolipoma and who are asymptomatic should be followed at 6- to 12-month intervals with CT and/or renal ultrasonography. Patients who develop symptoms or in whom the lesion enlarges should be advised to undergo elective radiographic embolization or in situ partial nephrectomy as described above.

SUGGESTED READING

Blute ML, Malek RS, Segura JW. Angiomyolipoma: clinical metamorphosis and concept for management. J Urol 1988; 139:20–24.

Earthman WJ, Mazer MJ, Winfield AC. Angiomyolipomas in tuberous sclerosis: subselective embolotherapy with alcohol, with long-term follow-up study. Rad 1986; 160:437–441.

Malone MJ, Johnson PR, Jumper BM, et al. Renal angiomyolipoma: six case reports in literature review. J Urol 1986; 135:349–353.

Oesterling JE, Fischman EK, Goldman SM, Marshall FF. The management of renal angiomyolipoma. J Urol 1986; 135:1121–1124.

Sant GR, Ayers DK, VanKoff MS, et al. Fine needle aspiration biopsy in the diagnosis of renal angiomyolipoma. J Urol 1990; 143: 999–1001.

TRANSITIONAL CELL CARCINOMA OF THE RENAL PELVIS

JAMES G. McCOY, M.D.
RICHARD D. WILLIAMS, M.D.

Urothelial cancers of the renal pelvis and ureter account for 5 percent to 9 percent of renal tumors and 5 percent of all urothelial tumors, the vast majority being in the bladder. Transitional cell carcinoma (TCC) indicates the presence of a field defect of the urothelium with risk of synchronous or metachronous tumor developing in the opposite kidney (2 to 4 percent) and in the bladder (30 to 50 percent). More than 90 percent of urothelial tumors are TCC. The disease is three times more common in men than in women and has a peak incidence in the sixth to seventh decades. Risk factors for the development of TCC include cigarette smoking, ingestion of caffeine, and exposure to the aromatic amines used in the rubber and textile industries.

Patients diagnosed with upper-tract TCC present with gross or microscopic hematuria in 60 to 75 percent of cases. Thirty to forty percent have flank pain and less than 15 percent have a flank mass, usually indicating high-stage disease. Fifteen percent are asymptomatic and diagnosed incidentally during evaluation for other reasons.

Standard evaluation for hematuria consists of intravenous urography (IVU) and cystoscopy with urinary cytology. Intravenous urography reveals an abnormal filling defect in 50 to 75 percent of renal urothelial tumors. Nonvisualization of a renal unit occurs in 10 percent of cases and, when due to a ureteral tumor, is associated with muscle invasion in 60 percent. Retrograde pyelograms are indicated when the upper tracts are inadequately visualized on IVU. Once a lesion that is suspicious for urothelial cancer is identified, the diagnosis should be confirmed with upper-tract urine cytology. However, false-negative results range from 30 to 60 percent, most occurring from low-grade lesions. Brush biopsy may be helpful in obtaining a more conclusive specimen. If the diagnosis cannot be confirmed with a blind approach, direct visualization and biopsy with a flexible ureteropyeloscope can definitively establish the diagnosis. Computed tomography (CT) scanning can be useful in distinguishing filling defects due to "radiolucent" stone, which has an attenuation value of greater than 70 Hounsfield units (HU), and urothelial tumors, which typically have attenuation values of 30 to 50 HU. However, CT does not distinguish tumors from other soft tissue densities, and tumors occasionally contain calcifications. Magnetic resonance imaging (MRI) offers no demonstrated advantage over CT in detection or staging of TCC of the upper tract. Staging systems for upper-tract urothelial neoplasms are not completely satisfactory, but for the most part they rely on depth of tumor penetration into the kidney or ureter. The commonly used system adapted from Grabstald and Cummings is shown in Figure 1.

THERAPEUTIC ALTERNATIVES

Therapeutic options have expanded with the advent of promising chemotherapy for TCC and the development of endoscopic techniques for instrumentation and therapeutic manipulation of the upper tract. The standard therapy for localized TCC of the upper tract continues to be radical nephroureterectomy with resection of a cuff of bladder. Resection of the local lesion only, with preservation of the ipsilateral renal unit, results in a 30 to 40 percent local recurrence rate over 2 to 5 years. The radical approach, including removal of the adrenal and Gerota's fascia, is advocated because 5-year survival has been shown to be 84 percent compared with 51 percent for simple nephroureterectomy. This improved survival is due to a reduction in the 30 to 40 percent local recurrence rate in the renal bed. Lymphadenectomy is of prognostic, not therapeutic, value in these patients, and thus only a limited node dissection is recommended.

Prognosis is highly dependent on stage and grade, and thus patients with low-stage, low-grade tumors do very well with any kind of complete tumor excision. A parenchyma-preserving approach is appropriate in patients with a solitary kidney, renal insufficiency, or bilateral lesions or in those with low-grade, low-stage lesions, negative cytology, and confirmed absence of multicentric disease. In all patients for whom parenchyma-sparing surgery is contemplated, meticulous follow-up is essential. Patients with locally advanced (C to D1) disease should be considered for cisplatin–based chemotherapy (CMV or MVAC), with subsequent surgical exploration if repeat clinical staging suggests downstaging to a level amenable to surgical resection. Radiation therapy has little role in this disease with the

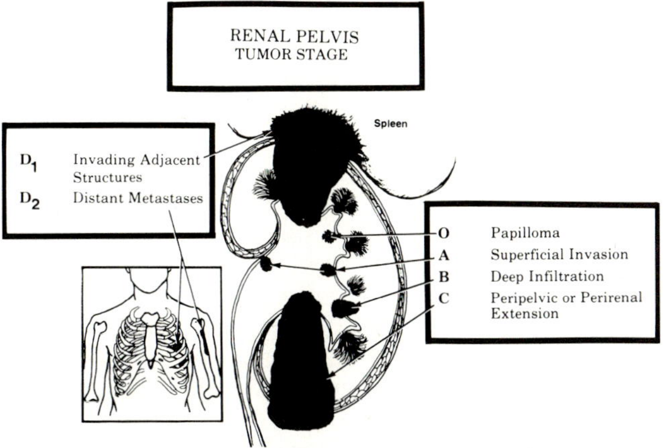

Figure 1 Staging system for transitional cell carcinoma of the renal pelvis.

exception of treatment for symptomatic metastasis resistant to chemotherapy.

PREFERRED APPROACH

Patient Selection

There is a close association of stage and grade in upper-tract urothelial carcinoma. High-grade lesions have an 80 percent incidence of positive cytology while low-grade lesions have a false-negative cytology rate of 30 to 40 percent. The patient with a small papillary lesion on pyelography and a low-grade cytology may not require abdominal CT to complete staging if a standard nephroureterectomy with bladder cuff resection is planned. For all other patients, abdominal CT should be performed. The sensitivity and specificity of CT for parenchymal invasion are 75 and 43 percent, respectively, with sensitivity and specificity for fat invasion 67 and 44 percent, respectively. Therefore, CT is not absolutely accurate for local staging. A CT scan will not detect microscopic lymph node metastasis but will identify enlarged nodes due to either tumor or inflammation. Enlarged nodes noted on CT may be aspirated percutaneously or excised laparoscopically to assess for lymph node metastasis. If liver or other distant lesions are noted and if there is any question about their identity, needle aspiration cytology should be performed. A bone scan should also be performed with plain film correlation of any areas of abnormal uptake. A chest radiograph or chest CT should be obtained to rule out pulmonary involvement. After a thorough assessment of the patient's tumor stage (Fig. 1), the most appropriate therapy can be determined as discussed above. Most patients with localized disease are best served by radical nephroureterectomy with bladder cuff resection.

Preoperative Preparation

A mechanical bowel preparation with Go-lytely is administered the day before surgery to decompress the bowel and facilitate exposure. The patient is hydrated intravenously overnight and inflatable peristaltic stockings are placed on the legs before transfer to the operating room. If there is carcinoma in situ of the bladder so that tumor spill is possible with cystotomy, 500 to 1,500 rads of external beam irradiation is administered on the morning of surgery to inhibit viable tumor cell implantation.

Choice of Procedure

For radical nephroureterectomy with bladder cuff resection, a two-incision approach is preferred with transection of the renal vessels and mobilization of the kidney, adrenal, and Gerota's fascia through a transperitoneal half-chevron incision (Fig. 2). The entire specimen is then pushed inferiorly and the distal ureter is mobilized down to the bladder. The entire renal unit is removed in continuity through a Gibson incision. Early

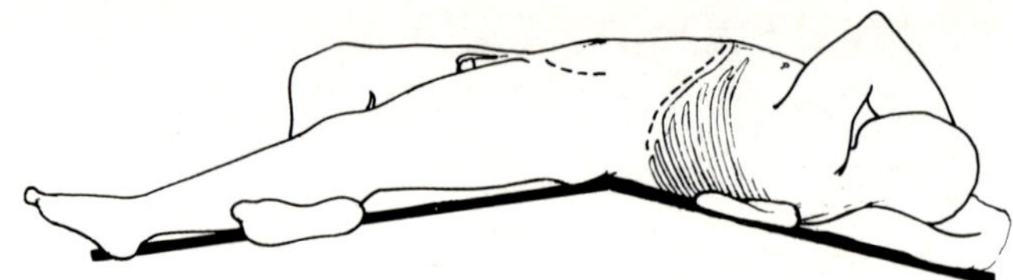

Figure 2 Patient positioning for a radical nephroureterectomy through two incisions: an anterior subcostal incision (dotted line at costal margin) and a lower Gibson incision.

ligation of the ureter (without division) below the tumor may prevent tumor cell seeding into the bladder. A 1- to 3-cm margin of urothelium around the orifice is removed. This can be accomplished by an anterior cystotomy with direct incision around the orifice. An equally acceptable, perhaps preferable, approach is to dissect out the intramural ureter down to the trigone extravesically and then open the bladder immediately around the orifice, excising a 1- to 3-cm cuff of bladder epithelium.

A limited pericaval (right-sided tumor) or periaortic (left-sided tumor) node dissection adds very little morbidity to the procedure and should be included in the treatment of healthy patients to determine the prognosis and the need for possible adjuvant chemotherapy. No therapeutic benefit should be ascribed to the lymphadenectomy, however.

Patients with biopsy-proved low-grade, low-stage solitary distal (lower third) ureteral tumors can be treated with distal ureterectomy and ureteroneocystostomy with a psoas hitch or Boari flap. A freely refluxing anastomosis is performed to facilitate future direct ureteroscopic inspection of the affected renal unit. Distal ureterectomy is performed extraperitoneally through a Gibson incision.

In a patient with a solitary kidney, renal insufficiency, or bilateral tumors, surgery is individualized according to tumor location. It is essential that all areas of the urothelium in these patients be visually inspected preoperatively. One must be aware of the imperfections of current clinical staging techniques, and the alternative of radical resection and dialysis should be considered if the tumor is not unequivocally low grade and low stage. Patients with upper or middle third ureteral tumors can be managed with segmental ureterectomy and ipsilateral ureteroureterostomy. Patients with low-grade caliceal, infundibular, or renal pelvis tumors may be amenable to partial nephrectomy. Arteriography is essential in these patients preoperatively to devise a strategy for vascular control and to determine the boundaries of the resection. These patients are approached through a half-chevron incision. The arterial supply is identified and tagged with vessel loops. Segmental arteries to the portion of the kidney to be removed are ligated. The kidney is then incised sharply in the previously determined plane, hemostasis being achieved by digital compression on the parenchyma adjacent to the transection. No major artery is clamped and renal cooling is not required. There is essentially no warm ischemia time.

Some patients may require brief clamping of the renal arteries, however. The parenchymal vessels are oversewn with figure-of-eight 4-0 PDS suture. The renal collecting system is carefully inspected for residual tumor, and if none is seen and the margins are pathologically (via frozen section) clear, the edges are oversewn with 4-0 PDS suture. A Jackson-Pratt suction drain is left in place near the closure of the collecting system but not in direct contact with it. In the future it may be possible to treat small renal urothelial tumors with laser ablation through a flexible ureteroscope. Percutaneous endoscopic therapy may also be appropriate in patients with small papillary lesions in the renal pelvis and negative cytologic results. However, use of these limited ablation techniques may be compromised by the presence of carcinoma in situ of the collecting ducts in 35 percent of patients with caliceal tumors.

Postoperative Course

Patients found to have positive lymph nodes, positive margins, high-grade tumor invasive into fat, or unresectable disease may benefit from adjuvant chemotherapy with MVAC or CMV. A substantial percentage of patients with measurable residual disease have had tumor regression with either of these regimens, but it is currently unknown whether such treatment affords any survival advantage. Radiation for patients with local residual disease is of minimal benefit. The usefulness of radiation therapy is limited to control of focal pain from tumor resistant to chemotherapy.

Complications and Sequelae

Significant bleeding from adrenal vessels, the renal vascular pedicle, or the spleen, although rare, may occur for up to several days postoperatively. Bleeding can also occur from the cut surface of the kidney after partial nephrectomy. Primary management of these problems consists of meticulous attention to hemostasis at the time of operation. Suture ligature of the renal artery and vein with 4-0 Prolene, as well as free ties with 0 silk, ensures pedicle control. Although it is preferable to identify and ligate the adrenal arteries individually, hemostatic clips can routinely be placed on the tissue medial and superior to the adrenals before transection. Despite these precautions, a high index of suspicion for hemorrhage must be maintained if the patient develops unexplained symptoms and signs of volume depletion postoperatively. The incidence of wound infection can be reduced with prophylactic perioperative antibiotics. A first-generation cephalosporin to cover skin flora is most appropriate. Prolonged urinary leakage at the cystotomy site will resolve with catheter drainage. A prolonged leak from the upper tract after a parenchyma-sparing procedure may require placement of a ureteral stent. Retroperitoneal lymphocele may complicate the limited node dissection; these are usually asymptomatic and eventually resolve spontaneously. The above complications are uncommon.

Follow-up

As previously stressed, TCC represents a field defect of the urothelium, and thus affected patients require careful follow-up to eliminate the possibility of recurrence. When a standard radical nephroureterectomy with bladder cuff resection is performed, the patient should undergo cystoscopy with urine cytology every 3 months for the first year, every 6 months for the second year, and annually thereafter unless the tumor recurs. An IVU should be performed annually. In patients who have undergone limited resection, retrograde pyelography or visual inspection of the affected renal unit and selective urine cytology should be performed on each follow-up visit. This may be accomplished using a flexible ureteropyeloscope with the patient under intravenous sedation. Patients at increased risk for local recurrence (those with high-grade invasive tumors) may benefit from CT every 6 months the first year and annually for 3 to 5 years thereafter.

SUGGESTED READING

Barron RL, McClennan RL, Lee JKT, Lawson TL. Computed tomography of transitional cell carcinoma of the renal pelvis and ureter. Radiology 1982; 144:125–130.

Batata M, Grabstald H. Upper urinary tract urothelial tumors. Urol Clin North Am 1976; 3:79–86.

Cummings KB. Nephroureterectomy: rationale in the management of transitional cell carcinoma of the upper urinary tract. Urol Clin North Am 1980; 7:569–578.

Droller MJ. Transitional cell cancer: upper tracts and bladder. In: Walsh PC, Gittes RF, Perlmutter AD, Stamey TA, eds. Campbell's urology. 5th ed. Philadelphia: WB Saunders, 1986:1343–1440.

Fraley EE. Cancer of the renal pelvis. In: Skinner DG, deKernion JB, eds. Genitourinary cancer. Philadelphia: WB Saunders, 1978: 134–149.

Huffman JL. Endourologic diagnosis and treatment of upper tract urothelial tumors. In: Williams RD, ed. Advances in urologic oncology. New York: MacMillan, 1987:89–110.

Johansson S, Wahlquist L. A prognostic study of urothelial renal pelvic tumors: comparison between the prognosis of patients treated with intrafascial nephrectomy and perifascial nephroureterectomy. Cancer 1979; 43:2525–2531.

McLaughlin JK, Blot WJ, Mandel JS, Schuman LM, Mehl ES, Fraumeni JF. Etiology of Ca of renal pelvis. J Natl Cancer Inst 1983; 71:287–291.

Richie JP. Management of ureteral tumors. In: Skinner DG, de Kernion JB, eds. Genitourinary cancer. Philadelphia: WB Saunders, 1978:150–165.

Schmauz R, Cole P. Epidemiology of cancer of the renal pelvis and ureter. J Natl Cancer Inst 1974; 52:1431–1434.

Sternberg CN, Yagoda A, Scher HI, et al. M-VAC for advanced transitional cell carcinoma of the urothelium: efficacy and patterns of response and relapse. Cancer 1989; 64:2448–2458.

Williams RD. Renal, perirenal, and ureteral neoplasms. In: Gillenwater JY, Grayhack JT, Howard SS, Duckett JW, eds. Adult and pediatric urology. 2nd ed. Chicago: Year Book, 1987:571–614.

Ziegelbaum M, Novick AC, Streem SB, et al. Conservative surgery for transitional cell carcinoma of the renal pelvis. J Urol 1987; 138:1146–1149.

RENAL ONCOCYTOMA

H. BARTON GROSSMAN, M.D.

Oncocytomas are tumors that arise in a variety of organs, including the salivary glands, thyroid, parathyroid, and others. These neoplasms exhibit a common morphology characterized microscopically by abundant eosinophilic cytoplasm, which on the ultrastructural level is found to contain numerous mitochondria with a paucity of other organelles. Although the existence of renal oncocytomas is not a recent event, only in the past decade have they been commonly recognized as a clinical entity. It is important to differentiate these neoplasms from the more usual renal adenocarcinoma because oncocytomas exhibit a much more benign natural history.

Renal oncocytomas represent approximately 5 percent of adult kidney neoplasms. Their average size is 6 cm with a broad distribution ranging from less than 1 to 25 cm or more in diameter. Most oncocytomas present as solitary lesions, but 4 percent are bilateral, and multifocal oncocytomas within a kidney have been reported. The presence of an oncocytoma associated with multiple renal masses is still cause for concern, because sporadic reports testify that renal oncocytomas can occur in conjunction with benign (angiomyolipoma) and malignant (adenocarcinoma) renal neoplasms. On gross appearance, oncocytomas typically exhibit a homogeneous mahogany-brown color and frequently contain a central scar. Nuclear grading has been applied by some investigators to characterize renal oncocytomas further. Only tumors with a nuclear grade of 1 (uniform, round nuclei) should be considered typical oncocytomas. These tumors behave in a benign fashion and have not been shown to metastasize. Metastasis has occasionally been documented in oncocytoma-like renal tumors with a nuclear grade of 2 (larger, more irregular nuclei). Because of this, renal oncocytomas with nuclear grades other than 1 should be followed as renal carcinomas.

Most renal oncocytomas are asymptomatic and detected during routine imaging studies—e.g., excretory urography, ultrasonography, computed tomography (CT), or magnetic resonance imaging (MRI). Just as with the more typical renal carcinoma, they appear as a solid mass. The preoperative diagnosis of renal oncocytoma is frequently difficult. Although "classic" angiographic features have been described, including a homogeneous nephrogram and a spokewheel pattern, these findings are neither unique to nor common among oncocytomas. Both ultrasonography and CT usually demonstrate a well-demarcated solid mass. A central scar is particularly suggestive of an oncocytoma, but this finding is frequently absent. Fine-needle aspiration cytology may be helpful when the radiographic findings are suggestive of an oncocytoma.

TREATMENT

Nephrectomy

The biggest problem influencing the treatment of renal oncocytomas is the difficulty in diagnosing them preoperatively. Most oncocytomas are excised by radical nephrectomy, the correct diagnosis being made only after histologic examination. Solid, vascular renal masses are usually indicative of renal carcinomas and therefore are commonly treated with radical nephrectomy. The unexpected diagnosis of a grade 1 renal oncocytoma presenting as an asymptomatic large solid renal mass is a good finding that has a favorable prognosis.

Large renal tumors are usually treated by nephrectomy with little consideration that the mass is anything but malignant. Small, solitary renal tumors with smooth, distinct margins are more problematic. However, the most conservative approach in the presence of a normal contralateral kidney is still radical nephrectomy. If preoperative imaging studies seriously suggest that the renal mass may be an oncocytoma, and if alternative therapy such as partial nephrectomy is being considered if the mass is a benign renal neoplasm, further diagnostic information may be obtained by fine-needle aspiration cytology.

Bilateral solid renal masses are always a significant clinical problem. While bilateral nephrectomy and subsequent renal transplantation are safest from the standpoint of excising all the neoplasm, the consequent renal failure, dialysis, and ultimate renal transplantation are associated with significant risk. Because of this, bilateral nephrectomy should be avoided whenever technically possible. Frequently, this clinical dilemma is managed by nephrectomy on the side of the largest neoplasm and partial nephrectomy on the other. When technically possible, however, I prefer bilateral partial nephrectomies. If the renal masses are suspected to be bilateral oncocytomas, partial nephrectomy rather than nephrectomy is the treatment of choice. Unfortunately, this is often an unexpected finding. Even when oncocytomas are considered unlikely and bilateral nephrectomy is being performed, it is prudent to send the first specimen for frozen section to document the true nature of the renal masses before proceeding with the second nephrectomy. In fact, the histologic picture can often be surmised by looking at the sectioned gross specimen. Oncocytomas exhibit a uniform brown appearance, whereas carcinomas usually are yellow in color. Frozen-section demonstration of an oncocytoma in the nephrectomy specimen suggests that the contralateral renal mass is the same and should be treated in a less aggressive fashion (i.e., partial nephrectomy). Whether radical or partial nephrectomy is performed, the goal is complete surgical excision of the renal mass.

Partial Nephrectomy

Partial nephrectomy is generally accepted as appropriate therapy for the multifocal renal carcinomas associated with von Hippel-Lindau disease and as a method for the diagnosis and treatment of complex cysts that have not been characterized as benign or malignant by less invasive diagnostic methods. Although the use of partial nephrectomy as definitive therapy for excising small renal carcinomas with normal contralateral kidneys has been reported to have good results, the routine use of this method of treatment is still controversial. However, partial nephrectomy is the treatment of choice for low-grade renal oncocytomas because they exhibit a benign natural history. The problem, of course, is accurately detecting oncocytomas preoperatively.

Partial nephrectomy is usually performed in situ, and only in exceptional circumstances are bench surgery and autotransplantation required. Peripheral renal masses can often be excised without vascular control. I employ arterial occlusion and in situ cooling only for larger and central renal tumors. Although partial nephrectomy appears intuitively to be a better surgical approach than enucleation as therapy for small renal masses, there is no convincing proof that the excision of greater amounts of normal kidney around a renal mass results in a clinically recognizable difference in tumor recurrence or patient survival. I frequently use the Cavitron Ultrasonic Surgical Aspirator in these dissections and believe that it facilitates the goals of a partial nephrectomy by excising renal masses intact while removing a minimal amount of surrounding normal renal parenchyma.

Patients who have had partial nephrectomy require periodic monitoring of the remaining renal parenchyma. I obtain a CT scan of the kidney several months postoperatively to provide a point of reference with which future diagnostic studies can be compared.

Observation

Because grade 1 renal oncocytomas behave in a benign fashion, it is tempting to leave them in situ with close monitoring by noninvasive imaging studies. Despite the paucity of information regarding the natural history of untreated oncocytomas, there is some evidence that their growth is exceedingly slow. However, it is important to bear in mind that this approach is fraught with increased risk to the patient. Renal oncocytomas have occurred in association with renal adenocarcinomas, and higher-grade oncocytomas have demonstrated their aggressiveness by developing metastases. Furthermore, there is always a low risk that an aspiration cytology consistent with a low-grade oncocytoma may not be representative of the entire renal mass. Observation can be considered as the primary method of treatment if a grade 1 oncocytoma is demonstrated by biopsy, and surgical therapy causes significant risk to the patient or results in decreased renal function requiring dialysis. If this approach is successful in these selected patients, observation may be applicable to a more general population in the future.

Although a relatively obscure neoplasm for many years, renal oncocytoma is now widely recognized as a distinct pathologic entity conveying a favorable prognosis. Its benign natural history appears to be limited to grade 1 oncocytomas, and care should be taken not to presume that renal carcinomas with oncocytic features or high-grade oncocytomas will behave in a similar fashion.

The biggest clinical problem with renal oncocytomas is making the correct preoperative diagnosis. Although this would theoretically result in a surgical approach designed to excise less normal renal parenchyma, this is often difficult. Even with a high index of suspicion, the radiologic findings are often equivocal. Renal carcinomas are much more common than oncocytomas, and therefore small encapsulated renal masses are more likely to be malignant adenocarcinomas than benign, grade 1 oncocytomas. Aspiration cytology can support the diagnosis of an oncocytoma. However, this approach is not often used in the face of a probable renal carcinoma, and even a positive cytologic diagnosis is representative of only a small portion of any mass and does not completely eliminate the low probability of an adjacent focus of carcinoma.

The bottom line is that well-encapsulated solid renal masses may occasionally represent what is probably a benign renal tumor (i.e., an oncocytoma) rather than the more common renal carcinoma. Since this unexpected event will eventually occur to most urologists, it seems prudent to inform patients of this possibility and remind them that a nephrectomy is still the most conservative form of treatment. The end result of this philosophy is that some kidneys will be lost that potentially could have been saved with a parenchyma-sparing procedure. However, this remains the safest way of dealing with solid renal masses in individuals with adequate renal function and a normal contralateral kidney.

The alternative approach is to perform a partial nephrectomy in peripheral, well-circumscribed renal masses. This treatment is frequently employed in individuals who would suffer significant impairment of renal function if a nephrectomy were performed. The broader application of this approach to patients with a normal contralateral kidney is becoming more acceptable as data documenting its safety are published. At this point, however, partial nephrectomy should be considered carefully before routinely employing it in the treatment of solitary renal masses in patients who are good surgical candidates and are not at increased risk for renal failure.

Although individuals with surgically excised (by either total or partial nephrectomy) low-grade renal oncocytomas have an excellent prognosis, the natural history of untreated oncocytomas is relatively unknown. The limited data available suggest that these neoplasms grow slowly and behave in a benign fashion. However, insufficient information is available to recommend routinely following these tumors in situ unless there are extenuating clinical circumstances, such as poor renal function or increased surgical risk.

SUGGESTED READING

Levine E, Huntrakoon M, Wetzel LH. Small renal neoplasms: clinical, pathologic, and imaging features. AJR 1989; 153:69–73.

Lieber MM, Tomera KM, Farrow GM. Renal oncocytoma. J Urol 1981; 125:481–485.

Novick AC, Streem S, Montie JE, et al. Conservative surgery for renal cell carcinoma: a single-center experience with 100 patients. J Urol 1989; 141:835–839.

Spring DB, Ulirsch RC, Starke WR, Brown S Jr. Renal oncocytoma followed for eighteen years without resection. Urology 1985; 26:389–392.

PRIMARY RETROPERITONEAL TUMOR

ROBERT A. BADALAMENT, M.D.
JOSEPH R. DRAGO, M.D.

ANATOMY OF THE RETROPERITONEAL SPACE AND ORGANS

The retroperitoneal space includes many organs, such as the adrenal, pancreas, kidneys, ureter, and bladder and parts of the duodenum, as well as parts of the prostate and seminal vesicles in males and internal genitalia in females. The retroperitoneal space is a large space extending from the respiratory diaphragm to the pelvic diaphragm. It is bounded by the posterior layer of parietal peritoneum, segments of the colon and duodenum, and the posterior surface of the liver. Its posterior boundary consists of the perivertebral fascia, the quadratus lumborum muscle, and the soleus muscle above the iliac crest.

Many tumors may arise from the organs in their retroperitoneal location; these are not called "retroperitoneal tumors" but are termed by their primary organs — e.g., adrenal carcinoma and renal carcinoma. The specific term "retroperitoneal tumor" refers to neoplasms arising from various structures in the retroperitoneal space, including lymphatic, vascular, supporting muscular, connective tissue, lipomatous, neural, and various embryonic remnants.

To date, no exogenous or other agents have been specifically identified as causing retroperitoneal tumors. Experimental evidence has shown that various sarcomas such as the liposarcoma can be experimentally induced in animals. These tumors, in general, are rare, making up 0.1 to 0.2 percent of the total number of malignancies. They usually occur with equal frequency between males and females, although some series show a female preponderance, and are noted more often in those 40 to 50 years of age. However, there are rhabdomyosarcomas and teratomas that more frequently occur in childhood.

Most of these masses (70 percent) prove to be malignant; these most commonly are liposarcomas and myosarcomas. All retroperitoneal mass lesions must be distinguished from primary retroperitoneal malignancy. In the differential diagnosis of such lesions and masses in the retroperitoneum, the following must be included: (1) hematoma; (2) abscess, either psoas or primary retroperitoneal; (3) metastatic disease; and (4) cysts, including those of pancreatic, renal, and adrenal origin. When faced with establishing a differential diagnosis of retroperitoneal masses, the clinician must be careful to include in their history a search for trauma, anticoagulation therapy, fever, and leukocytosis. Fever and leukocytosis help differentiate a large mass that may be benign from one that is an abscess in nature.

Primary retroperitoneal cysts are benign, rare, and generally found only at the time of exploration. They may arise from many structures, including urogenital and lymphatic structures or even the mesentery of the colon or stomach.

Early diagnostic signs of retroperitoneal tumors are the development of an abdominal mass and abdominal enlargement as well as weight loss. Most patients with retroperitoneal tumors present with an enlarging mass in the abdomen or flank or a vague sensation of abdominal fullness or pain. Occasionally they also have fever secondary to central tumor necrosis as the tumors grow large. In addition, patients may present with pain, lethargy, and anorexia secondary to the enlarging abdominal mass causing abdominal symptoms. Pain is the most frequent symptom in several large series, and is present in approximately 50 percent of patients. Initial findings may include nausea, vomiting, abdominal distention, obstipation, and symptoms that may mimic partial small bowel obstruction (Table 1). These abdominal symptoms are often secondary to invasion of the

Table 1 Chief Complaint of Patients Presenting with Retroperitoneal Tumors

Clinical Signs	Percentage
Abdominal pain	50
Abdominal mass	33
Gastrointestinal symptoms	25
Backache	7
Pain in leg or swelling in leg	7
Genitourinary symptoms	4
Weight loss	4
Fever	2

area of the celiac axis and stretching of the intestinal mesentery, which may mimic the signs of intestinal ischemia. These tumors, like all others, grow in the plane of least resistance, which is usually anterior toward the peritoneal surface and not posterior into the back muscles or vertebral column. This is why these masses may achieve a large size before they can be palpated. Most have no hormonal or endocrine function, and thus there are no early signs of endocrinopathy or hormone changes that might permit early detection.

These tumors may also present with signs such as those of vascular insufficiency due to compression of various and lymphatic channels in the pelvis, and may result in poor drainage, poor blood flow to the areas of the lower extremity, and edema or varices (Table 2). They generally achieve a significant size, causing neurologic compression symptoms, and may give rise to motor or sensory reflex changes, sphincteric changes, or back or leg pain. The urinary system may also be involved, especially in the pelvis from bladder pressure or in the upper urinary system from compression of the retroperitoneal tumors on the ureters or renal pelvis. Further symptoms such as obstruction and pyelonephritis may follow secondary to the size of the mass and the compression of the mass on the upper urinary tract.

LABORATORY STUDIES

Physical examination usually confirms an abdominal or flank mass in most patients. The mass may be tender in 10 to 20 percent of cases, and patients may present with fever secondary to central tumor necrosis. Plain x-ray films of the abdomen may help to show the general location of the mass and whether it contains fat or calcium. Other important studies include intravenous pyelography (IVP), computed tomography (CT), magnetic resonance imaging (MRI), and barium studies to determine gastrointestinal involvement. Arteriography and venography are occasionally necessary, and rarely lymphangiography. Biopsy under fluoroscopy or CT guidance is helpful and appropriate. Retroperitoneal pneumography was used in the past to outline some large retroperitoneal tumors, but with the advent of CT and MRI this invasive test has become largely one of historic interest.

The most common type of tumor found in the retroperitoneum is that of Hodgkin's disease; others

common in this area include liposarcoma, myelosarcoma, and fibrosarcoma. The advantages of CT or MRI for diagnosis of retroperitoneal tumors are twofold: (1) detection of the tumor and (2) for localization of the tumor and defining its relationship to adjacent structures, blood vessels, and lymph nodes. It also helps determine the presence of metastasis. MRI has been used most recently and has been shown to be as effective as CT in the diagnosis of retroperitoneal tumors in the early stages. The IVP is important in evaluation of patient status, particularly for the presence and function of the opposite kidney, because nephrectomy may be required in as many as 30 percent for complete surgical extirpation of the primary retroperitoneal tumor. The ultimate test, however, is that of exploratory laparotomy. Standard bowel preparation should precede this, and systemic antibiotics are used for prophylaxis.

SURGICAL APPROACHES: PATIENT SELECTION

The most appropriate surgical treatment consists of complete excision of the tumor along with any adjacent organs, if necessary, to ensure as wide a tumor-free margin as possible around the resection, thereby reducing the risk of local recurrence. The transperitoneal approach offers the best exposure for proper exploration with adequate incision, and can be effected by a midline or a chevron incision. Our personal preference is for an upper abdominal chevron incision, which allows for better healing in most patients and affords the opportunity to inspect both areas of the retroperitoneum clearly, especially lateral to the kidneys, and to perform any intra-abdominal manipulation that may be necessary. This is ideal for an upper abdominal retroperitoneal tumor. For the lower tumors, however, Pfannenstiel's midline incision is appropriate.

The operative treatment of these retroperitoneal tumors can be difficult for many reasons. Their origin often is well concealed, which allows them to undergo tremendous local growth and amass large volumes before symptoms occur or the mass becomes palpable. Because of this delay in diagnosis, there is a high likelihood (as much as 25 percent) of distant metastasis before the time of exploration. The vast majority of these tumors have a somewhat pseudoencapsulated wall, which does permit appropriate dissection, especially in their posterior aspects, and frees them off the great vessels. In planning the approach, early vascular access control must be gained. In most cases, the main organ of interest will be the area of the kidney and its accompanying ureter. If a preoperative decision has been made that the patient also needs an ipsilateral nephrectomy, early control of the blood vessels in the kidney and renal artery and vein must be obtained. In addition, there are many satellite and parasitizing vessels in these retroperitoneal tumors that must be individually ligated. The size of the draining retroperitoneal veins may be large and great care must be exercised in dissecting this area. If the tumor is a primary liposarcoma of the retroperitoneum involving the kidney, attention is initially directed toward

Table 2 Late Complications in Patients with Large Retroperitoneal Tumors

Clinical Signs	Percentage
Abdominal swelling	40
Weight loss	35
Gastrointestinal symptoms	30
Abdominal pain	15
Pain or swelling in leg	11
Fever	9
Back pain	4

the upper pole of the kidney, freeing this from the posterior peritoneum and taking the ipsilateral adrenal with it. On the left side, dissection is generally complicated by the spleen, which invariably is close to the line of resection. Great care must be taken in protecting the spleen from retractor or surgical injury. On the right side, care must be taken not to avulse the right adrenal vein, which is short and often concealed by the retroperitoneal tumor in this area. Once the anterior and superior surfaces of the tumor and kidney have been appropriately secured, the remainder of the dissection of the posterior plane can be taken much as in a retroperitoneal node dissection for testicular malignancy. Individual ligature and metallic clips are helpful in these instances. Often, major vascular invasion is seen with these retroperitoneal tumors, which may make them unresectable. With appropriate preoperative consultation and diagnosis, however, one may plan to resect segmentally a portion of aorta and replace this with a graft, which has proved successful in a few instances. If the tumor is not completely resected, there is a high risk of intraperitoneal and wound recurrences after surgery.

The thoracoabdominal approach, either a super eleventh or super twelfth rib incision, extending across the anterior or upper abdomen has also been found successful in treating patients with large retroperitoneal tumors. In an occasional patient it is even necessary to use a ninth rib thoracicoabdominal incision. In this case, the patient is placed at approximately 45 degrees on the operating table, and the incision extends from the tip of the rib, medially transecting the external oblique and rectus abdominis muscles. The peritoneum is easily retracted medially. We generally open the peritoneum to explore for intraperitoneal metastasis. This approach is suitable for most patients, but particularly for those with a large upper abdominal retroperitoneal tumor. Should the tumor be in the upper third of the kidney, a thoracoabdominal approach is made with the incision over the ninth or tenth rib from the posterior axillary line to the costochondral junction and extended obliquely to the lower quadrant of the abdomen. The size and location of the primary tumor help govern the choice of the most appropriate incision. Additional considerations are the need to explore other areas and the intra- or extraperitoneal base, and to resect or repair other areas of damage secondary to the primary retroperitoneal tumor.

Despite all of the above factors, complete tumor resection is possible in only 60 to 70 percent of patients. Most surgeons believe that partial resection is beneficial in relieving symptoms that may be caused by compression of adjacent organs in the gastrointestinal or genitourinary system, and that this debulking has resulted in a better response than that from radiation or chemotherapy.

RADIOTHERAPY

Radiotherapy may play a role as an adjunctive treatment for patients with these retroperitoneal tumors and has been used by several investigators, since at least 25 percent cannot be completely resected. In patients with lymphoma, both chemotherapy and radiotherapy have been shown to have a tremendous effect on tumor volume.

Chemotherapy has been applied to this disease when it has been far advanced and resection has not been possible, and reports in the literature describe dramatic responses to chemotherapy. No best agent has been found for specific histologic types, however, and the predictability of the chemotherapeutic response remains unclear. Nevertheless, innovative approaches with infusional chemotherapy or preoperative systemic therapy and radiation therapy to decrease the size of the mass may alter survival rates in this patient population. Chemotherapy given up front may actually aid the resection because of the pseudocapsule that usually is present after chemotherapy. It has been useful in patients who have been subject to combined preoperative chemotherapy and radiation therapy, and the follow-up arteriogram before surgery has shown considerable shrinkage of the mass. In most patients, the mass has attained a great size, and preoperative arteriography is essential for planning the operative approach. Swan-Ganz catheters are also useful in monitoring patients undergoing these potentially extensive operative procedures.

POSTOPERATIVE CARE AND COMPLICATIONS

Much of the care is standard as with any major surgical procedure. However, in the area of retroperitoneal tumor, as in the area of retroperitoneal lymphadenectomy for testicular malignancy, a large third space fluid loss occurs. Replacement of this with plasma is essential only in the early postoperative period, and even then only for the first 36 to 48 hours. After a thoracoabdominal incision, a chest tube is indicated in most patients, along with a nasogastric drainage or gastrostomy tube. The most common complications include infection, lymphocele, ureteral injury, and bowel fistulas. Fortunately, these occur in only a few patients, and appropriate early diagnosis and recognition is a key to patient survival in these circumstances (Table 3).

Five-year survival for patients with these large retroperitoneal tumors ranges from 5 to 30 percent. This is because (1) only 40 to 60 percent of all primary retroperitoneal tumors can be resected in total and (2) preoperative and postoperative chemotherapy and radiation therapy have not improved the early survivorship

Table 3 Common Complications

Clinical Signs	Percentage
Lymphocele	2
Ureteral injuries	< 1
Bowel fistulas	< 1
Injury to the renal polar artery	0.2
Wound infection	3

in the limited numbers of patients treated. Most recurrences of these tumors tend to be local, and many surgeons have adopted a second-look procedure. Careful follow-up is indicated, including CT three to four times per year for the first 2 years, every 6 months for the next year, and annually thereafter. Repeat surgical exploration with excision is necessary after recurrence.

SUGGESTED READING

Crawford ED, Borden TA. Genitourinary cancer surgery. Philadelphia: Lea & Febiger, 1982.
Culp DA, Loening SA. Genitourinary oncology. Philadelphia: Lea & Febiger, 1985.
DeVita VT Jr, Hellman S, Rosenberg SA. Cancer: principles and practice of oncology. Philadelphia: JB Lippincott, 1982.
Walsh PC, Gittes RF, Perlmutter AD, Stamey TA. Campbell's urology. 5th ed. Philadelphia: WB Saunders, 1986.

METASTATIC RETROPERITONEAL TUMOR

CHARLES B. BRENDLER, M.D.

Metastatic retroperitoneal tumors commonly assume urologic significance when they produce ureteral obstruction. This chapter focuses on the diagnosis and treatment of ureteral obstruction caused by metastatic cancers.

ETIOLOGY

Metastatic retroperitoneal tumors can produce ureteral obstruction either by direct extension of malignancy or as a result of metastases to retroperitoneal lymph nodes. Although in 60 to 70 percent of patients ureteral obstruction occurs within 2 years of the primary diagnosis, it may occur as much as 20 years later.

PATHOGENESIS

Ureteral obstruction secondary to metastatic tumors usually results from extrinsic obstruction by retroperitoneal lymph nodes. The distal or pelvic ureter is the most frequent site of obstruction, but any portion of the ureter may be involved. Table 1 lists the secondary retroperitoneal tumors that cause extrinsic obstruction of the ureter. Carcinomas of the cervix, prostate, bladder, and colon are the most common causes and account for 70 percent of cases. Lymphoproliferative disorders, including lymphoma and leukemia, may also produce ureteral obstruction.

Less commonly, ureteral obstruction results from direct invasion of the ureteral wall. True metastases to the ureter invade the ureter by intramural growth, are

Table 1 Secondary Retroperitoneal Tumors That Cause Extrinsic Obstruction of Ureter*

Cervix	
Prostate	— account for 70% of cases
Bladder	
Colon	
Ovary, uterus	
Stomach	
Breast	
Lymph nodes	
Pancreas	
Lung	
Gallbladder	
Testis	
Small bowel	

*Presented in order of decreasing frequency.
Republished with permission by Persky L, Kursh ED, Feldman S, Resnick MI. Extrinsic obstruction of the ureter. In: Walsh PC, ed. Campbell's urology 5th ed. Philadelphia: WB Saunders, 1986:605.

present in periureteral lymphatics, and do not involve the ureter by direct extension or contiguity. Metastases to the ureter are uncommon, being seen in only 0.1 to 4 percent of all cancer patients at autopsy. Ureteral metastases may occur at any level, are bilateral 25 to 60 percent of the time, and are more common in women than in men. Breast cancer is the most common nonpelvic tumor associated with ureteral obstruction, and autopsy studies of women who have died of breast cancer have found metastatic involvement of the ureters in up to 8 percent.

SYMPTOMS AND SIGNS

Patients with metastatic retroperitoneal tumors involving the ureter may present with classic symptoms of ureteral obstruction, including fever and flank pain. Often, however, ureteral obstruction is not suspected until the patient develops anuria and renal failure caused by obstruction of both ureters. Infrequently, metastatic ureteral obstruction may be the first evidence of malignancy. Physical signs and laboratory findings include flank tenderness, leukocytosis, pyuria, azotemia, and septicemia.

DIAGNOSIS

Since malignant ureteral obstruction frequently is asymptomatic, it is sometimes detected on intravenous pyelography done for other reasons. Once suspected, the diagnosis can be confirmed by ultrasonography or computed tomography (CT). Alternatively, magnetic resonance imaging (MRI) may be useful.

In extrinsic ureteral obstruction, the etiology may be established in more than 90 percent of cases by percutaneous needle aspiration with a 22- to 23-gauge Chiba needle under ultrasound, CT, or fluoroscopic guidance. Complications with this technique have been very low.

In metastatic intrinsic ureteral obstruction, urinary cytology frequently yields a diagnosis of malignancy. The specific cause may be determined either by ureteral brushing or by ureteroscopy and direct visual biopsy of the lesion. However, it is more difficult to establish the diagnosis with metastatic than with primary ureteral tumors because metastatic lesions involve the muscular wall of the ureter rather than the mucosa. Not infrequently, surgical exploration is required to establish the diagnosis and relieve the obstruction if possible.

TREATMENT

In cases of metastatic ureteral obstruction, the major dilemma facing the physician is whether to treat the patient at all. Ureteral obstruction is often a manifestation of far-advanced disease, and in general, the prognosis for bilateral ureteral obstruction secondary to carcinoma is poor. If no effective therapy can be offered to the patient, it may be better not to treat at all, because death from uremia is relatively painless. On the other hand, patients with a better prognosis deserve aggressive management. In particular, men with ureteral obstruction due to previously untreated metastatic prostatic carcinoma should be treated since, with hormonal therapy, they have a median survival of 3 years.

Patients who also may respond well to relief of ureteral obstruction include those with previously untreated malignancies. The prognosis in patients with malignant ureteral obstruction has increased with improved chemotherapy, and the mean survival in all cases after nonoperative urinary diversion is 10 months. Complete resolution of ureteral obstruction caused by metastatic breast cancer has been reported with combination chemotherapy and radiation. Patients with ureteral obstruction secondary to direct extension of tumor generally do better than patients with obstruction from retroperitoneal lymph nodes.

Until fairly recently, patients with metastatic ureteral obstruction who underwent urinary diversion did poorly: 40 to 50 percent of those who had nephrostomy tubes placed never left the hospital, and the mean survival was less than 6 months. Overall, patients spent 60 percent of their time hospitalized.

More recently, patients with metastatic ureteral obstruction have fared better, owing to improved methods of urinary diversion and better chemotherapy. Open surgical placement of nephrostomy tubes for relief of ureteral obstruction is done only rarely today. Alternative methods of treatment include placement of double-J silicone ureteral catheters and percutaneous nephrostomy. Silicone ureteral catheters are more comfortable for the patient and, because they are internal and nonreactive, are associated with a lower incidence of infection than percutaneous nephrostomies. However, they are frequently difficult to position above the point of ureteral obstruction.

Percutaneous nephrostomy has much less morbidity than open nephrostomy. The perioperative mortality rate is about 10 percent; the most common complication is dislodgment of the nephrostomy catheters, which occurs in about 40 percent of patients. Percutaneous nephrostomies have the additional advantage over open nephrostomy of being placed under local anesthesia in an outpatient setting.

Although formal surgical nephrostomy is seldom performed today to relieve ureteral obstruction, there are patients in whom supravesical diversion may be desirable, particularly to palliate distal ureteral obstruction caused by advanced pelvic malignancy. In such patients, it is better to avoid more complicated procedures that use intestine. Alternative procedures include cutaneous end or loop ureterostomy, perhaps in combination with transureterostomy.

SUGGESTED READING

Akmal M, Kaptein EM, Bertram J, Massry SG. Acute renal failure due to bilateral ureteral obstruction by metastases from breast cancer. Nephron 1986; 42:23.

Corwin HL, Murthy A, Pessis D, Bonomi P. Renal failure from metastatic breast carcinoma reversed by radiotherapy and chemotherapy. Arch Intern Med 1984; 144:1679.

Culkin DJ, Wheeler JS Jr, Marsans RE, et al. Percutaneous nephrostomy for palliation of metastatic ureteral obstruction. Urology 1987; 30:229.

Persky L, Kursh ED, Feldman S, Resnick MI. Extrinsic obstruction of the ureter. In Walsh PC, ed. Campbell's urology. 5th ed. Philadelphia: WB Saunders, 1986:579.

Schlegel PN, Epstein JI, Fishman EK, Brendler CB. Rapidly progressive bilateral ureteral obstruction. J Urol 1990; 144:957.

URETERAL TRANSITIONAL CELL CARCINOMA

STEVEN H. SELMAN, M.D., F.A.C.S.

Although transitional cell carcinoma of the ureter is an uncommon neoplasm, it is often considered in the differential diagnosis of patients who present with hematuria, a ureteral filling defect, or a nonfunctioning renal unit. Rare before 30 years of age the incidence of this carcinoma increases with advancing age. As in urothelial carcinomas of the bladder and renal pelvis, carcinoma of the ureter is more common in men. Most of these carcinomas arise in the distal ureter with a pathologic spectrum ranging from superficial low-grade tumors to those that are infiltrating and anaplastic. Bilaterality (which is rare), a solitary renal unit, compromised renal function, or associated medical problems may require individualization of therapy for the patient with carcinoma of the ureter.

The standard therapy for carcinoma of the ureter is nephroureterectomy with removal of a cuff of bladder. This approach has been advocated because of the multicentricity of these tumors, especially those arising in the upper two thirds of the ureter. However, less radical surgical approaches to the problem have also been advocated.

The patient with carcinoma of the ureter most commonly presents with hematuria or flank pain. Patients can present with a flank mass, but in my experience, this seems to be more closely associated with tumors of the renal pelvis. The development of ureteral tumors can be seen in patients with a history of carcinoma of the bladder. Persistent microhematuria subsequent to successful removal of an intravesical neoplasm should alert the clinician to the possibility of a carcinoma of the ureter or renal pelvis.

The intravenous pyelogram is the first diagnostic procedure I obtain in patients thought to have a ureteral neoplasm. A filling defect, ureteral obstruction, or nonfunctioning renal unit is the usual finding. At times, confusion with a nonopaque stone, blood clot, or benign ureteral polyp can arise. I perform cystoscopy and retrograde pyelography in all patients with a suspected ureteral tumor. Retrograde pyelography is performed in a cystoscopy suite equipped with fluoroscopy, since this offers the greatest versatility in obtaining a diagnosis.

Cystoscopy is done to rule out concomitant bladder tumors. In cases of distal ureteral tumors, the lesion may at times be seen protruding from the ureteral orifice, in which case biopsy can be performed. If the involved ureteral orifice appears normal, advance a bulb-tip (8 Fr) ureteral catheter into the ureteral orifice or slightly beyond. Depending on the situation, urine is collected by cytologic study and immediately sent to the cytology laboratory. It has been my practice to alert the cytopathologist before sending the specimen. I generally barbotage the ureter with normal saline and send the resulting specimen for cytologic study. With the aid of fluoroscopy, I can usually position the catheter near the area in question before beginning the barbotage. In selected patients, I have used the brush biopsy catheter to establish a diagnosis. I currently reserve the brush technique for patients in whom cytologic findings are negative and in whom the diagnosis has not been established by other techniques. Once the cytologic materials have been obtained, snugly engage the bulb tip into the ureteral orifice and obtain a retrograde ureterogram. When fluoroscopy is used as an adjuvant to retrograde pyelography, the physical characteristics (motion, presence of stalk) of the area in question can sometimes be observed. Obtain retrograde pyelograms for small ureteral tumors using dilute (30 percent) contrast media, since in some cases full-strength contrast media result in a "whiteout" and loss of detail. When I have had difficulty differentiating a ureteral tumor from a radiolucent calculus, computed tomography (CT) is used to differentiate the two. I have also used CT when encountering constricting lesions of the ureter, since it can help in differentiating instrinsic from extrinsic lesions.

A number of rigid and flexible ureterscopes have been recently introduced into our diagnostic armamentarium. They can be used to inspect the ureter as well as to obtain tissue for diagnosis. The new generation of small caliber (7.2 Fr) semirigid instruments are very useful, especially for the distal one third of the ureter.

Finally, antegrade pyelography is sometimes used to establish a diagnosis. This has been helpful when retrograde pyelography has been unsuccessful or yields incomplete information on the extent of the tumor. In the presence of a nonfunctioning renal unit, antegrade pyelography can be done under ultrasound guidance.

Once the diagnosis of transitional cell carcinoma is established, the patient undergoes an evaluation for metastatic disease. Currently, this includes a chest x-ray film, bone scan, and liver function tests. If there is no evidence of metastatic disease, surgery is recommended. My approach to the patient with normal bilateral renal function is to recommend nephroureterectomy. If the uninvolved renal unit is compromised or the patient has only one renal unit, I discuss a more conservative surgical approach with the patient. I have found split renal creatinine clearance levels to be the best predictor of the contribution of each renal unit to total renal function. This is helpful in determining whether nephrectomy can be tolerated.

If ureteral carcinoma arises in a solitary renal unit, the benefits of preserving that unit must be weighed against the risks of inadequate resection and the probability of future recurrences. Patient compliance and the ability to detect early recurrences are also included in the decision.

THERAPEUTIC ALTERNATIVES

Endoscopic Management

The increasing use of ureteroscopy will probably change the standard approach to superficial, low-grade ureteral tumors. Ureteroscopy implies that the natural history of these lesions is similar to that of those found in the bladder, a point that has not been firmly established. Also, as mentioned above, rigid ureteroscopy is not always technically possible. Biopsy as well as fulguration can be performed under direct vision through the working channel of the rigid ureteroscope.

Topical Chemotherapy

Intravesical chemoimmunotherapy seems to be of some benefit in the management of patients with low-stage, low-grade urothelial tumors of the bladder. In selected patients with ureteral tumors, topical chemotherapy can be tried as an alternative to surgery. A number of innovative techniques have been suggested to provide topical agents with direct access to the upper urinary tract urothelium, including placing double-J ureteral stents to create vesicoureteral reflux.

Unfortunately, most current reports on the use of topical antineoplastic agents are anecdotal. The dose, frequency of treatment, and best method of drug delivery are unknown.

Laser Ablation of Ureteral Tumors

The use of the laser in the management of patients with urothelial tumors has not been clearly defined. The fiberoptic delivery systems available for the Nd:YAG laser are well suited for the endoscopic ablation of ureteral tumors. However, its use at this time is still considered experimental.

Systemic Chemotherapy

Systemic chemotherapy generally is not used to treat patients with nonmetastatic carcinoma of the ureter. When the disease is no longer localized, systemic chemotherapy is the only nonpalliative therapeutic option. The cisplatin-based regimens seem to be the most promising for ureteral tumors. I have seen striking short-term urothelial tumor regression using the combination of cisplatin, methotrexate, doxorubicin (Adriamycin), and vinblastine. In patients with locally advanced ureteral tumors, I envision using this combination for preoperative chemocytoreduction followed by nephroureterectomy.

PREFERRED APPROACH

Nephroureterectomy

Nephroureterectomy is the standard procedure in most patients with transitional cell carcinoma of the ureter. I prefer the eleventh rib extrapleural extraperitoneal approach to the kidney and upper ureter, and a second Gibson incision for access to the lower ureter and bladder. To gain access to the kidney, position the patient in the flank position with the coronal plane rotated slightly posteriorly. Incise over the eleventh rib, curving slightly downward off the tip of the rib to the edge of the ipsilateral rectus. Once the rib is removed, I divide the internal oblique muscle to reveal the lumbodorsal fascia and transversus abdominis muscles. Incise the lumbodorsal fascia slightly anterior to the tip of the bed of the eleventh rib. Insert the index finger into this opening to push the peritoneum off the undersurface of the transversus abdominis and divide the transversus. All that remains is to divide the bed of the eleventh rib, which is begun anteriorly and completed by incising slightly above its lower margin. Avoid the pleura by first visualizing its caudal extension and gently elevating it away from the rib bed. Once this is completed, I use the Bookwalter self-retaining retractor to maintain the exposure of the retroperitoneum afforded by this incision.

For right-sided tumors, push the peritoneum anteriorly until the anterior surface of the vena cava is exposed. Elevate the right renal vein, then identify the renal artery and ligate it with 0 silk. At this point, I generally ligate and divide the renal vein, which better exposes the underlying renal artery and then divide the renal artery after it is secured by a second ligature. I routinely remove the ipsilateral adrenal gland and Gerota's fascia. For left-sided tumors, the approach is similar. Expose the renal vessels by separating the peritoneum from Gerota's fascia and sweeping it anteriorly. Exposure of the renal artery is best attained by dividing the adrenal vein, which allows the renal vein to be displaced inferiorly, exposing the underlying renal artery. When encircling the left renal vein, be cautious of lumbar veins entering to the left of the aorta.

Once the kidney is mobilized, free the ureter and a generous amount of periureteral tissue. Mobilize the ureter to the level of the iliac crest, then push the kidney and ureter caudally as far as possible. Close the wound, and place the patient in the supine position. Fill the bladder with 150 ml of sterile water and clamp the Foley catheter. After the entire abdomen is rewashed and draped, make a Gibson incision. Extend the medial aspect of the incision slightly beyond the midline. Once the muscles of the abdominal wall are divided, develop the preperitoneal space, exposing the iliac vessels, distal ureter, and bladder. In men, sharply freeing the spermatic cord from the peritoneum greatly facilitates development of this space. Carefully pack the wound with moist abdominal tapes to isolate the bladder. Make a cystotomy, identifying both ureteral orifices. Catheterize the orifice of the involved ureter with a 5 Fr Silastic tube that is secured in place with a 3-0 silk pursestring suture ligature placed around the orifice. The free ends of this ligature can be "bootstrapped" around this tube to obliterate the lumen. Incise a 2-cm diameter circle of mucosa around the orifice using electrocautery. With gentle traction on the feeding tube, dissect the ureter with attached cuff of bladder out of the bladder wall, then free the extravesical and pelvic portion of the ureter. A curved retractor can be used to lift the pelvic peritoneum to allow in-continuity removal of the kidney and ureter. After removing the specimen, close the bladder in three layers. Usually, I do not drain the wound. I have not routinely performed a lymphadenectomy for carcinoma of the ureter; however, this can be done as a staging maneuver if desired.

Postoperative Course

Leave a nasogastric tube in place for 24 to 48 hours. Withhold oral feedings until normal gastrointestinal motility resumes. Remove the Foley catheter on the fifth postoperative day. Patients usually can be discharged on the seventh postoperative day.

Sequelae

Since up to 20 percent of patients with carcinoma of the ureter eventually develop carcinoma of the bladder, I recommend that patients undergo observational cystoscopic study every 3 months for 2 years. If cytologic washings as well as cystoscopic examinations are negative during this period, examinations during the next year are performed every 6 months and are thereafter performed yearly. Intravenous pyelograms are performed yearly.

Distal Ureterectomy

In selected patients with ureteral carcinoma, I have performed a distal ureterectomy with resection of a bladder cuff and ureteral reimplantation. I have limited this procedure to patients with tumors of the distal ureter in whom nephroureterectomy would lead to severe renal impairment or dialysis.

I use a Gibson incision to gain access to the bladder and distal ureter as described above. Once the ureter has been dissected free of the bladder, ligate the ureter above and below the proposed line of ureteral transection. Transect the ureter and send it for frozen section. If pathologic examination is negative, open the proximal ureter. I have used the flexible 6.5-mm diameter nephroscope intraoperatively to ensure that the proximal ureter was free of disease. Once this is ascertained, reimplant the ureter into the bladder. Usually a psoas hitch is required. Do not attempt to use an antireflux reimplantation, since such a maneuver makes subsequent ureteroscopy more difficult. I stent all these reimplantations using a silicone rubber double-J stent. Close the bladder and wound as described above. Use a single Penrose drain at the operative site.

Postoperative Course

I do not routinely use a nasogastric tube after this procedure. The patient is not fed until normal gastrointestinal motility is restored. The Foley catheter is generally removed on the seventh postoperative day. If there is no evidence of urinary leakage from the wound, the drain can be removed. The ureteral stent is removed 3 weeks later as an outpatient procedure.

Sequelae

Observational cystoscopy as well as urinary cytologic examination are performed at the previously described time intervals. I have used the flexible nephroscope to examine the ureter at the time of interval cystoscopy. Retrograde pyelography also is performed at this time.

Other Procedures

Other surgical approaches can be applied in special situations. These include segmental ureteral resection with end-to-end ureterostomy, ureterectomy with small bowel replacement, or ureterectomy and renal autotransplantation.

With the introduction of cyclosporine, I have liberalized our age limits for potential transplant recipients. Currently, the oldest is 68 years old. In some patients with ureteral carcinoma, removal of a solitary renal unit and dialysis may be the safest treatment alternative. If the patient remains free of metastatic disease for 24 months, renal transplantation can be offered.

METASTATIC URETERAL CARCINOMA

JOEL SHEINFELD, M.D.
NEIL H. BANDER, M.D.

Carcinoma of the ureter is a rare malignancy, accounting for 1 percent of all genitourinary tumors. Ureteral tumors are more frequent in men than in women by a ratio of 2 to 3 : 1, with a peak incidence in the fifth and sixth decades of life, increasing progressively with advancing age.

Approximately 60 to 70 percent of ureteral tumors involve the distal third of the ureter. Histologically, more than 95 percent of these tumors are transitional cell carcinoma; squamous and glandular differentiation are rare. Benign tumors of the ureter are extremely rare and include fibroepithelioid polyp, leiomyoma, and angioma. Metastases within the ureteral wall may arise from the stomach, prostate, breast, lung, and cervix. Non-neoplastic ureteral lesions include endometriosis and ureteritis cystica.

CLINICAL PRESENTATION

Either gross or microscopic hematuria is the most common symptom, occurring in 70 to 90 percent of cases. Flank pain due to tumor obstructing the ureter is seen in approximately 10 to 40 percent. Symptoms of bladder irritability are seen in 5 to 10 percent and constitutional symptoms such as weight loss and anorexia usually indicate advanced disease. Physical examination is usually unremarkable except for an occasional palpable mass secondary to tumor or associated hydronephrosis.

The diagnosis of a ureteral tumor is often suspected on the basis of an intravenous pyelogram, since most are abnormal. Filling defects with or without hydroureter-onephrosis or nonvisualization are the most common radiographic findings. Retrograde pyelography, selective cytologic studies, brush biopsies, and computed tomography (CT) are useful adjuncts in distinguishing ureteral tumors from nonopaque stones, blood clots, or benign strictures. Ureteroscopy allows direct visualization and biopsy of the lesion and can provide useful information regarding the status of the apparently uninvolved ureter and the presence of associated carcinoma in situ.

Multiple reports in the literature indicate that survival for patients with transitional cell carcinoma of the upper tract is dependent on tumor grade and stage. The classic form of management has been nephro-ureterectomy with excision of a cuff of bladder; however, recent studies substantiate a favorable outcome in patients with early-stage and low-grade disease (stages 0 and A, grade I) with segmental resection of the ureter, particularly for tumors of the lower third of the ureter.

The prognosis for invasive (stages B or C) and high-grade tumors is poor, with 5-year survival rates ranging from 20 to 40 percent, while advanced disease (stage D) is almost invariably fatal without adjuvant therapy, with only anecdotal 2-year survivors.

Although many failures undoubtedly arise from the primary ureteral tumor, it is important to recognize that there is a 30 to 50 percent likelihood of a coexistent or subsequent transitional cell carcinoma of the bladder, and a 2 to 4 percent risk of development of a tumor in the contralateral collecting system.

PATIENT SELECTION

The most common metastatic sites of transitional cell carcinoma of the ureter are the regional lymph nodes, liver, lung, and bone. Local recurrence in the retroperitoneum in the area of the primary tumor is also frequently seen. The likelihood of regional lymph node involvement and distant metastases is related to tumor stage. Approximately 15 percent of ureteral tumors present initially with advanced disease (stage D). Stage B (muscle invasion) disease accounts for approximately 10 percent of ureteral tumors and demonstrate metastases in 40 percent of cases, while stage C (penetration through the entire ureteral wall) constitutes 20 percent of ureteral tumors and has about a 75 percent likelihood of metastases.

The patients discussed in this chapter include those who present initially with metastatic transitional cell carcinoma of the ureter, those who develop metastases subsequent to surgical resection of a ureteral tumor, and those whose surgical specimens demonstrate regional lymph node involvement or periureteral involvement. Adjuvant therapy for patients at high risk for recurrence or metastases (high-grade stages B and C) remains controversial and has not been evaluated prospectively in a randomized fashion.

COMBINATION CHEMOTHERAPY

The treatment of advanced urothelial cancer consists of platinum-based combination chemotherapy. The most widely used regimens are the M-VAC protocol developed at Memorial Sloan-Kettering Cancer Center, the CMV protocol popularized by the Northern California Oncology Group, and the CISCA protocol used by the M.D. Anderson Cancer Center (Table 1).

Combination chemotherapy has clearly proved more effective than the various drugs administered singly. Furthermore, early trials with combinations of methotrexate and vinblastine and of cisplatin and doxorubicin (Adriamycin), with or without cyclophosphamide (Cytoxan), produced responses in 39, 48, and 46 percent, respectively, but fewer than 5 to 10 percent achieved complete response.

Ureteral cancer is rare and most trials of advanced urothelial cancer incorporate them with their bladder counterparts. Advanced transitional cell carcinoma of the upper tract is aggressive and heralds an unfavorable prognosis, but, like tumors of bladder origin, it is responsive to combination chemotherapy and clinically behaves in a similar fashion. Except for occasional anecdotal cases, nontransitional cell tumors, such as squamous cell carcinoma and adenocarcinoma, do not usually respond favorably to the combination chemotherapy protocols discussed below.

Methotrexate, Vinblastine, Doxorubicin, and Cisplatin (M-VAC)

Patients are evaluated by a complete history taking and physical examination, and the longest perpendicular diameters of all measurable lesions are recorded from appropriate CT scans, radiographs, and sonograms. Laboratory tests include automated blood and platelet counts, 12-channel biochemical screening profile, serum creatinine levels, and 12- or 24-hour creatinine clearance. Weekly blood counts are obtained.

Entry criteria include a two-dimensionally measurable indicator lesion, Karnofsky Performance Status greater than 30 percent, white blood cell (WBC) count greater than 3,500 cells per cubic millimeter, platelet count greater than 150,000 cells per cubic millimeter, serum creatinine greater than 1.7 mg percent, blood urea nitrogen (BUN) less than 30 mg per deciliter, and/or creatinine clearance greater than 50 ml per minute, and a New York Heart Association functional class less than III and bilirubin less than 1.5 mg percent.

Patients are hospitalized monthly for 3 to 5 days for appropriate laboratory and diagnostic tests, and for days 1 and 2 of the M-VAC protocol. Methotrexate (30 mg per m^2 intravenously) is given on day 1 followed by enough D_5 1/2 NS to obtain a urine output of 100 ml per hour. Vinblastine (3 mg per m^2), doxorubicin (30 mg per m^2), and cisplatin (70 mg per m^2) are administered 24 hours later. Intravenous mannitol (12.5 mg) is given prior to cisplatin. Antiemetics consist of metoclopramide, 2 mg per kilogram, diphenhydramine, 25 mg, and dexamethasone, 20 mg, intravenously 30 minutes before cisplatin and followed by 2 mg per kilogram metoclopramide intravenously 90 minutes later. Aggressive hydration is continued until pretreatment BUN and creatinine values are obtained. Methotrexate and vinblastine are administered on an outpatient basis on days 15 and 22 if the WBC is greater than 2,500 cells per cubic millimeter, platelets are greater than 100,000 cells per cubic millimeter, and there is no evidence of mucositis. One of the two interim doses is withheld if there is any evidence of toxicity. Occasionally the cisplatin dosage is split equally over days 2 and 3 if there is borderline renal function, and is stopped if the creatinine clearance is less than 40 ml per minute. The doxorubicin dose is decreased to 15 mg per m^2 in patients who received irradiation of more than 2,500 rads in 5 days or in whom two or more bone marrow–containing sites had been irradiated. Every effort is made to repeat the cycle on day 28 if the patient's clinical condition and the laboratory values permit.

Tumor regression secondary to M-VAC has been noted in all sites, including metastatic nodes, pelvic masses, pulmonary and hepatic lesions, subcutaneous masses or nodes, and osseous lesions. Complete regression has been more commonly observed in nodal, pulmonary, and local-regional lesions.

Of the first 83 adequately treated patients with measurable and evaluable disease, complete remission was seen in 37 percent and partial remission in 31 percent.

Most patients received five or six cycles of M-VAC. Toxicity is significant with approximately a 4 percent drug-related death rate, 20 percent nadir sepsis, 31 percent renal toxicity, and 41 percent mucositis. Nausea, vomiting, neurotoxicity, and hepatic toxicity are also occasionally seen. Administration of G-CSF (granulocyte colony stimulating factor) in doses greater than 3 mg per kilogram virtually negates the myelosuppression and significantly reduces the incidence of mucositis.

A small group of patients who initially are categorized as partial responders achieve complete remission after surgical resection of residual disease. Another small group are initially found to be unresectable, but after M-VAC chemotherapy are able to undergo successful surgical excision of the disease.

Table 1 Chemotherapy Regimens

M-VAC	*Day (mg/m²)*			
	1	2	15	22
Drug				
MTX	30		30	30
VIN		3		
ADR		30		
CIS		70		

CMV	*Day (mg/m²)*		
	1	2	8
Drug			
CIS		100	
MTX	30		30
VIN	4		4

CISCA	*Day (mg/m²)*	
	1	2
Drug		
Cytoxan	650	
ADR	50–60	
CIS		100

MTX = methotrexate; VIN = vinblastine; ADR = doxorubicin (Adriamycin); CIS = cisplatin; Cytoxan = cyclophosphamide.

Cisplatin, Methotrexate, and Vinblastine (CMV)

This combination is administered in 21-day cycles. Methotrexate, 30 mg per m^2, and vinblastine, 4 mg per m^2, are given intravenously on days 1 and 8, and cisplatin, 100 mg per m^2 is given on day 2 as a continuous four-hour infusion after aggressive prehydration. Dose modification of cisplatin and/or methotrexate in the face of renal dysfunction is as follows: no methotrexate is administered if the creatinine clearance (Cr Cl) falls below 45 ml per minute or if the serum creatinine level increases above 2 mg per deciliter. Full-dose cisplatin is given for Cr Cl greater than 60 ml per minute; it is reduced by 50 percent for a Cr Cl between 45 and 60 ml per minute and deleted if the Cr Cl falls below 45 ml per minute. Methotrexate and vinblastine dosages are also adjusted on the basis of WBC and platelet counts.

Of the first 62 evaluable patients in this protocol, 16 (26 percent) achieved a complete response, and an overall response rate (CR + CRs) of 34 percent was noted. Again, all sites of metastases responded to CMV, including bone and liver. As in the M-VAC experience, central nervous system relapses were noted in a group of patients responding at their systemic sites.

Moderate toxicity was seen with CMV. All patients had nausea, vomiting, and alopecia. Renal dysfunction and leukopenia were common. There were six episodes of bacteremia with two deaths; however, these occurred in the early phase of the trial when methotrexate (40 mg per m^2) and vinblastine (5 mg per m^2) were administered at higher doses.

Cyclophosphamide, Doxorubicin, and Cisplatin (CISCA)

The intravenous CISCA protocol consists of cyclophosphamide, 650 mg per m^2, and doxorubicin, 50 to 60 mg per m^2 on day 1, followed by cisplatin, 100 mg per m^2 on day 2 for patients with a Cr Cl of at least 75 ml per minute. Patients with Cr Cl in the range of 40 to 60 ml per minute receive 75 mg per m^2 of cisplatin. Again,

aggressive hydration and antiemetic medication are utilized. Renal function is monitored carefully with serial creatinine clearances. Side effects are similar to those seen with the MVAC and CMV regimens.

In summary, cisplatin-based combination chemotherapy is the treatment of choice for advanced urothelial carcinoma. Durable complete responses have been achieved with M-VAC, CMV, and CISCA. We favor M-VAC chemotherapy for advanced ureteral cancer of transitional cell histology. M-VAC is significantly less effective against nontransitional cell types such as adenocarcinoma or squamous carcinoma. It does not prevent de novo tumors in situ in other areas of the urothelium. Toxicity is significant, but the introduction of G-CSF ameliorates myelosuppression and mucositis. Aggressive hydration, forced diuresis, and appropriate dose modifications protect renal function.

SUGGESTED READING

Chong CDK, Logothetis CJ. Treatment of advanced transitional cell carcinoma of the renal pelvis and ureter. In: Johnson D, Logothetis CJ, von Esthenbach AC, eds. Systemic therapy for genitourinary cancers. Chicago: Year Book, 1989:94.

Droller MJ. Transitional cell cancer: upper tracts and bladder. In: Gittes RF, Perlmutter AD, Stancey TA, eds. Campbell's urology. 5th ed. Philadelphia: WB Saunders, 1986:1408.

Lo RK, Freiha FS, Torti FM. CMV for metastatic urothelial tumors. In: Johnson D, Logothetis CJ, von Esthenbach AC, eds. Systemic therapy for genitourinary cancers. Chicago: Year Book, 1989:59.

Logothetis CJ. CISCA chemotherapy for disseminated bladder carcinoma. In: Johnson D, Logothetis CJ, von Esthenbach AC, eds. Systemic therapy for genitourinary cancers. Chicago: Year Book, 1989:43.

Sternberg C, Yagoda A, Scher HI, et al. M-VAC (methotrexate, vinblastine, doxorubicin and cisplatin) for advanced transitional cell carcinoma of the urothelium. J Urol 1988; 139:461–470.

SUPERFICIAL TRANSITIONAL CELL CARCINOMA

ANGELO S. PAOLA, M.D.
DONALD L. LAMM, M.D., F.A.C.S.

Bladder cancer is the second most common urologic malignancy, with an estimated 49,600 new cases and 9,700 deaths occurring each year in the United States. With a male to female ratio of 3:1, transitional cell carcinoma accounts for approximately 90 percent of cases, squamous cell for 8 percent, and adenocarcinoma for approximately 2 percent.

Superficial transitional cell carcinoma—i.e., tumor confined to the mucosa (Ta or Tcis) or with invasion of the lamina propria (T1)—accounts for approximately 80 percent of cases at presentation. Up to 80 percent of patients undergoing initial endoscopic resection of superficial disease experience tumor recurrence, and 10 to 30 percent progress to muscle invasive disease. Factors that increase the risk of tumor recurrence include urothelial dysplasia, carcinoma in situ, lamina propria invasion, tumor multiplicity, rapid recurrence, size greater than 3 cm, and higher grades (II or III).

Intravesical therapy is designed to eradicate residual tumor if present (through treatment), and to delay or prevent subsequent recurrences (through prophylaxis). There are presently two well-established forms of intravesical therapy for superficial bladder cancer: chemotherapy and immunotherapy. Two additional forms of treatments, phototherapy and radiation therapy, are being developed. In this chapter we discuss the initial assessment and management of superficial transitional cell carcinoma (i.e., stage Ta or T1 disease), review the alternatives for intravesical therapy, and discuss our methods for approaching this disorder. Carcinoma in situ and its management are discussed elsewhere in this text.

INITIAL EVALUATION

All patients presenting with a bladder tumor require an excretory urogram to rule out concomitant upper tract lesions (1.7 percent risk). Hydronephrosis may signify superficial tumor growing over a ureteral orifice, but is usually a poor prognostic sign indicating muscle invasive disease.

Although the initial diagnosis of bladder cancer may be made at outpatient cystoscopy for hematuria or irritative voiding symptoms, definitive evaluation and tumor resection are performed in the operating room with the patient under spinal or general anesthesia (Table 1).

The endoscope is introduced under direct vision with the 30-degree lens, noting any abnormality of the urethra, especially the prostatic urethra. Once the bladder is entered, 90 to 120 ml of normal saline is injected and withdrawn multiple times with a Toomey syringe. This bladder barbotage specimen is sent for cytology and, if available, DNA flow cytometry. In patients with a low-grade tumor, the finding of high-grade tumor cells on cytology studies or flow cytometry may indicate that another tumor of higher grade may have been missed.

After bladder barbotage is completed, the entire bladder is examined systematically with both the 30- and 70-degree lenses. In patients with enlarged prostates, the 120-degree lens may be necessary to visualize the entire bladder neck area. After cystourethroscopy, random cold-cup bladder biopsies are obtained from the posterior and lateral walls, the dome, and the trigone, as well as any abnormal-appearing areas in the bladder. Biopsies of the prostatic urethra are also performed routinely. Random biopsies are performed, because there may be several areas not visible cystoscopically that harbor urothelial atypia or malignancy.

After random bladder biopsies, the cystoscope is removed and the urethra dilated using van Buren sounds. A rectoscope is then inserted and used to

Table 1 Initial Evaluation of Superficial Bladder Cancer

1. Excretory urogram (IVP)
2. Cystourethroscopy under anesthesia
3. Bladder barbotage for cytology and DNA flow cytometry (especially important in follow-up)
4. Biopsies of normal and suspicious bladder mucosa (including prostatic urethral biopsies)
5. Transurethral resection of tumor
6. Bimanual examination under anesthesia
7. Determine need for intravesical therapy (treatment or prophylaxis)

remove as much tumor as possible. Even with apparently highly superficial tumors, it is important to obtain specimens containing the muscle layer to ensure accurate histologic staging. After resection, the rollerball is used to fulgurate the base of the resection and the surrounding urothelium in order to increase the margin of tumor kill and obtain meticulous hemostasis. A final review of the bladder using the 70-degree lens is imperative to ensure adequate resection.

A thorough bimanual examination under anesthesia is an important part of the initial evaluation. It may be performed before prepping or at the end of the endoscopic resection. If a mass is palpable before resection, the examination should be repeated after resection. A palpable mass is a poor prognostic sign, usually indicating muscle invasive disease. A residual mass after aggressive transurethral resection usually indicates extravesical extension of tumor.

CANDIDATES FOR INTRAVESICAL THERAPY

After the pathology of the specimens obtained during resection has been reviewed, a decision regarding further management is made. Since up to 80 percent of superficial bladder tumors recur, with up to 30 percent progressing to a higher stage or grade, long-term follow-up is the rule ("eternal vigilance"). Patients have been helped considerably by the development of various modes of intravesical therapy that have been shown to decrease the number of recurrences, lengthen the time to recurrence, and in some instances, delay the need for cystectomy.

Patients with Stage Ta, grade 1 disease are at low risk for recurrence with progression (2 percent). However, patients with a high-grade tumor or one that invades the lamina propria have a 25 to 30 percent chance of developing a muscle invasive tumor. Patients with grade 1, Ta lesions can be safely followed with cystourethroscopy and cytology every 4 months for the first year, every 6 months for the next 2 years, and every year thereafter. We follow patients with stage Ta, grades II to III tumors and all patients with stage T1 tumors with cystourethroscopy and cytology every 3 months for 2 years, every 6 months for the next 2 years, and every year thereafter. Patients with Ta tumors who are at significant risk of recurrence owing to tumor multiplicity, size greater than 3 cm, or grade III staging, as well as all patients with stage T1 tumors (regardless of grade), are considered candidates for intravesical therapy.

INTRAVESICAL CHEMOTHERAPY

The most commonly used intravesical chemotherapeutic drugs are alkylating agents. Topical therapy offers the advantage of instilling an agent that will affect much of the urothelial surface and inhibit growth of preneoplastic lesions, as well as eradicate viable tumor cells that may have remained in contact with the urothelium following resection. Although resistance to one chemotherapeutic agent increases the likelihood of resistance to another, this rule is not absolute. The most commonly used intravesical agents include thiotepa, mitomycin C, doxorubicin, and epodyl (Table 2). VM26 (a podophyllin derivative), bleomycin, cisplatin, and mitoxantrone have each had equivocal responses as intravesical agents; 5-fluorouracil, actinomycin D, and methotrexate have been ineffective when given intravesically to treat bladder cancer.

Thiotepa

Thiotepa (triethylene thiophosphoramide) is an alkylating agent related to nitrogen mustard. It was the first approved intravesical chemotherapeutic agent and is still widely used. Most commonly employed regimens give 30 to 60 mg in an equal volume of water weekly for 4 weeks, then monthly for 1 year, but there is no convincing evidence that maintenance treatment is necessary. We usually initiate treatment within 48 hours of resection to prevent implantation, and repeat weekly treatments for 6 to 8 weeks. Patient age and size, bladder size, the extent of resection, and the amount of cystitis are considered when selecting dosages, but we generally prefer to use 30 mg since it has been found to be as effective as 60 mg. Tumor kill is proportional to drug concentration and duration of exposure. Patients are therefore asked not to drink liquids for 4 hours before treatment and, if possible, to retain the solution for 2 hours. Vesicoureteral reflux is not a contraindication to treatment but may increase systemic absorption.

Complete response rates in treating unresected tumors range from 20 to 55 percent with a mean complete response rate in all series of 29 percent. In six of ten controlled studies, prophylactic thiotepa significantly reduced the rate of tumor recurrence. On average, tumor recurrence is reduced from 62 to 45 percent with thiotepa after tumor resection.

Owing to its relative low molecular weight, drug absorption and systemic toxicity are more likely with thiotepa than with other agents. Myelosuppression has been more common with thiotepa than with other intravesical drugs, being noted up to 27 percent and an average of 9 percent of patients. Leukopenia and thrombocytopenia are the usual manifestations, and

Table 2 Common Intravesical Chemotherapeutic Agents and Suggested Dosage Schedule

Agent	Dosage	Treatment Schedules
Thiotepa	30 mg/30 ml water	Weekly for 6–8 weeks
Mitomycin C	40 mg/40 ml water	Weekly for 6–8 weeks
Adriamycin	50 mg/50 ml water	Weekly for 6–8 weeks
Epodyl*	1 gm/100 ml water	Weekly for 12 weeks then monthly for 1 year

*Not available for use in the United States.

therefore the white blood cell (WBC) and platelet counts should be monitored before treatment. Since absorption can approach 100 percent after transurethral resection, early intravesical administration should be limited to systemically tolerated doses of 0.5 mg per kilogram. Local toxicity consisting of chemical cystitis with irritative voiding symptoms is the most common side effect of thiotepa, but is rarely severe enough to warrant discontinuing treatment.

Mitomycin C

Mitomycin C is an antitumor antibiotic that inhibits DNA synthesis by acting as an alkylating agent. The dosage used in various studies has ranged from 20 to 60 mg, and frequency of treatment from one to three times per week. We prefer a dosage of 20 to 40 mg in an equal volume of water given weekly for 6 to 8 weeks.

Considerable experience has demonstrated that mitomycin C is highly effective in decreasing the incidence and frequency of recurrences of bladder carcinoma. The mean complete response has been 47 percent with a range of 39 to 78 percent. Mitomycin has a higher complete response rate than thiotepa in treating unresected tumors, but is not superior to thiotepa in preventing tumor recurrence. It should be noted, however, that failure with one intravesical chemotherapeutic agent does not preclude success with another. Mitomycin is also more expensive than most other agents.

Toxicity with mitomycin is generally believed to be the least of any intravesical chemotherapeutic agent, which is probably due to its larger molecular weight and resultant decreased absorption. Myelosuppression has not been seen in most studies, and we do not routinely follow leukocyte or platelet counts with therapy. Blood counts should be taken when mitomycin is given within 48 hours of tumor resection or when increased absorption due to cystitis or existing tumor is expected. The most common side effect seen with mitomycin, as with all other intravesical agents, is chemocystitis, occurring in approximately 10 percent of patients. Unique to mitomycin is a desquamating palmar, genital, or diffuse rash that occurs in approximately 6 percent of patients. It is believed to be contact dermatitis, and meticulous washing of the hands and genitalia after each instillation and initial voiding is recommended. Decreased bladder capacity can occur as with any intravesical agent, even to the point of requiring supravesical urinary diversion for a severely contracted bladder.

Doxorubicin

Considerable experience, much of which comes from Japan, has shown that doxorubicin (Adriamycin) is an effective intravesical chemotherapeutic agent in the treatment of superficial bladder cancer. Dosages have ranged from 10 to 100 mg given daily to monthly. Even though the dosage has not been standardized, a review of the data has led us to favor 50 mg in an equal volume of water weekly for 6 to 8 weeks.

Complete responses observed with doxorubicin range from 20 to 67 percent with a mean of 38 percent. Studies have shown that patients with previous thiotepa or bacillus Calmette-Guérin (BCG) failure may respond to intravesical doxorubicin. Although doxorubicin is superior to surgery alone, it has not been found to be superior to thiotepa in preventing tumor recurrence.

The toxicity of intravesical doxorubicin has not been a major problem. Cystitis has been reported in approximately 26 percent of patients, but relatively few require cessation of therapy because of irritative symptoms. Decreased bladder capacity has been noted in 9 percent of patients and is especially common in those who have received previous radiotherapy. Systemic absorption through the bladder wall appears to be insignificant, and therefore the systemic toxicity (myelosuppression and cardiac toxicity) seen with intravenous administration of doxorubicin has not been a problem with intravesical therapy. Routine WBC counts can therefore be safely omitted in most patients.

Epodyl

Epodyl (triethylene glycol diglycerol ether) has been used extensively for the treatment of superficial bladder cancer in Europe. It is a tumor-inhibiting diepoxide. Treatment usually consists of 1 g in 100 ml of normal saline given weekly for 12 weeks followed by monthly instillations for 1 year.

Complete responses have ranged from 33 to 75 percent with a mean of 55 percent. Recent controlled studies have demonstrated its value in preventing tumor recurrence, but this agent is not currently available in the United States.

Systemic toxicity with epodyl is uncommon. Chemical cystitis has been noted in approximately 30 percent of patients, 16 percent having to discontinue treatment because of this side effect. Decreased bladder capacity has also been reported in up to 21 percent of patients treated with epodyl.

IMMUNOTHERAPY

In recent years, immunotherapy for bladder cancer has gained increasing popularity. It has been classified into two categories: active, in which administered immunostimulants induce the host's immune system to respond to tumor antigens; and passive, which transfer immunologically active reagents (serum, cells, or cell products) directly to the host in an attempt to mediate an antitumor response. Each of these immunotherapies can be further divided into specific and nonspecific immunostimulants on the basis of their mechanisms of action (Table 3). Currently the most successful form of immunotherapy for human malignancy is the bacillus Calmette-Guérin (BCG), which has been especially successful in the treatment of superficial bladder cancer. Its dramatic success in this area has prompted the search for different forms of immunotherapy.

Bacillus Calmette-Guérin

Since the first trial of intravesical BCG was reported by Morales in 1976, its efficacy in preventing tumor recurrence has been confirmed in many other studies. Its mechanism of action is still largely unknown, but it is known to be a potent nonspecific immunostimulant.

Animal studies have suggested that BCG may have decreased effectiveness when tumor burden exceeds 100,000 cells. Therefore, even though BCG has been remarkably effective in the treatment of residual bladder cancer, we suggest that efforts be made to resect *all* tumor before initiation of BCG immunotherapy.

The best protocol for BCG immunotherapy remains undefined. Preparations that have been demonstrated to be effective intravesically include Armand-Frappier, BCG-RIVM, Connaught, Evans (Glaxo), Pasteur, Tice, and Japanese. Although the optimal doses have not been established, commonly used effective intravesical doses are listed in Table 4. In the United States the Connaught and Tice preparations are commercially available. On the basis of experience, we recommend 50 mg of Tice BCG or 120 mg of Connaught (three ampules) in 50 ml of normal saline weekly for 6 weeks, resting for 6 weeks, then weekly for 3 weeks, with subsequent single treatments at 6 months, and every 6 months thereafter for up to 4 years (first course). Many patients who have recurrence of tumor after BCG respond to a second course as follows: weekly for 2 weeks, then every other week for three treatments, then monthly for 4 months, and then every 6 months for 4 years (second course). Although the necessity of maintenance immunotherapy is still debatable, increasing evidence suggests that a single 6-week course of BCG is highly effective yet suboptimal for many patients. We assess response by performing cystourethroscopy washings for cytology every 3 months for 2 years, then every 6 months for the next 2 years, and every year thereafter. Therapy is usually started within 2 weeks of tumor resection to provide optimal juxtaposition of BCG and any residual tumor. Treatments should be delayed 1 to 2 weeks after extensive resections to decrease the risk of absorption and sepsis. Other treatment schedules reported can be found in Table 4. Neither percutaneous nor oral BCG administration have been shown to improve antitumor response over intravesical therapy alone, and we therefore believe that intravesical instillation alone is sufficient.

Since BCG's mechanism of action is different from that of the chemotherapeutic agents, cross resistance has not been identified. Therefore, patients who have failed intravesical chemotherapy often respond to BCG, and vice versa.

BCG has been shown to be more effective than thiotepa in preventing tumor recurrence. A prospective study recently completed by the Southwest Oncology Group has demonstrated that BCG immunotherapy is superior to doxorubicin chemotherapy. In a preliminary evaluation of a comparison of BCG-RIVM with mitomycin C, no advantage of either agent was apparent. Concern has been raised about the efficacy of the RIVM preparation, however, and a subsequent comparison of Pasteur BCG and mitomycin C found BCG to be superior. Dramatic reductions in tumor progression have also been reported with BCG compared with surgery alone, the overall progression being reduced from 95 to 53 percent, progression to stage T2 from 46 to 28 percent, cystectomy from 42 to 25 percent, and deaths from 32 to 14 percent.

Life-threatening and even fatal complications of BCG therapy have been reported. These are rare, however, and most patients tolerate therapy well. The most common side effect noted with intravesical BCG, occurring in approximately 90 percent of patients, is granulomatous cystitis with irritative voiding symptoms of frequency and dysuria. Symptoms usually begin after the second or third instillation and persist for about 2 days. Phenazopyridine hydrochloride (Pyridium) (200 mg) and oxybutynin hydrochloride (Ditropan) (5 mg)

Table 3 Immunotherapy for Bladder Cancer

Active Therapy

Specific
  Vaccines
Nonspecific
  BCG, KLH
  Lymphokines: interferon, interleukin-2 (IL-2), tumor necrosis
    factor
  OK-432

Passive Therapy

Specific
  Monoclonal antibodies
Nonspecific
  LAK cells generated by IL-2 expansion.

BCG = bacille Calmette-Guérin; KLH = keyhole-limpet hemocyanin; LAK = lymphokine-activated killer.

Table 4 BCG Doses and Treatment Schedules

Treatment Schedules

Morales: Intravesical and percutaneous weekly × 6
Brosman: Intravesical weekly × 6, then monthly
Lamm: First course: intravesically weekly for 6 weeks, then
     weekly for three instillations at 3 months, then at 6
     months, and every 6 months for up to 4 years.
    Second course: intravesically weekly for 2 weeks, every
     other week for three treatments, monthly for 4 months,
     then every 6 months for 4 years.

Effective Vaccine Doses

Armand-Frappier: 120 mg
Connaught: 120 mg
Pasteur: 75–150 mg
Tice: 50 mg
Japanese: 40 mg

orally three times daily have been useful to minimize these symptoms. For severe irritative symptoms, 300 mg of oral isoniazid taken the day before treatment and for 2 days afterward has reduced discomfort. Approximately 25 percent of patients experience constitutional symptoms such as low-grade fever, malaise, or nausea. Granulomatous prostatitis has been reported to occur in 1.3 percent of patients and cannot be distinguished from carcinoma of the prostate without a biopsy specimen. Systemic BCG infection involving the lungs or liver has occurred in approximately 1 percent. This usually responds to isoniazid and rifampin, but in some cases of acute septic or anaphylactic shock cycloserine and prednisone should be added to the usual antituberculosis regimen. Cycloserine inhibits BCG growth within 1 day, while isoniazid and other antibiotics take up to 1 week to act. Also, since the shock may be partly due to a cell-mediated immune response, corticosteroids may be beneficial. In cases of life-threatening infections, therefore, we suggest 250 to 500 mg of cycloserine twice daily and 40 mg of prednisone (or its equivalent) daily in addition to isoniazid and rifampin.

Other rare complications of BCG therapy have included ureteral obstruction due to cystitis, bladder contracture, epididymo-orchitis, and pancytopenia (all less than 1 percent). The side effects and complications of BCG therapy should not be minimized, but the benefits of this therapy far exceed its risks, and the vast majority of patients have no significant side effects.

Keyhole-Limpet Hemocyanin

Keyhole-limpet hemocyanin (KLH) is a complex protein found in the marine mollusk Megathura crenulata and is one of the most immunogenic of antigens. Olsson was the first to report a marked reduction in tumor recurrence in patients immunized with subcutaneous KLH.

Dosages for KLH have ranged from 10 to 30 mg in an equal volume of normal saline given intravesically with a 1-mg intradermal injection given weekly for 4 weeks and then monthly.

KLH has been found to be superior to mitomycin C and equal to epodyl. It is therefore potentially more effective than BCG. No toxicity has been reported to occur with KLH, but more controlled studies are needed before its beneficial effect can be firmly established.

Other Immunotherapeutic Agents

Several other agents are currently being investigated for their ability to enhance the body's immune response selectively. These include various lymphokines such as interferon, interleukin-2, and tumor necrosis factor; monoclonal antibodies; lymphokine-activated killer (LAK) cells, maltose tetrapalmitate, poly I:C, irradiated tumor vaccine, and butanol-extracted antigen. All the above have been shown to have some antitumor activity, and although more controlled studies are being conducted to confirm their effectiveness, the preliminary results from many of these have been promising.

PHOTOTHERAPY

Laser therapy and phototherapy have recently been applied to urology in the management of superficial bladder cancer. Two approaches have been used: (1) direct destruction of tumors with a focused laser beam and (2) the use of light to excite photosensitive molecules within malignant tissue.

Of the three most commonly used lasers (carbon dioxide (CO_2), argon, and neodymium:YAG), the CO_2 laser cannot be used intravesically because its output of light is readily absorbed by water. The argon laser will coagulate and vaporize tissue to a depth of 1 mm, and therefore only very superficial neoplasms (Ta or Tis) are suitable for treatment with this laser. The neodymium: YAG laser is also water transmissible and penetrates tissue to a depth of 5 mm. It has been used in the treatment of Ta, Tis, T1, and even some muscle-invasive tumors. With laser, tissue is not removed but coagulated.

Treatment of superficial bladder tumors with neodymium:YAG lasers can be favorably compared with transurethral resection. Advantages of lasers include the ability to perform the procedure with the patient under local anesthesia; reduced bleeding, since vessels are coagulated, obviating the need for catheter drainage; and a decreased risk of bladder perforation. Disadvantages include bowel perforation caused by excessive energy; lack of tissue available for histologic study and accurate staging, since tissue is not resected; and uncertainty regarding the depth of tumor destruction. It has been suggested that cold cup biopsies, with incorporation of the muscle layer, be performed before laser therapy to obtain tissue for histologic study. Controlled studies comparing laser and electrosection have not yet been completed.

Phototherapy has also been used with compounds that sensitize tissue to light. Hematoporphyrin derivatives (HPD) have proved most useful. HPD is a mixture of several hematoporphyrins that are preferentially absorbed by malignant tissues (including superficial bladder tumors) when injected intravenously. When sensitized by certain wavelengths of light, HPD has a cytotoxic effect in absorbed tissue. Initial studies in bladder cancer were reported by Kelley and Snell, and since then it has been used experimentally in the treatment of Tis, Ta, T1, and T2 tumors.

Local side effects of HPD are minimal since absorption is preferentially limited to epithelium. Irritative voiding symptoms and reduced bladder capacity have been reported. These effects are generally transient, but bladder contracture has been noted, as have third-degree burns in patients exposed to excessive sunlight. Patients must therefore be advised to use sunscreen on all exposed skin and to avoid direct sunlight for 1 month after injection of HPD.

HPD phototherapy is still experimental, and further studies must be performed to determine a standard therapeutic protocol and compare its efficacy with other forms of intravesical therapy.

RADIATION THERAPY

External beam radiation therapy has been used to treat noninvasive bladder cancer with poor results. Russell and colleagues reported combined intracavitary and external beam radiation to be an attractive option in patients with superficial bladder cancer resistant to the standard intravesical therapies. Further controlled studies are required to determine whether this mode of therapy can be recommended as an alternative before resorting to cystectomy in patients with superficial tumors refractory to conventional intravesical agents.

DISCUSSION

The initial endoscopic evaluation of the patient with transitional cell carcinoma of the bladder is important in designing the subsequent treatment plan, which will depend on the stage and grade of the resected tumor, and other risk factors for recurrent disease. For example, a patient who has a grade I, stage Ta tumor, no history of tumor, and a normal cytologic study following resection would not be a candidate for intravesical therapy. On the other hand, patients with tumors larger than 3 cm in diameter, multiple tumors, grades II to III histology, lamina propria invasion, or carcinoma in situ require intravesical therapy.

Owing to the apparent lifelong risk of recurrent disease, we believe that follow-up must be aggressive and long term. We follow all patients who have undergone transurethral resection of tumors, regardless of subsequent intravesical therapy, with cystoscopy and cytology every 3 months for the first 2 years, every 6 months for the next 2 years, and every year thereafter. Any patient who has suspicious cytology despite a normal cystoscopy will undergo endoscopy with random bladder and prostatic urethral biopsies and possibly ureteral washings for cytology, to detect the source of abnormal cytologic results at the next scheduled follow-up (3 months).

Some authors advocate that patients with low-grade, noninvasive tumors can be followed with infrequent endoscopy and a reliance on cytologic studies. This is a viable alternative in patients with low-grade stage Ta tumors.

Studies have suggested that once the need for intravesical therapy has been established, BCG is the most effective agent available. It is relatively inexpensive compared with mitomycin C or doxorubicin. In patients who need intravesical therapy (prophylactic or therapeutic), we initiate BCG. If they develop a subsequent tumor after an initial course of BCG, we generally attempt a second course of BCG. Failure with this regimen usually prompts us to use thiotepa, doxorubicin, or mitomycin C. In patients who develop systemic symptoms of BCG infection, we usually use isoniazid with or without rifampin (depending on the severity of symptoms), and the BCG therapy is discontinued. Patients with severe systemic symptoms are subsequently treated with intravesical chemotherapy rather than BCG.

If tumors persist or recur despite treatment with BCG plus thiotepa, doxorubicin, or mitomycin C, cystectomy is considered. In patients with grade III or lamina propria invasive tumor despite treatment with BCG and intravesical chemotherapy, cystectomy is recommended. The advent of highly successful intestinal bladder reconstructive procedures, which permit normal voiding and sexual function, has greatly increased patient acceptance of cystectomy.

SUGGESTED READING

Heney NM, Ahmed S, Flanagan MJ, et al. Superficial bladder cancer: progression and recurrence. J Urol 1983; 130:1083.

Herr HW, Laudone VP, Whitmore WF Jr. An overview of intravesical therapy for superficial bladder tumors. J Urol 1987; 138:1363–1368.

Kelley JF, Snell ME. Hematoporphyrin derivative: a possible aid in the diagnosis of carcinoma of the bladder. J Urol 1976; 115:150.

Kowalkowski TS, Lamm DL. Intravesical therapy of superficial bladder cancer. In: Resnick M, ed. Current trends in urology. Vol IV. Baltimore: Williams & Wilkins, 1988.

Russell KJ, Koh WJ, Russell AH, et al. J Urol 1989; 141:30.

Smith JA. Treatment of invasive bladder cancer with a neodymium: YAG laser. J Urol 1986; 135:55.

Solloway MS. Diagnosis and management of superficial bladder cancer. Semin Surg Oncol 1989; 5:247–254.

Sosnowski JT, Lamm DL. Immunotherapy of bladder cancer. Urology Annual 1990; 4:123.

MINIMALLY INVASIVE TRANSITIONAL CELL CARCINOMA (T1 AND T2)

J . BRANTLEY THRASHER, M.D.
E. DAVID CRAWFORD, M.D.

The treatment of patients with minimally invasive transitional cell carcinoma (TCC) of the bladder remains one of the most controversial areas in urology. Included in this stage are lesions that invade the lamina propria (T1) as well as those that superficially invade the bladder musculature (T2). The nomenclature "minimally invasive" would seem to imply that these lesions are minimally aggressive. However, Skinner reported that 17 percent of patients thought to have T1 disease of the bladder were found to have pelvic lymph node metastases. Other series have revealed that 20 to 35 percent of patients with clinically localized bladder cancer actually have nodal metastases, lending credence to the theory that minimally invasive TCC of the bladder may exert a very aggressive behavior and therefore at times demands an aggressive approach to treatment.

THERAPEUTIC STRATEGY

Our current treatment algorithm for patients with minimally invasive TCC is predicated on (1) overall assessment of the tumor; (2) the patient's age and general health; and (3) the status of the entire bladder urothelium. Table 1 outlines the initial approach to therapy. Aggressive therapy is defined as radical cystectomy. High-grade tumors usually exhibit a tentacular extension into the bladder wall (Fig. 1) and frequently invade lymphatics and blood vessels. The remaining urothelium associated with such tumors often exhibits areas of dysplasia. These tumors require an aggressive treatment approach. Conversely, if the tumor is well differentiated, it often invades with a broad front of cells, which appears to imply a lesser likelihood of shedding of

cells for dissemination (Fig. 2). The remaining urothelium frequently exhibits minimal atypia or appears normal. These tumors evoke a more conservative treatment approach. The patient's age and general health status also play a part in the treatment strategy.

DIAGNOSIS AND PREOPERATIVE EVALUATION

Patients usually present with hematuria or irritative voiding symptoms. After urinary infection is first excluded, voided urine is obtained for cytology, and intravenous pyelography (IVP) is performed to exclude upper-tract lesions. This is followed by cystoscopy. The advantage of performing an IVP before cystoscopy is that if the upper urinary tracts were not visualized adequately, retrograde ureteropyelography can be performed at the time of cystoscopy.

The cystoscopic demonstration of bladder cancer or a report of positive cytology with radiographically normal upper tracts prompts the scheduling of transurethral resection of the bladder tumor and/or multiple biopsies with the patient under anesthesia. Also at this time, a chest x-ray examination and liver function tests are performed as a part of staging. If the tumor appears invasive or involves a large portion of the bladder, a preoperative computed tomographic (CT) scan of the abdomen and pelvis with contrast enhancement is obtained. The CT scan determines bladder wall thickening and aids in the staging of the bladder cancer, as well as acts as a baseline for later comparison. Several recent studies have advocated magnetic resonance imaging (MRI) as a more sensitive mode of staging for

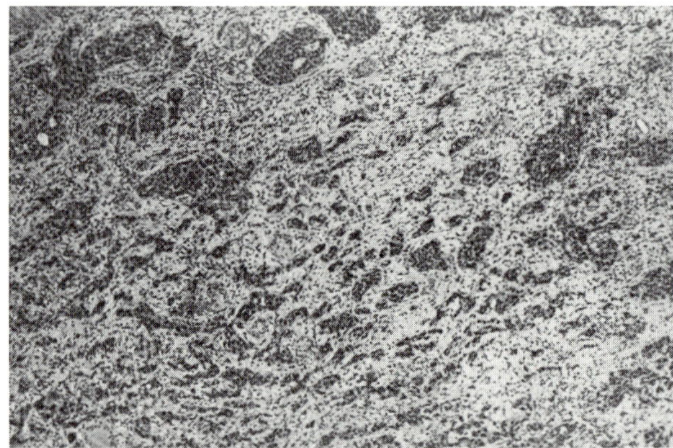

Figure 1 Tentacular infiltration of the bladder wall. In progressing to infiltration, finger-like projections of dysplastic cells can be seen to extend through the bladder wall. The clustering of such cells is smaller than in the papillary form of infiltration. In addition, it is not uncommon to see involvement of the bladder wall lymphatics at the time that muscle or lamina propria infiltration are diagnosed histologically. (Republished with permission from Droller MJ. Transitional cell cancer: upper tract and bladder. In: Walsh, Gittes RF, Perlmutter AD, Stanley, eds. Campbell's urology. 5th ed. Philadelphia: WB Saunders, 1986:1343.)

Table 1 Factors Affecting Therapeutic Approach in Minimally Invasive TCC

Aggressive	*Conservative*
Poorly differentiated neoplasm	Well to moderately differentiated neoplasm
Vascular or lymphatic permeation	No lymphatic or vascular involvement
Moderate to severe dysplasia of remaining urothelium	Absent or minimal atypia of remaining urothelium
Tentacular extension of tumor into bladder wall	Broad front of cells advancing into bladder wall

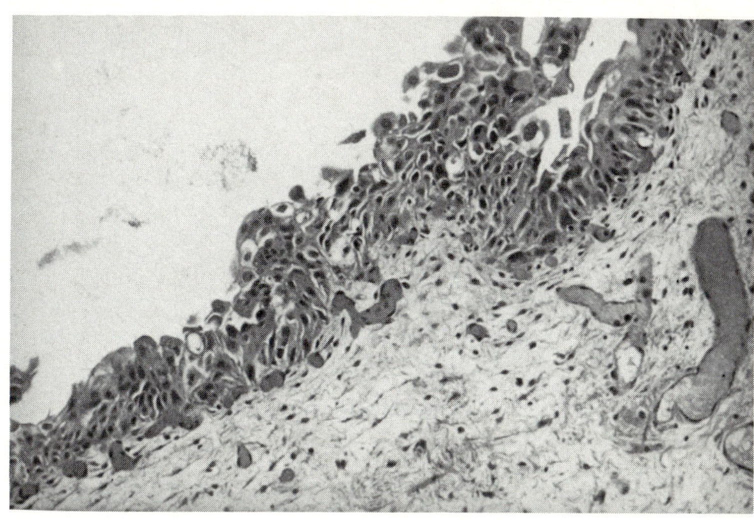

Figure 2 Papillary invasion of transitional cell cancer. Notwithstanding the depth of infiltration of the transitional cell bladder carcinoma shown in this figure, the papillary architecture and infiltration into the muscle by broad clusters of cells imply a cohesiveness in what may be interpreted as a generally proliferative process. This in turn implies the likelihood that this tumor, although infiltrative within the detrusor muscle, has remained regionally confined and amenable to local therapies. (Republished with permission by Droller MJ. Transitional cell cancer: upper tract and bladder. In: Walsh, Gittes RF, Perlmutter AD, Stanley, eds. Campbell's urology. 5th ed. Philadelphia: WB Saunders, 1986: 1343.)

bladder cancer. Other investigators have found no significant advantage of MRI over CT for staging purposes. Although previous surgery or radiation therapy may lead to overestimation of neoplasm extension, the reliability of CT increases with progression of the disease. We continue to use CT as our primary radiographic tool for staging.

TREATMENT AND FOLLOW-UP

Once the patient is anesthetized, a vaginoabdominal or rectoabdominal examination is performed to determine the mobility of the bladder and the extent of the tumor. A palpable tumor, and certainly one that renders the bladder immobile, generally indicates deep muscle infiltration. Conversely, a nonpalpable tumor suggests superficial infiltration. The bimanual examination is repeated after the transurethral resection. The cystoscope is introduced under direct vision. The bladder is methodically inspected with the 70-degree lens; a 120-degree lens is occasionally used to visualize the anterior bladder wall. A 30-degree lens is used to review the floor of the bladder and the entire urethra at the termination of endoscopy.

Multiple cold cup biopsies are obtained from the urothelium lateral to each ureteral orifice, the posterior midline, the dome, and the prostatic urethra. In addition, any suspicious or erythematous regions are biopsied. The lesion is resected and submitted for pathologic evaluation. In a lesion that is small and papillary with a distinct stalk, the entire lesion is resected and the remaining bed delicately resected to assess the depth of invasion. The cutting current is used to avoid cautery artifact. Lesions that appear sessile or occupy large segments of the bladder are evaluated before surgery with CT. If the preliminary CT scan has shown a thickened bladder wall in the region of the tumor, the tumor is resected and sent for pathologic evaluation separately. An attempt is made to resect into deep muscle to assess the level of invasion. In all cases, care

is taken to avoid bladder perforation, which could result in dissemination of the carcinoma beyond the bladder wall into the perivesical space.

The histologic grade and extent of neoplastic diathesis, and the patient's age, medical condition, and availability for follow-up examinations, are all integral factors involved in the decision for subsequent therapy. Therapeutic options are presented to the patient based on the integration of the above factors (Figs. 3 and 4).

Bladder tumors that infiltrate the lamina propria (stage T1) are included under the category of minimally invasive bladder carcinoma owing to the difference in their biologic behavior relative to tumors confined to the mucosa (T0). These neoplasms exhibit a more aggressive biologic capability, which makes them more closely categorized with bladder tumors that superficially invade the bladder musculature (stage T2). Recently, studies by Jacobsen and colleagues and Wolf and colleagues found progressive disease in 30 percent of patients treated with transurethral resection of T1 lesions. Wolf and colleagues reported a 25 percent true recurrence rate in T1 lesions with a 5-year survival of 20 percent in this group.

These studies and the experience at our institution confirm the aggressive nature of T1 lesions, mandating compulsive surveillance after transurethral resection. When multiple tumors are found at the time of surgery or when the remaining urothelium is found to harbor carcinoma in situ or moderate-to-severe atypia, we institute intravesical chemotherapy. We implement the same treatment when these patients are noted at follow-up visits to have recurrence of the tumor or positive voided urine cytology specimens.

Mitomycin C (40 mg per 40 ml distilled water in eight weekly instillations) is our first-line chemotherapeutic agent unless the lesion is associated with carcinoma in situ at which time bacille Calmette-Guérin (BCG) (120 mg Connaught in 60 ml of saline) is used. We have also switched to BCG in cases in which the tumor recurred while the patient was receiving mitomycin C. The patient is instructed to retain the chemotherapeutic agent for 2 hours and to change positions

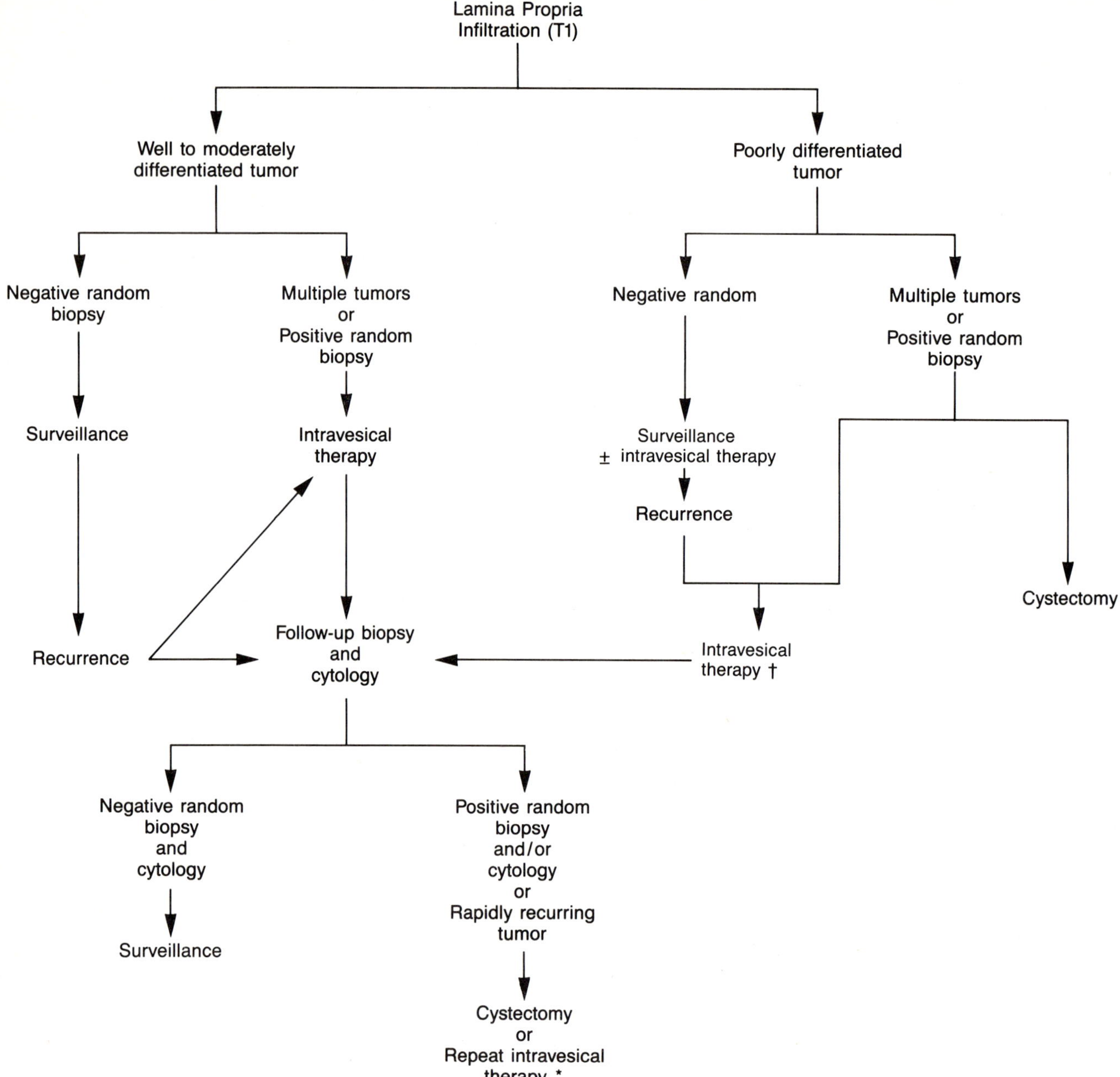

Figure 3   Algorithm for the treatment of tumor infiltrating the lamina propria. *Only poor surgical candidates or those who refuse cystectomy. †Preferred initial treatment.

frequently to subject as much of the bladder urothelium as possible to the agent. Six weekly treatments are instilled with repeat cystoscopy, urine cytology, and cold cup biopsy performed 6 weeks after the last treatment. If the biopsy or urine cytology study reveals recurrent tumor, a radical cystectomy is recommended. This same treatment is generally recommended for patients initially found to have superficial ductal neoplastic involvement of the prostatic urothelium.

The approach to patients who show minimal muscle infiltration (T2) at their initial clinical presentation represents less of a dilemma. These patients are offered radical cystectomy as the standard approach in the management of their disease process with relatively few exceptions. If the histologic review discloses very superficial penetration of a low-grade tumor into the muscularis, and the rest of the urothelium appears uninvolved, the patient may be given the option of very close surveillance, which involves repeat cystoscopy, urine cytology, and biopsies 2 months later. If any tumor is found on follow-up, the patient is urged to undergo radical cystectomy. However, if the biopsy specimen, urine cytology, and cystoscopy all remain negative, the patient is followed with cystoscopy and urinary cytologic

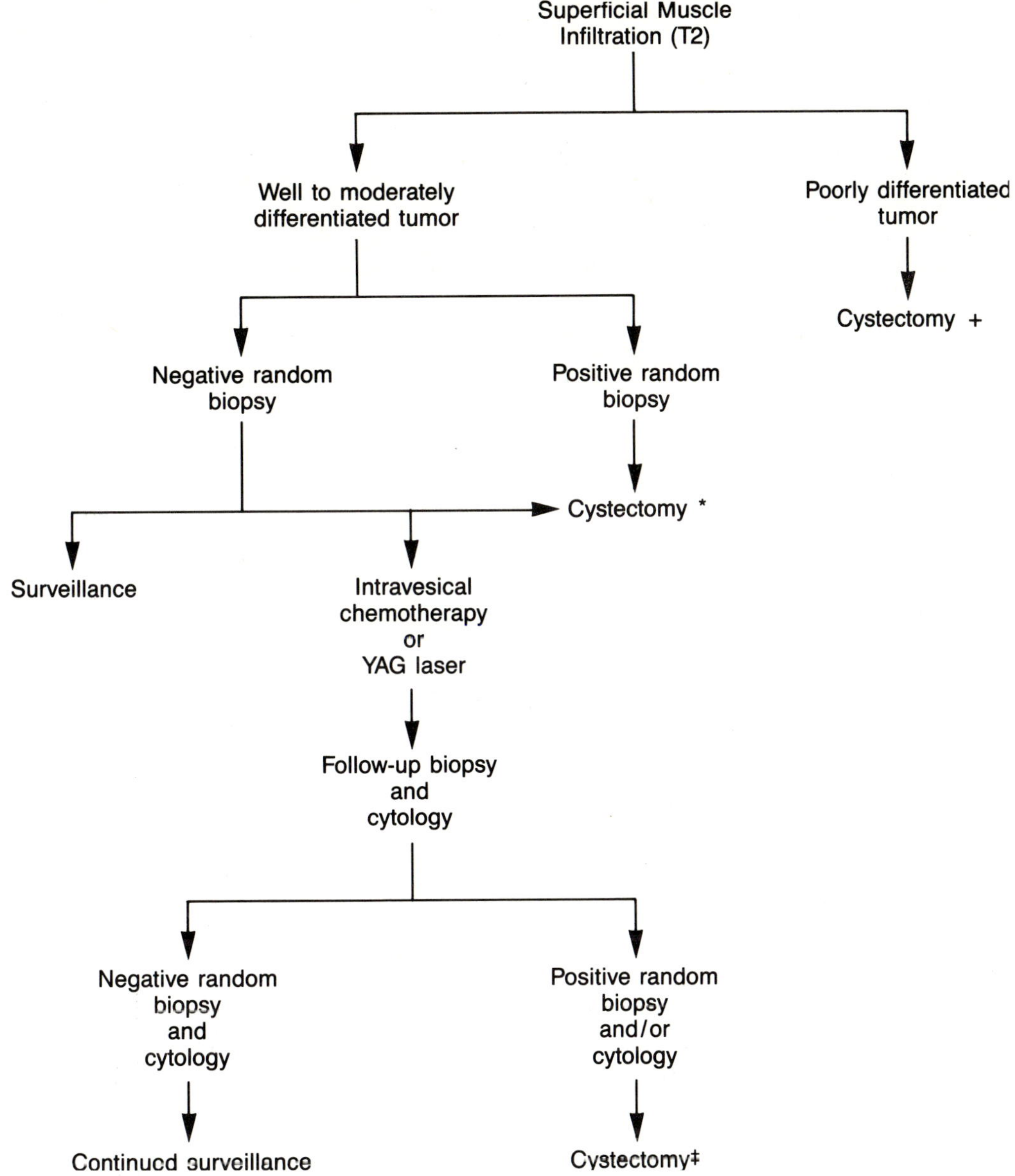

Figure 4 Algorithm for the treatment of tumor infiltrating the superficial bladder musculature. *Preferred initial treatment. †Poor surgical candidates may be considered for systemic chemotherapy plus radiation therapy. ††Poor surgical candidates may be considered for systemic chemotherapy with or without repeat transurethral resection if recurrent tumor is noted.

studies every 3 months for 2 years, changing to semiannually for 2 more years and then yearly. CT is performed on a semiannual basis.

Recently, several studies have advocated conservative therapy for patients with minimal muscle invasive bladder carcinoma. The rationale for this treatment is based on an attempt to preserve bladder function and sexual potency. Conservative therapeutic options include segmental cystectomy, external beam irradiation, interstitial irradiation, and various combinations of the three. A few of these studies have reported 5-year disease-free survival of up to 50 percent. However, critical review of these data is difficult owing to differences in patient selection for various protocols as well as inherent differences between groups. We therefore believe that radical cystectomy with or without adjuvant chemotherapy offers the best chance of cure for localized bladder cancer.

We do not employ radiation therapy in most patients with minimally invasive TCC of the bladder. However, van der Werf-Messing has reported that low-dose radiation therapy offers some protection against local tumor implantation in the event of an inadvertent spill during open-bladder surgery. We have found that attention to detail at surgery has avoided the need for adjunctive radiation therapy. In patients who are medically unfit to undergo cystectomy, we generally advocate repeat transurethral resection, systemic chemotherapy, or external beam radiation therapy.

Our experience with the use of laser in controlling

minimally invasive disease has been limited. The neodymium:yttrium-aluminum-garnet (Nd:YAG) laser is utilized to treat tumors confined to the mucosa; however, the treatment of minimally invasive disease becomes difficult. The first challenge is the well-recognized incidence of clinical understaging of this disease. The second is the inability to accurately predict or control the depth of thermal injury that results from Nd:YAG laser treatment. We feel that this limits the use of this modality in minimally invasive disease to patients who are poor candidates for radical surgery or who refuse cystectomy.

The treatment of minimally invasive TCC of the bladder must be individualized on the basis of several factors. The age of the patient, tumor pathology and architecture, and the status of the remaining bladder urothelium must be assessed. In patients whose tumors appear to have aggressive malignant potential, an aggressive approach (i.e., cystectomy) is the preferred treatment. In patients whose tumors appear less aggressive or whose overall medical status does not permit radical surgery, a more conservative position can be taken. However, these patients should be followed with compulsive surveillance as an integral part of the treatment of their diathesis.

In the near future, adjuvant chemotherapy may play an important role in conjunction with surgery in the treatment of minimally invasive TCC of the bladder. Considering that the high failure rate associated with radical cystectomy is due primarily to distant metastases rather than to local recurrence, neoadjuvant chemotherapy emerges as a viable option. A multicenter phase III study is presently under way comparing M-VAC (methotrexate, vinblastine, doxorubicin [Adriamycin], and cisplatin) followed by radical cystectomy with radical cystectomy alone in locally advanced bladder cancer. Participating intergroups include SWOG (Southwest Oncology Group), ECOG (Eastern Cooperative Oncology Group), and CALGB (Cancer and Leukemia Group B). It is too early in the study to draw conclusions relative to response rates and survival. However, the study is progressing well and should soon shed light on the advantages and disadvantages of neoadjuvant chemotherapy in the treatment of locally advanced bladder cancer.

DEEPLY INVASIVE TRANSITIONAL CELL CARCINOMA

MARC S. ERNSTOFF, M.D.
THOMAS HAKALA, M.D.

Bladder cancer affects approximately 50,000 Americans per year, and about 10,000 die of the disease. Most patients present with superficial bladder cancers and have an excellent prognosis. Once it is invasive, however, bladder carcinoma has a high degree of metastatic potential, with 5-year survival rates ranging from 50 to 90 percent for T2 lesions and 10 to 40 percent for T3b tumors. Although radical cystectomy controls local disease, patients die as a result of metastases, which raises questions about the role of adjuvant strategies, including radiotherapy and chemotherapy.

Therapy for invasive bladder cancer should be planned using a multidisciplinary approach, including surgery, radiotherapy, systemic chemotherapy, and possibly local chemo- and immunotherapy. In general, patients with invasive transitional cell carcinoma of the bladder (T2, T3, T4a) who are healthy enough to undergo cystectomy and chemotherapy are considered for clinical trial. A multicooperative group study evaluating the role of preoperative (neoadjuvant) chemotherapy, using three cycles of methotrexate, vinblastine, doxorubicin (Adriamycin), and cisplatin (M-VAC), has been initiated and has evaluated approximately 144 patients to date. This study is designed to determine whether chemotherapy and cystectomy will improve both disease-free and overall survival. Until this question is answered, the case for adjuvant chemotherapy should be considered unproved.

PATIENT SELECTION

When considering patients with invasive bladder cancer for definitive therapy, the physician should take into account their overall medical condition, with specific attention to renal, pulmonary, and cardiac function. Comorbid diseases such as diabetes, hypertension, and nutritional disorders that might impact on overall survival should be weighed carefully. Radical cystectomy with an ileal loop diversion or bladder reconstruction remains the treatment of choice for patients with invasive bladder cancer in 1991, and is the foundation from which additional treatment recommendations are made. Combination endoscopic surgery, radiotherapy, and systemic chemotherapy may allow bladder preservation in a select group of patients and is currently undergoing evaluation in clinical trials. These bladder-sparing techniques are currently considered for patients unable or unwilling to undergo cystectomy.

All patients should have a full endoscopic evaluation, including a bimanual examination under anesthesia and a deep biopsy of tumor-suspected areas to include muscularis propria and a bladder barbitage. The pathologic review should identify muscle in the specimen, the histologic appearance, and the cytologic grade. Prognostic categories to consider include histologic variants such as squamous cell carcinoma and adenocarcinoma, which tend to respond poorly to chemotherapy; cytologic and nuclear grade; depth of muscle invasion; and lymphatic or vascular invasion. We routinely review all pathologic specimens, and if insufficient material exists, we repeat a TURB.

Patients with invasive bladder cancer stages T2, T3, and T4a are considered for adjuvant therapies if they have adequate cardiac and renal function.

TREATMENT

Although questions related to adjuvant chemotherapy and bladder-sparing approaches will probably receive partial answers during the next decade, practitioners are faced with a multiplicity of problems when discussing these options with patients.

Patients with squamous cell carcinoma or adenocarcinoma of the bladder (including urachal tumor) do poorly and require different strategies from the one outlined here for transitional cell carcinoma. Patients with invasive transitional cell carcinoma of the urinary bladder, who are candidates for adjuvant chemotherapy, are considered for entry in the multigroup preoperative chemotherapy plus cystectomy protocol (Intergroup protocol 0080). After appropriate staging procedures, patients are randomized to receive either cystectomy alone or three cycles of M-VAC followed by cystectomy.

The rationale for preoperative chemotherapy includes: (1) treatment of microscopic metastatic foci at the earliest opportunity, (2) improvement in tolerance of chemotherapy, and (3) reduction of tumor bulk and downstaging of the primary tumor.

Preoperative radiotherapy downstages the primary tumor, but does not appear to change overall survival rates. Preoperative chemotherapy may improve overall survival by controlling micrometastases that have occurred at the time of diagnosis and treatment. Our own experience with postoperative chemotherapy employing M-VAC does not suggest any significant improved tolerance of these drugs compared with patients receiving preoperative chemotherapy. Finally, preoperative tumor reduction and downstaging may improve the surgical approach, particularly for larger, bulky primary tumors.

Although M-VAC has been shown to be superior to cisplatin alone in a randomized clinical trial, it may produce only a 20 to 30 percent complete and durable response in patients with metastatic disease. The use of neoadjuvant chemotherapy delays definitive surgery for about 3 months. As almost 40 percent of patients will not have local responses to M-VAC, a delay of cystectomy in these patients may be clinically detrimental. Furthermore, if the detriment from delay in cystectomy is equivalent to the benefit from neoadjuvant chemotherapy, there may be no overall survival advantage from administering chemotherapy before surgery. Thus, adjuvant (postoperative) chemotherapy must be tested as well. The question in the 1990s is not whether preoperative M-VAC is better than postoperative chemotherapy, but whether adjuvant therapy will improve overall survival at all in this high-risk group of patients.

A related question is whether drug resistance, either on a cellular level or a drug distribution level, plays in chemotherapy failures. If cellular drug resistance has a significant part in chemotherapy failures, then strategies directed at modulating cellular causes of drug resistance may improve the clinical outcome.

If the patient decides against enrollment in a clinical trial, alternative options are considered. The decision to recommend adjuvant chemotherapy is again based on the medical condition of the patient and the estimated risk of relapse from the tumor. With deeply invasive transitional cell cancers of the bladder, we usually favor chemotherapy either before or after cystectomy. Whether pre- or postoperative treatment is given is decided by symptoms, the estimated difficulty of surgery, and an estimation of the patient's compliance and performance status. Preoperative chemotherapy is initiated with standard M-VAC. Patients are restaged with cystoscopy and biopsy after the second course of chemotherapy, because this appears to be the most accurate technique in evaluating response. If a patient is found to be a responder, a third cycle of M-VAC therapy is given. After the return of hematologic parameters to normal, a cystectomy is performed. If a patient shows no response to two cycles of M-VAC therapy, chemotherapy is aborted and the patient undergoes a cystectomy at that time. Postoperative adjuvant chemotherapy is usually begun no earlier than 2 weeks after surgery and no later than 4 weeks if possible. We begin chemotherapy with M-VAC as soon as the patient has recovered from surgery and is able to maintain a normal diet. We have been administering two cycles of M-VAC treatments in the postoperative adjuvant setting.

For patients who refuse cystectomy or are medically unable to undergo surgery, combination chemotherapy and radiotherapy is employed. We have been following a protocol described by Prout and colleagues. Two cycles of methotrexate, vinblastine, and cisplatin are administered before and after low-dose cisplatin and radiotherapy to the bladder. Patients are restaged at the completion of the first two cycles of chemotherapy. Responding patients continue with treatment as outlined; nonresponders are again considered for surgical treatment or definitive radiotherapy.

Patients who show a poor response to preoperative chemotherapy or radiotherapy tend to do poorly, with a survival of about 2.5 years. Although cystectomy does not appear to influence survival for large tumors (stages T3b, T4) that do not respond to chemotherapy initially, we still advocate cystectomy to determine accurate staging and local control.

Bladder-sparing therapy has the attraction of maintaining an intact genitourinary system, although bladder capacity may be impaired. Alternative approaches include partial cystectomy and bladder reconstruction combined with chemotherapy and radiotherapy. A particular disadvantage of bladder-sparing procedures is the risk of second primary cancers developing in the remaining bladder mucosa, necessitating repetitive cystoscopy and biopsy. If superficial tumor occurs, management with transurethral resection of the bladder and intravesical chemo- and immunotherapy is instituted. The development of a second invasive bladder tumor would force consideration of cystectomy again.

RISKS AND BENEFITS

We continue to emphasize that the standard approach to invasive bladder cancer remains cystectomy. The depth of invasion of the tumor and other prognostic categories such as lymphatic and blood vessel invasion, grade, and histotype are discussed with the patient and family, with specific reference to overall prognosis. Neoadjuvant chemotherapy is presented to the patient and family as a first investigative approach. The benefits and risks associated with chemotherapy are discussed at length.

The benefits from multidrug chemotherapy include prevention of tumor recurrence (disease-free survival) and possible prolonged overall survival. Although benefit from adjuvant chemotherapy is currently unproven for bladder cancer, other cancers such as breast cancer may provide a reasonable human model allowing some guarded predictions. Complete response rates for chemotherapy-treated metastatic breast cancer are 30 to 50 percent. Definitive cures are not seen. Complete response rates for M-VAC in metastatic cancer are 20 to 30 percent, and cures are not seen. Adjuvant chemotherapy for patients with lymph node–positive breast cancer is accepted as standard care and has a survival advantage of 5 to 15 percent. A similar advantage might be expected for locally invasive bladder cancer treated with adjuvant M-VAC.

The risks from chemotherapy with M-VAC include hair loss; leukoneutropenia with significant risk of a febrile episode and hospitalization; gastrointestinal toxicity including nausea, vomiting, and mucositis; and a decrease in overall performance status. Recognized as a common toxicity is loss of appetite and weight loss, necessitating careful observation and nutritional support as needed in the form of high calory supplements and counseling. Death has occurred from a complication of combination chemotherapy and may be related to cardiac, renal, or bone marrow factors. Other toxicities may occur but are rare and do not usually complicate the administration of chemotherapy.

DISCUSSION

Several therapeutic choices regarding the management of invasive transitional cell cancer of the bladder are currently available. Cystectomy remains the treatment of choice, with participation in clinical trials designed to assess the role of adjuvant chemotherapy (given pre- or postoperatively) or bladder-sparing approaches. For patients unwilling to enter clinical trials, we consider adjuvant chemotherapy as part of their treatment under specific circumstances. Bladder-sparing approaches are attractive, but they raise secondary questions in the management of invasive transitional cell cancer that need to be answered through clinical trials.

SUGGESTED READING

Bahnson RR, Ernstoff MS, Miller RJ, O'Donnell WF. Toxicity comparison of neoadjuvant versus adjuvant methotrexate, vinblastine, doxorubicin, and cisplatin (M-VAC) in radical cystectomy patients. J Surg Oncol 1990; 45:143.

Herr HW, Whitmore WF, Morse MJ, et al. Neoadjuvant chemotherapy in invasive bladder cancer: the evolving role of surgery. J Urol 1990; 144:1083.

Scher HI, Yagoda A, Herr HW, et al. Neoadjuvant M-VAC (methotrexate, vinblastine, doxorubicin, and cisplatin) effect on the primary lesion. J Urol 1988; 139:470.

Yagoda A. Progress in the treatment of advanced urothelial tract tumors. J Clin Oncol 1985; 3:1448.

METASTATIC TRANSITIONAL CELL CARCINOMA

ARMEN G. APRIKIAN, M.D.

WILLIAM R. FAIR, M.D.

Muscle invasive transitional cell carcinoma of the bladder continues to pose a significant problem in management. Survival rates for patients with locally advanced cancers have remained at approximately 50 percent, with the majority of deaths occurring secondary to unrecognized micrometastases at the time of presentation. Distant spread in this group of patients usually appears within 12 to 18 months, regardless of the initial treatment modality. The outlook for these patients is uniformly poor, with the median survival time for untreated cases being less than 6 months.

During the past decade, the management of metastatic urothelial cancers has undergone significant change due to the application of investigational chemotherapy programs. With the introduction of cisplatinum as systemic therapy for disseminated transitional cell carcinoma, survival rates have improved. Currently a variety of combination chemotherapy regimens are under investigation around the world with encouraging results. These regimens are the result of numerous careful phase II studies of single-agent cytotoxic therapy.

Single-agent chemotherapy for transitional cell carcinoma has proven to be effective in inducing clinical responses (Table 1). A number of cytotoxic agents administered alone have achieved response rates of approximately 30 percent. The most active agents are methotrexate and cisplatinum. Methotrexate was one of the first drugs applied to the management of advanced bladder cancer. Response rates are seen in approximately 30 percent of patients for a median duration of approximately 6 months. Cisplatinum-induced response rates range between 30 and 40 percent, with a median survival time of 6 to 8 months. Other agents, including doxorubicin, vinblastine, and cyclophosphamide, produce lower response rates when given alone. Despite these figures, one must realize that the majority of reported responses achieved by single-agent therapy are partial and are not durable. Rarely do patients achieve complete remission and benefit from relatively long-term relapse-free survival.

Because single agents have shown some activity in the regression of systemic disease, it is logical to expect combined therapy to possibly be superior. Cisplatinum has formed the nucleus of multidrug regimens for metastatic transitional cell carcinomas. The most popular current programs are: (1) CMV (cisplatinum, methotrexate, vinblastine) developed by the Stanford University-Northern California Oncology Group; (2) CISCA (cisplatinum, cyclophosphamide, doxorubicin), popularized at the University of Texas-M.D. Anderson Cancer Center; and (3) M-VAC (methotrexate, vinblastine, doxorubicin, cisplatinum), realized at the Memorial Sloan-Kettering Cancer Center (MSKCC).

Use of CMV chemotherapy has yielded good results. In one uncontrolled study, 16/62 (26 percent) of treated patients achieved a complete response. Complete responders received a median of six cycles of cytotoxic therapy. Four additional patients attained complete response status after surgical resection of residual disease. Combining the two groups, an overall complete response rate of 34 percent is reported. However, the median survival time of complete responders was 14 months. Toxicity from therapy was reported as being moderate. There were two deaths associated with nadir sepsis, however, these occurred prior to the implementation of a dose modification protocol.

CISCA chemotherapy has been studied extensively since 1977. A retrospective analysis of the M.D. Anderson Cancer Center experience has identified a high overall response rate of 64 percent (complete response: 36 percent; partial response: 28 percent. In approximately half of the complete responders, survival has been in excess of 100 weeks. In an attempt to identify variable predictors of response, subgroup analysis was performed yielding several findings. It appeared that histologic subtype influenced response rates; pure transitional cell carcinomas were more responsive than those of mixed histology. Patients with nodal disease only attained complete remission with greater frequency than

Table 1 Single-Agent Trials in Previously Treated and Untreated Patients with Advanced Urothelial Tract Tumors

Drugs	*No. of Patients*	*Percent Complete and Partial Remission**
Amsacrine (AMSA)	61	12 (4–20)
Bisantrene	13	0 (0–23)
Bleomycin	79	5 (0–10)
Carboplatin	80	11 (7–15)
Cisplatin	320	30 (25–35)
Cyclophosphamide	26	7 (0–17)
10-Deazaaminopterin	15	20 (0–40)
Diaziquone (AZQ)	16	0 (0–17)
Doxorubicin	248	17 (12–23)
Etoposide (VP-16-213)	47	2 (0–4)
5-Fluorouracil	105	15 (18–22)
Gallium nitrate	26	27 (11–48)
Hexamethylmelamine	24	13 (0–31)
Methotrexate	236	29 (23–35)
(high dose)	57	45 (32–50)
Mitomycin-C	42	13 (3–23)
Mitoxantrone	28	0 (0–10)
Neocarcinostatin	19	5 (0–19)
PALA	18	0 (0–16)
Teniposide (VM-26)	64	11 (3–19)
(intravesical)	148	13 (8–18)
Vinblastine	38	16 (4–28)
Vincristine	42	14 (3–25)

*Numbers in parentheses indicate range of 95 percent confidence intervals.

patients with visceral metastases (45 percent vs 20 percent). However, only patients achieving complete response demonstrated a survival advantage. The most important predictor of survival was the response to CISCA chemotherapy. In the group of complete responders, no differential factor could be identified between the durable and nondurable responses. Thus, although patients with nodal metastases only, and patients with pure transitional cell tumor histology were more likely to respond to therapy, no differential impact on rates of disease-free survival was noted. Of the entire patient population receiving CISCA therapy, 19 percent achieved a durable complete response lasting longer than 100 weeks.

Extensive experience with M-VAC chemotherapy has been acquired at MSKCC. This multidrug regimen is based on considerable experience with active single agents (Table 1). Based on these experiences, methotrexate, vinblastine, doxorubicin (Adriamycin) and cisplatin were combined into the M-VAC regimen. Sternberg and colleagues have reported the results of a phase II trial that includes a minimum follow-up of 3 years. Using the MSKCC Response Criteria (Table 2), an overall response rate of 72 percent (87/121) was achieved. Of more importance, complete tumor regression occurred in 36 percent of patients after a mean of six cycles of therapy; 13/44 complete responses were achieved surgically after four cycles of M-VAC. The median survival of complete responders was greater than 39 months, compared with 11 months in the partial and minimal response groups. Patients who manifest only a partial or minimal response to treatment had no survival advantage over nonresponders. Survival rates of those achieving clinical complete response were significantly greater than those achieved surgically (39 months vs 25 months).

Total regression was observed more frequently in

Table 2 Memorial Sloan-Kettering Cancer Center Response Criteria for Urothelial Tract Tumors

Complete remission (CR): Complete disappearance of all evidence of tumor by physical examination, radiographs, radionuclide scans, computed tomography scans, sonography, tumor-related biochemical and biological marker parameters, urine cytology, cystoscopy, and biopsy (including no T_{is}) for more than 1 month.

   $_cCR$ = clinically proven, defined by criteria listed above
   $_pCR$ = pathologically proven by laparotomy, thoracotomy, or biopsy of previous sites of known disease
   CR_s = surgical removal of all residual disease required to attain CR status

Partial remission (PR): more than 50% decrease in the summed products of the longest perpendicular diameters of all measured lesions without simultaneous increase in size of any lesion or appearance of new lesions for more than 1 month (PR is used for CR with positive cytology or T_{is}).

   Minor response (MR): 25–49% decrease in tumor size for more than 1 month
   Stabilization (STAB): less than 25% change in tumor size more than 3 months
   Progression (PROG): more than 25% increase in tumor size, STAB less than 3 months, appearance of new lesions, or mixed response

the lung, abdominal lymph nodes, and bone. Hepatic metastases did not respond well. The toxicity associated with this regimen was significant. Mucositis was evident in half the patients. A 25 percent nadir sepsis rate was encountered, as well as a 3 percent treatment-related mortality rate. Although M-VAC chemotherapy is associated with substantial toxicity, its ability to induce relatively long-term disease-free survival in a subgroup of patients is clear.

The experience discussed above solidly establishes the fact that some metastatic transitional cell carcinomas are responsive to chemotherapy. However, several problems exist when attempting to draw clinically relevant conclusions from comparisons of various phase II trials. Patient selection bias creates the major obstacle to proper comparative evaluations. This bias is the result of fundamental differences in patient populations examined. Such differences include the ratios of histological subtypes, clinical stages, number and location of metastases, performance status, and type of prior therapy. A number of institutional factors must also be observed. Differences in drug dosages and eligibility criteria are significant. In terms of remission rates, one must critically examine the response criteria employed, as well as the aggressiveness with which staging was performed.

These issues cause great difficulty in providing answers to important clinical questions. Does combination chemotherapy, with its inherent additive toxicity, offer an advantage over single-agent therapy? If so, which regimen is more effective? Which regimen is the least toxic? Such relevant questions can only be answered by properly conducted prospective randomized trials.

The results of several randomized studies comparing multidrug therapy to single-agent therapy have not demonstrated a significantly greater clinical benefit from the former. These results stimulated much skepticism throughout the oncologic community over the advantage of combinaiton chemotherapy in advanced urothelial cancers. Recently, a large intergroup randomized trial comparing M-VAC chemotherapy to DDP (cisplatinum) alone, with survival as the end-point, reaffirmed the position of combined cytotoxic treatment: 239 patients were effectively randomized and complete response rates for M-VAC and DDP groups were 15 percent and 3 percent, respectively. Overall response rates were 36 percent and 11 percent in favor of M-VAC (p = 0.01). The median survival time for M-VAC treated patients was 13.5 months; DDP-treated patients had a significantly shorter survival time (7.4 months). Although the response rates were lower than those observed in single-institution studies, these results support the continued investigation and employment of combination chemotherapy in advanced urothelial cancer.

Randomized trials comparing different multidrug regimens are few. A recent phase III study evaluating M-VAC and CISCA chemotherapy with 110 patients was conducted at the M.D. Anderson Cancer Center. The complete and partial response proportions were greater in the M-VAC arm, although the differences did not achieve statistical significance. The combined total response rate, however, statistically favored the M-VAC-treated group. The median survival time between the two groups was also statistically distinct, with the M-VAC-treated patients surviving longer (62.6 weeks vs 40.4 weeks). Toxicity was not significantly different between the two groups. Therefore, it appears that in similar groups of patients, M-VAC chemotherapy achieves a significantly greater overall response rate and longer overall survival time compared with CISCA chemotherapy.

Do better regimens exist? In view of the considerable toxicity associated with M-VAC therapy, less toxic, yet hopefully similarly effective, combination programs are being tested. One such alternate regimen was introduced recently, and consists of replacing cisplatinum and doxorubicin by their less toxic counterparts, producing a combination of methotrexate, vinblastine, mitoxantrone and carboplatin (MVMJ). The early published results give a 27 percent complete response rate and a 36 percent partial response rate. The median duration of complete response was in excess of 9 months. Toxicity with this treatment was relatively low. Neutropenic fever was encountered in 22 percent of subjects. No evidence of renal toxicity was described. No mortalities resulted from this therapy; although these findings are preliminary, and the number of patients evaluated relatively small, they remain encouraging. Whether this regimen will prove to be as effective as M-VAC remains to be shown.

The outlook for patients failing to respond to M-VAC or similar combination chemotherapy regimens is dismal. However, some activity has been observed in 30 percent of such patients with the combination of fluorouracil and recombinant human interferon α, with a median duration of response of 6 months. These findings warrant further investigation.

Certain features common to several studies deserve mention. It is apparent that combination chemotherapy possesses activity against the primary bladder carcinoma in those patients who have not undergone cystectomy. This has prompted many institutions to initiate neoadjuvant chemotherapy programs for localized bladder cancers in an attempt to sterilize occult distant metastases and thus improve survival, as well as down-stage the local cancer and hopefully preserve the bladder. Care must be exercised in extrapolating the encouraging results obtained with chemotherapy in metastatic TCC to the state-of-the-art treatment on all patients with invasive urothelial cancer in the neoadjuvant setting. It is clear that only a minority of patients will respond completely, and overall significant survival benefit can be expected in no more than 10 to 20 percent of patients. For the others receiving combination chemotherapy, an appreciable potential for toxicity exists with no demonstrated survival advantage. Thus, the known hazards of toxicity must be weighed against the uncertainty of benefits denied. Combination chemotherapy in the neoadjuvant setting should be explored in randomized

studies, but is not yet correct standard practice. The value of this approach to apparently localized bladder carcinoma is still unclear, and clinical understaging of the bladder lesion after chemotherapy remains a significant problem.

Relapses after cytotoxic therapy–induced remissions occur not infrequently in the central nervous system. Because of its privileged nature in relation to chemotherapy, routine evaluation of this area for disease is mandatory.

As the number of patients benefiting from continent urinary reservoirs and intestinal neobladders after radical cystectomy increase, one must be aware of the potential augmented toxicity of cytotoxic systemic therapy, particularly with methotrexate. These patients should receive chemotherapy after establishing continuous drainage of the reservoir to prevent increased reabsorption from the intestinal surface.

Last, toxicity induced by current systemic therapy continues to present great difficulty to both the individual patient and the treating physician. Myelosuppression, with its resultant consequences, is by far the greatest factor contributing to morbidity and mortality. Also, leukopenia frequently delays the administration and alters the dosage of the scheduled treatment regimen, possibly affecting tumor response adversely.

With the advent of recombinant DNA technology and a finer understanding of the molecular biology of the hematopoietic system, human recombinant granulocyte colony-stimulating factor (rhG-CSF) was introduced. Colony stimulating factors are glycoproteins involved in the regulation of granulocyte and macrophage proliferation. Gabrilove and colleagues at MSKCC evaluated the ability of rhG-CSF to prevent chemotherapy-induced neutropenia or to promote its recovery and therefore permit full-dose administration of cytotoxic therapy as scheduled. This phase I-II study consisted of 27 patients with metastatic transitional cell carcinoma receiving a course of rhG-CSF before M-VAC chemotherapy. Depending on the neutrophil response, patients were chosen for a second course of growth factor to be employed during the first cycle of M-VAC. The patients' second cycle of M-VAC served as the control experiment. The results were impressive. A significant reduction in severity and duration of neutropenia was achieved. All patients treated with rhG-CSF were able to receive the full-dose regimen of M-VAC as scheduled. Interestingly, the incidence of mucositis was significantly reduced (11 percent vs 44 percent), implying rhG-CSF protection of mucosal barriers. Whether this occurs secondary to increases in neutrophil count or as a direct effect is still unclear. Thus, administration of rhG-CSF enables patients to undergo full-dose chemotherapy with lower morbidity. Whether these results will translate into improved survival awaits further study. Whether intensification of cytotoxic therapy results in increased survival is controversial. However, the reduction in morbidity associated with rhG-CSF might enable clinical testing of this issue.

It appears that the outlook for patients with metastatic transitional carcinoma is improving. Further laboratory research at the molecular level will help us to better understand the heterogeneous biological behavior of these tumors and provide prognostic information to help select patients for appropriate therapy. Improving patient survival will require continued investigation of new therapeutic strategies tested with carefully structured clinical trials.

SUGGESTED READING

Gabrilove JL, Jakubowski A, Scher HI, et al. Effect of granulocyte colony-stimulating factor on neutropenia and associated morbidity due to chemotherapy for transitional cell carcinoma of the urothelium. N Engl J Med 1988; 318:1414–22.

Harker WA, Meyers FJ, Freiha FS, et al. Cisplatin, methotrexate, and vinblastine (CMV): an effective chemotherapy regimen for metastatic transitional cell carcinoma of the urinary tract. A Northern California Oncology Group Study. J Clin Oncol 1985; 3:1463–1470.

Khandekar JD, Elson PJ, DeWys WD, et al. Comparative activity and toxicity of cis-diamminedichloro-platinum (CDDP) and a combination of doxorubicin, cyclophosphamide and DDP in disseminated transitional cell carcinoma of the urinary tract. J Clin Oncol 1985; 3:539.

Loehrer PJ Sr, Elson P, Kuebler JP, et al. Advanced bladder cancer: a prospective intergroup trial comparing single agent cisplatin (CDDP) versus M-VAC combination therapy. Proc Am Soc Clin Oncol 1990 (in press).

Logothetis CJ, Dexeus FH, Chong C, et al. Cisplatin, cyclophosphamide and doxorubicin chemotherapy for unresectable urothelial tumors: the M.D. Andersen experience. J Urol 1989; 141:33–37.

Logothetis CJ, Dexeus FH, Finn L, et al. A prospective randomized trial comparing MVAC and CISCA chemotherapy for patients with metastatic urothelial tumors. J Clin Oncol 1990; 8:1050–1055.

Logothetis CJ, Hossan E, Sella A, et al. Fluorouracil and recombinant human interferon alpha-2a in the treatment of metastatic chemotherapy—refractory urothelial tumors. J Natl Cancer Inst 1991; 83:285–288.

Soloway MS, Einstein A, Corder MP, et al. A comparison of cisplatin and the combination of cisplatin and cyclophosphamide in advanced urothelial cancer. Cancer 1983; 52:767.

Sonza LM, Boone TC, Gabrilove J, et al. Recombinant human granulocyte colony-stimulating factor: effects on normal and leukemic myeloid cells. Science 1986; 232:61–65.

Sternberg CN, Yagoda A, Scher HI, et al. Methotrexate, vinblastine, doxorubicin and cisplatin for advanced transitional cell carcinoma of the urothelium. Cancer 1989; 64:2448–2458.

Troner MB, Birch R, Omura GA, et al. Phase III comparison of cisplatin alone versus cisplatin doxorubicin and cyclophosphamide in the treatment bladder (urothelial) cancer. A Southeastern Cancer Study Group trial. J Urol 1987; 137:660–662.

Waxman J, Abel P, James N, et al. New combination chemotherapy programme for bladder cancer. Br J Urol 1989; 63:68–71.

Whitmore WF. Management of invasive bladder neoplasms. Semin Urol 1983; 1:4–10.

Yagoda A. Chemotherapy of urothelial tract tumors. Cancer 1982 (suppl); 60:574–585.

Yagoda A. Chemotherapy for advanced bladder cancer. In: Yagoda A, ed. Bladder cancer—future directions for treatment. New York: John Wiley & Sons, 1986:87.

CARCINOMA IN SITU

DAVID L. McCULLOUGH, M.D.

Carcinoma in situ (CIS) is a form of transitional cell carcinoma (TCC) of the urinary bladder. Its behavior is unpredictable, but it should be treated as a potentially aggressive and progressive cancer that, if left alone, often results in muscle invasive and metastatic disease.

CIS resides only in the mucosal layer. No basement membrane invasion is present. Lesions may be discrete and diffuse, have poorly defined margins, and on occasion look grossly normal on cystoscopy. It detaches from the basement membrane easily, and cells often exfoliate readily because of weak intercellular bridges to adjacent cells. About 95 percent of cases have positive urinary cytologic examinations. CIS may coexist with papillary superficial or invasive TCC. This discussion focuses on flat CIS not associated with invasive TCC.

Biopsy proof of the lesion (usually cold-cup biopsy) is normally required before institution of intravesical instillation therapy. The cystoscopic appearance is often that of a flat patch or diffuse areas of a reddish, velvety nature.

SIGNS AND SYMPTOMS

Presenting signs and symptoms include one or more of the following: gross or microscopic hematuria, dysuria, frequency, urgency, and nocturia. Such symptoms are often identical to those of interstitial cystitis. CIS *must* be ruled out in anyone thought to have interstitial cystitis. One should be especially suspicious of CIS in a male believed to have interstitial cystitis. I have observed several cases of delayed diagnosis of patients harboring CIS who were thought to have interstitial cystitis. Approximately 25 percent of patients with CIS are asymptomatic, but most have microhematuria.

DIAGNOSTIC STRATEGIES

A positive urine cytology is often obtained before a biopsy. In such cases a careful search must be conducted for the site of origin of the malignant cells. A very-high-quality intravenous urogram (IVU) is a first step, or retrograde pyelography may be indicated. If there is doubt whether the cells originate in the urothelium above the bladder level, collection of urine from the upper tracts, with or without retrograde ureteroscopy and pyeloscopy and possible biopsy, is sometimes necessary.

Biopsies of any suspicious areas of the bladder are indicated, and random biopsies of the bladder dome, base, lateral walls, trigone, bladder neck, and prostatic urethra should be performed. About 20 percent of patients with bladder CIS have positive prostatic urethral biopsies.

If the prostatic urethral biopsies are positive, deeper prostatic biopsies are indicated to ascertain whether superficial gland or deeper gland/stromal involvement is present. If CIS is detected only in the urethra or very superficial glands, a transurethral resection of the prostate (TURP) with subsequent bladder instillation of bacille Calmette-Guérin (BCG) is indicated. If deeper areas are involved, strong consideration of cystoprostatectomy is warranted. The primary focus of this section is on treatment of CIS of the bladder.

THERAPEUTIC ALTERNATIVES

If the CIS bladder involvement is focal or localized, one may occasionally achieve successful control by simply performing a transurethral resection/fulguration of the lesion. In my experience, this is rare. If such therapy is contemplated or performed, follow-up cytologies and biopsies are mandatory within 6 to 12 weeks. If these are positive, intravesical instillation (induction) therapy with an active agent is indicated. If the initial biopsies or cystoscopy reveal multifocal or diffuse disease, intravesical instillation therapy should be initiated as soon as the bladder heals.

Intravesical Instillation Agents

Thiotepa is less effective than mitomycin C, which in turn appears to be less effective than BCG. Mitomycin is much more expensive than thiotepa or BCG. BCG is my first-line therapy for CIS. Doxorubicin has also been used by some for CIS treatment.

Preferred Approach

Once the diagnosis of bladder CIS has been made, it is desirable to wait several weeks after biopsy before beginning BCG therapy. It is preferable to have few or no red blood cells in the urinalysis. Attempts are made to avoid having BCG enter the bloodstream, with its attendant risk of sepsis. If the patient has been traumatically catheterized and gross blood is noted, one should delay BCG therapy for a week and attempt a nontraumatic catheterization before initiating therapy. Five deaths have been reported as a result of systemic BCG sepsis.

Several strains of BCG are available: Armand Frappier, Connaught, and the Tice substrain. My choice is Tice, which is a live attenuated culture of the BCG strain of *Mycobacterium bovis;* its mechanism of action appears to be a localized, cell-mediated immune response.

CONTRAINDICATIONS AND COMPLICATIONS

Instillation BCG therapy is contraindicated in immunosuppressed patients or those with congenital or acquired immune deficiencies, whether due to concurrent disease (e.g., AIDS, leukemia, lymphoma) or cancer therapy with cytotoxic drugs or radiation. Asymptomatic HIV-positive patients or those on large doses of corticosteroids are at risk for developing systemic BCG sepsis, and intravesical therapy in such patients should be avoided.

A concurrent febrile illness, a urinary tract infection, or gross hematuria also precludes such therapy. Pregnant or lactating females should also not receive BCG. Some antibiotics may inhibit the clinical effectiveness of BCG, and treatment should be delayed until such therapy has been completed.

After each intravesical treatment, patients should be monitored for signs and symptoms of side effects. Flu-like symptoms and febrile episodes lasting for more than 48 hours, fever of greater than 103°F, systemic manifestations increasing in intensity with repeated instillations, or persistent liver function test abnormalities suggest systemic BCG infection and require anti-tuberculosis therapy.

Reduced bladder capacity has been associated with an increased rate of severe local reactions, and this should be considered prior to BCG therapy. No attempt should be made to deliver BCG under high pressure.

The most common side effect (60 percent) is bladder irritation. If this is severe, the interval between treatments may be extended to 2 weeks. Systemic side effects often mimic those of a limited viral illness, with fever and malaise evident for 24 to 48 hours after BCG instillations. When such symptoms persist longer than 24 to 48 hours, isoniazid (INH) (300 mg) per day plus vitamin B_6 should be considered. More severe systemic symptoms should be treated with rifampin (600 mg per day), cycloserine (250 to 500 mg twice daily), and ethambutol hydrochloride (15 mg per kg per day). Five unexplained deaths after BCG therapy have been reported, as mentioned above. The report of Rawls and colleagues and other authoritative articles should be consulted before patients who have BCG reactions and sepsis are treated.

Table 1 lists the local and systemic adverse effects in patients receiving intravesical BCG for superficial TCC, including some with CIS.

TECHNIQUES OF INTRAVESICAL BCG THERAPY

An ampule of Tice BCG is mixed with approximately 50 ml of normal saline and instilled under

Table 1 Summary of Adverse Effects Seen in 674 Patients With Superficial Bladder Cancer, Including 153 With Carcinoma In Situ

Adverse Effects	Number of Patients	Percent (%)	Toxicity by Grade (%)*			
			Mild	Moderate	Severe	Not Stated
Local						
Dysuria	401	59.5	28.2	18.1	10.7	2.5
Urinary frequency	272	40.4	17.2	15.7	7.4	—
Hematuria	175	26.0	8.2	9.6	7.4	0.8
Cystitis	40	5.9	1.6	2.4	1.9	—
Urgency	39	5.8	1.2	1.8	1.3	1.5
Nocturia	30	4.5	1.3	1.8	0.6	0.7
Cramps/pain	27	4.0	0.9	1.3	0.9	0.9
Urinary incontinence	16	2.4	0.4	0.9	—	1.2
Urinary debris	15	2.2	0.2	1.0	0.4	0.6
Genital inflammation/abscess	12	1.8	0.3	0.4	0.4	0.6
Urinary tract infection	10	1.5	0.2	0.3	0.9	0.2
Urethritis	8	1.2	0.3	0.6	—	0.3
Pyuria	5	0.7	0.2	0.1	0.1	0.3
Epididymitis/prostatitis	2	0.3	—	—	—	0.3
Urinary obstruction	2	0.3	—	—	—	0.3
Contracted bladder	1	0.2	—	—	—	0.2
Orchitis	1	0.2	—	—	—	0.2
Systemic						
Flu-like syndrome†	224	33.2	9.3	10.9	9.0	4.0
Fever	134	19.9	6.1	5.3	7.6	0.9
Malaise/fatigue	50	7.4	2.7	3.1	—	1.6
Shaking/chills	22	3.3	0.2	1.5	1.0	0.6
Nausea/vomiting	20	3.0	1.0	1.5	0.3	—
Arthritis/myalgia	18	2.7	0.3	1.0	0.4	0.9
Headache/dizziness	16	2.4	0.3	0.9	—	1.2
Anorexia/weight loss	15	2.2	0.4	1.3	0.1	0.5
Allergic	14	2.1	0.6	0.7	0.4	0.3
Cardiac	13	1.9	—	0.3	1.3	0.3
Respiratory (unclassified)	11	1.6	0.4	0.4	0.2	0.6
Abdominal pain	10	1.5	—	0.5	0.6	0.3
Anemia	9	1.3	0.2	0.5	0.1	0.1
Diarrhea	8	1.2	0.2	0.5	0.1	0.3
Pneumonitis	8	1.2	0.2	—	0.6	0.4
Gastrointestinal (unclassified)	7	1.0	0.2	0*	—	0.7
Neurologic	6	0.9	0.1	—	0.3	0.4
Rash	4	0.6	—	0.4	0.2	—
BCG sepsis	3	0.4	—	—	0.4	—
Coagulopathy	2	0.3	—	—	0.3	—
Leukopenia	2	0.3	0.2	0†	—	—
Thrombocytopenia	2	0.3	0.2	0†	—	—
Hepatic granuloma	1	0.2	—	—	0.2	—
Hepatitis	1	0.2	—	—	0.2	—

Republished with permission by Organon Teknika, Durham, NC.
*Grade was determined using the ECOG scale of toxicity criteria: mild, grade 1; moderate, grade 2; severe, grade 3 or 4.
†Flu-like syndrome includes fever, shaking chills, malaise, and myalgia.

low-pressure gravity drainage through a catheter tip syringe attached to a bladder catheter. No additional pressure should be exerted. The solution is retained for 1 to 1½ hours if possible. It is then voided, and oral fluids should be forced for several hours to flush out the bladder. The standard course consists of six weekly treatments.

RESULTS

One can expect about a 70 percent response rate with an initial course of six weekly instillations of BCG (induction therapy) without subsequent maintenance therapy. Controversy exists over whether maintenance therapy on a monthly basis for 12 months is worthwhile, in view of the potential complications arising therefrom. If the initial 6-week course is unsuccessful, another 6-week course is given.

FOLLOW-UP

Four to six weeks later, at which time therapy is completed, repeat specific and random biopsies and urine cytology should be performed. If CIS persists after 2 courses of BCG, cystectomy is advised.

Patients should be told that disease progression may

occur during the first or second course of BCG therapy, and they should understand that BCG is being used as a bladder-sparing attempt.

After the initial post-BCG biopsy and cytology, office cystoscopy under local anesthesia and cytologic studies are performed every 3 months for 2 years. IVU is performed every 12 to 24 months. If the above studies are normal during the third year, the interval for cystoscopy and cytology is increased to every 4 months. During the fourth and fifth years, evaluation is performed at 6-month intervals and yearly after that. IVU is performed every 2 to 3 years. One cannot be too dogmatic about the proper intervals. However, any sign of gross or microscopic hematuria or recurrence of symptoms warrants immediate re-evaluation.

BCG is effective in 50 + percent of patients in whom thiotepa or mitomycin C has failed. As noted above, the risk of progression of the disease during sequential courses of intravesical agents should be kept in mind.

SUGGESTED READING

Brosman SA. The use of bacillus Calmette-Guérin in the therapy of bladder carcinoma in situ. J Urol 1985; 134:36–39.

DeKernion JB, Huang MY, Linder A, et al. The management of superficial bladder tumors and carcinoma in situ with intravesical bacillus Calmette-Guérin. J Urol 1985; 133:598–601.

Guinan P, Richardson C, Hanna M, et al. BCG in the management of superficial bladder cancer. Prog Clin Biol Res 1989; 303:447–553.

Kavoussi LR, Torrence RJ, Gillen DP, et al. Results of 6 weekly intravesical bacillus Calmette-Guérin instillations on the treatment of superficial bladder tumors. J Urol 1988; 139:935–940.

Rawls WH, Lamm DL, Lowe BS, et al. Fatal sepsis following intravesical bacillus Calmette-Guérin administration for bladder cancer. J Urol 1990; 144:1328–1330.

Sarosdy MF, Lamm DL. Long term results of intravesical bacillus Calmette-Guérin therapy for superficial bladder cancer. J Urol 1989; 142:719–722.

Soloway MS, Perry A. Bacillus Calmette-Guérin for treatment of superficial transitional cell carcinoma of the bladder in patients who have failed thiotepa and/or mitomycin C. J Urol 1987; 137:871–873.

ADENOCARCINOMA

JEFFREY M. IGNATOFF, M.D., F.A.C.S.

Adenocarcinoma of the bladder is an uncommon tumor, with an incidence estimated between 0.5 and 3.9 percent of all bladder tumors. Adenocarcinoma may be of urachal or nonurachal origin, tumors of nonurachal origin outnumbering urachal tumors by a ratio of approximately 1.5:1.

The occurrence of adenocarcinoma in the bladder is not surprising in view of the embryologic derivation of this organ and the potential of bladder epithelium to differentiate into colonic-like mucosa, as seen in exstrophy. This potential may persist into adult life and may be further manifested by proliferative changes of cystitis cystica and glandularis. There are several predisposing factors in the development of primary bladder adenocarcinoma. Vesical schistosomiasis has been associated with a higher incidence of adenocarcinoma, although squamous carcinoma is a more frequent sequela of this infestation. Bladder exstrophy and epispadias have an observed association with vesical adenocarcinoma. In addition, adenocarcinoma has been observed in the defunctionalized bladder.

The etiology and pathogenesis of urachal carcinoma remain poorly understood. Along the urachal cord, including the umbilicus, enteric-type glandular structures may be encountered that may give rise to adenocarcinoma. It seems implausible that this anaplastic event in the urachus is related to a urine-borne carcinogen, since urachal reflux of urine is an unlikely occurrence.

Primary vesical adenocarcinoma is seen most commonly between the sixth and eighth decades of life, with men more frequently involved (the ratio of men to women being 2.5:1). Urachal carcinoma tends to occur in a somewhat younger population, with two-thirds of cases seen between 40 and 70 years of age. Clinical presentation of either primary bladder adenocarcinoma or urachal carcinoma is most commonly with gross hematuria, in at least 75 percent of cases. Dysuria and irritative bladder symptoms occur less frequently (25 percent), and mucus production in the urine is occasionally seen (4 percent).

The diagnosis of primary vesical adenocarcinoma and the majority of urachal carcinomas rests on cystoscopic identification and biopsy. Approximately 88 percent of urachal tumors are cystoscopically visible. The distinction between primary vesical and urachal carcinoma can be difficult, since at least 15 percent of primary vesical adenocarcinomas are confined to the dome or anterior wall of the bladder. Tumors of urachal origin should show a sharp demarcation between tumor and surface epithelium, and the epithelial surface should be free of glandular or polypoid proliferation. Tumors involving the bladder dome may also result from local invasion or metastasis from adenocarcinoma of the rectum, endometrium, cervix, prostate, ovary, or breast; a metastatic origin of adenocarcinoma involving the bladder is, in fact, a more common occurrence than is a primary bladder origin of adenocarcinoma. Preoperative assessment of patients presenting with adenocarcinoma in the bladder should therefore include evaluation of the gastrointestinal tract, and in women, a careful gynecologic examination. Computed tomography (CT) is helpful for the diagnosis and staging of urachal carcinoma and may show the typical midline anterior supravesical mass extending into the bladder dome. Magnetic resonance imaging (MRI) may further complement staging because of the advantage of multiple imaging planes.

Once the diagnosis is confirmed, therapy should achieve total extirpation of the tumor, with the understanding that most treatment failures occur because the tumor is not controlled locally by the original operative procedure. The decision to proceed with surgical therapy depends both on tumor stage and on standard patient selection criteria for a major operative procedure. Furthermore, selection of a surgical procedure must be predicated on the knowledge that 90 percent or more of all bladder adenocarcinoma is deeply invasive at diagnosis. Transurethral resection as curative treatment is appropriate only in rare instances when a superficial tumor of nonurachal origin is encountered. Most patients with primary vesical adenocarcinoma without metastatic disease are best treated by radical cystectomy, including pelvic lymphadenectomy and urinary diversion. I include excision of all potential urachal remnant tissues cephalad to the bladder routinely in a radical cystectomy, both because of neoplastic potential and also to avert entry into the bladder dome in the course of cystectomy. The field change appearance of cystitis cystica and glandularis in some bladders harboring adenocarcinoma suggests that a partial cystectomy may leave a bladder remnant with continued risk of oncogenesis, although this is not a settled issue. In addition, the occurrence of a linitis plastica type of bladder wall involvement has been described, making it difficult to secure a satisfactory tumor-free margin by partial cystectomy.

Urachal adenocarcinoma is best treated by either radical cystectomy or wide-margin partial cystectomy, with en bloc resection (in either case) of contiguous peritoneum and all soft tissue of the lower midline abdominal wall between the umbilical ligaments, encompassing urachal structures up to and including the umbilicus. Total cystectomy has been advocated by most authors, except for lower-stage urachal adenocarcinoma,

or sarcoma, in which extended partial cystectomy, including the urachal structures, is sufficient if wide margins can be satisfactorily achieved. However, if the ability to safely encompass a urachal tumor with wide margins by a bladder-sparing procedure is in doubt, the local recurrence rate of 15 to 50 percent should argue in favor of radical cystectomy. As it may be difficult to determine the origin of bladder adenocarcinoma arising on the dome or anterior bladder wall, tumors in this location should be approached initially as if they were of urachal origin.

Although preoperative radiation therapy has been suggested by some, most of these tumors are resistant to radiation therapy, and its role remains undefined for either primary vesical or urachal adenocarcinoma. Systemic chemotherapy has likewise shown little effect against these tumors. The lack of response to cytotoxic therapy suggests no role for these agents in an adjuvant or neoadjuvant setting. Consideration might be given, however, to systemic or intra-arterial infusion chemotherapy in large-volume pelvic disease in an effort to downstage a lesion and permit surgical extirpation. Agents that have shown some response include 5-fluorouracil, methotrexate, mitomycin C, and doxorubicin.

The prognosis for adenocarcinoma of bladder of urachal origin is poor overall, with a 6 to 33 percent 5-year survival reported. This limited outlook has been related to the late appearance of symptoms, especially from tumors originating in the bladder dome or urachus. Most reports cite a worse outlook for urachal adenocarcinoma than for primary vesical adenocarcinoma.

Less common types of adenocarcinomas seen in the bladder include signet-ring cell carcinoma, usually reported as a separate entity and associated with a poor prognosis, and clear cell adenocarcinoma, an even less common tumor of debatable origin, also referred to as mesonephric adenocarcinoma. At least some of the reported clear cell carcinomas, most of which are seen in women, arise from urethral sites, and recent evidence suggests that they may derive from female periurethral glandular epithelium. Therapy for these rare tumors is generally limited to radical cystectomy and urinary diversion if distant metastatic involvement is not present.

SUGGESTED READING

Johansson SL, Anderstrom CR. Primary adenocarcinoma of the urinary bladder and urachus. In Williams CJ, Kirkorian JC, Green MR, Raghavan D, eds. Textbook of uncommon cancer. Chichester: John Wiley & Sons, 1988:275.

Sheldon CA, Clayman RV, Gonzales R, et al. Malignant urachal lesions. J Urol 1984; 131:1–8.

Skinner DG, Lieskovsky G. Techniques of radical cystectomy. In: Skinner DG, Lieskovsky G, eds. Genitourinary cancer. Philadelphia: WB Saunders, 1988:607.

SQUAMOUS CELL CARCINOMA

JOHN M. FITZPATRICK, M.Ch., F.R.C.S.I.

This condition is uncommon in the Western world but very common in areas where schistosomiasis is endemic. In my experience, squamous cell tumors appear de novo, without having progressed through either squamous metaplasia of normal urothelium or squamous change in a transitional cell tumor. Squamous metaplasia is a regular finding, particularly in females, but does not seem to have any significance in relation to squamous cell carcinoma of the bladder.

There has been considerable interest in this condition for some years, but the combined experience in the Western world is small. The role of radiotherapy and chemotherapy is therefore uncertain, although it is widely suggested that these forms of treatment are unhelpful. Because the prognosis of squamous cell carcinoma of the bladder is poor in the West, some additional therapy is required as an adjunct to surgery. A careful evaluation of the value of chemotherapy and immunotherapy is thus required, along with a re-evaluation of radiotherapy, which is successful in the management of squamous cell tumors in other parts of the body but relatively unhelpful in similar tumors of the bladder.

PATIENT EVALUATION

There are many methods of presentation in this condition. In areas where schistosomiasis is endemic, the index of suspicion is already high, and bladder irritative symptoms require careful assessment. In other parts of the world, because the condition is so uncommon, it may be that it will not be suspected by the clinician. Such symptoms as hematuria, chronic bladder irritation, and a bloody urethral discharge from the defunctioned bladder are all possible indicators of disease. It is particularly important not to assign symptoms such as frequency, nocturia, and perineal pain necessarily to chronic infection in the older age groups, as they may indicate the presence of either a squamous cell carcinoma of the bladder or indeed carcinoma in situ.

Routine evaluation with urine culture, urine cytology, and intravenous urography is important. Cystourethroscopy will show the presence of a tumor in the bladder, which in the case of squamous cell carcinoma is usually exophytic and nodular. As with other bladder tumors, it should be resected with the resectoscope, ensuring that all the tumor is sent for evaluation. At the end of the resection, I take cold cup biopsies from the bed of the resected area, and routine cold cup biopsies from normal mucosa throughout the bladder. The biopsies from the tumor bed will make clear whether there is deep invasion into the muscle layers, which may

be difficult to assess on resected tissue that may be charred by the heat of the resection. A catheter is then put into the bladder and a careful bimanual examination performed with the patient still relaxed.

Before a decision is made regarding the next stage of treatment, a chest x-ray and a computed tomography (CT) scan of the abdomen and pelvis should be performed. Routine pedal lymphography is unhelpful in this condition. Magnetic resonance imaging (MRI) has not proved especially helpful in detecting lymph node metastases within the pelvis, and the bladder image may be distorted if the imaging is carried out soon after the initial resection.

The classic association between squamous cell carcinoma of the bladder and schistosomiasis is well known, and exists particularly in Egypt and south-central Africa. In these areas the vast majority of squamous cell carcinomas are caused by chronic bladder infection with *Schistosoma haematobium,* and these cancers occur in patients younger than those who have such tumors in the Western world. There have been some interesting contributions to the literature, some of which are listed at the end of this chapter, suggesting that the squamous cell carcinoma that occurs after chronic infection with *S. haematobium* is more often of low grade, and also has a lesser incidence of deep invasion and metastatic disease.

When schistosoma is not the causative agent, as in the West, the prognosis is less likely to be favorable. It is of interest that whereas 80 percent of bladder cancers in Egypt are squamous cell tumors, only 1 percent of bladder cancers in the British Isles are of this kind.

In areas where schistosomiasis is not common, there has been considerable interest in this disease. Unfortunately, it is impossible under these circumstances to conduct a randomized trial with sufficient numbers to achieve statistical significance. The outcome is that although radiotherapy and chemotherapy for squamous cell carcinoma of the bladder are considered to be unhelpful, it is difficult to say that this is absolutely the case.

In this condition it is essential that, when radical surgery is being contemplated, either a continent urinary diversion or a bladder substitution procedure is performed. As these operations are gaining more universal acceptance, procedures involving ureterosigmoidostomy or a rectal bladder are no longer considered appropriate.

CHOICE OF PROCEDURE

The references at the end of this chapter deal with the management of squamous cell carcinoma of the bladder in the United States and the United Kingdom, and in areas where schistosomiasis is endemic. In these latter areas, the experience in the management of squamous cell tumors is considerable, and there appears to be a difference in the presentation of this condition in the two areas. In countries such as Egypt there is a much higher incidence of patients who present with low-grade and lower-stage tumors. In spite of this, it is interesting to note that the 5- and 10-year survival rates are similar in both areas. It is clear that it will take some time before the collective world experience is large enough for us to be sure of the exact roles, both individual and complementary, of surgery, radiotherapy, and chemotherapy.

SURGICAL TECHNIQUE

Partial Cystectomy

Partial cystectomy is sometimes an acceptable option in the management of squamous cell carcinoma of the bladder. This is more often the case in this condition than in transitional cell carcinoma of the bladder, in which widespread urothelial dysplasia or carcinoma in situ would preclude such a procedure.

It is an absolute rule in both these conditions, particularly when partial resection is being considered, that multiple random mucosal biopsies of seemingly normal urothelium be taken and sent for histologic examination. The size of the tumor is also important, because it is clear that tumors on the dome or anterior surface of the bladder are more suitable for partial cystectomy than are those on the base. This procedure is possible as long as a 2- to 3-cm margin of normal bladder around the tumor can be removed at the same time, but if it appears that the residual bladder capacity would be too small, the more radical operation is preferable.

The patient is laid flat on the table and should be in a moderate Trendelenburg position. A lower midline incision is performed and the peritoneum opened. Before the bladder lesion is dealt with, a pelvic lymphadenectomy should be carried out on the side of the lesion, but if the tumor is in the midline, a bilateral procedure is more appropriate. The dissection should proceed as far forward on the external iliac vein as possible and then extend backward to the bifurcation of the common iliac vessels. The lateral margin is the external iliac artery, and inferomedially the dissection should extend to the obturator fossa, leaving the obturator nerve and vein standing out free from the side wall of the pelvis.

The Trendelenburg position can be increased after the node dissection, and at that stage, the small bowel should be packed into the upper abdomen. The parietal peritoneum should be cut in the midline down to its reflection onto the base of the bladder, and the bladder itself can be freed up anteriorly by gently sweeping the finger on either side, so that it falls away from the posterior surface of the pubic bone. It is not necessary at this stage to extend this dissection anteriorly down to the apex of the prostate; when it is intended to open the bladder, care should be taken that the prostate in the male and bladder neck in the female should be seen clearly, and that the pelvic veins on either side of the midline at this level are avoided.

Two 2-0 chromic catgut sutures should be inserted into the bladder on either side of the midline, which should then be opened between these. The incision is carried backward to the tumor, which is then circumscribed with a 2- to 3-cm cuff of normal bladder. It is advisable to put a stay suture every 2 inches on either side of the incision, to help the aligning of the bladder when it is being closed. Bleeding vessels in the wall of the bladder should be undersewn. If the tumor is involving a ureteric orifice, the ureter must be reimplanted into the bladder, either by a direct reimplant using a nipple technique or by a Leadbetter-Politano procedure. If the tumor is lying close to a ureteric orifice but not involving it, it is advisable to place a ureteric catheter in position and then assess the necessity for a ureteric reimplantation as the operation proceeds, remembering the requirement to remove a cuff of normal bladder with the tumor specimen.

A No. 22 Fr hematuria catheter of the Foley type should be inserted perurethrally into the bladder, which should then be closed in two layers using 2-0 chromic catgut. It is inadvisable to use a suprapubic cystostomy tube, because of the possibility of seeding from the bladder along the track thus formed. I leave the urethral catheter in place for 12 days postoperatively. A pelvic drain should be used to drain the prevesical space postoperatively. I prefer a tube drain to a suction drain when the urinary tract is opened.

Radical Cystectomy

If the patient undergoing radical cystectomy is regarded as a good operative risk with a significant life expectancy, a bladder substitution or continent urinary diversion should be considered. In all other cases, a standard ileal conduit should be performed. I do not consider a ureterosigmoidostomy because of the metabolic complications and the long-term possibility of the development of bowel cancer.

Whatever procedure is chosen, a mechanical bowel preparation must be performed for 48 hours before the operation. Prolonged antibiotic cover preoperatively is not required, but I generally use prophylactic antibiotics, giving the first dose with the premedication and continuing for 5 days postoperatively. Ampicillin and an aminoglycoside with metronidazole cover the vast majority of aerobic and anaerobic bowel organisms. It is essential that the patient be seen by the stoma therapist before the operation, examining the patient in several positions, in order that two possible sites for a diversion be marked on the abdominal wall; it is impossible to pick an optimal site at the time of surgery with the patient lying flat on the table. In patients with squamous cell carcinoma of the bladder, it is unlikely that the urethra will need to be removed, so the patient may be placed supine on the operating table in a moderate Trendelenburg position. I prefer to use a left lower paramedian incision, which can be extended upward if required. This means that the incision is kept as far away as possible from the stoma on the right side of the abdomen, ensuring that ostomy bags do not encroach on the wound. The peritoneum is opened and the intraperitoneal organs are palpated.

In men, the peritoneum should be incised over the right ureter, and this is then freed up as far distally toward its insertion into the bladder as possible. This procedure is carried out in the same way on the left side. The pelvic parietal peritoneum is swept away from the pelvis on either side and the bladder is freed up anteriorly as far down as the prostate. The peritoneum is then cut on either side close to the pelvic wall down to the previous incision over the ureters. This is carried medially across to the opposite side. It is then easy to develop a plane between the posterior surface of the bladder and the anterior surface of the rectum as far down as the base of the prostate.

The internal iliac vessels are dissected free on either side, and first the obliterated umbilical artery and then the superior and inferior vesical pedicles are clipped and ligated. There are no other vessels of significance laterally or posteriorly, so any other pieces of tissue may be diathermized or clipped.

When the lateral vascular attachments of the bladder have been clipped and divided, attention may be diverted to the apex of the prostate, and the dissection here is exactly the same as for a radical prostatectomy. The endopelvic fascia on either side is incised and a finger may be passed round to the other side under the urethra. The deep dorsal vein of the penis is undersewn after the puboprostatic ligaments have been divided. With the completion of these maneuvers, the apex of the prostate may be mobilized cranially and a considerable amount of the proximal urethra brought into view. The urethra is transected at the apex of the prostate, and the catheter clamped and cut. This will act as a useful retractor and help to bring the apex of the prostate even farther cranially. Any other attachments of the prostate may then be clipped and divided. The entire specimen consisting of bladder prostate and seminal vesicles is removed en bloc. If it is intended to perform a potency-sparing operation in males, the dissection along the lateral sides of the prostate may be brought as far away from the pelvic side wall and rectum as possible, to avoid damaging the neurovascular bundle.

In women, the initial approach to the ureter is made by dividing the broad ligament on either side. This ensures that the fallopian tubes and ovaries may be brought medially and included in the specimen to be removed. The peritoneum is then divided on either side in the same way as in men, the round ligament being ligated and divided instead of the vas deferens.

The peritoneal incision is continued medially from both sides, in the same way as in men. The cervix is easily palpable above this incision. There is no need to dissect between the vagina and the rectum: it is sufficient to remove only the upper third of the vagina with the specimen. The dissection continues as in men, and when all lateral attachments have been divided the urethra is transected and the vagina divided. The vagina is closed with 2-0 chromic catgut.

In men, a No. 24 Fr Foley catheter is passed up through the urethra and 40 ml of saline put in the balloon. The catheter is attached to a drainage bag into which 400 ml of saline is placed; the bag is then allowed to hang over the end of the operating table to facilitate hemostasis. In both men and women, a pelvic drain is inserted. As stated previously, I prefer a tube drain to a section drain.

If it is possible to avoid a urinary diversion such as an ileal or colonic conduit in which the patient must wear an ostomy bag, a continent urinary diversion or bladder substitution procedure is indicated. In the case of a continent diversion, I prefer the Indianapolis pouch; for bladder substitution I have found the Mainz bladder satisfactory, with a relatively low incidence of complications. It is important to check the residual urine in these patients on a regular basis; if it is high, it may be necessary for the patient to self-catheterize.

If performing an ileal conduit, I prefer the Wallace ureteroileal anastomosis, with the ureters being spatulated and anastomosed side-to-side before being anastomosed onto the end of the ileal loop. The incidence of ureteroileal stenosis is extremely low. I routinely use No. 8 Fr ureteral catheters, which are left in situ for 8 days. I do not intubate the conduit itself. The abdomen is closed in the standard manner.

CHOICE OF TREATMENT

Traditionally there are three types of treatment for patients with transitional cell carcinoma of the bladder, depending on the stage of the disease. In patients with superficial disease, intravesical chemotherapy or intravesical immunotherapy may have a role to play in patients with recurrence or with risk factors that may lead to the development of multiple superficial recurrences or invasive bladder cancer. Unfortunately, in squamous cell carcinoma of the bladder, superficial disease is uncommon and thus intravesical agents do not fulfill any valuable role; squamous cell carcinoma has not been shown to be responsive to these agents.

Many squamous cell tumors throughout the body have been shown to be sensitive to radiotherapy; for example, such tumors of the skin, which in most cases respond by complete disappearance. The results of radiotherapy to squamous cell carcinoma of the bladder are very poor indeed and I consider that it has virtually no role to play in this condition. Until recently, very few studies supported the role of radiotherapy, but within the last few years, two studies (one from Mansoura in Egypt and the other from the M.D. Anderson Cancer Center) have suggested that preoperative radiotherapy prior to radical cystectomy may be important in improving survival from this disease. These observations raise the question of neoadjuvant or adjuvant chemotherapy.

The conventional wisdom has been that these tumors are not chemosensitive; and so there has been no prospective trial to determine whether this form of treatment may be helpful. Another factor militating against such trials is that this disease is so uncommon that the length of time required to raise the numbers prospectively for a trial would be intolerably great.

The choice therefore remains between partial cystectomy and radical cystectomy, depending on the size of the tumor. If it is thought that the entire tumor can be removed with a cuff of normal bladder of 2 to 3 cm surrounding the tumor without sacrificing too much bladder capacity, a partial cystectomy may well be deemed appropriate. It must also be remembered that the bladder has the ability to increase its capacity over a period of some months after removal of some of its volume. If the tumor is too large but lies above the trigone, a supratrigonal cystectomy and substitution cecocystoplasty may be indicated, given that in the squamous cell carcinoma a "field lesion" is very uncommon.

It is likely that the best operation in most cases is a radical cystectomy. In this instance, a urinary diversion such as an ileal conduit may be required, or in optimal circumstances, a continent urinary diversion or bladder substitution may be possible.

It is to be hoped that future studies will address the possibility of combining preoperative radiotherapy or chemotherapy with radical surgery, and that the ideal combination of drugs will become clear. Unfortunately, the numbers in any one center (outside Egypt) being small, it may be difficult to find the answer to these questions.

SUGGESTED READING

Ghoneim MA, Ashamalla A, Gaballa MA, Ibrahim EI. Cystectomy for carcinoma of the bilharzial bladder: 126 patients 10 years later. Br J Urol 1985; 57:303.

Ghoneim MA, Ashamalla A, Awaad HK, Whitmore WF Jr. Randomized trial of cystectomy with or without preoperative radiotherapy for carcinoma of the bilharzial bladder. J Urol 1985; 134:266.

Ghoneim MA, Mansour MA, El-Boulkany MN. Radical cystectomy for carcinoma of the bilharzial bladder. Br J Urol 1972; 44:461.

Richie JP, Waisman J, Skinner DG, Dretler SP. Squamous carcinoma of the bladder: treatment by radical cystectomy. J Urol 1976; 115:670.

Rundle JSH, Hart AJL, McGeorge A, et al. Squamous cell carcinoma of the bladder; a review of 114 patients. Br J Urol 1982; 54:522.

Swanson DA, Liles A, Zagars GK. Preoperative irradiation and radical cystectomy for stages T2 and T3 squamous cell carcinoma of the bladder. J Urol 1990; 143:37.

LEUKOPLAKIA AND PREMALIGNANT CONDITIONS

JONATHAN FLEISCHMANN, M.D., M.M.S., F.A.C.S.

Sometimes the urologist views an abnormality of the bladder that is not recognized immediately and the clinical significance of which is unknown. A biopsy is the straightforward method of addressing this problem, but the urologist must be aware that between the obviously benign and the frankly malignant resides the "premalignant." Premalignant lesions of the bladder are uncommon, and the pathologist may not be aware that some non-neoplastic lesions are a cause for concern.

Transitional epithelium has the potential to differentiate into epithelial carcinomas of the squamous or transitional cell types, or may transform into adenocarcinoma. Carcinomas of the bladder may be heralded by benign lesions, and these premalignant disorders reflect the varieties of mucosal inflammation. Both the type of inflammation and the antecedent status of the transitional epithelium influence the subsequent morphology of the carcinoma. For example, adenocarcinoma is the long-term complication of bladder exstrophy in 3 to 5 percent of affected patients, but squamous carcinoma is the usual consequence of unresolved bladder calculi, even though both groups of patients may have experienced similar bacterial infections. Conversely, patients who underwent enterocystoplasty require periodic cystoscopic and cytologic surveillance for either adenocarcinoma or transitional cell carcinoma. An appreciation of both the "at-risk" patient and the herald lesion, therefore, may reduce patient morbidity. These herald lesions are described below.

LEUKOPLAKIA

Leukoplakia appears as a plaque of keratinized epithelium, gray or white, surrounded usually by inflamed mucosa. Floating keratinaceous debris is often seen at cystoscopy. Squamous metaplasia, a condition caused by chronic nonspecific or bacterial inflammation, commonly coexists with leukoplakia, and some believe that it is the precursor of leukoplakia because of the similar pathology. Leukoplakia differs from squamous metaplasia with respect to keratinization, intracellular bridges, and an occasionally observed stratum granulosum. The diagnosis of leukoplakia precedes the development of carcinoma in 10 to 25 percent of affected patients.

Any patient with chronic bacterial cystitis is at risk

for acquiring leukoplakia, and the most common cause of chronic bacterial cystitis is an indwelling catheter. It has been estimated that at least three quarters of the patients managed by chronic indwelling catheterization for 10 years or more will contract this disease. Consequently, the 10-year risk for developing carcinoma is approximately 5 to 20 percent among these patients. There has been some debate over whether it is the foreign body or the chronic infection that provokes a malignant transformation. For countries in which endemic diseases include schistosomiasis (bilharziasis) and systemic tuberculosis, there is an increased risk of vesical leukoplakia and subsequent carcinoma. Any type of epithelial carcinoma may occur after the formation of leukoplakia, but it is usually a squamous carcinoma.

In the management of leukoplakia, one must first attempt to correct the underlying cause, such as a bilharzial, tubercular, or "routine" infection associated with catheter dependence or a bladder calculus. Unfortunately, addressing the underlying cause of leukoplakia often does not prevent its recurrence. The insidious nature of leukoplakia must be factored into its treatment, which is dependent on the extent of the disease. A small patch of disease can be resected, after which the patient must undergo a surveillance schedule similar to that for superficial bladder cancer: regular cystoscopic examinations with urine cytology and, if indicated, mucosal biopsy to rule out carcinoma. Disease too extensive for complete resection is best managed by cystectomy, since carcinoma may brew undetected beneath a plaque.

CYSTITIS FOLLICULARIS, CYSTITIS CYSTICA, AND CYSTITIS GLANDULARIS

A spectrum of cystic mucosal abnormalities engendered by infection or by foreign body irritation are represented by the cystites: follicularis, cystica, and glandularis. Cystitis follicularis is distinguished by delicate mucosal bubbles, occasionally punctuated by bright yellow inclusions at the end of a gossamer stalk. Without correction of the underlying mucosal irritation, cystitis follicularis can progress to cystitis cystica, which has a bullous appearance. Neither cystitis follicularis nor cystitis cystica are known to progress to carcinoma. In contrast, cystitis glandularis is distinguished by sessile mucosal adenomatous glandular formation that can progress to adenocarcinoma. Although cystitis glandularis is not as worrisome as leukoplakia, its management includes eradication of the underlying cause, judicious

biopsies to rule out carcinoma, and periodic cystoscopic surveillance with urinary cytologic studies.

INVERTED PAPILLOMA

An inverted papilloma is a benign, rare entity usually observed in the trigone or bladder neck. It is characterized as a sessile nubbin, covered by normal mucosa, which has fingers of normal transitional epithelium extending into the submucosa. Since it cannot be distinguished grossly from a carcinoma, it is managed initially by transurethral resection. Follow-up cystoscopic and cytologic surveillance is required because papillomas can recur and are often associated with a new carcinoma.

NEPHROGENIC ADENOMA

Nephrogenic adenoma is a metaplastic collection of mesonephric tubules in the lamina propria. The clinical presentation (irritative voiding symptoms, hematuria) and cystoscopic appearance of a nephrogenic adenoma mimics the presentation of a sessile bladder carcinoma. In many instances there is antecedent trauma. The lesions can be single or multiple and may be surrounded by erythematous mucosa. Although uniformly benign, nephrogenic adenomas are known to recur in most patients and have been associated with adjacent carcinomas. A simple transurethral resection is the usual method of treatment, but more extensive lesions or lesions that cause debilitating voiding symptoms may require partial or total cystectomy.

SUGGESTED READING

Berger BW, Bhagavan BS, Reiner W, et al. Nephrogenic adenoma: clinical features and therapeutic considerations. J Urol 1981; 126:824–826.

Dubeau L, Jones PA, Rideout WM III, Laug WE. Differential regulation of plasminogen activators by epidermal growth factor in normal and neoplastic human urothelium. Cancer Res 1988; 48:5552–5556.

Filmer RB, Spencer JR. Malignancies in bladder augmentations and intestinal conduits. J Urol 1990; 143:671–678.

Kaufman JM, Fam B, Jacobs SC, et al. Bladder cancer and squamous metaplasia in spinal cord injury patients. J Urol 1977; 118:967–971.

Mortensen PB, Jensen KEJ, Nielsen K. Adenocarcinoma development in the trigone 34 years after trigonocolonic urinary diversion for exstrophy of the bladder. J Urol 1990; 144:980–982.

Waisman SS, Banko J, Cromie WJ. Single polypoid cystitis cystica and glandularis presenting as benign bladder tumor. Urology 1990; 36:364–366.

SARCOMA, PHEOCHROMOCYTOMA, AND BENIGN TUMORS

ROBERT C. FLANIGAN, M.D., F.A.C.S.

Tumors arising from the urothelium of the bladder (transitional cell carcinoma, squamous cell carcinoma, and adenocarcinoma of the bladder) constitute the vast majority of neoplastic lesions of this organ. The tumors described in this chapter are less common tumors, which are nonepithelial in origin. Nonetheless, a clear understanding of these tumors and their management is essential for the urologist.

ADULT SARCOMAS

The signs and symptoms of adult sarcomas include hematuria, irritative urinary symptoms, urinary retention, and a pelvic mass. An intravenous pyelogram (IVP) may be helpful in making the diagnosis, since nearly one half of the patients studied in several trials have shown evidence of upper tract obstruction at the time of initial presentation. In addition, most patients have demonstrated filling defects during the cystogram phase of the IVP.

Leiomyosarcoma has been the most common histologic type reported, followed by fibrous histiocytic sarcoma, osteogenic sarcoma, and chondrosarcomas. Most of the tumors reported have been of high histologic grade.

The initial evaluation of these tumors begins with physical examination, including a bimanual examination to assess for size, extent, and fixation of tumor. Biopsies of the mass can be obtained either transurethrally or transrectally, using needle aspiration or core biopsy techniques. I prefer the latter technique when possible because of the potential difficulty for the cytopathologist in distinguishing between a high-grade sarcoma and a highly undifferentiated tumor of epithelial origin. When the bladder is involved with tumor, transurethral biopsies of the bladder, bladder neck, and prostatic urethra are important, even if these areas appear to be endoscopically normal. In addition, transsrectal or transvaginal biopsies of perivesical tissues (prostate, urethrovaginal septum, and cervix) may provide useful information regarding the extent of local disease and may help predict the feasibility of surgical excision.

The current treatment of bladder sarcomas in adults is complete excision of the primary tumor when the patient presents with apparently localized disease. Depending on the nature and degree of involvement, this may necessitate partial cystectomy, or more commonly, radical cystectomy. In patients with advanced pelvic disease, urinary diversion may be palliative. Conservative endoscopic surgery (transurethral resec-

tion) has also been reported in combination with chemotherapy.

Experience suggests that most adult patients with bladder sarcoma have localized disease at initial presentation and that the disease is often extensive locally before metastasis occurs. The extent of surgery therefore depends on the size and location of the tumor. It is important to remember that because of the insidious ability of sarcomas to develop nests of tumor away from the primary tumor mass, a generous 4- to 5-cm normal margin of full-thickness bladder wall should be obtained in patients undergoing partial cystectomy. Furthermore, the urachus and perivesical fatty tissue involving the upper hemisphere of the bladder should be completely removed. For any patient undergoing surgery aimed at a cure, I recommend bilateral pelvic lymphadenectomy.

Although adjunctive therapy trials, including radiotherapy or chemotherapy, have been small and nonrandomized, several concepts of management appear to be increasingly clear. Postoperative radiotherapy alone, when used to consolidate control of an incompletely resected locally extensive bladder sarcoma, has generally been unsuccessful, associated with high local recurrence rates and toxicity (generally involving the small bowel). Combination radiotherapy and chemotherapy appears to hold more promise. The current recommendation is therefore complete surgical resection for apparently localized disease. If surgical margins are negative, the patient is observed. If surgical margins are positive or lymph node metastases are present, adjuvant external beam radiotherapy (4,500-5,000 cGy), and chemotherapy (60 mg per square meter doxorubicin and 100 mg per square meter cisplatin every 3 weeks times 2) are given. In patients presenting with bulky or transmural disease, cytoreductive chemotherapy (doxorubicin plus cisplatin) with or without radiotherapy is employed before exenterative surgery.

RHABDOMYOSARCOMA

Sarcomas arising in the soft tissues are the third most common solid tumor of childhood, after central nervous system tumors and neuroblastoma. Rhabdomyosarcoma originates histologically from the same embryonal mesenchyme that gives rise to striated skeletal muscle and is the most common soft tissue sarcoma, making up about 50 percent of these lesions. It is more common in whites than in blacks, with incidences of 4.4 and 1.3 per million, respectively. The male to female ratio is 1.4:1. The peak age for presentation is between 2 and 6 years, with a second peak at approximately 15 to 19 years of age. Almost three quarters of patients present before the age of 10. There appears to be a potential genetic component to rhabdomyosarcoma. Familial aggregations of these tumors have been reported and an increased incidence has been seen in patients with neurofibromatosis.

The bladder is the second most common site of

rhabdomyosarcoma, most frequently involving the trigone of the bladder. The natural history of these tumors is one of rapid growth with invasion of adjacent tissues. The tumor tends to be unencapsulated and infiltrative, as is typical of other sarcomatous lesions. When metastases are destined to occur, approximately 75 percent manifest themselves within 6 months of diagnosis, and over 80 percent within 1 year. Therefore, before the development of effective chemotherapy, 70 to 80 percent of patients with rhabdomyosarcoma died with widespread metastases in spite of local surgical removal and radiotherapy.

Grossly, rhabdomyosarcomas tend to be nodular and firm. They often appear at surgery to be deceptively well circumscribed. Only in cases of sarcoma botryoides, which looks like a cluster of grapes, are any remarkable gross features of rhabdomyosarcoma present. Histologically, these tumors can be divided into several classifications, depending on the degree of mesenchymal differentiation. Embryonal rhabdomyosarcoma, the most common type, morphologically resembles developing skeletal muscle, as seen in the 7- to 10-week fetus. Sarcoma botryoides is a polypoid form of embryonal rhabdomyosarcoma. Alveolar rhabdomyosarcoma histologically resembles skeletal muscle in the 10- to 21-week fetus. This tumor type is more frequent in adolescents and young adults and is relatively less common in the genitourinary tract. The pleomorphic type of rhabdomyosarcoma is a rare lesion, accounting for approximately 1 percent of these tumors, and is usually found in adulthood. Again, it is highly uncommon in the genitourinary tract. Rhabdomyosarcomas are often highly undifferentiated. Approximately 10 to 20 percent are classified as histologically mixed.

The signs and symptoms of rhabdomyosarcoma of the genitourinary tract depend on the exact site of origin. When the bladder is involved, the child typically presents with strangury due to lower urinary tract obstruction. From the bladder base, the tumor typically extends submucosally to involve the bladder neck, prostate, and prostatic urethra in boys. In girls it may extend posteriorally into the wall of the vagina and cervix. This may lead to urinary retention and secondary incontinence or infection. Hematuria may occur if the tumor breaks through the lining of the genitourinary tract, although this tends to be a late event.

Children with rhabdomyosarcoma may present with a large abdominal mass whose primary site is initially difficult to determine. Diagnostic imaging usually involves intravenous urography, computed tomography (CT), and/or ultrasound examinations. The combination of cystoscopy (and vaginoscopy in the female child) is often useful in delineating the site of the primary tumor. If the mucosa of the bladder, prostatic urethra, or vagina is clearly abnormal, an endoscopic biopsy is useful to confirm the presence of tumor and to demonstrate its histologic type. Careful manual examination during cystoscopy or vaginoscopy is important in delineating the extent of the tumor. When endoscopic biopsy is not possible, a percutaneous needle biopsy may help determine the histology of the tumor. Approximately 20 percent of genitourinary rhabdomyosarcomas will have spread to the retroperitoneal lymph nodes at the time of first diagnosis; careful inspection of these areas with CT is therefore useful.

The clinical staging systems used for rhabdomyosarcoma have generally relied significantly on the resectability of the primary tumor and the status of the draining lymph nodes. The Intergroup Rhabdomyosarcoma Study clinical grouping classification is shown in Table 1.

After information developed suggesting that both radiation therapy and chemotherapy were effective in rhabdomyosarcoma, interest developed in the *primary* use of these modalities in order to avoid unnecessarily exenterative surgery. At the present time, therefore, primary surgical treatment has been restricted largely to tumor biopsy. After this, intense chemotherapy with repetitive monthly courses of pulse-VAC (vincristine, actinomycin D, and cyclophosphamide) is begun. After 8 weeks of treatment, a re-evaluation is completed. If a complete or partial response has occurred, chemotherapy is continued until week 16. At that time, a similar re-evaluation is followed by surgical exploration (biopsy or partial cystectomy) to determine the extent of residual disease. If, after surgical resection, gross or microscopic residual disease remains, the patient receives adjuvant radiotherapy and continues on pulse-VAC chemotherapy for 2 years. If no residual tumor is present after surgery, radiotherapy is omitted, but the patient is maintained on pulse-VAC chemotherapy for 2 years. If at the 8-week re-evaluation no response to therapy or progressive disease is found, radiotherapy is added. At 16 weeks, surgical exploration is performed. If no residual disease is found, pulse-VAC alternating

Table 1 Intergroup Rhabdomyosarcoma Study Classification

1. Group I. Localized disease; completely removed; regional nodes not involved
   A. Confined to muscle or organ or origin
   B. Contiguous involvement with infiltration outside the muscle or organ of origin, as through fascial planes

   Inclusion in this group includes both gross impression of complete removal and microscopic confirmation of complete removal

2. Group II
   A. Grossly removed tumor with microscopic residual disease; no evidence of gross residual tumor; no evidence of regional node involvement
   B. Regional disease; completely removed (regional nodes involved or extension of tumor into an adjacent organ; no microscopic residual disease)
   C. Regional disease with involved nodes; grossly removed, but with evidence of microscopic residual disease

3. Group III. Incomplete removal or biopsy with gross residual disease

4. Group IV. Distant metastatic disease present at onset

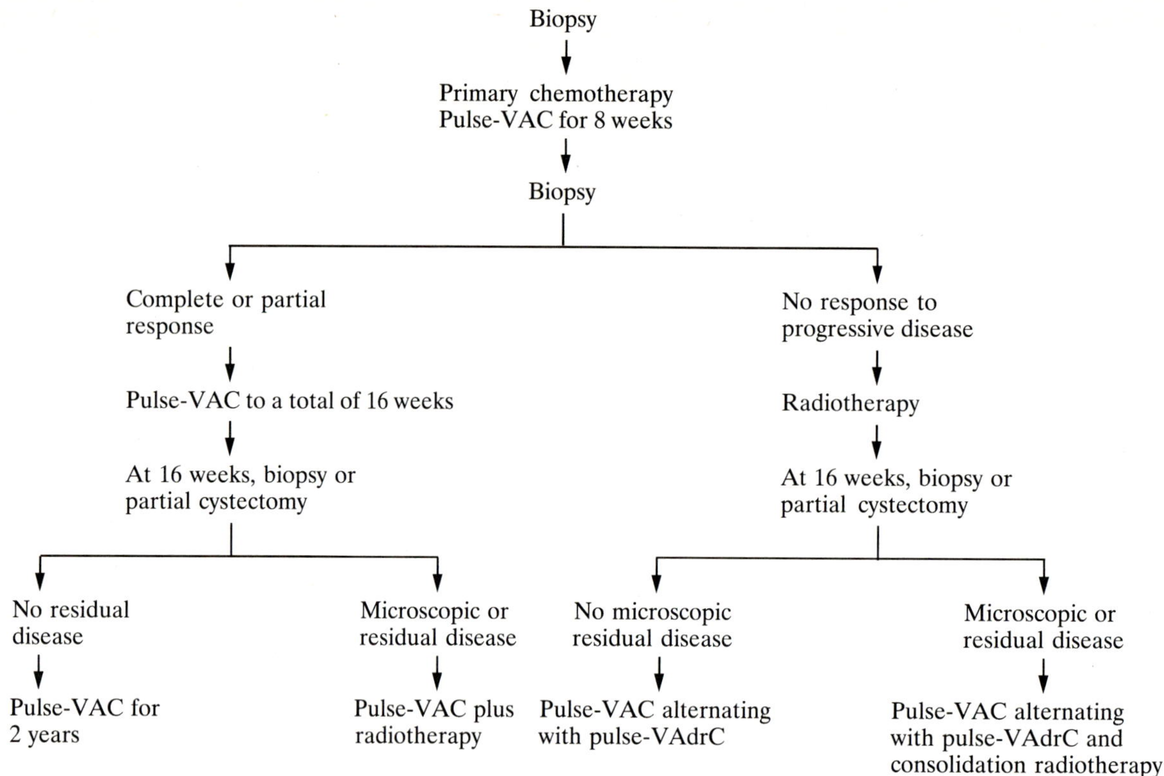

Figure 1 Modified from Kramer SA. Urologic oncology. Urol Clin North Am. 1985; 12:31–42.

with pulse-VAdrC therapy is continued for 2 years. If microscopic or residual disease is found, pulse-VAC alternating with pulse-VAdrC therapy is continued for 2 years with completion of radiotherapy to tolerable limits.

The initial hope that primary chemotherapy would avoid the need for radiation therapy and radical surgery has, in general, not been realized. Only about 10 percent of patients have achieved relapse-free survival with chemotherapy alone. Three quarters of bladder or prostate tumors have required radiotherapy. On the other hand, with a combination of chemotherapy, radiotherapy, and more limited surgical resection, approximately two-thirds of patients have been able to maintain their bladder and are alive and relapse free with a median follow-up of 2.7 years, a result somewhat better than that seen with primary surgical treatment alone. Two-thirds of patients with vaginal rhabdomyosarcoma have required partial vaginectomy to remove residual tumor.

PHEOCHROMOCYTOMA

Pheochromocytoma (paraganglianoma) involving the urinary bladder is an extremely rare lesion accounting for only 0.4 percent of cases of bladder tumors reported to the Armed Forces Institute of Pathology. Most pheochromocytomas of the bladder are benign, with only rare malignant pheochromocytomas described. Patients may present with symptoms of throbbing headache, faintness, or pain associated with micturition, gross hematuria, or hypertension. There is often a long history of attacks that appear to occur infrequently. Micturitional attacks may be the only significant manifestation, and frequently their significance is not appreciated until after surgery. Pheochromocytomas of the bladder generally are located submucosally but often present with significant intravesical extension. Ulceration of the underlying mucosa with associated hemorrhage is common. The measurement of levels of serum and urinary catecholamines and their metabolites, especially vanillylmandelic acid (VMA), dihydroxyphenylalanine (DOPA), and dopamine, are critical to the diagnosis of pheochromocytoma. Approximately 60 percent of cases analyzed with these tests preoperatively have been reported to be positive. Elevated DOPA or dopamine levels are more commonly associated with malignant pheochromocytoma.

The distinction between multifocal and malignant tumors is often difficult. A diagnosis of malignancy cannot rest on cellular characteristics of the tumor or its infiltration of bladder muscle. To confirm malignancy, secreting cells must be demonstrated at a site where chromaffin tissue does not occur—for example, in the regional lymphatics.

The management of pheochromocytoma of the bladder is surgical. A partial cystectomy is typically satisfactory. Lymphadenectomy, I believe, should be performed on a routine basis because between 7 and 20 percent of these tumors can be shown to be malignant by demonstration of regional lymphatic metastases. The perioperative management of these patients is extremely important to the successful outcome of surgical intervention. Preoperative CT and MIBG scanning are used to determine metastases, tumor size, and location. A negative metastatic work-up, however, does not preclude the possibility of lymphatic metastases. Preoperative management in these patients may consist of the use of alpha blockers, beta blockers, calcium channel blockers, inhibitors of catecholamine synthesis, and magnesium sulfate. Most commonly, prazosin, a selective alpha$_1$ antagonist, is begun in a dosage of 0.5 mg per day with increases to levels necessary for alpha blockade and control of hypertension. Propranolol may then be used for beta blockade in patients with tachycardia. Although more selective beta antagonists such as esmolol and metoprolol may avoid the increase in systemic vascular resistance seen with beta-2 blockade, preoperative beta blockade in patients with catecholamine-producing tumors is controversial and should be accomplished only after treatment with alpha antagonists.

Nifedipine, a potential vasodilator, may also be useful in selected patients because of its properties of suppressing catecholamine release.

Intraoperative problems, including hypertension, may occur because of noxious stimuli or tumor manipulation. Careful hemodynamic monitoring is therefore essential.

SUGGESTED READING

Ahlering TE, Weintraub P, Skinner DG. Management of adult sarcomas of the bladder and prostate. J Urol 1988; 140:1397–1399.

Crist W, Garnsen L, Beltangady MS, et al. Prognosis in children with rhabdomyosarcoma: a report for the Intergroup Rhabdomyosarcoma Studies I and II. J Clin Oncol 1990; 8:443–456.

Flanigan RC, Whitman RP, Huhn R, Davis CJ. Malignant pheochromocytoma of the urinary bladder. Urology 1980; 16:386–388.

Maurer HM, Beltangady M, Gehan EA, et al. The Intergroup Rhabdomyosarcoma Study. 1: A final report. Cancer 1988; 61:209–220.

Splinter W, Milne B, Nickel C, Loomis C. Perioperative management for resection of a malignant nonchromaffin paraganglioma of the bladder. Can J Anaesth 1989; 36:215–218.

MALACOPLAKIA

MITCHELL C. KAYE, M.D.
ERIC A. KLEIN, M.D.

Malacoplakia was first described by Michaelis and Gutmann in 1902. This rare, acquired, granulomatous disease may affect any organ. Approximately 200 cases of malacoplakia are documented in the literature. Stanton and Maxted reviewed 153 of these cases and noted that 80 percent involved the genitourinary tract. Occurrence within the urinary system is most often seen in the bladder (40 percent), followed by the renal parenchyma (16 percent), ureter (11 percent), renal pelvis (10 percent), and prostate (10 percent). The gastrointestinal tract and retroperitoneum each account for 12 percent of cases. Long and Althausen noted bladder involvement in 70 percent of cases, with isolated upper tract lesions in 15 percent and combined upper and lower tract disease in 15 percent. Typically, malacoplakia involving the urinary system is seen in females with a 4:1 preponderance. The usual age is in the fifth decade, but the disease has been reported in patients aged from 6 months to 85 years.

PATHOLOGY

The term "malacoplakia" is of Greek origin and refers to the characteristic lesion, a soft *(malakos)* plaque *(plakos)*. Cystoscopically, the gross lesion consists of variably sized yellow-brown plaques, often with a central umbilication or ulceration and a peripheral hyperemia. In the bladder, the transitional cell epithelium initially remains intact before eroding. Perivesical extension may occur with progressive disease. In the kidney, malacoplakia may be unifocal or multifocal. Multifocal involvement is seen in 75 percent of cases, and in approximately 50 percent of cases parenchymal involvement is bilateral. Extension to perinephric fat may also occur.

Microscopically, malacoplakia is characterized by dense aggregates of large mononuclear histiocytes referred to as von Hansemann cells, admixed with intracellular and extracellular Michaelis-Gutmann (MG) bodies in a scanty connective tissue stroma infiltrated by varying numbers of lymphocytes and plasma cells (Fig. 1). The MG bodies are also known as calcified residual bodies, calcospherules, calcospherites, and siderocalcific bodies. They arise within phagolysosomes and appear as sharply demarcated intracellular or extracellular spherical structures, composed primarily of calcium hydroxyapatite with variable amounts of iron, ranging in diameter from 5 to 10 microns, with a concentric "owl's-eye" appearance. MG bodies stain Gram negative, positive for PAS, Prussian blue, and alizarin red; they stain Sudan black negative and black with von Kossa's stain.

In 1965 Smith divided the morphogenesis of urinary tract malacoplakia into three phases: early, granulomatous, and healing. The early phase is characterized by plasma cells and von Hansemann cells in an edematous connective tissue stroma. In the granulomatous phase,

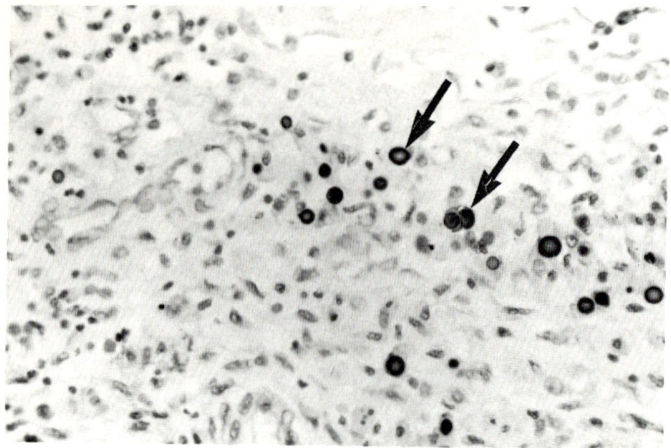

Figure 1 Typical histologic appearance of malacoplakia involving the bladder. Michaelis-Gutmann bodies are evident (*arrows*).

MG bodies and large histiocytes with occasional giant cells and lymphocytes are seen. The healing phase is evidenced by fibrosis around histiocytes with only a rare MG body.

PATHOGENESIS

A clear association between malacoplakia and urinary tract infection has been established, 80 to 90 percent of affected patients having cultures positive for bacilliform organisms. Approximately 75 percent of these isolates are *Escherichia coli*, although other associated organisms include *Proteus mirabilis, Aerobacter aerogenes, Klebsiella pneumoniae, Enterobacter,* and *Pseudomonas.* An enzymatic defect resulting in faulty phagolytic activity has been postulated as the underlying cause of malacoplakia, with MG bodies representing incomplete bacteriolysis. Other disorders such as carcinoma, autoimmune diseases, and immune deficiency syndromes have been noted in up to 40 percent of affected patients. Whether these syndromes are primary causes of malacoplakia, or whether malacoplakia associated with these results from alterations in the immune system, is unknown.

CLINICAL PRESENTATION

The site of malacoplakia affects the clinical presentation. In the bladder, irritative voiding symptoms and hematuria in association with persistent urinary tract infection are most commonly seen. Evaluation with urinary cultures and cytology, intravenous pyelography (IVP), and cystoscopy with biopsies help to establish the diagnosis and rule out carcinoma and tuberculosis. Histiocytes with MG bodies may be revealed in the urinary sediment. Pelvic computed tomography (CT) or transrectal ultrasonography is helpful in delineating perivesical extension. Retrograde pyelography searching for ureteral defects and strictures may be necessary to further investigate abnormal findings on IVP. Ureteral malacoplakia radiographically appears similar to the appearance of a patient with multiple tumors or ureteropyelitis cystica, and hence selective brush biopsies or ureteroscopy may be indicated. Symptoms of obstruction secondary to significant ureteral narrowing or isolated ureteropelvic junction obstruction may occur rarely. With renal parenchymal involvement, presentation is often with urinary tract infection, fever, chills, and flank pain. Perinephric extension may be appreciated as a palpable mass. Radiographically, the kidneys are typically enlarged with cortical defects and perhaps a discrete mass or masses. A CT scan is necessary to delineate the extent of any perinephric process and aid in distinguishing carcinoma. Angiographically, renal malacoplakia generally manifests as cortical defects, as hypovascular masses with peripheral neovascularity, or occasionally with a vascular pattern suggestive of neoplasm.

Malacoplakia of the prostate is often an incidental finding at the time of a transurethral resection (TURP) or autopsy, although symptoms of outlet obstruction or chronic prostatitis may exist. Physical examination may reveal a prostatic nodule or induration that necessitates biopsy to rule out adenocarcinoma. Testicular malacoplakia typically presents as an acute epididymo-orchitis, although it has been found incidentally in orchiectomy specimens from patients with prostate cancer.

TREATMENT

The therapeutic approach to malacoplakia is site dependent in the realization that upper tract involvement often heralds more aggressive disease. Lower tract involvement permits more conservative measures. When the bladder or prostate alone is involved, antibiotic therapy is initiated to sterilize the urine. The use of an agent that enhances intraphagocytic killing of bacteria is preferable. Appropriate choices include trimethoprim and rifampin, although apparent cures have also been reported with para-amino-salicylate, streptomycin, isoniazid, and penicillin. Additional therapy with agents that alter the intracellular ratio of cyclic guanine monophosphate and enhance microtubular metabolism and lysosomal function, and hence bactericidal activity within the phagocyte, may be required if symptoms are not relieved by antibiotics alone. Appropriate drugs include ascorbic acid (500 mg four times per day) and anticholinergics such as bethanechol (10 to 25 mg four times per day). More severe bladder involvement, including perivesical extension, usually can be treated conservatively; surgical therapy should be a last resort.

With ureteral malacoplakia the principal approach is conservative management as above. If ureteral involvement is complicated by obstruction, temporary relief with a stent or nephrostomy tube is warranted to allow for an appropriate trial of antibiotics, anticholinergics, and ascorbic acid. Refractory disease or residual stricture and obstruction may need to be managed surgically. Depending on the clinical situation, balloon dilatation, segmental ureteral resection with or without reimplantation, pyeloplasty, ureteral substitution, or autotransplantation may be required.

Renal parenchymal involvement by malacoplakia, owing to a high associated mortality rate, commands a more aggressive approach. With unilateral involvement in a patient with a normal contralateral kidney, nephrectomy is indicated. When malacoplakia involves both kidneys or a solitary kidney, an aggressive trial of medical therapy should be initiated. Failure of conservative management may necessitate a surgical approach even in the solitary kidney. Malacoplakia involving the transplant kidney may initially be managed with long-term antibiotic therapy and the reduction or withdrawal of azathioprine, early graft nephrectomy to increase survival being reserved for patients with deterioration of renal function.

Malacoplakia of the testicle typically presents as an epididymo-orchitis that fails to respond to antibiotic therapy. This presentation usually results in inguinal exploration and orchiectomy, intended both for cure and for differentiation from malignancy.

SUGGESTED READING

Long JP Jr, Althausen AF. Malacoplakia: a 25-year experience with a review of the literature. J Urol 1989; 141:1328–1331.

McClure J. Malakoplakia. J Pathol 1983; 140:275–330.

Smith BH. Malacoplakia of the urinary tract: a study of 24 cases. Am J Clin Pathol 1965; 43:409–417.

Stanton MJ, Maxted W. Malacoplakia: a study of the literature and current concepts of pathogenesis, diagnosis and treatment. J Urol 1981; 125:139–146.

Streem SB. Genitourinary malacoplakia in renal transplant recipients: pathogenic, prognostic and therapeutic considerations. J Urol 1984; 132:10–12.

NEOBLADDER CONSTRUCTION USING THE KOCK POUCH

EILA C. SKINNER, M.D.
GARY LIESKOVSKY, M.D.
STUART D. BOYD, M.D.
DONALD G. SKINNER, M.D.

The field of reconstructive urology has undergone tremendous development over the past 20 years, and nowhere is this more evident than in the area of urinary diversion. A wide variety of continent forms of urinary diversion have now been investigated in many different centers, and new adaptations are continually being made.

In 1982, on the basis of the elegant animal and human studies of Dr. Nils Kock, we began performing Kock continent cutaneous diversions in patients with bladder cancer and benign conditions requiring diversion. In 1986, we adapted the Kock pouch to be reanastomosed directly to the urethra in males. This chapter discusses our recent review of 126 such patients treated from 1986 to February 1990.

PATIENT SELECTION

The Kock urethrostomy is currently our diversion of choice for men undergoing radical cystoprostatectomy for malignant disease, as well as those undergoing continent diversion for neurogenic bladder, fibrosis due to radiation or chemotherapy, or other benign conditions. The following criteria, however, must be fulfilled:

1. In patients with transitional cell carcinoma of the bladder, the prostatic urethra must be free of carcinoma in situ or invasion of the prostatic stroma by cancer. We routinely recommend a loop biopsy of the prostatic urethra as part of the staging work-up of such patients. If a prostatic urethral biopsy has not been done, a frozen section should be performed at the time of cystectomy.
2. The external sphincter mechanism must be fully functional. This must be carefully assessed in patients with neurogenic bladder or who have undergone previous lower urinary tract surgery.
3. Often, for patients who are wheelchair bound or nonambulatory, who may have difficulty emptying the neobladder, a cutaneous form of diversion should be used. For the most part, however, body habitus is not a real concern. In fact, obese patients do better with a Kock urethrostomy than with a cutaneous continent diversion, because it obviates the difficulty of creating a catheterizable stoma through a thick abdominal wall.

Occasionally, patients request conversion from an ileal conduit or other form of diversion to a Kock urethrostomy months to years after cystectomy. We have done this in a few cases; the success depends on the status of the urethral stump and may result in a higher incidence of anastomotic stricture and incontinence than a primary reconstruction. If all or part of the prostate was left in situ at the first operation, such conversions were very successful.

OPERATIVE TECHNIQUE

Details of construction of both the cutaneous and the urethral Kock pouch have been reported previously and are available on videotapes. Construction of the Kock urethrostomy is identical to that in the cutaneous Kock except that the 17-cm segment that would form the efferent limb (the most distal segment) is omitted. The two 22-cm segments are opened and sewn together to form the pouch, and the proximal 17-cm segment is intussuscepted to form the afferent nipple valve (Fig. 1).

Several technical points warrant emphasis. The urethral stump is prepared in a manner identical to that used during a radical prostatectomy. We routinely place the eight anastomotic sutures of 2-0 chromic catgut circumferentially around the urethra at the time it is

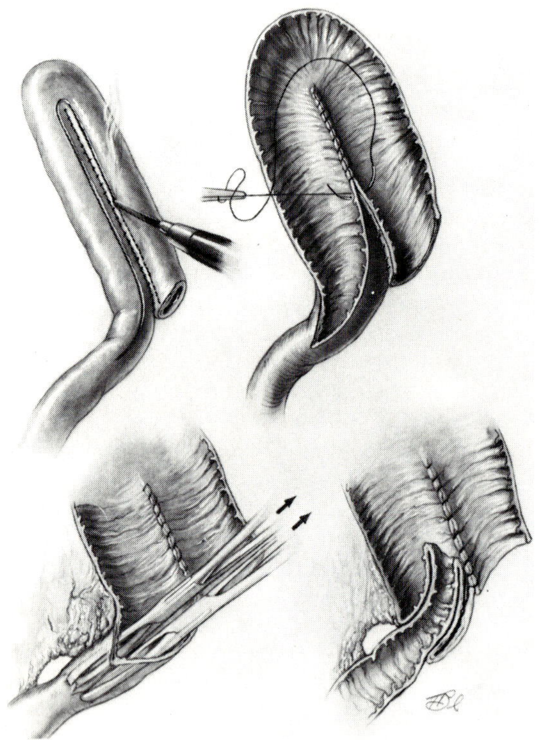

Figure 1 Technique of construction of the Kock neobladder. Two 22-cm segments are opened longitudinally and sewn together with two layers of running PGA suture. The afferent nipple is intussuscepted and fixed with three rows of staples, with the third row fixing the nipple to the back wall alongside the mesentery. (Republished with permission by Skinner DG, Boyd S, Lieskovsky G, et al. Lower urinary tract reconstruction following cystectomy: experience and results in 126 patients using the Kock ileal reservoir with bilateral uretero-ileourethrostomy. J Urol (in press). Copyright by Williams & Wilkins.)

divided, and these are tagged and protected under a towel during pouch construction.

Maintenance of the intussuscepted ileal valve is critical to the prevention of reflux and the ability of the pouch to expand up to an adequate volume. Approximately 8 cm of mesentery is stripped off the serosa of the ileum adjacent to the pouch, according to the method originally described by Hendren. At least one or two vascular arcades are left intact, and a 2-cm wide strip of polyglycolic acid mesh (PGA) soaked in tetracycline (250 mg in 10 ml saline) is passed through the next window of Deaver. With intussusception, the PGA mesh will be brought up adjacent to the pouch wall, where it is fixed to the seromuscular wall with interrupted 2-0 chromic catgut sutures. This technique helps to fix the valve in place and prevent extussusception.

Three rows of 4.8 mm-stainless steel, nonhemostatic, and noncrushing staples must be used to further fix the intussusception. It is important to use the pin of the stapling device to avoid misaligned staples, but the pinhole must be carefully closed with 2-0 chromic catgut to prevent a fistula at the base of the nipple valve. Alternatively, a stapling apparatus that does not use a pin can be used, avoiding this potential complication. We use either the PI-55 automatic stapler or the PL450 Proximate with manufacturer-provided custom cartridges in which the six most proximal staples have been removed (plus two of the four rows of the PL450 Proximate). The staples at the end of the nipple do not contribute to maintenance of the intussusception and may form a nidus for stone formation.

The third row of staples fixes the intussuscepted nipple valve to the back wall of the pouch. The anvil of the stapling device is passed between the walls of the intussuscepted nipple from outside the pouch. Only two bowel layers are included in the staple line, and these staples will not be exposed to urine. A full cartridge is used here to ensure fixation of the base of the nipple.

The pouch is closed transversely, leaving a 2-cm opening at the end of the suture line in the corner opposite the afferent limb. The ureters are anastomosed to the afferent limb in a single-layer mucosa-to-mucosa anastomosis using 4-0 PGA suture. No. 8 infant feeding catheters are placed in the ureters before the anastomoses are completed and are passed into the pouch and out the opening. They will be secured to the urethral catheter with a 3-0 nylon suture before completion of the urethral anastomosis.

The pouch is then rotated down to the urethral stump, with the suture line anterior and the mesentery posterior. The ureters make a gentle turn and should lie without any acute angulation (Fig. 2). The previously placed 2-0 chromic sutures are then positioned circumferentially around the new "bladder neck," and a No. 24 French soft Simplastic hematuria catheter is placed before the sutures are tied down.

The pelvis is routinely drained with a large Hemovac suction catheter, which is removed in 24 hours, and a large Penrose drain. We leave the urethral catheter and Penrose drain for 3 weeks after surgery, removing them

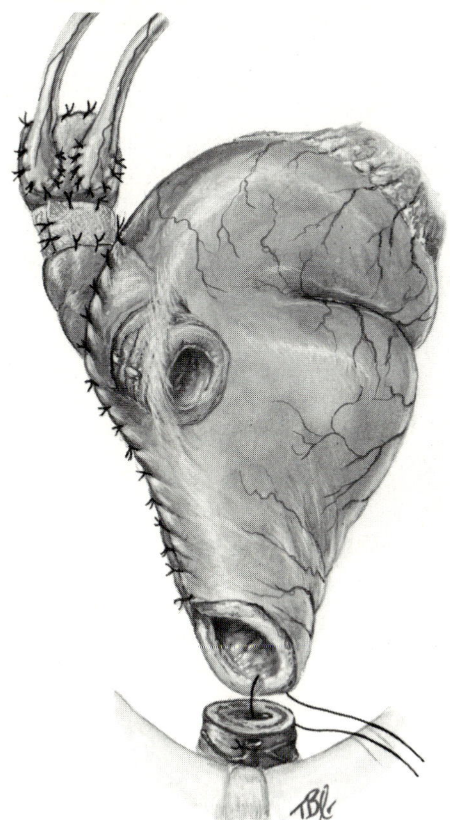

Figure 2 Completed pouch as it lies in the pelvis. The mesentery is posterior and the suture line anterior. (Republished with permission by Skinner DG, Lieskovsky G, Boyd S. Continent urinary diversion. J Urol 1989; 141:1323. Copyright by Williams & Wilkins.)

with the attached ureteral stents after a Kock-o-gram demonstrates no leakage from the pouch. If leakage is seen, we typically remove the catheter and stents and then replace a catheter for an additional week or until the Penrose drainage stops.

RESULTS

Complications

Early complications occurred in 14 of the 126 patients (11.1 percent), with two postoperative deaths. Complications included fatal cardiac arrhythmia (one), fatal stroke (one), prolonged ileus (two), myocardial infarct (one), pelvic bleeding (four), leak from a gastrostomy tube site (one), fascial dehiscence (one), urinoma requiring drainage (one), pyelonephritis due to an obstructed stent (one), and rectoreservoir fistula requiring temporary colostomy (one). Average postoperative stay was 8 days for patients with no complications and 18 days for those with nonfatal complications.

Late complications requiring rehospitalization have been relatively few. We have not yet observed any ureteroileal anastomotic strictures, although we expect

these to occur in approximately 3 percent of patients on the basis of previous experience. Most patients have sterile urine (as opposed to most cutaneous Kock pouch patients who have chronic bacterial colonization), and pyelonephritis has not been observed. To date, only one patient has developed a stone in the pouch, which was managed endoscopically. Metabolic electrolyte abnormalities have also not been seen so far. However, we anticipate that some patients may require vitamin B_{12} supplementation owing to the amount of distal ileum used for the pouch.

Continence

Patients void by Valsalva maneuver and typically have considerable incontinence when the catheter is initially removed. They are carefully instructed in Kegel exercises, and patient motivation is clearly a factor in the speed of achieving continence. All patients are taught intermittent catheterization preoperatively and are sent home with a No. 18 French coudé catheter to be used in case of retention. Four patients have required chronic intermittent catheterization because of incomplete emptying of the reservoir, and three others catheterize occasionally because of mucus or a sensation of poor emptying.

Information regarding continence was available from 117 of the 124 patients who survived the operation. The remaining seven died of metastatic disease before information was obtained. The results are detailed in Table 1.

Overall daytime continence was excellent in 93 percent, satisfactory in 2 percent, and poor in 5 percent. Nighttime continence was excellent in 18 percent, satisfactory in 68 percent, and poor in 14 percent. Only three patients chose to have an artificial urinary sphincter implanted, all because of nighttime incontinence. These patients generally activate it only at night and have experienced no complications relating to the sphincter.

Pelvic Recurrence

Pelvic recurrence of malignancy has occurred in five patients to date (4 percent), 4 to 8 months after surgery. A change in voiding pattern, with a new onset of difficulty in emptying the reservoir, was the initial symptom in all five patients. In spite of aggressive therapy with radiation, surgery, and/or chemotherapy in four patients, none has been cured of the malignancy, and four have died within 8 to 16 months of metastatic disease. This is similar to our past experience with locally recurrent invasive bladder cancer. Although the management of pelvic recurrence may be complicated by involvement of the reservoir, the incidence of such recurrence does not seem to be increased by this form of diversion.

In patients with carcinoma in situ of the bladder or prostatic urethra in the cystectomy specimen, we recommend regular surveillance with urethral washings for cytology. We expect a 7 to 10 percent incidence of

Table 1 Continence after Urethral Kock Pouch Urinary Diversion (N = 117)

Daytime	
Completely dry (no protection)	109 (93%)
by 3 months	42
by 6 months	58
after 6 months	9
Occasional accidents	2 (2%)
Incontinent or frequent accidents	6 (5%)
Nighttime	
Completely dry	21 (18%)
by 3 months	11
by 6 months	7
after 6 months	3
Dry with wakening 1–3 times/night	79 (68%)
or <3 accidents/night:	
by 3 months	11
by 6 months	58
after 6 months	10
Incontinent	17 (14%)

carcinoma in situ developing in the urethra in such patients, requiring urethrectomy and conversion to a cutaneous form of diversion. We have not seen this complication so far. If carcinoma in situ is noted to be present preoperatively on prostatic urethral biopsy, the patient undergoes en bloc urethrectomy at the time of cystectomy, with cutaneous urinary diversion.

REMARKS

Our experience with this adaptation of the Kock pouch has been extremely positive, with excellent patient acceptance and very few postoperative complications. Early concerns about inability to empty such a low-pressure reservoir have not been justified. Similarly, the efficacy of the cancer operation does not appear to be compromised in properly selected patients. The biggest drawback to the operation continues to be nighttime incontinence, which often requires that the patient get up once or twice during the night to remain dry. However, this appears to be remarkably well tolerated in men in this age group.

Lower urinary tract reconstruction with the urethral Kock pouch is currently our diversion of choice for men undergoing cystectomy in whom the above-mentioned conditions are satisfied. We consider it a very important addition to the options available to the urologist undertaking reconstructive surgery.

SUGGESTED READING

Kock NG, Nilsson AE, Nilsson LO, et al. Urinary diversion via a continent ileal reservoir: clinical results in 12 patients. J Urol 1982; 128:469.

Skinner DG, Boyd SD, Lieskovsky G. Technique of continent lower urinary tract reconstruction with Kock pouch urethrostomy following cystectomy. Videotape. St. Paul: Marketing Communications, 3M Medical-Surgical Division.

Skinner DG, Lieskovsky G, Boyd SD. Technique of creation of a continent internal reservoir (Kock pouch) for urinary diversion. Urol Clin North Am 1984; 11:741.

Skinner DG, Lieskovsky G, Boyd SD. Continent urinary diversion. J Urol 1989; 141:1323.

STAGE A1 PROSTATIC ADENOCARCINOMA

H. BALLENTINE CARTER, M.D.
PATRICK C. WALSH, M.D.

Stage A prostate cancer is defined as cancer discovered at the time of simple prostatectomy for benign prostatic hyperplasia (BPH) in a man who reveals no suspicion of cancer on rectal examination. These cancers are thought to arise anteriorly in the periurethral glands where BPH begins, compared with most prostate cancers, which arise peripherally and closer to the rectum. This explains why stage A cancers are not palpable and are discovered during surgery for benign disease. Approximately 10 percent of patients who undergo simple prostatectomy for BPH are found to harbor prostate cancer, and stage A cancers account for around 20 percent of the 100,000 newly diagnosed prostate cancers each year. Currently there is no universally agreed upon method of subdividing stage A cancers into stages A1 and A2; however, the distinction is important because the natural histories of stages A1 and A2 differ. Since recommendations for therapy must be based on knowledge of the natural history of a disease, this chapter discusses what has been learned about the natural history of stage A1 prostate cancer, using the definition proposed at Johns Hopkins Hospital, and then discusses current thinking with regard to the management of stage A1 disease.

DEFINITION AND NATURAL HISTORY

In 1975, Hugh J. Jewett proposed that stage A cancers be subdivided into focal, low-grade tumors (stage A1) and diffuse, high-grade tumors (stage A2), basing his proposal on the observation that diffuse, high-grade tumors behave aggressively compared with focal, low-grade tumors. Although this was an important observation, the limitation of this categorization was the lack of a quantitative method for distinguishing stage A1 from stage A2 prostate cancer. In 1981, studies at Johns Hopkins Hospital showed that the morphometric deter-

mination of the percentage of specimen involved with tumor was the most accurate predictor of disease progression in stage A cancer. If 5 percent or less of the simple prostatectomy specimen is involved with tumor, 2 percent of patients followed longer than 4 years progress if untreated, and if more than 5 percent of the specimen is involved with tumor, one third of patients have disease progression if untreated. Thus, we believe that determination of the percentage of the simple prostatectomy specimen involved with cancer is a good method of distinguishing stage A1 from stage A2, using a 5 percent cut-off. The grade of the tumor, if not poorly differentiated, does not help predict which men will have tumor progression. However, if the tumor is poorly differentiated (Gleason score of 8–10), this portends a greater risk of progression even if 5 percent or less of the specimen is involved with cancer. Therefore, if 5 percent or less of a simple prostatectomy specimen is involved with tumor and the tumor is not of high grade (Gleason score of 2–7), we believe that this tumor should be staged as A1 prostate cancer. If more than 5 percent of the specimen is involved with tumor no matter what the grade, or if the tumor is of high grade no matter what percentage of the specimen is involved with tumor, we believe the tumor should be staged as A2.

This definition suggests that stage A1 prostate cancer behaves in a benign fashion. However, the long-term outcome for men with stage A1 prostate cancer is an important question, since the peak age of prostate cancer in the United States is 70 to 74 years and the life expectancy of a 70-year-old American male is 11 years. Studies addressing this question at Johns Hopkins Hospital and elsewhere have shown that approximately 16 percent of men with stage A1 prostate cancer who are untreated and remain at risk long term (8 to 10 years) have progression of disease. In the Johns Hopkins series, 75 percent of the men with progression died of prostate cancer. Thus, men with stage A1 prostate cancer are not entirely risk free, but most of these do not need therapy. How then does one select appropriate treatment for a man with stage A1?

CHOICE OF TREATMENT

With regard to the selection of appropriate therapy for a man with stage A1 prostate cancer, two questions need to be answered: (1) which men will progress and therefore may benefit from further therapy?; and (2) what is the best therapy for localized prostate cancer?

In trying to answer the first question, we have attempted to predict progression in untreated men with stage A1 prostate cancer using the percentage of the simple prostatectomy specimen involved with tumor, the tumor volume (grams of tumor) removed at the time of simple prostatectomy, and the tumor grade determined from the simple prostatectomy specimen. In 50 percent of our patients who progressed without therapy, less than 1 percent of the simple prostatectomy specimen was involved with tumor, and in 75 percent there were well-differentiated tumors (Gleason score of 2–4). Therefore, the percentage of specimen involved with tumor and tumor grade are not predictive of disease progression. Tumor volume or grams of tumor removed at the time of simple prostatectomy do not predict progression any better than percentage of specimen involved with tumor. Therefore, there are currently no pathologic predictors of tumor progression in stage A1 prostate cancer. For this reason, we believe that men who have stage A1 and whose age and state of health place them at risk in the long term (8 to 10 years) should be offered definitive treatment. Men who meet the above criteria are usually younger than 70 years of age and are otherwise healthy. If age and coexisting medical problems (e.g., cardiovascular disease, pulmonary disease) make it unlikely that a man with stage A1 prostate cancer will be at risk long term, observation is a reasonable course of action.

The best therapy for any localized cancer is one that completely eliminates all cancer cells with the lowest morbidity. Options for treatment in a man with stage A1 prostate cancer include radiation therapy and radical prostatectomy. Unfortunately, there are no well-randomized prospective studies comparing these different forms of therapy for men with stage A1 prostate cancer. However, removal of the prostate gland is the only therapy available that ensures eradication of all cancer cells if the cancer is truly organ confined.

Radiation therapy for localized prostatic cancer is associated with positive prostatic biopsies after completion of treatment in up to 90 percent of patients. The significance of residual cancer after radiation therapy has been demonstrated by a greater prevalence of disease progression in men with positive prostate biopsies compared with those without positive biopsies. This suggests that prostatic cancers are heterogeneous with respect to radiation sensitivity, and that some men who have organ-confined disease will demonstrate disease progression from residual radioresistant cancer. At present there is no way to predict which cancers will be treated successfully by radiation therapy. Furthermore, if this form of therapy fails to eradicate the tumor, removal of the prostate after radiation results in greater morbidity than extirpation of the gland in a nonradiated field. Finally, radiation therapy for prostate cancer is associated with a 4 to 5 percent prevalence of significant complications involving the urinary tract and bowel.

Sexual dysfunction is thought to occur in around 40 percent of men after radiation therapy.

Radical prostatectomy, or removal of the entire prostate gland and seminal vesicles, offers the greatest chance for cure in men with organ-confined disease, since no cancer cells remain after therapy. Approximately 92 percent of men diagnosed with stage A1 prostate cancer after simple prostatectomy have the disease pathologically confined to the prostate, and therefore most of these should be cured by surgery. In experienced hands, this form of therapy is extremely well tolerated and associated with a mortality rate of less than 1 percent. Virtually all men are continent 9 months after surgery, and in stage A1 disease, approximately 90 percent of men retain potency as a result of the modifications of radical prostatectomy that preserve the nerves responsible for erection.

In summary, since there are no pathologic predictors of progression in stage A1 prostate cancer, we believe that men who remain at risk for long-term progression should be offered additional therapy after simple prostatectomy. We also believe that radical prostatectomy offers men with organ-confined prostate cancer the best chance of cure with low morbidity. Our experience with this form of management in 66 men with stage A1 prostate cancer has reinforced our bias. We have found in reviewing the prostatectomy specimens from these 66 men that the majority (more than 90 percent) have residual tumor remaining after simple prostatectomy, which is usually located anteriorly. This suggests that a repeat transurethral resection after diagnosis of stage A1 disease, as advocated by some, will not remove all remaining tumor and will not predict the presence of residual tumor because of an inaccessible location.

FUTURE DIRECTION

Because of our inability to predict which individuals will progress if untreated, we currently recommend treatment for a large number of men with stage A1 disease who do not need therapy. Prostate-specific antigen (PSA), a protein produced by prostatic epithelial cells only and detectable by serum assay, may be helpful in choosing appropriate therapy for men with stage A1 disease. It has been found that serum PSA levels correlate with prostate cancer volume. However, since PSA is produced by both benign and malignant prostatic epithelium, a single PSA level does not reflect cancer volume alone. Recently we have evaluated the ability of PSA to predict residual tumor volume in 22 stage A1 prostate cancer patients. In these men, a significant portion of benign prostatic epithelium had been removed by simple prostatectomy, and thus one would anticipate that the correlation between PSA and tumor volume would be greater than if the benign epithelium were present. We found that if the serum PSA was 1 ng or less per milliliter after simple prostatectomy, all men had a residual tumor volume of less than 0.5 ml, and that if the serum PSA was greater than 10 ng per milliliter, all men had a residual tumor volume of more than 0.5 ml. A serum PSA level between 1 and 10 ng per milliliter was not helpful in predicting residual tumor volume in these patients. The significance of a residual tumor volume of less than 0.5 ml in a man with prostate cancer is that the volume of cancer has to more than double to reach a volume associated with the risk of aggressive behavior (e.g., capsular penetration).

The ability to predict residual tumor volume in stage A1 prostate cancer would be beneficial only if there were a means of detecting tumor growth should it occur. Several clinical observations suggest that serial PSA measurements can detect the growth of residual tumor: (1) it is known that serum PSA increases with increasing tumor volume, (2) the contribution of cancer to serum PSA is estimated to be ten times greater than that of BPH on a volume-for-volume basis, and (3) the doubling time of prostate cancer is estimated to be 50 to 200 days compared with the doubling time of BPH, which is estimated to be 100 times longer. On the basis of these observations, one would anticipate that the slope of the curve representing serial measurements of PSA over time would be greater for stage A1 patients with progressive tumor growth than for stage A1 patients with residual BPH tissue and small-volume cancer in whom the disease remained quiescent.

In conclusion, serum PSA may be useful in stage A1 prostate cancer to select a group of patients who have minimal residual disease after simple prostatectomy. Serial PSA measurements may be useful in following these men in order to detect disease progression early at a curable stage.

SUGGESTED READING

Epstein JI, Walsh PC. The classification and prognosis of untreated stage A1 and A2 prostate cancer with a comparison of their histologic findings at radical prostatectomy. In: Coffey DS, Resnick MI, Dorr FA, Karr JP, eds. A multidisciplinary analysis of controversies in the management of prostate cancer. New York: Plenum Press, 1988:41.

Stamey TA. Prostate cancer: some basic clinical and morphometric observations. Monogr Urol 1989; 10:79–91.

Walsh PC, Oesterling JE, Lepor H. Radical prostatectomy for the treatment of localized prostatic cancer. In: Coffey DS, Resnick MI, Dorr FA, Karr JP, eds. A multidisciplinary analysis of controversies in the management of prostate cancer. New York: Plenum Press, 1988:123.

STAGE A2 PROSTATIC ADENOCARCINOMA

KEVIN T. McVARY, M.D.
JOHN T. GRAYHACK, M.D.

Adenocarcinoma of the prostate is the most common cancer among American males. It has achieved parity with colorectal carcinoma as the second most common cause of cancer death in males. Unsuspected carcinoma is identified in about 30 percent of autopsy specimens in men older than 50 years of age. This incidence increases progressively, reaching more than 90 percent of males in the ninth decade of life. In a recent American College of Surgeons survey of practice patterns in the United States, carcinoma of the prostate was unsuspected clinically in 25 percent of the patients in whom it was identified. The diagnosis in these patients was made on the basis of histologic examination of the tissue removed at the time of prostatectomy to relieve bladder neck obstruction from presumed benign disease.

NATURAL HISTORY OF STAGE A PROSTATE CARCINOMA

The prevalence of clinically unsuspected prostate cancer far exceeds its clinical incidence. Clearly, the failure to identify a cancer relates to the nature of the diagnostic techniques available and employed, the restricted period for tumor growth and patient observation, and the biologic characteristics of the cancer. Whether the transition from a clinically unsuspected to a clinically manifest lesion is a function of the duration of observation or a change in the genetic or phenotypic phenotype status of the cancer cells is unknown.

Carcinoma of the prostate recognized histologically but unsuspected clinically is designated stage A. It represents a diagnostic error discovered on evaluation of tissue removed to correct obstruction of the bladder outlet with a clinical diagnosis of benign prostatic hyperplasia (BPH). Its incidence in this setting is roughly half of that anticipated from reported autopsy experiences in the corresponding age groups. Failure to identify a carcinoma that is present may be related to its peripheral location, its size, the extent of the prostatectomy performed, or the completeness of histologic evaluation of resected material. The relationship between clinically occult (stage A) carcinoma recognized by an operation designed for benign disease and biologically significant cancers is an important unknown. Since most prostatic cancer is believed to originate in the peripheral prostate, the possibility that a surgical procedure designed to remove periurethral tissue might not identify or completely remove cancer cells prone to clinical progression warrants concern. Morphologic studies from radical prostatectomy specimens in stage A patients suggest that residual stage A cancers are located anteromedially and apically. Clinically suspected tumors (stage B) tend to be in the periphery near the rectal surface. In both instances, a high incidence of multicentric lesions has been noted. Stage A tumors tend to invade the anterior fibromuscular stroma and BPH nodules, with limited involvement of the posterior, peripheral, readily palpable portion of the gland (Fig. 1). Whether cancers originating in different anatomic locations of the prostate have differences in biologic potential is not known. Clearly, some clinically unrecognized carcinomas grow and metastasize as indicated by pelvic node involvement and progression of disease.

PREDICTION OF BIOLOGIC ACTIVITY

Identification of patients with biologically aggressive (A2) versus biologically indolent (A1) stage A

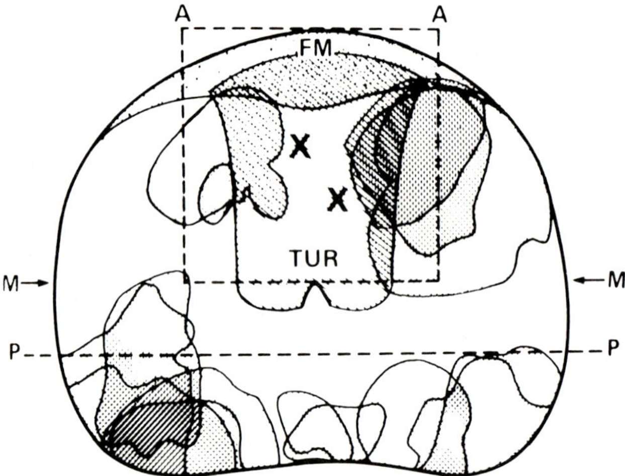

Figure 1 Transverse plane through the midportion of the prostate shows posterior locations of ten stage B carcinomas of less than 1.2 ml (posterior to line P-P), compared with anteromedial locations of residual carcinoma at prostatectomy in seven small stage A cancers (within box A-A). The outline of maximal transurethral resection (TUR) tissue defect in these seven cases is indicated by crosshatching. X = presumed locations within the transurethral resection defect of two completely resected cancers; FM = anterior fibromuscular stoma; M = midline of glandular prostate. (Republished with permission by McNeal JE, Price HM, Redwine EA, et al. Stage A versus stage B adenocarcinoma of the prostate: morphological comparison and biological significance. J Urol 1988; 139:61–65. Copyright by Williams & Wilkins.)

tumor is important clinically to help guide the selection of treatment. Both cellular characteristics and an assessment of tumor mass or volume are currently used in this attempt. Light microscopic evaluation of cellular characteristics (grade) is an established method of attempting to predict biologic behavior. Various criteria have been employed, including acinar pattern and various aspects of cellular detail. At the extremes (for example, Gleason score sums 2 to 4 versus 8 to 10), grading can usually separate indolent from aggressive lesions. However, most cases are in the intermediate grade groups (e.g., Gleason sums 5 to 7) where prediction of biologic activity is clearly equivocal. Subjectivity of histologic grades increases the risk of error. The assessment of ploidy by flow cytometry or individual cell assessment is currently being explored to aid in predicting biologic activity, and seems to hold enough potential to supply useful information to warrant consideration for use.

Staging is an attempt to identify the phase of the natural history that is present in a clinical setting. One aspect of stage is an assessment of the local tumor mass. Available data indicate that it is unusual for tumors less than 1 cm in diameter to metastasize. Attempts to assess tumor mass in stage A tumors currently include counting the number of chips involved, attempting to assess the percentage of resected tissue that is malignant, and trying to reconstruct the resected tumor to calculate volume.

At this time, clinically unsuspected tumors are divided into two subcategories (A1 and A2) based on tumor mass and tumor grade. Patients with stage A1 carcinoma are judged to have minimal risk of clinically significant progression of disease within a 10-year period, but those with A2 are judged to have neoplasms with a biologic potential comparable with those of prostatic carcinomas that have produced palpable changes. Patients with poorly differentiated tumors (Gleason score sums 8 to 10) are universally excluded from the A1 substage. In contrast to some authors, we also exclude patients who have tumors with Gleason sums 5 to 7, reserving this substage for patients with well-differentiated tumors (Gleason sums 2 to 4). However, the criteria for evaluating mass vary. Some limit the stage A1 designation to individuals with carcinoma in no more than three resected fragments; others propose that the designation be based on a tumor volume of less than or equal to 1 ml. We have taken involvement of 5 percent or less of the removed tissue, as proposed by Cantrell and associates, as a criterion to separate A1 and A2 substages. Our practice has also been to exclude from the stage A1 group any patient who has had all or almost all of a sizable fragment replaced by malignancy, because of the high probability that an existing intragland lump (Fig. 2) has been only partially sampled. In an enucleated adenoma, the relationship of the carcinoma to the margin of the resected tissue is an important consideration.

ADDITIONAL EVALUATIVE PROCEDURES

Recognition of an unsuspected carcinoma reinforces the need to examine the entire prostatectomy specimen histologically. A histologic grade should be assigned, and either the percentage of involvement or volume of the disease should be calculated. Staging studies, including measurements of serum acid, alkaline phosphatase, and prostate-specific antigen (PSA), bone scan, and x-ray examination should be performed as for any prostate cancer patient. These studies may indicate disseminated tumor, thus excluding a patient from stage A classification.

The propensity of transurethral resection of the prostate (TURP) to understage incidental cancers is another point of controversy. Some reports advocate repeat TURP to identify patients with more extensive disease. However, many judge that the low incidence of upstaging does not support the routine use of repeat resection. It is not our practice to employ routine repeat TURP for staging purposes. Recently, routine re-evaluation of patients with stage A carcinoma by transrectal ultrasonography has been advocated. The experience with this procedure has been insufficient to allow critical evaluation. Selective employment of prostatic ultrasonography and possible biopsy is worth considering. Patients who are designated stage A, on the basis of initial or repeat evaluation, require clinical re-evaluation including a history, digital rectal examination, and blood marker studies two to three times per year. We still undertake acid phosphatase and PSA determination at these return visits. Serial observations of PSA may aid in identifying patients in whom secondary imaging and tissue sampling techniques may be needed. Identification of residual tumor indicates the probability of increased potential for a biologically active (stage A2) tumor.

The failure to recognize regional lymph node metastases on clinical evaluation clearly does not exclude their presence. On surgical staging, stage A2 lesions have approximately a 25 percent chance of lymph node metastasis, whereas stage A1 lesions have a 2 percent chance of disease in the nodes. This observed difference in the incidence of regional node involvement confirms the validity of the separation of stage A into substages.

TREATMENT AND OUTCOME

In our opinion, once the histologic and staging assessment is complete, the practice of categorizing patients into those with a high probability of a biologically aggressive tumor (stage A2) requiring serious consideration of active intervention, and those with a high probability of a biologically indolent carcinoma (stage A1) often amenable to assessment over time is appropriate. As for patients with clinically recognizable carcinoma, age and general health status should be taken into account in formulating a treatment plan for the individual patient. Lowe and Listrom constructed

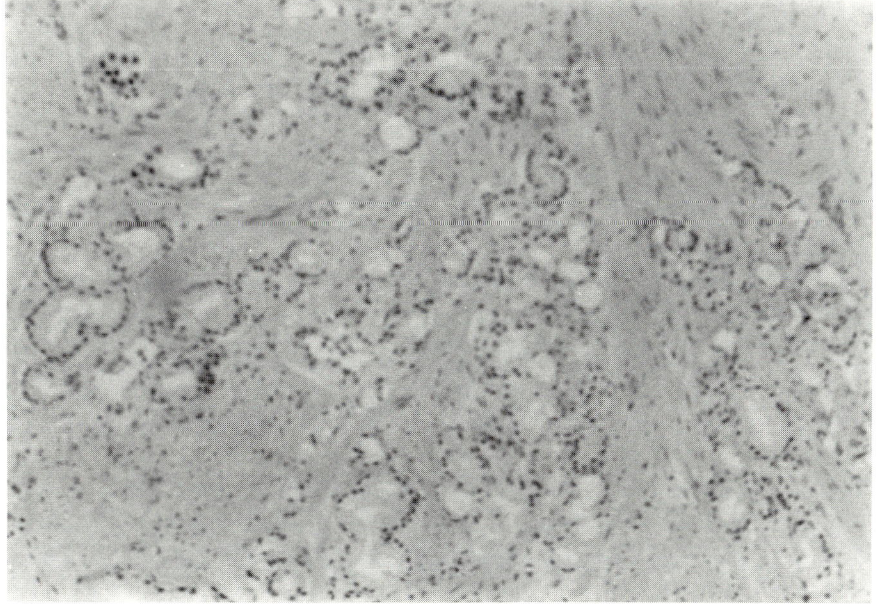

Figure 2 Photomicrograph of prostate tissue resected for presumed benign disease in a 66-year-old man. Note the relatively large lump of low-grade adenocarcinoma (Gleason sum = 1 + 1). The patient was noted to have 4 percent of resected material involved with cancer. He underwent radical retropubic prostatectomy. Examination of the specimen revealed multifocal and diffuse involvement with similarly low-grade lesions (magnification of originals, 40×).

probability tables for disease progression at 5 and 10 years based on increasing age, Gleason score, and percentage of tumor involvement (Tables 1 and 2). These tables assist one in recommending definitive local therapy in high-risk patients.

Generally, therapy for patients with stage A disease centers on attempts to achieve a cure by surgical excision (radical prostatectomy) or radiation therapy. Our assessment of the available data and our own experience leads us to prefer radical retropubic prostatectomy (RRP) to irradiation because of its inherent advantages in long-term tumor-free survival and quality of life. We consider both approaches as potentially curative, although with appreciable differences in tumor-free survival in patients with low-stage disease. In our opinion, the younger the patient, the greater the relative advan-

tage of radical prostatectomy. Patients with a less than 10-year expected survival are rarely encouraged to proceed with RRP. To reduce periprostatic tissue reaction, we advise patients to allow post-TURP healing to occur (6 to 8 weeks) before either RRP or radiation therapy is initiated.

Although most patients have a relatively uneventful hospital course and a satisfactory surgical result, RRP has been associated with complications of varying degrees of severity. On the basis of available data, a mortality rate of 1 percent or less seems to be a reasonable expectation. With regard to intraoperative complications, the risk of ureteral or rectal injury may be slightly increased in patients subjected to RRP after TURP compared with those who undergo only a biopsy. Unequivocal identification of the ureteral orifices, their

Table 1 Probability Table for Disease Progression at 5 Years for Individual Patients of a Given Age, Gleason Score, and Extent

Age at Diagnosis	Grade	Extent	Probability of Progression to Disease
		Time to Progression 5 years	
60	2,3	<1	0.03
	2,3	1–5	0.08
	4	<1	0.06
	4	1–5	0.14
	4	>5	0.31
	5,6	1–5	0.24
	5,6	>5	0.49
	7,8,9	1–5	0.39
	7,8,9	>5	0.70
65	2,3	<1	0.04
	2,3	1–5	0.09
	4	<1	0.07
	4	1–5	0.16
	4	>5	0.35
	5,6	1–5	0.27
	5,6	>5	0.54
	7,8,9	1–5	0.43
	7,8,9	>5	0.75
70	2,3	<1	0.05
	2,3	1–5	0.11
	4	<1	0.08
	4	1–5	0.18
	4	>5	0.39
	5,6	1–5	0.31
	5,6	>5	0.59
	7,8,9	1–5	0.48
	7,8,9	>5	0.80
75	2,3	<1	0.05
	2,3	1–5	0.12
	4	<1	0.09
	4	1–5	0.21
	4	>5	0.44
	5,6	1–5	0.35
	5,6	>5	0.65
	7,8,9	1–5	0.54
	7,8,9	>5	0.85

Table 2 Probability Table for Disease Progression at 10 Years for Individual Patients of a Given Age, Gleason Score, and Extent.

Age at Diagnosis	Grade	Extent	Probability of Progression to Disease
		Time to Progression 10 years	
60	2,3	<1	0.06
	2,3	1–5	0.15
	4	<1	0.11
	4	1–5	0.25
	4	>5	0.51
	5,6	1–5	0.41
	5,6	>5	0.72
	7,8,9	1–5	0.61
	7,8,9	>5	0.90
65	2,3	<1	0.07
	2,3	1–5	0.17
	4	<1	0.13
	4	1–5	0.29
	4	>5	0.56
	5,6	1–5	0.46
	5,6	>5	0.77
	7,8,9	1–5	0.67
	7,8,9	>5	0.93
70	2,3	<1	0.08
	2,3	1–5	0.19
	4	<1	0.15
	4	1–5	0.32
	4	>5	0.62
	5,6	1–5	0.51
	5,6	>5	0.82
	7,8,9	1–5	0.72
	7,8,9	>5	0.95
75	2,3	<1	0.10
	2,3	1–5	0.22
	4	<1	0.17
	4	1–5	0.36
	4	>5	0.67
	5,6	1–5	0.56
	5,6	>5	0.86
	7,8,9	1–5	0.77
	7,8,9	>5	0.97

Republished with permission by Lowe BA, Listrom MB. Incidental carcinoma of the prostate: an analysis of the predictors of progression. J Urol 1988; 140:1340–1344. Copyright by Williams & Wilkins.

Republished with permission by Lowe BA, Listrom MB. Incidental carcinoma of the prostate: an analysis of the predictors of progression. J Urol 1988; 140:1340–1344. Copyright by Williams & Wilkins.

relationship to the bladder neck as assessed with preoperative cystoscopy, and the use of intraoperative chromogenes reduce the risk of ureteral injury (reported to be approximately 1.5 percent). Ensuring a complete incision through the posterior bladder wall to facilitate separation of the seminal vesicles and bladder also lowers the risk of ureteral injury. The risk of rectal injury can be minimized by judicious use of a combination of sharp and blunt dissection under vision to establish the proper plane between the rectum and Denonvilliers' fascia; at times this is difficult in these patients.

Postoperatively, stress urinary incontinence of varying degrees is noted commonly, but this resolves within 8 to 10 weeks in about 80 percent of patients. The remainder take up to 6 months to regain satisfactory control. Permanent two-pad or more urinary incontinence is infrequent, approximating 2 percent. Current experience indicates that this incidence is not increased as a result of the preceding TURP. Postoperative potency is inversely correlated with the age of the patient and with preservation of one as compared to two nerve bundles. Potency rates approximating 60 to 70 percent have been reported in stage A patients undergoing RRP. Selective nerve sacrifice, as we now commonly recommend for palpably identifiable carcinoma of the prostate, is usually not feasible in patients with clinically nondetectable lesions. The advantages and disadvantages with regard to potency and surgical excision of the neoplasm need to be presented to the patient to help him determine his priorities. Current experience indicates that radical prostatectomy can be performed with limited risk and a high probability of maintenance of a satisfactory quality of life in patients with stage A carcinoma of the prostate. Comparative survival rates with and without evidence of neoplasm with regard to surgical excision, radiation therapy, and observation are not available. The limited retrospective observations of Lowe and Listrom indicate an advantage for treatment and an advantage of surgical over radiation approaches. However, most patients with stage A disease are probably best managed by careful observation. Identification of those who have significant potential for progressive disease (stage A2) and therefore are prime candidates for active intervention is the foremost challenge in the management of individuals with histologically documented and clinically unsuspected disease. When the need for treatment (either immediate or delayed) is determined by a high probability of progressive disease, it can be advised in the knowledge of its limited risk and the likelihood of a disease-free survival.

FUTURE EFFORTS

The most logical way to reduce the presence of unsuspected carcinoma is to have an increased awareness of the possibility. The role of digital rectal examination, imaging studies including transrectal ultrasonography, and blood, urine, and prostate fluid tumor markers attempting to achieve this goal continues to evolve. The problem of recognition and identification of biologically aggressive as opposed to biologically indolent tumors is persistent and challenging. The increasing sophistication of histologic, genetic, and biochemical techniques in assessing clinical material holds promise of progress in this endeavor.

SUGGESTED READING

Blute ML, Nativ O, Zincke H, et al. Pattern of failure after radical retropubic prostatectomy for clinically and pathologically localized adenocarcinoma of the prostate: influence of tumor deoxyribonucleic acid ploidy. J Urol 1989; 142:1262–1265.

Bridges CH, Belville WD, Insalaco SI, Buck AS. Stage A prostatic carcinoma and repeat transurethral resection: a reappraisal 5 years later. J Urol 1983; 129:307–308.

Cantrell BB, DeKlerk DP, Eggleston JC, et al. Pathological factors that influence prognosis in stage A prostatic cancer: the influence of extent versus grade. J Urol 1981; 125:516–520.

Carroll PR, Leitner TC, Yen TSB, et al. Incidental carcinoma of the prostate: significance of staging transurethral resection. J Urol 1985; 133:811–814.

Lowe BA, Listrom MB. Incidental carcinoma of the prostate: an analysis of the predictors of progression. J Urol 1988; 140: 1340–1344.

Lowe BA, Listrom MD. Management of stage A prostate cancer with a high probability of progression. J Urol 1988; 140:1345–1347.

McNeal JE, Price HM, Redwine EA, et al. Stage A versus stage B adenocarcinoma of the prostate: morphological comparison and biological significance. J Urol 1988; 139:61–65.

STAGE B1 PROSTATIC ADENOCARCINOMA

HERBERT LEPOR, M.D.
PATRICK C. WALSH, M.D.

DEFINITION OF STAGE B1

Stage B adenocarcinoma of the prostate refers to disease that is confined within the prostatic capsule on rectal examination with no evidence of systemic metastases. It can be subdivided into two biologically meaningful subclasses based on local tumor burden: stage B1 and stage B2. Stage B1 represents tumor occupying less than one entire lobe of the prostate, and stage B2 represents tumor occupying one lobe or greater. This subclassification of stage B disease was devised by Jewett on the basis of a retrospective study of a large group of patients who underwent radical prostatectomy at The Johns Hopkins Hospital. In the most recent review of that series, only 6 percent of patients with B1 disease had involvement of the seminal vesicles, and the 15-year tumor-free survival rate was 51 percent, similar to the long-term survival rate in an age-matched group of patients without cancer. In stage B2 disease, 56 percent of patients had involvement of the seminal vesicles, and the 15-year tumor-free survival rate in this group was only 25 percent. Thus, the clinical finding of induration involving less than one entire lobe of the prostate identifies a group of patients who are likely to have organ-confined disease, and thus likely to achieve long-term tumor-free survival after appropriate therapy.

DIAGNOSIS

Men with stage B1 disease often have no symptoms, and thus the disease is usually diagnosed during a carefully performed rectal examination as part of a routine physical examination. During digital palpation of the prostate, the examiner should estimate the percentage of the prostate involved with induration and the presence of extension or fixation to the lateral pelvic side walls or to the seminal vesicles. Suspicious lesions are biopsied using core biopsy techniques or fine-needle aspiration. Core-needle biopsy not only confirms the presence of cancer, but gives additional information on the histologic grade of the tumor. It is unlikely that a high-grade clinical stage B1 lesion will prove to be pathologically confined to the prostate.

Once a diagnosis of adenocarcinoma of the prostate is confirmed pathologically, evaluate the patient for the presence of systemic metastases to pelvic lymph nodes or bone. Metastatic disease in pelvic lymph nodes has been reported to occur in 11 to 23 percent of patients with B1 tumors. Because the metastatic deposits in lymph nodes are frequently microscopic, it is difficult to identify them with lymphangiography or computed tomography (CT). For accurate staging of the pelvic lymph nodes, perform a diagnostic pelvic lymphadenectomy before a planned radical prostatectomy. To evaluate patients for the presence of systemic metastases, perform serum acid phosphatase and prostate specific antigen determinations and bone scans. Because persistently elevated serum acid phosphatase levels usually indicate extensive local and/or metastatic disease, we exclude such patients from consideration for definitive local therapy.

RATIONALE FOR RADICAL PROSTATECTOMY

The cure of prostatic cancer requires excision or destruction of all viable tumor cells. Since stage B1 disease is usually pathologically confined to the prostate, these patients are ideal candidates for radical prostatectomy. Although the optimal management of men with stage B1 carcinoma remains controversial, there is no evidence that any treatment other than radical prostatectomy produces better control of the primary tumor and of distant metastases. For this reason, radical prostatectomy remains the treatment of choice for men with stage B1 disease who are otherwise healthy and have a 10- to 15-year projected life span.

To demonstrate the value of radical surgery in the cure of patients with prostatic cancer, long-term tumor-free survival without adjunctive hormonal therapy should be demonstrated in patients who are carefully staged. Only two institutions have reported 15-year follow-up data on men undergoing radical prostatectomy for stage B1 disease that meet the above mentioned criteria. The 15-year tumor-free survival in the Johns Hopkins Hospital and Mason Clinic reports were 51 and 50 percent, respectively. The survival data for men with stage B1 disease in both series are identical to those for age-matched controls selected from the general population.

Radical prostatectomy may be performed perineally or retropubically. Advocates of the perineal approach emphasize the advantages afforded by the direct approach to the prostate and the ease of performing the urethrovesical anastomosis. They also emphasize that blood loss is less than with the retropubic approach. However, to gain this advantage the dissection is performed immediately adjacent to the prostatic capsule and inside the confines of the lateral pelvic fascia, which contains Santorini's plexus. The primary disadvantages of the perineal approach are the inability to perform a simultaneous staging pelvic lymphadenectomy, the risk to the patient's sexual function, and the skimpy soft tissue margins surrounding the prostate owing to the intrafascial dissection that is necessary to avoid injury to Santorini's plexus, and the need to separate the anterior and posterior layers of Denonvilliers' fascia in order to avoid rectal injury.

Because of unfamiliarity with the male perineum and increasing experience with pelvic surgery, many urologists have turned to the retropubic method for removal of the prostate. During this procedure, pelvic lymph nodes clinically involved with cancer can be recognized. Although the accuracy of frozen section analyses of lymph nodes has been questioned by several authors, a review of 310 staging pelvic lymphadenectomies at our institution demonstrated that frozen section evaluations were accurate in 299 (96.5 percent) of the cases. In a small number of patients in whom tumor was not identified by frozen sections, the average size of the metastatic focus not identified on frozen section was 1.4 mm. Because of the minimal volume of tumor in these patients, we feel that radical prostatectomy was not performed unnecessarily owing to the potential value for excellent local control with low morbidity. In our limited experience with radical prostatectomies performed in men with false-negative frozen sections, 75 percent of the patients who have been followed for longer than 6 years are free of disease. In addition to the ability to perform a simultaneous staging pelvic lymph node dissection, radical retropubic prostatectomy provides a wider berth in the dissection. The prostate is approached from outside the lateral pelvic fascia, and the dissection plane includes all layers of Denonvilliers' fascia. This provides wider margins of excision. In addition, the neurovascular bundles, which contain the branches of the pelvic plexus that innervate the corpora cavernosa, can be identified and preserved where indicated to preserve sexual function postoperatively. We reviewed the first 100 consecutive patients who underwent nerve-sparing radical prostatectomy at The Johns Hopkins Hospital. Based on careful pathologic evaluation of the specimens, there was no indication that the nerve-sparing modification compromised the adequacy of removal of the cancer, which is determined primarily by the extent of the tumor rather than the operative technique. Critics of the retropubic operation state that it is a more major procedure, that blood loss during or after the operation is greater, and that reconstruction of the vesical neck and anastomosis of the bladder to the urethra are generally more difficult. However, if the anatomy of the dorsal vein of the penis and Santorini's plexus is well understood, blood loss should be minimal. In addition, through the use of epidural anesthesia, bulldog clamps on the hypogastric arteries, and autotransfusion, the transfusion of heterologous blood should occur very rarely. Furthermore, because the urogenital diaphragm is not violated, the incidence of postoperative incontinence should approach zero.

In a personal series of 290 radical retropubic prostatectomies performed at the Johns Hopkins Hospital between 1982 and 1985, the in-hospital mortality was zero. There were no rectal injuries or other bowel complications. One patient sustained a ureteral injury that was easily corrected at the time of surgery with no sequelae. Three of the first 100 patients developed pulmonary emboli, and one died 3 weeks postoperatively while at home. In the next 170 patients there have been no recognized cases of thrombophlebitis or pulmonary emboli. No patient who has been followed for 1 year or longer is totally incontinent, no patient wears a urinary appliance, and no patient has undergone anti-incontinence surgery. Fewer than 5 percent of the patients wear a small pad in their trousers that may be changed once or twice daily. Impotence following radical prostatectomy prevented the wide-spread application of this very effective and safe treatment for localized prostatic cancer. However, using the newly described nerve-sparing technique, it is now possible to preserve sexual function in most patients. In 64 patients with stage B1 disease who were potent preoperatively, who have sexual partners, and who have been followed 1 year or longer, 81 percent are potent.

RATIONALE FOR RADIOTHERAPY

Since the cure of prostatic cancer requires the excision or destruction of all viable tumor cells, radiation therapy is a theoretical alternative to radical prostatectomy. Bagshaw reported the only series of patients with localized carcinoma of the prostate treated with radiation therapy, with 15-year survival data. The projected 15-year survival for stage B disease was 37 percent. Only six patients with B1 disease were at risk for 15 years. It is unclear in this report, however, what percentage of patients were treated with adjunctive hormonal therapy and what percentage were disease free. Although 15-year tumor-free survival data are not available for patients treated with interstitial implantation of radioactive seeds, the 5-year tumor-free survival rate for patients with clinical stage B1 disease (tumor occupying less than one entire lobe) following interstitial implantation of ^{125}I is 66 percent. These data are based on a very generous definition of tumor-free survival; i.e., if the patient has palpable tumor, but does not require a transurethral resection for the treatment of outlet obstructive symptoms, he is considered tumor free. The 5-year tumor-free survival rate following radical prostatectomy in comparable patients is 85 to 90 percent.

The value of radiotherapy for local control has been challenged owing to the high incidence of positive postradiation biopsies. Freiha and Bagshaw reported that the incidence of positive biopsies after external beam radiation in men with stage B disease was 50 percent. The presence of a positive biopsy after radiation therapy indicated a greater tendency for disease progression. Freiha and Bagshaw reported disease progression in 72 percent of men with positive biopsies compared with 24 percent of men with negative biopsies. A similar incidence of positive biopsies has been reported following interstitial irradiation.

For years radiotherapists have stressed the low morbidity of radiation therapy in the management of patients with prostatic cancer. This has been the major rationale for employing this technique in patients with stage B1 disease. The Patterns of Care Outcome Study reported a 4.5 percent incidence of major complications requiring readmission to the hospital; 2.6 percent required surgical intervention, and 1 of 619 patients died. The Joint Committee on Radiation Therapy reported on its large experience with external beam radiotherapy for prostatic cancer and described a 4.8 percent incidence of significant complications. The exact incidence of sexual dysfunction following external beam radiotherapy is unclear but is estimated to be approximately 50 percent. However, Goldstein and colleagues reported that sexual dysfunction occurred in 79 percent of patients treated with external beam radiotherapy. Many patients have selected radiotherapy in an effort to avoid the side effect of impotence. If the nerve-sparing technique of radical prostatectomy had been developed 20 years ago, it is unlikely that many patients with stage B1 disease would have been treated with radiotherapy.

The morbidity following interstitial implantation of ^{125}I has been reported. The incidence of major complications was pelvic abscess, 2 percent; pulmonary embolus, 1 percent; myocardial infarction, 1 percent; bladder neck contracture, 3.3 percent; urinary incontinence, 2.2 percent; and proctitis, 3 percent. Major rectal ulcer and/or prostatic urethrorectal fistula occurred in 3.2 percent. Potency was preserved in 78 percent of patients who survived 5 years without receiving adjunctive hormonal therapy. These early and late complications after interstitial implantation were thought to be fewer than those in a similar group of patients treated with external beam radiotherapy at their institution.

RATIONALE FOR OBSERVATION

Although long-term tumor-free survival has been demonstrated following prostatectomy for the treatment of localized prostatic cancer, some have attributed these results to the favorable natural history of prostatic cancer rather than to the therapeutic influence of surgery. In an effort to evaluate this possibility, the Veterans Administration Cooperative Urological Research Group (VACURG) undertook a randomized multicenter study comparing placebo and radical prostatectomy in patients with clinical stage A and B disease. Based on median follow-up intervals of 6.8 and 7.7 years for stages A and B, respectively, they concluded that survival and disease progression were similar in patients treated with either radical prostatectomy or placebo. This study has been criticized because of excessive protocol violations in the placebo group, the absence of staging pelvic lymphadenectomies and bone scans, the fact that 40 percent of stage A patients were stage A1, the short follow-up interval, and the failure to include progression of the primary lesion in the analysis of progression rates. Although treatment was stated to have been randomly assigned, six of the six poorly differentiated lesions (Gleason grade 8 to 10) in the stage B group were assigned to radical surgery. Indeed, the majority of disease progressions in the prostatectomy group occurred in these poorly differentiated tumors. We agree with Byar's impression that most treatment failures resulted from metastases that occurred before randomization. This study is of historical interest only, since today no one would subject a patient to radical prostatectomy without obtaining a bone scan or performing a staging pelvic lymphadenectomy. In view of the above-mentioned deficiencies of protocol design, it is unlikely that the VACURG study will ever provide meaningful insight into the management of patients with localized prostatic cancer.

DISCUSSION

Men with stage B1 adenocarcinoma of the prostate are ideal candidates for radical prostatectomy. Radical prostatectomy is a safe procedure that can be performed by the experienced surgeon with the assurance of preserving continence and the likelihood of preserving potency. The alternatives to radical prostatectomy are radiation therapy or no treatment. Historically, advocates of radiotherapy have contended that long-term survival and local control were comparable with those from radical surgery and that radiotherapy was better tolerated. These claims can no longer be substantiated. The long-term survival of men with stage B1 disease following radical prostatectomy is comparable with that of age-matched controls. Insufficient follow-up data are available to make a similar comparison with radiotherapy. However, at best, radiotherapy should be able to equal the effectiveness of surgery only in patients with B1 disease. The observation that only 50 percent of men with stage B lesions have persistent or viable tumor after radiotherapy, and the finding that these men are at increased risk of progression to systemic disease, raise questions on the potential of radiotherapy to achieve control of local and distant disease. The only randomized study that compares radical surgery and definitive radiotherapy in stages A2 and B disease has shown a significantly lower incidence of disease progression in the radical surgery group. The major complication rates for radical prostatectomy and definitive radiotherapy, when performed by experienced surgeons and radiotherapists, are comparable, and when radical prostatectomies are performed using the nerve-sparing technique it is likely that potency rates will be higher than in men treated with external beam radiotherapy. The decision to select radiotherapy in patients with stage B1 disease is no longer justified on the basis of survival, local control, or relative morbidity. Thus, the ability to perform radical prostatectomy with preservation of sexual function without compromising the efficacy of the procedure should encourage more physicians to offer this option to the young, healthy, sexually active patient, who is often the ideal candidate for the procedure.

STAGE B2 PROSTATIC ADENOCARCINOMA

PAUL C. PETERS, M.D.

This chapter is concerned with the management of pathologic stage B2 carcinoma of the prostate. This stage is defined as palpable disease with a nodule of 1.5 cm or greater confined to one lobe histologically, or disease involving both lobes but with negative lymph nodes and no invasion of the seminal vesicles or extension through the prostate capsule.

I am not aware of 15-year survival rates for the disease as defined. In my opinion, a lesion that has extended through the prostate capsule is a stage C lesion and should be so classified in outcome research. Walsh, in reviewing the experience at Johns Hopkins Hospital, reported only one patient surviving 15 years with clinical stage B2. Some of these were probably D1, because lymphadenectomy as done today was not performed in these patients and staging was less accurate. I prefer radical prostatectomy as the treatment of choice for pathologic stage B2. Nerve sparing is done only on the side opposite the palpable disease, and on neither side if it appears grossly that the lesion is extensive on both sides, especially near the apex of the prostate. External beam therapy is a second choice for treatment. In my experience, radiotherapists have more difficulty in controlling the larger lesions, and because of this, surgery is offered as the first alternative. The lesion is usually understaged. In 39 radical prostatectomies at our institution this year thought to be clinical B2 or B in which prostate-specific antigen (PSA) was less than 40, the acid phosphatase level was normal (less than 5.1 U), and the bone scan was negative, the lesion was more extensive in the prostate in 34 patients than thought clinically. Two of the cases showed seminal vesicle invasion microscopically. One was really a D1 (positive pelvic lymph node) and only two actually had about the amount of disease thought to be present by ultrasonography, digital rectal examination, PSA, acid phosphatase, and bone scan results.

Commonly, what is thought to be stage B2 clinically is really a stage C pathologically with extension either into the seminal vesicles microscopically or through the capsule of the prostate into the periprostatic fat. It is my practice to recommend external beam radiotherapy to supplement surgery in such cases, with patients receiving 5,500 to 7,500 rad to the prostate and 4,500 rad to the internal iliac obturator areas. This additional therapy is controversial, but Bagshaw has suggested a 5-year 14 percent local recurrence rate in patients so staged and treated, versus a 68 percent local recurrence rate in individuals with extension into the periprostatic fat if no additional therapy is given. The significance of local recurrence is that it is soon followed by distant metastatic disease if its course is not altered by therapy.

If the lesion truly is a pathologic stage B2, the survival rate should be as good as for stage B1 and A2 tumors appropriately *pathologically* staged. Figures reported by Smith were 91 percent 5-year and 52 percent 10-year disease-free survival for stage B1 tumors; for stage B2 tumors, 5-year and 10-year disease-free survival was 81 and 50 percent, respectively. In conversation with Dr. Richard Middleton, I learned that a few of these stage B2 tumors did have extension through the capsule of the prostate into either the seminal vesicle or periprostatic fat, but that they all had negative nodes and negative bone scan results. This, however, would make a few of these patients a clinical stage C, and therefore one might have expected an even worse survival rate than for the clinical stage B1 tumors.

On the horizon is a clinical trial of preoperative or preradiation therapy to diminish the volume or bulk of the disease before radical prostatectomy or radiation therapy is performed. If these lesions are not staged accurately pathologically before surgery, it will be difficult to make any sense from the results obtained and it will be 10 to 15 years before failure of this form of treatment is accepted. A 25-year retrospective study in patients who had advanced prostate cancer, probably not confined to the prostate, was reported by Scott and Boyd. Lesions thought to be just beyond the prostate capsule were downstaged by estrogen therapy, and the patients were then subjected to radical prostatectomy. Of 39 patients studied who underwent a radical prostatectomy and were available for 15-year follow-up, nine were found to be alive (23 percent). In addition, it is known only that nine patients were alive and not whether they were all alive free of disease or whether some of them still had disease. It should be remembered that Barnes demonstrated a 33 percent 15-year survival rate in patients with carcinoma of the prostate treated by orchiectomy and estrogens alone. A carefully controlled randomized prospective study will be needed to determine whether downstaging before radiotherapy with modern agents is any better than radical prostatectomy or radiation therapy alone.

STAGE C PROSTATIC ADENOCARCINOMA

OLOF E. SOHLBERG, M.D.
PAUL H. LANGE, M.D.

The therapy for prostate cancer is fraught with controversy, and this is certainly true of those prostate cancers that are of larger volume but still apparently localized. We will discuss the various therapeutic options available for this type of tumor, which usually is categorized as stage C disease.

DIAGNOSIS AND EVALUATION

One must distinguish between clinical stage (cC) and pathologic stage (pC) disease, since they may be prognostically and perhaps biologically different. Clinical stage C prostate cancer is defined as tumor that appears to have locally extended beyond the prostate on digital rectal examination or imaging studies in the setting of an otherwise negative metastatic evaluation (e.g., a negative bone scan). Clinical stage C disease can be further divided into disease that appears to be minimally extended beyond the gland (C1) and disease that seems significantly beyond the prostatic capsule (e.g., that which extends to the pelvic side wall or significantly into the seminal vesicles).

When the digital rectal examination suggests cC1 disease, imaging studies have significant false-negative and some false-positive rates. In cC2 disease as appreciated by rectal examination, imaging studies such as transrectal ultrasonography (TRUS), pelvic computed tomography (CT), or magnetic resonance imaging (MRI) usually provide only confirmatory information. In cC1 disease we routinely do not obtain imaging studies except in equivocal situations such as when anatomic constraints limit the palpability of the prostate. In cC2 disease, we usually obtain pelvic CT scans to evaluate the pelvic lymph nodes (see later), and therefore prostatic images are also available. Recently, some investigators have proposed purposeful TRUS biopsy of extracapsular prostatic sites to prove or discover tumor extension. We are not yet convinced that this maneuver provides important information for making therapeutic decisions.

The role of pretreatment prostate-specific antigen (PSA) levels in the evaluation of stage C disease is uncertain. There is a linear relationship between PSA level and both surgical and clinical stage, but the "scatter" is so great that it is difficult to make definitive decisions based on any one PSA value. In general, PSA levels greater than 50 predict a high likelihood (>50 percent) of disease that has extended significantly beyond the capsule or into the lymph nodes. An elevated prostatic acid phosphatase level (particularly when determined by enzymatic methods) is almost always associated with extracapsular disease and/or positive lymph nodes, but normal serum acid phosphatase levels are often present in these circumstances.

Pathologic stage C disease is appreciated and so defined only after a radical prostatectomy, and can be further divided into C1 disease (that through the prostatic capsule only), C2 disease (that extending to the "inked" surgical margin), and C3 disease (that extending into the seminal vesicles). Techniques for increased scrutiny of the pathologic prostate specimen have now become popular and are necessitating even further subdivisions for prognostic purposes. In general, however, only C2 and C3 disease have adverse prognostic implications.

TREATMENT

Patients with clinical stage C prostate cancer have many options for treatment, but currently available therapies are rarely considered curative. In stage cC2 disease, observation is probably not a viable choice in patients who have more than 5 to 10 years of life expectancy. A key point in considering therapeutic options for the stage C patient is the role of pelvic lymph node dissection before the selection of therapy. Although node dissections may have no therapeutic benefit, as many as 60 to 70 percent of patients with clinical stage C2 disease have involvement of the pelvic lymph nodes (stage D1). We do not believe that radiation therapy improves survival in D1 disease, and although it may be palliative in patients with bladder outlet obstruction, it is probably no better than TURP with or without androgen ablation therapy (see later). We advise a diagnostic pelvic lymph node dissection in stage C patients who are candidates for radiation therapy. The morbidity from this surgical procedure can be minimized provided that certain precautions are observed, including preservation of lymphatic tissue lateral to the external iliac vessels.

Radiation therapy has been widely applied to patients who are clinical stage C2 after lymphadenectomy. In this chapter, we discuss only external beam radiation therapy because we believe interstitial radiation therapy in stage C disease given transabdominally has proved disappointing and because radiation therapy administered perineally with ultrasonographic guidance is still experimental. Although recent evidence indicates that the tumor is unlikely to be "sterilized" by radiation in cC2 disease, radiation still carries a substantial survival advantage over no treatment. The standard radiation dose is 7,000 rads of wide-field external beam radiation, usually given in fractions of approximately 120 rads, with 5,000 rads to the whole pelvis, and the final 2,000 rads cGy coned down to the prostate only. Complications include fatigue, and some diarrhea in most patients; serious complications rarely occur. Impotence occurs in the immediate posttreatment period in 20 to 40 percent, but the long-term impotence rate is substantially higher.

The application of radiation therapy in patients with cC2 disease who have severe symptoms of bladder outlet obstruction or total retention requires special comment. If retained urine is not a problem, radiation therapy is usually given in the expectation that transurethral resection of the prostate (TURP) will not be necessary. Indeed, TURP performed after radiation therapy is fraught with a high incidence of bladder neck contracture. If there is retained urine, alternative therapy is necessary. A TURP can be performed initially, but radiation therapy must be delayed at least 6 to 8 weeks to avoid excessive scarring. Alternatively, the patient can be managed by intermittent catheterization or even by a suprapubic tube, in which case attempts to place a small-bore tube tunneled superiorly outside the radiation field may be advantageous in order to avoid the potential healing problems of the tube exit site.

We do not believe that TURP increases the likelihood of subsequent metastasis, as suggested in some reports. However, it is probably true that stage C2 patients with significant symptoms of bladder outlet obstruction have a more aggressive tumor than those who do not have such symptoms. There are no data to suggest that concurrent radiation and hormonal therapy offer any advantage over initial radiation therapy and subsequent hormone manipulation if and when the patient fails. However, this approach is currently being studied in clinical trials.

Hormone therapy is an excellent therapeutic choice, especially for the older clinical cC2 patient with significant symptoms of bladder outlet obstruction. This therapy is palliative but clearly prolongs life as compared to no treatment, but whether it improves survival over and against observation and hormone treatment when symptoms occur is still controversial. We prefer to give hormone therapy early unless the patient has concerns about potency. If bladder outlet obstruction is a problem, TURP can be performed simultaneously, before, or after hormone therapy. In approximately 30 to 50 percent of patients, previous hormone therapy may obviate the need for TURP; this can usually be determined within 3 to 4 months.

The established treatment for stage cC1 disease is the same as for stage cC2: a modified pelvic lymphadenectomy to establish lack of lymph node involvement, followed by radiation with hormone therapy with or without TURP, reserved for special circumstances. Currently this is our recommended approach, but special comments should be made about other experimental approaches now being contemplated.

The treatment of stage cC1 disease is controversial because of the increasing realization that although radiation therapy may be better than observation with regard to local progression, time to recurrence, and possibly even survival, radiation rarely sterilizes the tumor within the gland. It is also true that while most digital rectal examinations understage the extent of local disease, the tumor is pathologically confined within the prostatic capsule in 10 percent of cC1 disease. Thus,

some investigators are contemplating initial endocrine therapy (e.g., neoadjuvant endocrine therapy) for 2 to 3 months to see if the tumor can be made to shrink, followed if so by extirpative surgery in the form of radical prostatectomy or even radical cystoprostatectomy. Although we believe these therapies show promise, they should be tested first in formal trials and cannot be recommended as established therapy.

The patient who after radical prostatectomy is categorized as having pC2 and pC3 disease has significant risks of "recurrence" (which is really a euphemism for persistent disease). This fact prompted the use of adjuvant radiotherapy or endocrine therapy in these patients, and many reports of uncontrolled adjuvant therapy series are in the literature. However, the availability of serum PSA assays has made these reports somewhat obsolete. For example, PSA should theoretically be undetectable if no malignant or benign prostatic tissue exists after radical prostatectomy. In practice, levels of PSA should be less than 0.4 to 0.6 ng per milliliter and should be stable if the patient is cured. Once postoperative PSAs are above this level and rising, persistent disease definitely exists and any therapies given are no longer adjuvant but really active treatment.

Radiation given after radical prostatectomy probably decreases local recurrence but may not increase survival. If the PSA level is elevated, radiation decreases it to undetectable levels in about 50 percent, but the durability of this suppression is probably short (12 to 36 months). We recommend radiation therapy (45 rads to the pelvis with a boost to 60 rads to the prostatic bed) for patients with pC2 and pC3 disease whose PSA level remains elevated after radical prostatectomy or who develop elevated PSAs within the first year. Radiation therapy is also recommended for pC2 and pC3 patients with normal postoperative PSA levels, but we give them a choice of observation until PSA levels become elevated, or immediate adjuvant radiotherapy. Observation is a particularly attractive option to men who have maintained significant potency after surgery. Post radical prostatectomy radiation therapy should not be given until the patient is fully continent and recovered, which is almost always at least 2 months after the surgery.

We are not convinced from the literature that adjuvant hormone therapy to pC2 and pC3 patients has significant effects in delaying recurrence or in increasing survival. We prefer to reserve hormone therapy until there is evidence of recurrence from symptoms, imaging studies, or serum marker levels.

SUGGESTED READING

Lange PH. Controversies in management of apparently localized carcinoma of the prostate. Urology 1989; 15:13–18.

Oesterling JE. Prostatic specific antigen: a critical assessment of the most useful tumor marker for adenocarcinoma of the prostate. J Urol 1991 (in press).

Smith JA Jr. Early detection and treatment of localized carcinoma of the prostate. Urol Clin North Am 1991; 17:689–891.

STAGE D1 PROSTATIC ADENOCARCINOMA

LESLIE M. RAINWATER, M.D.
HORST ZINCKE, M.D.

Patients with stage D1 (T0–4, N1–2, M0) adenocarcinoma of the prostate have positive lymph nodes confined to the pelvis and a negative bone scan. The incidence of metastasis to pelvic lymph nodes has been correlated with clinical staging: 20 to 30 percent of A2, 10 to 15 percent of B1, 25 to 35 percent of B2, and 50 to 65 percent of C cases have positive pelvic lymph nodes at lymphadenectomy. Attempts to determine involvement of pelvic lymph nodes with computed tomography (CT), magnetic resonance imaging (MRI), and lymphangiography have met with limited success. False-negative nodes appear to arise from microscopic metastases, and false-positive nodes from hyperplasia and fat replacement of the lymph nodes. Attempts to decrease the false-negative results have included combined lymphangiography and percutaneous biopsies of lymph nodes by fine-needle aspiration and, more recently, percutaneous pelvic lymphadenectomy. However, an open bilateral pelvic lymphadenectomy remains the most accurate means of assessing lymph node involvement.

The importance of determining lymph node involvement relates to the prognosis. Whether one performs an extended lymph node dissection or a limited external iliac and obturator space node dissection probably does not affect the prognosis because the node dissection is considered diagnostic only (except perhaps in the rare solitary micrometastasis $pN_{1.1}$); metastasis implies systemic disease. In our series, the number of pelvic lymph nodes involved had no significant impact on progression or survival: 30 to 40 percent nonprogression rates and 60 to 65 percent cause-specific survival rates at 5 and 10 years, respectively, for patients with one, two, or three or more nodes. Further, an extended node dissection is associated with increased morbidity, particularly if adjuvant radiation is included.

Historically, treatment has varied: observation with either early or late androgen ablation, external beam radiation, interstitial irradiation with ^{125}I or [198]Au, radical prostatectomy, radical cystoprostatectomy, and chemotherapy. Interestingly, all these monotherapies have resulted in similar progression rates of 60 to 75 percent at 5 years and survival rates of 10 to 20 percent at 10 years.

MONOTHERAPY

Bagshaw and colleagues at Stanford University have the largest experience with radiotherapy of the prostate, and survival rates in their series were less than 50 and 20 percent at 5 and 8 years, respectively. In addition, positive prostate biopsies after radiation therapy have been found in 50 to 60 percent of cases, raising the question whether radiation therapy can even control local disease long term. Indeed, Smith and associates at the University of Utah found symptomatic local disease in 51 percent of patients treated with pelvic irradiation compared with 65 percent of those having no treatment at 5 years. Memorial Sloan-Kettering Cancer Center has the largest experience with interstitial ^{125}I irradiation. Only 40 percent of patients with nodal disease were alive at 5 years and only 14 percent were tumor free. Paulson and colleagues at Duke University compared radical perineal prostatectomy, external beam radiation to the full pelvis and periaortic nodes, and delayed hormonal therapy. The median survival of the entire group was 39.5 months, and no treatment was superior in prolonging survival. The Uro-Oncology Research Group compared extended field irradiation with delayed androgen ablation in a randomized clinical trial. Although the median time to first evidence of treatment failure was twice as long in the radiation group, 23.9 months versus 12.2 months, the survival at 48 months was not significantly different. Zincke reported similarly poor results in patients treated with radical retropubic prostatectomy alone: 18 percent nonprogression rate at 5 years and 20 percent survival at 10 years.

On the basis of these and other reports, positive pelvic lymph nodes should be considered a systemic disease that will not respond to current monotherapy treatment aimed at local control. However, when we reviewed our patients who underwent a staging lymphadenectomy and orchiectomy alone (treating the systemic disease), a progression rate of 44 percent at 5 years and only 26 percent survival at 10 years was observed. Local or systemic treatment alone has a dismal prognosis. Thus, if an attempt is to be made at prolonging patient survival, therapy should consist of a combined multimodality approach treating not only the local disease but also the systemic disease.

COMBINATION THERAPY

Modern therapeutic approaches have combined hormonal manipulation via orchiectomy or luteinizing hormone–releasing factor antagonists with antiandrogens, or chemotherapy to achieve systemic control with radical retropubic prostatectomy or radiation therapy (either external beam or interstitial irradiation) to achieve local control. However, when the National Prostatic Cancer Project randomized patients treated with external beam radiation with or without adjuvant cyclophosphamide, no difference was seen in time to disease progression or overall survival. With limited follow-up, deVere White and associates reported on patients who had ^{125}I interstitial irradiation with or without adjuvant chemotherapy (cyclophosphamide and doxorubicin). At 36 months 33 percent of the patients who received chemotherapy had already progressed.

Similar poor results have been seen with external beam radiation or interstitial irradiation combined with hormonal manipulation, which may be related to the known poor results of local control with radiation: 50 to 60 percent of patients have positive prostate biopsies after radiation therapy with curative intent.

Can cytoreduction (radical retropubic prostatectomy) combined with adjuvant systemic therapy (hormonal manipulation or chemotherapy) improve the time to progression and ultimate survival of patients with node-positive adenocarcinoma of the prostate? Isaacs and Coffey at Johns Hopkins University have been instrumental in elucidating the biologic tumor behavior of the androgen-sensitive Dunning R-3327 H rat prostatic adenocarcinoma model. By flow-cytometric analysis of nuclear shapes and cell sizes, the tumor cell heterogeneity has been shown to consist of numerous well-differentiated to anaplastic tumor lines that have differing biologic behaviors with regard to growth rate, metastatic potential, and hormone responsiveness. Therefore, in dealing with a heterogeneous population of cells, treatment should consist of multimodality regimens in order to decrease the likelihood of a clone of cells escaping a chosen therapy. From Goldie's model of tumor heterogeneity, the larger the tumor volume, the greater the genetic instability and likelihood of clones resistant to chemotherapy. Isaacs further examined the most effective timing of hormonal manipulation and found significantly longer survivals when orchiectomy was performed early on minimal tumor volume (cytoreduction). In addition, with cytoreduction, early administration of chemotherapy (cyclophosphamide) further enhanced survival, especially when used in combination with androgen ablation.

In support of this experimental model, Zincke and colleagues reported significantly improved survival when radical retropubic prostatectomy (cytoreduction) was combined with early, as compared with late, androgen ablation. In a review of 93 patients followed for 5 years or more, immediate adjunctive orchiectomy resulted in 84 and 78 percent nonprogression rates at 5 and 10 years, respectively, compared with 46 and 35 percent (p = .0009) when immediate orchiectomy was not performed. Survival at 5 and 10 years was 87 and 77 percent for the early orchiectomy compared with 78 and 49 percent for the delayed orchiectomy group, respectively.

PLOIDY PATTERNS

The diversity in the biologic behavior of prostatic adenocarcinoma, as exemplified by 10 percent of patients showing no evidence of disease progression at 10 years' follow-up with local treatment alone and the varied response of tumors to hormonal manipulation, led us to search for a probe that would subclassify and further delineate this variability in tumor behavior. DNA ploidy patterns were determined by flow-cytometric analysis of paraffin-embedded tumor nuclei. Of 91 patients with stage D1 disease, DNA ploidy pattern was diploid in 42 percent of tumors, tetraploid in 45 percent, and aneuploid in 13 percent. Only 15 percent of DNA diploid tumors progressed locally or systemically, whereas 75 percent of tumors with a nondiploid pattern (tetraploid or aneuploid) progressed (p < .0001). None of the patients with a DNA diploid tumor died of prostate cancer; 43 percent of those with DNA tetraploid and 44 percent with DNA aneuploid tumors died of prostate cancer (p < .001). Nuclear DNA ploidy analysis of tumor nuclei appears to provide objective, prognostic information. In a subsequent analysis of 62 patients with long-term follow-up (range, 9.8 to 17.6 years), the effects of early versus late androgen ablation were determined. No patient with a DNA diploid tumor treated with a radical retropubic prostatectomy and adjuvant early hormone therapy has progressed or died of prostate cancer. In contrast, of patients with diploid tumors who did not receive early adjunctive hormone therapy, 56 percent have progressed, and 22 percent of these have died of prostate cancer. Patients with nondiploid tumors did not appear to benefit from early or delayed adjuvant hormonal manipulation; 50 percent of these patients who received early adjuvant hormonal treatment have progressed and died, whereas 68 percent of patients who received delayed treatment have progressed, and 40 percent of these have died of disease. Thus, patients with nondiploid tumors respond poorly to adjunctive hormonal treatment alone despite cytoreduction of tumor mass; however, tumors with a DNA diploid pattern (representing 40 percent of stage D1 tumors) respond favorably to cytoreduction (radical prostatectomy) and early adjunctive androgen ablation.

Cytoreduction, androgen deprivation, and adjuvant chemotherapy as suggested by Isaacs appear to be necessary for patients with nondiploid stage D1 tumors who otherwise are doomed to failure under present treatment regimens. Chemotherapy has not shown substantial promise in previous trials; however, the overwhelming tumor volume may have been the limiting factor. As suggested by Isaacs, Skinner and colleagues, and deVere White, adjunctive therapy of cyclophosphamide with or without doxorubicin may be of benefit in low-volume residual disease and seems to be well tolerated with minimal morbidity.

Previously, progression of disease was monitored crudely with bone scan, CT, and acid phosphatase. By measuring the level of prostate-specific antigen (PSA), progression of disease can be noted months to years before it is clinically detectable. Therefore, failure to respond to multimodality therapy can now be monitored with greater acumen, and alterations in therapy can be initiated earlier when the tumor volume is minimal and potentially more responsive to other forms of treatment (e.g., chemotherapy).

SUMMARY

A new era in the treatment of prostate cancer has arrived. Previously, the urologist thought that patients

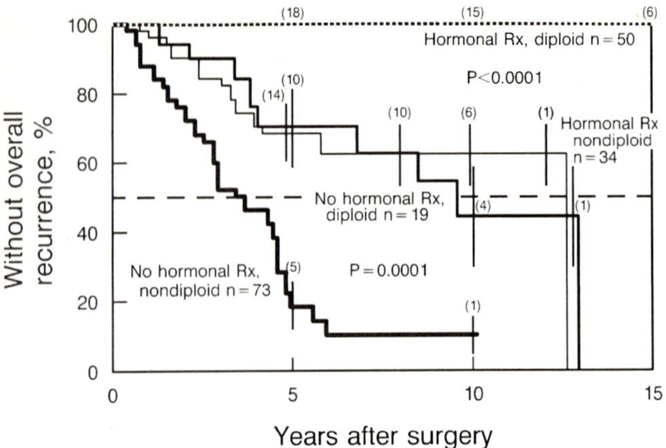

Figure 1 Kaplan-Meier curves of overall survival without recurrence in 176 patients with stage D1 prostate cancer who underwent radical prostatectomy according to adjuvant treatment and tumor nuclear DNA ploidy pattern. The numbers in parentheses represent patients under observation at that time. (Republished with permission of W.B. Saunders Company. Combined surgery and immediate adjuvant hormonal treatment for stage D1 adenocarcinoma of the prostate: Mayo Clinic experience. Semin Urol 1990; 8:175–183.)

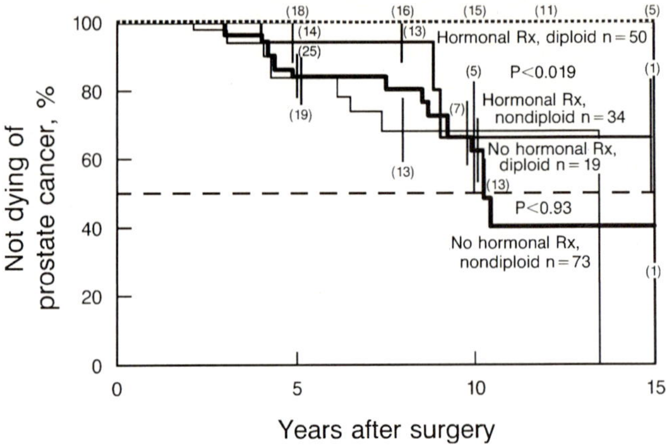

Figure 2 Kaplan-Meier curves of cause-specific survival in 176 patients with stage D1 prostate cancer who underwent radical prostatectomy according to adjuvant treatment and tumor nuclear DNA ploidy pattern. The numbers in parentheses represent patients under observation at that time. (Republished with permission of W.B. Saunders Company. Combined surgery and immediate adjuvant hormonal treatment for stage D1 adenocarcinoma of the prostate: Mayo Clinic experience. Semin Urol 1990; 8:175–183.)

would die with prostate cancer rather than of prostate cancer. However, prostate cancer is the most common cause of cancer in men in the United States; 122,000 new cases are predicted in 1991, resulting in 32,000 expected deaths. Some of these patients, with stage D1 disease and a DNA diploid tumor (40 percent), can expect 10 years of disease-free survival if treated aggressively with radical prostatectomy and *immediate* adjunctive androgen ablation. Delayed use of hormonal manipulation in patients with DNA diploid tumors has proved to be ineffective; 30 percent of those who progressed died of disease despite immediate treatment on progression (Figs. 1 and 2). The remaining patients with nondiploid tumors (60 percent) should not be neglected, but treated aggressively with multimodality therapy in a prospective setting in hopes of improving on the present 40 to 50 percent 10-year disease-free survival presently achieved with cytoreduction and adjuvant hormone therapy.

SUGGESTED READING

Bagshaw MA, Ray GR, Cox RS. Radiotherapy of prostatic carcinoma: long- or short-term efficacy (Stanford University experience). Urology 1985; 25 (suppl):17–23.

Benson MC, Coffey DS. Prostate cancer research: current concepts and controversies. Semin Urol 1983; 1:323–330.

Carter GE, Lieskovsky G, Skinner DG, et al. Results of local and/or systemic adjuvant therapy in the management of pathological stage C or D1 prostate cancer following radical prostatectomy. J Urol 1989; 142:1266–1271.

DeVere White R, Babayan RK, Krikorian J, et al. Adjuvant chemotherapy for stage D1 adenocarcinoma of prostate. Urology 1983; 21:270–272.

Isaacs JT. The timing of androgen ablation therapy and/or chemotherapy in the treatment of prostatic cancer. Prostate 1984; 5:1–17.

Paulson DF, Cline WA Jr, Koefoot RB Jr, et al. Extended field radiation therapy versus delayed hormonal therapy in node positive prostatic adenocarcinoma. J Urol 1982; 127:935–937.

Rainwater LM, Zincke H. Nuclear DNA ploidy and prostate cancer. In: Lepor H, Lawson R, eds. Urologic oncology. Vol 5. Norwell, MA: Kluwer Academic Publishers (in press).

Winkler HZ, Rainwater LM, Myers RP, et al. Stage D1 prostatic adenocarcinoma: significance of nuclear DNA ploidy patterns studied by flow cytometry. Mayo Clin Proc 1988; 63:103–112.

Zincke H. Bilateral pelvic lymphadenectomy and radical retropubic prostatectomy for stage C or D1 adenocarcinoma of the prostate: possible beneficial effect of adjuvant treatment. NCI Monogr 1988; 7:109–115.1

Zincke H. Combined surgery and immediate adjuvant hormonal treatment for stage D1 adenocarcinoma of the prostate: Mayo Clinic experience. Semin Urol 1990; 8:175–183.

Copyright 1990 Mayo Foundation.

STAGE D2 PROSTATIC ADENOCARCINOMA

JAMES L. MOHLER, M.D.

THE CLINICAL PROBLEM

In 1990, prostatic carcinoma became the most common male cancer with approximately 103,000 new cases and 29,500 deaths. Among newly diagnosed patients, approximately 50 percent present with bone metastases. Almost 30 percent present with regional metastases or local tissue invasion rendering cure unlikely, and most of these progress to stage D2 disease. The survival of patients with distant metastatic disease averages 2.5 years, and thus the treatment of disseminated prostatic carcinoma constitutes a major public health concern.

BIOLOGY

Prostatic carcinoma follows a gompertzian growth curve typical of all carcinomas. Tumor doubling times may be as long as 3 years in incidental prostatic carcinoma, but by the time clinically localized or metastatic disease can be appreciated, tumor doubling time may be as short as 3 months. Successful radiation or chemotherapy depends on rapid cell growth that occurs among solid tumors only in testicular cancer. A more fruitful treatment approach in prostatic carcinoma may be the acceleration of cell death instead of reduction of cell proliferation. The mechanism of prostatic cell death by androgen ablation appears to be directed by premature activation of the normal processes that govern cell death. Upon androgen ablation, intracellular heat shock proteins appear, TRPM-2 gene is activated, and intracellular calcium and calcium-magnesium endonucleases increase. An irreversible commitment to death is signaled by DNA fragmentation. Soon the nucleus becomes pyknotic, cell shape changes, adenosine triphosphate (ATP) diminishes, membrane integrity is lost, and death rapidly ensues. This process, termed "apoptosis," results in the death of nonproliferating cells and presents an opportunity to impact on metastatic prostatic carcinoma.

All cancers are characterized by genetic heterogeneity that results in subpopulations of cells with varying characteristics. Prostatic carcinomas contain a subset of hormone-independent cells that grow in the absence of androgen. Whether these cells exist before androgen deprivation or are capable of rapid adaptation to androgen absence remains unclear. However, other cells are completely androgen dependent and die when androgen concentrations drop below a critical threshold. Other cells appear hormone sensitive and become quiescent but do not die when androgens decline. The relative number of these three cell types determines a patient's initial response to androgen deprivation. Although the critical level for testosterone is unknown in man, extrapolation of animal data would demonstrate maximal cytotoxicity at androgen levels corresponding to 70 ng per deciliter. Further lowering of serum testosterone in rats bearing Dunning tumors or in humans appears to be without benefit. After initial androgen withdrawal, hormone-independent cells continue to grow and may render additional hormonal manipulation fruitless.

Luteinizing hormone–releasing hormone (LHRH) from the anterior hypothalamus stimulates secretion of luteinizing hormone (LH) by the anterior pituitary. LH stimulates testicular Leydig cells to produce testosterone. Testosterone directly suppresses LHRH production by the hypothalamus. In parallel fashion, the hypothalamus produces corticotropin-releasing factor (CRF), which stimulates the anterior pituitary to produce adrenocorticotropic hormone (ACTH). ACTH stimulates production of the weak adrenal androgens androstenedione and dihydroepiandosterone. These represent approximately 3 percent of the total amount of circulating androgen, the remainder being produced by Leydig cells. Adrenal androgen production is negatively affected by modulation of the pituitary secretion of ACTH by adrenally produced cortisol. Five percent of circulating testosterone occurs free and is available for uptake in affector cells and conversion to dihydrotestosterone (DHT) by the enzyme 5-alpha-reductatase. The remaining 95 percent of circulating testosterone is bound to sex steroid binding globulin and plasma albumin. DHT enters the nucleus and interacts with the androgen receptor that was recently identified and cloned and now may be recognized directly by specific antibodies.

TREATMENT OPTIONS

Treatment options include orchiectomy, medical castration, chemotherapy, and radiation therapy, among others (Table 1).

Orchiectomy

Huggins received the Nobel Prize for work in the 1940s that demonstrated that both the benign and the malignant prostate was androgen dependent, and bilateral orchiectomy resulted in regression of carcinoma with symptomatic improvement. Bilateral orchiectomy is a simple procedure that can be performed under local anesthesia in an outpatient setting. It produces prompt resolution, often within minutes, of bone pain from metastatic prostatic carcinoma by rapidly eliminating production of kallikreins. Eighty percent of patients respond to androgen ablation by orchiectomy, with half demonstrating tumor regression and half stable disease by objective parameters. Among patients who respond to androgen ablation, mean life expectancy is approximately 3.5 years, in contrast to nonresponders, who live

Table 1 Available Treatment for Stage D2 Prostatic Adenocarcinoma

Method	Dose	Action	Toxicity (in order of frequency)	Response	Monthly cost*
Orchiectomy	–	Irreversible elimination of testicular androgens	Impotence, hot flashes, psychological	80%	$78†
Estrogen (DES)	1–3 mg daily	↓ LH, ↑ SBG, ↓ DHT	Painful gynecomastia, nausea and vomiting, fluid retention, stroke, deep vein thrombosis, myocardial infarction	80%	$5–8‡
LHRH analogs					
Goserelin acetate	3.6 mg monthly	Desensitization of pituitary to endogenous LHRH→ ↓ LH	Hot flashes, impotence, fluid retention, flare reaction	80%	$322
Leuprolide	7.5 mg monthly				$373
Flutamide	750 mg daily	Nonsteroidal, DHT-receptor blockade	Gynecomastia, hot flashes, diarrhea, occasional impotence	80%	$282
Ketoconazole	1,200 mg daily	Cytochrome P450 inhibitor, blocks adrenal and testicular androgen production	Hepatotoxicity, nausea, adrenal insufficiency	80%	$303
Aminoglutethamide	500–1,000 mg daily	General and incomplete impairment of steroidogenesis	Nausea, vomiting, rash, ataxia, dizziness, drowsiness	20%	$54–$106
Corticosteroids (prednisone)	120 mg	↓ Adrenal androgens, euphoria		20%	$10

*University of North Carolina Hospitals as of June 1, 1991 rounded to nearest dollar; cost per month normalized for mean life expectancy 2½ years.
†Outpatient local anesthesia including one postoperative check-up.
‡Add $110 per month for prophylactic breast irradiation.
DES = diethylstilbesterol, LH = luteinizing hormone, SGB = sex steroid binding globulin, DHT = dihydrotestosterone, LHRH = luteinizing hormone releasing hormone.

an average of 6 to 9 months. Whether the average survival of approximately 2.5 years in treated patients exceeds that of untreated patients is controversial and has been addressed only through historical and indirect comparisons.

Orchiectomy produces irreversible elimination of the major source of circulating androgens. It results in near-universal impotence, although many patients who are highly motivated maintain potency after castration. Hot flashes affect as many as 60 percent of patients and can be treated in most with low-dose estrogen (diethylstilbestrol 1 mg per day), progestational agents, or alpha-adrenergic blockers. The primary toxicity of significance to many patients and physicians is the psychological effect of castration. Proper patient education may serve to minimize the trauma of body image alteration, because the commonly perceived changes of personality and energy level are probably more fiction than fact. The psychological trauma of castration may be lessened by subcapsular orchiectomy that produces equivalent post-treatment serum testosterone levels compared with total orchiectomy. Testicular prostheses may be appropriate in some patients, although they increase the cost of the procedure and carry a small risk of infection. When orchiectomy is used following medical androgen ablation, 5 to 15 percent of patients respond subjectively, but objective tumor regression and improvement in survival in the absence of medical noncompliance probably does not occur. Orchiectomy without additional therapy during the remaining lifetime of the patient would involve an average monthly cost of $78, although this may vary widely throughout the United States.

Medical Castration

The patient with metastatic prostatic carcinoma and the physician may choose from a wide range of therapeutic alternatives to bilateral orchiectomy, which differ in their action, toxicities, and costs but probably differ little in their response rates. Diethylstilbestrol (DES) can produce safe chemical orchiectomy in most patients. When DES is administered at 1 mg per day, approximately two thirds of patients have castrate serum testosterone levels. The life expectancy of patients with metastatic prostatic carcinoma so treated exceeded that of placebo-treated patients in the second Veterans Administration Cooperative Urological Research Group (VACURG) study, and cardiovascular toxicity was not found. DES acts centrally to diminish the production of LH, with resultant loss of testicular testosterone production. In addition, it increases sex steroid binding globulin, which decreases free testosterone. It may also impair the conversion of testosterone to dihydrotestosterone intracellularly and thus directly affect prostatic carcinoma cells. The most frequent side effect is painful gynecomastia, which occurs in approximately 70 percent of patients receiving 3 mg of DES daily. It can be prevented by pretreatment breast irradiation. Once gynecomastia has occurred, radiation therapy may eliminate the pain, but it rarely causes regression of breast size. More serious is fluid retention and hypercoagulability, which may result in myocardial infarction, cerebravascular accident, and deep vein thrombosis with pulmonary embolism. These side effects, with the possible exception of gynecomastia, appear to be dose dependent; they probably occur rarely, if at all, at a dose of 1 mg daily but seriously affect about 5 percent of patients taking 3 mg daily. Risks of estrogen therapy can be diminished by cessation of therapy after 3 years, as most patients remain castrate. Response rates are equivalent to those with orchiectomy, although secondary treatment probably benefits fewer patients because noncompliance does not occur after orchiectomy. DES itself is very inexpensive. However, prophylactic breast irradiation and the cost of myocardial infarction, stroke, and deep vein thrombosis, especially when used at 3 mg daily produce total costs that far exceed those of orchiectomy.

The LHRH analogs goserelin acetate and leuprolide are now available and should be administered in depot form to ensure maintenance of castrate levels of testosterone. They overwhelm pituitary receptors for LHRH, rendering them insensitive to endogenous LHRH, and produce castrate androgen levels in approximately 2 weeks. From day 3 to 10 a flare in symptoms may occur owing to initial Leydig cell stimulation with increased levels of circulating testosterone. The flare response may be blocked by concomitant administration of antiandrogens, although whether the flare has a deleterious effect on survival is uncertain. The primary toxicities of LHRH analogs are hot flashes, impotence, and fluid retention. Response rates are similar to those with orchiectomy or DES, but the risk of cardiovascular and thromboembolic catastrophies is diminished and the psychological effects of castration are avoided. The monthly costs of depot formulations of goserelin acetate and leuprolide are $322 and $377, respectively. Office visits for intramuscular depot placement add to the expense of therapy unless the patient is willing to self-administer the medication.

Flutamide is a nonsteroidal anilide decapeptide that produces its antiandrogenic action through competition with the intracellular DHT receptor. Because flutamide is nonsteroidal, testosterone levels remain unchanged or increase mildly, so that potency is preserved in most patients. The incidence of gynecomastia and hot flashes is similar to that with other therapy. Tolerable diarrhea occurs in 15 percent of patients, but another 15 percent have severe diarrhea necessitating discontinuation of medication. Cardiovascular and thromboembolic complications have not been described. Response rates are similar to those with other therapies, and when flutamide is used secondarily or in patients in whom elevated testosterone levels occur after orchiectomy, responses occur rarely. Flutamide costs $282 per month. Combined with LHRH analogs or orchiectomy, a treatment program costs about $630 or $360 per month, respectively. Used alone it appears to produce equivalent responses to combination therapy, but the durability of response is not yet known. Supranormal or normal levels of testos-

terone may overcome receptor blockade when flutamide is used alone. Flutamide therefore has not been approved for monotherapy by the Food and Drug Administration.

Ketoconazole is a broad-spectrum antifungal agent that in high doses inhibits cytochrome P450, blocking adrenal and testicular androgen production. Castrate androgen levels are obtained within 16 hours. With prolonged administration, hepatoxicity occurs in many patients, but is usually mild; severe hepatoxicity occurs rarely and can be fatal. Nausea is usually self-limiting, and mild adrenal insufficiency must be recognized and treated. Response rates are similar to those with orchiectomy. Subjective secondary responses after orchiectomy occur in as many as 50 percent of patients, but objective response is rare and prolongation of survival has not been demonstrated. This drug is best used in the short term when rapid achievement of castrate androgen levels is required and orchiectomy cannot be performed immediately or is declined by the patient.

Chemotherapy

The role of chemotherapy in the treatment of prostatic carcinoma remains unclear. The low proliferative rate of prostatic carcinoma renders it poorly susceptible to standard chemotherapeutic agents, which produce alterations in DNA that are lethal only if followed promptly by cell division. The National Prostate Cancer Project thoroughly evaluated chemotherapeutic agents used alone or in combination with estrogenic compounds in patients with metastatic prostatic carcinoma. Ten to 15 percent of patients responded, although the duration of response was short and survival benefit over standard or no therapy was not clearly shown. Among agents tested, cyclophosphamide, 5-fluorouracil, and methotrexate are the most likely candidates for beneficial effect, although treatment with these or any other agents should not be conducted outside a protocol setting, because side effects are great and benefit is small.

Radiation Therapy

Radiation therapy may be used for palliation as well as prophylaxis in patients with metastatic prostatic carcinoma. Pain due to discrete bone involvement responds to 3,500 rads with improvement or resolution in 80 percent of patients. When bone metastases are diffuse, hemibody irradiation delivered to the involved half or sequentially to both halves produces similar responses. The duration of pain relief is short, averaging 5 months, but may cover most of the remaining life expectancy of the patient. Prophylactic irradiation may prevent pathologic fracture, although this is unproved. Radiation also plays a role in the treatment of acute cord compression when coadministered with high-dose steroids and androgen ablation, if not already performed. There is often recovery of function when neurologic deficits are incomplete. However, when paralysis is complete and even of short duration, recovery is unusual. More rapid decompression can be achieved by laminectomy, which should generally be performed by an anterior approach because cord compression most frequently results from extension from the vertebral body. Results from surgical decompressions may be superior to those from nonsurgical treatment, but patients must be selected carefully.

Other Therapies

Surgical adrenalectomy or medical or surgical hypophysectomy no longer has a place in the treatment armamentarium for prostatic carcinoma. Multiple agents exist that ablate the effects of testicular and andrenal androgens without the need to resort to these dangerous therapies. Intravenous diethylstilbestrol can no longer be recommended for rapid induction of castrate testosterone levels since the availability of ketoconazole. Early results with immunotherapy, including adoptive transfer of immune cells, alpha-interferon, and coumarin, appear disappointing. Aminogluthethimide generally and incompletely impairs steroidogenesis and has many, often severe side effects. Response rates are low and may result from coadministration of corticosteroids to prevent rebound ACTH elevations. Corticosteroids reduce adrenal androgen production through central mechanisms, but their activity is more likely to be related to the euphoria induced. Responses are primarily subjective and occur in about 20 percent of patients.

TREATMENT ISSUES

Delayed Versus Early Treatment

In asymptomatic patients with metastatic disease the timing of androgen ablation is controversial. Studies in animal models suggest that early androgen ablation prolongs survival. However, tumor burdens necessary to demonstrate survival advantages are less than those that correspond to clinically detectable disease in humans. Historical data from the 1940s are difficult to interpret. Evidence from the placebo-controlled VACURG trial of 1967, in which patients treated with androgen ablation upon failing placebo showed survival similar to those treated with androgen ablation at enrollment, seems to refute the theoretical advantages of initiating treatment at low tumor volumes demonstrated in the animal studies and reported in some human studies. Because androgen deprivation is palliative and not curative, and because there is uncertainty regarding the proper timing of treatment in patients who are potent and whose potency is of importance to them, these individuals may be best served by delayed androgen ablation. Flutamide represents a hedge on this bet, although its long-term equivalence to orchiectomy has not been shown, and the incidence of severe diarrhea necessitating cessation of flutamide is significant.

Surgical Versus Medical Castration

The choice between surgical and medical castration remains a difficult problem for most patients. Rates of acceptance of orchiectomy vary from state to state and country to country. Many patients have been disserviced by as yet unsubstantiated claims of the superiority of medical castration and especially total androgen ablation. Orchiectomy remains the standard of therapy against which all others must be compared. It is simple and cost effective. Most of the psychological issues of castration can be dealt with by appropriate counseling and patient selection. For the patient who cannot overcome reticence regarding castration, a variety of medical alternatives exist. However, whether the health care system can afford the financial burden of medical androgen ablation becoming the standard of therapy remains unclear. Combination therapy with LHRH analogs and antiandrogens would add $1 billion annually compared with orchiectomy. This eightfold increase over the cost of orchiectomy fails to include for medical therapy the cost of noncompliance, orchiectomies in patients for whom side effects prevent continued medical therapy, or orchiectomies performed as secondary therapy after failure of medical androgen ablation.

Ethical Considerations

The American health care system continues to value the physician-patient relationship above all issues of personal, third-party, or national health care expense. Each of us has urologic colleagues who have responded to a diagnosis of metastatic prostatic carcinoma with androgen ablation followed by crossover to orchiectomy or medical castration upon failure, and then to ketoconazole, aminoglutethimide, steroids, or chemotherapy for secondary treatment. Some proceed to surgical treatment of pathologic fractures, intravenous diethylstilbestrol, and even surgical adrenalectomy before death. Studies of intensive care unit treatments for severe disease indicate that most patients and their families do not regret, and would pursue again, aggressive medical therapy in spite of all psychological, physical, and financial costs. Thus, as physicians of individual patients in the current health care system, it may be inappropriate to raise concerns of cost benefit analysis and the results of clinical studies when counseling individual patients.

TREATMENT

Patients may be divided into those who present without symptoms but biochemical evidence of metastatic disease (elevated enzymatic prostatic acid phosphatase, stage D0), asymptomatic patients with documented metastatic disease (stage D2), and symptomatic patients with stage D2 disease. In addition, patients treated initially progress to hormone-insensitive prostatic carcinoma (stage D3) unless death occurs from other causes. The role of the urologist is to produce a high quality of life for as long as possible. This role should not be subjugated to that of a family physician, medical oncologist, or radiation oncologist. A hopeful outlook must be maintained, but it is inappropriate not to deal with average life expectancy realistically and the results of treatment alternatives through frank and honest discussion. Patients require time to adjust to their diagnosis and the almost certain outcome of death from disease, and to prepare their loved ones psychologically, physically, and financially for life without them. The goal of my treatment program with all patients is to (1) make them physically unaware of their prostatic carcinoma for as long as possible; (2) counsel them about treatment alternatives with regard to efficacy, side effects, and cost; and (3) provide a personal recommendation if I have one.

Androgen ablation should be instituted immediately when metastatic prostatic carcinoma presents with bone pain, ureteral obstruction, or neurologic deficits. In addition, bladder outlet obstruction in the face of significant skeletal metastases warrants androgen ablation; two thirds of patients resolve the bladder outlet obstruction without requiring transurethral resection. Impotent patients are treated initially with orchiectomy unless psychologically they are unable to tolerate castration. Serum testosterone levels are measured 4 weeks after orchiectomy and at the time of progression. In 10 percent of patients, the levels exceed 70 ng per deciliter. In these patients antiandrogens are offered, although there are no data demonstrating their efficacy.

If orchiectomy is declined, I offer DES, 1 mg daily, with serum testosterone at 1 month. Before treatment with DES, LHRH analogs, or flutamide, all patients are offered prophylactic breast irradiation in view of the high incidence of gynecomastia. If the serum testosterone level remains greater than 50 ng per milliliter, DES is increased to 2 mg daily and serum testosterone measurement is repeated 1 month later. If serum testosterone remains greater than 50 ng per milliliter, I advise the patient that increase of DES to 3 mg daily is associated with a small but significant risk of fatal cardiovascular or thromboembolic events. If they do not choose castration at this time, I offer goserelin acetate in depot form without flutamide, because no flare should occur after 2 months of DES therapy. This regimen renders all patients anorchid with minimal toxicity and at reasonable expense.

To my knowledge, there are no data available from human trials or experiments conducted in animal models that warrant flutamide use in view of its cost and side effects. However, flutamide represents an opportunity to maintain potency when used as monotherapy if the patient accepts the uncertainties regarding its long-term equivalence to orchiectomy, and if escape from receptor blockade is monitored by serial PSA measurements. If depot therapy is chosen for first-line treatment without previous low-dose DES, it must be coadministered with flutamide for the first 10 days of therapy to prevent flare reactions, which may manifest as increased bone pain or possible neurologic injury.

In D2 disease that is asymptomatic, symptoms of bladder outlet obstruction are indications for androgen ablation unless skeletal metastases are minimal and tumor growth is slow (e.g., if serial PSA demonstrates a doubling time of 6 months or greater). I do not routinely employ prophylactic radiation therapy to weight-bearing areas because I am uncertain whether an irradiated but tumor-free bone is any stronger than an unirradiated tumor, and the incidence of pathologic fractures is small.

Stage D0 and asymptomatic D2 patients are followed every 3 months for the first year and every 6 months thereafter. Patients treated with androgen ablation are seen at 1 month and androgen ablation response is assessed with serum PSA. If PSA has declined to normal levels or by greater than 90 percent, patients are followed at 6-month intervals; otherwise they are followed at 3-month intervals. Follow-up consists of measurements of PSA for monitoring of tumor burden, serum creatinine levels to detect asymptomatic renal impairment, and hematocrit to recognize asymptomatic anemia. Other studies, including bone scans, are performed only if indicated clinically.

Relapse after androgen ablation is usually preceded by rising PSA, which is a signal to decrease follow-up to every 3 months. Upon development of symptomatic recurrence, patients are counseled that life expectancy is about 9 months and referred to home health services or a hospice program. Palliative radiation therapy is delivered to focal areas of bone pain, and the need for hemibody irradiation has been small. If patients have been managed with medical androgen ablation, orchiectomy is offered, although it is recommended only if serum testosterone exceeds 50 ng per deciliter. Chemotherapy should be considered only in a protocol setting and after extensive counseling. Ureteral obstruction can be managed with ureteral stents, which can be placed retrograde successfully 50 percent of the time, or by percutaneous nephrostomy. Urinary diversion is left up to the patient, although I routinely advise against it in the face of metastatic disease, since a uremic death usually minimizes suffering. Bladder outlet obstruction is treated by transurethral resection of the prostate, which usually requires repeating within 6 months, and if performed again needs repeating within 2 months.

Pain is managed initially with nonsteroidal antiinflammatory medications. Narcotics are used liberally to ensure maximal pain relief. Steroids may be used to induce euphoria, but have rather marked side effects in these debilitated patients. Final options for severe pain control include chronic indwelling epidural catheters and intravenous patient-controlled analgesia.

Patients who present with neurologic deficits that are incomplete or less than 24 hours in duration are (1) managed with high-dose steroids and immediate orchiectomy or short-term ketoconazole, (2) evaluated by MRI, and (3) treated by appropriate neurosurgical, orthopedic, or radiation oncologic intervention. Diffuse vertebral disease should be managed with radiation therapy, whereas focal deficits are often treated by anterior laminectomy. When incomplete neurologic deficits occur in patients who have failed androgen ablation, they are managed with short-term high-dose steroids and radiation therapy, because approximately 10 percent resolve. If systemic disease is extensive, intervention is not recommended.

The success of the treatment of metastatic prostatic carcinoma has changed little since Dr. Huggins demonstrated the androgen responsiveness of prostatic carcinoma. However, urologists have a varied armamentarium that can be tailored to the needs and choices of their patients with metastatic prostatic carcinoma. The hallmarks of successful treatment are compassion with realism, treatment guidance with patient selection, treatment supervision with extensive assistance from the patient's personal physician, consultants when necessary, and above all home health and hospice caretakers. Significant impact on prostatic carcinoma awaits the development of new therapies that will cause the death of nonproliferating cells that are androgen independent.

PROSTATIC TRANSITIONAL CELL CARCINOMA

ROBERT C. FLANIGAN, M.D., F.A.C.S.

Although 95 percent or more of prostatic malignancies are adenocarcinomas, transitional cell carcinoma of the prostate (TCCP) has been recognized with increased frequency since its first description in 1952 by Melicow and Hollwell. TCCP accounts for 1.5 to 5 percent of prostatic cancers, underscoring the need for better understanding of the clinical presentation, diagnosis, and therapeutic management of these patients.

Histologically, TCCP, whether in situ or invasive, may be classified as one of three neoplastic processes: (1) *primary* (no antecedent or simultaneous cancer found elsewhere in the urothelium); (2) *secondary* (TCCP associated with a synchronous or metachronous urothelial tumor—a synchronous lesion may be contiguous, as in direct extension from bladder neck to prostate, or noncontiguous); or (3) *mixed* (a combination of prostate adenocarcinoma and TCCP that may occur simultaneously or, more typically, in a setting of apparent androgen insensitivity of a previously diagnosed prostate adenocarcinoma). The relative frequency of these neoplastic processes reported in the literature are secondary (65 percent), primary (25 percent), and mixed (10 percent).

TCCP may occur by direct extension of a bladder neck carcinoma or may arise from the prostatic periurethral ducts that form as evaginations of the embryonic urethra. More specifically, primary TCCP is believed to arise from the reserve (or indifferent) cells located between the surface columnar cells and the basement membrane at the transformation zone in the prostatic duct between columnar and transitional epithelium. Despite the fact that TCCP and prostatic adenocarcinoma can occur simultaneously, there is little evidence to support the transformation of adenocarcinoma to TCCP. Rather, adenocarcinoma is believed to maintain its initial histologic pattern throughout the life of the host.

TCCP has a marked tendency for intraductal growth. Histologic changes within the prostatic duct, from normal to hypertrophy to atypia to carcinoma in situ, have been demonstrated. Ultimately, TCCP may proceed to invasion of the prostatic stroma by penetration of the basement membrane and hence to local extension and distant metastases.

PRESENTING FEATURES AND EVALUATION

The distinction between TCCP and prostatic adenocarcinoma is generally made histologically. Patients with TCCP present at a slightly younger age (63 to 70 years) than is typical for prostatic adenocarcinoma. Signs and symptoms of bladder neck obstruction predominate (79 percent), with hematuria (41 to 44 percent), retention (25 percent), bone pain (14 percent), weight loss (7 percent), and rectal pain (4 to 6 percent) occurring less frequently. Prostatic enlargement on rectal examination is reported in 90 percent of patients, but the prostate may be palpably benign in 33 to 50 percent of patients.

The keys to early and correct diagnosis may be provided by cystoscopy and urinary cytology. Cystoscopic examination will reveal an obstructing or infiltrating tumor in about 85 percent of patients, with a polypoid mass protruding into the urethra in nearly one third of patients. Transurethral biopsy is the method of choice for diagnosing TCCP and should be combined with a careful inspection of *all* urothelium, including random bladder biopsies. Results of transrectal or transperineal biopsies are seldom diagnostic. Urinary cytology is positive for malignancy in 90 percent of cases and thus may be very helpful in distinguishing between TCCP and prostatic adenocarcinoma. Recently, transrectal ultrasound studies have demonstrated its ability to detect involvement of the prostate by bladder cancer. In many of these cases the prostatic involvement may not be accessible by cystoscopic examination.

The alkaline phosphatase level is elevated in roughly one third of patients, whereas acid phosphatase elevation is rare except in the mixed histology pattern. Forty percent of patients become azotemic at some point in their course, and excretory urography reveals hydronephrosis in 25 percent of patients. As opposed to prostatic adenocarcinoma, more than 70 percent of metastatic bone lesions are lytic.

As in the diagnosis of prostatic adenocarcinoma, I employ computed tomographic (CT) scanning and/or bipedal lymphangiography for further clinical staging of these tumors. It is important to obtain CT scans if possible before any significant prostatic biopsy or resection occurs, because postoperative changes make interpretation of capsular invasion, for example, very problematic. In this regard, I would not preclude surgical exploration and resection on the basis of CT or lymphangiography alone, except for the case of histologically confirmed (thin-needle biopsy) lymph node metastases at or above the aortic bifurcation.

PATIENT SELECTION

At the time of initial evaluation it is critical to determine which of the above-mentioned neoplastic processes (primary, secondary, or mixed) is being dealt with. A careful urologic history, including documentation of previous urothelial tumors, is mandatory. Correct clinical staging of the patient is also critical in defining further therapeutic alternatives.

Staging of TCCP has in the past been varied and confusing. Many authors cite the Whitmore-Jewett staging system commonly employed for staging prostatic adenocarcinomas. Still others stage the lesion according to the presence or absence of prostatic stromal invasion. My concept is to consider primary TCCP as I would any other urothelial tumor, and to stage it using a modification of the Jewett-Strong staging or TNM systems commonly employed for bladder and ureteral cancers (Table 1). In this regard, it is important to note that stage A tumors do not exist, since no well-defined submucosal layer is present between the glandular epithelium and the fibromuscular stroma. This staging system therefore serves to emphasize the early "invasiveness" and metastatic potential of these tumors.

On the basis of the two factors of neoplastic process and stage, one can delineate a treatment plan. Although it is true that the relatively small number of patients reported in the literature and the combinations of treatment used in these patients make it difficult to judge the efficacy of any treatment, I have attempted to describe my treatment choices by neoplastic process type and clinical stage.

PRIMARY OR SECONDARY TCCP IN SITU (STAGE O)

There is evidence in the literature to support the use of transurethral resection of the prostate (TURP) for the treatment of TCCP in situ. Several centers have reported 5-year survivors with this technique. In my experience, these patients most commonly present with prostatic "recurrences" after or during intravesical chemotherapy for superficial transitional cell cancers (stages O, A) of the bladder. If the prostatic lesion does not penetrate the basement membrane and is not diffuse in the prostate, I favor TURP with a repeat resection at the 3-month follow-up examination. If the process is diffuse within the prostate at the initial resection or if any residual cancer is found at repeat TURP, I recommend cystoprostatectomy with urethrectomy even if penetration of the basement membrane has not occurred.

PRIMARY TCCP INVADING PROSTATIC STROMA (STAGE B)

Once prostatic stromal invasion occurs, the risk of development of metastatic disease is extremely high. I therefore typically proceed to radical prostatectomy or radical cystoprostatectomy with lymphadenectomy and urethrectomy in these patients. I reserve radical prostatectomy for patients whose disease is clinically confined to the prostate and clearly away from the bladder neck.

There is considerable disagreement in the literature concerning the role of radiation therapy in these patients. There is evidence that radiation therapy can reduce the local recurrence rate in patients with advanced disease. I am not convinced, however, that there is reliable experience to conclude that TCCP is a radiocurable lesion, and I therefore reserve radiation therapy for patients who are not suitable surgical candidates.

SECONDARY TCCP WITH PROSTATIC STROMAL INVASION (STAGE D1 BLADDER CANCER BY JEWETT-STRONG STAGING)

This lesion is fairly common and carries a dismal prognosis. Because it results from a bladder primary lesion, the presence of prostatic stomal invasion denotes

Table 1 Proposed Staging for Transitional Cell Prostatic Cancers

Jewett-Strong Stage	TNM Stage	Description
0	TIS, Ta	In situ tumor not penetrating basement membrane
A*	T1	
B	T5	Invasion of prostatic fibromuscular stroma (penetrating basement membrane) but palpably confined to prostate
C	T3	Extending beyond prostatic capsule
D1	T4 N+	Extending to regional lymphatics below aortic bifurcation
D2	T4 N+ M+	Distant metastases

*Stage A does not exist because of the absence of a submucosal layer.

a D1 Jewett-Strong stage. Most series in the literature of patients in this category report a 5-year survival rate of approximately 20 percent despite cystoprostatectomy, lymphadenectomy, and preoperative radiation therapy. Despite this dismal prognosis and because of notable advances in the treatment of metastatic transitional cell cancers using combination chemotherapy, preoperative chemotherapy with or without concomitant radiation therapy is beginning to be used in these patients, followed by radical cystoprostatectomy, urethrectomy, and lymphadenectomy.

PRIMARY OR SECONDARY TCCP WITH EXTENSION BEYOND THE PROSTATE OR MINIMAL INVOLVEMENT OF REGIONAL LYMPHATICS (STAGES C AND MINIMAL D1)

My approach to patients with this stage of TCCP is to use combination therapy. If CT or lymphangiography does not reveal evidence of lymph node involvement, but the prostatic lesion is judged to be outside the prostatic capsule, I proceed to combination preoperative chemotherapy and radiation therapy followed by cystoprostatectomy and lymphadenectomy. If at exploration the tumor is believed not to be resectable because of nodal involvement above the aortic bifurcation or fixation to the pelvic side wall, I proceed to completion of the full course of radiation therapy to include lymph nodes above those known to be involved.

PRIMARY OR SECONDARY TCCP WITH DISTANT METASTASES (STAGE D2)

Little information is available regarding the treatment of advanced (metastatic) TCCP except for the clear message that *hormonal therapy is of no value*. Certainly this disease follows a course similar to invasive transitional cell cancer of the bladder with early metastatic disease to bone, lung, and liver. Isolated reports of single patients treated with combination chemotherapy have detailed partial objective responses with significant symptomatic improvement of short duration (5 to 6 months). More encouraging are the results of several clinical trials of combination chemotherapy for metastatic urothelial cancers. The Northern California Oncology Group, for example, reported complete responses in 35 percent (13 of 37 patients) and partial responses in 22 percent (8 of 37 patients) to cisplatin, methotrexate, and vinblastine. Complete responses have also been found with MVAC (methotrexate, vinblastine, adriamycin, cisplatin) chemotherapy, even in patients with nodal metastases. Most important, some of these responses are of significant duration. Because of the paucity of clinical experience with TCCP and the fact that any single institution is unlikely to see a significant number of these patients, it would seem prudent that clinical protocols be developed for multi-institutional (perhaps national) use in the future.

RHABDOMYOSARCOMA OF THE PROSTATE

THOMAS H. STANISIC, M.D.
JOHN J. HUTTER, Jr., M.D.
J. ROBERT CASSADY, M.D.

Rhabdomyosarcomas are highly malignant lesions that constitute the most common soft tissue sarcomas of childhood. About 25 to 35 percent arise in the genitourinary tract. Prostate and bladder lesions are generally considered as a unit, since early invasion of contiguous structures is so common that accurate determination of origin (prostate or bladder) is difficult except in the small minority of cases arising in the bladder dome. The tumor typically arises in the connective tissue stroma of its organ of origin. Local extension is common early in the disease process, and distant hematogenous and lymphatic metastases are frequently noted at autopsy or surgical exploration. When the tumor protrudes into the bladder lumen, it generally assumes a classic polypoid or botyroid form. A high percentage of these children have "favorable" embryonal histopathology, in contrast to the higher incidence of the "unfavorable" alveolar subtype seen in trunk or extremity primary lesions.

The median presenting age is in the mid-preschool years, and initial signs and symptoms include hematuria, irritative bladder symptoms, urinary obstruction, abdominal pain, and/or mass and constipation. Tissue diagnosis is by transurethral or perineal needle biopsy, and the tumor is staged using standard x-ray examination, computed tomography (CT), magnetic resonance imaging (MRI), and ultrasonography to delineate tumor extent in the pelvis, abdomen, and chest. Complete blood count (CBC) and SMAC-20 determinations provide rough indicators of organ involvement. Although bone metastases are unusual, many centers recommend bone scans and bone marrow biopsy as part of the initial staging evaluation. Bimanual examination under anesthesia at the time of biopsy is also helpful in estimating tumor extent and resectability. Because of the high frequency (41 percent) of lymphatic spread documented in children with prostatic primary cancers clinically limited to the pelvis, some centers include surgical staging of the pelvic lymph nodes in their initial evaluation when the results of such biopsies might significantly influence treatment planning.

The clinical group schema of the Intergroup Rhabdomyosarcoma Study (IRS) is currently used most commonly in staging patients and is used here in discussing therapeutic options (Table 1).

THERAPEUTIC ALTERNATIVES

During the past two decades, it has become clear that successful treatment of this tumor involves a multidisciplinary team approach combining surgery, radiotherapy, and chemotherapy. There is no question that current survival rates from combination therapy far exceed those resulting from radical surgery alone, which was the cornerstone of therapy before the early 1970s. However, there is no general agreement currently regarding the precise role in terms of magnitude, order, or timing of each therapeutic modality in an optimal treatment plan as might be applied to the individual patient. The reasons for this lack of consensus are understandable. Most important, the tumor is uncommon. Because of this, over a given time, when a single combination treatment regimen might be employed, no single individual or institution generally accumulates enough experience to justify firm conclusions and

Table 1 Intergroup Rhabdomyosarcoma Study Clinical Group Scheme

Group I:	Localized disease completely resected with regional nodes not involved
	a. Confined to organ of origin
	b. Contiguous involvement outside organ of origin
Group II:	a. Grossly resected tumor, microscopic residual
	b. Regional disease with complete resection
	c. Regional disease, grossly resected, microscopic residual
Group III:	Incomplete resection or biopsy with gross residual disease
Group IV:	Metastatic disease present at onset

Modified from Hays DM, Raney RB Jr, Lawrence W Jr et al. Bladder and prostatic tumors in the Intergroup Rhabdomyosarcoma Study (IRS-I): results of therapy. Cancer 1982; 50:1473.

definitive, absolute recommendations. On the basis of small sample sizes, different institutions have reported divergent experiences with similar treatment combinations and have made opposing recommendations in the literature.

The two cooperative Intergroup Rhabdomyosarcoma Studies (IRS-I and -II) provide useful data from large numbers of patients enrolled since 1972, but several basic issues remain unanswered at this time. IRS-I demonstrated that for localized nonmetastatic disease, radical surgery (generally cystoprostatectomy) followed by chemotherapy with or without radiotherapy cured most patients so treated (23 of 25, 92 percent). However, survival with this type of treatment was associated with substantial body image problems and sexual dysfunction secondary to radical cystoprostatectomy and urinary diversion. Simultaneously, in this same study, a smaller number of patients with localized disease were treated with primary chemoradiotherapy (PCR) after incisional biopsy. Seven of 17 such patients maintained bladder function and remained disease free without radical surgery.

Results in this small group of patients and similar reports from other institutions led to an approach in IRS-II in which children with nondisseminated disease were treated with initial incisional biopsy and subsequent "pulse-VAC" chemotherapy (vincristine, actinomycin D, and cyclophosphamide) in an effort to limit radical surgery and radiation to chemotherapy failures. As IRS-II progressed, it became apparent that chemotherapy alone would not obviate the need for radiotherapy or surgery. Less than 10 percent of patients with pelvic rhabdomyosarcomas achieved relapse-free survival with VAC alone. Radiotherapy or extirpative surgery was necessary to achieve cure in a vast majority of patients. Of 39 patients with localized bladder and prostatic rhabdomyosarcoma enrolled and reported on in 1984, 25 (64 percent) experienced a relapse-free survival overall, while 16 (41 percent) retained the bladder and remained disease free. However, only three of these children did not require either radiation or surgery after chemotherapy, and two of the three had previously undergone partial cystectomy. A later update reported an overall relapse-free survival for prostate-bladder of about 55 percent at 2-year follow-up. Because varying radiation dosages, including some now considered suboptimal, were used, particularly early in IRS-II, these studies did not produce data on which to base firm recommendations regarding radiation doses and timing. Similarly, while subsequent anecdotal reports have described poorly functioning bladders and sphincter mechanisms as sequelae to more intense radiotherapy regimens, no systematic review of intermediate and long-term toxicity from chemoradiotherapy has been published. Thus, basic questions regarding the magnitude of lower genitourinary tract changes that can result from radiotherapy are not clearly answered either.

Urologists treating a child with localized prostate-bladder rhabdomyosarcoma should be aware of this historical background. Specifically, they should recognize that an initial radical cystoprostatectomy, when possible, offers a high chance (90+ percent) of cure when followed with adjunctive chemoradiotherapy. However, a bladder-sparing option employing primary chemoradiotherapy can be used successfully in a substantial number of patients, although this approach is potentially associated with somewhat increased mortality. Also, some children in whom organ salvage and disease control with this approach is attempted ultimately require secondary cystoprostatectomy, either because of local failure or because of adverse normal tissue consequences of chemoradiotherapy. Parents must understand that treatment of this tumor is not "cut and dried" and should be involved in the therapeutic decision-making process as much as possible.

PREFERRED APPROACH

After biopsy confirmation, the staging studies outlined above separate the relatively few patients with distant metastases from the vast majority with tumor localized to the pelvis. As discussed later, treatment of metastatic disease is relatively straightforward, although disappointing. Those treating localized disease, on the other hand, must deal with complex and controversial issues that warrant considerable discussion.

Localized Disease

On the basis of the IRS experience, we believe that an attempt at an organ-sparing approach initially, using primary chemotherapy followed by radiation and/or surgery, is appropriate in most patients with localized disease. Many patients with disease limited to the pelvis are found to have local tumor extent that precludes initial total tumor removal by radical cystoprostatectomy or prostatectomy. In this group, a neoadjuvant approach provides an opportunity for initial cytoreduction that may make subsequent treatment with surgery or radiation more effective. Even when disease is more limited, when an initial radical extirpation followed by adjuvant chemotherapy with or without radiotherapy is possible and provides a maximal chance of cure, we believe many families will wish to combine an attempt at organ preservation with definitive treatment once they are aware that this is a realistic option with a substantial chance of cure.

It is important that frank discussions take place at the outset of such an approach so that all involved recognize that a disease-free status will be combined with functional organ preservation in a minority of patients so treated. Prompt recognition of the indications of failure of conservative management is necessary as treatment progresses, to allow for appropriate initiation of aggressive surgical management when indicated to maximize patient survival. Our approach to treatment is broadly based on the therapeutic schema used in the IRS, and the rationale for many therapeutic decisions is based on data derived from these studies and other similar approaches. However, treatment plans must be flexible and individualized since all questions about treatment of this disease are certainly not answered at this time. Certainly, tumor size must be carefully re-evaluated after each course of therapy in children receiving primary chemotherapy, to allow for early aggressive surgical intervention in patients who do not demonstrate good partial or complete responses.

Currently, standard primary chemotherapy consists of pulse-VAC as detailed in Table 2. This can often be administered in the ambulatory setting. Children receiving high doses of cyclophosphamide must be well hydrated to minimize the risk of hemorrhagic cystitis from this agent. Other potential complications from pulse-VAC chemotherapy include myelosuppression, mucositis, and vincristine neurotoxicity. Dose modifications may be necessary if these complications are severe. Institutions participating in the IRS-IV Clinical Group III Pilot Study may offer patients the choice of taking part in another primary chemotherapy regimen currently being evaluated in this clinical trial.

After two courses of pulse-VAC, clinical assessment, including CT, MRI, ultrasonography, repeat cystoscopy, bimanual examination, and biopsy, dictates further management. In the event of a complete or substantial (greater than 50 percent) clinical response, two more courses of pulse-VAC are administered. After this, at 16 weeks another complete clinical reassessment is indicated, which may include surgical exploration and tumor-nodal biopsy if clinical staging provides inadequate information about the disease status. In the IRS studies, only a small minority (less than 10 percent) of children with localized disease obtained a sustained pathologic complete response from chemotherapy alone. Durable responses require that either local-regional radiotherapy or surgery be included in the

<table>
<tr><td colspan="2" align="center">**Table 2** "Pulse" VAC Chemotherapy</td></tr>
<tr><td>A. Induction (12 weeks):</td><td>1. Vincristine 2 mg/m^2 (maximum dose 2 mg) IV q week × 12
2. Dactinomycin 0.015 mg/kg (maximum dose = 0.5 mg) IV daily × 5 days (days 1 through 5)
3. Cytoxan 10 mg/kg/day IV × 3 days (days 1, 2, 3)
4. Cytoxan 20 mg/kg IV day 21, day 42, day 63</td></tr>
<tr><td>B. Maintenance (beginning week 12 and administered q 4 weeks up to 2 years):</td><td>1. Vincristine 2 mg/m^2 (maximum dose 2 mg) IV
2. Dactinomycin 0.015 mg/kg (maximum dose 0.5 mg) IV daily × 5 days
3. Cytoxan 10 mg/kg IV × 3 days</td></tr>
</table>

treatment plan for most children at this point. Certainly, when residual disease is present after four courses of pulse-VAC, additional therapy with surgery or radiation is essential. Whichever is chosen, pulse-VAC or other appropriate chemotherapy is continued for 2 years as maintenance therapy.

When radiation therapy is chosen to augment the initial care and chemotherapeutic response in this setting, it is reasonable to expect a good result. In IRS-II, several patients achieved long-term disease-free status with intact bladders by means of chemotherapy and subsequent radiotherapy. None had initial complete clinical responses to chemotherapy alone. The initial prechemotherapy tumor volume and involved node volumes should be included in treatment fields. Recent data indicate that radiation doses of 4,000 rads are sufficient to control microscopic disease of embryonal type. A four-field approach is advisable with weighting of the anterior and posterior fields to limit proximal femoral dosage to 1,500 rads or less to minimize growth arrest. The optimal radiation dose for gross residual tumor is controversial, and no IRS report has simultaneously reviewed adequacy of treatment volumes and dose and correlated these with local control. We recommend a 5,000 to 5,500 rad minimal tumor dose to gross residual tumor within the constraints of normal tissue tolerances. Small bowel is the most common dose-limiting normal tissue, especially considering the radiation-enhancing effects of doxorubicin (Adriamycin) and actinomycin D. Toxicity expectations should be realistic. Some degree of growth arrest of bony or soft tissue (muscle) structures is virtually inevitable, depending on the age of the patient. There is also a small but real risk of resultant bowel, bladder, and/or sphincter dysfunction. Finally, there is a risk of second tumors, since most of these children have been noted to have consistent chromosomal abnormality at the 11p locus (embryonal subtype). Finally, in our experience, although a response of rhabdomyosarcoma to irradiation is regularly seen, peristent mass effect on imaging studies may be noted for some time. This does not necessarily denote treatment failure in the absence of tumor progression. Biopsy of such areas, most commonly performed in children with head and neck primary lesions, has frequently revealed a stromal pattern and no evidence of rhabdomyosarcoma.

If surgery is employed to augment the initial chemotherapeutic response, either radical prostatectomy or cystoprostatectomy may be indicated, depending on tumor location and extent. The goal of such surgery is complete tumor excision. At the time of operation, frozen sections may be employed in an attempt to evaluate resection margins, but interpretation is notoriously difficult and the potential for error is substantial. If radical cystoprostatectomy is employed, continent urinary diversion is preferable to the standard ileal conduit. Continent diversion allows for a much more active life-style and enhanced body image, and provides a much higher level of patient satisfaction and function. The Indiana reservoir uses standard techniques familiar to most urologists and is the preferred method of continent diversion at our institution. The efferent limb can be brought to either the abdominal wall or the distal urethra for intermittent catheterization. An umbilical stoma minimizes cosmetic deformity if an abdominal site is chosen. We generally employ a mechanical bowel preparation using an oral electrolyte solution (Colyte), delivered per nasogastric tube intermittently over 6 to 8 hours the day before surgery until stools are clear. At surgery we use a GIA stapler to narrow the efferent ileal limb over a red rubber catheter, and drain the reservoir with both a large Malecot, via an abdominal stab wound, and a Foley catheter through the ileal limb. The use of two tubes facilitates postoperative irrigation, which is done on a regular basis at increasing intervals of 2 to 4 hours until 3 to 4 weeks postoperatively. At that time, we perform a "pouchogram" to check suture line integrity, remove both catheters, and initiate a program of clean, intermittent catheterization and self-irrigation at gradually increasing intervals. The procedure generally adds about 2 hours to the time required for a standard ileal conduit, and hospital stay is about 10 to 14 days. Continent diversion techniques have evolved rapidly and successfully in recent years, and many institutions are reporting success with various techniques using both large and small bowel. Clearly, any of several alternative techniques can provide acceptable results in experienced hands, as long as the family are responsible and committed to an intermittent catheterization program. If the native urethra is incorporated into the reconstruction, biopsies are indicated preoperatively, using permanent sections to allow for careful evaluation of the bulbomembranous urethra to detect tumor involvement.

When microscopic or gross tumor residual remains after attempted surgical extirpation, postoperative adjuvant radiotherapy is indicated. The question of what doses are appropriate is controversial in this setting. However, we favor approximately 4,000 to 4,400 rads for treatment of potential residual microscopic disease and larger doses of 5,000 to 5,500 rads to treat gross residual disease. Intraoperative interstitial approaches should be kept in mind for prostatic rhabdomyosarcoma, particularly as an adjunct to attempted surgical extirpation, either primarily or for recurrent or residual disease after attempted conservative treatment. These approaches confine moderate or high doses of radiation to a relatively small volume and offer real advantages in normal tissue preservation and retention of growth potential. Whether surgery, radiation, or both are used to treat initial responders, pulse-VAC is continued for 2 years on a maintenance schedule, assuming that no evidence of tumor cell resistance to these agents has arisen.

When there is a less than 50 percent response after two courses of pulse-VAC induction therapy, or if there is disease progression, a decision must be made at this point whether to employ radiation therapy or extirpative surgery as an adjunct. More intense chemotherapy with other potentially effective agents such as cisplatin, doxorubicin, and ifosfamide may also be considered. The rationale employed in the decision-making process is the same as that outlined above for individuals who initially respond to pulse-VAC at 8 weeks but still have residual disease after two more courses of chemotherapy. Frankly, proponents of radiation or surgery in this situation can find supportive evidence in the literature suggesting that their point of view is a reasonable one. Ultimately, the choice of therapy at this point may well be based on subjective factors, such as how much weight the parents place on quality of life issues and body image, how comfortable they feel with intermittent catheterization and the concept of continent diversion, and how they balance these factors with the risk of disease recurrence. As indicated previously, if surgery is utilized at this point, and if microscopic disease remains afterward, adjunctive postoperative radiation therapy is recommended. In individuals who have not responded well to the first two courses of pulse-VAC, after radiation or surgery is completed, maintenance chemotherapy generally involves more intense chemotherapeutic regimens with additional agents. Maintenance chemotherapy in such patients should be designed to include those agents that have produced the most effective clinical response for the individual patient's tumor. In such patients, attempts are made to keep the treatment intervals between courses of maintenance therapy as short as possible in order to maximize any chemotherapeutic benefit.

Metastatic Disease

Little has been said about the treatment of Group IV disease. Results with standard pulse-VAC chemotherapy have been poor, with less than 30 percent long-term survivors. The primary therapeutic approach at this time should be a systemic one. Since the results of treatment of children with Group IV disease have been so poor, we recommend enrollment in clinical trials such as the current IRS pilot study for Group IV disease. This is evaluating ifosfamide-doxorubicin chemotherapy for induction and subsequent use of these agents in combination with VAC as maintenance chemotherapy. In addition to the chemotherapy question, this study is evaluating the feasibility and toxicity of a hyperfractionated radiation therapy regimen following induction chemotherapy.

Local radiation and surgery may be used on a case-by-case basis to palliate symptoms or to treat or excise tumor remaining after an initial chemotherapy response. This may be particularly useful in a small subset of children who are classified Group IV solely by virtue of nodal extension (i.e., high para-aortic or supraclavicular disease), who fare better than their cohorts with visceral disease. Palliation of bone, spinal cord, or other local problems for the child in whom cure is not possible is often attainable with local fields delivering 3,000 rads per 10 fractions or 4,000 rads per 20 fractions.

ADVANTAGES AND DISADVANTAGES

Initial treatment with radical surgery may offer the best chance of disease-free survival, and when combined with continent urinary diversion, provides an opportunity for an active life-style and a positive body image. Isolated reports of malignancies occurring in bowel mucosa used in urinary reservoirs are worrisome; such events appear to be infrequent but require careful actuarial assessment. In the short term, the adverse effects of continent diversion on renal function seem minimal, but long-term follow-up will be necessary to allow firm conclusions regarding the safety of this new advance. On the other hand, initial treatment of localized tumor with primary chemotherapy provides an opportunity for genitourinary organ preservation in some children. However, recurrences are frequent when primary chemotherapy is the sole modality, and adjunctive radiation and surgery are necessary to eradicate disease fully in most cases. Persistent disease-free survival appears less with this approach, but the small numbers reported make firm conclusions regarding this point hazardous. Variations in timing and increased dosages of radiation may be important in increasing survival with this conservative regimen, but precise optimal treatment schedules remain undefined pending further investigation. Adverse long-term side effects of chemoradiotherapy have been reported anecdotally: fibrotic nonfunctional bladders, secondary malignancies in the field of radiation, and adverse effects of chemoradiotherapy on reproductive function. It will be necessary for more survivors to grow into adulthood and provide an opportunity for long-term follow-up before more detailed information is available about the adverse sequelae of these treatment regimens.

SUGGESTED READING

Hays DM, Mauer HM, Soule EH, et al. Rhabdomyosarcoma of bladder, prostate, and vagina. Dialogues in Pediatric Urology Vol 7, No. 4, April 1984.

Hays DM, Raney RB Jr, Lawrence W Jr, et al. Bladder and prostatic tumors in the Intergroup Rhabdomyosarcoma Study (IRS-I): results of therapy. Cancer 1982; 50:1472–1482.

Hays DM, Raney RB Jr, Lawrence W Jr, et al. Primary chemotherapy in the treatment of children with bladder-prostate tumors in the Intergroup Rhabdomyosarcoma Study (IRS-II). J Pediatr Surg 1982; 17:812–819.

Hensle TW, Connor JP, Burbige KA. Continent urinary diversion in childhood. J Urol 1989; 143:981.

Kramer SA, Kelalis MD. Pediatric urologic oncology. Yearbook Medical Publishers, Inc., In: Gillenwater, Grayhack, Howards, Duckett, eds. Adult and pediatric urology, Vol 2. Chicago: Year Book, 1987:2001.

Loughlin KR, Retik AB, Weinstein HJ, et al. Genitourinary rhabdomyosarcoma in children. Cancer 1989; 63:1600.

PREMALIGNANT LESIONS OF THE PROSTATE

MICHAEL K. BRAWER, M.D.

Premalignant changes have been identified in many organs. In general, the criteria for a lesion to be considered premalignant include increased incidence, the severity and extent of the entity in organs harboring invasive carcinoma, similar morphology to invasive carcinoma, a spatial relationship between the premalignant change and invasive cancer, and focal invasive cancer observed arising from the putative premalignant change. Finally, serial biopsy over time should show progression from a premalignant lesion into invasive carcinoma.

A premalignant lesion of the prostate was identified in 1926. Since then, two conditions—prostatic intraepithelial neoplasia (PIN) and atypical adenomatous hyperplasia (AAH)—have emerged as the most likely candidates for premalignant change in the human prostate.

PIN fulfills most requirements for a premalignant lesion. Atypical AAH is somewhat controversial in this regard.

PATHOLOGY

Prostatic intraepithelial neoplasia, is a term used to describe atypical lesions arising from epithelial cells but confined to the lumens of prostatic ducts and acini, as well as similar lesions exhibiting microinvasion. PIN has been referred to in the literature by a number of synonyms, including atypical epithelial hyperplasia, atypical glandular hyperplasia, cytologic atypia, cellular atypia, duct-acinar dysplasia, glandular atypia, intraductal dysplasia, intraglandular dysplasia, and large acinar atypical hyperplasia. In part because of the significant confusion arising from the lack of standardization of nomenclature, not only in the literature but also in surgical pathology reports, a consensus conference was recently held. At this conference, it was decided that such lesions should be described as prostatic intraepithelial neoplasia. Grading and diagnostic criteria were also agreed upon.

PIN may be divided into three grades. Grade 1 consists of proliferation of the cells lining the prostatic ducts and acini. Instead of the normal basal and single luminal cell layer, there is piling up of the luminal cells. Associated with this are variations in nuclear size (anisonucleosis) and crowding and irregular spacing between cells. Nucleoli may be present although small. It is important to note that both architectural (piling up) and cytologic changes must be present for a diagnosis of PIN.

Grade 2 PIN is distinguishable from grade 1 in that most of the nuclei are markedly enlarged. Prominent nucleoli may be observed along with increased hyperchromasia. Grade 3 PIN, which is thought to be synonomous with carcinoma in situ, is distinguishable from the lower grades because of large prominent nucleoli. Cytologically, grade 3 PIN may be indistinguishable from the cells making up invasive carcinoma. Not infrequently, grade 3 PIN may exhibit luminal bridging reminiscent of cribriform Gleason grade 3 adenocarcinoma.

The major feature that distinguishes invasive carcinoma from grade 3 PIN is the presence of a basal cell layer in the latter. Basal cells, although at times disrupted, are always present in PIN but never in invasive carcinoma. This important histologic differentiation may be difficult to appreciate on standard hematoxylin and eosin–stained material, and cytokeratin immunohistochemistry may be needed.

Atypical adenomatous hyperplasia consists of clusters of small acinar structures lined by cuboidal to low columnar cells. Gland formation consists of small single structures discretely separated from the surrounding parenchyma. There may be peripheral budding of the acini into the surrounding tissue. Cytologically, the cells making up AAH are essentially identical to those of normal prostatic luminal epithelium. The nuclei appear bland and are basally oriented. On light microscopy, the basal cell layer is inconspicuous or even absent, unlike that seen in PIN. The major distinguishing feature between AAH and invasive carcinoma is the bland cytology of the former.

The differential diagnosis of AAH is primarily that of invasive carcinoma. PIN must be considered in the context of a number of other lesions, including seminal vesicles, Cowper's glands, paraganglionic tissue, benign hyperplasia, basal cell hyperplasia, atrophy and atrophy-associated hyperplasia, transitional metaplasia, infarction-induced atypia, inflammation-induced atypia, and radiation-induced atypia.

PREMALIGNANCY OF PROSTATIC INTRAEPITHELIAL NEOPLASIA

The data suggesting that PIN is a premalignant lesion are considerable. There is increased frequency of PIN in prostates with invasive carcinoma, as opposed to those without. In addition, higher-grade PIN is more commonly associated with invasive carcinoma. The extent of PIN is more common in organs with invasive cancer. Histologically, PIN is very similar to invasive carcinoma. Both are more commonly observed in the peripheral zone of the prostate. There may be disruption or loss of the basal cell layer in PIN, as in invasive carcinoma, but some basal cells are universally present. Invasive carcinoma may be seen to arise from foci of PIN and, significantly, there is juxtaposition of glands exhibiting PIN and invasive carcinoma. This latter observation is of particular importance, as discussed below.

Recently, several investigations have shown phenotypic similarity between invasive carcinoma and PIN. For example, antibodies against cytokeratins, vimentin, and blood group antigens, as well as the lectin Ulex europaeus, show phenotypic similarities between invasive carcinoma and PIN, but dissimilarities between PIN and benign epithelium.

Thus, PIN appears to fulfill most criteria for premalignant change. The one that has not been met—the ability to show over time with serial biopsies progression from PIN and into invasive carcinoma—probably will not be achieved. This stems from the fact that the prostate is a three-dimensional epithelial structure, and repeated biopsy of the same duct-acinar system is not possible. In two-dimensional epithelium organs, such as the urinary bladder, esophagus, respiratory tract, and uterine cervix, it is possible to visualize a lesion and biopsy the exact site over time. No imaging modality, including prostate ultrasonography, currently allows placement of a biopsy needle into the exact site on separate occasions.

CLINICAL SIGNIFICANCE OF PROSTATIC INTRAEPITHELIAL NEOPLASIA

The clinical relevance of PIN stems from three primary observations: (1) it may be associated with elevation of prostate-specific antigen (PSA), (2) it may appear indistinguishable from the most common presentation of adenocarcinoma on transrectal ultrasonography, and (3) patients who show PIN on prostate needle biopsy have a high likelihood of having concomitant invasive carcinoma.

PSA represents a major advance in the tumor marker armamentarium. It has proved usefulness in monitoring patients with established carcinoma, and may have applications in early detection and perhaps in staging. For PSA to be detectable in the serum, not only must there be PSA-secreting cells present, but this analyte must gain in access to the systematic circulation. Several potentially formidable barriers, including the prostatic basal cell, prostate basement membrane, intervening stroma, capillary basement membrane, and capillary endothelial cells, must all be crossed before this 34-kilodalton protein elaborated in the prostatic luminal cell can be detectable in the circulation. As noted above, invasive carcinoma is associated with loss of the basal cell layer and disruption or loss of the basement membrane. Similarly, disruption of the basal cell layer has been observed in PIN. Indeed, in high-grade PIN, the vast majority of acini and ductules exhibit some disruption of this barrier.

It has been observed that among men undergoing simple prostatectomy, the preoperative PSA was elevated in approximately half of those with incidental carcinoma, acute inflammation, or PIN, but was abnormal in only one of 26 men with simple benign prostatic hyperplasia (BPH) alone or BPH associated with chronic inflammation. Similarly, among men undergoing ultrasound-guided prostate needle biopsy for a palpable prostatic abnormality, PSA values in those with PIN was noted to be intermediate between those with benign histology and those with carcinoma. Whether this correlation is related to the high frequency of PIN in association with carcinoma, and in the sampling the carcinoma was missed, or whether PIN itself is the cause of the elevation of this analyte remains unknown. Of interest in this regard is a recent observation that, utilizing quantitative immunohistochemistry, it appears that both PIN and invasive carcinoma elaborate less PSA on a cell-by-cell basis than benign prostatic epithelium.

Transrectal ultrasonography has revolutionized our ability to image and perform biopsy of the prostate. Eight cases of PIN have been detected on biopsy of peripheral zone hypoechoic lesions—the most common presentation for invasive carcinoma. PIN without carcinoma has been reported in 11 to 14 percent of men undergoing ultrasound-guided biopsy of hypoechoic peripheral zone lesions.

Perhaps the greatest evidence that PIN is significant stems from our experience with 21 men who were shown to have PIN on biopsy of palpably abnormal prostatic lesions. We performed repeat ultrasound-guided biopsy and noted carcinoma in 12 (67 percent). This included two patients with an initial biopsy revealing PIN 1, and all patients with PIN 2 (eight) and PIN 3 (two). This finding correlates with the observation that PIN frequently is found adjacent to invasive carcinoma, which perhaps suggests a field affect in the area surrounding the transformed epithelium.

TREATMENT

The most important factor with regard to the management of PIN and AAH hyperplasia is the need for these conditions to be reported on simple prostatectomy or prostate needle biopsy specimens by the surgical pathologist. Urologists must encourage their pathologic colleagues to learn about these lesions and to refrain from simply making the diagnosis of "no evidence of malignancy."

Currently, neither PIN nor AAH is an indication for treatment. A cautionary note is in order. There have been several cases in which radical prostatectomy has been performed because of an erroneous interpretation of PIN, but no cancer was found in the specimen. It is important that a firm diagnosis of carcinoma be made before therapeutic decisions are rendered.

How do we manage men with a diagnosis of PIN or AAH? If the diagnosis is made on transurethral resection or simple open prostatectomy specimens, the surgical pathologist should embed all remaining tissue and section with levels the existing blocks. If invasive carcinoma is not found, I not only perform transrectal ultrasonography and biopsy of any suspicious hypoechoic peripheral zone lesions, but also biopsy in a random fashion areas adjacent to the resected area. The finding of transition zone carcinoma is problematic on transrectal ultrasonography because of the relative hypoechoic nature of the transition zone normally. If these biopsies are negative, the patient is followed clinically, and PSA levels are determined. If there is a significant change in the PSA, repeat ultrasonography is probably warranted.

When PIN is noted on a prostate needle biopsy and is grade 2 or 3, a repeat biopsy of the areas where the PIN was encountered is recommended. This is one example of the importance of labeling the specimens from the initial biopsy with the location within the prostate form where they are obtained (e.g., right base, left apex). The biopsy is then repeated only in the areas exhibiting PIN. As noted, a high percentage of the repeat biopsies reveal carcinoma. If these biopsies are negative, the patient is again followed clinically and with 6-month or yearly serum PSA determination. In a previous investigation with repeat biopsy of men with PIN, PSA levels stratified patients into those with invasive carcinoma and those without. Further investigations of the relationship of PSA to PIN are clearly indicated before definitive statements in this regard can be made.

With regard to grade 1 PIN, as noted, two of 11 patients on repeat biopsy were observed to have invasive carcinoma. The evaluation of men with low-grade PIN must be done within the clinical context. If the digital abnormalities or ultrasonographic findings raise suspicion or if the PSA level is elevated, repeat biopsy is recommended, particularly in a relatively young patient.

SUGGESTED READING

Bostwick DG, Brawer MK. Prostatic intraepithelial neoplasia and early invasion in prostate cancer. Cancer 1987; 59:788–794.

Brawer MK, Lange PH. Prostate-specific antigen and premalignant change: implications for early detection. CA 1989; 39:361–375.

Brawer MK, Rennels MA, Schifman RA, et al. Significance of serum prostate-specific antigen in men undergoing prostate surgery for benign disease. Am J Clin Pathol 1989; 92:760–764.

Brawer MK, Peehl DM, Stamey TA, Bostwick DG. Keratin immunoreactivity in the benign and neoplastic human prostate. Cancer Res 1985; 45:3663–3667.

Brawer MK, Rennels MA, Nagle RB, et al. Prostatic intraepithelial neoplasia: a lesion which may be confused with cancer on prostate ultrasound. J Urol 1989; 142:1510–1512.

McNeal JE, Bostwick DG. Intraductual dysplasia: a premalignant lesion of the prostate. Hum Pathol 1986; 17:64–71.

BENIGN PROSTATIC HYPERPLASIA

HERBERT LEPOR, M.D.

Twenty-five percent of the urologist's work load and 40 percent of major urologic surgery are related to the management of benign prostatic hyperplasia (BPH). Prostatectomy has become the standard treatment for BPH, because the surgical procedure is rarely associated with life-threatening complications and most patients achieve a highly satisfactory outcome. Nonsurgical alternatives for the treatment of BPH are presently receiving much attention. The possibility that the most common surgical procedure performed by the urologist may be replaced by medical therapy, a urethroplasty catheter, metallic stent, or hyperthermia probe has engendered a great deal of concern regarding the future well-being of our specialty. Nonsurgical treatment for BPH cannot be ignored, since the media has effectively stimulated an awareness of these alternatives, resulting in a well-informed public. Unfortunately, the limitations of prostatectomy and the effectiveness of nonsurgical treatment have not always been presented objectively. Nevertheless, urologists are under increasing pressure to offer these innovative treatment modalities. There are no reliable clinical data to justify incorporating many of these new treatment alternatives into the treatment strategy for BPH. The main objective of this chapter is to provide a practical overview of surgical and nonsurgical alternatives for the treatment of BPH. The treatment of BPH is presently in a state of evolution. The chapter represents an effort to present a practical and objective state-of-the-art overview.

INDICATIONS FOR TREATMENT

The indications for surgical and nonsurgical treatment of BPH are highly variable. Absolute indications for treatment require expeditious intervention. Urinary retention, recurrent urinary tract infection, and renal insufficiency secondary to BPH are generally accepted as absolute indications for treatment. Relative indications for intervention include moderate postvoid residual and annoying symptoms of prostatism. The symptoms of prostatism such as nocturia, urgency, urge incontinence, and postmicturition dribbling may significantly impair the quality of life without jeopardizing overall life expectancy. Approximately 80 percent of individuals undergo prostatectomy for relative indications, and there are many variations in treatment patterns among urologists. The decision to offer surgical, nonsurgical, or no treatment for individuals in whom there are relative indications should reflect the impact of symptoms on quality of life; the expectations, general medical condition, and treatment preferences of the patient; and the relative effectiveness, cost, and morbidity of available treatment options.

The effectiveness of treatment for BPH must be based on the ability to achieve the desired outcome. Unfortunately, most clinical reviews have not assessed outcome on the basis of the pretreatment severity of clinical or urodynamic obstruction. For example, the results of multicenter randomized, placebo-controlled studies often exclude patients with large postvoid residuals, urinary retention, and renal insufficiency. Therefore, conclusions from these studies cannot be extrapolated to patients with absolute indications for treatment. The data on the outcome of prostatectomy are similarly deficient. In interpreting the available clinical evidence, this important omission must be recognized.

PROSTATECTOMY

Prostatectomy is performed as an open enucleation (retropubic, suprapubic, perineal) or transurethral prostatectomy (TURP). The choice between these is based on the size of the gland and the abilities of the surgeon. Most urologists will resect 50-g adenomas. In the United States, 90 percent of prostatectomies for BPH are performed transurethrally and approximately 400,000 TURPs are performed annually. Prostatectomy has gained widespread acceptance for the treatment of BPH, since this procedure is relatively free of life-threatening complications, and in most patients a satisfactory outcome is achieved.

Despite the large numbers of patients who have undergone TURPs, data on results have been reported for only 414 surgical patients. Unfortunately, symptom score questionnaires have not been used routinely to assess the outcome of prostatectomy. Most investigators in reporting global patient satisfaction after TURP have used highly subjective and qualitative measures. Approximately 20 percent of patients do not achieve satisfactory relief of their presenting symptoms of prostatism after TURP. Unfortunately, there are no clinical or urodynamic parameters that are predictive of the outcome of TURP. Uroflowmetry has been used to measure objective urodynamic improvement after treatment for infravesical obstruction. Peak uroflow rates improve by approximately 95 percent after TURP. The magnitude of the increase in peak uroflow rates after prostatectomy exceeds that for all other treatment options.

The intraoperative and postoperative complications associated with TURP include bleeding requiring transfusion (6 percent), impotence (10 percent), incontinence (3 percent), infection (8 percent), and death (< 1 percent). Approximately 10 percent of men require additional surgical intervention within 10 years of prostatectomy. Roos and associates reported that patients undergoing TURP are at greater risk of cardiovascular death than individuals undergoing open prostatectomy. Comorbidity, as captured in the claims data in this retrospective chart review, did not account for the observed survival differences. The methodology and conclusions derived from retrospective outcome surveys have been criticized. Although there is no physiologic explanation for the increased cardiovascular-related morbidity and mortality, the urologic community cannot ignore these

preliminary observations. The American Urological Association (AUA) is presently organizing a multicenter clinical study to compare cardiovascular-related morbidity and mortality after TURP compared with open prostatectomy and other treatment options.

TRANSURETHRAL INCISION OF THE PROSTATE

Transurethral incision of the prostate (TUIP) is an operative procedure popularized by Orandi. It may be achieved by means of incisions of various lengths, depths, and locations. Advocates of this procedure have suggested using a single incision at the 6 o'clock position, or two incisions at the 5 and 7 o'clock positions or the 4 and 8 o'clock positions. The neurovascular bundle mediating erectile function originates from the lateral pedicles, and courses posterolaterally along the prostate. Thermal injury to the neurovascular bundle may result from incisions at the 4 and 8 o'clock positions. I prefer to make the incisions at the 6 o'clock position, or the 5 and 7 o'clock positions, in order to minimize procedure-related erectile dysfunction. The incisions are most commonly made with a Collings knife. The incisions are most commonly made from the level of the ureteral orifices to the verumontanum. Several authors suggest extending the incisions through the bladder neck into the perivesical fat. On the basis of an extensive experience with TUIP, Orandi concluded that prostate adenomas of less than 20 g are suitable for this procedure. The median weight of prostate adenomas resected by American urologists is approximately 15 g. Most men currently undergoing TURP are therefore candidates for TUIP.

TUIP has been associated with a much lower morbidity rate than TURP. Bladder neck contractures develop in approximately 5 percent of men after TURP and are most likely to occur after resection of smaller glands. Such contractures rarely, if ever, occur after TUIP. TUIP performed at the 6 o'clock position, or the 5 or 7 o'clock positions, should not result in impotence. Approximately 50 percent of men develop retrograde ejaculation after TURP. Although the impact of retrograde ejaculation has not been critically examined, it has been assumed that patients are rarely bothered by postprostatectomy retrograde ejaculation, which occurs in approximately 20 percent of patients after TUIP. A small subset of patients who are definite candidates for TUIP are those with infravesical obstruction secondary to BPH who wish to preserve their fertility potential or those who express concern regarding retrograde ejaculation.

Several investigators have compared the outcomes of TUIP and TURP in randomized clinical studies, which were limited to men with prostatism and estimated prostate volumes between 20 and 30 g. Overall, patient satisfaction and uroflowmetry after TURP and TUIP were comparable. On the basis of relative efficacy and morbidity, TUIP is a reasonable surgical alternative for the relief of prostatism secondary to relatively small adenomas. The primary limitation of TUIP is that a tissue diagnosis is not obtained.

ALPHA-BLOCKERS

The rationale for using alpha-blockers to treat BPH was based on the observation that the contractile properties of prostate smooth muscle are mediated by $alpha_1$ adrenoceptors. Caine and associates reported in 1976 that phenoxybenzamine (a nonselective alpha-blocker) was effective in the treatment of BPH. Over the past 14 years, 18 clinical trials evaluating alpha-blockers for the treatment of BPH have been reported. Most of these studies were deficient in protocol design and criteria for enrollment, and assessments of efficacy were not standardized. Sixteen of the 18 reported clinical studies confirmed Caine's observation that alpha-blockers are effective in the treatment of BPH. The two studies reporting lack of efficacy were designed to evaluate the effectiveness of low-dose alpha-blockade. The lack of both efficacy and side effects in these studies indicated that the low dose of alpha-blocker was insufficient to achieve alpha-adrenoceptor blockade. Although the protocol designs for evaluating alpha-blockers for BPH have been variable, the improvements in urinary flow rates have been highly consistent. Overall, urinary flow rates improve approximately 50 percent after administration of alpha-blockers. The degree of symptomatic improvement after alpha-blockade is difficult to ascertain, since quantitative symptom score questionnaires have not been consistently used as outcome parameters. The toxicity associated with the commercially available alpha-blockers is variable. The incidence and severity of adverse reactions associated with the nonselective alpha-blockers, such as phenoxybenzamine, are far greater than the toxicity of selective alpha-blockers such as prazosin and terazosin. The implication of the clinical experience with alpha-blockers for BPH is that efficacy is dependent on $alpha_1$-adrenoceptor blockade, whereas toxicity is related to $alpha_2$-adrenoceptor blockade.

Terazosin is the only selective long-acting $alpha_1$-adrenoceptor antagonist that is presently FDA (Federal Drug Administration) approved for the treatment of hypertension. The primary advantage of terazosin over all the other commercially available alpha-blockers is that its longer half-life allows for a once-a-day dosage regimen. The preliminary experience with terazosin in the treatment of BPH has been encouraging. We recently reported an open labeled study evaluating the safety and efficacy of terazosin in 45 normotensive males between 50 and 80 years of age with symptomatic BPH. The dose of terazosin was titrated to 5 mg over a period of 1 month. Orthostatic hypotension was observed in only one patient during the dose titrations. The evaluation of the efficacy of terazosin was based on improvement in urinary flow rates, obstructive and irritative symptom scores, and the patient's global assessment of improvement. Thirty-nine patients completed the

2-month dose-titration study; five were excluded owing to relatively minor and reversible adverse reactions, and one was unable to return for follow-up visits. The baseline clinical and urodynamic parameters confirmed that the patients enrolled in the study had bladder outlet obstruction. Overall, the mean systolic and diastolic blood pressures were not significantly affected by any dose of terazosin administered. The improvement in peak and mean urinary flow rates was 42 and 48 percent, respectively, and in the obstructive and irritative symptoms, 63 and 35 percent, respectively. The efficacy of terazosin has been maintained over a mean follow-up interval of 15 months. The durability and compliance of alpha-blockade requires further investigation.

ANDROGEN SUPPRESSION

The reduction of prostate volume after castration in males with BPH was observed 100 years ago. Castration never gained widespread acceptance for the treatment of BPH owing to the psychological impact of removal of the testes and the subsequent development of impotence, loss of libido, and hot flashes resulting from the imbalance of androgens and estrogens. Medical castration can be achieved by drugs that block the action, or synthesis, of testosterone. The primary limitation of testosterone-lowering drugs such as diethylstilbestrol (DES), progestational agents, and gonadotropin-releasing hormone (Gn-RH) analogs is again the resulting impotence, loss of libido, and hot flashes. The morbidity associated with castration and testosterone-lowering drugs is often greater than the therapeutic response for men with BPH.

Alternative approaches for achieving androgen suppression in BPH have been the use of 5-alpha–reductase inhibitors and blockade of androgen action at the cellular level of the prostate. The maintenance of prostate volume is dependent on tissue levels of dihydrotestosterone (DHT). Pharmacologic agents that selectively inhibit the action or synthesis of DHT without altering serum testosterone levels reduce prostate volume without causing impotence, loss of libido, and hot flashes. Testosterone is converted to DHT by the enzyme 5-alpha–reductase. MK906 (Proscar) inhibits the synthesis of DHT by blocking 5-alpha–reductase. Flutamide inhibits the binding of androgen to the androgen receptor. Therefore, MK906 and flutamide achieve reduction of prostate volume without producing impotence, loss of libido, and hot flashes, since serum testosterone levels are not lowered.

Seven studies evaluating androgen suppression for BPH have been reported in the peer-reviewed literature. Most of these studies enrolled small numbers of patients, and only one study was randomized and placebo controlled. Symptomatic improvement was evaluated using a standardized symptom score questionnaire in only one study. There have been no compelling data supporting the role of androgen suppression in the treatment of BPH. Experience with this therapy has consistently shown a 30 percent reduction in prostate volume. The degree of clinical efficacy also appears to be independent of the specific pharmacologic agents. The optimal hormonal pharmacotherapy for BPH will be based on relative cost and drug-related toxicity. Flutamide and MK906 are the only drugs currently under investigation in the United States that do not result in impotence, loss of libido, and hot flashes. When coadministered with Lupron in stage D2 carcinoma of the prostate, flutamide has been associated with diarrhea (10 percent) and gynecomastia (10 percent). Reversible hepatocellular damage, manifested by an elevation of liver function enzymes, has been observed in approximately 1 percent of men receiving flutamide. The preliminary experience with MK906 indicates that this drug causes no adverse side effects. Flutamide is presently approved by the FDA for the treatment of prostate cancer, whereas MK906 has not been approved for any clinical indication. MK906 will most likely be the drug of choice in the hormonal treatment of BPH.

BALLOON DILATATION

Deistling reported in 1956 that avulsion of the prostate with a urethral sound improved the symptoms of prostatism. Castanada and associates subsequently described the use of a balloon catheter to dilate the prostatic urethra. Several investigators have since advocated this therapeutic approach to BPH.

Unfortunately, the effectiveness of balloon dilatation has not been reviewed in the urologic literature. Although advocates of balloon dilatation report that this technique relieves symptoms of prostatism, the parameters for assessing efficacy have been highly subjective and poorly defined. The data presented at the 1990 AUA meeting in New Orleans indicated that balloon dilatation does not provide long-term resolution of prostatism. The failure to demonstrate objective urodynamic improvement suggests that a significant component of symptomatic relief achieved following balloon dilatation may be attributed to a placebo effect. We are presently conducting a double-blind, randomized, placebo-controlled study comparing cystoscopy and transurethral dilatation of the prostate in the hope of clarifying the role of balloon dilatation in the treatment of BPH.

TREATMENT OF CHOICE

There is little argument that prostatectomy represents the most established and effective treatment for BPH. Absolute indications for intervention such as urinary retention, renal insufficiency, and urinary tract infection warrant definitive intervention. It is conceivable that alpha-blockers, hormonal therapy, and balloon dilatation may relieve urinary retention, reverse renal insufficiency, and eradicate infections. There are no data demonstrating the effectiveness of these alternative therapies for the recognized absolute indications for treatment. Until then, prostatectomy must be the preferred treatment for males with absolute indications for intervention.

The vast majority of individuals seeking urologic consultation for BPH do not have absolute indications for intervention. I inform these patients about all reasonable treatment alternatives for symptomatic BPH. In general, this discussion includes my interpretation of the available clinical data and the recognized complications of the treatment options. Several phase II and III studies evaluating alpha-blockade (terazosin, doxazosin, and YM617) and androgen suppression (flutamide and MK906) are under way. Until these multicenter randomized, placebo-controlled studies are reported, the practicing urologist may counsel patients that pharmacotherapy for BPH is presently under investigation. Similarly, there is no objective evidence that balloon dilatation is effective to treat BPH. The preliminary experience with alpha-blockade in the treatment of BPH has been encouraging. Urologists may reasonably offer pharmacologic agents such as terazosin according to their interpretation of the available literature.

My approach to the treatment of BPH is based on an extensive experience with nonsurgical treatment alternatives and a comprehensive review of the literature. The literature has consistently demonstrated the effectiveness of alpha-blockade in BPH. The compliance and durability of treatment requires longer follow-up. The literature on androgen suppression has been far less extensive and consistent. Although several studies have demonstrated lack of efficacy, some investigators have concluded that approximately one third of patients may benefit from hormonal therapy. Yet are these the same one third who respond favorably to placebo? The agents commercially available for androgen suppression are extremely costly. It is my impression that androgen suppression will play a limited role in the treatment of BPH since these drugs are costly, only a small proportion of patients achieve symptomatic relief, and the clinical improvement is realized 6 months after treatment is initiated. The enthusiasm for balloon dilatation appears to be diminishing. The randomized, double-blind, placebo-controlled study presently under way in Milwaukee will provide an objective assessment of balloon dilatation.

In light of the above considerations, I offer males with symptomatic BPH the alpha-blocker terazosin provided there is no absolute indication for intervention. Patients are counseled that they are embarking on a life-long commitment to medical management. It has been my experience, based on 2-year follow-up data, that over 80 percent of patients who respond favorably to alpha-blockers remain under medical management. I offer those individuals who fail medical management flutamide, balloon dilatation, no treatment, or a prostatectomy. I share with these patients my limited enthusiasm for flutamide and balloon dilatation. According to the severity of symptoms and the impact of these symptoms on quality of life, these patients either are followed conservatively or undergo prostatectomy.

The treatment of BPH is evolving and will continue

to do so as we develop a more comprehensive understanding of the relative efficacy and morbidity of surgical and nonsurgical alternatives for this condition. Prostatectomy represents the most definitive therapy for BPH and therefore will play a prominent role in its treatment in the foreseeable future. Nonsurgical alternatives such as alpha-blockade, hormonal therapy, and balloon dilatation are likely to assume some role in the management of BPH. The future challenge is to identify those clinical and urodynamic parameters that will aid in the selection of the most effective treatment for individuals with symptomatic BPH.

SELECTED READING

Lepor H., ed. New approaches in the treatment of benign prostatic hyperplasia. Prostate Suppl 1990; 3:1–93.

Lepor H. Nonsurgical management of benign prostatic hyperplasia. J Urol 1989; 141:1283–1289.

Lepor H, Walsh PC. Benign prostatic hyperplasia. Urol Clin North Am 1990; 17:461–684.

LOCALIZED SQUAMOUS CELL CARCINOMA OF THE PENIS

GARY R. WALTON, M.D.
CARL A. OLSSON, M.D.

Carcinoma of the penis is an uncommon disease in the United States affecting 0.1 per 100,000 males. Penile carcinoma represents a significant portion of male cancer in many other parts of the world, including South America (6.6 per 100,000 in Brazil) and Africa (7 per 100,000 in Rhodesia). Almost 99 percent of primary penile carcinomas are squamous cell carcinoma. The incidence of penile carcinoma increases with age, and the average age of diagnosis in the United States is 60 years.

Because of the relative rarity of the disease, it has not been studied as thoroughly as other malignant conditions. Although the precise etiologic agents are as yet unknown, there is a definite link between cancer of the penis and the presence of a foreskin. Penile carcinoma is extremely rare among populations who practice neonatal circumcision. Less than 15 cases have been reported in men circumcised in infancy. Inadequate circumcision or circumcision performed in late childhood is far less protective. Other known risk factors include a history of phimosis, which occurs in more than 50 percent of patients, and balanitis. Penile carcinoma has been associated with poor hygiene. Possible etiologic agents suggested include smegma and human papillomavirus. Epidemiologic data have failed to show a correlation between penile carcinoma and venereal infection, but have recently linked penile cancer to cigarette smoking.

There is controversy over the treatment of the primary lesion and nodal disease. This chapter focuses on treating localized penile carcinoma. Investigation and treatment of lymph node metastasis is discussed elsewhere in this text.

DIAGNOSIS

Symptoms

The initial penile lesion may appear as an indurated lesion or area of erythema in about 15 percent of patients. In 35 percent, an ulcer or sore is noted; a small nodule or exophytic mass is seen in approximately 50 percent. Less than 1 percent of penile carcinomas are found incidentally at adult circumcision. The primary lesion is seldom very painful. It arises predominantly on the glans or foreskin, but rarely may appear on the penile shaft. At the time of diagnosis, 60 percent of lesions are greater than 2 cm in diameter.

The symptoms depend on whether the patient is circumcised or not, as well as on the degree of phimosis, if present. If the foreskin is easily retracted, the primary lesion can be noted initially as a wart or sore. Significant phimosis can obscure the lesion, and such patients may present with a foul discharge reflective of secondary infection, with bleeding from the obscured primary lesion or with actual erosion of the tumor through the foreskin. Inguinal adenopathy may be the primary complaint. Occasionally, patients present with weakness or weight loss secondary to a chronic suppurative process. Urinary symptoms are rare.

Penile cancer is known for its delayed presentation to the physician. The average interval from initial symptoms to presentation is 10 months. Up to 50 percent of patients delay seeking medical attention for more than 1 year, possibly because of embarrassment, or ignorance as well as neglect of the problem.

Untreated lesions advance to involve eventually Buck's fascia, which serves as a temporary barrier to invasive disease. Continued progression may lead to autoamputation. Metastases are common and occur almost exclusively via the lymphatics, with initial involvement of the inguinal nodes, after which the iliac and hypogastric nodes may be affected. Patient survival is exquisitely dependent on nodal stasis. Death occurs within 2 to 3 years in most untreated cases and is commonly secondary to uncontrolled lymphatic spread, leading to death by inanition. Other sequelae of lymphatic spread may include skin necrosis with subsequent sepsis, or erosion of the femoral vessels with hemorrhage.

Differential Diagnosis

The differential diagnosis of penile squamous cell carcinoma includes inflammatory lesions, benign tumors, premalignant lesions, other primary malignancies, and metastatic tumors. Inflammatory lesions include

Table 1 Jackson Staging System for Penile Cancer

Stage I	Tumor confined to glans and/or prepuce
Stage II	Invasion into shaft or corpora
Stage III	Tumor confined to shaft with node metastases
Stage IV	Invasion from shaft with inoperable inguinal metastases or distant metastases

chancre, chancroid, syphilis, herpes, lymphogranuloma venereum (LGV), granuloma inguinale, and tuberculosis. Possible benign tumors are condyloma acuminatum (genital warts), molluscum contagium, sebaceous cysts, fibromas, and angiomas. Premalignant lesions include leukoplakia, erythroplasia of Queyrat, Bowen's disease, balanitis xerotica obliterans, and the so-called Buschke-Löwenstein tumor. Basal cell carcinomas, melanomas, sarcomas, and metastatic tumors may also involve the penis.

Serologic tests may help diagnose particular inflammatory agents, but any penile lesion of undetermined origin demands biopsy in order to obtain a diagnosis. Empiric treatment without biopsy may delay a diagnosis of cancer or cause confusion. Treatment of genital warts with podophyllin produces a histologic picture not unlike squamous cell carcinoma.

Staging

Discussion of treatment alternatives requires an adequate knowledge of staging. The Jackson staging

Table 2 Tumor Node Metastasis (TNM) Classification for Staging Penile Cancer

Tumor Staging

T0	No evidence of primary tumor
T1	Tumor 2 cm or less in its largest dimension, strictly superficial or exophytic
T2	Tumor more than 2 cm, but no more than 5 cm in its largest dimension with minimal infiltration
T3	Tumor more than 5 cm in its largest dimension, or tumor of any size with deep infiltration, including urethra
T4	Tumor invading neighboring structures (T = primary tumor; TIS = carcinoma in situ)

Node Staging

N0	No palpable nodes
N1	Movable unilateral nodes (N1a = not considered to contain growth; N1b = considered to contain growth)
N2	Movable bilateral nodes (N2a = not considered to contain growth; N2b = considered to contain growth)
N3	Fixed nodes (N = regional lymph nodes)

Metastasis Staging

M0	No evidence of distant metastases
M1	Distant metastases present (M = distant metastases)

system (Table 1) was popular in earlier literature, but the tumor node metastasis (TNM) system of the Union Internationale Contre Cancer (UICC) (Table 2) describes the extent of disease more accurately. When the initial penile lesion is secondarily infected, the patient should be treated with antibiotics after appropriate cultures are obtained, especially if inguinal adenopathy is present, in order to determine better the true stage of the tumor. A more complete discussion of lymph node staging may be found elsewhere in this text.

TREATMENT

Any squamous cell carcinoma of the penis is potentially lethal. The initial tumor must be eradicated to prevent local recurrence and, more important, to prevent metastases, because the prognosis is much worse when there is lymph node involvement. With adequate local treatment, metastases are rare after 3 years. However, the impact of this therapy on the patient should not be underestimated. Sacrifices include the loss of sexual function, inability to void in the upright position, and not least, the loss of body image. The psychological impact of such sacrifices, especially on the younger male, has promoted organ-preserving local therapies. Historically in the United States, the standard for local treatment has been partial or total penectomy. The treatment of localized disease has become more controversial with the increasing number of modalities available.

Special Considerations

Patient selection for organ-sparing alternative therapies should be limited to younger, highly motivated patients with confined lesions. A low threshold for biopsy is required.

Although the treatment of premalignant penile disease is discussed elsewhere in this text, several of the therapeutic modalities mentioned below, along with topical chemotherapy, are acceptable forms of treatment for these lesions. It is our opinion that biopsy should be used liberally for evaluation of treated premalignant lesions.

The so-called Buschke-Löwenstein tumor is a voluminous condyloma that is locally destructive. It does not respond well to radiotherapy, and surgical removal is appropriate.

Laser Therapy

Laser therapy of penile carcinoma is considered only for superficial lesions of the TIS, T1, and T2 stages (see Table 2). This modality is still in its infancy, and the largest reported experience with biopsy-proved penile squamous cell carcinoma is by Boon. Of 16 patients with cancer in situ (TIS), T1, and T2 lesions treated with the Nd-YAG laser, there were three recurrences during a follow-up of 4 to 36 months. One patient required a meatoplasty owing to stenosis. A tourniquet is used to control bleeding so as not to compromise the power of the laser beam. Exophytic lesions are excised, and the base is necrosed in a controlled fashion.

The cosmetic results have been good and complications few, but aggressive close follow-up is required in order to detect the 20 percent of patients who experience recurrence. Again, this technique is limited to superficial lesions and to younger patients in whom penile preservation is important. Patient selection also demands that only those individuals willing to undertake compulsive follow-up examinations be treated by laser technology.

Micrographic Surgery

Penile cancer may extend beyond the clinically visible palpable margins of the tumor. The concept of micrographic surgery is based on removal of tumor under complete microscopic control. The tumor is removed by layers, and the entire undersurface of each layer is examined under the microscope to look for residual tumor. The process is continued until clear margins are obtained. Hemostasis is obtained by means of previous treatment of the tumor with a fixative (chemosurgery), or previous placement of a tourniquet and subsequent cautery. The procedure conserves as much penile tissue as possible.

The largest series is described by Mohs and colleagues. In this report, the cases were classified by the Jackson staging system, which does not afford the reviewer sufficient information about the lesions treated. Local recurrence occurred in one of 16 stage I and one of seven stage II tumors; both were high grade. Treatment lasted for 1 to 7 days and was performed on an outpatient basis, and complications were rare.

Although local recurrence (10 percent) is less than that for laser treatment, meticulous follow-up is still required. As for laser treatment, this approach is also more appropriate for smaller, low-grade lesions, especially in younger, motivated patients.

Radiotherapy

Squamous cell carcinoma is characteristically radioresistant, so that high doses are required, especially to eradicate larger tumors. Infection of the target area decreases the efficacy of external radiation. The major advantage of radiotherapy is the preservation of penile anatomy and function. Circumcision should precede treatment in order to allow infected areas to heal and prevent sclerosis and phimosis of the foreskin. The survival rates for patients treated with radiotherapy or surgery have been similar; however, irradiated patients experience higher incidences of local recurrence (approximately 50 percent in studies before the 1970s) and complications. The European community has had much more experience with radiotherapy using varied schedules and delivery systems.

External Mold Radiotherapy

The external mold is a radiotherapy technique commonly used in the past in England. A cylindric mold containing a radiation source, typically iridium, is placed over the penis for 6 to 8 hours a day for about a week. The radiation hazard to those exposed is considerable and the patient must be isolated during treatments. Recent experience reported by El-Demiry and colleagues from London revealed a 22 percent recurrence rate for Jackson stage I and 75 percent for Jackson stage II lesions. Tissue necrosis complications requiring further surgery are few.

External Beam Radiotherapy

Megavoltage x-rays can be produced via present-day linear accelerators for treatment of penile carcinoma. Recurrence rates for T1 and T2 lesions have varied from 10 to 30 percent. Local reactions can take weeks to months to heal and may cause problems in determining what to biopsy. Telangiectasia, patchy pigmentation, and fibrotic skin are also commonly persistent after treatment. In Duncan and Jackson's study, 10 percent of patients required amputation for penile necrosis and 30 percent had urethral strictures.

Persistent follow-up is required because of the high recurrence rate, and biopsy decisions may be difficult because of postradiation changes. Only smaller lesions should be treated with this modality.

Interstitial Radiotherapy

Interstitial implantation of iridium-192 wires is a common treatment in France for the management of primary penile lesions. The implants are placed via hypodermic needles under general or spinal anesthesia. Edema and acute mucocutaneous reactions occur but regress spontaneously after about 3 months. A series reported by Mazeron and colleagues included 50 patients; recurrence was seen in 11 percent of T1 lesions, 22 percent of T2 lesions, 29 percent of T3 lesions, and 50 percent of all tumors larger than 4 cm. Of patients with T1 and T2 lesions, 20 percent developed urethral strictures while 7 percent had penile necrosis. Penile anatomy was preserved in most cases, but with more than 20 percent local recurrence and 20 percent urethral stricture rates, the importance of follow-up and the likelihood of multiple procedures is obvious.

Surgery

Circumcision

Small tumors limited to the prepuce can be treated successfully by circumcision. However, there may be local recurrences after this treatment, and it should be limited to low-grade lesions on the distal portion of the foreskin, allowing for an adequate histologic margin. Again, close follow-up with a low threshold for subsequent biopsy is required.

Excision

Local excision of glandular lesions has resulted in a 30 to 40 percent recurrence rate and should be performed only if more appropriate therapy is adamantly refused.

Partial Penectomy

The standard of treatment for distal penile tumors is partial amputation of the penis at a point 2 cm proximal to the lesion, with frozen sections confirming a tumor-free margin. Local tumor recurrence is rare (0 to 5 percent). If the remaining penile stump is too short for sexual intercourse or for directed standing micturition (at least 3 cm), a total penectomy is indicated. Partial penectomy is indicated for tumors that are large, invasive, or high grade. Recurrent tumors, postradiation necrosis, and poorly compliant patients who are unlikely to cooperate with follow-up should also be treated with partial penectomy.

Certain aspects of the surgical procedure should be stressed. The patient should be placed in the extended lithotomy position in case total penectomy with perineal urethrostomy is required. After appropriate prepping and draping, the tumor should be isolated from the field with a glove or adherent drape to prevent seeding of the wound. A circumferential skin incision is marked 2 cm proximal to the tumor, and a tourniquet is placed at the penile base. After the skin incision the corpora cavernosa are divided and the dorsal vasculature is ligated. The urethra is divided at least 5 mm distal to the amputated corpora, and a proximal urethral margin is submitted for frozen section. The urethra is spatulated to prevent stricture formation. The corpora are closed with interrupted absorbable sutures, including the intervening septum, and the urethral margins are sutured to full-thickness skin edges. Simple skin approximation dorsally closes the rest of the wound, and an indwelling catheter is left in place to prevent urine from contaminating the wound.

Total Penectomy

Total penectomy is indicated for local control of any lesion in which a partial penectomy leaves less than a 3-cm penile stump. These lesions are usually larger and generate the least amount of controversy, as any other modality provides poor local control. Laser therapy, micrographic surgery, and interstitial radiation are usually relatively ineffective in the management of these larger lesions. The dose of external radiation required often leads to tissue necrosis and stricture.

Again, the patient is placed in the extended lithotomy position and the tumor is isolated from the field with an occlusive dressing. A vertical, elliptic incision is made at the base of the penis, the penile suspensory ligament is divided, and the dorsal vessels are ligated. The urethra is divided in the bulbar region and dissected sharply from the corpora. The corpora are then divided at the ischial rami and the specimen is removed. After the corporeal stumps are sutured, an ellipse of skin is removed from the perineal body, and a tunnel is created bluntly through the subcutaneous perineal tissues. The urethra is grasped and transposed without angulation to the perineum. The urethra is spatulated and anastomosed circumferentially to the perineal skin. Drains are placed and the primary incision is closed transversely to provide elevation of the scrotum away from the urethrostomy.

SUGGESTED READING

Boon TA. Sapphire probe laser surgery for localized carcinoma of the penis. Eur J Surg Oncol 1988; 14:193–195.

Duncan W, Jackson SM. The treatment of early cancer of the penis with megavoltage x-rays. Clin Radiol 1972; 23:246–248.

El-Demiry MIM, Oliver RTD, Hope-Stone HF, Blandy JP. Reappraisal of the role of radiotherapy and surgery in the management of carcinoma of the penis. Br J Urol 1984; 56:724–728.

Hellberg D, Valentin J, Eklund T, Nilsson S. Penile cancer: is there an epidemiological role for smoking and sexual behavior? Br Med J 1987; 1295:1306–1308.

Mazeron JJ, Langlois D, Lobo PA, Huart JA, Calitchi E, Lusinchi A, Raynal M, Le Bourgeois JP, Abbou CC, Pierquin B. Interstitial radiation therapy for carcinoma of the penis using iridium 192 wires: the Henri Mondor experience (1970–1979). Int J Radiat Oncol Biol Phys 1984; 10:1891–1895.

Mohs FE, Snow SN, Messing EM, Kuglitsch ME. Microscopically controlled surgery in the treatment of carcinoma of the penis. J Urol 1985; 133:961–966.

METASTATIC SQUAMOUS CELL CARCINOMA OF THE PENIS

MICHAEL F. CARTER, M.D.

In patients with squamous cell cancer of the penis, the diagnosis, treatment, and timing of therapy for lymph node metastases presents an unusual challenge because of the rare nature of this condition. Penile cancer accounts for less than 0.5 percent of all cancers in men in the United States, and about 30 percent of these have metastases at the time of initial diagnosis. Most of these metastases are to the regional (superficial and deep subinguinal) lymph nodes or the pelvic nodes; only 2 percent of penile cancers demonstrate hematogenous metastases at initial presentation. Cancer of the penis is one of the few cancers that can be cured by excision of the regional lymph nodes containing metastatic carcinoma. Because of the high mortality rate in patients with untreated or inadequately treated metastatic penile cancer, it is important to understand the principles involved and the necessity for aggressive management of this condition.

THERAPEUTIC ALTERNATIVES

The only effective treatment of inguinal lymph node metastases from penile cancer is inguinal lymph node dissection. This is generally accomplished when the nodes are palpably enlarged and technically resectable. Without this surgical therapy, 95 percent of these patients will die of their disease within 3 years. This should be compared with a 5-year survival rate of 50 percent when lymph node dissection is performed for grossly positive nodes.

Since about 60 percent of patients with penile cancer present with enlarged inguinal lymph nodes and only about 50 percent of these enlarged nodes harbor cancer, it becomes important to select those patients who will benefit from node dissection. Fortunately, infection is often the cause of the lymphadenopathy. Excision of the primary penile lesion, which in 90 percent of cases is associated with suppuration, plus a 4- to 6-week course of antibiotics will allow differentiation of nodes that are enlarged as a result of infection from those enlarged by cancer. Persistent lymphadenopathy implies metastatic cancer, which should be treated by immediate lymphadenectomy. In patients who present with inguinal skin ulceration due to cancerous nodes, a short course of antibiotics followed by node dissection is indicated rather than waiting several weeks to determine response.

Of equal concern is the fact that 20 percent of normal-feeling lymph nodes harbor microscopic metastases. The options for these patients are close observation, delaying lymphadenectomy until nodal enlargement occurs, or early lymphadenectomy, particularly in patients at high risk for metastases. Some authors have shown similar survival rates for patients treated by early lymph node dissection and for those treated by delayed dissection when lymph node enlargement occurred. Others have been concerned by poor patient compliance as well as an inability to detect early enlargement reliably, and thus believe that early lymph node dissection is preferable.

The role of lymph node biopsy as advocated by Cabanas is controversial. In an attempt to identify patients with occult metastases to groin nodes without performing complete lymphadenectomy with its attendant complications, early biopsy of the so-called sentinel nodes was performed. These lymph nodes are on the anteromedial aspect of the superficial epigastric vein just above and medial to the epigastric-saphenous junction and are thought to be the primary site of metastases from penile cancer. The sensitivity in determining the presence of occult nodal metastases has been reported to be as high as 88 percent, but other studies have been more discouraging. Most consider that the value of lymph node biopsy has yet to be proved.

In Jackson stage III patients (Table 1) with unilaterally palpable nodes, ipsilateral groin dissection should be performed, and if those nodes are positive, the contralateral groin dissection will be necessary, since there is a 50 percent incidence of occult metastases to contralateral groin nodes. Some authors advocate pelvic lymph node dissection before the groin dissection, but if the groin nodes are positive, pelvic lymphadenectomy should at least be done subsequently. If there are bilaterally palpable nodes (after antibiotic treatment), we perform a pelvic node dissection and bilateral inguinal node dissection simultaneously. Most believe that extensive metastases above the external iliacs are incurable.

Radiation therapy and chemotherapy have been largely ineffective and currently are not used in the management of lymph node metastases. However, cisplatin and 5-fluorouracil (5-FU) have been used before lymphadenectomy as neoadjuvant therapy with minimal side effects and a 40 percent response in one small study.

In summary, the therapeutic options for lymph node metastases in penile cancer are as follows:

1. Immediate lymphadenectomy. This is used for high-stage and high-grade tumors when nodes obviously contain cancer and local infection is not an issue. It is also a consideration in patients with

Table 1 Jackson Staging System for Cancer of the Penis

Stage I	Tumor confined to glans and/or prepuce
Stage II	Invasion into shaft or corpora
Stage III	Tumor confined to shaft of penis and lymph node metastasis
Stage IV	Invasion beyond shaft with inoperable inguinal or distant metastasis

stage II disease who have clinically negative nodes but moderate- to high-grade cancer, in view of the high incidence of microscopic metastases in this subset.

2. Early lymphadenectomy. This treatment is advisable for enlarged inguinal nodes that do not resolve with a 4- to 6-week course of antibiotics, as well as for most patients with stage II disease.
3. Delayed lymphadenectomy. This therapeutic modality is imperative when clinically negative nodes become enlarged on follow-up examination.
4. Observation. This is reserved for stage I disease and perhaps some selected low-grade, small-volume stage II lesions.
5. Biopsy of sentinel nodes only (Cabanas), limited dissection (superficial nodes only) or complete dissection (including pelvic nodes).
6. Chemotherapy as neoadjunctive therapy.

PREFERRED APPROACH FOR LYMPH NODE METASTASES

Patient Selection

Patients with Jackson stage III tumors are unequivocal candidates for lymphadenectomy. Controversy exists over the management of stage II cancers. My preference is to perform early lymph node dissection in patients with penile cancer who do not have palpable lymphadenopathy on initial presentation, as well as those whose lymphadenopathy responds to antibiotics *if* they are at high risk for developing metastases. This includes pathologic findings of moderate-to-poor differentiation in the primary lesion (40 percent incidence of positive nodes), the presence of vascular invasion in the primary lesion, and most stage II disease patients, since approximately two thirds of these have positive nodes. Other important considerations that, in my opinion, prompt early lymphadenectomy include patients who are thought to be unreliable about careful follow-up (unwilling or unable to come for the bimonthly evaluations), those in whom my ability to detect early lymph node enlargement may be limited by the patient's obesity or scarring from previous inguinal surgery, and younger patients without medical contraindications to surgery.

Timing of Surgery

Following treatment of the primary penile lesion and after review of the pathology and metastatic work-up, the timing of lymphadenectomy can be assessed. For high-stage, high-grade tumors in which the inguinal lymph nodes are obviously cancerous and local infection is not an issue, immediate lymphadenectomy should be considered if the patient is medically ready. This should also be a consideration when the nodes are clinically not involved but when moderate- to high-grade stage II disease is present since it is associated with a high incidence of microscopic metastases to the regional lymph nodes.

Enlarged nodes that do not resolve with a 4- to 6-week course of antibiotics, or disease with a high metastatic potential despite response to a course of antibiotics, should be considered for early lymphadenectomy.

In patients in whom observation is chosen because the inguinal nodes are clinically negative, and whose nodes become enlarged during this period of observation, delayed lymphadenectomy is performed.

Preoperative Preparation

The patient should be in optimal condition, since lymphadenectomy is a significant operative procedure in which wound healing is particularly important. I attempt to achieve bacterial sterilization of the lymph nodes with a 4- to 6-week course of antibiotics before lymphadenectomy, if the penile lesion is associated with suppuration, to avoid compromised wound healing.

Computed tomography (CT) of the pelvis may help in staging; if para-aortic, paracaval or common iliac nodes are seen, one should consider a preliminary staging laporotomy. I do not perform lymphangiography because of a 20 percent false-negative staging error and because the contrast agent may produce enough lymphatic reaction to complicate the node dissection. Pelvic and femoral angiography should be considered if there are large fixed inguinal nodes, since the femoral artery may have to be resected with the tumor. If arterial resection is necessary, it should be replaced with saphenous vein or other autologous material, because prosthetic grafts are prone to infection in this area.

In preparation for surgery, the patient should be fitted for full-length surgical elastic stockings that will be available at the time of surgery. Open wounds, rashes, or infected areas over the groin need to be cleared before surgery. A mechanical bowel preparation is given the day before surgery in preparation for prolonged bed rest postoperatively. If nutrition is poor, serious consideration should be given to hyperalimentation preoperatively, and it should be continued postoperatively to aid in the crucial stages of wound healing. Intravenous hydration and intravenous antibiotics are begun the night before surgery.

Surgical Approach

The patient is placed on the operating table in the supine position with the thigh abducted and the knee bent and externally rotated. A sandbag or rolled towel is used to support the knee, and pressure points should be well padded. The elastic stocking is pulled up to the knee; it will be used to cover the thigh postoperatively. The penis and scrotum are draped out of the field. An oblique incision is made 4 cm below and parallel to the inguinal ligament. It is advisable to excise the biopsy incision if the patient had a previous biopsy of cancer-bearing lymph nodes in this area. Skin flaps 4 to 5 mm in thickness are raised and dissected laterally to the sartorius muscle, medially to the adductor longus muscle, superiorly to a point approximately 2 cm above the inguinal ligament, and inferiorly past the apex of the femoral triangle. These few millimeters of subcutaneous fat contain the skin's blood supply, and it is important to leave the skin flaps thick to maintain tissue viability. The skin edges need to be handled atraumatically and kept moist. Skin hooks, delicate retraction, and avoidance of tissue drying are also critical for viability.

Lymph node dissection is initiated 2 cm above the inguinal ligament by incising down to the external oblique aponeurosis. The fatty tissue and nodes are dissected off the fascia, as well as the spermatic cord distal to the external inguinal ring, and carried down to Poupart's ligament bluntly; sharp dissection is necessary to remove this tissue from the inguinal ligament. Blood vessels are ligated with absorbable sutures or cauterized. The dissection is carried on to the thigh; the lateral extent of this portion of the dissection is the lateral border of the sartorius muscle, and the medial margin is the adductor longus muscle. Inferiorly, the apex of the femoral triangle forms the distal extent of the operation. The fascia lata over these structures is incised, beginning just below the inguinal ligament, in order to gain access to the proper plane deep to the fascia lata. Care is taken to avoid injury to the lateral femoral cutaneous nerve, which lies over the lateral portion of the sartorius muscle just below the inguinal ligament. All tissue below the skin flaps and the plane deep to the fascia lata is excised between absorbable sutures along the lateral, medial, and inferior margins of the dissection. The saphenous vein will be encountered along the inferior margin of dissection and superficial to the fascia lata. It will probably be necessary to ligate and divide this vein with 2-0 silk sutures at this level, as well as where it joins the femoral vein about 1 inch below the inguinal ligament. When possible, sparing this vein may help avoid or reduce the degree of postoperative lymphedema. Moving from the margins of dissection centrally, the femoral sheath will be encountered and is incised to expose the femoral vessels and the deep inguinal lymph nodes. Care should be taken at this point to avoid injury to the femoral nerve, which lies lateral to the artery. The deep nodes are then removed by skeletonizing the femoral vessels anteriorly and laterally and dividing all the superficial branches of both vessels with nonabsorbable sutures. However, one should be careful to preserve the profunda femoris artery, which lies deep to the femoral artery. The fibrofatty nodal package, containing both superficial and deep nodes, is dissected from the apex of the femoral triangle to the femoral canal where the lymphatics enter and drain into the pelvic nodes. The lymphatics are divided between metal clips and the package is removed. The metal clip serves to identify the distal point of dissection if pelvic lymphadenectomy is necessary.

Wound closure is initiated by detaching the origin of the sartorius muscle from its origin on the anterior iliac spine, taking care to preserve its blood supply and transposing it to cover the femoral vessels. The origin of the sartorius is sutured to the inguinal ligament with 2-0 Prolene, and the lateral edges of the sartorius are preferably sutured to surrounding thigh musculature with absorbable sutures to cover the vessels completely. Closure of the femoral canal with nonabsorbable sutures prevents a femoral hernia and should be completed before the sartorius is sutured in place. Two 7-mm Jackson-Pratt drains are brought through separate incisions in the upper thigh and allowed to lie on either side of the sartorius muscle. At this point the skin edges are gently brought together, but there is often excess skin because so much subcutaneous tissue has been removed. If the skin edges do not look healthy, and particularly if there is excess skin, it is wise to resect 4 to 5 mm from each edge to reach viable tissue. Most commonly, the edge of skin on the distal flap is at greatest risk of compromise. If there is any question about the viability of the skin, intravenous fluorescein can be given; viable skin will fluoresce under an ultraviolet lamp. The subcutaneous tissue is then approximated with interrupted 4-0 Dexon and the skin is closed without tension. Clear occlusive dressings are applied to allow frequent inspection of the wound edges, and the elastic stockings are rolled up over the wounds.

If the inguinal nodes are positive for malignancy, contralateral inguinal dissection is necessary, since the incidence of positive contralateral nodes, even when palpably normal, is 50 percent. I generally prefer to stage these procedures because of their magnitude and associated morbidity.

Preliminary pelvic lymphadenectomy is performed if lymph node involvement is extensive clinically. The presence of bilateral multiple nodes or large fixed nodes suggests pelvic nodal metastases. In addition, if involvement of the femoral artery that may require resection or large pelvic nodes is seen on diagnostic studies such as CT, preliminary pelvic lymphadenectomy is indicated. In the absence of the above-mentioned risk factors, I usually concentrate on the inguinal lymph node dissection first and perform the pelvic lymph node dissection and contralateral groin dissection 2 weeks later only if the first inguinal nodes are positive.

Pelvic lymphadenectomy is performed through a vertical midline incision extending from umbilicus to midpubis. The rectus fascia is opened longitudinally and the rectus muscles are separated sharply. Dividing the transversalis fascia allows entry into the prevesicle space without injury to the inferior epigastric vessels. Division of this fascia superiorly, as well as the posterior rectus sheath, frees the rectus muscles from the peritoneum anteriorly for better exposure. The bladder is retracted medially to enter the desired iliac fossa, and the peritoneum is retracted cephalad to expose the external and internal iliac vessels. To expose the common iliac vessels, it is necessary to retract the spermatic cord medially and follow the plane lateral to the cord up along the lateral peritoneum. The transversalis fascia and obliterated umbilical artery can then be seen and incised cephalad to free the peritoneum and allow further medial retraction of the peritoneum for exposure of the common iliac artery and vein. Early identification and medial retraction of the ureter where it crosses the distal common iliac artery will help prevent its injury during node dissection. Total lymphadenectomy is recommended and includes common and external iliac nodes from the aortic bifurcation to the inguinal ligament, as well as the nodes in the femoral canal down to the point of proximal groin dissection if that procedure was performed first. The lateral margin of dissection will be just medial to the genitofemoral nerve, and the medial margin is the obturator nerve. Occasionally it may be necessary to resect the obturator nerve if involved by tumor. While this could cause some difficulty with ambulation, it has not been a significant long-term problem in my experience. The node dissection is begun by incising the endopelvic fascia medial to the genitofemoral nerve from the inguinal ligament to a point high on the common iliac artery. An en bloc dissection is performed, skeletonizing the vessels. The inguinal ligament is sutured to Cooper's ligament with nonabsorbable sutures for closure of the femoral canal and to prevent a hernia. A suction drain is left in the obturator fossa and brought out through a separate stab incision lateral to the midline incision. Wound closure is accomplished by approximation of the rectus muscles, and closure of the anterior rectus fascia with interrupted sutures.

Postoperative Course

Postoperatively, the patient is kept at bed rest for approximately 1 week with the thigh slightly flexed to minimize tension on the sartorius muscle as well as the skin. The foot of the bed should be raised to minimize swelling, and the patient should be encouraged to exercise his legs by flexion and extension of the ankles. The suction catheters are usually maintained for 5 to 7 days and removed when drainage is minimal. Ambulation is allowed after skin flaps become fixed to underlying tissue at 7 to 10 days, but sitting with thighs flexed is discouraged except at mealtime during the first month postoperatively. The elastic stockings that were fitted before surgery should be worn for at least 3 months postoperatively except for showers. Although there is some risk of deep venous thrombosis, I do not routinely use anticoagulants, but I do encourage leg exercises. Sodium warfarin (Coumadin) may be advisable in patients prone to venous thrombosis; heparin has been associated with formation of lymphoceles. Perioperative antibiotics are continued for several days, and a Foley catheter is used until the patient can sit up to void and keep his wounds dry.

Complications and Sequelae

The most common complication of the surgery is chronic lymphedema, which occurs in approximately 30 percent of patients; about 15 percent consider this incapacitating. Local tissue breakdown has been reported to occur in up to 60 percent of cases, but is less of a problem if the incision avoids the inguinal skin crease; in more contemporary reports, the incidence approaches 10 to 15 percent. When it occurs, it usually involves the midportion of the inguinal skin flaps and becomes apparent between the 4th and 12th days postoperatively. It is treated by debridement and split-thickness skin grafting. Inguinal or femoral hernias rarely occur unless the inguinal ligament is divided in its midportion or the femoral canal is not closed.

Continued lymph drainage is uncommon, but when it occurs it is treated by leg elevation and continued suction. Accumulation of lymph or serum under skin flaps occurs in about 10 percent of patients and is treated by aspiration and pressure dressings.

Hemorrhage from the femoral vessels can result from infection or skin flap necrosis and may be fatal. This is rarely a problem if the sartorius muscle is used to cover the femoral vessels after completion of the groin dissection. Thrombophlebitis is an infrequent complication, occurring in about 5 percent of patients and requiring anticoagulation. Attempts at prevention, as discussed earlier, are of greatest importance.

Minor wound complications are frequent and can usually be managed conservatively without significant sequelae.

PREFERRED APPROACH FOR DISTANT METASTASES

Of patients with high-stage carcinoma of the penis, only one half to two thirds are cured by aggressive lymph node dissection. The other patients eventually experience progression of the disease with recurrences locally, and ultimately metastatic disease. Untreated, 95 percent of patients with stage III disease will be dead within 3 years. Palliative local resections may be indicated to avoid such complications as arterial erosion, and severe local infection that could result in sepsis. Radiotherapy has been used for palliation but is rarely associated with cure.

Distant metastases to bone, liver, lung, and other sites are rarely if ever cured by any means, although chemotherapy may result in temporary remission for an average of several months. Methotrexate, cisplatin, and bleomycin alone or in combination have been most effective against squamous cell carcinoma, with methotrexate achieving a response rate of 50 to 60 percent, which is approximately twice the response rate of cisplatin or bleomycin alone. The duration of these responses has been brief, however, ranging from 2 to 11 months. In one study, a combination of methotrexate, cisplatin, and bleomycin resulted in a 100 percent response rate, with one complete responder still under control at 17 months and eight partial or minor responses lasting 3 to 8 months. In this latter study, methotrexate 200 mg per square meter per day intravenously on days 1, 15, and 22 with leucovorin rescue at 24 hours (25 mg orally or intravenously every 6 hours for 72 hours) was combined with bleomycin, 15 mg per day continuous infusion for 5 days, and cisplatin, 20 mg per square meter per day for 5 days. The main complication from bleomycin is pulmonary fibrosis; early evidence of pulmonary toxicity necessitates withdrawal of this agent. We are far from finding an effective form of treatment for distant metastases from squamous cell cancer of the penis, and at present even multiple drug regimens have been disappointing because of the limited durability of the responses achieved.

SUGGESTED READING

Cabanas RM. An approach for the treatment of penile carcinoma. Cancer 1977; 39:456–466.

Fraley EE, et al. The role of ilioinguinal lymphadenectomy and significance of histological differentiation in treatment of carcinoma of the penis. J Urol 1989; 142:1478.

McDougal WS, et al. Treatment of carcinoma of the penis: the case for primary lymphadenectomy. J Urol 1986; 136:38.

Mukamel E, deKernion JB. Early versus delayed lymph-node dissection versus no lymph-node dissection in carcinoma of the penis. Urol Clin North Am, 1987; 14:707.

ERYTHROPLASIA OF QUEYRAT AND BALANITIS XEROTICA OBLITERANS

R. BRUCE BRACKEN, M.D.
CHARLES L. HEATON, M.D.

ERYTHROPLASIA OF QUEYRAT

Erythroplasia of Queyrat is a clinical term used to designate a unique presentation of carcinoma in situ when it occurs on the glans penis (Figs. 1 to 3). A number of clinical designations have been used to describe carcinoma in situ of mucous membranes. This has led to some confusion among clinicians and has often resulted in unnecessary mutilating therapies. Terms such as *leukokeratosis, erythrokeratosis, Bowen's disease, bowenoid papulosis,* and *erythroplasia of Queyrat* are used to designate variations in the clinical appearance of lesions that *may* contain carcinoma in situ. Red, hyperkeratotic lesions appearing in the mouth that are histologically carcinoma in situ are frequently referred to as *erythrokeratosis. Leukokeratosis* may or may not represent a malignant lesion (Fig. 3). Friction on mucous membranes may result in hypertrophy of the epithelium and a white appearance. The term *Bowen's disease* is usually reserved for lesions of non–mucous membrane surfaces that are carcinoma in situ. *Bowenoid papulosis* is a new term used to designate dark lesions on the genitalia that are produced by human papillomavirus types 5, 10, 16, 18, and 31 (Fig. 4). The histology of carcinoma in situ may be misleading in these cases. Lesions produced by human papillomavirus types 5 and 10 rarely undergo malignant change, whereas those produced by types 16, 18, and 31 are regularly associated with invasive neoplasms. Cofactors such as ionizing radiation to these lesions may precipitate frank, aggressive, invasive neoplasia. The term *Erythroplasia of Queyrat* has been used to designate carcinoma in situ of the glans penis, and is in fact an erythrokeratosis with abnormal changes within the epithelium. These red tumors of carcinoma in situ have been described not only on the glans penis but also on the clitoris and in the adjacent mucous membranes of the genitalia of both sexes.

Although the precise cause of erythroplasia of Queyrat is unknown, the disorder is seen only in uncircumcised males. The current literature suggests that there is a strong association between this carcinoma in situ and human papillomavirus types 5, 10, 16, 18, and 31. Types 16, 18, and 31 appear to be most frequently associated with invasive neoplasms, but their precise role in carcinoma in situ remains to be delineated. Since the database is small, one would be remiss in concluding that erythroplasia of Queyrat is simply an unusual wart or that all warts may lead to malignant neoplasia.

The presence of elevated red, white, or dark lesions on the mucous membranes of the genitalia requires biopsy without exception. The lesions may in fact be carcinoma in situ, invasive carcinoma, balanitis circumscripta plasmacellularis, an inflammatory granuloma, or metastatic prostatic carcinoma, which may produce red papulonodules on the glans. Other differential diagnostic possibilities include Bowen's disease, extramammary Paget's disease, and Zoon's balanitis. On histologic study, erythroplasia of Queyrat exhibits epidermal hyperplasia, large hyperchromatic and polymorphic nuclei, and multinucleated keratinocytes. Numerous abnormal mitotic figures are usually present, as well as scattered dyskeratotic scales. The basement membrane remains intact, which indicates that the tumor has not spread beyond the epithelium, thus negating the need for radical amputation.

Therapeutic Alternatives

Therapy for carcinoma in situ of the glans penis is in a state of transition and re-evaluation. Historically, amputation of the distal portion of the penis was considered the treatment of choice. Partial penectomy

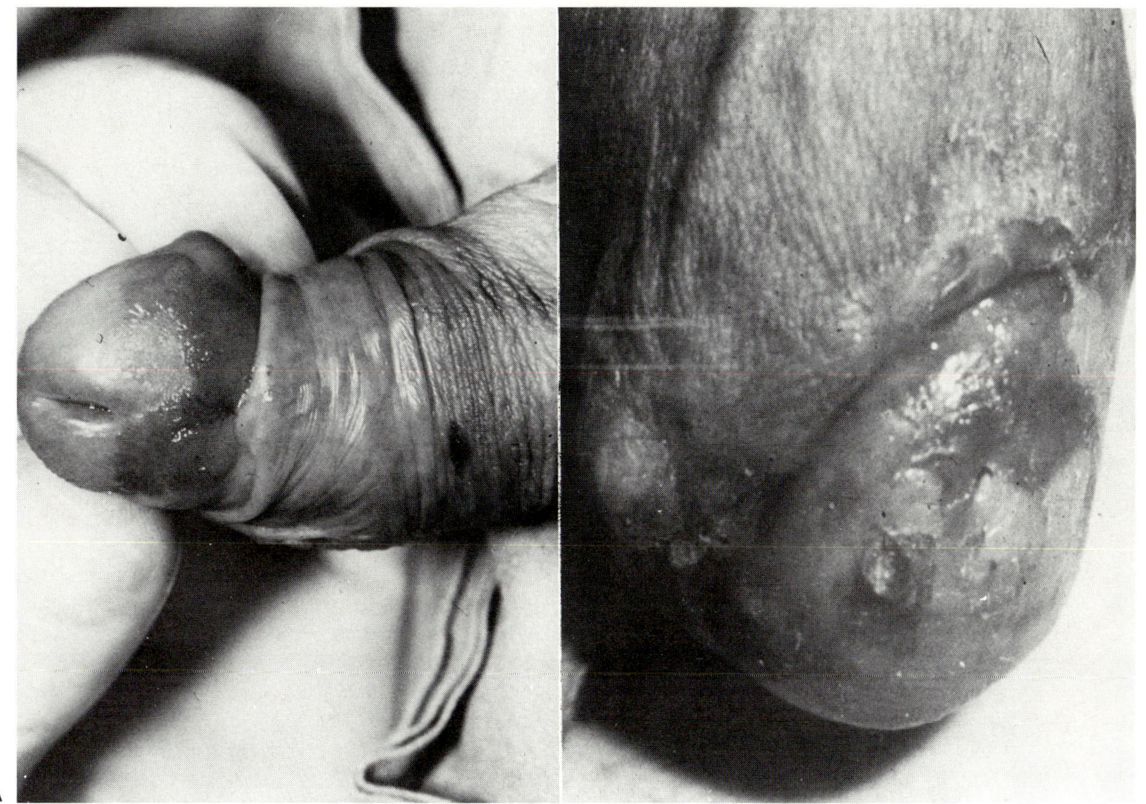

Figure 1   *A* and *B,* Erythroplasia of Queyrat on the glans penis.

controlled these neoplasms locally in virtually all cases. Unrecognized areas of invasive cancer are completely controlled by this method as well. Microscopically controlled Mohs fresh tissue surgery has been used to excise all tumor while preserving the glans and distal urethra. Mohs surgery is effective only when the neoplasm is limited to the epithelium. Cosmetic and functional results are good, and the tumor can be controlled. However, if invasive cancer is encountered, partial penectomy is indicated. Tumor vaporization by the laser in hopes of preserving the penis is to be condemned. This method destroys the tissue and thus fails to provide histologic evidence of microinvasion if present. Partial penectomy may then inappropriately be withheld. Circumcision is recommended when erythroplasia of Queyrat is confined to the foreskin. Microinvasion, which is present in 30 percent of cases of erythroplasia of Queyrat, dictates partial penectomy.

Other forms of therapy include topical 5-fluorouracil and intralesional bleomycin (2 mg per 0.1 ml) if the tumor is not invasive. Several injections of bleomycin may be required for cure. Because these injections are painful, local anesthesia is desirable. Locally administered chemotherapy produces an intense, exudative, erosive balanitis lasting several weeks to several months. This reaction heals when the neoplasm has been eliminated.

BALANITIS XEROTICA OBLITERANS

Balanitis xerotica obliterans is the term applied to lichen sclerosus et atrophicus of the glans penis, the prepuce, and occasionally the fossa navicularis. It is predominantly a disease of middle-aged males, but prepubertal boys have occasionally been described with these lesions. The urologist often encounters asymptomatic patients who require endoscopy for an unrelated complaint. Phimosis and the development of petechial and ecchymotic hemorrhages into the lesions on the glans penis are the usual presenting complaints. Despite the name, obliteration of the urethral meatus is usually insufficient to impede normal voiding; however, a relative meatal stenosis that restricts the routine passage of urologic instruments is the common reason for performing meatotomy in patients with this disease. Circumcision has classically been the treatment for the phimosis, but since this procedure may be complicated by a persistent erosive balanitis postoperatively, it should not be employed indiscriminately and should be combined with postoperative application of testosterone cream. Malignant change in balanitis xerotica obliterans is rare but has been reported. Ectopic nongenital lesions may occur but are more frequent in females than in males. Prepubertal lesions generally resolve at puberty without either specific medical or surgical therapy.

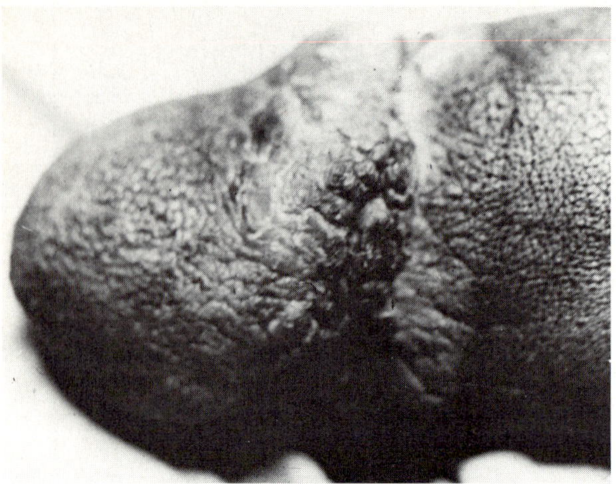

Figure 2   Erythroplasia of Queyrat on the foreskin.

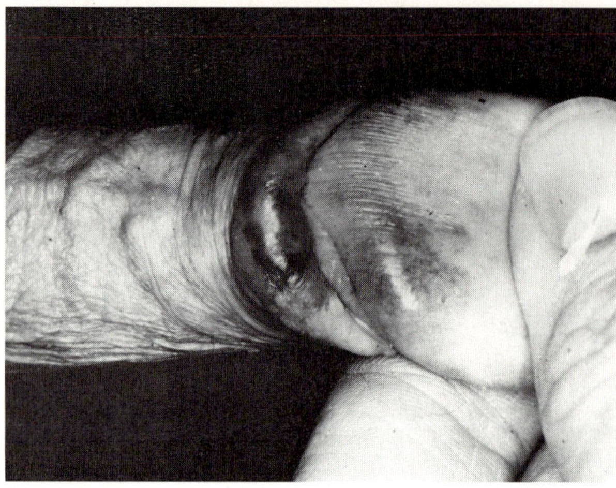

Figure 4   Bowenoid papulosis in the coronal sulcus.

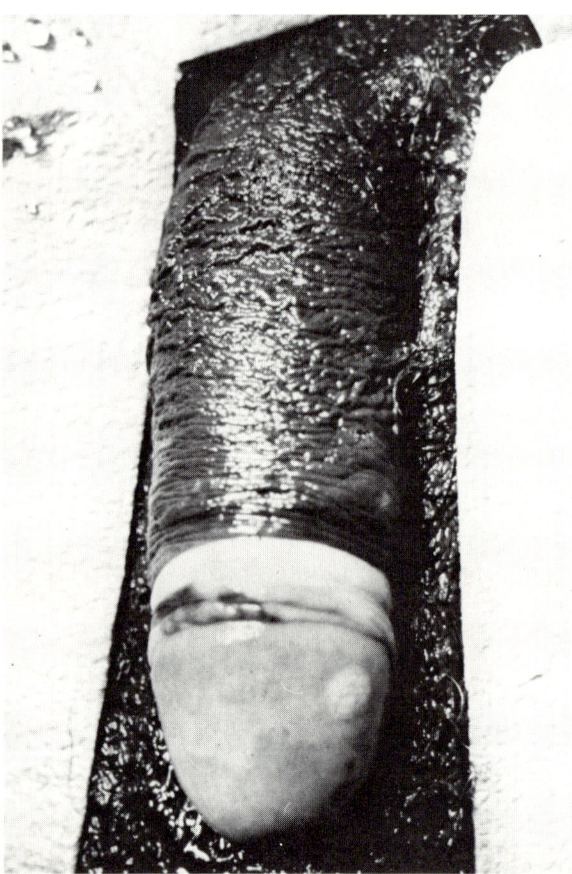

Figure 3   Leukokeratosis on the glans penis in a patient with squamous cell carcinoma in situ.

Biopsy confirmation of the diagnosis of balanitis xerotica obliterans is strongly recommended because these lesions may mimic those of localized scleroderma. More important, all areas of leukokeratosis and erythrokeratosis should be excised and examined histologically because these are the areas likely to contain squamous cell carcinoma. Although rare, such lesions should be given first priority, since all subsequent therapy will depend on a benign or malignant diagnosis. Biopsy is simple and creates little morbidity. Multiple small biopsies of all sites of questionable involvement are advised.

On histologic section, there is mild epithelial hyperkeratosis and marked atrophy of the epithelium. Homogenization and edema of the collagen of the upper portion of the dermis are characteristic. There is a band of inflammatory cells beneath the damaged dermal collagen in the mid-dermis that disappears late in the course of the disease.

Therapeutic Alternatives

Patients who present with petechiae and simple atrophic changes in the skin of the glans without constrictive phimosis or a history of recurrent balanitis should initially receive medical management. Topical testosterone, 5 percent, in xipamide (Aquaphor) applied for a year or more two to three times a day will halt the progression of the disease in a significant number of patients. Cutaneous blood vessel fragility will diminish, and the texture of the atrophic skin will improve. A decision to perform circumcision in patients with balanitis xerotica obliterans implies that the risk of development of postoperative problems is distinctly less than in the preoperative patient status. If circumcision is required to control symptoms of phimosis and recurrent balanitis, topical treatment with testosterone, 5 percent, in Aquaphor for a year or more two to three times a day decreases the possibility of postcircumcision erosive balanitis.

Patients who develop persistent erosive balanitis after circumcision require further therapy. Destruction of the diseased genital epithelium with a CO_2 laser in the defocused mode has resulted in dramatic improvement. Within 3 to 6 weeks after laser treatment the glans will re-epithelialize and the new epithelium will be normal in texture and resistance to trauma. The reason for this normalization without recurrence of disease is unknown. If regrowth of epithelium is delayed after laser therapy, small pinch grafts taken from nearby genital or thigh skin may be placed on the denuded areas. This results in rapid reseeding of the denuded area with epithelial cells. The end product is both cosmetically and functionally acceptable and is more desirable than the severe form of the basic disease process.

Topical chemotherapeutic agents such as 5-fluorouracil and bleomycin should *not* be used in the treatment of balanitis xerotica obliterans, since they simply produce ulcerations that do not heal.

Preferred Approach

If there is no obstructive phimosis or symptomatic urethral stenosis, hormonal therapy is the treatment of choice. It is atraumatic, and the patient obtains acceptable cosmetic and functional results. Either circumcision or meatotomy may result in failure of complete uncomplicated healing and thus should be undertaken only if specifically indicated. If these operations are required, postoperative hormone therapy to the involved skin is the next treatment of choice.

Laser therapy is useful only in cases in which hormone therapy has failed and persistent erosive balanitis is present.

Incisional surgery with elliptical excision of small patches of lichen sclerosus et atrophicus is regularly and routinely associated with recurrence. For that reason, this form of therapy should be excluded for the treatment of the benign process and should be reserved for carcinoma in situ or invasive squamous cell carcinoma.

SUGGESTED READING

Chalmers RF, Burton PA, et al. Lichen sclerosus et atrophicus. A common and distinctive cause of phimosis in boys. Arch Dermatol 1984; 120:1025–1027.

Friedrich EG, Kalra PS. Serum levels of sex hormones in vulvur lichen sclerosus, and the effect of topical testosterone. N Engl J Med 1984; 310:488–91.

Ross SA, Sanchez JL, et al. Spirochetal forms in the dermal lesions of morphea and lichen sclerosus et atrophicus. Am J of Dermatopathol 1990; 12:357–62.

Ridley CM. Lichen sclerosus et atrophicus. Arch Dermatol 1987; 123:457–461.

SARCOMA OF THE PENIS

KENNETH B. CUMMINGS, M.D., F.A.C.S.
JOSEPH G. BARONE, M.D.

Sarcoma of the penis is an uncommon malignancy. The incidence is highest in adults between the ages of 45 and 55 years and in children between the ages of 5 and 10 years. There are 60 different histologic types of sarcoma, leiomyosarcoma being the most common penile variety. There are no obvious etiologic factors for the development of this tumor, with the exception of penile Kaposi's sarcoma in acquired immunodeficiency syndrome (AIDS) patients. Patients typically present with a painless, slow-growing penile mass. In some cases the tumor presents with priapism or a corporal calcification that is grossly indistinguishable from a Peyronie's plaque.

A complete history, physical examination, and biopsy will establish the diagnosis. Further work-up should include computed tomography (CT) of the chest, abdomen, and pelvis along with a complete blood count and liver function studies in order to stage the tumor (Table 1).

TREATMENT OPTIONS

Since penile sarcoma is so unusual, there are no prospective randomized clinical trials for its treatment. Experience with sarcomas in other anatomic locations provides much of the information needed for treating this tumor. Although much effort has been devoted to differentiating tumors according to histologic type or level of invasion, tumor grade is the single most important prognostic factor in treatment planning. The American Joint Committee has developed a system that grades all malignant soft tissue sarcomas according to the number of mitoses per high-power field (Table 2). Because the system does not consider tumor histology or anatomic location, it has prognostic significance for planning treatment.

Surgery

Unlike pelvic or retroperitoneal sarcomas, which present late and may be unresectable at the time of diagnosis, the location of penile sarcoma should make early detection and diagnosis possible. Surgery therefore plays a major role in the treatment of local disease. The goal of surgery is total tumor eradication with microscopically negative surgical margins. Grade I lesions are

Table 1 American Joint Committee Staging of Soft Tissue Tumors

Stage I

(G1, T1, N0, M0) Ia	Grade I less than 5 cm, no regional or distant metastasis
(G2, T2, N0, M0) Ib	Grade II more than 5 cm, no regional or distant metastasis

Stage II

(G2, T1, N0, M0) IIa	Grade II less than 5 cm, no regional or distant metastasis
(G2, T2, N0, M0) IIb	Grade II more than 5 cm, no regional or distant metastasis

Stage III

(G3, T1, N0, M0) IIIa	Grade III less than 5 cm, no regional or distant metastasis
(G3, T2, N0, M0) IIIb	Grade III more than 5 cm, no regional or distant metastasis
(G1–3, T1–2, N1, M0) IIIc	Any grade with regional metastasis without distant metastasis

Stage IV

(G1–3, T3, N0–1, M0) IVa	Any tumor grossly invading bone, major vessel, or nerve without distant metastasis
(G1–3, T1–3, N0–1, M1) IVb	Distant metastasis

Modified from Beahrs OH, ed. Manual for staging of cancer. 3rd ed. Philadelphia: JB Lippincott, 1988.

Table 2 Tumor Grade Based on Mitosis Per High-Power Field (hpf)

Grade	Number of Mitoses per hpf	5-Year Survival (%)
I	0–1	100
II	1–4	73
III	75	46

Modified from Coindac JM. Reproducibility of a histopathologic grading system for adult soft tissue sarcoma. Cancer 1986; 58:306.

low grade and have successfully been treated with local excision or partial penectomy. Grades II and III are high-grade lesions that usually require partial or total penectomy to achieve adequate local control because of their aggressive biologic behavior.

If regional lymph nodes are palpable in a patient with nonmetastatic disease, most surgeons would agree that ileoinguinal lymphadenectomy is warranted; if this is positive, a pelvic lymphadenectomy and contralateral ileoinguinal dissection is performed. The role of prophylactic lymphadenectomy is not established, but some authors favor it for stage II or III lesions because there is up to a 20 percent chance of microscopic nodal disease.

Radiation

Sarcomas are not highly radiosensitive tumors. Radiation failure rates range from 19 to 100 percent. McNeer has determined that a small tumor (2 cm) that receives a large radiation dose (6,000 rads) is most likely to respond. At least 3,000 rads is needed for a minimal response. The use of hyperfractionation (more than one fraction daily) may provide slightly better results, but toxicity is increased.

Radiation is seldom used alone to control local disease for penile sarcoma because doses of 6,000 rads are required, response rates are poor, and complications include soft tissue necrosis and lower extremity edema. Preoperative radiation has been used, but there is no conclusive evidence that local tumor recurrence rates are reduced, and morbidity can be significant if high doses (>5,000 rads) are used. Postoperative radiation may be indicated when disease remains after surgery.

Chemotherapy

Chemotherapy has been used for both adjuvant therapy and for treating metastatic disease. Doxorubicin (Adriamycin) is the most effective single agent and is given in intravenous doses of 50 to 70 mg per square meter every 3 to 4 weeks. Sixteen to 36 percent of patients respond, median response rates lasting 12 to 36 months. Toxicities include myelosuppression, alopecia, nausea, vomiting, and stomatitis. Cardiac toxicities occur at cumulative doses exceeding 550 mg per square meter.

Dacarbazine (DTIC) is an imidazole that has been used alone and in combination with doxorubicin; as a single agent it produces 18 percent response rates. The major toxicities are gastrointestinal. The Eastern Cooperative Oncology Group reported a slight advantage in response rates, but not survival, with doxorubicin plus DTIC compared with doxorubicin alone.

Various combination regimens have been used to treat sarcoma. Perhaps the best studied regimen after doxorubicin-DTIC is the CYVADIC regimen developed at the M.D. Anderson Hospital for the treatment of metastatic sarcoma. This consists of cyclophosphamide (500 mg per square meter) intravenously and doxorubicin (50 mg per square meter) intravenously on day 1 and DTIC (250 mg per square meter) intravenously and vincristine (1.5 mg per square meter) intravenously on days 1 to 5. Response rates of 17 to 30 percent have been reported, the duration of response lasting up to 63 weeks. Major toxicities include vomiting, congestive heart failure from doxorubicin, and hemorrhagic cystitis (from cyclophosphamide). An effective regimen for children consists of vincristine (2 mg per square meter) intravenously and actinomycin D (0.015 mg per kilogram per day, maximal dose of 0.5 mg) intravenously on days 1 to 5 and cyclophosphamide (10 mg per kilogram per day) intravenously on days 1 to 3. For adjuvant therapy, a combination of intravenous cyclophosphamide, intravenous vincristine, and intravenous actinomycin D alternated with intravenous vincristine and intravenous DTIC showed a significant (p < 0.001) decrease in the

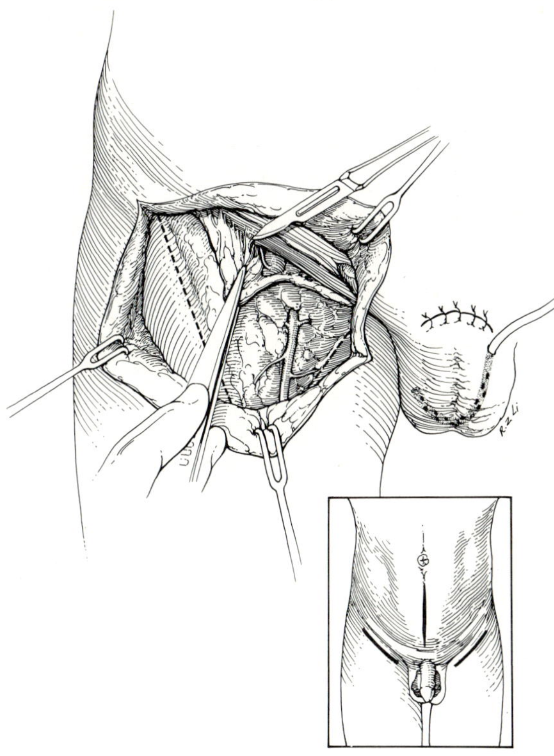

Figure 1 The anatomic boundaries of inguinal lymphadenectomy are indicated by dotted lines. Insert illustrates skin incisions.

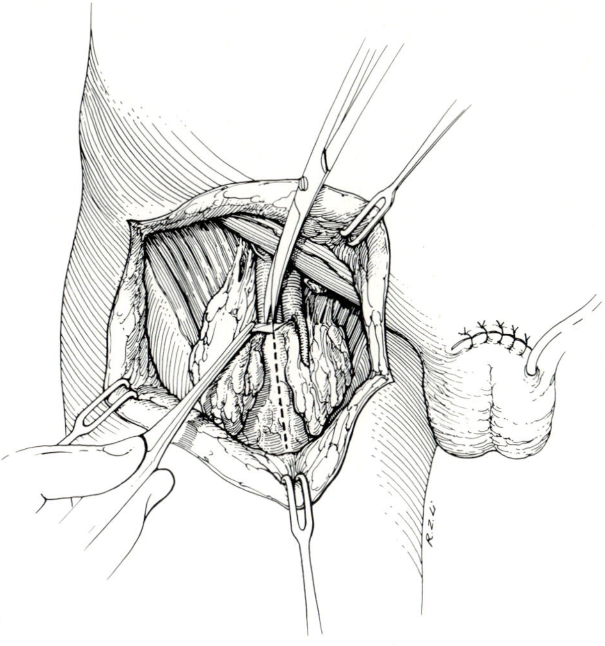

Figure 2 Dense fibrous connective tissue forming the femoral sheath must be sharply incised to allow dissection of the deep inguinal nodes.

incidence of metastasis after 2 years in patients who received surgery plus chemotherapy compared with that of patients who received surgery alone.

ROBERT WOOD JOHNSON APPROACH

Stage I

We use tumor grade and stage to plan treatment. Stage I tumors are grade I lesions and have a good prognosis. They are treated by local excision or partial penectomy, depending on their location and size. Every effort is made to preserve the penis to allow the patient to stand to void. However, if the lesion is large and if less than a 3-cm stump remains after resection, a total penectomy with perineal urethrostomy may be preferable to a urinary stream that has no directional control. Prophylactic lymphadenectomy is not indicated.

Stage II

Stage II disease represents a high-grade lesion (grade II) and local excision is rarely definitive. Partial or total penectomy is more appropriate, depending on the location and size of the tumor. The issue of prophylactic lymphadenectomy is not defined. Appropriate assessment of nodal disease is best obtained as

guided by the anatomic and clinical studies of Cabanas, with sentinel node biopsy performed bilaterally. If this is negative, observation is appropriate.

The procedure can be accomplished through a small incision two fingerbreadths lateral and inferior to the pubic tubercle. These nodes are superomedial to the femoral and saphenous vein junction and rest between the medial branches of these veins (superficial external pudendal and superficial epigastric veins).

Stage III

Stage III lesions are high grade (grade III) and are treated with partial or total penectomy, depending on location and tumor size. Large lesions may require excision of the scrotum, urethra, urogenital diaphragm, and even bladder to achieve local regional control. If complete tumor excision is not possible, we suggest suspending the small bowel and sigmoid colon out of the pelvis, employing an absorbable mesh. This permits postoperative radiation up to doses of 6,000 rads without causing unacceptable intestinal morbidity.

After successful extirpation of the local disease surgically, it should be anticipated that there is regional lymph node involvement even in the clinical N0 patient.

Our approach starts with a meticulous pelvic lymphadenectomy. In the absence of significant pelvic lymph node involvement, we proceed with one side of the superficial and deep ileoinguinal node dissection.

The incision is two to three fingerbreadths beneath and parallel to the inguinal ligament. Skin flaps are developed with meticulous care, preserving their vascu-

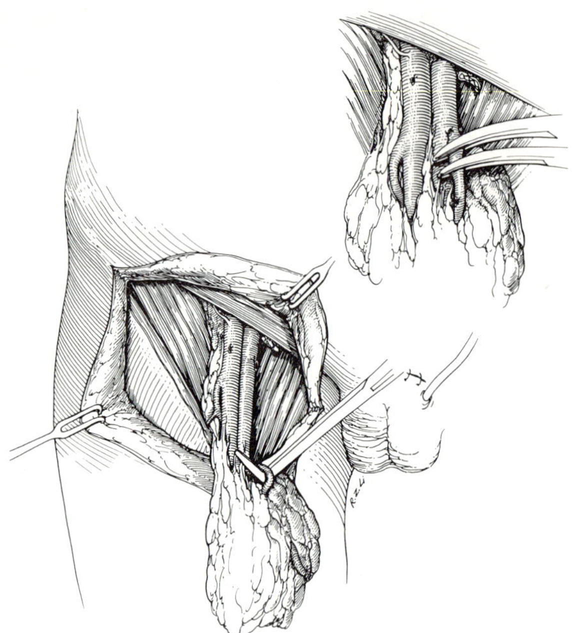

Figure 3 Skeletonization of the femoral artery and vein to the apex of the femoral triangle.

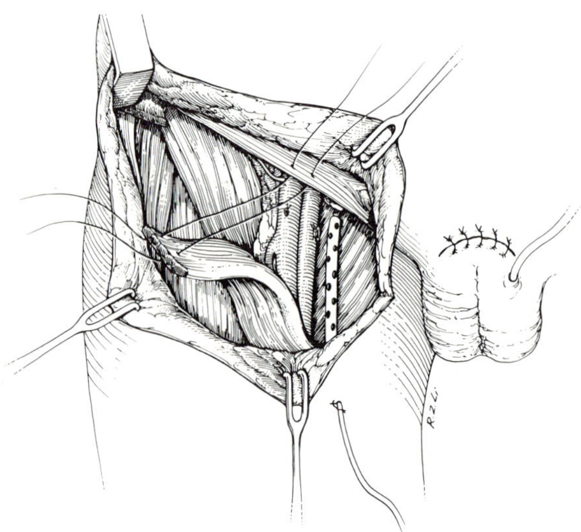

Figure 4 After lymphadenectomy, the sartorius muscle is transposed over the femoral vessels.

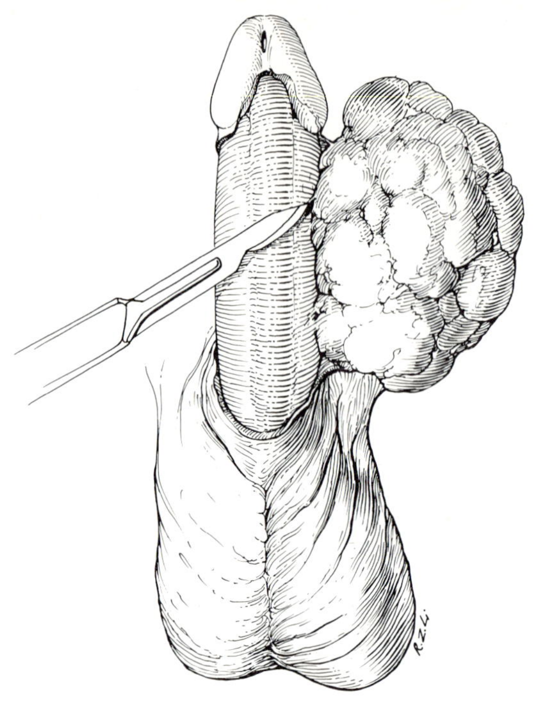

Figure 5 Total tumor excision and denudation of the penis.

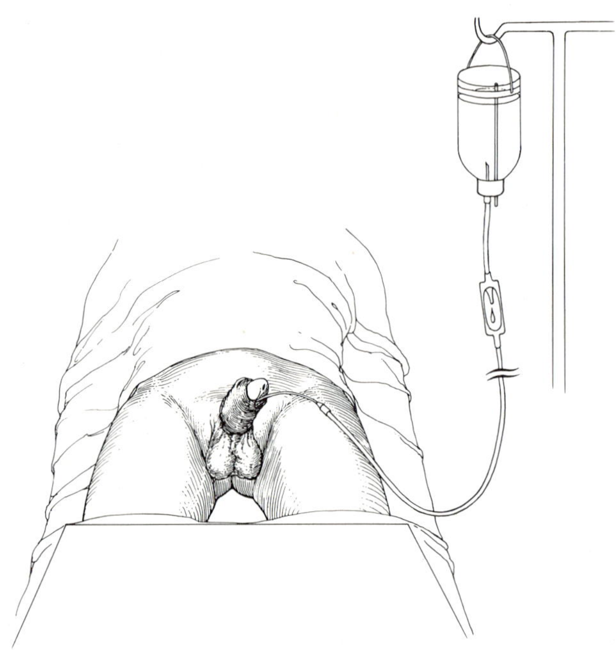

Figure 6 Denuded penile shaft prepared for skin grafting by use of a constant saline drip.

larity in the subcutaneous fat. This incision is ample to expose the entire site of the dissection as outlined in the dotted lines in Figure 1. Sharp dissection is initiated cephalad above the inguinal ligament on the aponeurosis of the external oblique muscle, the sartorius muscle laterally, medially over the adductor magnus, and inferiorly to the apex of the femoral triangle. The dissection is then directed centripetally toward the

femoral vessels. The superficial branches of these vessels are ligated with absorbable suture. In the absence of gross disease, the saphenous vein is preserved to reduce postoperative leg edema. If there is gross disease, the saphenous vein may need to be controlled initially distal to the fossa ovalis.

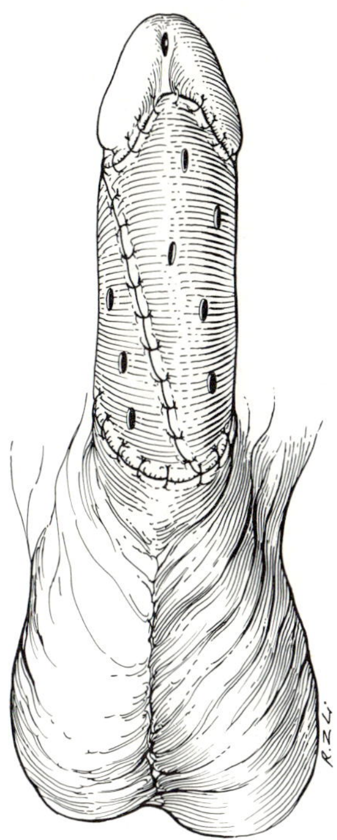

Figure 7 Meshed split-thickness skin graft covers the penile shaft.

When the femoral sheath is visualized, it is incised (Fig. 2) to allow entrance through this dense fibroconnective tissue to the deep inguinal nodes, which are delivered by skeletonizing the femoral vein and artery. Care must be exercised not to damage the profunda femoris artery or the femoral nerve. As the dissection proceeds toward the apex of the femoral triangle, the saphenous vein is ligated at its origin. Delivery of the dissected specimen en bloc from the apex of the femoral triangle is completed with division of the remaining fibrolymphatic attachments (Fig. 3).

The femoral vessels are protected by transposition of the sartorius muscle from its tendinous origin onto the inguinal ligament with nonabsorbable sutures (Fig. 4). Suction catheter drainage (Jackson-Pratt) via a stab wound is continued in the first postoperative week.

Wound closure must be meticulous with resection of up to 1 cm of skin from the free margins. Skin viability can be evaluated with intravenous floracene.

The remaining groin dissection is deferred for 2 to 3 weeks, in part to allow ambulation after the week of postural confinement required following the initial operation. The risk of thromboembolism is real, and minidose heparin or warfarin and also pneumatic boots have their role to play.

For patients with positive nodes, it is reasonable to administer adjuvant chemotherapy postoperatively. As of this writing, the CYVADIC regimen appears appropriate.

Stage IV

Patients with metastatic disease are treated with the CYVADIC regimen. Local disease is treated with surgery if this can be accomplished, or by a combination of surgery and radiation therapy. Effective palliation can frequently be achieved with radiation dosages not in excess of 4,000 rads over a 4-week period.

KAPOSI'S SARCOMA OF THE PENIS

Experience with massive Kaposi's sarcoma has established complete excision of tumor and the involved skin of the penile shaft as an acceptable surgical therapy (Fig. 5). The denuded shaft is then prepared for grafting by a slow (normal saline) drip on a gauze-wrapped operative bed (Fig. 6). When the site is appropriately prepared, skin grafting can provide an excellent cosmetic result (Fig. 7). It has not been shown that chemotherapy has a role as an adjuvant to surgery for Kaposi's sarcoma.

PROGNOSIS

The prognosis for patients with a grade I lesion is excellent, with 5-year survival rates approaching 100 percent. Patients with grades II and III lesions have a rather dismal 5-year survival rate despite aggressive surgery, radiation, and chemotherapy.

CONDYLOMATA ACUMINATA

AUGUST ZABBO, M.D.
BARRY S. STEIN, M.D., F.A.C.S.

Condylomata acuminata result from anogenital infection with certain types of human papillomavirus (HPV). The infection is sexually transmitted, with an infectivity rate of approximately 65 percent. The incubation period is variable, from 3 weeks to 9 months, before infection is detectable. Malignancies of the female genital tract have been associated with HPV infection, leading to the referral of male sexual partners of women with HPV-related lesions to urologists for evaluation and treatment. There is controversy over which men should be evaluated and treated, given (1) the high prevalence of HPV infection (up to 30 percent in sexually active women studied by molecular biologic techniques in some series), (2) a high failure rate with all reported treatments (20 to 75 percent), and (3) that most men are asymptomatic. The partners of sexually active women with HPV-related lesions should be treated in order to prevent recurrence of these lesions in the current sexual partner; prevent HPV-associated disease in future sexual partners; treat the symptoms and psychologic distress caused by the infection; and detect and treat penile intraepithelial neoplasia, which has been associated with HPV infection in men.

EVALUATION

Patients rarely complain of symptoms from condylomata acuminata. Occasionally, a man complains of urethral discharge or burning or hematuria when a urethral condyloma is present. Among patients with obvious lesions, only about half recognize them as genital warts.

When first seen, the patient is given a brochure that describes in layman's terms the disease process, the risk of neoplasm in women, and the reasons for which men should be treated. Most men do not recognize that they are infected with HPV, and written information that they can return to for reference and reassurance has been found very helpful. The brochure sheet also describes the evaluation that they will be undergoing as well as the possible need for biopsy and treatment.

Evaluation of the male patient begins with inspection of the anogenital area. The foreskin must be fully retracted and all surfaces inspected. The meatus is spread and gentle pressure applied just below the fossa navicularis to attempt to extrude any distal meatal condylomata. A pediatric nasal speculum is helpful in inspecting the first 1 to 2 cm of the urethra to the fossa navicularis. A cytology specimen is obtained to screen for intraurethral condylomata. Voided urine has generally been sufficient for this screening, while some authors have recommended sampling the urethra with a calcium

aginate swab and preparing a Papanicolaou smear. Only patients with positive cytologic results (approximately 5 percent) then undergo urethroscopy. Urethroscopy is also performed in patients with obvious meatal condylomata to check for lesions further within the urethra. Inspection must include the anal area, and when external perianal lesions are found, anoscopy is recommended to rule out higher involvement in the anal canal. Next the genitalia are incubated with 3 to 5 percent acetic acid–soaked sponges for at least 5 minutes. It is important to retract the foreskin and make certain that the acetic acid has made contact with all surfaces. Areas of involvement with subclinical HPV infection appear as acetowhite plaques, which are discrete areas of grayish-white discoloration of the skin. This reaction, however, is not specific for condylomata acuminata, and any inflammatory lesion, as well as many other benign skin conditions, may result in an acetowhite reaction. Large patches of acetowhite discoloration usually result from benign irritations such as that from scratching, particularly on the scrotum. It is common to find large areas of acetowhite in the presence of fungal infections, particularly under the foreskin. If such areas are found, treatment with antifungal creams and reinspection after 1 month are indicated. Biopsies are obtained of (1) acetowhite lesions, because this is not specific; (2) obvious lesions that are not definitely condylomatous in nature; and (3) lesions suspicious for intraepithelial neoplasia (brownish-to-purple papules typical of bowenoid papulosis or other long-standing hyperkeratinized areas). The biopsy is accomplished with the patient under local anesthesia with 2 percent plain lidocaine. A disposable, 2-mm skin-punch biopsy is used to obtain the specimen, and the base of the biopsied area is cauterized with a silver nitrate stick. A small amount of bacitracin ointment is applied to the biopsy site, and the patient is instructed to apply this ointment twice per day for 3 days after the biopsy. Minimal scarring is evident after healing and no complications have resulted from this technique.

TREATMENT

Treatment is based on the extent and location of involvement. Single small lesions can be removed by excision, which can often be accomplished with the skin-punch biopsy. Circumcision is recommended when there is involvement of the foreskin beyond a few small lesions. In most cases, however, the patient has already been circumcised and there are only a few small scattered lesions on the shaft of the penis. Treatment with lasers is preferred to other local therapies because more precisely controlled destruction of the lesions can be accomplished and because it is safe and effective. There are minimal complications when the laser is properly applied, and there have been fewer recurrences in the area of treatment.

The current lasers used are the carbon dioxide, Nd:YAG, and KTP lasers. All can be used with the patient under local anesthesia in an office setting if the lesions are limited. A smoke evacuator is required to remove the plume during laser therapy, which might include infectious viral particles. When lesions are extensive or if there is a large perianal condyloma, it is best to handle these with the patient under regional or general anesthesia in the outpatient operating room or in multiple office sessions. Urethral lesions can also be treated in an office setting, using a pediatric cystoscope for urethroscopy and a small laser fiber from either the KTP or Nd:YAG laser without the need for anesthesia.

The lasers differ in their depth of penetration of energy and thermal effects, which must be taken into account with the use of the specific lasers. In general, the carbon dioxide laser is useful for treating external and meatal lesions; intraurethral lesions require the cystoscopic fibers of either the Nd:YAG or KTP laser.

Treatment with the carbon dioxide laser is generally done with a power setting of 2 to 5 watts and a focused beam. Larger lesions may require higher power settings. The surface of the lesion and a 2- to 3-mm surrounding area are laser photocoagulated, which causes carbonization of the surface tissue. The laser beam is applied in three directions: horizontally, vertically, and obliquely, since the carbon dioxide laser has a U-shaped area of tissue destruction and since there may be intervening ridges that are untreated if the same direction is used constantly. Tissue vaporization leaves behind a black eschar, which is wiped free with a dry gauze, and the remaining condylomatous lesion is treated again. Repeat application of the laser and removal of the carbonized area is done until the basal layer is reached, which shows as a shiny, opalescent, flat area. A small amount of bacitracin ointment is applied, and the patient is instructed to treat the lasered area with this ointment twice per day for 3 days after treatment.

Perianal warts that are limited in size and number can be treated with the patient under local anesthesia in the office, using similar technique in the knee-chest position. However, most perianal warts are extensive, and it is best to treat these in the outpatient operating room with the patient under regional general anesthesia, using the Nd:YAG or KTP laser.

Urethral meatal warts, if they can be everted completely, can be treated in the office with the patient under local anesthesia. The anesthetic is administered to the base of the wart or to the periurethral area just inside the meatus, and the lesion is treated as previously described. The patient is given a prescription for adjunctive intraurethral 5-fluorouracil cream to be inserted once per day for 2 weeks. Urethroscopy is performed at the next visit if the meatal lesion has resolved.

Intraurethral warts require either the KTP or Nd:YAG lasers. These lasers are also preferred when the lesions are very large, and for perianal warts. These lasers can be used interchangeably, but it must be recognized that the depth of penetration of the KTP laser is 1 to 2 mm, while that of the Nd:YAG is 4 mm using a focused beam. Use of the sapphire contact tip with the Nd:YAG laser allows direct contact with surface warts and less penetration of energy. With large warts and anal warts, the sapphire contact tip is used with a light erasing motion over the condyloma to vaporize its surface. When all visible condylomata have been removed, the bare fiber is used with a slightly defocused beam to photocoagulate the base of the condylomata using a power of 25 watts. The KTP laser can be used similarly, but given its lower depth of penetration, actual contact with the laser fiber is possible. The KTP laser is very satisfactory for intraurethral condylomata done through a pediatric cystoscope. The lesions are visualized and a focused beam at 1 to 2 watts is used to photocoagulate the condyloma and its base, which will give a whitish discoloration through the cystoscope. Again, any intraurethral condyloma is treated adjunctively with 5-fluorouracil cream.

Healing generally takes 1 to 2 weeks and patients are instructed to use a condom for sexual intercourse; however, they are warned that this will protect only against contact with the area under the condom, and the remainder of the genital and pubic areas are still at risk. The importance of follow-up examination is stressed, as the recurrence rate will still be approximately 50 percent. Follow-up is done 6 to 8 weeks later, at which time urethroscopy is performed if the patient has had a positive screening cytologic study or intraurethral warts. Urethroscopy is done with a pediatric cystoscope down to the level of the external sphincter; it is not advanced farther than this for fear of iatrogenically spreading the urethral warts into the bladder.

Repeat visits are made every 6 to 8 weeks until the HPV lesions are completely cleared. At this time, a 6-month follow-up is arranged, because late recurrences have been known to occur. Repeat examination in 6 months is also recommended in patients who have an initial negative examination, because the incubation period is potentially long. This approach has resulted in approximately 60 percent elimination of condylomata with a single treatment. However, it seems that a certain percentage of recurrence persists with each subsequent treatment, and therefore a subset of patients will require multiple treatments. Whether this is because of subclinical infection that is not detected at the initial setting or because of re-exposure to the virus through sexual partners is unknown. There have been minimal complications and scarring has not been a problem, except with the most extensive lesions.

ALTERNATIVE THERAPIES

Many alternative therapies for condylomata acuminata have been advocated. All have a significant recurrence rate and potential local and systemic side effects. The fact that so many therapies are still in vogue confirms that we have not yet found the ideal therapy for this viral infection.

Cryotherapy has been used, particularly by dermatologists, in treating condylomata acuminata. Recurrence rates are similar to those with other forms of treatment. Inadequate control of the depth of penetration of the freezing may result in large ulcers and scarring.

Electrocoagulation has been used to treat condylomata acuminata, but this treatment is associated with a lack of control of the depth of penetration. Local anesthesia needs to be more extensive, as there is arcing of the current, and scarring is generally more severe than with lasers. Particular caution is necessary in using electrocautery for urethral meatal or intraurethral warts, or urethral stricture may result.

Podophyllin is a resin available in 10 and 25 percent strengths in benzoin solution, applied directly to the warts with a cotton-tipped applicator and allowed to dry. It is washed off 4 to 6 hours later. The agent is toxic to the myocardium, neurologic system, and kidneys if absorbed in sufficient amounts. Given the limited nature of most penile lesions, this is unlikely in male patients, but it may occur if large perianal or vaginal lesions are treated with this agent. Topical administration of podophyllin causes a blanching of the affected area, with sloughing in 2 to 4 days. Repeat applications are required every 7 days until resolution of the lesion is complete. The success rate is approximately 25 percent.

Bichloracetic and trichloroacetic acids have been popularized by gynecologists for treating external genital lesions in the female. The acids are used as a 50 to 85 percent solution in 70 percent alcohol. Topical application results in a chemical cauterization of the lesions and intense skin irritation, which lasts 3 to 5 minutes. If the irritation is too intense or if a wider application is administered than was intended, the acids can be neutralized with diluted sodium bicarbonate. The patient can be taught self-administration, to be repeated every 2 to 4 days. The effectiveness of these acids is equivalent to that of podophyllin, but their use, especially in female patients, is safer.

5-fluorouracil is an antineoplastic antimetabolite that has shown activity in condylomatous disease. It is available as a 5 percent cream. Daily application causes erythema and vesiculation owing to chemical dermatitis. It is therefore important to apply the cream only to the intended area and to protect the untreated areas, particularly the scrotum. The cream may be applied by patients themselves, but again caution must be used to prevent application of the cream in unattended areas.

Alpha-interferon injected intralesionally three times per week for 3 weeks has been advocated as immunotherapy for condylomata resistant to other therapies. This agent has recently been released by the Federal Drug Administration for this purpose. Side effects include a 26 percent incidence of leukopenia as well as a lower incidence of fever, chills, myalgias, and headaches, making this a less desirable mode of treatment, certainly for the initial therapy.

SUGGESTED READING

Krebs HB. Genital HPV infections in men. Clin Obstet Gynecol 1989; 32:180–190.

Malloy TR, Zderic SA, Carpiniello VL. External genital lesions in lasers in urologic surgery. Chicago: Year Book Medical Publishers, 1989:23.

Stein BS. Laser treatment of condylomata acuminata. J Urol 1986; 136:593–594.

URETHRAL CARCINOMA IN MALES

WILLIAM R. FAIR, M.D.
CHI-REI YANG, M.D.

Approximately 600 cases of primary carcinoma of the male urethra have been reported. The disease is unusual among genitourinary tract neoplasms in that it occurs more commonly in females than in males. Carcinoma of the urethra has been reported in males as young as 13 years and as old as 91 years of age, although most cases occur in the fifth to the seventh decades. No racial predisposition has been recorded. The etiology is undetermined; it has been suggested that the frequent presence of infection and chronic irritation may be contributing or promoting factors.

For clinical convenience, patients with carcinoma of the urethra are classified into three groups according to location of the lesion: penile, bulbomembranous, or prostatic urethral carcinoma. In published reports 59 percent of tumors occurred in the bulbomembranous urethra, 34 percent in the penile urethra, and only 7 percent in the prostatic urethra. Histologically, 78 percent of male urethral carcinomas were squamous cell carcinoma compared with 15 percent transitional carcinoma, 6 percent adenocarcinoma, and 1 percent undifferentiated carcinoma. Squamous cell carcinoma occurred most commonly in the penile and bulbomembranous urethra, and transitional cell carcinoma more often in the prostatic urethra. Adenocarcinoma, which is almost always found in the bulbomembranous or prostatic urethra, is presumed to arise from periurethral glands.

Male urethral carcinoma tends to spread by direct extension to adjacent structures and usually involves the vascular spaces of the corpus spongiosum and periurethral tissue. Carcinoma of the bulbomembranous urethra often extends to the urogenital diaphragm, prostate, perineum, and scrotal skin. Hematogenous spread is uncommon except in advanced disease. Metastasis occurs by lymphatic embolization to regional lymph nodes. The lymphatics from the anterior urethra drain into the superficial and deep inguinal lymph nodes and occasionally to the external iliac nodes. Lymphatics from the posterior urethra drain into the external iliac, obturator, and hypogastric nodes. Tumors of the anterior urethra metastasize generally to the inguinal nodes, and tumors of the posterior urethra metastasize to pelvic nodes; however, there are some exceptions. At Memorial Sloan-Kettering Cancer Center, 33 percent (five of 15) of patients with penile urethral carcinoma had groin metastases, whereas 19 percent (4 of 21) of patients with bulbomembranous urethral carcinoma had pelvic metastases, and 14 percent (three of 21) had groin metastases or groin metastases combined with distant spreading.

Urethral obstruction, palpable mass, and urethral discharge or bleeding are common symptoms in urethral carcinoma. Not infrequently, some patients were treated for benign urethral strictures for a long period before diagnosis. Urethral stricture or bleeding in a patient without a history of trauma, stricture, perineal abscess, or fistula in an elderly male should suggest the possibility of urethral carcinoma.

The evaluation should include careful inspection and palpation of the external genitalia and perineum, and cystourethroscopy and bimanual examination with the patient under anesthesia. Urethroscopic or needle biopsy is the most efficient way to make the diagnosis. Cytologic studies of voided urine may be helpful for diagnosis in some patients (Table 1). The lymphangiogram is sometimes useful to evaluate pelvic and para-aortic nodes before a surgical decision is made, but it is not routinely required. The staging system of Memorial Sloan-Kettering Cancer Center as proposed by Ray and associates is defined in Table 2.

Table 1 Sensitivity of Urine Cytology for the Diagnosis of Carcinoma of the Male Urethra (1949–1984)

Location	Positive	Negative	Not Done	Sensitivity
Penile urethra	7	3	4	70%
Bulbomembranous urethra	5	1	14	83%
Prostatic urethra	4	2	2	67%
Totals	16	6	20	73%

Table 2 Staging System for Carcinoma
of the Male Urethra

0	Confined to mucosa only (in situ)
A	Into but not beyond lamina propria
B	Into but not beyond substances of corpus spongiosum or into but not beyond prostate
C	Direct extension into tissue beyond corpus spongiosum (corpora cavernosa, muscle, fat, fascia, skin, direct skeletal involvement) or beyond prostatic capsule
D1	Regional metastasis including inguinal and/or pelvic lymph nodes (with any primary lesion)
D2	Distant metastasis (with any primary lesion)

Modified from Ray B, Canto AR, Whitmore WF Jr. Experience with primary carcinoma of the male urethra. J Urol 1977; 117:591–594.

GENERAL TREATMENT PHILOSOPHY

Based on past experience and a review of the literature, surgery, with or without combined radiation therapy, is the treatment of choice. The extent of surgery depends on the location and stage of the tumor. In general, anterior urethral carcinoma seems more amenable to surgical control than posterior urethral carcinoma, and the prognosis for anterior urethral carcinoma is better than for those tumors originating posteriorly. Although some instances of tumor control by irradiation have been reported, we believe that this treatment is appropriate only for patients with early lesions of the anterior urethra who refuse surgery. Radiation therapy has the advantage of preserving the penis but may result in urethral stricture, chronic edema, and, rarely, penile atrophy. In general, the response of patients with metastatic urethral cancer to chemotherapy has been disappointing, especially in those with squamous cell carcinoma, adenocarcinoma, or undifferentiated tumors. A few patients with metastatic transitional cell tumors have shown encouraging responses to combination chemotherapy using methotrexate, vinblastine, doxorubicin (Adriamycin), and cisplatin (M-VAC), but the results are too preliminary to make any definitive statements concerning results. Based on the response to M-VAC chemotherapy in bladder and upper tract urothelial tumors, however, continued investigation into its use in transitional cell carcinoma of the urethra is warranted.

Penile Urethral Carcinoma

Carcinoma of the penile urethra may be treated by transurethral resection, local excision, partial amputation, or radical amputation with or without emasculation. For superficial, papillary, or in situ tumor, transurethral resection may be sufficient. For tumor infiltrating the corpus and localized to the distal half of the penis, a partial amputation with a 2-cm margin proximal to any visible or palpable lesion is the generally accepted form of treatment. If the infiltrating tumor is located in the proximal penile urethra or involves the entire penile urethra, radical amputation should be done. Emascula-

tion is indicated only when the scrotal skin is involved. Unlike carcinoma of the penis, clinically palpable adenopathy in the groin of patients with penile carcinoma usually represents metastasis and is not often the result of reactive inflammation. Ilioinguinal node dissection is indicated only if the inguinal nodes are palpable. There is no evidence of benefit from prophylactic groin dissection. After excision of the primary tumor, the patients should be followed with careful examination of the inguinal areas for evidence of lymphadenopathy, and a groin dissection should be done on the finding of metastatic disease.

From 1949 to 1984, there were eight cases of carcinoma of the fossa navicularis or urethral meatus managed at Memorial Sloan-Kettering Cancer Center (Table 3). All tumors were epidermoid carcinoma. One patient died of metabolic encephalopathy 2 weeks after ilioinguinal node dissection (negative nodes). Of the remaining seven patients, six survived free of disease (two more than 10 years, three more than 5 years, and one more than 2 years). Three patients underwent partial penectomy and were found to be free of disease for more than 5 years. A patient with a superficial lesion treated by irradiation also survived with a good functional result. Bilateral groin dissection was performed prophylactically in one patient, and ilioinguinal node dissection was done therapeutically in two other patients. The former patient subsequently developed lung and liver metastases and died. The latter two patients had positive nodes: one survived more than 13 years, and another one treated 30 months ago remains alive and well.

In seven patients seen at Memorial Sloan-Kettering Cancer Center during the same period, the tumor involved the middle or entire penile urethra (Table 4). Of two patients with superficial lesions, one was treated by transurethral resection and another by distal urethrectomy. The former survived more than 5 years without disease; the latter patient is alive with disease at 30 months. In two patients with locally invasive disease, one underwent partial penectomy and remains alive after 7 years, and another patient treated by total penectomy was lost to follow-up 1 month after surgery. Clinically palpable inguinal nodes were found in three patients. Two patients had ilioinguinal node dissections after penectomy; one survived more than 10 years and another died of lung metastases. One patient with inguinal lymphadenopathy without node dissection developed lung metastases and died.

For patients followed for more than 5 years, the overall survival rate for those with middle or entire penile urethra carcinoma was 60 percent (3 of 5). For those with carcinoma of the fossa navicularis or urethral meatus, the result was 71 percent (5 of 7). Even in the presence of regional lymph node metastases, cure is still possible in some cases.

Bulbomembranous Urethral Carcinoma

Transurethral or segmental resection with end-to-end anastomosis may be adequate for treatment of the

Table 3 Carcinoma of the Male Urethra—Meatus or Navicularis Fossa

Patient	Age	Date of Treatment	Histology	C/Stage	P/Stage	Treatment	Complication	End Result
C.R.	75	10/30/50	Squamous GIII	B	A	Partial penectomy		NED at 5 years Died 3/57
S.J.	47	10/14/62	Epidermoid GII	D1	D1	Partial penectomy and ilioinguinal node dissection	Lymphedema Cellulitis	NED 13 years Last follow-up 1975
G.A.	49	4/17/66	Epidermoid	A	A	Excisional biopsy Irradation, 5,250 rads	Stricture of meatus	NED 5 years
I.F.	51	11/09/69	Epidermoid GIII	B	B	Partial penectomy		NED 13 years
B.B.	59	11/03/71	Epidermoid GII	A	A	Partial penectomy		NED 66 months
M.J.	53	10/29/73	Epidermoid GII	B D2	B	Partial penectomy and groin dissection (bilateral)		Died 3/23/74 Lung and liver metastasis
K.B.	47	3/18/78	Epidermoid GII	D1	A	Distal urethrectomy and perineal urethrostomy Ilioinguinal node dissection	Metabolic encephalopathy Pelvic abscess	Died 2 weeks post-operation
C.V.	72	10/14/83	Squamous GII	D1	D1	Partial penectomy and ilioinguinal node dissection		NED 30 months

NED, no evidence of disease.

Table 4 Carcinoma of the Male Urethra—Midpenile or Whole Penile

Patient	Age	Date of Treatment	Histology	C/Stage	P/Stage	Treatment	Complication	End Result
F.E.	71	5/12/64	Epidermoid GII	B1 D1	B D1	Total penectomy (5/64) Ilioinguinal node dissection (5/67)	Stricture of meatus	NED 10 years Died 3/22/82
L.G.	54	1/8/67	Epidermoid GII	D1	D1	Total penectomy No lymphade-nectomy		Node biopsy and lung metastasis Died 7/7/67
A.D.	51	2/22/76	Epidermoid	C	C	Total penectomy		Lost to follow-up
S.A.	67	5/29/78	Epidermoid GII	B	B	Partial penectomy		NED 7 years
M.E.	62	9/12/78	Papillary Ca in situ	A	O	Distal urethrectomy and perineal urethrostomy		NED 5 years
S.J.	66	3/27/83	Epidermoid GI	A	A	Transurethral resection and fulguration		Alive with disease
R.L.	57	5/20/84	Epidermoid GIII	D1	D1	Transurethral resection (6/83) Partial penectomy (5/23/84) Ilioinguinal node dissection		Lung metastasis Died 1/18/86

NED, no evidence of disease.

early superficial tumors over this portion of the urethra, but these cases are rare. At Memorial Sloan-Kettering Cancer Center, only one patient with papillary epidermoid carcinoma of the bulbous urethra was treated successfully by repeated transurethral resections. Most patients presented with infiltrating bulky tumor with invasion of surrounding structures. In our series, 90 percent of patients were diagnosed as having stage C or D disease when treated. About one third of clinical stage C patients were understaged and later proved to have pelvic node metastases. The survival of patients in this group was poor despite a distinctly radical surgical approach. The postoperative mortality rate was also excessive. In a previous report from Memorial Sloan-Kettering Cancer Center of patients treated between 1940 and 1969, ten patients had radical surgery, including radical cystectomy, radical penectomy with or without total emasculation, bilateral pelvic node dissection, and formation of an ileal conduit. Of these ten patients, four died postoperatively. Of the six patients who survived radical surgery, five died with local recurrence and/or distal metastases, and only one is alive with no evidence of disease 17 years postoperatively.

The experience suggests that when local control of the tumor can be achieved, overall long-term results are favorable. When the lesion recurs locally, metastatic disease develops within a short period. In an attempt to reduce the frequency of local recurrence, patients with infiltrating posterior urethral carcinomas treated at Memorial Sloan-Kettering Cancer Center after 1970 were designated to undergo preoperative irradiation, radical cystectomy, radical penectomy, and inferior pubic ramus resection, the latter to improve surgical margins around the urogenital diaphragm in bulky tumors. Between 1970 and 1981, five patients with clinical stage C (one patient later proved to have pelvic nodes metastases) were treated in this manner (Table 5). Preoperative external radiation therapy consisted of 2,000 rads delivered over 5 days to large anterior and posterior portals and, on one occasion, with a supplemental perineal port. The operation included anterior exenteration, routine bilateral pelvic lymph node dissection, total penectomy and total emasculation in selected cases, and excision of the inferior ischiopubic rami. There were no postoperative deaths in this experience, but morbidity exceeded 50 percent. Of four patients with pathologic stage C disease, two survived their cancer, remaining free of disease for more than 5 years. One patient died of pulmonary insufficiency at 39 months after surgery, but no evidence of recurrence or metastasis was detected at autopsy. Although we have no concurrent controls, the limited data suggest that this approach is as effective as radical surgery alone. In five patients with pathologic stage C disease treated by radical cystectomy, bilateral pelvic node dissection, and total penectomy with or without emasculation between 1949 and 1969, only one patient survived more than 5 years.

Prostatic Urethral Carcinoma

Carcinoma arising from the prostatic urethra is rare and accounts for only 7 percent of urethral carcinomas. Between 1949 and 1984 we collected eight cases of primary carcinoma of prostatic urethra: six patients had epidermoid carcinoma and two had adenocarcinoma. The diagnosis was based on the finding of a solitary tumor in the prostatic urethra without associated coexisting or pre-existing urothelial tumors elsewhere (such as bladder, ureter, or renal pelvis) on initial diagnosis, and of carcinoma in situ arising in prostatic ducts or periurethral glands.

There are no characteristic symptoms of this lesion. In our eight patients, four had hematuria and five had obstructive symptoms at initial presentation. Prostatic

Table 5 Results of Treatment of Patients with Stage C Carcinoma of Bulbomembranous Urethra

Result	Group I (5 Cases)	Group 2 (4 Cases)
Postoperative mortality	1	0
Postoperative morbidity	2	2
Local recurrence	2	0
Distant metastasis	2	1
NED 3 years	1	3*
NED 5 years	1	2

Group 1: Patients were treated by radical surgical excision between 1949 and 1969. Group 2: Patients were treated by preoperative irradiation (2,000 rads) coupled with radical surgical excision and inferior pubic rami resection between 1970 and 1981.

*One patient died of pulmonary insufficiency 39 months after operation, clinically NED (no evidence of disease).

induration detected by rectal examination represented far-advanced disease. The serum acid phosphatase value was normal. Diagnosis depends on transurethral biopsy of the prostate.

Superficial lesions of the prostatic urethra have been successfully managed by transurethral resection in more than half of the patients. However, such tumors are uncommon. In most instances the tumor involves the bulk of prostate with variable extension to the bulbomembranous urethra or to the bladder neck and trigone. In this situation, radical prostatectomy only may not provide a tumor-free margin, and anterior exenteration is the treatment of choice.

Of eight patients with prostatic urethral carcinoma, one with epidermoid carcinoma was treated by transurethral resection and remains alive without current evidence of disease despite three recurrences. Two patients who presented with pelvic node metastases proved by exploration or lymphangiography underwent radiation therapy and died within 15 months. Two patients were treated by radical radiation therapy after transurethral resection of the prostate; one developed lung metastases 6 months later, and another developed pelvic and liver metastases 4 years later. Two patients with local invasive disease were treated by preoperative irradiation (2,000 to 4,000 rads) followed by radical cystectomy and prostatectomy; one survived more than 10 years, and the other died of recurrence. One patient with epidermoid carcinoma invading the prostatic sinus was treated with local resection and three courses of M-VAC chemotherapy. He remains free of disease and with negative cytology 16 months after therapy. A prostatic urethral biopsy 4 months after initial therapy was free of tumor.

The overall 5-year survival rate for patients with prostatic urethral carcinoma was poor (2 of 7). The case responding to M-VAC chemotherapy is encouraging, and this therapy may play an important role in future management of these diseases.

URETHRAL CARCINOMA IN FEMALES

MICHAEL J. DROLLER, M.D.

Primary urethral carcinoma is rare in both males and females. It is unique among genitourinary malignancies in being the only one that has a substantially higher incidence in females than in males. Although urethral cancers in males often appear to be related to transitional cell cancer of the bladder (particularly those that involve only the prostatic urethra), urethral cancer in females appears to be a distinct entity unrelated to the occurrence of malignancies elsewhere in the urinary tract.

The first report of urethral cancer appeared in 1856. Since then, only about 1200 cases of urethral carcinoma have been reported in the literature. The vast majority of these have been found to have an ominous prognosis, probably because a substantial proportion of patients have had metastatic disease at the time of initial presentation. With a high index of suspicion for the diagnosis and the possibility of discovery of this condition at an earlier stage, prognosis might not be uniformly so ominous (see below). Notwithstanding the variety of treatments attempted (radiation therapy, extensive surgery, and chemotherapy), patients in advanced stages have usually died of their disease.

The rarity of this entity makes it impossible to ascertain any common etiology or to prescribe a standard approach to treatment. However, several features permit a discussion that may allow the physician to become alerted to this problem, to recognize it at an earlier stage, and to address its treatment with an improved prospect for cure and perhaps a better chance of preserving the integrity of the urinary tract and the quality of urinary function.

HISTOPATHOLOGY

Urethral carcinoma in females consists of a variety of disease entities, depending on the site of origin of the particular cancer. The proximal one third of the urethra is lined by transitional epithelium. Primary development of carcinoma at this site is uncommon. Generally, cancer here is associated with transitional cell carcinoma of the bladder and is most often seen when the bladder cancer involves the bladder neck and presumably has extended directly to involve the epithelial lining of the adjacent urethra. In this setting, transitional cell carcinoma of the urethra shares the histopathologic features seen in transitional cell carcinoma involving the bladder.

When transitional cell carcinoma of the urethra is primary, its staging appears to depend on the depth of penetration of the urethral wall. As far as can be determined, the histologic appearance of these tumors is identical to that seen in transitional cell carcinoma of the bladder.

Occasionally, urethral cancers of the posterior urethra take the form of adenocarcinoma. Although this may reflect the malignant transformation of adenomatous rests occasionally seen in the proximal urethra (similar to what is sometimes seen in the trigone), some authors have suggested that transitional cell carcinoma may occasionally take the form of a glandular architecture and possibly develop into an adenocarcinoma. The fact that many of these lesions are found to be associated with metastatic disease at the time of their initial diagnosis is compatible with their possible origin in subepithelial rests.

Carcinoma of the distal two thirds of the urethra in females is generally squamous cell type. This reflects the histology of the normal urethra at that site. Occasionally, transitional cell elements are seen in these malignant conditions. Adenocarcinomas are rarely seen.

The staging of these types of cancers can be considered similar to the staging of carcinomas of the proximal urethra, but must also take into account the possibility of involvement of adjacent structures with a different potential drainage pattern, requiring a concomitant different approach. This is needed both to assess the extent of disease and to define the extent of treatment that may be necessary.

It is more common to see a pronounced inflammatory component in cancers of the distal urethra, presumably because of the association of these types of cancers with chronic inflammation and irritation, a factor that may contribute to their pathogenesis (see below). The same is not necessarily true of cancers in the proximal urethra.

PATHOGENESIS

The pathogenesis of transitional cell carcinoma of the proximal urethra in females probably involves the same factors that may be causative in cancer of the bladder. A variety of carcinogens have been described in this regard, including prolonged exposure to high concentrations of aromatic amines ("industrial" carcinogens), cigarette smoking, previous treatment with cyclophosphamide, abnormalities in tryptophan metabolism, ingestion of high doses of phenacetin, and possibly chronic infections with bacteria that can convert nitrates and nitrites to nitrosamines. All of these substances are promoters rather than initiators in the process of carcinogenesis. However, they all stimulate mitogenesis, which may then indirectly lead to mutagenesis if exposure to these agents is in sufficiently high doses.

The fact that the urethra is not as commonly susceptible to prolonged contact with urine as is the bladder (in both males and females) may explain the relative rarity of this particular entity. Indeed, it is probably more likely that a random event occurs to account for spontaneous malignant transformation of the transitional epithelium of the urethra, and that exposure to promotional agents as the cause of the cancer is more relevant when transitional cell carcinoma in the urethra occurs in the presence of bladder cancer.

On the other hand, squamous cell carcinoma of the distal urethra has been linked to the occurrence of chronic irritation as an etiologic factor. Irritative factors have been associated with mutagenesis and malignant transformation at other sites. In the urethra, the strongest of such associations have been seen in the presence of urethral diverticula, urethral strictures, and urethral caruncles, each of which has been shown to predispose not only to chronic inflammation, but also to retention of urine, to increased concentrations of carcinogens in pools of stagnant urine, to development of infection with bacteria that may contain carcinogen-producing enzymes, and to continuous stimulation of cell proliferation.

Because of the rarity of urethral carcinoma, however, specific etiologic factors have never been clearly characterized. Whether exposure to certain viruses in the context of the above factors may predispose to the development of these conditions (much as appears to be the case with cervical carcinoma), and what role possible sexual activity or hygiene may play in the process of carcinogenesis in this setting, remain to be determined.

DIAGNOSIS

Symptoms

The most common symptoms that characterize the development of carcinoma in either the anterior or posterior urethra in females are voiding irritability and the appearance of blood in the urine (or on the toilet tissue used to clean the perineum after voiding). In the case of transitional cell carcinoma (generally of the proximal urethra), an increased sense of urgency with urinary frequency may represent the earliest symptom of the development of malignancy. As the tumor grows, obstructive symptoms may begin to appear. Diminished force of the urinary stream, increased urinary dribbling, hesitancy, and possibly a sense of urinary retention may all appear to some extent. A mass may actually be palpable when the patient cleans the perineum after voiding. Pain is generally not a concomitant of urethral cancer; dysuria is. Urinary incontinence is generally not seen unless the cancer has become far advanced and a fistula has developed between the urethra/bladder and the anterior vaginal wall.

Symptoms are similar in cancer of the distal urethra. Unfortunately, these symptoms are not pathognomonic of cancer but are more indicative of the presence of the chronic irritation that may be seen in association with a urethral caruncle or a urethral diverticulum. The diagnosis of urethral cancer in this setting therefore needs to be based on a high index of suspicion when a patient has had a prolonged history of urethral stricture and chronic infection, urethral diverticulum, or urethral caruncle

that has worsened with time and is producing increasing symptoms of irritability.

Physical Findings

The physical findings of cancer in the proximal urethra may consist only of the sensation of a fullness or mass on vaginal or perineal palpation. Carcinoma of the distal urethra may be masked by a concomitant urethral diverticulum and by scarring that may create the sensation of palpable induration without cancer being present. It is critical to consider the possibility of cancer in these instances, so that earlier diagnosis can be made and potentially life-saving treatments applied at earlier stages of disease.

It is also important to perform careful palpation of the inguinal lymph nodes. Urethral cancers are accompanied by metastases to the inguinal lymph nodes in at least 15 to 20 percent of instances. This is most commonly seen in cancers of the distal urethra. Its frequency probably reflects the later diagnosis of this entity because of the long-term presence of benign inflammatory processes that may have led to the development of cancer, but at the same time masked its occurrence.

Diagnostic Procedures

Diagnosis generally depends on endoscopy with deep biopsy of the presenting lesion. The necessity of deep biopsy cannot be overemphasized. The chronic inflammation that may have led to the development of the cancer is often located most superficially, while the cancer itself is deep to the inflammatory process. Because so much scarring may be present, the depths of any presenting mass or induration must be sampled for adequate pathologic review. This is most important for cancers of the distal urethra where chronic inflammation is likely to be greater. Indeed, cancers of the proximal urethra may be recognized earlier both because of their endoscopic appearance and also by the appearance of malignant cells in a urine specimen analyzed for abnormal cytology.

Adjunctive diagnostic studies are used to gauge the extent of the disease. Since 15 to 20 percent of urethral cancers have concomitant regional lymphatic involvement, and because malignant involvement is found in up to 80 percent of patients with palpable inguinal nodes (in contrast to what is seen in penile cancer), needle aspiration or node biopsy is generally indicated in this setting.

In cancers of the proximal urethra, which may drain to the external iliac, obturator, and hypogastric nodes, computed tomography (CT) may be useful in determining the extent of the disease. Distant metastatic sites for both types of urethral cancer include lung, liver, and bone. The latter is also often the site of involvement of a primary adenocarcinoma of the mesonephric type, which may be found in the posterior urethra. Bone scans, CT scans of the chest and abdomen, and sonography of the liver may therefore each be indicated in determining the extent of disease once a diagnosis of urethral cancer has been made.

TREATMENT

The prognosis for urethral cancer is generally not good. This probably reflects the fact that most of these cancers at the time of initial clinical discovery are diagnosed at later stages in their evolution, predisposing to extensive regional involvement, or even metastases. It is also possible that when these cancers develop, they occur in a more aggressive form to begin with; since their occurrence is usually masked by the variety of etiologic factors that contribute to their development, they have time to progress before diagnosis is made.

Attempts to treat these cancers while preserving normal voiding function have relied on the use of either radiation therapy or regional excision. The results of these approaches have generally been best in cancers of the distal urethra. Even in these instances, however, 5-year survival rates have been no greater than 50 percent, and generally much less. Although this has prompted many to employ radical exenterative surgery, further improvements in disease-free survival have generally not been seen. The best results appear to have been obtained from a combination of preoperative radiation therapy and extensive exenterative surgery. Attempts to perform only urethrectomy in these instances have generally had little success. Therefore, the entire urethra and bladder have been removed. Actuarial 5-year survival rates from these approaches for cancers of the anterior urethra have been less than 50 percent.

Five-year survival rates for similar approaches in treatment of cancers of the proximal urethra have been only 10 to 15 percent. This reflects the different histopathologies of these diseases, as well as their stage at initial diagnosis and their intrinsic progressive potential.

The clinical involvement of lymph nodes is an ominous finding. Because of its morbidity, so-called "prophylactic" inguinal lymph node dissection is generally not performed. However, since 80 percent of clinically palpable lymph nodes generally are found to reflect the presence of metastases, a unilateral inguinal lymph node dissection is generally done in the setting of palpably positive lymph nodes, in association with the exenterative surgery described above, in an attempt to obtain even a small chance of cure. Some authors have suggested that radiation therapy may enhance the results of such surgery in providing for better control of disease, but the risks associated with radiation in increasing the morbidity of the associated inguinal lymph node dissection need to be considered.

Bilateral lymph node dissection is not necessarily performed unless clinically palpable nodes are present bilaterally. In these instances, however, survival is virtually nil. The same is true when the deep pelvic lymph nodes are involved, as may be the case with transitional cell cancers of the proximal urethra or adenocarcinomas at this site.

Some promising results have been obtained with various chemotherapeutic regimens, especially in treating transitional cell cancers of the posterior urethra. Both partial and complete responses have been described, but durability of response and efficacy in terms of survival have not been reported.

SUGGESTED READING

Benson RC Jr, Swanson SK, Farrow GM. Relationship of leukoplakia to urethral malignancy. J Urol 1984; 131:507.

Bracken RB, Johnson DH, Miller LS, et al. Primary carcinoma of the female urethra. J Urol 1976; 116:188.

Cuatico W, Cheving CH, Sy F. Molecular evidence of viral-like, biochemical activities in human genitourinary malignancies. J Urol 1980; 123:895.

Desai S, Libertino JA, Zinman L. Primary carcinoma of the female urethra. J Urol 1973; 110:693.

Droller MJ. Bladder cancer. Curr Prob Surg 1981; 18:205.

Grabstald H. Tumors of the urethra in men and women. Cancer 1973; 32:1236.

Grabstald H, Hilaris B, Henschke U, Whitmore WF Jr. Cancer of the female urethra. JAMA 1966; 197:835.

Hopkins SC, Grabstald H. Benign and malignant tumors of the male and female urethra. In: Walsh PC, Gittes RF, Perlmutter AD, Stamey TA, eds. Campbell's urology. Philadelphia: WB Saunders, 1986:144.

Hopkins SC, Vider M, Nag SK, et al. Carcinoma of the female urethra: reassessment of modes of therapy. J Urol 1983; 129:958.

Levine RL. Urethral cancer. Cancer 1980; 45:1965.

McCrea LE. Malignancy of the female urethra. Urol Surv 1952; 2:85.

Monaco AP, Murphy GB, Dowling W. Primary cancer of the female urethra. Cancer 1958; 11:1215.

Pointon RC, Poole-Wilson DS. Primary carcinoma of the urethra. Br J Urol 1962; 40:682.

Prempree T, Amornmarn R, Patanaphan V. Radiation therapy in primary carcinoma of the female urethra. II. An update of results. Cancer 1984; 54:729.

Richie JP, Skinner DG. Carcinoma in situ of the urethra associated with bladder carcinoma. The role of urethrectomy. J Urol 1978; 119:80.

Roberts TW, Melicow MM. Pathology and natural history of urethral tumors in females. Urology 1977; 10:583.

Sabin AB, Tarro G. Herpes simplex and herpes genitalia viruses in etiology of some human cancers. Proc Natl Acad Sci USA 1973; 70:3225.

Sarosdy M. Urethral carcinoma. AUA Update Series, Vol VI, Lesson 13, 1987.

Schellhammer PF. Urethral carcinoma. Semin Urol 1983; 1:83.

Shuttleworth KED, Lloyd-Davies RW. Radical resection for tumours involving the posterior urethra. Br J Urol 1969; 41:739.

Sullivan J, Grabstald H. Management of carcinoma of the urethra. In: Skinner DG, deKernion JB, eds. Genitourinary cancer. Philadelphia: WB Saunders, 1978:419.

Taggart GG, Castro JF, Rutledge FN. Carcinoma of the female urethra. Am J Roentgen 1972; 114:145.

Tines SC, Bigongiari LR, Weigel JW. Carcinoma in the diverticulum of the female urethra. Am J Radiol 1982; 138:582.

Weems WL. Surgical management of carcinoma of the male and female urethra. In: Crawford ED, Borden TA, eds. Genitourinary cancer surgery. Philadelphia: Lea & Febiger, 1982:324.

Zeigerman JH, Gordon SF. Cancer of the female urethra. Obstet Gynecol 1970; 36:785.

URETHRAL CARUNCLE

JØRN AAGAARD, M.D.
REGINALD BRUSKEWITZ, M.D.

Urethral caruncle is a benign tumor seen only in females. It is noted primarily in postmenopausal women, seldom during the child-bearing years, and rarely during childhood.

ETIOLOGY

Urethral caruncles probably develop from an ectropion of the posterior urethral wall, incidental to postmenopausal shrinkage of the vaginal mucosa.

Other possible causes for development of a caruncle are chronic irritation and infection. An association of chronic cystitis, urethritis, cystocele, and rectocele with this condition has also been mentioned. These are all conditions seen more frequently among postmenopausal women and may be explained at least in part by lack of estrogen.

SYMPTOMS

Patients with a caruncle may present with symptoms of dyspareuria, dysuria, hematuria, deviation of the urinary stream, urethral bleeding, frequency, or urgency, but in most cases the caruncle is completely asymptomatic and is recognized on routine pelvic examination.

CLINICAL FINDINGS

Urethral caruncles are red, round, polypoid tumors in the distal portion of the urethral mucosa, usually at the posterior lip of the urethral meatus, and are seldom larger than 1 to 2 cm. They may be pedunculated or sessile. They have an irregular surface and a vascular consistency, are often sensitive to touch, and may be inflamed or ulcerated.

MICROSCOPIC APPEARANCE

Caruncles consist of loose connective tissue, dilated blood vessels, and inflammatory cells covered with an epithelial layer. Three forms have been described: papillomatous, angiomatous, and granulomatous. The classification depends on the degree of inflammatory reaction, hyperemia and proliferation, and infolding of transitional or squamous epithelium.

DIFFERENTIAL DIAGNOSIS

Because there is a wide variation in the clinical appearance of urethral caruncles, the following benign conditions may be misdiagnosed as caruncles: hemangiomas, condylomatous polyps, papillomas, varicose veins, and prolapse of the urethral mucosa. However, urethral carcinoma may also be indistinguishable from urethral caruncles; tenderness and induration are more common with urethral carcinoma.

The literature on caruncles and urethral carcinoma repeatedly mentions that development of carcinoma may develop in previously benign urethral caruncles, and coexistence of a caruncle and carcinoma are well documented. In reports by Hess and by Walther, the reported incidence of carcinoma found in caruncles was 14 and 40 percent, respectively. In both studies, however, the histologic examination was carried out in less than half of the patients, suggesting that there may be a selection bias and that the true incidence may be less than that stated.

McCrea published a series of 546 cases of urethral carcinoma in which there were six cases of caruncles coexisting with malignant lesions. Marshall studied 394 patients with urethral tumors, 376 of which invaded in patients whose tumors were clinically diagnosed as caruncles. However, in 20 out of 376 patients, the histologic examination differed from that of a caruncle, and in nine patients, a malignant tumor was found. In one instance a caruncle and a malignant tumor coexisted in the same specimen. Approximately one in 40 patients in this series with a clinical diagnosis of urethral caruncle had a malignant urethral neoplasm.

These studies do not address the question of whether a urethral caruncle is a premalignant lesion or whether urethral carcinoma and caruncles coexist. It is difficult to distinguish clinically between caruncle and urethral carcinoma.

The fact that a large number of caruncles and few urethral carcinomas are seen indicates that malignant degeneration in a urethral caruncle is not a common occurrence. A Medline Search covering the last 20 years identified no research concerning urethral caruncles. Only single case reports about carcinoma, degeneration, and heteropia in caruncles without clinical relevance have been reported.

Before guidelines for diagnostic and therapeutic procedures are prescribed, one must take the following into consideration:

1. The peak incidence of urethral carcinoma and urethral caruncle is between the fifth and seventh decades.
2. Approximately half of all urethral malignant tumors in females arise in the distal third of the urethra.
3. Primary carcinoma of the urethra in the female is uncommon. The treatment in early stages is effective, but the carcinoma becomes refractory to treatment and lethal if recognition is delayed.

PHYSICAL EXAMINATION

Inspection is mandatory and should include careful examination of the urethra, labia, vagina, and inguinal areas and palpation, including bimanual examination of the pelvis. Cystoureteroscopy should also be performed routinely.

BIOPSY

If the nature of the lesion is questionable, a sufficient specimen should be removed for histologic study to establish the diagnosis.

TREATMENT

The primary objective of treatment is to afford symptomatic relief, and this should be accomplished by the simplest method available. Topical application of estrogen cream to the vagina and urethra, or sub-bleeding dosages orally, should be tried before surgical correction is attempted. If surgery on caruncles becomes necessary, the specimen removed should be suitable for histologic examination. This excludes such methods as cauterization and fulguration, in which the specimen would be destroyed such that structural relations could not be determined microscopically. Furthermore, the method of removal must avoid excessive scar formation and stricture of the urethra.

The procedure can be carried out with the patient under local analgesia. Because in many cases of urethral caruncles the meatus is contracted, dilatation of the urethra is recommended. A traction suture is passed deeply through the base of the caruncle, which is then brought into view. An electrocautery knife or loop is brought into contact with the base of the lesion, and the growth is completely removed. After excision, a Foley catheter is left indwelling for 24 to 48 hours.

TUMORS OF THE SCROTUM

SAM D. GRAHAM, Jr., M.D.

Tumors of the scrotum make up a very small percentage of the malignancies seen in urology. Carcinoma of the scrotum, however, was the first malignancy linked to environmental carcinogenesis by Percival Pott in 1775. Pott described a malignancy of the scrotum that had a high incidence in chimney sweeps and was related to the accumulation of soot in their clothing. It was also observed that this disease was relatively uncommon in coal miners, leading to the conclusion that the disease was caused by carcinogens in the products of combustion of the coal. Until relatively recently, this tumor was more common and was linked to exposure to a variety of potential carcinogens such as tar, paraffin, machine oil, metal products associated with lubricating oils, cotton, and wool spinners. The incidence of this tumor is significantly lower now, presumably owing to the awareness of environmental hazards and better working conditions. The current incidence quoted for carcinogen exposure–related carcinoma of the scrotum is 26 percent, as opposed to the incidence of 65 to 100 percent cited in earlier reports.

Carcinoma of the scrotum is most frequently diagnosed in the sixth and seventh decades and affects whites more frequently than blacks. The latency period following environmental exposure is 10 to 25 years. Approximately 50 to 75 percent present with metastases to the lymph nodes.

PATHOLOGY

Benign Tumors

A variety of inflammatory and other benign lesions may be found in the scrotum. Venereal lesions such as herpes, condylomata, and lymphogranuloma venereum are covered in other chapters and are not discussed here. A relatively uncommon inflammatory lesion, sclerosing lipogranuloma, is due to direct injection of petroleum lipids and waxes; it is more common in younger patients. Presenting symptoms are usually a tender subcutaneous mass. The overlying skin may be attached or ulcerated, and the diagnosis is made by identifying lipid vacuoles in the excisional biopsy. Sebaceous cysts, nevi, and other relatively common cutaneous lesions are also common on the scrotum. Benign mesenchymal lesions of the scrotum include hemangiomas and lymphangiomas, both of which are very rare.

Premalignant Lesions

Although far more common on the penis than on the scrotum, premalignant lesions such as in Bowen's disease may be found on the scrotum. The typical appearance is that of a barely raised, sharply outlined, red plaque. Extramammary Paget's disease is another uncommon premalignant lesion of the scrotum. This is most common in the sixth to eighth decades of life and presents as a slowly enlarging indurated plaque. Diagnosis is made by excisional biopsy, demonstrating the typical PAS-positive cells with abundant cytoplasm and vacuolization in the epidermis and epidermal-dermal border. Spread of the disease is by local infiltration of the neighboring skin and direct invasion of the dermis and lymphatics.

Malignant Lesions

By far the most common malignancy of the scrotum is squamous cell carcinoma. Other malignant lesions include basal cell carcinoma, melanoma, Buschke-Löwenstein tumors, hemangioepitheliomas, Kaposi's sarcoma, and a variety of sarcomas including fibrosarcomas, leiomyosarcomas, angiosarcomas, rhabdomyosarcomas, and liposarcomas. Most of the sarcomas are actually sarcomas of the scrotal contents and very rarely originate in the scrotum.

Squamous cell carcinoma of the scrotum is usually an insidious lesion that grows slowly and begins to ulcerate as it enlarges. The most common presentation is ulceration; it may be distinguished from other ulcerative lesions such as herpes progenitalis by being relatively large and a single lesion. In McDonald's series, the interval between patient awareness of a lesion and diagnosis was 3.3 years. Owing to the ulcerative condition and resultant inflammatory response seen with these lesions, there is a high incidence of enlarged inguinal lymph nodes at presentation. Diagnosis is made by excisional biopsy, and staging should include a pelvic computed tomographic (CT) scan. A staging system proposed by Ray and Whitmore is shown in Table 1.

A less frequent malignancy of the scrotum is basal cell carcinoma, despite its being so common in other cutaneous areas. Diagnosis is made by excisional biopsy, and the microscopic appearance is identical to that of basal cell carcinomas of the head and neck. This lesion rarely metastasizes, although it may be locally aggressive.

Melanoma of the scrotum is also very rare, although in males this is the next most common site after the penis and urethra. These lesions are biologically the same as melanomas of other areas and are diagnosed by wide excisional biopsy. As opposed to nevi of other areas (e.g., the head, trunk, or extremities), nevi are relatively uncommon on the scrotum. Any nevus of the scrotum should therefore be carefully watched or excised if it raises any suspicion at all.

TREATMENT

Benign Tumors

Most benign symptomatic lesions of the scrotum are treated by surgical excision. The scrotal skin can easily be brought together in most cases to cover the defect. In most patients, the indications for surgery are discomfort or deformity, and most lesions can be managed by observation only. Some lesions, such as sclerosing lipogranulomas, may frequently recur. Special attention should be directed toward nevi of the scrotum because these are more frequently associated with melanoma than nevi of the trunk and extremities.

Premalignant Lesions

Treatment of extramammary Paget's disease consists of wide excision of the lesion. The prognosis depends on the natural history of the disease, including regional spread and associated malignancies.

Malignant Lesions

Regardless of the type of lesion, the initial therapy is wide surgical excision. This is usually curative in basal cell carcinomas. Squamous cell carcinomas may require additional therapy, depending on the stage.

Patients with enlarged nodes on physical examination or CT scan should be initially treated with antibiotics and observation after excision of the primary lesion. If the nodes do not resolve, a node dissection is indicated. Lymphatic drainage of the scrotum, like the penile shaft,

Table 1 Staging System for Scrotal Tumors

Stage	Site
A1	Localized to Scrotum
A2	Extending to adjacent structures
B	Regional metastases (resectable)
C	Regional metastases (nonresectable)
D	Distant

From Ray B, Whitmore WF Jr. Experience with carcinoma of the scrotum. J Urol 1977; 117:741.

is via the pudendal vessels to the superficial and deep inguinal nodes and onto the external iliac nodes. If a lymph node dissection is performed, it should include all tissue in the triangle from the inguinal ligament to the sartorius muscle to the adductor longus. The femoral artery, vein, and nerve should be dissected clean of lymphatics in the deep node dissection. Ray and Whitmore advocated extending the dissection up the iliac vessels, because in five of 13 patients, they found positive inguinal and iliac nodes. None of these five survived, which signifies that extensive positive nodes indicate systemic disease. In patients with clinically unilateral lymphadenopathy, there is a relatively high rate of contralateral disease, but the role of simultaneous bilateral node dissection in this setting is controversial.

Treatment of locally advanced disease with either radiation or chemotherapy has not been generally successful. There have been anecdotal reports of combined radiation and surgery resulting in cures, and additional reports of successes with chemotherapy.

SUGGESTED READING

Hagan KW, Braren V, Viner NA. Extramammary Paget's disease in the scrotal and inguinal areas. J Urol 1975; 114:154.

McDonald MW. Carcinoma of the scrotum. Urology 1982; 19:269–274.

Melicow MM. Percival Pott (1713–1788) 200th anniversary of first report of occupation-induced cancer of the scrotum in chimney sweepers (1775). Urology 1975; 6:745.

Oka M, Saita B. Simultaneous prostatic carcinoma and genital Paget's disease associated with subjacent adenocarcinoma. Br J Urol 1979; 51:49.

Pott P. Chirurgical observations relative to the cataract, polypus of the nose, the cancer of the scrotum, the different kinds of ruptures, and the mortification of the toes and feet. London: Hawes L, Clarke W, Collins R, 1775. Quoted by McDonald MW. Urology 1982; 19: 269–274.

Ray B, Whitmore WF Jr. Experience with carcinoma of the scrotum. J Urol 1977; 117:741.

Vermillion CD, Page DL. Paget's disease of the scrotum: a case report with local lymph node invasion. J Urol 1972; 107:281.

TESTICULAR SEMINOMA

EDWARD M. MESSING, M.D.

HISTOLOGIC CLASSIFICATION

Seminomas are the most common germ cell tumor of the testicle, making up 40 to 50 percent of all such tumors. An additional 12 to 15 percent of testicular tumors contain both seminomatous and nonseminomatous elements. These mixed tumors are treated as "nonseminomas" and are described elsewhere. Approximately 15 percent of pure seminomas are subcategorized, based on histologic appearance, as "anaplastic" or "spermatocytic." Anaplastic seminomas have three or more mitotic figures per high-power microscopic field without any trophoblastic elements, and account for 10 percent of all seminomas. Although survival rates are somewhat poorer for anaplastic than for "standard" seminomas, the explanation appears to be that a higher percentage of anaplastic seminomas are diagnosed only after metastases develop, because on a stage-for-stage basis survival is the same for both types of seminomas. There is also no evidence to indicate that anaplastic seminomas (1) have a different pattern of metastases than does their standard counterpart, (2) have different predisposing risk factors (see below), (3) arise in different populations (see below), or (4) have different responsiveness to therapies. Finally, on the basis of ultrastructural studies, it is not clear that the "anaplastic" designation is of histologic significance; an opinion supported by its clinical behavior (Janssen and Johnston).

Approximately 5 percent of seminomas are spermatocytic. These tumors are somewhat softer and more cystic than the usually homogeneous standard or anaplastic seminomas. It appears likely that spermatocytic seminomas arise from more differentiated spermatogonia than other germ cell tumors (Rosai and colleagues). This impression would be consistent with differences in clinical behavior, since spermatocytic seminomas are uncommon in individuals younger than 50 years of age, almost never metastasize (Schoborg and colleagues), and do not appear to be associated with cryptorchidism. There is little evidence to indicate that treatment other than radical orchiectomy is required for spermatocytic seminomas.

EPIDEMIOLOGY

Seminomas, like all germ cell tumors, occur primarily in young adults, but the peak age is 5 to 10 years older than for nonseminomatous and mixed tumors. Seminomas are also the most common tumor in cryptorchid patients (and are also found in the normally descended testicle of patients with unilateral cryptorchidism). Roughly two thirds of all testicular tumors associated with cryptorchidism are seminomas, while less than half of all germ cell testicular tumors are seminomas. No other predisposing factors have clearly been identified, although, as with other germ cell tumors, seminomas occur less commonly in non-Caucasians.

PRESENTATION AND DIAGNOSIS

Like other germ cell tumors, most seminomas are first recognized as painless scrotal masses. Because fewer seminomas have metastasized before diagnosis than nonseminomas, constitutional symptoms or those caused by masses in distant sites are proportionately less common. In addition, gynecomastia is rarely seen because secretion of human choronic gonadotropin (hCG) is less common as well. Roughly 2 percent of all testicular tumors arise bilaterally, often in a metachronous fashion. Seminomas are the most likely tumor to arise in the contralateral testis even when the first tumor is a nonseminoma.

All scrotal masses must be evaluated for the possibility of a testicular neoplasm. When any uncertainty arises, the threshold for performing an inguinal exploration of the testicle should be quite low. Scrotal ultrasonography may be useful in a patient in whom a hydrocele makes satisfactory testicular examination impossible, but otherwise is primarily of value to confirm a clinical impression that a scrotal lesion is *not* intratesticular. As with any suspected testicular mass, normality of testis tumor markers (beta-hCG, alpha-fetoprotein, and lactic dehydrogenase [LDH]) should also not dissuade one from recommending surgical exploration. However, blood for these determinations should be drawn preoperatively. At the time of operation, radical inguinal orchiectomy should be performed; the testicle *must* be removed unless an unequivocal diagnosis other than testicular neoplasm can be established with intraoperative inspection and/or "frozen section" histopathologic evaluation. If at the time of inguinal exploration there is little doubt, based on palpation, that the mass lies within the testicle, we do not incise through the tunica vaginalis to inspect further, but instead proceed with ligating the spermatic cord and removing the testicle and its tunics. Long, nonabsorbable sutures are left on the proximal end of the spermatic cord in case retroperitoneal lymphadenectomy is required in the future.

CLINICAL STAGING

Because the management of seminomas and nonseminomas is different, extremely careful histopathologic inspection of the entire tumor is critical to make certain that nonseminomatous elements are not present. Moreover, in the absence of severe liver dysfunction, an elevated serum alpha-fetoprotein provides unequivocal evidence of a nonseminomatous component, even if this cannot be histologically confirmed. Elevated beta-hCG before orchiectomy occurs in 5 to 10 percent of pure seminomas, although in the absence of histologic evidence of trophoblastic components this test result should raise serious concern about the possibility of missed nonseminomatous elements, and thus mandates repeat sectioning and examining of tissue.

SUBSEQUENT METASTATIC EVALUATION

Once the diagnosis of pure testicular seminoma is secure, the staging evaluation includes postorchiectomy markers (if any were elevated preoperatively), abdominal computed tomography (CT), and (at least) chest radiography. The presence of retroperitoneal adenopathy, persistent elevation of beta-hCG after orchiectomy, or suspicious lesions on chest x-ray mandate a more detailed chest evaluation with CT. Because lymphatic metastases occur far more frequently with seminoma than do hematogenous ones, the finding of pulmonary or hepatic metastases in the absence of substantial adenopathy should make one strongly suspect the presence of mixed germ cell elements in these metastases. Although initially these metastatic lesions would be treated with systemic chemotherapy regardless of specific histology, the management of a residual mass, particularly in the retroperitoneum, would be quite different for seminomas and nonseminomas. Thus, histologic sampling of those visceral metastases occurring without sizeable adenopathy should be done before any therapy is begun. Bipedal lymphangiography can detect small-volume nodal metastases not causing lymphadenopathy (and hence, not visible on CT), provides a guide for radiotherapeutic planning, and facilitates posttreatment follow-up. Although almost half of the patients who die of seminoma have bony metastases (Johnson and co-workers) in the absence of extensive disease, we do not routinely obtain bone scans.

On the basis of this evaluation, the following staging system is routinely used. Stage 1, disease confined to the testis; stage 2A, retroperitoneal disease less than 2 cm in diameter on CT or elevation of beta-hCG in the absence of radiographic evidence of metastases; stage 2B, retroperitoneal disease 2 to 5 cm in diameter; stage 2C, retroperitoneal disease greater than 5 cm in diameter; stage 3, supradiaphragmatic lymphatic disease; stage 4, extralymphatic disease. Both the prognosis and management of seminoma depend on disease volume and stage.

TREATMENT: GENERAL PRINCIPLES

Standard and anaplastic seminomas are far more sensitive to external beam radiotherapy than are nonseminomas. Furthermore, the metastatic routes of seminomas via retroperitoneal lymphatics are even more predictable than those of nonseminomas. Seminomas are also very sensitive to the chemotherapeutic regimens pioneered for nonseminomatous tumors. Awareness of these principles offers an excellent outlook for all seminoma patients except those with the most widely advanced disease.

Stage 1

Probably no more than 10 percent of clinical stage 1 seminoma patients have microscopic retroperitoneal metastases (Maier and colleagues). Traditionally, clinical stage 1 seminomas have been treated by administration of 2,500 to 3,000 rads external beam radiotherapy to the ipsilateral iliac nodes and to the aortocaval chains superiorly to the diaphragmatic crura. This treatment seems justified not only because it is so well tolerated, but also because CT and lymphangiographic staging cannot detect micrometastases and because most seminomas do not produce elevations of any testicular tumor marker (although Peckham reported in a preliminary study that nearly 90 percent of nonsmokers with seminoma have elevated serum placental alkaline phosphatase) levels, thus requiring a greater volume of cancer for metastases to be recognized. The involved hemiscrotum should also be treated if a scrotal incision was made at the time of orchiectomy or if there was local extragonadal extension of the original tumor.

Currently there is considerable interest in surveillance management for men with clinical stage 1 nonseminomatous testicular tumors. On the surface, arguments used for these patients can be extended to those with seminomas. After all, because fewer than 10 percent of patients with clinical stage 1 seminomas would be found to have microscopic metastases if they underwent retroperitoneal lymphadenectomy (Maier and co-workers), 90 percent who receive prophylactic retroperitoneal radiotherapy are undergoing unnecessary treatment. Also, those clinical stage 1 seminoma patients who do progress can usually be successfully treated by chemotherapy or radiation therapy (Duchesne and colleagues). Except in extremely well organized surveillance regimens, however, patients have been very difficult to follow, largely because this young and mobile population is not very compliant with rigorous follow-up schedules. Furthermore, because of the absence of useful testicular tumor markers (at least until placental alkaline phosphatase is completely evaluated), very frequent radiographic imaging needs to be maintained. These standard problems with surveillance regimens are compounded in the case of seminoma because prolonged follow-up is almost certainly required (Duchesne and colleagues). Thus, expense, inconvenience, and the risk of losing initially compliant individuals probably outweighs the disadvantage of the potential morbidity associated with retroperitoneal radiotherapy. Currently, therefore, all of our clinical stage 1 seminoma patients receive abdominal radiotherapy as outlined.

Stages 2A and 2B

Patients with disease Stages 2A and 2B also have an excellent outlook when traditionally managed by 3,000- to 3,500-rad abdominal radiotherapy (as for stage 1 seminoma) and prophylactic mediastinal and supraclavicular doses of 2,000 to 3,000 rads. However, most individuals who have small retroperitoneal metastases and fail when supradiaphragmatic radiation is withheld usually relapse in extralymphatic sites rather than in the mediastinal or supraclavicular areas (Peckham). In such patients, cisplatin-based chemotherapeutic regimens must be administered (currently I favor etoposide and cisplatin with or without bleomycin [EP or BEP]). If both the retroperitoneum and mediastinum have been irradiated, however, bone marrow suppression may occur, often limiting the dosages of chemotherapeutic agents and resulting in unmanageable problems. Furthermore, if bleomycin is used, the likelihood of developing clinically significant pulmonary fibrosis is considerably enhanced in patients who have also received chest irradiation (even if directed primarily at the mediastinum). I thus believe that, certainly for stage 2A patients and probably for 2B patients as well, radiotherapy should be limited to the retroperitoneum. This will undoubtedly result in higher clinical failure rates, but will permit life-salvaging chemotherapy to be delivered effectively, and ultimately improve long-term disease free remission rates approaching those for similar-stage nonseminomatous tumors managed by primary retroperitoneal lymphadenectomy with or without postoperative chemotherapy (Williams and colleagues).

Stages 2C, 3, and 4

Traditionally, bulky retroperitoneal disease has also been managed by therapeutic abdominal and prophylactic mediastinal/supraclavicular irradiation. A dose of 3,500 to 4,000 rads is administered to the retroperitoneum and 2,500 to 3,000 rads above the diaphragm. However, even in the most optimistic series, relapse rates of 20 to 30 percent are seen (Smalley and colleagues), and salvage chemotherapy is extraordinarily difficult to administer in such patients. Thus, I believe that stage 2C patients should be initially managed as similarly staged nonseminoma patients, with three cycles of bleomycin, etopicide, and cisplatin (BEP) or four of EP.

The treatment of stage 3 and 4 disease is also the same as for nonseminomatous tumors. The use of initial chemotherapy for bulky seminomatous metastases has generally been regarded as an important advance over treatment by initial radiotherapy. When treated in the latter fashion, stages 2C, 3, and 4 seminoma patients experience long-term cure rates below 50 percent even with subsequent chemotherapeutic salvage, whereas nonseminoma patients of similar stages of disease, treated initially with chemotherapy, experience cure rates of 70 to 90 percent. Patients with similar-stage seminomas treated initially with chemotherapy now achieve results the same as or better than those of nonseminoma patients (Smith).

The management of advanced seminoma patients after initial chemotherapy is still in evolution, however. Complete response rates in patients with bulky seminomas currently are only about 15 percent after chemo-

therapy (Peckham). Originally, such patients were managed as individuals with nonseminomatous tumors in whom postchemotherapy masses remained: they underwent surgical removal. However, in seminoma patients such surgery was often very difficult because of exuberant fibrosis, and in most series (and my experience) residual tumor was rarely found (Smith, 1988; Morse and colleagues).

Thus, although one group claimed that over 40 percent of bulky seminoma patients will have residual tumor found in postchemotherapy masses (Motzer and colleagues), I currently do not advocate surgery in such patients unless the initial tumor produced beta-hCG or the mass enlarged during or after chemotherapy. Furthermore, because the few tumors found in postchemotherapy masses often contained nonseminomatous elements, the practice of administering radiotherapy to postchemotherapy masses that are not enlarging is also of questionable value. Currently, I advocate simply observing patients with these masses, and so far there is little evidence to show that relapse rates are any higher in individuals undergoing observation than in those who receive postchemotherapy surgery or radiotherapy (Smith). However, this practice, while clearly reducing initial morbidity, provokes far greater physician and patient uncertainty, and continued close follow-up is needed. The additional problem created by this approach is that it is difficult to interpret results of clinical studies in which few patients actually achieve radiographic complete responses, especially in a disease in which progression may not occur until years later.

The appropriate intensity, frequency, and duration of follow-up of individuals with stages 2C to 4 seminomas with stable masses after chemotherapy is also uncertain. I currently obtain chest radiographs, complete blood counts, renal and hepatic function studies, testis tumor markers, and physical examinations every 6 weeks, and abdominal CT (thoracic CT scans as well if disease was originally supradiaphragmatic or if the chest x-ray becomes abnormal) every 3 months for the first 2 years after the completion of chemotherapy. Thereafter, chest x-rays, laboratory tests, and physical examinations are done every 3 months for the next 3 years, while CT of appropriate areas is performed on a semiannual basis. Recommendations for follow-up after 5 years are still in evolution, but experience with nonseminomatous tumors suggests that this probably should be carried out semiannually or annually indefinitely.

Treatment of Recurrent Seminoma

The treatment of recurrences depends on the site(s) of relapse, the previous site(s) of disease, and the previous treatment(s) patients have received. In general, men who originally had stages 1, 2A, or 2B seminomas who received only abdominal radiation will relapse either in the mediastinum or, more commonly, in the lungs. Extralymphatic metastases undoubtedly require systemic chemotherapy, and EP or BEP is usually administered. Although mediastinal recurrences could theoretically be managed by radiotherapy alone, they rarely arise exclusively in this site (even if the mediastinum is the only location where disease is detectable on CT at the time recurrence is recognized). Moreover, administration of mediastinal and supraclavicular radiation will again complicate subsequent chemotherapy, which will probably be needed eventually. Thus, I also treat these patients as if they have extralymphatic disease as well.

Although it is unusual because most patients receiving radiotherapy have complete responses (radiographically) in the fields treated, management is far more problematic if, in the patient initially treated with abdominal radiotherapy, recurrence is exclusively in the retroperitoneum. Even if these recurrences are not accompanied by elevated testis tumor markers, the possibility of nonseminomatous disease must be entertained and is actually more likely than radioresistant seminoma.

Furthermore, since bilateral tumors occur metachronously in 2 percent of germ cell tumor patients, the possibility of a second testicular primary in the remaining gonad must be strongly considered. Scrotal ultrasonography is thus mandatory. Because it is unlikely that recurrent retroperitoneal metastases would be detected until they are fairly sizeable, it is justifiable to treat these individuals again with EP (4 cycles) or BEP (3 cycles) therapy. However, if there is not a complete response to this chemotherapy on CT, retroperitoneal lymphadenectomy is mandatory because of the possibility of residual (particularly nonseminomatous) germ cell tumor, or malignant degeneration of a persistent teratoma. This is a different approach from that taken for a persistent retroperitoneal mass after primary chemotherapy for seminoma, which I would normally observe closely.

For individuals with initial stages 2C, 3, or 4 seminomas who are treated by primary EP or BEP chemotherapy and relapse with disseminated disease, salvage regimens are employed as for chemotherapy failures with nonseminomas (currently vinblastine, iphosphamide, and cisplatin). However, if the only site of relapse of a bulky tumor is detected by growth of a retroperitoneal mass (which may or may not have initially shrunk with chemotherapy), surgical therapy (if feasible) is probably warranted. This is advocated rather than retroperitoneal radiotherapy because the possibility of residual teratoma is significant and this can only be managed surgically. Furthermore, the dosage of radiation necessary to be delivered to an original stage 2C tumor that has actually enlarged is often higher than the 2,500 to 4,000 rads normally delivered to the retroperitoneum. The likelihood of intestinal or renal injury, depending on the tumor's size and location, is significant. If surgery is deemed not feasible technically, however, and if needle or laproscopic biopsy reveals no nonseminomatous elements or teratoma, radiation therapy or salvage chemotherapy must be administered.

The removal of postchemotherapy or postradiotherapy masses can be a formidable undertaking, and a variety of preoperative radiographic imaging studies, including angiography and venacavography, as well as visualization of the gastrointestinal tract, are often needed. It may be necessary to remove contiguous structures. In two postchemotherapy seminoma patients with enlarging or recurring retroperitoneal masses (each of whom had residual seminoma and teratoma), I had to remove the ipsilateral kidney in each and the subrenal inferior vena cava in one.

Isolated recurrences in the mediastinum or extralymphatic sites need to be managed individually. The principle of performing surgical excision or at least biopsy rather than proceeding immediately with radiotherapy should be adhered to because of the likelihood of there being radioresistant (usually nonseminomatous) elements.

SPECIAL CONSIDERATIONS

Primary Extragonadal Seminomas

Primary germ cell malignancies that arise in extragonadal sites are invariably detected at stage 2C, 3, or 4. Although patients with extragonadal primary tumors generally fare worse than those with germ cell malignancies of the same metastatic stage that have arisen from a known testicular primary tumor, this is not true for seminomas (Motzer and colleagues). The reason for this is uncertain, but the management of primary extragonadal seminomas requires special attention.

Even before treatment is started, it must be remembered that a small or burned-out focus hidden in the testicle that has been overlooked can continue to metastasize. Tumors in testicular locations are relatively protected from the effects of chemotherapy, and a very small gonadal focus can go undetected. Hence, with any presumed primary extragonadal germ cell neoplasm, careful sonographic as well as palpatory examination of the testicles is crucial. Abnormal findings or a suspicious history (e.g., that of cryptorchidism), despite a normal examination, may mandate surgical exploration and even orchiectomy. However, it is currently believed that if findings on history, examination, and ultrasonography are negative, bilateral groin explorations or orchiectomies are unnecessary. In such individuals, aggressive scrutiny of the testicles must be continued throughout follow-up.

Because the vast majority of patients with extragonadal germ cell malignancies have undergone only small incisional or needle biopsies, sampling artifacts make a diagnosis exclusively of seminoma highly suspect. Initial treatment remains EP or BEP chemotherapy, as would be administered for similar-stage tumors that have metastasized from gonadal primaries. However, it is far more troubling in a patient who has only had a scant amount of tissue sampled to be followed after an incomplete radiographic response to chemotherapy, as are individuals who have metastases from primary gonadal seminomas. Because of the possibility of the patient originally having had nonseminomatous elements that were unrecognized owing to sampling issues, whether or not the tumor initially produced beta-hCG (which has descended after chemotherapy), I advocate complete surgical removal with retroperitoneal lymphadenectomy. If necrotic or scar tissue only is found, remaining supradiaphragmatic and extralymphatic suspicious lesions should be followed only with careful surveillance. Alternatively, if residual disease is pure seminoma, I treat other sites with further cycles of salvage chemotherapy as would be done for residual nonseminomatous cancers after primary chemotherapy. An acceptable alternative approach is to use radiation therapy, particularly for mediastinal masses. If residual tumor is primarily teratoma, surgical removal of remaining disease beyond the retroperitoneum is mandatory. Finally, if residual disease is nonseminomatous germ cell cancer or malignant degeneration of a teratoma, further salvage chemotherapy is indicated.

HIV-Positive Patients

There have been several reports of testicular cancers arising in men infected with the human immunodeficiency virus (HIV). Whether this is a coincidence has not been established. Seminomas appear to be particularly common in this group, perhaps because of the ages of patients usually recognized as being HIV positive (these patients are usually slightly older than those who develop nonseminomatous tumors). In such individuals, management paradigms become problematic, not only because of the almost invariable presence of retroperitoneal adenopathy, but also because of the unknown effects of chemotherapy and radiotherapy on the progress of the immunodeficiency disease. Furthermore, management strategies that increase the likelihood of later treatment with systemic agents should probably be avoided because it is probable that by the time recurrences are finally recognized, the toxic effects of chemotherapy in the face of progressive immunodeficiency may present insurmountable problems. Because many HIV-infected patients have sizable lymphadenopathy, most will be considered to have stage 2C or 3 at diagnosis of their testicular tumor. They will therefore be initially treated with EP or BEP. Those who do not show a complete radiographic response (in my limited experience, virtually everyone) probably should undergo retroperitoneal lymphadenec-

tomy, since surgery would have less damaging long-term effects on the progression of the HIV infection than would mere observation and the possible need for radiotherapy or chemotherapy in the future. An alternative approach is immediate administration of radiotherapy; however, radiographic complete responses would be unlikely because of virus-infected nodes. Observation of postchemotherapy or postradiotherapy residual masses seems fraught with difficulties because it is likely that adenopathy would increase over time, even if due entirely to HIV infection. This would lead to certain further treatment, probably chemotherapy, in the future at a time when the patient would be less likely to tolerate its toxic effects.

SUGGESTED READING

Duchesne GM, Honvich A, Dearnaley DP, et al. Orchidectomy alone for stage I seminoma of the testis. Cancer 1990; 65:1115–1118.

Janssen M, Johnston WH. Anaplastic seminoma of the testis: ultrastructural analyses of three cases. Cancer 1978; 41:538–544.

Johnson DE, Appelt GR, Samuels ML, Luna M. Metastases from testicular carcinoma: study of 78 autopsied cases. Urology 1976; 8:234–239.

Maier JG, Mittemeyer BT, Sulak MH. Treatment and prognosis in seminoma of the testis. J Urol 1988; 99:72–78.

Morse M, Herr H, Sogani P, et al. Surgical exploration of metastatic seminoma following VABG chemotherapy. Proc Am Soc Clin Oncol 1983; 2:C559.

Motzer RJ, Bosl GJ, Geller NL, et al. Advanced seminoma: the role of chemotherapy and adjunctive surgery. Ann Intern Med 1988; 108:513–518.

Peckham MJ. Presentation at the Second Urological Cancer Symposium, USC School of Medicine, Los Angeles, CA, January 18, 1985.

Rosai J, Silber I, Khodadoust K. Spermatocytic seminoma: II. Ultrastructural study. Cancer 1969; 24:103–116.

Schoborg TW, Whittaker J, Lewis CW. Metastic spermatocytic seminoma. J Urol 1980; 124:739–741.

Smalley SR, Earle JD, Evans RG, Richardson RL. Modern radiotherapy results with bulky stages II and III seminoma. J Urol 1990; 144:685–689.

Smith RB. Testicular seminoma. In: Skinner DG, Lieskovsky G, eds. Diagnosis and management of genitourinary cancer. Philadelphia: WB Saunders, 1988:508.

Williams SD, Stablein DM, Einhorn LH, et al. Immediate adjuvant chemotherapy versus observation with treatment at relapses in pathological stage II testicular cancer. N Engl J Med 1987; 317: 1433–1438.

NONSEMINOMATOUS GERM CELL TUMOR

RICHARD S. FOSTER, M.D.
JOHN P. DONOHUE, M.D.

PRESENTATION AND DIAGNOSIS

Approximately 95 percent of all cases of testicular cancer represent tumors of germ cell origin. Such tumors are conveniently divided into nonseminomatous and seminomatous germ cell tumors. The rationale for this division is the extreme sensitivity of seminomas to radiotherapy and chemotherapy as contrasted with a much lower sensitivity of nonseminomas to radiation therapy. The incidence of testicular cancer in young white males in the United States appears to be rising, with an age-adjusted incidence of approximately four per 100,000.

A nonpainful mass in the involved testicle of increased firmness compared with normal testicular tissue is the most common presentation. After determination of serum alpha-fetoprotein and beta-hCG, radical inguinal orchiectomy is the treatment of choice to confirm the diagnosis. Transscrotal orchiectomy is to be condemned because of the potential of contaminating another site of lymphatic drainage, the inguinal region. Since testicular cancer is one of the few malignancies surgically curable when metastatic disease is present, it is preferable to limit the potential sites of metastatic spread.

STAGING

Various staging systems are available to subclassify nonseminomatous testicular tumors. Both the TNM and Indiana classification systems are useful, but perhaps the most functional and clinically useful system divides nonseminomatous disease into stage I (or A), referring to tumors confined to the testis; stage II (or B), denoting metastatic disease to the retroperitoneum without visceral or pulmonary involvement; and stage III (or C), indicating metastasis to the viscera or above the diaphragm. Abdominal and chest computed tomography (CT) are the primary tools used to stage the patient. Lymphangiography is limited by its low sensitivity (75 percent) and specificity. Other radiologic modalities (e.g., head CT) are not routinely recommended but are ordered only as history and physical examination warrant. Standard CT-based staging results in an understaging error of approximately 30 percent and a small but definite overstaging error rate. These inaccuracies in clinical staging further support the concept of surgical staging.

Elevations in serum alpha-fetoprotein and/or beta-hCG indicate active carcinoma. However, the absence of elevation of either of these markers does not preclude the presence of carcinoma. Therefore, if a surveillance policy is contemplated in a clinical stage I patient, these markers are extremely useful for diagnosis. If, however, a surgical staging policy is planned, initial serum levels of hCG and alpha-fetoprotein are not as pertinent.

TREATMENT

The therapies for the treatment of nonseminomatous germ cell tumors are listed in Table 1.

Clinical Stage I

Since approximately 30 percent of clinical stage I patients are indeed pathologic stage II, the traditional approach to clinical stage I has been retroperitoneal lymph node dissection (RPLND). Because germ cell testicular cancer predictably spreads via lymphatics, the removal of retroperitoneal lymph nodes accurately stages the patient. Another advantage of lymphadenectomy in clinical stage I patients who are pathologic stage II is its therapeutic benefit. About 70 percent of patients found to have metastatic disease to the retroperitoneum who are followed closely after RPLND remain disease free without the need for subsequent chemotherapy.

The major objection to RPLND has been the attendant loss of emission and ejaculation accompanying full bilateral RPLND. Mapping studies performed by Donohue and colleagues approximately 10 years ago led to the adoption of various modified dissections in which lymphatic tissue was dissected only in those regions of the retroperitoneum at high risk for microscopic metastasis. These modified procedures preserved ejaculation in some but not all patients.

Subsequently, the development of the nerve-sparing RPLND has allowed 99 percent of patients subjected to initial RPLND to retain the ability to ejaculate. In this procedure, the efferent sympathetic fibers of the retroperitoneum are dissected prospectively and preserved (unilaterally or bilaterally), and this is followed by en

Table 1 Management of Nonseminomatous Germ Cell Cancer at Indiana University

Clinical stage I	Nerve-sparing RPLND
Clinical stage II	
Low volume	RPLND
Moderate volume	RPLND/primary chemotherapy
High volume	Primary chemotherapy/ postchemotherapy RPLND
Clinical stage III	Primary chemotherapy/ postchemotherapy RPLND

RPLND = retroperitoneal lymph node dissection.

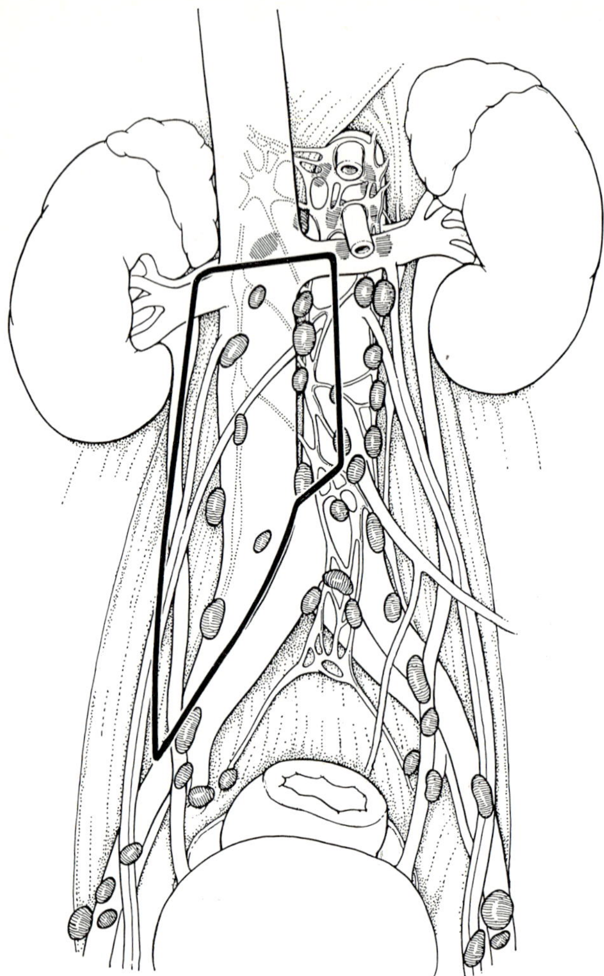

Figure 1 Template for right-sided, nerve-sparing RPLND for clinical stage I patients.

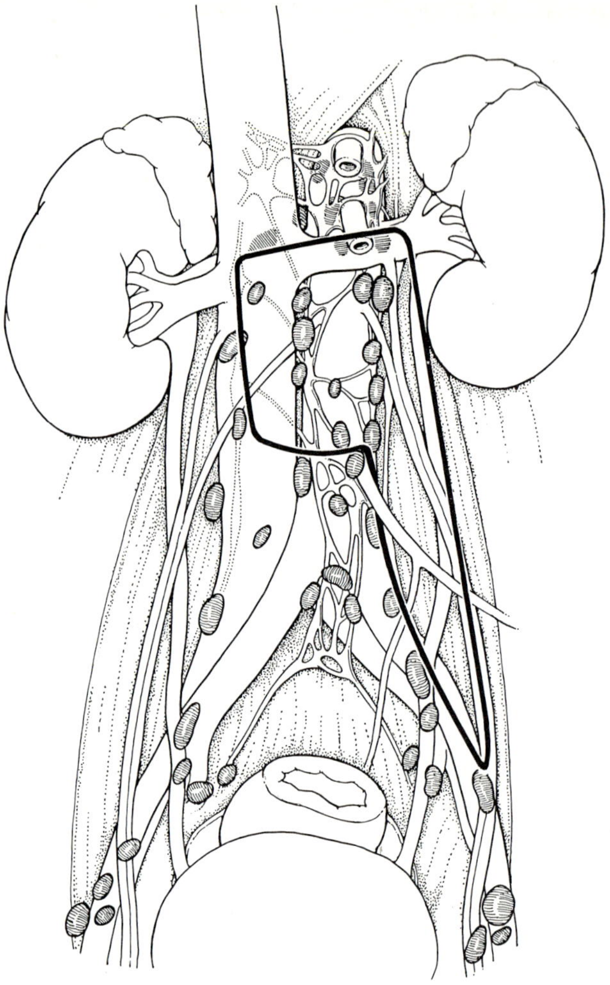

Figure 2 Template for left-sided, nerve-sparing RPLND for clinical stage I patients.

bloc RPLND of the areas of the retroperitoneum at high risk for microscopic metastasis (Figs. 1 and 2). Long-term follow-up of a large series of patients at Indiana University managed in this fashion has resulted in a 99 + percent chance of cure with a concomitant 99 percent rate of preservation of emission and ejaculation.

Long-term follow-up of the Indiana University series of initial RPLND for clinical stage I nonsemi-nomatous testicular cancer has shown this approach to have several advantages. First, the overall chance for cure is 99 percent or greater. Second, patients who relapse after RPLND do so either serologically or in the lungs, two sites that can be monitored with great sensitivity (with standard chest films and serum marker determinations) to identify relapse early. Third, patients who were thought to be clinical stage I but found to be pathologic stage II after RPLND have a 70 percent chance of cure with surgery alone, thereby avoiding chemotherapy. Fourth, patients are accurately staged soon after diagnosis. Finally, close follow-up is necessary for only 2 years after RPLND.

The strategy of surveillance after radical orchiectomy in clinical stage I nonseminomatous testicular cancer is based on several factors. Perhaps the most important of these has been the development of platinum-based chemotherapy, a powerful means of eradicating low-volume metastatic disease. Similarly, the loss of ejaculation and emission after traditional full bilateral RPLND was a major impetus toward development of the surveillance strategy.

If CT scans of the chest and abdomen are normal and serum markers normalize after radical orchiectomy, the patient is followed at regular intervals with CT, chest x-ray examinations, marker determinations, and/or lymphangiography. Although the optimal schedule of follow-up studies has not been determined, various investigators adept in urologic oncology have now reported results of this method of management in approximately 1,000 patients worldwide. Of the approximately 30 percent who have relapsed (as pathologic stage II or III), over 7 percent died (having failed chemotherapy rescue); 94 percent are disease free, and the overall survival is 97 percent. This means that a relapsing patient managed initially by surveillance has a higher risk of dying of testicular cancer than patients managed by primary RPLND.

There are controversial issues concerning surveillance. First, the optimal schedule and type of follow-up has not been determined. Second, patient compliance is of utmost importance. Studies have shown that some patients still relapse in the third to fourth year of follow-up after orchiectomy. Therefore, a patient committed to surveillance must be willing to comply for a much longer period of intensive follow-up than the 2 years needed for patients undergoing initial RPLND. Third, on the basis of currently available data, the risk of dying of testicular cancer is higher with a surveillance strategy than with immediate RPLND. Fourth, monitoring of the retroperitoneum with CT for recurrence is not as sensitive as monitoring the chest for recurrence after RPLND.

Clinical Stage II

Patients who undergo RPLND for clinical stage I disease and are found to have pathologic stage II disease have an approximately 50 to 70 percent chance of long-term cure without the need for subsequent chemotherapy. The testicular cancer intergroup study randomized pathologic stage II patients to either close follow-up or two immediate postoperative courses of platinum-based chemotherapy. No survival advantage was demonstrated with either regimen. Therefore, patients who have undergone RPLND for low-volume pathologic stage II disease are offered either close follow-up or two adjuvant courses of platinum-based chemotherapy.

The management of clinical stage II disease is controversial. The traditional treatment has involved full bilateral RPLND with attendant loss of emission and ejaculation. Surgical cure in this situation is approximately 50 percent. It should be stressed that the surgeon contemplating performing a limited dissection who palpates obvious gross retroperitoneal disease should abandon the limited dissection and perform full bilateral RPLND. This is because it is impossible to predict sites of microscopic disease in the face of gross adenopathy in the retroperitoneum. Full bilateral dissection is therefore performed. We as well as others have performed nerve-sparing dissections in highly selected pathologic stage II patients with good results and low local recurrence rates. This method of management, however, should be considered experimental at this time.

Other investigators have reported results of primary chemotherapy in clinical stage II patients, 96 percent of whom achieved a complete remission status. However, 20 to 30 percent of patients treated with initial chemotherapy require postchemotherapy RPLND with its concomitant increased morbidity compared with initial RPLND.

The best management for these patients with low-volume clinical stage II disease remains to be determined. The toxicities of immediate RPLND versus primary chemotherapy plus or minus subsequent postchemotherapy RPLND are currently under considerable discussion. The development of nerve-sparing techniques has certainly lowered the morbidity of RPLND. Current management should probably be based on the experience of the physician and the desires and needs of the individual patient. At Indiana University, we proceed with RPLND in these low-volume stage II patients.

The presence of large-volume abdominal disease not amenable to surgical removal indicates the need for primary platinum-based chemotherapy. Whether a patient is judged surgically resectable on the basis of the staging CT scan depends on the discretion and experience of the surgeon. If there is any doubt whether the patient is resectable, primary chemotherapy should be given.

Clinical Stage III

Appropriate management for patients presenting with clinical stage III disease consists of primary platinum-based chemotherapy. About 70 percent of patients presenting with disseminated disease are "good risks." They have either serum marker elevation only or small-volume infra- or supradiaphragmatic involvement (or both) without visceral metastasis. At Indiana University, these patients are given three courses of bleomycin, etopicide, and cisplatin (BEP). The remaining one third of patients presenting with "poor-risk" disease receive four courses of BEP. About 70 percent of all clinical stage III patients experience a complete remission (no radiographic evidence of disease and serum alpha-fetoprotein and beta-hCG normal), and 30 percent experience a partial remission (serum markers normal, radiographic disease remaining). Most of this 30 percent then undergo postchemotherapy RPLND. An exception to this rule is made in patients who had no teratoma in the orchiectomy specimen and who experience a greater than 90 percent volumetric reduction in radiographic disease during chemotherapy. These patients have a very high likelihood of having only necrosis at RPLND and therefore are followed clinically.

The technique of postchemotherapy RPLND has been well described. Briefly, patients are cautiously hydrated 24 to 36 hours before the procedure, because we believe that sudden changes in intravascular volume may predispose to bleomycin-induced noncardiogenic pulmonary edema. The type of incision is determined by the volume and site of disease and may be transabdominal, thoracoabdominal, thoracic, or median sternotomy. A full bilateral RPLND is routinely employed, although in highly selected patients we have used a unilateral nerve-sparing approach to preserve ejaculation. All lumbar arteries and veins are divided and the retroperitoneum is swept clean of lymphatic tissue and tumor. Specialized approaches such as the transthoracic approach to the retrocrural area are sometimes employed. Vascular surgical techniques are required, along with a commitment from the surgeon to a sometimes long and intensive procedure. Postoperative management usually includes an overnight stay in the intensive care unit so that fluid status and pulmonary function may be monitored.

After initial chemotherapy, teratoma will be found in the resected material in about 45 percent of patients, fibrosis in approximately another 45 percent, and cancer in 10 percent. The presence of cancer indicates the need for two postoperative courses of platinum-based chemotherapy, with a resultant chance for cure of approximately 60 to 70 percent. Resection of teratoma is therapeutic, although after resection of large-volume teratoma, the patient must be monitored for locally recurrent teratoma. Patients who have multiple recurrences of teratoma sometimes develop various types of sarcoma in the recurrence and are not surgically salvageable. Finally, the presence of fibrosis in the resected material indicates that an adequate dose of chemotherapy has been administered.

SUGGESTED READING

Bihrle R, Donohue JP, Foster RS. Complications of retroperitoneal lymph node dissection. Urol Clin North Am 1988; 15:237.

Donohue JP, Foster RS, Rowland RG, et al. Nerve-sparing retroperitoneal lymphadenectomy with preservation of ejaculation. J Urol 1990; 144:287.

Roth BJ, Nichols CR, Einhorn LH. Neoplasms of the testis. In: Holland, Frei, eds. Cancer medicine. 3rd ed. Philadelphia: Lea & Febiger, 1991.

TESTICULAR TUMORS IN INFANTS AND CHILDREN

WILLIAM E. KAPLAN, M.D.

Testicular tumors in children are the seventh most commonly occuring solid neoplasms in childhood and represent 2 to 3 percent of all testicular neoplasms. There are distinct differences between childhood testicular neoplasms and their adult counterparts. Whereas germ cell tumors represent more than 90 percent of adult neoplasms, only 60 to 75 percent of pediatric testicular tumors are of germ cell origin. Despite the often aggressive and malignant behavior of many of these childhood tumors, there is a larger proportion of testicular neoplasms in the pediatric population that are benign than there are in adults.

Some of the confusion between the adult and pediatric tumor type has been lessened since a workable classification scheme was accepted in 1983 by the Urology Section of the American Academy of Pediatrics. This system emphasizes the tumors that are peculiar to children, such as pure yolk sac carcinoma (Table 1).

CLINICAL FEATURES

The most common presentation is a painless scrotal swelling. The tumors are firm, are nontender, and do not transilluminate. These features should distinguish a tumor from epididymitis, hydrocele, or early torsion. However, in 10 to 15 percent of cases, hydroceles can be seen in association with a neoplasm. Late or neglected torsion can also present as an enlarged nontender mass. The symptomless quality of a testicular tumor and

Table 1 Classification of Prepubertal Testicular Tumors

   I. Germ cell tumors
    A. Yolk sac
    B. Teratoma
    C. Yolk sac tumor and teratoma (teratocarcinoma)
    D. Seminoma
  II. Gonadal stromal tumors
    A. Leydig cell
    B. Sertoli cell
    C. Intermediate forms
 III. Gonadoblastoma
 IV. Tumors of supporting tissues
    A. Fibroma
    B. Leiomyoma
    C. Hemangioma
  V. Lymphomas and leukemias
 VI. Tumor-like lesions
    A. Epidermoid cyst
    B. Hyperplastic nodules secondary to congenital adrenal hyperplasia
VII. Secondary tumors
VIII. Tumors of adnexa

Republished with permission by Kaplan GW. Testicular tumors in children. AUA Update Series, 1983.

possible presence of fluid can, however, cause a delay in a correct diagnosis. The hormonally active nongerminal tumors (Leydig or Sertoli cell) may aid in an early diagnosis by the presence of sexual precocity. Beyond a careful physical examination, ultrasonography or isotopic scanning of the scrotum may aid one in deciding on an exploration. If the diagnosis is clear, serum markers are obtained prior to surgical excision.

The definitive step regardless of eventual pathologic type is a surgical exposure through the inguinal approach. Noncrush clamping of the cord prior to testicular manipulation is essential and is my standard practice if there is any doubt about the diagnosis.

Once the testis is delivered, a high ligation of the

cord and orchiectomy is performed. A simple enucleation or resection of the tumor has been suggested for the prediagnosed teratoma or gonadal stromal tumors. This has not been my practice. After orchiectomy, the pathologist must carefully examine the severed cord to be certain that no local tumor remains. I have seen some children who underwent percutaneous biopsy or had an open biopsy without orchiectomy through either the scrotum or the inguinal approach. If the subsequent diagnosis is of a germ cell type, a simultaneous hemiscrotectomy is advised.

After the orchiectomy and certain diagnosis, a metastatic and staging process should proceed. Blood samples for serum markers of human chorionic gonadotropin (hCG) and especially alpha-fetoprotein (AFP) should be drawn. Computed tomography (CT) of the lung and retroperitoneum and chest roentgenography should be performed. Lymphangiography is not helpful in this population.

The serum marker AFP is especially significant when dealing with a patient with a yolk sac carcinoma. AFP is an amino acid produced by fetal yolk sac cells. By 3 months of age, AFP is normally less than 20 ng per milliliter.

However, there is a strong (90 percent) association between the yolk sac tumor and AFP. Tumors with yolk sac elements can have extremely high (>100 ng per milliliter) AFP levels. The only caution in following this marker is that its half-life is 6 days. Thus, when the initial level is quite high, it may take weeks following orchiectomy to normalize. If, however, the AFP level does not diminish, or starts to fluctuate upward, metastatic disease is surely present.

The serum hCG level is not usually elevated in pediatric patients with tumors unless an embryonal cell component is present.

SPECIFIC TUMOR TYPES: DIAGNOSIS AND MANAGEMENT

Germ Cell Tumors

Yolk Sac Carcinoma

Yolk sac carcinoma (Fig. 1*A*) is the most common pathologic type of testicular tumor in childhood. It is known by a variety of terms, most commonly endodermal sinus tumor, orchidoblastoma, embryonal adenocarcinoma, and embryonal carcinoma. However, the pure yolk sac tumor is quite distinct pathologically and behaviorally from the embryonal carcinoma of the adult. Tellum's concept was that these tumors of germ cell origin had selective overgrowth of yolk sac elements. Histologically, the most distinctive finding is the presence of periodic acid–Schiff (PAS)-positive inclusions in the cytoplasm. Immunochemical techniques will confirm that these inclusions contain AFP.

Perivascular Schiller-Duvall bodies (embryoid bodies) are also prominent (Fig. 1*B*).

The fact that this tumor can contain embryonal elements, and in the past has incorrectly been termed an embryonal carcinoma, is the reason for the confusion in the management of these patients. The clinical behavior of the pure yolk sac tumor is distinctly different from that of the adult variety, embryonal type. The initial therapy is as described previously: radical

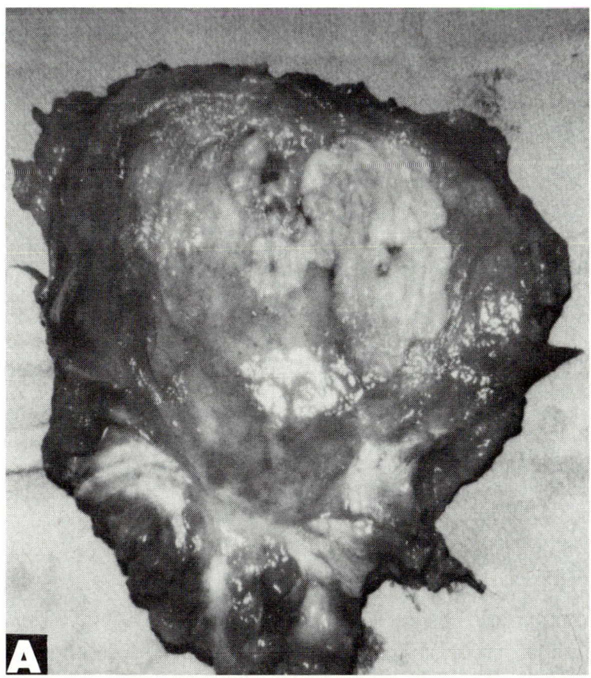
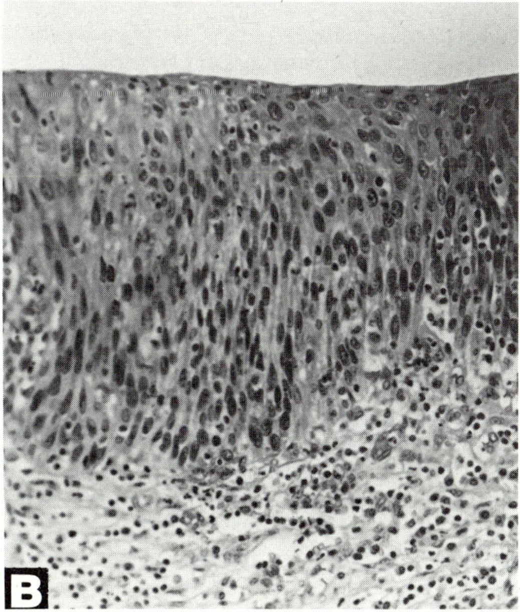

Figure 1 *A*, Yolk sac carcinoma. *B*, Perivascular Schiller-Duvall bodies.

orchiectomy, serial serum marker determination, and metastatic work-up.

The history of treatment of this disease is similar to that of others in oncology. It is recognized that less may be better and that modern chemotherapy can often obviate against radical surgery or significant radiation therapy. In the 1960s when retroperitoneal lymph node dissection was shown to be effective for adult patients with testicular tumor, pediatric centers began to treat childhood tumors in a similar fashion. Survival statistics improved from 50 percent for orchiectomy alone to 80 percent for orchiectomy with lymph node dissection. However, after reviews from other centers, it was noted that only 6 to 10 percent of node dissections resulted in the findings of nodal disease.

It became common acceptance that this disease was "benign" in the young child (under 2 years of age) and did not have significant nodal metastasis. Hematogenous metastasis was still known to occur, but probably not in the child under 2 years of age.

I have studied 12 children with pure yolk sac tumor. Ten were under 2 years of age. I expected to find in a retrospective review that few, if any, had nodal metastasis. In fact, I found three of ten with nodal disease, and in a fourth boy, who was 3 years of age, both lymphatic and pulmonary spread were noted. The child that prompted the review was an 8-month-old who had bulky nodal disease in the ipsilateral renal hilum. It was clear that although the spread may be primarily hematogenous, lymphatic spread occurred early. It was my initial impression that all children regardless of age should have a thorough extended unilateral lymph node dissection. I now look on that study as a warning that this is an aggressive disease. However, my conclusions and method of management have changed owing to increased reliance on CT and magnetic resonance imaging (MRI) and on the success of chemotherapy.

Currently, my routine is to perform a radical orchiectomy. Postoperatively, serum markers (AFP) are drawn and followed. CT of the chest and retroperitoneum is performed. If the AFP falls to normal and there is no metastatic disease, the child is followed with chest roentgenograms at 1 and 3 months and AFP determination for 2 years. This regimen applies to the child under 1 year of age. In the older child, although this course can be followed, it is definitely with some risk. My experience has not included an older child with stage A disease but only those who presented with higher stages of disease. If evidence for metastasis is present, either in the form of elevated markers or by imaging techniques, I am following the pilot study, which uses high-dose, short-duration, four-drug chemotherapy. I no longer believe the vincristine-doxorubicin (Adriamycin) cyclophosphamide regimen is as effective as any combination that includes platinum.

Thus, once the diagnosis is made, a regimen that includes vinblastine (Velban), bleomycin, cisplatin, and etoposide is administered over a 6-day period. It is then repeated every 3 weeks for six cycles (Fig. 2).

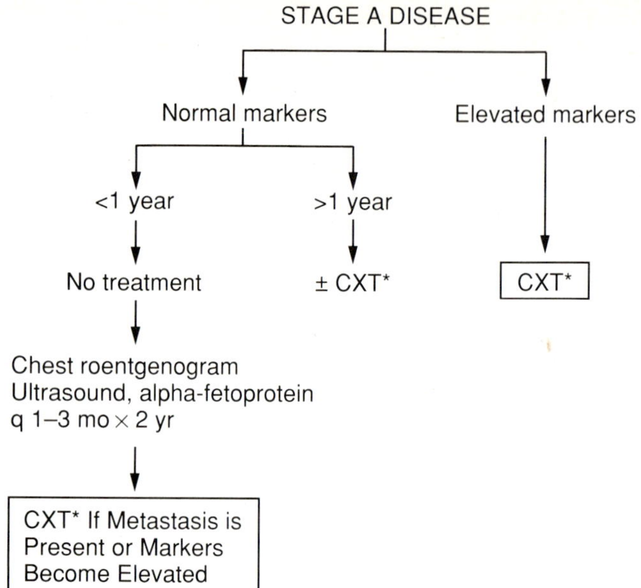

Figure 2 Testicular yolk sac tumor in children: stage A. *Chemotherapy with vinblastine, bleomycin, cisplatin, and etoposide.

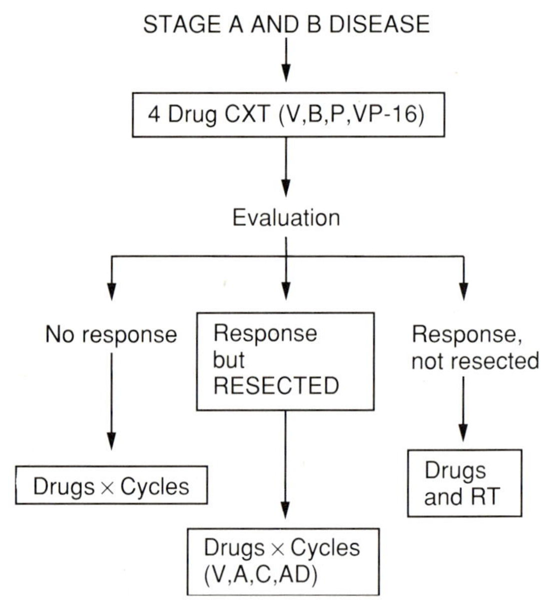

Figure 3 Testicular yolk sac tumor in children: stages B and C.
CXT, Chemotherapy; V, vinblastine; B, bleomycin; AD, doxorubicin (Adriamycin); NR, no response; R, response; RT, radiation therapy; P, cisplatin; A, dactinomycin (actinomycin D); C, cyclophosphamide.

For higher-stage tumors, the four-drug chemotherapeutic regimen is initially given. An evaluation and/or staging is then performed, and if there is no residual tumor, triple therapy with vinblastine, cisplatin, and etoposide is administered every 3 weeks for four cycles.

Table 2 Therapy and Prognosis of Pediatric Testicular Tumors

Tumor Type	Therapy	Prognosis (2 yr)
Yolk sac carcinoma	O, CXT ±, RLND ±	80–90%
Teratoma	O	Excellent
Teratocarcinoma	O, CXT, RLND ±	80%
Seminoma	O, RT	Good
Gonadal stromal	O	Excellent
Gonadoblastoma	O before puberty	Excellent
Lymphomas/leukemias	CXT, RT	Heralds relapse of primary
Rhabodmyosarcoma	O, CXT, RLND	90%

O, Orchiectomy; CXT, chemotherapy; RLND, retroperitoneal lymph node dissection; RT, radiation therapy.

Table 3 Endocrine Studies to Differentiate Leydig Cell Tumors from Congenital Adrenal Hyperplasia

Tumor Type	17-Ketosteroid	Dexamethasone	Urinary Pregnanetriol	17-Hydroxyprogesterone	Testosterone
Leydig cell tumor	± elevated	No effect on 17-ketosteroid		↑ mild	↑
Congenital adrenal hyperplasia	↑↑ maximal	↓ 17-ketosteroid	↑ moderate	↑ moderate	↑

If at the evaluation viable tumor is noted but is completely resected, combination chemotherapy that includes vinblastine, cyclophosphamide, dactinomycin, and doxorubicin (Adriamycin) is given every 6 weeks for six cycles. No chronic maintenance therapy is given. If at the evaluation viable tumor is noted and not completely resected, radiation therapy is added to the above regimen (Fig. 3; Table 2).

The entire question of chemotherapy and specific protocols is an evolving one, and certainly modifications in the future are expected.

Teratoma

Teratomas account for the second largest portion of germ cell tumors (10 to 15 percent). The vast majority of patients are treated before the age of 2 years. These tumors contain elements from the three germ cell layers and thus on cut section they may contain bone, skin, and neural tissue. In the prepubertal child they are benign and only require orchiectomy.

Teratocarcinoma

Teratocarcinoma is treated the same as in the adult. Eighty percent survival can be achieved when combination therapy with cisplatin, bleomycin, and vinblastine is used.

Seminoma

Seminoma is seen in the postpubertal child and is treated the same as in the adult.

Nongerminal Tumors

Gonadal Stromal Tumors

The gonadal stromal tumors are the most common nongerminal testicular tumors in children. Histologically, they may be composed of Leydig or Sertoli cells or be a combination of both types. The Leydig cell tumor occurs both prepubertally (under age 10) and again in the late 20s. The diagnosis is suggested by the presence of a scrotal mass and precocious puberty. Leydig cell tumor may also be associated with gynecomastia in 10 to 15 percent of cases.

The main differential diagnostic dilemma is whether the precocious puberty and testicular enlargement is due to a Leydig cell tumor or "adrenal rest" tissue located within the testis, which may occur in patients with congenital adrenal hyperplasia (CAH). A distinction is important because if the cause is CAH, the testicular nodules will regress with glucocorticoid treatment and no orchiectomy is needed. An orchiectomy alone, however, is appropriate treatment for Leydig cell tumors. CAH is genetically transmitted, and thus a family history will be of some help. Endocrinologic studies (Table 3) should include the following:

1. Dexamethasone suppression test. In CAH, urinary 17-ketosteroid production is significantly elevated, but in patients with Leydig cell tumors, 17-ketosteroid production can be variable. When, however, it is significantly elevated, dexamethasone will help to differentiate these two diseases by suppression of the urinary 17-ketosteroid in CAH alone.
2. Urinary pregnanetriol and 17-hydroxyprogesterone. In patients with CAH due to 21-hydroxylase deficiency, the 17-hydroxyprogesterone and its urinary excretory product pregnanetriol will be moderately elevated. In patients with Leydig cell tumors, however, the 17-hydroxyprogesterone level will be elevated, but to a much lesser extent, and the urinary pregnanetriol level will not be detectable.

Testosterone values alone will not be helpful in distinguishing between the conditions.

Sertoli Cell Tumors

Sertoli cell tumors usually occur earlier than Leydig cell tumors and are more likely to produce estrogen than testosterone. One reported case of metastasis required monitoring of the child's retroperitoneum on a 6-month to yearly basis with ultrasonography.

Gonadoblastomas

Gonadoblastomas are rare tumors that develop in children with dysgenetic gonads. The karyotype of these children always contains a Y chromosome. Most of these children display a female phenotype. The risk of tumor development increases at the time of puberty. Gonadectomy before this time is advised. Bilateral involvement is present one third of the time.

Lymphomas and Leukemia

The testis acts as a repository for tumor cells in patients with these neoplasms because of a blood-gonad barrier that prevents chemotherapy from reaching these errant cells. Approximately 10 percent of patients show evidence for testicular involvement during therapy, and 30 to 40 percent subsequently develop tumors after therapy stops. Bilateral occurrence is high. It is thus important to perform an open testicular biopsy before cessation of therapy. If tumor cells are present, combination chemotherapy and radiation therapy (2,400 rads) is advised. After this treatment sexual maturation is not affected, but patients will surely be sterile. Testicular disease often presages medullary or metastatic disease, and those with a relapse in the testis often fare poorly.

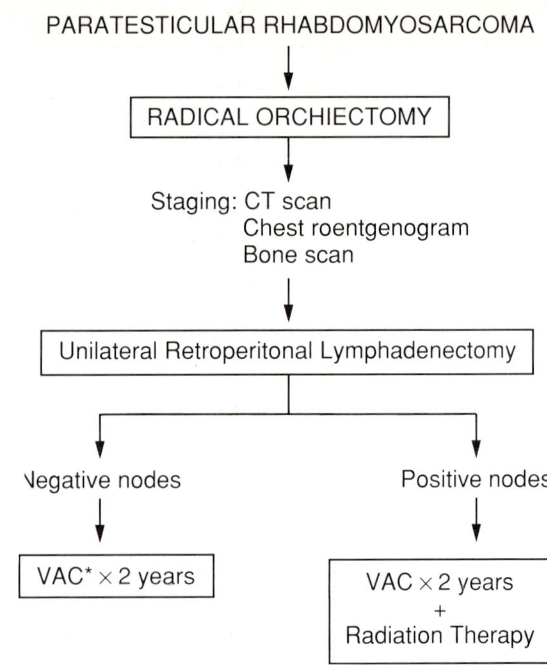

Figure 4 Treatment of paratesticular rhabdomyosarcoma. *VAC, Combination therapy with vincristine, dactinomycin (actinomycin D), and cyclophosphamide.

Paratesticular Tumors

Paratesticular rhabdomyosarcoma arises in the spermatic cord, grows rapidly, and metastasizes early to the retroperitoneum. In an Intergroup Rhabdomyosarcoma Study, 40 percent of patients had positive nodes in the retroperitoneum. The tumor is characterized by three cell types: (1) anaplastic, (2) monomorphous round cell, and (3) mixed. The mixed type provides for the best prognosis. The therapy begins with a radical orchiectomy (Fig. 4). If the scrotum was violated in making the diagnosis, a hemiscrotectomy is indicated. All patients then undergo a staging (not therapeutic) extended unilateral retroperitoneal lymph node dissection. If the nodes are negative, combination therapy with vincristine, dactinomycin (actinomycin D), and cyclophosphamide (VAC) is employed for 2 years. If the nodes are positive, radiation therapy and chemotherapy are used. If bulky disease is present, preoperative radiation therapy of 3,000 to 4,000 rads in 3 to 4 weeks can be given to help shrink the mass. Surgery can then be accomplished.

With this aggressive program of combined chemotherapy and radiation therapy, disease-free survival for 2 years can be expected in nearly 90 percent of patients.

INTERSTITIAL TESTICULAR CELL TUMOR

STEPHEN C. JACOBS, M.D.

Interstitial testicular cell tumors, also known as Leydig cell tumors, are uncommon malignancies of the testis and very rarely of extragonadal sites such as the spermatic cord or retroperitoneum. The cell of origin is the Leydig cell, and if the neoplastic cells can still produce sex steroids, signs and symptoms of excess androgens or estrogens may be present. The systemic effects of such sex steroid excess are easier to detect in prepubertal males, who represent about 25 percent of the patients.

The vast majority of testicular tumors arise from the germinal epithelium and present as seminoma, embryonal carcinoma, teratocarcinoma, or choriocarcinoma. The other testicular tissues from which malignancies can arise are the testicular interstitium (Leydig cells, Sertoli cells) and the mesenchymal interstitium (e.g., smooth muscle, vascular endothelium). Leydig cell tumors certainly represent less than 1 percent of primary testicular neoplasms, although there are several factors conspiring to make a truly accurate picture of the incidence difficult. Because most of these tumors are benign, they are not accumulated by institutions likely to report series. Enough cases have been reported, however, to make single case reports unlikely.

The etiology of Leydig cell tumors is totally unknown. There have been several case reports associated with undescended testis or estrogen administration, but most have no such identifiable possible etiologic factors. In rodents, interstitial testicular cell tumors can result from diethylstilbestrol (DES) exposure, but the human lesion has not been seen, even though many men have been exposed to DES.

The Leydig cells synthesize and secrete testosterone, and some of the tumors retain the ability to do so. Reinke's crystals can be seen histologically in the normal Leydig cell and in about 40 percent of Leydig cell tumors. In prepubertal males, this excess testosterone may lead to precocious virilization, but in adult males excess virilization is difficult to detect. The tumor cells may retain the ability to convert testosterone to estradiol, leading to the possible gradual appearance of gynecomastia and diminished libido.

The incidence of Leydig cell tumors is low and the age range broad, so that distinguishing the Leydig cell tumor patient from the vast background of germ cell neoplasm patients preoperatively is difficult, if not impossible. Prepubertal males tend to present after age 4 years and are detected because of their precocious virilization. The differential diagnosis includes adrenal hyperplasia and exogenous steroid administration. Most Leydig cell tumor patients have a palpable testicular mass, but testicular ultrasonography is useful in suspected cases without a palpable mass.

Adult patients are most commonly in the fourth and fifth decades of life, but can present even later. On presentation there is a testicular mass, which can be painful if recent interstitial hemorrhage has occurred (Table 1). If any hormonal effects are present, they have been of an insidious onset and are not usually prominent to the patient. The serum LH and FSH levels may be suppressed and the serum testosterone may be elevated, but these are not usually obtained before orchiectomy. The serum alpha$_1$-fetoprotein (AFP) and beta-human chorionic gonadotropin (beta-hCG) are always drawn before orchiectomy, and are normal.

The initial treatment of interstitial testicular cell tumors consists of inguinal orchiectomy. In most cases, the orchiectomy is diagnostic. Some have advocated a limited testicular resection for Leydig cell tumors, but intraoperatively it is almost impossible to be certain that a germ cell tumor or mixed tumor is not present. Consequently, these tumors need to be treated by orchiectomy, even if this represents overkill. The inguinal approach also is mandated by the probability that a testicular mass is of germ cell origin.

On gross inspection of the orchiectomy specimen, the Leydig cell tumor is a soft, yellow to deep brown tumor that is well defined or even encapsulated. If the patient has experienced bleeding previously, fibrosis and even calcification can be present. Necrosis is distinctly unusual. Histologically, broad sheets or tumor cells with intervening fibrous trabeculae are found. The polygonal tumor cells are not arranged in any particular manner. Reinke's crystals, eosinophilic, rectangular cytoplasmic inclusion bodies that contain steroids, are found in only 40 percent of the tumors. In most Leydig cell tumors, mitoses are very rare.

Malignant Leydig cell tumors tend to be larger and mitoses are seen. Invasion of vascular structures or the testicular capsule is seen in three out of four malignant Leydig cell tumors. No single finding is a guarantee of benignity or malignancy, with the exception of metastasis (Table 2).

After orchiectomy, testosterone levels should return to normal. Persistent serum testosterone elevation would probably represent persistent disease, and these levels are generally used for follow-up. If AFP and

Table 1   Signs and Symptoms of Interstitial Testicular Cell Tumors

Finding	Cause	Approximate Incidence (%)
Testicular mass	Neoplasm	99%
Testicular pain	Hemorrhage	10%
Bilateral testicular mass	Multicentricity	<10%
Precocious virilization	Testosterone	25%
Diminished libido	Estradiol	<20%
Gynecomastia	Estradiol	<20%
Eunuchoid habitus	Estradiol	<20%
Extratesticular mass only	Metastasis	<1%

Table 2 Benign versus Malignant Leydig Cell Tumors

	Benign	Malignant
Incidence	90%	10%
Prepubertal	100%	0%
Virilization	25%	0%
Feminization	20%	10%
Average age	35 yrs	60 yrs
Age range	4–70 yrs	29–82 yrs
Histopathology		
>5 cm	+	+ +
Reinke's crystals	40%	0%
Mitotic figures	–	+ +
Capsular invasion	0%	75%
Vascular invasion	0%	75%
Cytologic pleomorphism	–	–
Fibrosis	–	–
Necrosis	–	–
Metastasis	0%	100%

+, present; + +, present (moderately heavy); –, not present.

beta-hCG levels have been normal, they need not be followed; if these levels were elevated, the diagnosis of Leydig cell tumor is in error.

Only 10 percent or less of interstitial testicular cell tumors are malignant. These are exclusively in adult, not prepubertal, patients. Metastatic work-up for Leydig cell tumor patients usually includes the standard abdominal computed tomographic (CT) scan, chest x-ray examination, bone scan, and liver function tests. The detection of metastases is important for patient information, but if these are present, the outlook is bleak. Retroperitoneal lymphadenectomy should be attempted for resectable disease. As there is not an established effective radiotherapy or chemotherapy alternative, a complete resection without field modification or regard to nerve sparing should be carried out.

Radiation therapy for metastatic disease has been uniformly unsuccessful.

Chemotherapy in either an adjuvant or a curative setting has not been effective. Anecdotally, cisplatin has been infrequently effective. Others have advocated the use of mitotane, even though it is remarkably toxic and has shown only a few short-lived partial responses. Mitotane is a derivative of the insecticide DDT and alters synthesis and metabolism of steroids. Adrenocortical steroid support must be given when trauma, shock, or infection appear. Mitotane may well control symptoms of sex steroid excess when elevated androgens or estrogens are a problem. However, most cases of malignant Leydig cell tumors do not demonstrate high sex steroid levels. Other agents that have been ineffective include bleomycin, methotrexate, cytoxan, vinblastine, vincristine, actinomycin D, doxorubicin, and corticosteroids alone. Patients with metastatic disease generally succumb to the disease in less than 1 year.

SUGGESTED READING

Peterson RO. Urologic pathology. Philadelphia: JB Lippincott, 1986.

GONADAL STROMAL TUMOR

MICHAEL J. YOUNG, M.D.
W. BEDFORD WATERS, M.D.

Gonadal stromal tumors make up approximately 5 to 10 percent of all testicular tumors. They have been described under a host of different names, including sex cord–stromal tumors, androblastomas, granulosa cell tumors, interstitial cell tumors, and Sertoli cell tumors. It appears that the cell type, architecture, and degree of differentiation of these tumors may closely duplicate the supporting tissues in the gonads of either sex. Although it is thought that these cell types might perhaps arise from a primitive gonadal stromal mesenchyme or undifferentiated precursor cell, embryologically, their origin is unknown. Thus, considerable debate persists regarding the proper classification and nomenclature of these tumors.

The World Health Organization (WHO) classification of these tumors is listed in Table 1. These tumors present with a bimodal age distribution, occurring between the ages of 6 to 10 and 26 to 30 years, and constitute a greater proportion of testicular tumors in children (20 percent). They have also been reported in older men.

The Leydig cell tumor (interstitial cell) is the most common of the gonadal stromal tumors and makes up between 1 and 3 percent of all testicular tumors. Approximately 25 percent present before puberty with no specific cause identified. Unlike germ cell tumors, they do not appear to be associated with cryptorchidism.

Table 1 World Health Organization (WHO) Classification of Gonadal Stromal Tumors

Well-differentiated tumors
  Leydig cell
  Sertoli cell
  Granulosa cell

Mixed forms

Incompletely differentiated forms of gonadal stroma

The manifestations of Leydig cell tumors are varied. Because of their endocrine capability, these tumors may present in the prepubertal period with precocity and prominent genital and hair growth. Testosterone levels are generally elevated, with normal to elevated urinary 17-ketosteroids. Because of the similar embryologic origin of interstitial cells and adrenocortical cells, the occurrence of adrenal rests complicates the diagnosis. Virilizing congenital adrenal hyperplasia must therefore be included in the differential diagnosis. 17-OH-ketosteroids, 17-OH-progesterone, plasma cortisol (pre- and post-ACTH stimulation) should be obtained. Feminization may occur in boys with Leydig cell tumors, but this is always superimposed on virilism.

In adults, most cases present with an endocrine imbalance, which may precede the finding of a palpable gonadal mass. Twenty-five percent of Leydig cell tumors in adults are hormonally active and produce estrogen. Patients may have symptoms of a feminizing nature with an increase in plasma and urinary estrogens. Laboratory endocrine studies should include evaluation of testosterone, estrogen, follicle-stimulating hormone (FSH), and luteinizing hormone (LH) levels. Other considerations in the adult include Klinefelter's syndrome and the feminizing testicular disorders. However, the diagnosis of a gonadal stromal tumor can rarely be made before orchiectomy. These tumors can also occur in association with a germ cell tumor, necessitating alpha-fetoprotein and beta–human chorionic gonadotropin determinations.

Metastasis may be the presenting symptom in patients with malignant disease. It generally follows the embryologic origin of the testis, with the retroperitoneal space as the primary landing site. Metastases to the lung and liver have also been reported.

The pathognomonic feature for the Leydig cell tumor is the Reinke inclusion crystal, which is present in 40 percent of cases. Unfortunately, the ultrastructural features of the Leydig cell tumor do not make it possible to distinguish between benign and neoplastic cells. There are no consistent histologic criteria established to make this judgment.

Initial treatment for this disease is radical inguinal orchiectomy. The metastatic work-up after orchiectomy should include a chest, abdominal, and pelvic computed tomographic (CT) scan. The use of a lymphangiography is debatable and has generally fallen out of favor. As stated, there are no defined histologic criteria other than the evidence of metastic disease to define malignancy. Fortunately, only 10 percent of all cases in adults are malignant, and no case of metastasis has been reported in the prepubertal age group. Upon microscopic examination of the tumor, however, if there is evidence of vascular or lymphatic invasion, large tumor size, or severe anaplasia, further therapy is recommended. These tumors appear radioresistant, and no effective chemotherapeutic agent has been identified. Therefore, retroperitoneal lymph node dissection is the procedure of choice in this select group of patients.

Preoperative care includes placement of a central venous access line and a complete bowel preparation, if visceral involvement is noted on the CT scan. Our lymph node dissection is performed through a thoracoabdominal incision, allowing excellent exposure and ability to dissect suprahilar, if necessary. Given the low potential for metastatic disease, we perform a nerve-sparing modified lymph node dissection if at all possible. These templates have been well described in the literature, with preservation of sympathetic ejaculatory function in over 75 percent of patients. Generally, patients do well postoperatively, with removal of the chest tube on day 3 and advancement of diet and activity as with any major abdominal procedure. Follow-up studies should include a chest x-ray examination and CT scans of the abdomen and pelvis every 2 to 3 months for the first 2 years. Patients should also obtain hormonal studies and tumor markers routinely during this time. Overall, there is an excellent prognosis, with most relapses occurring within the first 2 years after orchiectomy.

Sertoli cell tumors, also referred to as androblastomas when incompletely differentiated, make up less than 1 percent of testicular tumors. They can present at any age, including infancy, and have a wide range of presenting signs and symptoms. Generally, patients note a nonpainful testicular mass; approximately 30 percent show evidence of gynecomastia or other feminizing characteristics.

The etiology of this tumor is unknown, with no identifiable contributing factor or specific tumor marker. Initial therapy includes radical orchiectomy followed by staging CT scans of the chest, abdomen, and pelvis. Microscopic examination reveals a well-circumscribed mass in benign lesions. However, as with the Leydig cell tumor, there are no definite histologic criteria to define malignancy. The invasion of paratesticular structures or the presence of severe anaplasia suggests possible metastatic disease necessitating further therapy. Retroperitoneal lymph node dissection, as previously described, is the indicated procedure for suspected malignancies. Once again, the prognosis is excellent: less than 10 percent of these tumors are malignant.

Granulosa cell tumors and mixed forms are rare tumors that have a similar pattern of endocrine disturbances associated with a testicular mass. Radical orchiectomy followed by retroperitoneal lymph node dissection is indicated for lesions that raise suspicion.

SUGGESTED READING

Campbell CM, Middleton AW Jr. Malignant gonadal stromal tumor: case report and review of the literature. J Urol 1981; 125:257.

Kaplan GW, Cromie WJ, Kelalis PP, et al. Gonadal stromal tumors: a report of the prepubertal testicular tumor registry. J Urol 1986; 136:300.

Masterson JST, McCullough AR, Smith RRL, Jeffs RD. Neonatal gonadal stromal tumor of the testis: limitations of tumor markers. J Urol 1985; 134:558.

McClennan DS, Rocher A. Intrascrotal tumors in the older male. Int Surg 1986; 71:51.

White JM, McCarthy MP. Testicular gonadal stromal tumors in newborns. Urology 1982; 20:121.

SERTOLI CELL TUMOR

RAY E. STUTZMAN, M.D.

Primary testicular tumors arise from either germ cells or the supporting elements of the stroma. Approximately 95 percent of testicular tumors originate from spermatogenic or germ cells, and 5 percent are classified as gonadal stromal tumors, which include Sertoli cell tumors (Table 1). Sertoli cell neoplasms constitute less than 1 percent of all testicular tumors and may occur in any age group, including infancy. It is a rare neoplasm in humans. It is the most common testicular tumor in dogs and is frequently feminizing owing to estrogen production by the neoplastic Sertoli cells. Most Sertoli cell tumors are benign, but approximately 10 percent have been proved malignant by the presence of metastases.

Leydig and Sertoli cells are derived from the same precursor cell, the former differentiating into cells capable of steroid elaboration, particularly androgen, and to a lesser extent, estrogen. Sertoli cells differentiate as nutrient cells sustaining spermatogenesis, and in a large measure lose their capacity for steroidogenesis. The association of endocrine disorders with Sertoli cell tumors is well documented, however, occurring in approximately one third of patients. Gynecomastia and hyperestrinism may be manifest. Testosterone and estradiol have been demonstrated in Sertoli cell tumors by immunochemical and biochemical methods.

Sertoli cell tumors can further be classified as well differentiated, moderately or poorly differentiated, and large-cell calcifying variant. Large-cell calcifying Sertoli cell tumors have been associated with complex endocrine abnormalities, including sexual precocity, adrenocortical nodular hyperplasia, pituitary adenoma, cardiac myxoma, pigmented skin lesions, endocrine overactivity, and testicular nodules of Leydig or adrenocortical cell origin. Large-cell calcifying Sertoli cell tumors of the testis differ histologically from pure Sertoli cell tumors by the composition of large cells with abundant eosinophilic cytoplasm, and a diffuse and trabecular pattern of growth with characteristic and often laminated calcifications. It is a rare neoplasm with fewer than 20 reported cases. Metastases have been rare with this lesion.

Table 1 World Health Organization (WHO) International Classification of Sex Cord–Stromal Tumors

Well-differentiated forms
  Leydig cell tumor
  Sertoli cell tumor
  Granulosa cell tumor

Mixed forms

Incompletely differentiated forms of gonadal stroma

Ten to fifteen percent of Sertoli cell tumors are malignant. The distinction between benign and malignant tumors cannot be made on macroscopic or microscopic inspection alone. Malignant tumors are usually larger than the benign neoplasms and also are moderately to poorly differentiated. The absolute criteria for malignancy, however, is the presence of metastases, this being the only unquestioned proof. Malignant Sertoli cell tumors tend to metastasize in a pattern similar to that observed with germ cell testicular neoplasms. Metastases usually are evidenced within the first 2 years after orchiectomy.

Sertoli cell tumors are typically small, 1 to 2 cm in diameter, but if they are neglected over a period of years, they may grow to 15 to 20 cm. Most patients are in the 20- to 50-year age range, but these tumors may be found from childhood to old age. On gross section, the tumor is usually yellowish-white, yellowish-gray, or yellowish-tan in appearance. It tends to be well delineated and slightly raised from the surrounding testicular tissue. Cystic degeneration may occur in large tumors, but the smaller ones are typically solid and firm. Most of the malignant neoplasms are large, 7 to 15 cm, with histologically demonstrated pleomorphism and mitotic activity and occasional evidence of lymphatic involvement. No single feature or combination of gross and microscopic findings has been predictive of biologic malignancy. The large cell calcifying tumors are typically yellow on section and are often gritty, owing to nodules or plaques of calcification, and mitoses are generally lacking.

The signs and symptoms of Sertoli cell tumors are not unlike those of germ cell tumors of the testis. Testicular enlargement without pain is the common symptom, with evidence of a firm mass within the testis. There also may be endocrine manifestations, particularly gynecomastia and loss of libido. The treatment of any patient with a testicular neoplasm consists of radical inguinal orchiectomy. A germ cell neoplasm is usually first suspected on the basis of the clinical presentation. Histologic evaluation confirms the correct diagnosis. The diagnosis of a Sertoli cell tumor can rarely be made definitively before orchiectomy, except possibly in the case of the large cell calcified variant.

All patients should undergo a thorough postorchiectomy evaluation after histologic confirmation of the tumor. Laboratory studies should include testosterone, estrogen, luteinizing hormone (LH), and follicle-stimulating hormone (FSH) determinations. Sex cord–stromal tumors, including Sertoli cell tumors, do not produce tumor markers, human chorionic gonadotropin, and alpha-fetoprotein, although these markers should be drawn. Sex cord–stromal tumors have been reported to occur in association with germ cell tumors. Computed tomography (CT) of the chest and abdomen is recommended to assess possible metastases to the retroperitoneal lymph nodes, liver, and lungs.

Radical orchiectomy alone with observation is recommended if there is no evidence of metastatic disease. If the tumor is large and there is microscopic suggestion of poorly differentiated or anaplastic cells and/or lymphatic and vascular invasion, retroperitoneal lymph node dissection for staging seems indicated. Node dissection is particularly indicated if on CT there is evidence of retroperitoneal lymphadenopathy.

The prognosis is excellent in patients having a tumor with no evidence of metastases. Close observation and surveillance is imperative, particularly during the first 2 to 3 years after diagnosis. Follow-up chest radiographs, abdominal CT scans, and hormone studies are appropriate every 3 months for 2 years. Since late metastases have been reported, continued annual evaluation is recommended.

The rarity of malignant and metastatic sex cord–stromal tumors and Sertoli cell tumors has precluded an in-depth study of the pathologic and clinical features in a large series. Therefore, no extensive data are available on management and prognosis. Retroperitoneal lymph node dissection for staging and treatment has been reported to improve survival in patients with suspected or confirmed malignant tumors. Radiation therapy alone and in conjunction with surgery has had variable results. Chemotherapy, so effective in germ cell tumors, has had little success in the management of sex cord stromal tumors.

SUGGESTED READING

Buchino JJ, Buchino JJ, Uhlenhuth ER. Large-cell calcifying Sertoli cell tumor. J Urol 1989; 141:953–954.

Eble JN, Hull MT, Warfel KA, Donohue JP. Malignant sex cord–stromal tumor of testis. J Urol 1984; 131:546–550.

Gabrilove JL, Freiberg EK, Leiter E, Nicolis GL. Feminizing and non-feminizing Sertoli cell tumors. J Urol 1980; 124:757–767.

Waxman M, Damjanov I, Khapra A, Landau SJ. Large cell calcifying Sertoli tumor of the testis. Cancer 1984; 54:1574–1581.

Wheeler JE. Testicular tumors. In: Hill GS, ed. Uropathology. New York: Churchill Livingstone, 1989:1047.

SPERMATIC CORD TUMOR

JACKSON E. FOWLER, Jr., M.D.

Tumors of the spermatic cord usually present as nontender, firm, paratesticular masses that can be separated from the testis and testicular adnexa during careful palpation. Most spermatic cord tumors are benign, encapsulated lipomas. Malignant lesions are almost uniformly sarcomatous in nature and arise from either the striated cremasteric muscle or the fibrofatty tissue that invests the vas deferens, gonadal vessels, and lymphatics. The former are rhabdomyosarcomas, whereas the latter make up a bewildering array of histologic types, including fibrosarcomas, leiomyosarcomas, liposarcomas, fibromyxosarcomas, and malignant fibrous histiocytomas.

RHABDOMYOSARCOMAS

Approximately 7 percent of rhabdomyosarcomas arise from the spermatic cord. The mean age of affected patients is 11 years, and the tumor is rarely seen after the age of 20 years. Rhabdomyosarcomas have a propensity for rapid lymphatic and hematogenous dissemination. Data generated by the Intergroup Rhabdomyosarcoma Study suggest that about 60 percent of patients with tumors of the spermatic cord present with localized, completely resectable lesions (group I), and that about 20 percent have grossly resectable disease but positive surgical margins or regional lymph node metastases (group II). In 20 percent of patients, the primary tumor is not resectable (group III) or there are visceral metastases (group IV). The systematic administration of locoregional radiation therapy and combination chemotherapy in addition to wide excision of the primary tumor, either before or after adjuvant therapies, has markedly improved the possibilities of cure. A 2-year disease-free survival can be anticipated in 90 percent of properly managed patients in groups I and II and in about 50 percent of those in groups III and IV.

ADULT SARCOMAS

Sarcomas of the spermatic cord in adults are far less common than analogous neoplasms arising at other sites. The usual age of affected patients is 40 to 60 years. Reliable data concerning the natural history and optimal treatment are not available, and therapeutic philosophies generally parallel those for soft tissue sarcomas of the same histologic type at other locations.

Most adult tumors are clinically localized at the time of diagnosis, but infiltration of adjacent tissues is the rule. The growth rate is characteristically slow and the propensity for dissemination limited. Some patients report palpable masses for years before seeking medical attention, and residual disease after excision of the primary tumor may not be manifested for years. Death from uncontrollable local or metastatic disease may not occur for as long as 10 to 20 years after diagnosis.

Adjuvant radiation therapy and chemotherapy have no defined role in the management of adult sarcomas, and curative therapy for unresectable or disseminated tumors is not available. Complete surgical excision of the primary lesion is the foundation of appropriate management.

Surgery for the Primary Tumor

Inguinal orchiectomy with removal of the entire spermatic cord is the minimal initial intervention for malignant tumors of the spermatic cord. Diagnostic uncertainty before exploration of small masses is not infrequent, and excisional biopsy, excision of the tumor only, or simple scrotal orchiectomy are common management errors. Intraoperative aspiration biopsy of lesions with the gross appearance of a carcinoma, and extension of a scrotal incision or the addition of a separate inguinal incision to permit removal of the testis and entire spermatic cord, obviate these therapeutic miscalculations.

The diameter of many childhood and adult sarcomas exceeds 5 cm, and malignancy is suspected before surgery. In these cases, the lesion is always approached through an inguinal incision. The contents of the hemiscrotum with the surrounding tunica vaginalis are freed from the tunica dartos and delivered into the wound, and the spermatic cord is mobilized from the inguinal canal and transected at the internal inguinal ring. The vas deferens and gonadal vessels are ligated individually, with the sutures cut long to permit identification during subsequent lymphadenectomy. If there is any suggestion of local tumor invasion due to adherence of the mass to the dartos muscle or induration of the scrotal skin, a hemiscrotectomy is performed.

Most spermatic cord tumors are situated distal to the external inguinal ring, and infiltration of the fibromuscular components of the inguinal canal is unusual. Tumors arising proximal to the external ring, however, are less easily detected by palpation and tend to be large at presentation. Wide excision of the overlying skin, subcutaneous tissue, and aponeurosis of the external oblique and of the underlying internal oblique is advisable when the lesion is bulky or grossly invasive. This is particularly important with adult sarcomas, but should be considered only when the prospect for complete removal of a childhood sarcoma is good. Unresectable rhabdomyosarcomas are treated with chemotherapy and radiation therapy first, and residual disease is removed at a later date. Partial excision of large rhabdomyosarcomas has *no* therapeutic value and may unnecessarily delay the administration of adjuvant therapies.

An extensive, ulcerating, malignant fibrous histiocytoma arising from the inguinal spermatic cord is shown in Figure 1. The surgical specimen, which includes the tumor, surrounding skin, subcutaneous tissue and fascia, and the spermatic cord and testis is shown in Figure 2. Primary closure of the skin and fascia after surgery of this magnitude is not generally possible, but satisfactory coverage of the defect can be achieved with a myocutaneous flap. I prefer the tensor fascia lata myocutaneous flap for this purpose. This flap, which receives its blood supply from the lateral circumflex femoral artery, is rotated from the lateral thigh and can be made as long as 35 cm and as wide as 15 cm. The defect of the thigh is closed primarily or with a split-thickness skin graft. The appearance of bilateral tensor fascia lata myocutaneous flaps used to cover the denuded groins after inguinal surgery for metastatic penile cancer is shown in Figure 3.

When an excisional biopsy has been performed, a hemiscrotectomy is recommended, in addition to an inguinal orchiectomy, to reduce the risks of local recurrence. For rhabdomyosarcomas, inguinal radiation

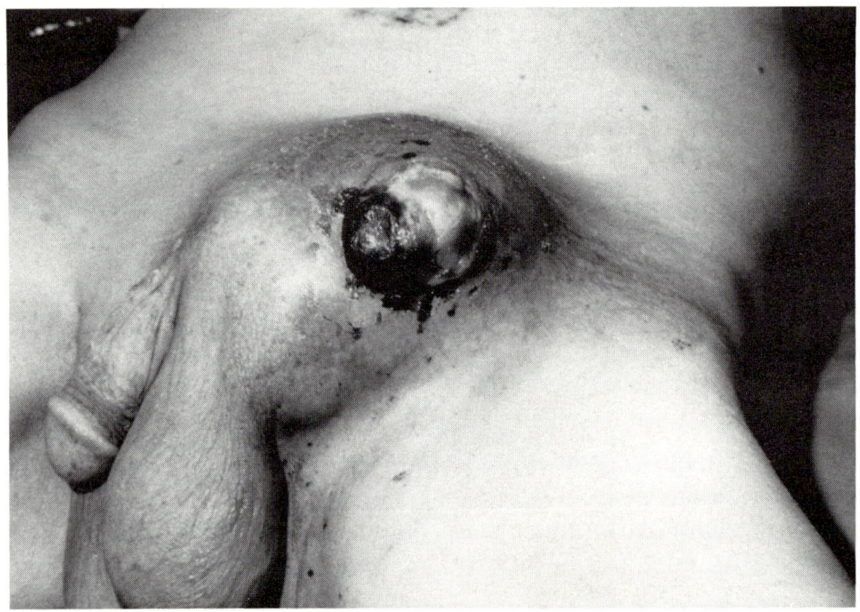

Figure 1 Gross appearance of an infiltrating malignant fibrous histiocytoma arising from inguinal spermatic cord.

therapy is also advisable. The inguinal spermatic cord is routinely removed when a simple scrotal orchiectomy is the initial management. This secondary procedure is indicated even if the surgical margins are tumor free.

Local recurrences develop in more than 50 percent of adults with spermatic cord sarcomas, and periodic, lifelong examination to identify residual malignancy is mandatory. Unlike many solid tumors that are resistant to chemotherapy and radiation therapy, recurrence does not necessarily imply incurability, and excision is always warranted. However, as sequential local recurrences are not unusual, a conservative approach to this intervention is inappropriate. A wide excision that may necessarily include extensive portions of skin, subcutaneous tissue, and fascia is the treatment of choice.

Local recurrence of rhabdomyosarcomas is unusual if the initial management includes chemotherapy and, when appropriate, radiation therapy. This reflects the activity of adjuvant therapies against rhabdomyosarcomas, as well as the lethal course of tumors that are not amenable to complete excision and are refractory to adjuvant therapies.

Surgery for Lymphatic Metastases

Most of the lymphatic channels within the spermatic cord traverse the retroperitoneum adjacent to the spermatic artery. They drain into the infrarenal para-aortic nodes and nodes clustered around the take-off of the renal arteries. In addition, lymphatics emanating from the vas deferens drain to the external iliac nodal chain. Unlike tumors of the testicular parenchyma, therefore, the pelvic lymph nodes are a potential site of early dissemination.

There is no unanimity of opinion concerning the advisability of lymphadenectomy among children or adults who show no evidence of lymph node metastases. Considerations that favor lymphadenectomy for rhabdomyosarcomas include the inaccuracy of computed tomography (CT) and lymphangiography in detecting retroperitoneal metastases, and the potential curability of the disease if properly staged and treated according to existing therapeutic guidelines. More specifically, treatment of the retroperitoneum with radiation therapy is recommended in the presence, but not the absence, of retroperitoneal metastases.

The rationale for lymphadenectomy in adults with

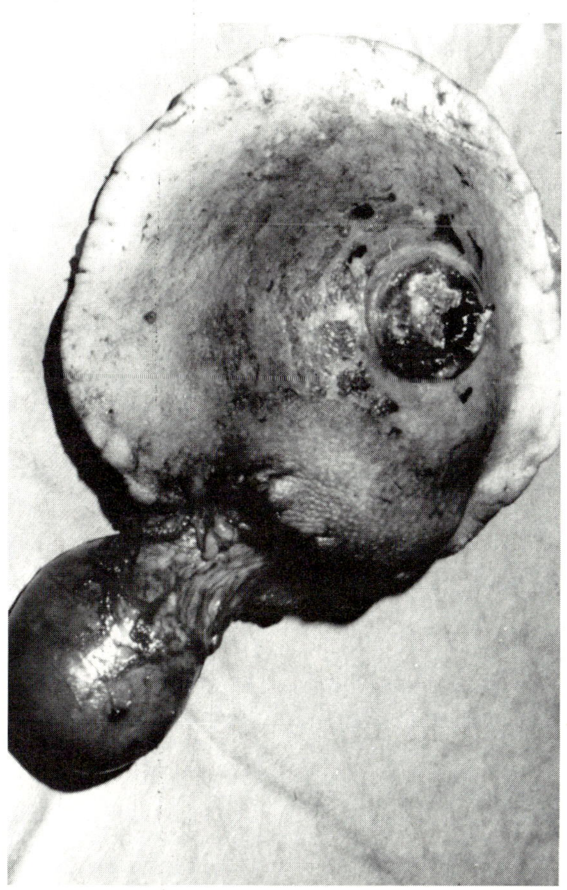

Figure 2 Appearance of the surgical specimen after wide excision of the tumor shown in Figure 1.

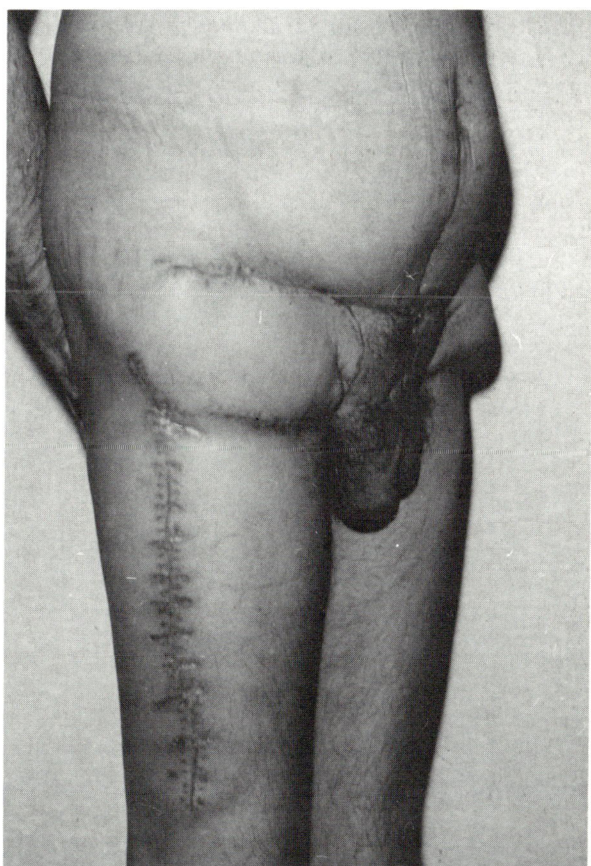

Figure 3 Another patient after excision of large bilateral inguinal metastases and coverage of the surgical defect with a tensor fascia lata myocutaneous flap. (Republished with permission by Fowler JE Jr. Mastery of surgery: urology. Boston: Little, Brown & Co.; in press.)

no clinical evidence of lymphatic dissemination is less compelling. On the one hand, nodal metastases are not particularly common and there is no convincing evidence that their excision has a favorable impact on survival possibilities. In addition, atherosclerosis of the aorta may create fibrous adherence of lymphatic tissues to the adventitia and increase the risks of difficult-to-control arterial bleeding. This technical consideration, as well as nonspecific complications inherent in major abdominal surgery in older patients, are potent arguments against routine lymphadenectomy in the elderly. On the other hand, the morbidity of lymphadenectomy in otherwise healthy middle-aged men probably parallels that in young men, and the potential complication of infertility due to the absence of seminal emission is of no clinical importance.

Lymphadenectomy should always be considered in children and adults with documented and seemingly resectable retroperitoneal metastases. With rhabdomyosarcomas the possibilities of cure with coordinated treatment regimens are clearly enhanced by the removal of all macroscopic tumor. The benefit of such surgery in adults is unquantifiable, but alternative therapies that may prolong life do not exist.

Children with seemingly unresectable retroperitoneal disease are treated with chemotherapy and radiation therapy initially, and are explored to document and remove residual tumor if there is a favorable response. Radiation therapy is probably advisable in men with unresectable retroperitoneal malignancy.

A systematic retroperitoneal and ipsilateral pelvic lymphadenectomy is performed using the techniques described elsewhere in this text. In children the paravertebral sympathetic chain and sympathetic fibers coursing anterior to the aorta below the inferior mesenteric artery are preserved if this is technically feasible. These maneuvers generally prevent infertility due to the absence of seminal emission. The most proximal para-aortic lymphatic tissue is marked for identification by the pathologist. Patients treated with the Intergroup Rhabdomyosarcoma Study protocols are considered to have positive surgical margins if there is involvement of the most proximal para-aortic node or nodes. In both children and adults, the entire ipsilateral gonadal vein and a generous portion of the pelvic vas deferens are removed. The margins of previous transection are identified by the long sutures applied during the inguinal orchiectomy. In middle-aged or elderly men, the inferior mesenteric artery and lumbar arteries are purposefully preserved to avoid the potential hazards of colonic or spinal cord ischemia due to inadequate collateral circulation.

Radiation therapy to the retroperitoneum is routinely delivered after lymphadenectomy in children with nodal metastases. Information on the benefit of postoperative radiation therapy or chemotherapy in adults is not available, and recommendations concerning adjuvant therapies must be individualized.

The lymphatics of the scrotum and of the inguinal skin and subcutaneous tissues drain directly to the superficial inguinal nodes. In addition, aberrant lymphatic drainage of the scrotal contents may develop after such procedures as orchidopexy or inguinal herniorrhaphy. Metastatic involvement of the inguinal nodes may be seen in patients with histories of previous inguinal or scrotal surgery, or in patients with infiltrating primary tumors. Enlargement of the inguinal nodes can be detected with ease by physical examination, and diagnostic aspiration or excisional biopsy of the superficial nodes is a straightforward procedure. Inguinal lymphadenectomy is never indicated in the absence of histologically documented metastatic disease.

SUGGESTED READING

Blitzer PH, Dosoretz DE, Proppe KH, et al. Treatment of malignant tumors of the spermatic cord: a study of 10 cases and a review of the literature. J Urol 1981; 126:611.

Mauer HM, Moon T, Donaldson M. The Intergroup Rhabdomyosarcoma Study. A preliminary report. Cancer 1977; 40:2015.

Raney RB, Hays DM, Lawrence W Jr, et al. Paratesticular rhabdomyosarcoma in childhood. Cancer 1978; 42:729.

Sogani PC, Grabstald H, Whitmore WF Jr. Spermatic cord sarcoma in adults. J Urol 1978; 120:301.

EPIDIDYMAL TUMOR

GABRIEL P. HAAS, M.D.
J. EDSON PONTES, M.D.

Lesions of the epididymis have received considerably less attention in the urologic literature than testicular tumors. The vast majority of epididymal abnormalities are due to either acute or chronic sequelae of epididymitis, and the incidence of epididymal malignancy is much smaller than the incidence of cancer in a testicular mass. Nevertheless, cancer of the epididymis does occur, and unless it is diagnosed and treated early the prognosis is poor. In addition, lesions of the epididymis may be the first manifestation of underlying systemic disease.

Most patients present with complaints of either pain or an intrascrotal mass. The urologist should differentiate between a lesion arising from the testicle, epididymis, spermatic cord, or (rarely) scrotal wall. In most cases this can be accomplished by physical examination and scrotal ultrasound examination, but occasionally only surgical exploration can reveal the origin of the mass.

Acute epididymitis presents as a very tender, enlarged, boggy epididymis, and the medical history usually suggests the cause of the infection. Sexually transmitted diseases are most common in individuals 15 to 40 years of age, and bladder outlet obstruction with consequent urinary tract infection is the usual etiology in patients older than 50 years of age. Acute epididymitis should be treated with the appropriate antibiotics, after which treatment the patient is re-examined for complete resolution of the symptoms.

Chronic inflammatory changes in the epididymis may be the results of recurrent infections and manifested by spermatoceles and epididymal calcifications. On physical examination, the lesions are irregular, consisting of cysts and firm nodules a few millimeters in diameter, and are either painless or accompanied by only moderate discomfort. Although much less likely to be encountered today, tuberculous epididymitis should be entertained in the differential diagnosis. Other granulomatous systemic diseases, such as sarcoidosis, may also involve the epididymis and should be considered in the differential diagnosis.

BENIGN LESIONS

Epididymitis nodosa is an infrequently encountered benign mass of the epididymis. Fifty percent of patients present with unremitting postvasectomy pain; the remainder have a history of trauma and/or recurrent epididymitis. The mass may reach several centimeters in size and is tender on examination. Ultrasonography shows a combination of cystic and solid components.

Pathologic findings include localized proliferation of small ductules lined by cuboidal or low columnar epithelial cells infiltrating haphazardly the interstitium of the epididymis. Spermatozoa in the ductules, sperm extravasation, sperm granulomas, and focal fibrosis and slight chronic inflammation are seen. Vascular or perineural invasion is not observed. When based on the patient's history, the proper preoperative diagnosis can be made; transscrotal epididymectomy will result in symptomatic improvement.

The most common neoplasm of the epididymis is the adenomatoid tumor, which accounts for 30 percent of all paratesticular tumors. The patients with the highest incidence are those between 45 and 70 years of age. The lesion presents as a small, solid, nontender mass that consists of tubules of various size in fibromuscular stroma. Although the lesion is benign, occasional cellular atypia suggests the possibility of local invasion.

Leiomyoma is the second most common tumor seen in the epididymis. It usually presents as an asymptomatic mass, and occasionally the patient complains of a dull ache. It is seen in children and adults alike, the youngest patient reported being 3 years of age. Local excision is adequate treatment.

Approximately 30 cases of papillary cystadenoma have been reported in the literature, accounting for 4 percent of epididymal tumors. Mostly diagnosed in the 20- to 40-year-old age group, the lesion consists of 1- to 2-cm nodules composed of cystic spaces lined by tall columnar ciliated epithelium. One third of the cases are bilateral and are associated with von Hippel-Lindau (VHL) disease. A patient in whom VHL has not yet been diagnosed at the time of presentation with the epididymal lesion should be screened for other manifestation of this disease, including renal cell cancer.

Fibromas, also called fibrous pseudotumors or giant pseudotumors, are rare, often very large masses of dense, hyalinized fibrous tissue. Although most of these lesions arise from the tunica vaginalis, 10 percent originate from the epididymis. Thirty percent are associated with a history of trauma and 50 percent with a hydrocele. The histologic appearance is of generalized, well-circumscribed fibrosis, and the lesion is uniformly benign.

MALIGNANT TUMORS

Malignant tumors of the epididymis may be primary or metastatic in origin. Primary tumors usually present between the ages of 20 to 40 years, frequently as a painful mass that is first thought to represent epididymitis. Some of the tumors may be masked by a hydrocele.

The most common malignant tumors of the epididymis are sarcomas. The most common cell type is the leiomyosarcoma, followed by fibrosarcomas and rhabdomyosarcomas. The last-named are most commonly seen in the younger age population. All sarcomas are extremely malignant in nature and should be treated with aggressive surgery, including retroperitoneal lymph node dissection, followed by radiation and chemotherapy.

Cystadenocarcinoma is a malignant variant of the benign cystadenoma. About 25 cases have been reported in the literature. The histologic picture is not unlike that of the benign cystadenoma, but areas of increasing atypia and anaplasia are present. Patients with tumors confined to the epididymis have a good prognosis, but those with metastatic disease do very poorly in the absence of any effective radiation or chemotherapy. Patients with metastatic disease at presentation rarely survive 1 year. Because of the poor prognosis of metastatic disease and the poor response to either chemotherapy or radiation therapy, it is important to establish the status of the retroperitoneal lymph nodes, and retroperitoneal lymphadenectomy is recommended.

Both Hodgkin's and non-Hodgkin's lymphomas have been reported to arise from the epididymis. These lesions are problematic because the extent of testicular involvement cannot be determined unless an orchiectomy is performed. Most of these patients are therefore treated by orchiectomy followed by chemotherapy.

Melanotic neuroectodermal tumors (also called retinal anlage tumors, retinoblastic teratomas, melanotic hamartomas, or melanotic progonomas) of the epididymis typically present in infancy or early childhood. The most common site is the maxilla, but ten cases reported had an epididymal origin. The lesions arise from neural crest tissue as very hard, often large masses. The reported cases were mostly benign lesions for which orchiectomy is curative, but there is malignant potential in at least 3 percent of these cases. The 24-hour vanilmandelic acid (VMA) analysis is elevated in some cases and may be followed as a marker for recurrence or metastases. At least one case of elevated alpha-fetoprotein was also reported in a patient in whom the level normalized after removal of the tumor. There have not been enough cases reported to enable an assessment of the role of radiation or chemotherapy in the management of metastatic disease. At the present time, radical orchiectomy with close follow-up appears to be the most reasonable approach to this rare lesion.

Metastatic tumors are most common in the older population. In most cases, the primary lesion is already known; only in extremely rare instances is epididymal metastasis the presenting symptom. Metastases to the epididymis are more common than to the testis itself. The extent of metastases to the scrotum is probably under-reported, because patients often have disseminated disease by the time the epididymal mass is discovered and it may not be worked up. Occult metastases at autopsy may also not be reported. Occasionally, special stains have to be applied to the neoplasm to differentiate a metastasis from an epididymal primary lesion. The most common source of the metastasis is the prostate, followed in decreasing frequency by kidney, stomach, and colon.

APPROACH TO THE UNDIAGNOSED EPIDIDYMAL MASS

History taking, physical examination, and scrotal ultrasonography are performed to differentiate among testicular, epididymal, and spermatic cord masses. If the lesion appears to be an inflammatory mass, it should be treated with antibiotics first and the patient should be followed for resolution of the symptoms. Granulomatous epididymitis due to systemic tuberculosis or sarcoidosis should be considered in masses that do not resolve with conventional antibiotic therapy. If the diagnostic workup is suggestive of spermatocele, epididymitis nodosa, or bilateral papillary cystadenoma, scrotal exploration with either local excision or epididymectomy may be performed. Otherwise, it is safest to proceed with an inguinal exploration and atraumatic clamping of the cord before opening the tunica vaginalis. The epididymis should be inspected and excisional biopsy of the entire lesion submitted for frozen section examination. Given the diagnosis of a benign lesion, the testicle may be preserved. In case of a diagnosis suggestive of malignancy or a tumor with a malignant potential, high ligation of the cord is completed. Once the diagnosis of a primary malignancy such as a sarcoma, cystadenocarcinoma, or malignant neuroectodermal tumor is confirmed in the final pathology report, we recommend a retroperitoneal lymph node dissection, since despite aggressive radiation therapy and chemotherapy, the prognosis for metastatic disease is very poor.

SURGICAL APPROACH

When the nature of the epididymal mass is unclear, an inguinal approach to the epididymis should be carried out. The incision is made above the inguinal ligament and carried down to the fascia of the external oblique muscle. The fascia is opened along the direction of its fibers from the external ring, and the underlying ilioinguinal nerve is identified and preserved. The spermatic cord is identified and gently dissected free of its surrounding structures, and an atraumatic, rubber-shod clamp is placed across the vascular pedicle. The testicle can then be delivered out of the scrotum. The gubernaculum is divided and hemostasis obtained. The testicle is carefully draped off the operating field, and the tunica vaginalis is opened. The testicle and epididymis are carefully palpated and examined. If possible, the mass is carefully dissected off the epididymis and submitted for frozen-section examination. If the mass is malignant or has malignant potential, a standard radical orchiectomy is performed. If the mass is benign, the site of excision is examined for the presence of proper hemostasis and the testicle is replaced in the scrotum in its anatomic position. A transscrotal drain is left in case of extensive dissection.

When the mass involves most of the epididymis, a partial or complete epididymectomy may be in order. The tunica albuginea is opened over the area of the rete testis, and the epididymis is carefully dissected free. Tubules of the rete testis are identified, divided, and cauterized or tied with fine absorbable sutures. The vascular pedicle to the testicle is encountered near the junction of the middle and upper thirds of the testis, and care must be taken to preserve the blood supply. Only the branches to the epididymis are ligated. On completion of the dissection, the vas is identified and divided and the epididymis is submitted as a specimen. The tunica albuginea is loosely reapproximated over the area of excision. Potential complications specific to this type of surgery are testicular atrophy if the vasculature is compromised, and postoperative hematoma. The latter can be reduced by meticulous hemostasis, a scrotal drain, and a pressure dressing.

SUGGESTED READING

Beccia DJ, Krane RJ, Olson CA. Clinical management of non-testicular intrascrotal tumors. J Urol 1976; 116:476–479.

Dovides KC, King LM, Paat F. Primary leiomyosarcoma of the epididymis. J Urol 1975; 114:642–644.

Gogus O, Bulay O, Yudakul T, Beduk Y. A rare scrotal mass: fibrous pseudotumor of the epididymis. Urol Int 1990; 45:63–64.

Golden A, Ash JE. Adenomatoid tumors of the genital tract. Am J Pathol 1945; 21:63.

Gruber MB, Healey GB, Toguri AG, Warren MM. Papillary cystadenoma of the epididymis: component of von Hippel-Lindau syndrome. Urology 1980; 26:305–306.

Murayama T, Fujita K, Ohashi T, Matsuhita T. Melanotic neuroectodermal tumor of the epididymis in infancy: a case report. J Urol 1989; 141:105–106.

CALICEAL DIVERTICULUM

RICHARD K. BABAYAN, M.D.

Caliceal diverticula are eventrations of the pyelocaliceal system into the renal parenchyma that are lined with nonsecretory transitional epithelium. These cystic cavities are usually solitary, small (< 1 cm in diameter), with a predominance in the upper pole calices. They contain urine and communicate directly to the collecting system via a narrow neck. Caliceal diverticula are often asymptomatic and found in both adults and children on routine radiologic assessment (excretory urography), with a reported incidence of 0.21 to 0.45 percent. Many of these asymptomatic diverticula are thought to be congenital in origin, although a number of specific etiologic factors have been suggested. There is a marked increased incidence in children with vesicoureteral reflux. In patients with a history of urinary tract infections, cortical renal abscesses, or obstructing caliceal calculi, inflammatory stenosis of the infundibular neck is a likely causative factor in the subsequent formation of the caliceal diverticulum.

Although most caliceal diverticula are small and asymptomatic, larger ones, especially those found in association with renal calculi, may be the source of pain, recurrent upper tract infection, or hematuria. Longstanding, large caliceal diverticula may be associated with significant overlying parenchymal loss or scarring. In the absence of concomitant caliceal stones, gross hematuria is rarely seen.

Surgical intervention for a caliceal diverticulum is indicated only for persistent symptoms, such as pain, infection, hematuria, or progressive renal deterioration. Intervention is most commonly undertaken in those caliceal diverticula containing calculi.

OPEN SURGICAL PROCEDURES

Until recently, the traditional surgical intervention for a symptomatic caliceal diverticulum was open surgical exploration with either wedge resection and marsupialization of the area, or partial nephrectomy if the diverticulum was in the polar portion of the kidney. Whenever diverticular excision is performed, a careful attempt should be made to identify and obliterate the opening between the diverticulum and the pelvis. Since the early 1980s, however, with the advent of endourologic procedures and the availability of extracorporeal shock wave lithotripsy, the need for open surgical measures has virtually disappeared except in individuals with severe parenchymal scarring and loss of surrounding functional renal tissue.

ENDOUROLOGIC APPROACHES

In the last decade, three minimally invasive techniques have been successfully employed in the treatment of caliceal diverticula: (1) direct percutaneous puncture, (2) retrograde ureteroscopic manipulation, and (3) extracorporeal shock wave lithotripsy (ESWL).

Direct Percutaneous Puncture

The direct percutaneous approach to the treatment of symptomatic caliceal diverticula (Fig. 1) was a natural extension of percutaneous nephrostolithotomy. In so far as stones are commonly found within symptomatic diverticula, percutaneous techniques were a logical means of eliminating the calculi without having to resort to open surgery. It was soon discovered that a number of simple endourologic manuevers could be employed to eliminate recurrent symptoms.

The simplest and most commonly used endourologic technique is direct percutaneous puncture of the diverticulum in question. If the caliceal diverticulum is large and contains stones, direct skinny needle puncture of the cystic cavity can be performed under fluoroscopy, with or without ultrasonic guidance. Once urine is obtained to ensure proper placement of the needle, contrast material can be instilled to distend the diverticulum and allow proper placement of a guidewire. Alternatively, before the puncture, flexible cystoscopy can be performed and an occlusion balloon catheter placed at the level of the ureteropelvic junction. Contrast material is injected retrograde through this catheter to allow filling of the caliceal diverticulum. This latter technique is sometimes

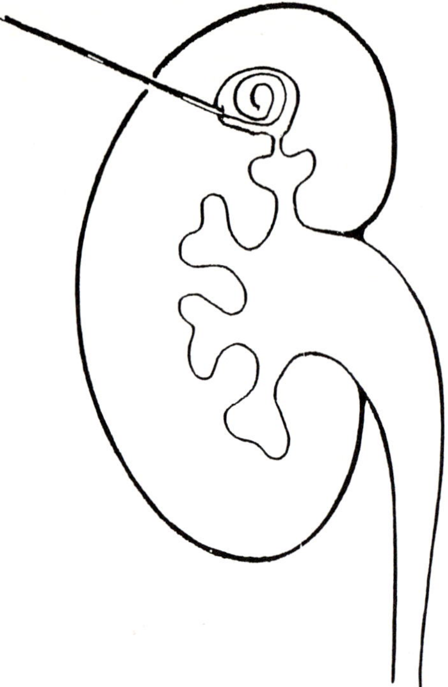

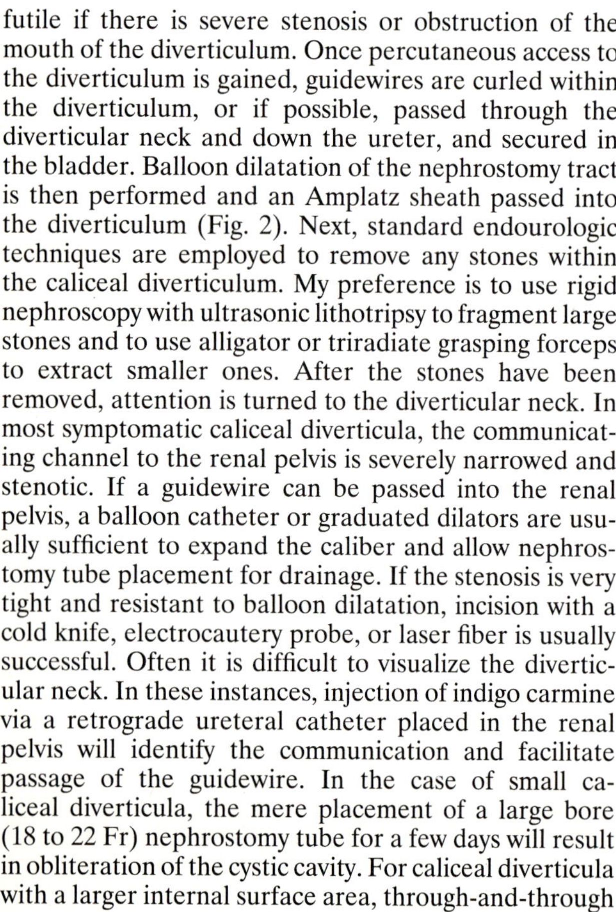

Figure 1 Upper pole caliceal diverticulum: direct percutaneous puncture.

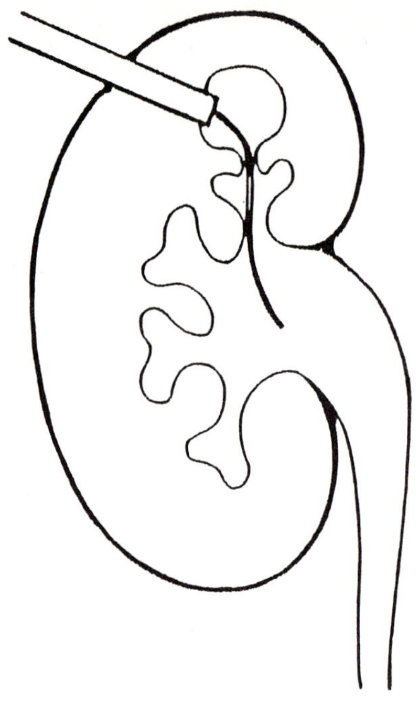

Figure 2 Amplatz sheath placed into the diverticulum with the guidewire passing into the renal pelvis.

futile if there is severe stenosis or obstruction of the mouth of the diverticulum. Once percutaneous access to the diverticulum is gained, guidewires are curled within the diverticulum, or if possible, passed through the diverticular neck and down the ureter, and secured in the bladder. Balloon dilatation of the nephrostomy tract is then performed and an Amplatz sheath passed into the diverticulum (Fig. 2). Next, standard endourologic techniques are employed to remove any stones within the caliceal diverticulum. My preference is to use rigid nephroscopy with ultrasonic lithotripsy to fragment large stones and to use alligator or triradiate grasping forceps to extract smaller ones. After the stones have been removed, attention is turned to the diverticular neck. In most symptomatic caliceal diverticula, the communicating channel to the renal pelvis is severely narrowed and stenotic. If a guidewire can be passed into the renal pelvis, a balloon catheter or graduated dilators are usually sufficient to expand the caliber and allow nephrostomy tube placement for drainage. If the stenosis is very tight and resistant to balloon dilatation, incision with a cold knife, electrocautery probe, or laser fiber is usually successful. Often it is difficult to visualize the diverticular neck. In these instances, injection of indigo carmine via a retrograde ureteral catheter placed in the renal pelvis will identify the communication and facilitate passage of the guidewire. In the case of small caliceal diverticula, the mere placement of a large bore (18 to 22 Fr) nephrostomy tube for a few days will result in obliteration of the cystic cavity. For caliceal diverticula with a larger internal surface area, through-and-through

transit of the postprocedure nephrostomy tube may be insufficient trauma to the epithelial lining to result in its complete elimination. In these cases, it is prudent to fulgurate the entire epithelial lining with a roller or bugby electrode to ensure its subsequent collapse and obliteration. In this latter event, it is often wise to leave the nephrostomy tube in place longer than the usual 24 to 48 hours after the procedure.

Retrograde Ureteroscopic Manipulation

In rare instances, direct percutaneous puncture of a caliceal diverticulum is technically difficult owing to anatomic variations or anomalies. In these patients, a retrograde ureteroscopic approach may be taken. During the last 5 years, a number of narrow-caliber ($<$ 10 Fr), flexible, deflectable ureterorenoscopes have been manufactured that allow excellent visualization and access to the entire upper collecting system via retrograde transurethral, transvesical passage of the instrument up the ureter into the renal pelvis. As mentioned previously, the mouth of a caliceal diverticulum may be very difficult to see, even with the best available optical imaging systems. It is therefore important to use direct injection of dilute contrast through the ureterorenoscope along with C-arm fluoroscopy to aid in localization of the diverticular opening. Once it is found, the same principles as used in the antegrade approach are applied. A guidewire is passed into the diverticulum and the neck is dilated with a balloon catheter. In rare instances, it may be necessary to incise a stenotic diverticular ostium with a Greenwald electrode to allow entry into the cavity. Since ultrasonic lithotripsy probes cannot be passed through the small flexible ureterorenoscopes, it is necessary to use laser or electrohydraulic lithotripsy probes to fragment large stones and allow their evacuation down the collecting system. A retrograde stent is left in place at the completion of the procedure.

Extracorporeal Shock Wave Lithotripsy

ESWL has a limited though sometimes effective role in the management of symptomatic caliceal diverticula. If the neck of the diverticulum is not stenotic and the presence of stones within it is the primary cause of symptoms, it is possible to provide symptomatic relief with ESWL treatment alone. It is important to administer a sufficient number of shocks to pulverize the stones into very fine particles in order to facilitate egress from the diverticulum. Some proponents of ESWL argue that fragmentation alone provides symptomatic relief and that complete elimination of the fragments is not necessary.

A number of surgical options are available for the treatment of symptomatic caliceal diverticula. The choice of treatment must be individualized to each patient and is dependent on the technical expertise of the urologic surgeon. The trend in management is clearly moving away from open surgery toward less invasive management techniques.

SUGGESTED READING

Hulbert JC, Reddy PK, Hunter DW, et al. Percutaneous techniques for the management of caliceal diverticula containing calculi. J Urol 1986; 135:225–227.
Hulbert JC, Lapointe S, Reddy PK, et al. Percutaneous endoscopic fulguration of a large-volume caliceal diverticulum. J Urol 1987;138:116–117.
Middleton AW Jr, Pfister RC. Stone containing pyelocaliceal diverticulum: embryogenic, anatomic, radiologic and clinical characteristics. J Urol 1974; 111:2–6.
Puppo P, Buttino P, Germinale F, et al. Management of caliceal stones resistent to extracorporeal shock wave lithotripsy. J Endourol 1989; 3:367–373.
Wolfsohn MA. Pyelocaliceal diverticula. J Urol 1980; 123:1–8.

SIMPLE RENAL CYSTS

JOHN A. BELIS, M.D.
D. FRANKLIN MILAM, M.D.

Renal cyst is the most common renal mass. Intravenous urography (IVU) or computed tomography (CT) of the abdomen often incidentally demonstrate renal cysts. Simple renal cysts do not communicate with the renal collecting system and are unilocular, but multiple simple cysts may occur in either kidney. With increasing age, both the number of renal cysts and their diameter increase. Most simple renal cysts are benign, and surgical intervention is seldom indicated. Surgery for simple renal cysts should be reserved for those that become symptomatic or have radiologic features that do not meet the criteria for simple cysts.

DIAGNOSIS

The initial evaluation of a renal mass found on IVU is to perform diagnostic ultrasonography (Fig. 1). If the mass meets the ultrasonographic criteria for a simple cyst, surgery is not indicated. The criteria for simple cyst on ultrasonography is that the cyst is anechoic, has a smooth posterior wall, has posterior wall enhancement, and has a spherical or oval shape. No further evaluation or therapy is necessary when all these criteria are met.

If these criteria are not met, CT is used to differentiate with high accuracy a cystic mass from a solid mass. The criteria for simple renal cyst on CT are water density, no enhancement with contrast media, a thin smooth wall with a round or oval shape, and smooth interaction with surrounding renal tissue. If calcification is present, it should be confined to the thin cyst rim.

If the diagnosis of a simple cyst cannot be made at this stage in the evaluation, renal arteriography and cyst puncture with aspiration, cytology, and cystography may be performed. These procedures may also fail to clarify the issue. It is therefore reasonable to proceed with surgery after ultrasonography and CT.

There are two main indications for surgical treatment of simple renal cysts. First are renal masses that cannot be diagnosed radiographically as simple renal cysts, and second are simple cysts that are symptomatic. The indications for surgery of symptomatic renal cysts include obstruction of the collecting system, pain, drainage of infected cysts (rare), and preservation of renal parenchyma when expansion of cysts may cause atrophy of parenchyma in patients with diminished renal function. Hemorrhage into a cyst may cause sudden onset of back or abdominal pain, and hematuria may occur if there is bleeding into the renal collecting system. Hemorrhage may also produce difficulty in definitive radiologic diagnosis and may appear hyperdense on CT.

Although the diagnostic accuracy of ultrasonography and CT for simple renal cysts exceeds 95 percent, a few patients will require surgical exploration for diagnosis. The most important indicators for surgery are radiographic findings that have any deviation from clear

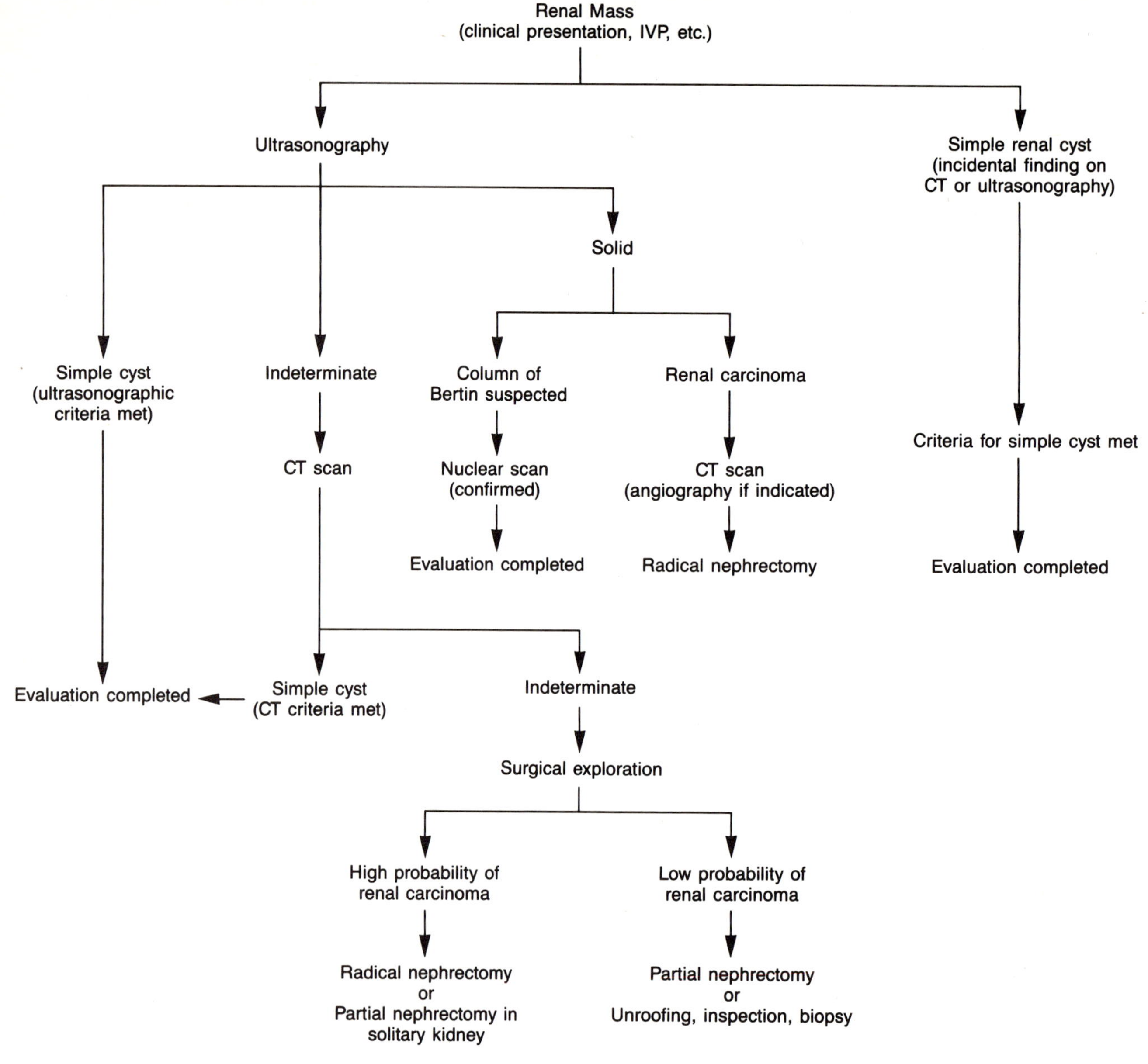

Figure 1   Evaluation of renal mass.

criteria for a simple renal cyst, or clinical symptoms that make the physician suspicious of a renal carcinoma. Some of the radiographic findings are a complex mass on ultrasonography, irregularity of the cyst wall, indeterminate density on CT scan, and calcifications within the mass. The rare incidence of a simultaneous renal cyst and renal tumor should be considered if atypical radiologic features are present. This would include a cystic lesion that has a thick wall as seen on ultrasonography. Aspiration, cytology, and cystography may be misleading, and surgery is indicated.

If suspicion of a tumor is high, radical nephrectomy should be performed; if suspicion is low, partial nephrectomy with a good surgical margin is sufficient. If patho-

logic examination reveals a tumor in the specimen, radical nephrectomy should be performed. A renal cyst associated with an enlarging mass, pain, or hematuria should raise suspicion of a tumor. Surgical exploration is also indicated if cyst aspiration demonstrates bloody fluid, since there is a significant incidence of tumor associated with hemorrhage into a renal cyst.

Although the most common problem is differentiation between renal carcinoma and simple renal cyst, there may be difficulty in distinguishing between multiple simple cysts and multilocular cysts (multilocular cystic nephroma). If ultrasonography, CT, and angiography suggest multilocular cysts, appropriate therapy is nephrectomy, or partial nephrectomy in a solitary kidney. If one is unable to differentiate a small multilocular lesion from multiple single cysts, partial nephrectomy is a reasonable approach. Partial nephrectomy is adequate only after the surgeon has determined that there is no tumor in the resected mass.

An incidental cyst found in the operating room and appearing as a classic cyst is probably best treated by surgical unroofing. This is preferable to performing a postoperative diagnostic evaluation with possible repeat surgery at a later date.

SURGICAL PROCEDURE

Percutaneous decompression of renal cysts can be performed, but cyst fluid often reaccumulates. Percutaneous internal drainage of a renal cyst into the renal collecting duct may also be performed, but the potential for causing a poorly drained appendage to the collecting system generally makes such procedures less desirable than open surgery. Percutaneous resection of a renal cyst wall has also been described, but its efficacy remains to be demonstrated and its potential use appears limited to symptomatic cysts where there is no evidence of tumor. Definitive surgical therapy is advisable if the patient can tolerate the procedure.

The choice of surgical procedure should be related to the possibility of tumor. For lesions with malignant features, a radical nephrectomy or a partial nephrectomy in a solitary kidney should be performed. For lesions with primarily benign but equivocal features, including hemorrhagic simple cysts and complex cysts with hemorrhage, partial nephrectomy with a good surgical margin should be performed followed by pathologic evaluation. For benign-appearing lesions with symptoms, the following surgical procedures for renal cysts may be carried out.

An extraperitoneal flank or anterior subcostal extraperitoneal incision is made. The fascia is entered and the area of the renal cyst exposed. The surgical area is packed off and the cyst aspirated. The wall of the cyst is excised near its junction with normal renal tissue, leaving a rim of cyst wall. Further resection into renal tissue is not necessary and may cause troublesome bleeding. The rim may be fulgurated or sutured as needed to control bleeding.

If the cyst is deep within renal parenchyma, a window of renal tissue may be removed to perform a marsupialization of the cyst. Hemostasis of the renal parenchyma is obtained with 4-0 chromic interrupted sutures. If possible, the renal capsule is sutured to the wall of the cyst with 4-0 chromic continuous suture.

The interior of a cyst should be inspected and any suspicious areas biopsied and sent for frozen section. The inner lining of the cyst otherwise should not be violated. Care must be taken to avoid large dilated vessels in the base of the cyst. The area should not be biopsied unless suspicious for tumor. If opened, the renal collecting system must be closed with a watertight suture.

A peripelvic cyst may be large and may require a more extensive surgical procedure. The cyst may be accessible through the renal sinus or through a pyelotomy. A vein retractor can be used to retract renal tissue and facilitate access into the renal sinus. One must be careful to avoid renal vessels. Occlusion of the renal artery on a short-term basis may be helpful to soften the renal parenchyma and permit further exposure to the renal sinus. Warm renal ischemia should be limited to 20 minutes; ice slush should be used if longer ischemic intervals are needed. If it is confirmed that the mass lesion is a cyst, the fluid again is aspirated and the anterior cyst wall is excised. Internal inspection is performed as described above. The cyst may be marsupialized externally or into the renal pelvis.

A drain is placed in the area of the cyst bed and brought extraperitoneally through a separate stab wound. The incision is closed in layers in the usual fashion. The drain is removed when postoperative drainage is minimal.

SUGGESTED READING

Abt AB, Demers LM, Schochat SJ. Cystic nephroma: an ultrastructure and biochemical study. J Urol 1979; 122:539.

Dalton D, Neiman H, Grayhack JT. The natural history of simple renal cysts: a preliminary study. J Urol 1986; 135:905.

Hulbert JC, Hunter D, Young AT, Castaneda-Zuniga W. Percutaneous intrarenal marsupialization of a perirenal cystic collection—endocystolysis. J Urol 1988; 139:1039.

Madewell JE, Goldman SM, Davis CJ Jr, et al. Multilocular cystic nephroma: a radiographic-pathologic correlation of 58 patients. Radiology 1983; 146:309.

AUTOSOMAL DOMINANT POLYCYSTIC KIDNEY DISEASE

LILLY BARBA, M.D.
PETER N. BRETAN, Jr., M.D.

Occasionally the practicing urologist is consulted for complications arising in patients with autosomal dominant polycystic kidney disease (ADPKD). Although symptoms associated with ADPKD most commonly present in the fourth or fifth decade of life, cyst formation may be identified in utero. Cyst formation is caused by progressive proliferation of epithelial cells, and while most are predominantly renal in origin, many cysts are observed in the liver, spleen, and pancreas. ADPKD is the most common form of cystic disease of the kidney, affecting one in 500 patients, and approximately 500,000 Americans. Progressive renal failure is not uncommon with ADPKD, and this contributes 8 to 10 percent to the incidence among those with end-stage renal disease. When preoperative assessment is sought, associated potentially complicating entities must be ruled out, such as manifestations of mitral or aortic insufficiency, hiatal hernia, and diverticulosis. During the course of development of associated signs and symptoms of ADPKD, the urologist may be consulted on the management of hematuria, infection, pain, renal calculi, or possible neoplasm. The purpose of this chapter is to outline suggested therapies.

HEMATURIA AND HEMORRHAGE

Hematuria is frequently observed microscopically or macroscopically and usually is not related to trauma but occurs spontaneously. Given the potential for enlarged kidneys, patients should be cautioned against participating in contact sports that may lead to traumatic cyst rupture and subsequent hemorrhage. An individual patient may note gross hematuria that may be associated with pain, and may seek medical attention. Most cases of hemorrhage are self-limited and can be treated conservatively with bed rest, hydration, and analgesics. The associated hematuria may abate within days, as in the case of gross hematuria, or be unrelenting, as in the case of microscopic hematuria. Intervention may be warranted in patients in whom significant blood loss or obstruction occurs.

The most frequent cause of hematuria is rupture of a cyst into the renal pelvis. On occasion, obstruction related to clot formation in the pelvis or ureter may develop. These patients commonly have pain. Induced diuresis may be helpful in alleviating the obstruction. Infrequently, catheter decompression may become necessary, but this carries the risk of infection. Surgical intervention is rarely required.

Intraparenchymal or subcapsular hemorrhage may also occur secondary to trauma or to blood vessel rupture into a cyst. Occasionally, significant bleeding into the retroperitoneal space may occur. These forms of bleeding may not be associated with gross hematuria. The patient, however, may note pain and abdominal fullness, or may become symptomatic from blood loss. The diagnosis is usually established clinically and by computed tomography (CT). Conservative and supportive treatment should be instituted when possible. In the azotemic patient under hemodialysis, desmopressin acetate may be helpful. Also, heparin dosage should be modified during hemodialysis treatments. When bleeding is unrelenting, segmental arterial embolization or percutaneous arterial infarction may become necessary. Nephrectomy should be reserved for when the patient becomes hemodynamically unstable.

INFECTION

Urinary tract infections are common in patients with polycystic kidney disease and may pose serious threats. Infections usually occur in an ascending order and may present as cystitis, pyelonephritis, and cystic infections. Pyuria may be seen and does not always signify infection. It is often difficult to distinguish pyelonephritis from cyst infection. The latter should be considered when a patient with ADPKD has fever, new or worsening flank pain, and pyuria without white cell casts. Urine and blood cultures may be helpful if positive. Failure to respond to standard antibiotic therapy for pyelonephritis remains the best clinical indicator of cyst infection.

Radiographic studies, especially when they are dependent on renal function, may not be helpful in identifying cyst infections. CT may be unable to differentiate a hemorrhagic from an infected cyst. An infected cyst, however, may appear to be thick walled on CT. A gallium scan may be helpful when positive, but many false-negative results are seen. Recently, indium-111 leukocyte imaging has proved helpful in localizing an infected cyst; its advantage lies in the lack of bowel or renal excretion and its nondependence on renal function. Cyst aspiration is not advised, given the great number of cysts and the possibility of infecting noninvolved renal tissue.

A course of parenteral antibiotics is warranted when a urinary infection is suspected and supported clinically. The urine culture may not be diagnostic. Coliforms, bacteroides, and staphylococcal organisms are common. Initial antibiotic therapy should consist of an aminoglycoside and a cephalosporin or penicillin. However, these antibiotics may not penetrate the infected cyst. Lipid soluble antibiotics such as chloramphenicol, clindamycin, tetracycline, trimethoprim, erythromycin, and metronidazole have been shown to enter cysts. The fluoroquinolones ciprofloxacin and norfloxacin have also been shown to penetrate infected cysts. Lipid-soluble antibiotics should be instituted when conventional antibiotic therapy fails. Intravenous antibiotic therapy should be followed by oral antibiotic administration for weeks to ensure eradication of the infecting organism. When a renal calculi is present, it may be impossible to treat an infection effectively without removing the stone. In cases of intractable, symptomatic cyst infection, nephrectomy may be required. An extraperitoneal incisional approach is advocated.

PAIN

As nephron cystic enlargement and eventual renal distention occur, a patient with ADPKD may experience unrelenting and disabling abdominal and flank pain. As with all acute attacks of pain, the pain of ADPKD must be distinguished from cyst infection, calculus formation, hemorrhage, or tumor. The pain may be treated with analgesics and narcotics, but care should be taken not to prescribe potentially nephrotoxic agents such as nonsteroidal anti-inflammatory agents.

Percutaneous aspiration and drainage of large symptomatic cysts may be attempted if an identifiable cyst can be correlated with pain. However, this generally is not helpful for long-term pain control. Surgical decompression, first described by Rovsing, has recently been revived for patients with poorly controlled pain. Concern regarding the reduction of renal mass with surgical decompression caused disfavor for this procedure, but it merits closer examination. Finally, nephrectomy remains an option for patients with intractable pain. Large kidneys are removed more safely via an anterior approach. Bilateral nephrectomies are readily accomplished by means of a Chevron (bilateral subcostal) incision.

NEPHROLITHIASIS

Renal calculi have been described in about 15 to 20 percent of patients with ADPKD. Stone composition includes uric acid, calcium oxalate, calcium phosphate, and struvite. Most stones are in intrarenal or intracaliceal locations; less common sites are the ureter and renal pelvis. Radiographically, the stones may have an opaque, a faintly opaque, or a bull's eye appearance. Uric acid and calcium oxalate stones are most frequently seen.

Anatomic obstruction of the renal collecting system is thought to be the most important determinant for the formation of stones. Nevertheless, metabolic factors may also be important. For example, patients with ADPKD have a tubular defect in the excretion of ammonium, resulting in acidic urine and decreased solubility of other excreted substances. The decreased excretion of citrate, probably secondary to a mild acidosis, also influences the excretion of calcium. Generally, renal calculi should be evaluated as with other stone formers. On occasion, they may become symptomatic, depending on the location. Stones may be retrieved cystoscopically or may require surgical intervention. Nephrectomy may be needed, if there is unrelenting infection or pain or if the patient is awaiting kidney transplantation.

NEOPLASM

Renal cell carcinomas are difficult to detect and evaluate in patients with ADPKD, given the large renal size and number of cysts. The incidence of neoplasia is unknown, but it has been seen in hemodialysis-dependent patients and transplant recipients. Evaluation for a possible renal cell carcinoma should be prompted by a new or unusual pattern of hematuria, weight loss, increasing flank pain, or fever. Radiographic evidence includes discrepancy in renal size or a large hemorrhagic cyst. Contrast CT or angiography may be helpful in evaluating a potential carcinoma. Radical nephrectomy is the therapy of choice, especially in a hemodialysis-dependent patient, because of the association with acquired renal cystic disease and renal cell carcinoma.

SUGGESTED READING

Bennett WM, Elzinga L, Golper TA, Barry JM. Reduction of cyst volume for symptomatic management of autosomal dominant polycystic kidney disease. J Urol 1987; 137:620–622.

Bretan PN Jr, Price DC, McClure RD. Localization of abscess in adult polycystic kidney by indium-111 leukocyte scan. Urology 1988; 32:169–171.

Grantham JJ. Polycystic kidney disease: neoplasia in disguise. Am J Kidney Dis 1990; 15:110–116.

Torres VE, Erickson SB, Smith LH, et al. The association of nephrolithiasis and autosomal dominant polycystic kidney disease. Am J Kidney Dis 1988; 11:313–325.

RENAL DYSPLASIA, HYPOPLASIA, MULTICYSTIC KIDNEY, AND POLYCYSTIC KIDNEY DISEASE IN CHILDHOOD

JONATHAN ROSS, M.D.
JACK S. ELDER, M.D.

RENAL DYSPLASIA AND HYPOPLASIA

There is often confusion regarding the precise meaning of the terms used to describe renal maldevelopment. In 1987 the Section on Urology of the American Academy of Pediatrics adopted a report on the classification of these disorders (Table 1).

Renal dysgenesis refers to abnormal size, shape, or structure of kidney development. Examples include dysplasia, hypoplasia, hypodysplasia, aplasia, agenesis, and dysmorphism.

Renal dysplasia is a histologic diagnosis indicating abnormal metanephric differentiation, although the diagnosis also may be suggested by gross examination of the kidney, and its presence often can be predicted on the basis of the clinical and radiologic findings. Dysplastic changes usually affect the entire kidney, although sometimes they are focal. In patients with complete duplication of the collecting system with upper pole obstruction, as in ectopic ureterocele, the upper pole often is dysplastic. Renal dysplasia is characterized primarily by the presence of primitive ducts lined by columnar or cuboidal epithelium, and there may also be metaplastic cartilage. Primitive glomeruli, tubules, and ductules, as well as cysts, often are seen, but these also occur in other conditions and thus are not pathognomonic of dysplasia.

Table 1 Classification of Hypoplasia and Hypodysplasia

Hypoplasia
  Simple hypoplasia (oligonephronia)
    Normal ureteral orifice
    Abnormal ureteral orifice
  Oligomeganephronia
  Segmental hypoplasia

Hypodysplasia
  Normal ureteral orifice
    With obstruction
    Without obstruction
  Abnormal ureteral orifice
    Lateral ectopia
    Medial or caudal ectopia and ureteroceles
  Urethral obstruction
  Prune-belly syndrome

Modified from Glassberg KI, Stephens FD, Lebowitz RL, et al. Renal dysgenesis and cystic disease of the kidney: a report of the Committee on Terminology, Nomenclature and Classification, Section on Urology, American Academy of Pediatrics. J Urol 1987; 138:1085–1092. © by Williams & Wilkins.

Hypoplasia refers to a small kidney or segment of a kidney with fewer than normal nephrons, without dysplastic elements. If hypoplasia and dysplasia coexist, the term hypodysplasia is preferred. A synonym that may be used for hypoplasia is oligonephronia. This should not be confused with oligomeganephronia, which usually is bilateral, and in which not only is there a reduced number of nephrons in the affected kidney, but also each nephron is significantly increased in size, with glomerular volumes that may be seven to ten times normal and with proximal tubular lengths that are four times normal.

Normally the ureteral bud, a diverticulum of the mesonephric duct, induces the metanephric blastema to differentiate into the kidney at 5 to 6 weeks of gestation. The metanephric blastema differentiates into the nephron units, while the ureteral bud becomes the collecting system, including the collecting ducts, calices, renal pelvis, and ureter. Development of the collecting system is completed by 20 weeks of gestation, and nephrogenesis by 36 weeks.

An abnormality in the position or timing of the inductive process, or prolonged severe obstruction, may result in renal dysplasia. According to the theory of Mackie and Stephens, if the ureteral bud exits the mesonephric duct in an abnormal position, its interaction with the metanephric blastema may also be abnormal, resulting in disruption of nephrogenesis and possible dysplasia. Clinical examples in which dysplasia may occur include ectopic ureterocele and ureter, posterior urethral valves, prune-belly syndrome, urethral atresia, vesicoureteral reflux, ureteropelvic junction (UPJ) obstruction, and multicystic dysplastic kidney. When a kidney is dysplastic, by definition it does not function. The management of renal dysplasia is individualized to the particular clinical situation.

A ureterocele is an example of a disorder in which dysplasia may result because of early embryologic obstruction (delayed rupture of Chwalle's membrane) and/or medial and caudal ureteral ectopia. In children, ureteroceles are usually ectopic. Ectopic ureteroceles occur three to four times more commonly in girls. Complete duplication of the urinary tract occurs in more than 90 percent of girls with a ureterocele, whereas in boys, only 60 percent have a duplicated system. When a ureterocele occurs in a duplicated urinary tract, it always drains the upper pole. Most children with a ureterocele are diagnosed after a febrile urinary tract infection, although an increasing number are being discovered by antenatal ultrasonography. Evaluation of the upper urinary tract with ultrasonography and excretory urography and/or renal scan provides a guide to management. In a duplicated system, the obstructed upper pole usually has little or no function, and upper pole heminephrectomy is the initial form of treatment. If the upper pole demonstrates significant function, however, upper-to-lower pole pyelopyelostomy is preferred. Histologically, the upper pole usually shows severe dysplasia and pyelonephritic changes. In addition, many patients have foci of nodular renal blastema, which also is found in some kidneys with Wilms' tumor and has unknown malignant potential. In selected cases, on gross inspection the upper pole may appear to have thick parenchyma, and a biopsy with frozen section helps determine whether to preserve or remove the upper pole.

An ectopic ureter also usually drains the upper pole of a duplicated system, but the upper pole is more likely to function than with an ectopic ureterocele, in which the obstructive component is more severe. If the upper pole does not function, upper pole heminephrectomy is preferred.

In boys with posterior urethral valves, dysplasia occurs in two clinical settings. In the most severe cases of bladder outlet obstruction, the kidneys are totally dysplastic and there is no potential for renal function after decompression of the lower urinary tract. Antenatal ultrasonography shows bilateral hydroureteronephrosis and a distended bladder with oligohydramnios. Typically the kidneys are echogenic and small cysts, which are pathognomonic of dysplasia, may be apparent. Perinatal mortality is nearly 100 percent because of pulmonary hypoplasia. The other situation in which dysplasia occurs is the vesicoureteral reflux and dysplasia (VURD) syndrome, which occurs in approximately 15 percent of boys with valves. Radiologic evaluation demonstrates unilateral high-grade reflux into a nonfunctioning dysplastic kidney, usually on the left side. The significance of the VURD syndrome is that, despite the nonfunctioning kidney, nearly all boys ultimately have normal serum creatinine levels. The explanation for this phenomenon is that the refluxing kidney acts as a pop-off valve for the very high detrusor pressure, allowing nephrogenesis in the nonrefluxing kidney to proceed normally. Treatment consists of ablation of the valve leaflets and nephroureterectomy.

Renal dysplasia also occurs in association with vesicoureteral reflux. Kidneys or segments of kidneys associated with reflux may be scarred or small because of complications from pyelonephritis, or may be congenitally hypoplastic with or without dysplasia. The term "reflux nephropathy" refers to abnormal renal morphology in association with reflux, whether acquired or congenital. Nonfunction of these kidneys is rare. At times primary reflux is detected in the perinatal period during evaluation for antenatal hydronephrosis ("fetal reflux"), and reflux nephropathy may already be apparent, indicating the congenital nature of some renal scarring. Although scarring is an indication for correcting reflux in older children, in infants the rate of spontaneous reflux resolution is significant, even with grade 4 reflux. Consequently, most of these children should be placed on antimicrobial suppression for several years to determine whether the reflux will resolve as they grow. In addition, boys should undergo circumcision to minimize the likelihood of developing a urinary tract infection. If there is progression of scarring on follow-up evaluation or breakthrough infection, ureteral reimplantation should be performed. Some patients have massive reflux and a distended bladder without outlet obstruction; this is called the megacystis-megaureter syndrome. The distended bladder results from aberrant micturition, with most of the voided urine going into the upper tracts. Ultimate management is ureteral reimplantation, which allows the bladder to diminish in size. In infants, however, this procedure carries significant risk for complications, and temporary cutaneous vesicostomy is preferred, allowing the upper tracts to decompress, reducing ureteral caliber, eliminating upper tract stasis, and facilitating later ureteral reimplantation.

A form of reflux nephropathy is the Ask-Upmark kidney, a specific form of segmental hypoplasia. Most of these patients are hypertensive and nearly all have reflux. Females are affected more often than males, and most are over 10 years of age at the time of presentation. Proteinuria and mild-to-moderate renal insufficiency may occur if the disease is bilateral. Affected kidneys have one or more deep grooves on their lateral convexity, beneath which the glomeruli are replaced by "thyroid-like" tubules. Affected segments may be adjacent to areas with normal renal morphology. Although treatment of the reflux has no effect on the hypertension, proteinuria, or renal function, it should prevent further renal damage. If the lesion is unilateral, nephrectomy or partial nephrectomy may cure the hypertension if the contralateral kidney is normal.

MULTICYSTIC DYSPLASTIC KIDNEY

Multicystic dysplastic kidney (MCDK) is the most common renal cystic disease of childhood. These kidneys do not function. The condition occurs more often on the left side and is more common in boys. Some mistakenly refer to an MCDK as a polycystic kidney. Proper nomenclature is important, however, because the latter is a bilateral disease process that is hereditary and often results in renal failure, whereas MCDK generally is not considered to be an hereditary disorder and typically is unilateral.

MCDK usually consists of a central core of stroma surrounded by cysts of varying sizes. There is a tremendous variation in the size; some are extremely large, crossing the midline with minimal stroma, while others are small, with microscopic cysts and composed primarily of stroma. The cysts, which usually do not communicate, are often large and give the kidney a "cluster of grapes" appearance. Microscopically, the stroma contains typical elements of renal dysplasia. In addition, the upper ureter is atretic for a variable length.

The pathoembryology of MCDK is uncertain but presumably is related in some way to the ureteral atresia, which results in total obstruction of the collecting system and disordered nephrogenesis. The ureteral atresia may result from an abnormal ureteral bud, ureteral ischemia secondary to abnormal vascular development, or a defect in the timing or quality of the inductive interaction between the ureteral bud and the metanephric blastema. MCDK represents part of the spectrum termed "infundibulopelvic dysgenesis," in which focal or diffuse narrowing of the infundibulopelvic system can result in a variety of congenital anomalies including infundibulopelvic stenosis, UPJ obstruction, and caliceal diverticulum.

Before the widespread use of antenatal ultrasonography, most MCDKs were diagnosed at birth after palpation of an abdominal mass, and they are recognized as the most common cause of an abdominal mass in newborns. Currently, however, most MCDKs are detected by prenatal ultrasonography. Typically, ultrasonography shows cysts of varying sizes and no identifiable parenchyma. There is also a "hydronephrotic variant" of MCDK in which there is a central large cyst surrounded by smaller cysts of similar size, resembling a hydronephrotic kidney, again with absent parenchyma. Some prenatally diagnosed MCDKs continue to grow throughout gestation, many remain unchanged in size, and an occasional MCDK regresses completely before delivery.

The most important entity in the differential diagnosis is hydronephrosis secondary to a UPJ obstruction. In older children, a cystic Wilms' tumor and a multilocular cyst are also included in the differential diagnosis. The diagnosis of MCDK may be confirmed by a renal scan, which shows nonfunction, although in neonates the MCDK occasionally may demonstrate uptake of radionuclide on 24-hour delayed images. Conversely, it is rare for a hydronephrotic kidney secondary to UPJ obstruction to show nonfunction in neonates. If either test is equivocal, antegrade pyelography should be performed. Typically, the cysts in an MCDK do not communicate. In selected cases a percutaneous nephrostomy may be inserted and left in place for a few days to determine whether the abnormal kidney functions, or surgical exploration may be required to make the diagnosis.

Approximately 25 percent have a contralateral urinary tract anomaly, UPJ obstruction and vesicoureteral reflux being the most common. Consequently, all children with MCDK should undergo careful imaging of the contralateral kidney by ultrasonography and a voiding cystourethrogram. Assessment of glomerular filtration rate (GFR) is important in patients with contralateral anomalies that may affect overall renal function.

Before it became possible to diagnose MCDK accurately by radiologic criteria, these kidneys were explored through a large incision and removed. More recently, however, it has become apparent that most MCDKs are asymptomatic. Serial postnatal ultrasonography demonstrates that many of the cysts regress in size or disappear as the child grows. Indeed, many adults with a diagnosis of unilateral renal agenesis probably were born with a multicystic kidney. However, there have been several case reports of MCDK causing hypertension in infants or undergoing malignant degeneration into Wilms' tumor or renal cell carcinoma in children and adults. Furthermore, careful microscopic examination of the stromal component of MCDK reveals nodular renal blastema in 3 to 6 percent of cases and an occasional Wilms' tumorlet, both of which are lesions with unknown malignant potential. The potential complications of MCDK arise from their stromal and not their cystic component. Consequently, complete regression of the cysts does not mean that the MCDK is benign.

However, the few reports of hypertension and malignant degeneration represent a fraction of all untreated MCDKs, and the question of whether infants with MCDK deserve annual sonographic follow-up for 5, 10, 20 years, or even longer is unresolved. Currently, the Section on Urology of the American Academy of Pediatrics has a registry to study the natural history of MCDK and the morbidity of surgical therapy.

In neonates with MCDK in whom there is a large abdominal mass or hypertension or in whom the diagnosis is uncertain after radiologic evaluation, renal exploration is carried out during the first few weeks of life.

In neonates with asymptomatic MCDK, blood pressure is monitored every 3 months during the first year, and prophylactic antimicrobial agents are prescribed if there is contralateral vesicoureteral reflux. Repeat ultrasonography of the kidney is performed at 4 to 6 months of age. If the kidney is enlarging or the child is hypertensive, nephrectomy is recommended. If the kidney size remains unchanged or is smaller, however, our approach is to discuss candidly the options with the parents. If nephrectomy is selected, the kidney is removed through a 2.5- to 3.0-cm incision, decompressing the cysts to facilitate removal. In most cases, the anesthesiologist administers an intercostal block to minimize postoperative discomfort. In recent years, most of these procedures have been performed on an ambulatory basis. This form of surgical management obviates the need for long-term medical and sonographic follow-up, and the scar is barely visible. Nephrectomy is not recommended if the MCDK is not visible on ultrasonography. If nonsurgical management is chosen, our empiric recommendations are to check the blood pressure every 6 months and perform renal ultrasonography annually until the child is 10 years old or there is total regression of the cysts.

POLYCYSTIC KIDNEY DISEASE IN CHILDHOOD

There are two forms of polycystic kidney disease and both occur in childhood: autosomal recessive polycystic kidney disease (ARPKD, previously referred to as infantile polycystic kidney disease) and autosomal dominant polycystic kidney disease (ADPKD, also termed adult polycystic kidney disease). Terminology is important, because many nonurologists mistakenly refer to a multicystic kidney as a polycystic kidney.

Autosomal Recessive Polycystic Kidney Disease

ARPKD is uncommon, occurring in approximately one in 10,000 to 40,000 live births. Whereas ADPKD is a relatively common cause of end-stage renal failure in adults, only 0.5 to 2.1 percent of children with renal failure have ARPKD. All affected patients have renal and liver changes.

The renal lesion is characterized by cystic dilatation of the collecting ducts and tubules. Glomerular cysts, which are seen in ADPKD, are never present. There is no dysplasia of the renal parenchyma. Grossly, the kidneys are massively enlarged but retain their reniform shape. On cut section, they have a frothy appearance secondary to the myriad small cysts and have been referred to as "tapioca" kidneys. The remainder of the urinary tract is usually normal.

The hepatic lesion consists of proliferation and dilatation of the biliary ducts with periportal fibrosis. Although portal hypertension may occur eventually, the hepatocytes themselves are normal.

All children with ARPKD have both renal and hepatic involvement. However, manifestations of one system or the other may predominate, depending on the age at presentation. For example, when ARPKD is detected in neonates or infants, the renal lesion is the most severe, whereas in patients whose disease develops in childhood or adolescence there are primarily hepatic findings and less obvious renal manifestations. The latter entity has been referred/to as congenital hepatic fibrosis (with renal tubular ectasia). Many patients with congenital hepatic fibrosis have kidney abnormalities other than polycystic kidney disease, however. Previously it was thought that the perinatal and juvenile forms of ARPKD are distinct genetic lesions. More recently, however, it has become apparent that there is one genetic lesion with various phenotypes, and that the ages of onset and severity of the disease within a sibship may be dissimilar.

In the most severe cases, there is oligohydramnios secondary to the extensive renal involvement, and the neonate dies shortly after birth from pulmonary hypoplasia. With improved intensive care, however, some of these infants have survived. Usually the neonate has bilateral flank masses with poor urinary output. If respiratory function improves, so often does renal function, and although the infant may have mild renal insufficiency, the GFR usually is sufficient to allow the child to reach adolescence without needing dialysis. Hypertension can be severe in infants with ARPKD, and the condition usually responds to an angiotensin-converting enzyme inhibitor.

Older children with ARPKD tend to present with complications of hepatic fibrosis, such as hematemesis from bleeding esophageal varices secondary to portal hypertension. Hepatic and splenic enlargement are common on physical examination. Many have anemia, leukopenia, and/or thrombocytopenia secondary to hypersplenism. However, liver enzyme study results are normal. Many of these children have short stature.

The diagnosis of ARPKD is often made by ultrasonography, which shows enlarged, markedly hyperechoic kidneys owing to the reflection of echoes off the innumerable microcysts. In older children, ultrasonography may show foci of brightly increased echogenicity secondary to focal tubular cysts, mimicking nephrocalcinosis. Macrocysts in ARPKD are evident by ultrasonography only in older children. The liver also may show enhanced echogenicity. An intravenous pyelogram (IVP) typically reveals bilateral nephromegaly with persistent nephrograms and radial streaking of contrast material as a result of pooling of the medium in dilated cortical and medullary cysts, or retention of contrast in dilated medullary collecting ducts.

The natural history of ARPKD is variable. Survival depends on the age at presentation. With modern improvements in neonatal intensive care, as many as 50 percent of those presenting at or shortly after birth survive beyond 2 years of age. Renal function tends to improve during the first 2 years of life and then slowly deteriorates. If the individual survives infancy, end-stage renal failure rarely occurs before 4 years of age. However, nearly half of patients with ARPKD develop severe renal insufficiency by the time they reach adolescence, and renal failure is nearly universal in those reaching adulthood. Thus, it is important not to be too pessimistic about the prognosis in counseling parents of children with this disorder. The hepatic aspect of the disease is rarely life-threatening. Some patients may require intervention for portal hypertension, whereas others have subclinical hepatic disease detectable only by ultrasonography or biopsy. None develop liver failure.

In ARPKD, the offspring of heterozygotes carry a 25 percent risk of having the disease. Asymptomatic siblings of a child with ARPKD or congenital hepatic fibrosis should undergo evaluation for renal and hepatic disease.

In selected patients, antenatal diagnosis of ARPKD is possible with ultrasonography. The disease is characterized by enlarged echogenic kidneys, a small or nonvisualized bladder, and oligohydramnios. No cysts are visible. However, ADPKD, Meckel's syndrome, and glomerulocystic disease may have similar sonographic features. In one recent series, 50 percent of affected cases were correctly diagnosed during the second trimester, and most were apparent by 30 weeks of gestation.

Autosomal Dominant Polycystic Kidney Disease

The incidence of ADPKD is approximately one in 1,000, and the disorder accounts for 10 percent of cases of end stage renal failure in adults. Pathologically, ADPKD is characterized by cystic dilatation involving all segments of the nephron. Cysts are distributed randomly throughout the parenchyma, vary in size, and may contain pale fluid or blood. The liver may also contain a few cysts, but there is no portal fibrosis. Since inheritance is autosomal dominant, each offspring has a 50 percent chance of inheriting the gene. Expression among affected family members may vary with regard to age at presentation and severity of involvement.

Expression of ADPKD in childhood is variable. In many cases, the disease is detected during screening of offspring of parents with ADPKD, whereas some children are symptomatic with hematuria, a urinary tract infection, lumbar pain, or intracerebral hemorrhage secondary to a ruptured aneurysm of the circle of Willis (berry aneurysm) or have hypertension, proteinuria, or palpable enlargement of the kidneys. The vast majority of children with manifestations of ADPKD have close relatives with symptoms suggestive of the disease. In many children, renal involvement with ADPKD is asymmetric and occasionally is unilateral. Most neonates in whom the disorder is clinically apparent have bilateral nephromegaly or succumb to pulmonary hypoplasia.

The diagnosis is often made using ultrasonography to identify enlarged kidneys with bilateral renal cysts that are similar in size. Hepatic, pancreatic, and splenic cysts may also be seen. The differential diagnosis includes simple renal cysts, multicystic dysplastic kidney, and multilocular cyst; in infants, tuberous sclerosis and glomerulocystic disease must also be considered. A few small cysts in an at-risk child most likely represent ADPKD, since simple cysts are unusual in normal children. Often, renal imaging of the parents is necessary to establish the diagnosis. However, not all children with ADPKD have abnormal findings on renal ultrasonography. It has been estimated that ultrasonography detects 22 percent of affected individuals during the first decade of life and 66 percent during the second decade.

Antenatal detection is possible using either ultrasonography or molecular genetics. Ultrasonography may show enlarged kidneys with macrocysts, or densely echogenic kidneys that are indistinguishable from ARPKD. In the most severe cases, oligohydramnios is present. Genetic mapping has localized the gene for most cases of ADPKD (PKD1) to the short arm of chromosome 16, but recently a second locus has been identified that is not on chromosome 16 and is responsible for a clinically indistinguishable form of ADPKD. DNA probes have been used prenatally to identify the embryo or fetus with ADPKD in a few cases, but the technology currently is available only in selected centers and costs approximately $2,000.

The prognosis for ADPKD in children is variable and depends on the patient's age at presentation. Approximately half of patients with clinical manifestations at birth or in infancy die of respiratory failure or sepsis. Of cases detected later in childhood, the development of renal failure before adulthood is uncommon.

The treatment of ADPKD in children is essentially the same as in adults. Aggressive management of the complications, such as hypertension and infection, is important to prevent or forestall renal failure.

SUGGESTED READING

Dimmick JE, Johnson HW, Coleman GU, Carter M. Wilms tumorlet, nodular renal blastema and multicystic renal dysplasia. J Urol 1989; 142:484–485.

Elder JS, Klacsmann PG, Sanders RC, Jeffs RD. Flank mass in a neonate. J Urol 1981; 126:94–98.

Gagnadoux A-F, Habib R, Levy M, et al. Cystic renal diseases in children. Adv Nephrol 1989; 18:33–58.

Glassberg KI, Stephens FD, Lebowitz RL, et al. Renal dysgenesis and cystic disease of the kidney: a report of the Committee on Terminology, Nomenclature and Classification, Section on Urology, American Academy of Pediatrics. J Urol 1987; 138:1085–1092.

Kaplan BS, Kaplan P, Rosenberg HK, et al. Polycystic kidney disease in childhood, J Pediatr 1989; 115:867–880.

Susskind MR, Kim KS, King LR. Hypertension and multicystic kidney. Urology 1989; 34:362–366.

PRIMARY URETEROPELVIC JUNCTION OBSTRUCTION

LOWELL R. KING, M.D.

Clear-cut ureteropelvic junction (UPJ) obstruction is said to be present in patients with a dilated renal pelvis, and *caliectasis* in those in whom there is no reflux and the ureter is of normal caliber. Such obstruction must be distinguished from "megacalicosis" (i.e., caliectasis in the absence of obstruction), and disproportionate dilatation of the calices and renal pelvis in patients with reflux.

As many as one in 800 fetuses are found to have pyelocaliectasis. This may resolve spontaneously, or it may persist after birth (in approximately 50 percent of babies). When the condition is persistent, early evaluation with isotope renography differentiates an obstructed hydronephrotic kidney from a multicystic kidney, which seldom functions and never to a significant degree (Fig. 1). Cystography is performed to exclude reflux. Some dilated kidneys function normally and drain promptly, so no obstruction may be present even when caliectasis persists. These babies need follow-up with sonography to at least the age of 2 years, however, as do those with more equivocal drainage patterns, because unequivocal worsening and obstruction may still occur.

If the renal pelvis remains full after the isotope has been excreted, furosemide, 1 mg per kilogram, is given, and the rate at which isotope empties from the dilated renal pelvis is measured via the renogram. Such patients may be found to have obstruction or clearly no obstruction, or may fall into an equivocal group. The nonobstructed and equivocal groups are followed primarily with serial ultrasonography. Those with obstruction, if otherwise healthy, undergo operation as soon as possible, often at 7 to 10 days of age, because the normal neonatal ureter is then dilated relative to the size of the baby. This facilitates pyeloplasty in early infancy. There is no longer any measurable anesthetic risk in children of any age.

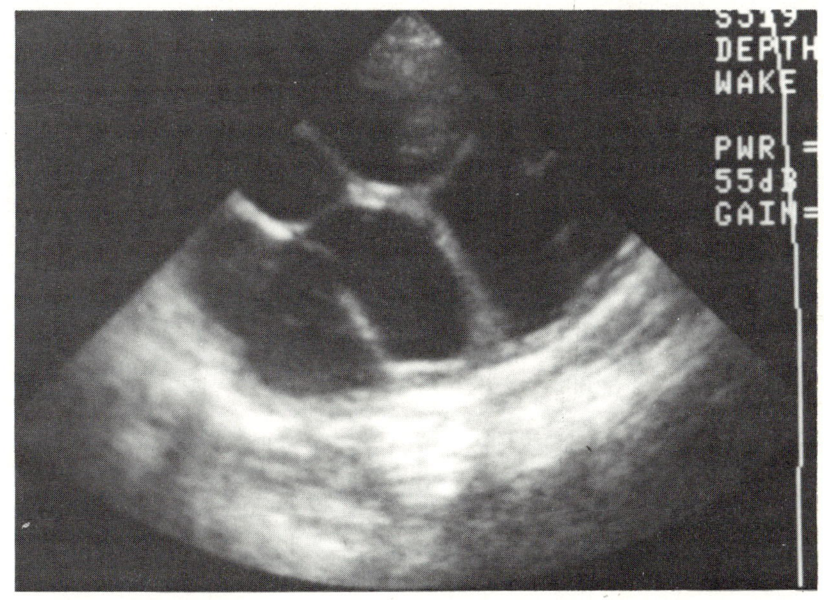

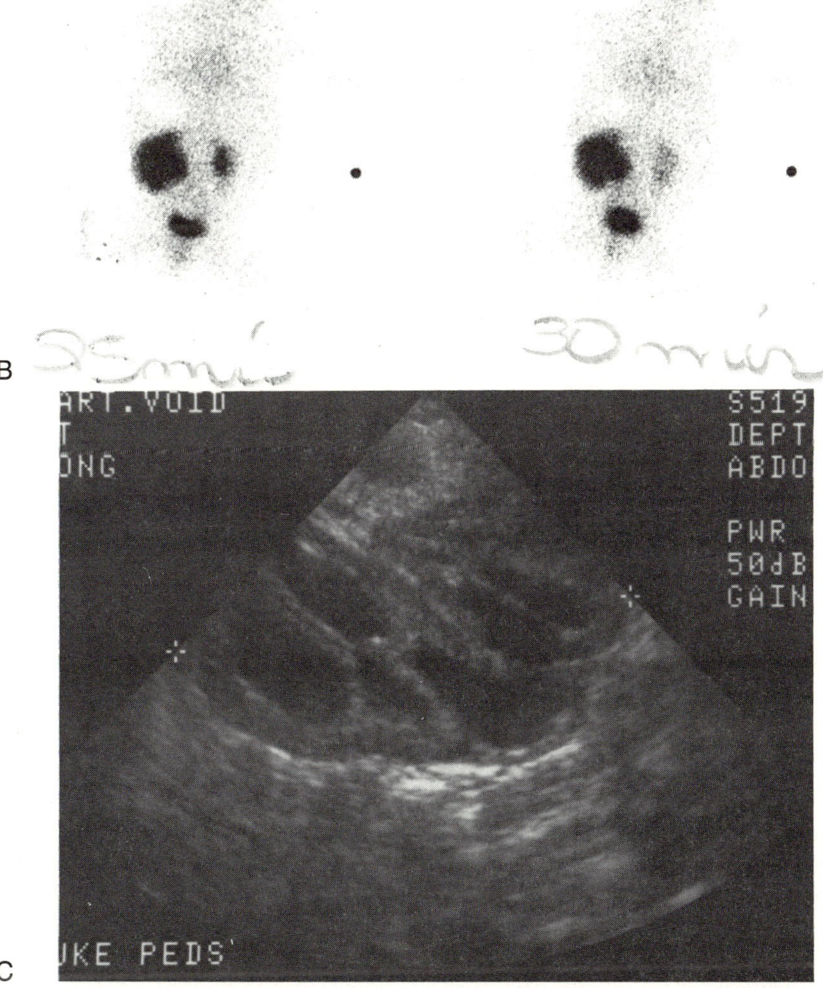

Figure 1 *A,* This ultrasonogram was read as a multicystic kidney, both before the patient's birth and after, by at least six radiologists. There are no apparent communications between the "cysts." The baby was not further evaluated until 3 months of age. *B,* A renal scan then clarified the diagnosis, revealing a typical ureteropelvic junction obstruction. Multicystic kidneys seldom function at all, whereas obstructed kidneys typically have good function in the neonatal period. *C,* Ultrasonogram 5 days following dismembered pyeloplasty, after wound drainage had ceased. Note the collapsed appearance of the dilated calices.

UPJ obstructions also present in infancy as palpable flank masses. In slightly older children, the most common presentation is with hematuria after minor trauma, urinary infection, or abdominal pain. However, urinary tract anomalies are found in only 3 to 4 percent of children with abdominal pain.

Older children and adults may present with any of these signs or symptoms. In those with pain, the initial intravenous pyelogram (IVP) is normal in about 4 percent of older patients with UPJ obstruction who manifest hydronephrosis only when well hydrated or if a diuretic is given during the examination. The pain is generally reproduced at this time.

ETIOLOGY

UPJ obstruction may be due to tight intrinsic stenosis, extreme tortuosity and kinking of the uppermost ureter, a tapering stenosis just below the UPJ, extrinsic bands that compress the ureter, compression between an artery and vein running to the lower pole of the kidney, a high insertion of the ureter into the renal pelvis, or any combination thereof.

Such obstructions are often bilateral and occur frequently with a contralateral multicystic kidney or in conjunction with reflux. Pyelography or renography must then be performed with a functioning catheter, keeping the bladder empty to ascertain whether the supposed obstruction is dilatation secondary to reflux. UPJ obstructions are common in horseshoe kidneys, incompletely rotated kidneys, and crossed-fused ectopia.

Since all causes of UPJ obstruction are amenable to pyeloplasty, no effort is made to determine the precise pathologic cause of the obstruction preoperatively. If a dilated ureter is not visualized on a renal scan, the ureter is probably normal. I consider UPJ obstruction to be diagnosable by IVP, and a cystogram to exclude reflux, when the appearance of the collecting system is typical, and do not obtain a scan on all patients. I then perform retrograde pyelography at the time of the pyeloplasty to be sure that multiple obstructions are not present; I do not routinely do this in male neonates, as urethral instrumentation may result in stricture even when the smallest instruments are employed and the urethra is not overdilated. The ureter can be calibrated intraoperatively by passing a feeding tube from the opened pelvis to the bladder.

The degree of hydronephrosis may remain stable for several years but may also worsen rapidly, so I tend to recommend repair soon after the diagnosis is made. I also try to preserve kidneys with any measurable function in children, because even a very poorly functioning hydronephrotic kidney excretes water well, and therefore should reduce the risk of eventual hyperfiltration glomerulopathy in even a completely normal contralateral kidney. In older adults, obstructed kidneys are often removed when they provide less than 10 percent of overall kidney function or when they are chronically infected. If at all possible, urinary infections should be eradicated before surgery.

PYELOPLASTY

Many have shown that pyeloplasty is successful when a careful procedure is performed using magnification and employing only a drain postoperatively. This is true for all age groups. The reported complication rate in neonates younger than 3 months of age, most often younger than 1 month old at the time of surgery, is less than 2 percent. Nephrostomy drainage is needed in those with inflammation at the time of surgery due to infection or stone, for example, because in this group the anastomotic site is likely to remain edematous for several weeks or months before free drainage to the bladder can be demonstrated at normal intrapelvic pressures. An internal stent does no apparent harm, but an externalized stent adds to postoperative morbidity and provides a pathway for the introduction of infection. I find the option of a double-J stent most attractive and use one in most older children and adults. The double-J is placed from above after the back half of the pyeloplasty is completed and the new anatomic relationships have been established. Such stents usually cause no symptoms and permit almost all pyeloplasty wounds to become dry 1 or 2 days after surgery, facilitating early discharge. A disadvantage is that the stent must be removed by cystoscopy, mandating a second general anesthetic in children 6 to 8 weeks after the initial procedure. However, the occasional prolonged hospitalization for urinary leakage or the need to place a percutaneous nephrostomy postoperatively is avoided.

Techniques of Pyeloplasty

Even in bilateral cases, a flank approach is generally performed. This obviates any risk of intraperitoneal urinary drainage postoperatively, because the peritoneum can usually be avoided, or closed if entered. Since I like to resect much of the dilated extrarenal pelvis, I prefer a subcostal incision to a lumbotomy, in which complete exposure of the extrarenal pelvis is sometimes difficult or impossible. A subcostal incision is always high enough, as the dilated kidney protrudes from beneath the ribs. I favor a relatively generous incision from the paraspinal musculature posteriorly to almost the lateral border of the rectus. The muscle layers are divided in the line of the incision, usually with cautery to minimize blood loss. The 12th intercostal nerve is preserved whenever possible by freeing it from the inferior margin of the rib and retracting it inferiorly. The transversalis muscle fibers are separated by blunt dissection after the lumbodorsal fascia has been incised. The peritoneum is retracted medially, and Gerota's fascia is opened in the posterior angle of the incision. The lower pole of the kidney then comes into view. A 2-0 silk suture is placed deeply into the lower pole as a traction suture to facilitate manipulation. Using blunt or sharp dissection, the kidney is then mobilized, although the upper pole does not need to be freed completely. The pelvis is usually identified as a tense cystic mass that can be cleared of fat as the lower pole is mobilized. The ureter will be seen on the inferior margin of the pelvis, medial to the pelvis, or can be identified below the pelvis, usually attached to the peritoneum. Tagging sutures are placed in the ureter 2 to 3 cm below the UPJ, and in the renal pelvis inferiorly and superiorly, at the 6 and 12 o'clock positions, at a distance of about 1 cm from the parenchyma. The pelvis is then transected in a straight line just distal to these two sutures (Fig. 2). Next, the ureter is transected obliquely just below the UPJ. The medial side of the ureter is left longer. In addition, the lateral edge of the ureter can be spatulated slightly to increase the area of the anastomosis. The entire UPJ is then sent intact for pathologic examination. The ureter is calibrated with a feeding tube at this point if it has not been imaged completely.

In patients of all ages, the anastomosis is performed with 5-0 chromic catgut sutures, all placed so that the knots are outside the lumen of the anastomosis. The first suture approximates the most dependent tip of the pelvis to the lateral margin of the ureter. This suture is then tied. If there is any sensation of tension, the ureter is mobilized for a distance of 4 to 6 cm, or the kidney is completely mobilized and pexed inferiorly, or both. When this stitch ties easily, the back row is completed. All sutures include only a minimal "bite" of tissue, including muscle, perhaps 1 mm on each side. The sutures are close together, perhaps 2 mm apart, and are a little more distant in the pelvis than in the ureter to flare the anastomosis.

After the back wall has been completed, the double-J stent (if one is to be employed) is inserted over a guidewire passed into the bladder. The anterior wall of the pyeloplasty is then completed. If a stent has not been used, the anastomosis is calibrated and inspected when the kidney has been dropped back into its normal position. The pelvis is then irrigated to wash out any clots and closed with 4-0 chromic gut. A drain is positioned over the anastomosis and anchored to the posterior angle of the incision before the wound is closed.

When a double-J stent is not employed, the duration of postoperative wound drainage is unpredictable, but it generally stops in 3 to 5 days. If it continues beyond 7 to 10 days, a percutaneous nephrostomy may reduce morbidity. Two weeks or more after surgery, the nephrostomy tract may be used for balloon dilatation of the repair and insertion of a double-J catheter to internalize drainage.

Other Surgical Options

Several different types of pyeloplasty work equally well or almost equally well. The greatest advance over the past decade has probably been the almost routine use of magnification to permit better suture placement. In the original dismembered pyeloplasty (Hynes-Andersen) a lip of inferior pelvis was preserved and folded down lateral to the spatulated ureter to increase both the dependency of the pelvis and the area of anastomosis. This works well, but is more difficult to visualize and is clearly unnecessary. The Foley Y-plasty is applicable for those with a smaller renal pelvis who do not need resection of excess tissue to reduce dead space. In this procedure, the limbs of the Y are widely separated, one on the anterior and one on the posterior aspect of the pelvis. The posterior aspect of the pelvis then drops inferiorly. The latter border of the ureter is opened through the UPJ at least 1 cm below the narrow point in the ureter. The midportion of the pelvic flap is sutured to the inferior margin of the ureterostomy, converting the incision to a V. Careful attention to suture placement is mandatory in all repairs.

When there is a high insertion of the ureter, and again when pelvic size is not excessive, an inverted U

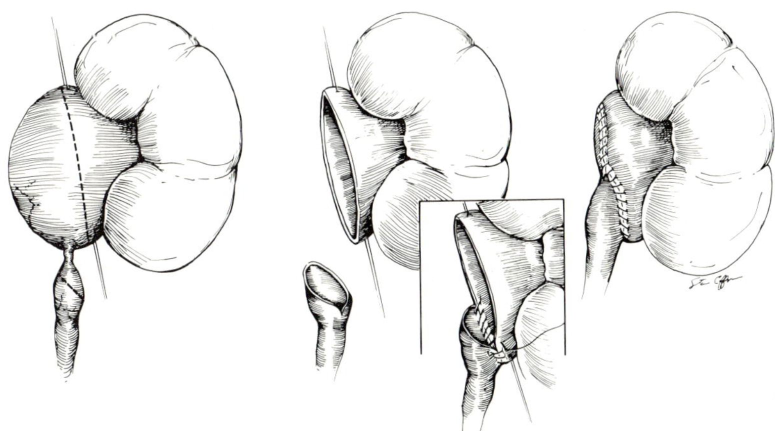

Figure 2 Steps in dismembered pyeloplasty. The pelvis is transected obliquely; the ureter is also transected obliquely, making the medial side longer; the ureter may be spatulated slightly. A precise anastomosis is carried out using 5-0 chromic suture. Knots are placed outside the lumen. The anastomosis is flared slightly by spacing the sutures more on the pelvis than on the ureter (*inset*). The pelvis is closed, and a drain is placed.

incision can be used to lower the UPJ to a dependent position. The medial wall of the pelvis abutting the ureter is opened linearly from the UPJ to the most dependent (inferior) point in the pelvis. The incision is carried through the UPJ and down the facing ureter. The ureteral edges are simply sewn to the adjacent edges of the pelvis, dropping the UPJ into a normal anatomic position.

A long flap of pelvis is occasionally needed when there is a long stricture of the upper ureter (mostly encountered in adults) or a ureteral stricture well below the UPJ, as is occasionally encountered in children. The length of such a flap is limited only by the size of the dilated pelvis. I have used an 11-cm flap successfully, and a longer one is feasible if necessary. The flap should be as broad as possible at the base, perhaps 2 cm, tapering slightly toward the tip. Obviously, the configuration of the vessels on the pelvis should be considered when the flap is planned. The ureter is simply opened through the UPJ to a point 1 cm below the inferior stricture. The flap is rotated alongside the opened ureter and anastomosed edge to edge, with interrupted sutures at the apex and running sutures along the edges.

Adjuncts to Successful Pyeloplasty

In patients with infection, especially, it is preferable to remove a very dilated lower caliceal group to facilitate optimal drainage of the kidney postoperatively. When hydronephrosis is severe, this partial nephrectomy is easily accomplished with minimal blood loss before the pyeloplasty is performed. The cut edges of the parenchyma are approximated with mattress sutures of 3-0 or 2-0 chromic catgut, and the capsule is closed with a running absorbable suture.

Percutaneous Techniques

Percutaneous pyeloplasties now enjoy a success rate of 80 to 85 percent. Usually both an incision through the UPJ and balloon dilatation are performed. A nephrostomy tract is established, usually through an upper pole calix, to facilitate visualization of the UPJ. A guidewire or ureteral catheter is placed from below, through the UPJ if possible. The nephrostomy tract is dilated. A visual urethrotome, typically a small resectoscope with a cold knife, is inserted. The incision through the UPJ is made completely through the ureter, until fat is seen. A second guidewire is placed if not done previously. A balloon catheter, typically 5 or 6 mm in diameter when inflated, is centered at the UPJ and inflated. Dilatation is continued until "wasting" (indentation into the balloon) disappears on fluoroscopy. A double-J catheter is then inserted and left in place for 6 to 8 weeks.

Excellent results have been achieved as both primary and secondary procedures, but these are not yet as good as with conventional open surgery. Also, conventional pyeloplasty is probably less costly in most institutions unless hospitalization is prolonged.

SUGGESTED READING

Chevalier RL, El Dahr S. The case for early relief of obstruction in young infants. In: King LR, ed. Urologic surgery in neonates and young infants. Philadelphia: WB Saunders, 1988:95.

Grignon A, et al. Urinary tract dilatation in utero: classification and clinical applications. Radiology 1986; 160:645.

Flake AW, et al. Ureteropelvic junction obstruction in the fetus. J Pediatr Surg 1986; 21:1058.

King LR, Hatcher PA. Natural history of fetal and neonatal hydronephrosis. Urology 1990; 35:443–448.

Smart WR. Surgical correction of hydronephrosis. In: Harrison JH, Gittes RF, Perlmutter AD, et al, eds. Campbell's urology. 4th ed. Vol 3. Philadelphia, WB Saunders, 1979:2047.

POSTSURGICAL URETEROPELVIC JUNCTION OBSTRUCTION

CULLEY C. CARSON, M.D.

The normal ureteropelvic junction (UPJ) provides a dependent, funnel-shaped exit for urine leaving the kidney and entering the ureter. Peristaltic activity that originates in the renal upper pole caliceal apex is conducted through the renal pelvis and down the ureter. Narrowing of the UPJ can occur as a result of extrinsic, intrinsic, or vascular defects producing a restriction of urinary flow. The resultant compensatory hypertrophy of the renal pelvic wall and renal pelvic dilatation leads to the symptoms of UPJ obstruction and, in some cases, a diminution in tubular function with alteration in urinary concentration and progressive renal failure. Urinary stasis in the renal pelvis can produce calculi or result in urosepsis.

PATIENT SELECTION

Selection of patients for treatment of UPJ obstruction is dependent on documentation of obstruction at the level of the UPJ and its association with symptoms and radiographic findings. Patients requiring treatment vary in age, but most are younger than 20 years old. The most common presenting symptoms include urinary tract infections, intermittent hematuria with or without a history of flank trauma, and intermittent flank pain. Neonates may present with a large flank mass, vague abdominal discomfort to palpation, or symptoms of vomiting and diarrhea often associated with urinary tract infections. Frequently, the symptoms of flank pain and hematuria are associated with increased fluid intake.

For patients in whom UPJ obstruction is suggested on presentation, excretory urography is usually the first procedure performed to document hydronephrosis and obstruction. Confirmation using furosemide to produce a renogram at high urinary flows may help select the patients by producing the flank discomfort and increased renal pelvic dilatation associated with UPJ obstruction during excretory urography. A more accurate and objective method for documenting obstruction is the furosemide-stimulated radioisotope renal scan. This diuretic renography, performed usually with DTPA and followed by administration of 0.3 to 0.5 mg per kilogram of furosemide in a well-hydrated patient, will document an obstructive-appearing renogram curve that remains flat for more than 20 minutes. However, this study may not be diagnostically valid in patients with severely compromised renal function, because the diuretic response will be inadequate.

Evaluation of the lower urinary tract is also imperative before surgical intervention in UPJ obstruction. It is important in children to eliminate the possibility of vesicoureteric reflux and to document a normal distal ureter. Voiding cystourethrography and retrograde or antegrade pyelography should be performed before definitive repair is undertaken.

PREOPERATIVE PREPARATION

Surgery should be performed only after adequate imaging studies have documented UPJ obstruction and eliminated the possibility of other ureteral abnormalities. Urine cultures must demonstrate sterile urine. If renal drainage is shown to be adequate, if calices are of normal caliber, and if the patient has no pain, pyuria, or renal calculi, repair of the UPJ is not appropriate. A period of observation and repetition of radiographic studies may be necessary to confirm the necessity for surgical intervention. When one or both kidneys demonstrate obstruction associated with symptoms, however, surgery is appropriate.

CHOICE OF SURGICAL PROCEDURE

The choice of surgical approach to UPJ obstruction must be on the basis of a combination of history and physical examination and a careful review of the preoperative imaging studies. When renal scan demonstrates minimal renal function and a satisfactory contralateral

kidney, consideration can be given to nephrectomy of the poorly functioning hydronephrotic sac. Similarly, a kidney with multiple cortical abscesses or long-standing pyonephrosis should be removed if the contralateral kidney appears normal.

Classic open repair with a dismembered pyeloplasty should be considered if a ureterovascular defect is identified radiographically suggesting a lower pole vessel crossing the UPJ. This defect is poorly treated with endopyelotomy. Two such cases performed in the Duke University experience have resulted in subsequent open surgical procedure as a result of failed endopyelotomy. While there was little morbidity and no damage to the lower pole crossing vessel associated with the endopyelotomy, the postoperative results demonstrated inadequate urinary flow.

The principles of endopyelotomy are modeled after the descriptions of Davis and Smart in the late 1940s. The Davis intubated ureterotomy was a method of open pyeloplasty and was first described in 1943 as a way to correct UPJ obstruction. The technique involved passing a silver probe down the ureter through a pyelostomy incision. Surgical incision over the probe allowed fine scissors to incise the stenotic UPJ. A large-caliber drainage catheter or stent was placed across the area of incision to the bladder. Separate nephrostomy drainage was maintained for 6 to 8 weeks. Davis's results were acceptable, but his surgical procedure was supplanted by flap and dismembered pyeloplasties. During the healing following Davis's procedures, however, smooth muscle and mucosa of the ureter were documented to regenerate over the large indwelling stent, providing excellent UPJ drainage. Using these principles endoscopically, endopyelotomy has been performed with great success and major open surgery avoided. Earlier results demonstrated that a cold-knife incision was preferable to electrocautery in producing better healing with less scarring and thermal injury. Cold-knife incision preserves ureteral blood flow with decreased tissue destruction.

SURGICAL TECHNIQUE

Adequate percutaneous nephrostomy access is critical to the success of endoscopic approach to the UPJ. This access must be placed so that vision and manipulation of the UPJ is optimal. The best percutaneous access is through the lateral kidney or upper pole calix; lower pole access provides inadequate visualization for endopyelotomy.

Once optimal percutaneous access is gained, an angiographic guidewire or catheter must be passed down the ureter to control incision and act as a safety device for later dilatation stent placement. In cases of severe stenosis or marked dilatation of the renal pelvis, however, antegrade guidewire passage may be impossible. In these situations, initial retrograde ureteral stent placement after retrograde pyelography may be necessary, and this allows retrieval through the nephrostomy tract before UPJ incision. An alternative method for access placement is through the use of retrograde nephrostomy techniques. After adequate positioning of a safety guidewire through the UPJ, the renal access tract is dilated in the standard fashion. The universal nephroscope is then inserted and the UPJ visualized and examined. If a retrograde safety guidewire has been passed, it is grasped by endoscopic forceps and retracted through the percutaneous access tract. This retrograde angiographic guidewire is exchanged for an antegrade guidewire using an open-ended ureteral catheter or safety wire catheter under fluoroscopic control. The guidewire is maintained in position for the entire procedure to guide incision and facilitate postincision stent passage.

If antegrade or retrograde passage of guidewires cannot be accomplished as a result of severe UPJ stenosis, more heroic techniques may be necessary. Methylene blue may be infused into the upper ureter via a ureteral catheter passed to the level of the obstruction. The area of obstruction may be observed with a nephroscope as methylene blue passes through the stenotic UPJ. The incision can be carried out through the methylene blue–defined tract. Because a safety guidewire is not present, however, this technique provides significant risk, and avulsion of the ureter or unsuccessful stenting is possible. If the methylene blue is visualized, however, initial incision should be followed by immediate, direct vision placement of a safety guidewire to maintain control of the incised ureter. Other possible procedures include retrograde placement of a fiberoptic light source or ureteroscope to the level of the UPJ. If a thin obstructing membrane is present at the UPJ, the light may be visible within the renal pelvis with the nephroscope light extinguished. Under these circumstances, a short incision may be carried out over the area of visible light and the connection established. Because this is also a poorly controlled technique without a safety guidewire present, ureteral avulsion and further stenosis are significant possibilities.

Once the UPJ is adequately visualized, clotted blood, debris, and any renal calculi can be removed before the incision is made. Cold-knife incision can be carried out using the direct vision endopyelotome, which is specially designed for endopyelotomy and provides excellent results. The endopyelotome consists of a working element and a scimitar-shaped hook blade knife that allows initial passage of the knife and incision with retraction toward the operator. The endopyelotome is not available in most hospitals, but excellent results can be obtained with a standard direct vision urethrotome. This instrument allows excellent visualization, control, and incision with a hook blade or semilunar urethrotomy knife (Fig. 1).

The incision is made by visualizing the angiographic guidewire passing through the UPJ. The cold knife is passed beside the angiographic guidewire and the incision made on the posterolateral aspect of the UPJ, to avoid damage to any aberrant lower pole vessels, which arise on the anterior surface of the UPJ in up to one third of patients with obstruction. The cold knife is advanced through the UPJ and withdrawn, producing a single full-

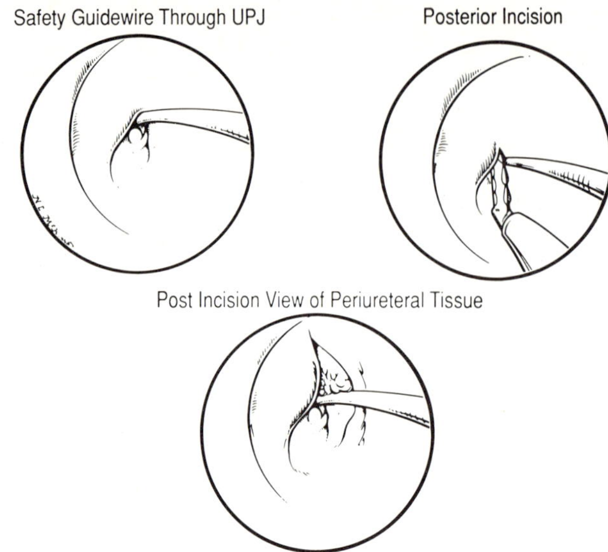

Figure 1 Endopyelotomy surgical technique.

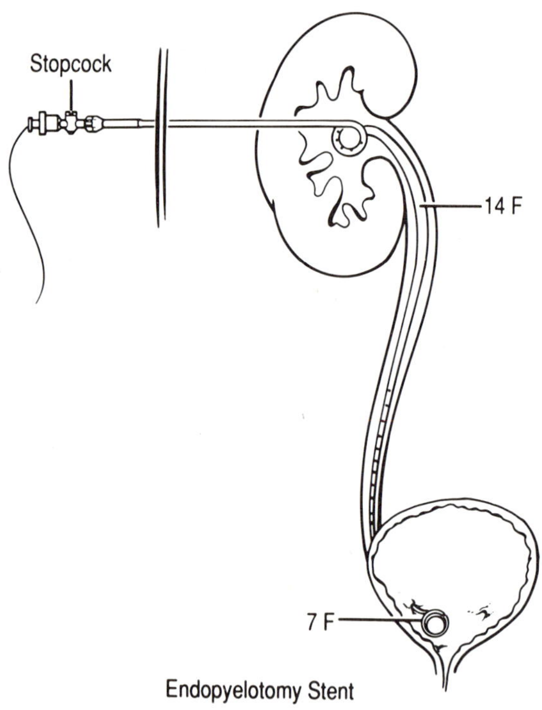

Figure 2 Postoperative stenting with endopyelotomy stent. Note the change in diameter from 14 Fr at the site of the endopyelotomy to 7 Fr at the bladder.

thickness incision through the ureteral mucosa and ureteral wall. Several passes of the cold knife may be necessary to accomplish adequate incision, especially in secondary endopyelotomies. A full-thickness incision is essential to ensure adequate incision. The incision is continued until periureteral adipose tissue is visualized.

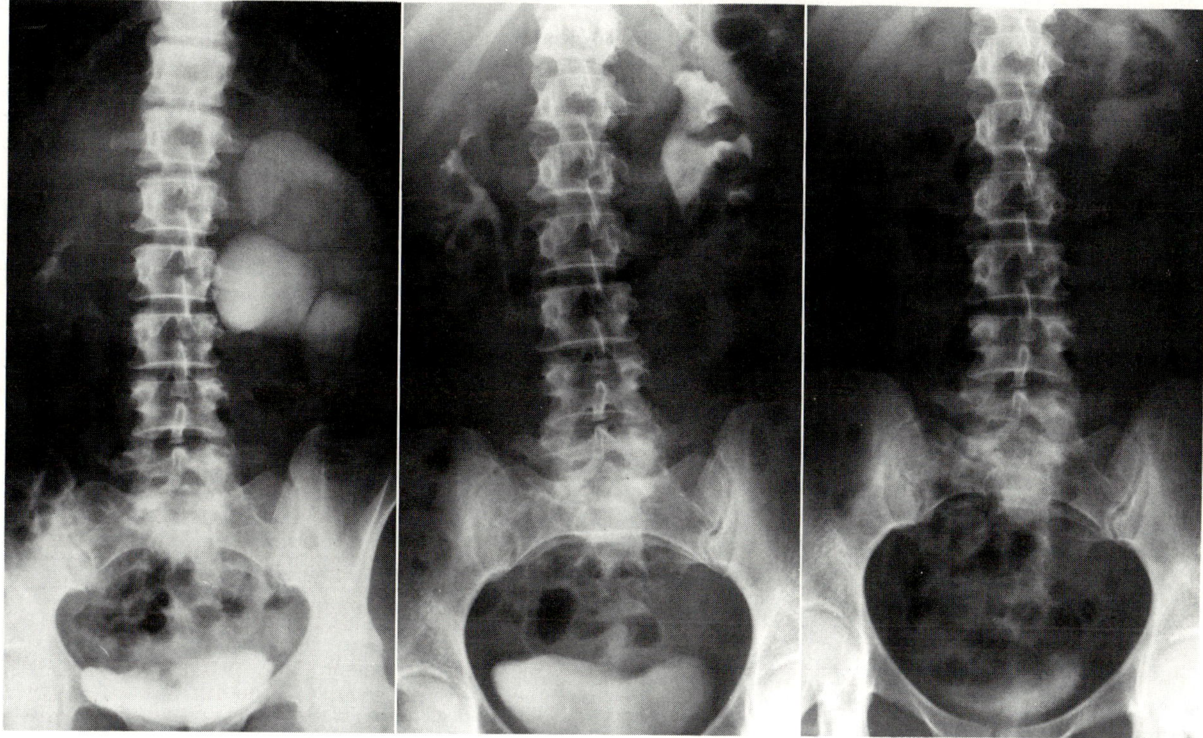

Figure 3 A 34-year-old woman with a history of persistent left flank pain and a dismembered pyeloplasty at age 6 years. *A,* Preoperative furosemide excretory urogram. *B,* Postoperative excretory urogram (15-minute film). *C,* Postoperative excretory urogram after furosemide administration.

Commonly, the UPJ will spring open when the incision is complete, allowing observation of normal ureter distally and the passage of the nephroscope beyond the stenotic UPJ into the normal ureter. The incision should be continued beyond the area of stenosis and into the most proximal portion of normal ureter to ensure satisfactory results. An incision approximately 2 cm in length, to include 0.5 to 1 cm of normal ureter, is generally necessary for adequate treatment. In order to evaluate results and ensure dilatation of periureteral scarring in secondary procedures, an angiographic dilatation balloon is placed through the UPJ over the angiographic safety guidewire after the incision is complete. Overdilatation to 15 to 18 Fr is then carried out with a high-pressure balloon, using an inflation syringe inflating to approximately 10 atmospheres. Fluoroscopic visualization of the balloon will confirm adequate incision if waisting at the UPJ junction is not pressure during dilatation. If waisting is observed, the balloon is removed and an additional incision carried out in that area. Balloon dilatation should be maintained for 5 to 10 minutes under fluoroscopic control. After the balloon is deflated and removed, the angiographic safety guidewire is used to pass a 12 to 14 Fr ureteral stent, which is advanced to the bladder. Special stents are available that measure 6 to 8 Fr distally and 12 to 14 Fr at the UPJ (Fig. 2).

Stents used after endopyelotomy must include fenestrations at a position that allows renal pelvis drainage externally or to the bladder. These stents are best controlled externally through percutaneous nephrostomy access. If drainage through the renal pelvis fenestrations is inadequate, an additional guidewire may be placed within the renal pelvis to position a self-retaining nephrostomy tube for additional drainage. This tube should remain for 24 to 48 hours to allow drainage of any blood or other debris before the patient's discharge from the hospital. The nephrostomy tube can then be removed if ureteral stent drainage is adequate. For adequate healing, the stent should remain in place for 6 to 8 weeks, during which the patient may resume normal activity. If there is no extravasation of contrast material and if the UPJ appears of adequate diameter at follow-up nephrostography, the ureteral stent is retracted into the renal pelvis to act as a nephrostomy tube. The tube is clamped for 24 to 48 hours to allow internal drainage through the repaired ureter. If drainage is adequate and the patient remains asymptomatic, the stent nephrostomy may be removed. Postincision follow-up intravenous pyelography is performed approximately 6 weeks later (Fig. 3). During the healing phase, patients should be maintained on antibiotic prophylaxis, which should be continued for approximately 72 hours after tube removal.

COMPLICATIONS AND SEQUELAE

The results of endopyelotomy demonstrate success in 82 to 86 percent of patients. The most common complication is restricture or repeat stenosis. Restricture can be demonstrated on the post-stent nephrostogram or on follow-up urography. It is thus important to follow patients with excretory urography, radioisotope renography, or nephrostography to confirm adequate postoperative results. Restricture or inadequate endopyelotomy will necessitate a secondary procedure. In some cases of failure, open pyeloplasty may be necessary.

Postoperative infection can not only adversely affect renal function, but can also lead to failure of endopyelotomy. Infection significantly increases the incidence of pyelitis, ureteritis, and foreign body inflammatory response. Furthermore, the leakage of infected urine through the area of incision may result in an increased incidence of periureteral cicatrization, prolonged incisional leakage, and possible retroperitoneal abscess formation. It is imperative, therefore, that patients undergoing endopyelotomy receive perioperative antibiotic prophylaxis, as well as postoperative antibiotic coverage during the time of healing. The antibiotics should be continued for 72 hours after all tubes are removed.

Postincision hemorrhage may occur but is more commonly associated with the presence of the nephrostomy tube. Since bleeding, hematoma, and persistent hemorrhage occur in 1 to 2 percent of patients undergoing percutaneous nephrostomy, this complication can be expected to occur in those undergoing endopyelotomy. One patient in the Duke University series required postnephrostomy tube removal, angiography, and embolization as a result of an arteriovenous fistula due to the initial percutaneous access placement.

With an open incision through the urinary tract, urinoma formation around the area of incision might be expected to be a common complication. With adequate nephrostomy drainage and ureteral stenting, however, this has not been identified to date. Extravasation during the immediate postoperative period is demonstrated in most patients, but adequate drainage results in resolution within 72 hours of incision. In one patient extravasation continued for 5 days, but ultimate resolution occurred simply with external drainage through the nephrostomy tube.

Hydronephrosis continues to be present in many patients after endopyelotomy or open pyeloplasty. Its importance and significance, however, can be measured only through diuretic urography or diuretic renography. If hydronephrosis persists and there is evidence of continued obstruction and inadequate flow, a repeat endopyelotomy may be warranted.

SUGGESTED READING

Carson CC. Percutaneous antegrade approach to ureteral calculi. Urol Clin North Am 1988; 15:399.

Carson CC. Endourology. In: Glenn JF, ed. Urologic surgery. 4th ed. Philadelphia: JB Lippincott, 1990.

deWeerd JH. Ureteropelvioplasty. In: Glenn JF, ed. Urologic surgery. 3rd ed. Philadelphia: JB Lippincott, 1983.

Karlin GS, Smith AD. Endopyelotomy. Urol Clin North Am 1988; 15:439.

King LR, Coughlin PWF, Ford KK, et al. Initial experience with percutaneous and transurethral ablation of postoperative ureteral strictures in children. J Urol 1984; 131:67.

ACQUIRED CYSTIC DISEASE OF THE KIDNEY

RALPH V. CLAYMAN, M.D.
PARAMJIT S. CHANDHOKE, M.D.
RALPH J. TORRENCE, M.D.

Acquired cystic disease of the kidney (ACDK) is defined as the development of multiple bilateral cysts in the kidneys of patients with chronic end-stage renal disease (ESRD) (Fig. 1). To confirm the diagnosis, more than three cysts should be present or more than 25 percent of the kidneys should be involved. Since its initial description by Dunhill and associates in 1977, who found 46.6 percent of patients on long-term hemodialysis to have acquired cysts within the kidneys on autopsy, ACDK has been the subject of over 100 publications. ACDK and its potential complications are now a well-recognized clinical entity. Over the last decade, this disease has also become more prevalent because patients with ESRD are living longer, are more likely to retain their native kidneys, and are undergoing more sensitive diagnostic imaging of the kidneys. The primary concern in patients with ACDK is the approximate 1 to 4 percent occurrence rate of renal carcinoma; whether this rate is significantly different from that in the normal population is still open to question.

PREVALENCE

The key factor in the development of ACDK is ESRD. Indeed, 8 percent of patients with ESRD are found to have ACDK at the initiation of dialysis. The continued development of ACDK is linked directly to the duration of dialysis. After 1 to 3 years of dialysis, 10 to 20 percent of patients develop ACDK; at between 3 and 5 years of dialysis, 40 to 60 percent of patients develop ACDK; after 5 to 10 years on dialysis, over 90 percent of patients have ACDK. ACDK affects patients on hemodialysis and peritoneal dialysis equally. Men and women have a similar prevalence of ACDK, but cancer

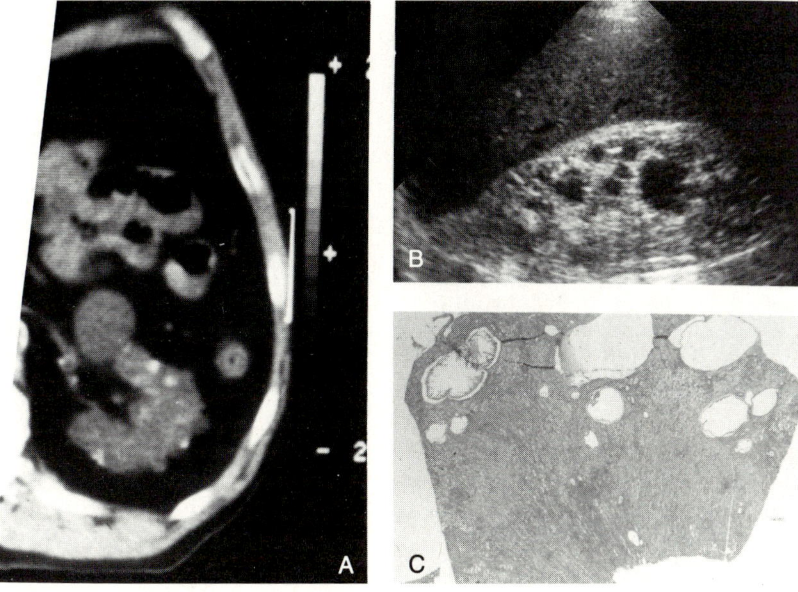

Figure 1 *A,* CT scan of a patient with ACDK; note the multiple small cortical cysts and solitary large anterior cyst. *B,* Ultrasonogram of the same patient; note the multiple "classic" cortical cysts of varying size. *C,* Histologic preparation of ACDK with H&E staining; note the thin-walled, multiple, small cortical cysts.

is more frequent in men (7:1 ratio). Age is not a factor, but race may be: blacks seem to be more likely than whites with ESRD to develop ACDK. Of all underlying kidney diseases, none protect ESRD patients from developing ACDK; however, nephrosclerosis appears to be more commonly associated with ACDK.

POSTULATED MECHANISMS OF ACDK DEVELOPMENT AND MALIGNANT TRANSFORMATION

The mechanism of renal cyst development or subsequent tumor formation is unproved. However, basement membrane alterations, intratubular or extratubular obstruction and endogenous or exogenous toxins/mutagens/mitogens, and growth factors within the circulation or cyst fluid have all been implicated in the development of cystic changes within the end-stage kidney. Of these, evidence to date points toward a circulating or intracystic renotropic or growth factor as the possible mechanism of both cyst formation and malignant transformation. In the patient with ESRD, high levels of a nondialyzable growth factor may be expected to cause an exaggerated hypertrophic and hyperplastic response in the proximal tubules of the few residual functioning nephrons. These hyperplastic nodules may lead to tubular obstruction. This hypothesis is supported by the finding that successful renal transplantation in patients with ACDK can lead to regression of cysts and reduction in size of the affected native kidneys. However, obstruction is only part of the formula for cyst development; the other half of the equation is the presence of impaired vascular inflow. As such, in the patient with ESRD due to glomerulosclerosis or arteriosclerosis, the combination of ischemia and tubular obstruction may result in formation of a cyst. In contrast, in the patient with an intact blood supply and constant uninterrupted delivery of growth factors, the overstimulated hyperplastic proximal tubular cells may undergo malignant transformation rather than cystic changes. This unifying hypothesis could explain the occurrence of both cysts and renal cancer in the patient with ACDK.

OCCURRENCE OF RENAL CANCER

It has long been established that patients with chronic renal failure have an increased incidence of malignancy, perhaps because of their immunosuppressed condition. In patients with ACDK, the occurrence of renal cancer is reportedly higher than in the general population. It is this association of ACDK with renal cancer that has attracted considerable clinical interest. In a careful review of the published data, the suggestion that ACDK is a necessary harbinger of renal carcinoma is open to challenge. First, the incidence of tumors in nondialyzed ESRD patients exceeds that in hemodialysis patients, even though the occurrence of ACDK is more than four times greater in dialysis patients. Second, renal cancer has occurred in dialysis patients without the appearance of concomitant ACDK.

The occurrence data of renal cancer are reported both as "autopsy series" and in "surveillance" form. Therefore, both rates should be compared uniformly between the normal population and ESRD patients.

Comparing autopsy series, the occurrence rate of adenomas is reported to be 7 to 25 percent in the normal population and 7 to 20 percent in ESRD patients, that of renal cancers about 1 to 2 percent in both patient populations, and that of unsuspected metastatic renal cancer 0.3 percent in the normal population and 0.5 percent in ESRD patients. Thus, autopsy data for renal cancer occurrence are similar in ESRD patients (average age 55 years) and in the general population (average age 66 years). If one selects only patients with ACDK, the incidences of adenoma, renal cancer, and metastatic renal cancer at autopsy are 25, 1 to 4, and 0 to 2 percent, respectively. Again, these figures are not that dissimilar from the corresponding data for patients with ESRD or the general population.

The currently available "surveillance" data (i.e., data derived from radiographic screening of ESRD patients) suggests an approximately 1 percent occurrence rate of renal cancer in ESRD patients and a 1 to 4 percent rate in ACDK patients (10 percent adenoma, 0.7 percent metastatic). However, similar data are not available for the general population because there are no comparable age-/sex-matched surveillance programs. Indeed, the detection of many renal cancers in ESRD patients is generally made by: ultrasonography or computed tomography (CT) as part of a surveillance program, as part of the evaluation before initiation of dialysis, or upon entry into a transplantation program. These tumors in the general population would be "silent" (i.e., asymptomatic). Therefore, comparison of surveillance-derived renal cancer occurrence rates in ESRD patients (0.1 to 0.18 percent per year) with clinically symptomatic incidence rates in the normal population (0.005 percent per year) is not valid. Accordingly, at present only autopsy data provide an acceptable comparison among ACDK patients, ESRD patients, and the general population. As such, renal cancer rates in ACDK and ESRD patients may not be increased over those in the normal population. All that can be stated is that cancer develops earlier in the ESRD patient's overall lifetime.

CLINICAL MANIFESTATIONS AND TREATMENT

ACDK is most commonly detected serendipitously as part of an initial ESRD evaluation or as part of a surveillance program. It is clinically silent in the vast majority of patients. Renal imaging (ultrasonography and CT) is the only available screening tool for ACDK. Usually a renal imaging study is done before the initiation of dialysis or is a part of the work-up for potential transplant candidates. CT is more sensitive than ultrasonography in identifying small tumors in end-stage kidneys, especially if they are intraparenchymal; hence, CT is preferable. Magnetic resonance imaging (MRI) may become the preferred modality in the future, because it can differentiate small solid from multiple small cystic masses better than CT.

Hematuria is the most common sign of a renal tumor, either in the form of macroscopic or microscopic hematuria. Bleeding into a cyst can occur, and if a communication between the cyst and pelviocalyceal system exists, this may manifest as macroscopic or microscopic hematuria. In addition, platelet dysfunction and heparinization for dialysis makes ESRD patients more prone to bleeding in general. Hematuria in ESRD patients should be evaluated with urinary cytology (if the patient is making any urine), cystoscopy, retrograde pyelography, and renal ultrasonography or CT.

Bleeding in the ACDK patient may become life threatening if it is associated with retroperitoneal hemorrhage. In these patients, flank or abdominal pain develops. An initial conservative approach is indicated: hydration, transfusion, and correction of coagulation indices. If the hematocrit fails to stabilize or hypotension develops despite these measures, emergency selective renal embolization may control the bleeding. Nephrectomy in this circumstance is undertaken as a last resort.

There are three basic clinical questions with regard to ACDK. First, is the risk of developing potentially malignant renal tumors so great among these patients that "preventive" native kidney nephrectomies should be performed in all ESRD patients on dialysis for more than 3 years? There are several points to consider in answering this question: (1) the value of the end-stage kidney to the patient, (2) the mortality and morbidity of native nephrectomy in dialysis patients, and (3) the nature of the potential renal tumors. The end-stage native kidneys of patients on chronic dialysis often provide substantial benefits by reducing dependence on dialysis, providing for easier fluid management and allowing some liberalization in fluid restrictions. Additional benefits can include a decreased need for blood transfusions (because of production of erythropoietin), and improved calcium balance (due to intact vitamin D metabolism). Also, the continued production of renin may preclude difficult-to-manage hypotension in the ESRD patient. Next, mortality and morbidity rates associated with native nephrectomy in a dialysis patient are not insignificant. Indeed, an overall operative mortality rate of 3.6 percent (11 percent in patients over the age of 50), with an associated major morbidity of 18 percent among ESRD patients undergoing bilateral nephrectomy, has been reported. Lastly, it should be noted that the vast majority of renal tumors found by the sensitive imaging tools presently available are small (<3 cm). The potential for metastatic renal cancer with lesions of this size is low (2.6 percent as reported by Bell in a 1937 necropsy series; hence, the appellation "adenoma"). Therefore, given (1) the benefits provided by the native kidneys, (2) the risks of bilateral nephrectomy, (3) the rarity of metastatic disease in this patient population, and (4) the overall low incidence (1 percent) of renal cell carcinoma in ESRD patients, "preventive" bilateral nephrectomies in ESRD patients cannot be recommended. Likewise, in patients with documented ACDK but no solid lesion, "preventive" nephrectomies cannot be recommended.

The second question relates to the management of

a solid renal lesion in the ESRD patient. Certainly, all *symptomatic* solid renal masses should result in unilateral radical nephrectomy. Likewise, *asymptomatic* solid lesions discovered by surveillance radiography should also lead to radical nephrectomy. Despite the oft-cited 3-cm rule, it is difficult to predict exactly at what size a renal "adenoma" will transform into a renal cancer and metastasize. As noted, even Bell recorded a 2.6 percent incidence of metastases with the under 3-cm lesion. There currently are no effective therapies for metastatic renal cancer, so the only opportunity for cure is to remove the cancer before it has metastasized. Therefore, removal of the kidney upon discovery of a solid lesion is recommended. However, only unilateral nephrectomy is necessary. Until more data become available, surveillance of solid renal lesions is to be discouraged.

The third question concerns the role of screening of ESRD patients for ACDK. It is of interest that in Ishikawa's large series, renal cancers were detected only after 5 years of dialysis. Thus, annual surveillance is an expensive but not helpful venture. There also are initial survival data now available for ESRD patients diagnosed with renal cancer. Interestingly, despite increased surveillance of ESRD patients over the last 10 years, the 5-year survival rate of ESRD patients with renal cancer is only 35 percent, no better than the 42 percent survival rate reported in 1989 for symptomatic renal cancer. Thus, surveillance appears to have had no significant impact on survival to date. These data are also consistent with the previously noted similar autopsy occurrence rates of adenomas, renal cancers, and unsuspected metastatic renal cancer in the normal population, ESRD patients, and ACDK patients. Furthermore, although all ESRD patients eventually develop ACDK, it is noteworthy that among all ESRD patients developing renal cancer, only one half to two thirds may have concomitant ACDK. Thus, currently available data suggest that while ACDK is a distinct clinical entity in the ESRD patient, the occurrence of renal cancer in the ACDK patient may be more of a coincidence than a consequence. In sum, it appears that the development of ACDK in patients with ESRD does not predispose them to an increased risk of developing or dying from renal carcinoma. Also, given the inherent limitations of imaging modalities in differentiating the low-grade, rarely metastasizing small "adenoma" from its more malignant counterpart, the cost of surveillance, the expense and morbidity of surgical intervention, and the lack of impact of current surveillance programs on subsequent survival, it seems that a screening or surveillance program for ACDK cannot be justified.

In conclusion, we believe that diagnostic screening tests, surveillance studies, and "preventive" nephrectomies are neither medically nor economically justifiable in ESRD patients. Rather, the urologist should be aware of the ACDK entity and its potential complications, but should reserve a full evaluation for patients presenting with definite signs and symptoms of ACDK or a renal tumor. Only among patients in whom a symptomatic or serendipitously detected solid renal mass is identified is unilateral radical nephrectomy indicated.

SUGGESTED READING

Basile JJ, McCullough DL, Harrison LH, Dyer RB. End-stage renal disease associated with acquired cystic disease and neoplasia. J Urol 1988; 140:938–943.

Bretan PN, Busch MP, Hricak H, Williams RD. Chronic renal failure: significant risk factor in the development of acquired renal cysts and renal cell carcinoma. Case reports and review of the literature. Cancer 1986; 57:1871–1879.

Gehrig JJ, Gottheiner TI, Swensen RS. Acquired cystic disease of end-stage kidney. Am J Med 1985; 79:609–620.

Grantham JJ, Levine E. Acquired kidney disease: replacing one kidney disease with another. Kidney Int 1985; 28:99–105.

Matson MA, Cohen EP. Acquired cystic kidney disease: occurrence, prevalence, and renal cancers. Medicine 1990; 69:217–226.

<h1 style="text-align:center">I URETER</h1>

URETEROVAGINAL FISTULA

HUGH A. G. FISHER, M.D., F.A.C.S.

A ureterovaginal fistula rarely occurs spontaneously and is most often a sequela of pelvic surgery involving removal of the uterus and upper portion of the vagina for carcinoma, of endometriosis, or as part of an en bloc dissection of a large pelvic tumor. Fistulas may occur in 1 to 2 percent of patients undergoing radical hysterectomy. Injury occurs either directly by ligation or transection of the ureter or as a result of ischemia secondary to compromise of the blood supply to the distal ureter. Vaginal drainage may occur immediately postoperatively if direct unrecognized injury has occurred or may begin days or weeks later with ischemic injury. Radiation administered pre- or postoperatively by combined external and internal techniques enhances the risk of fistula development, particularly if residual or recurrent tumor is present.

The site of ureteral injury during radical hysterectomy is usually deep within the pelvis at, or distal to, the uterine artery where the ureter passes beneath it and courses anteriorly and medially to enter the bladder adjacent to the apex of the vagina. In the pelvis, the accessory ureteral blood supply enters laterally and is derived from the branches of the hypogastric artery and from the overlying peritoneum. Ischemic injury occurs by interruption of these accessory vessels during mobilization combined with devascularization of the ureteral adventitia.

PREVENTION OF INJURY

Proper preoperative evaluation of potential ureteral involvement or anatomic distortion by the disease process may prevent iatrogenic ureteral injury. Intravenous urography or computed tomography (CT) may indicate hydronephrosis and define the relationship of the ureter to the surgical site. Placement of bilateral No. 5 or 6 Fr whistle-tipped catheters preoperatively in difficult cases involving previous pelvic surgery, endometriosis, or large cancers may assist in intraoperative identification of the ureters. Although these catheters are difficult to feel with extensive periureteral induration, they allow for immediate discovery of an inadvertent injury with intraoperative repair. They may be withdrawn at the end of the procedure, and if they are delivered easily, ureteral ligation will not have occurred. Intraoperatively, care must be taken to preserve the adventitia of the ureter during mobilization.

Prompt intraoperative recognition of ureteral injury and appropriate repair will obviate fistula development. Often the urologist is consulted intraoperatively by the gynecologist to investigate possible ureteral entry or devascularization. Loupe magnification is helpful. If there is any question of vascular compromise, a double-J stent placed immediately may avoid late stricture or fistula development. If mucosal penetration is suspected, 5 ml of indigo carmine or methylene blue may be given intravenously and the area observed for leak. If ureteral transection is present, immediate ureteroureterostomy or ureteroneocystostomy should be performed over a stent.

DIAGNOSIS

Postoperative identification of ureterovaginal fistula requires a high index of suspicion, particularly if the fistula is small and develops several weeks after surgery. Vaginal drainage may be scant or copious. Bimanual examination may reveal induration or mass. Vaginoscopy may reveal a fistulous opening and is facilitated by oral methylene blue or intravenous indigo carmine administration. Cystoscopy and methylene blue cystography are important to rule out a concomitant vesicovaginal fistula. A bulb retrograde study may reveal the site of the fistula, but often obstruction distal to the fistula does not allow passage of contrast material. Intravenous urography or CT with contrast may reveal hydronephrosis or may be normal because of decompression of the system by the fistula. If the above studies do not indicate the site of the fistula, an antegrade pyeloureterogram obtained through a percutaneous nephrostomy may be required.

TREATMENT

The approach to treatment depends on the timing of presentation relative to the injury; the severity of injury (complete or partial); the age and medical condition of the patient; the presence or absence of advanced carcinoma, radiation, or infection; and the status of the bladder and contralateral kidney.

If vaginal drainage occurs a few days postoperatively, intravenous urography, cystography, and retrograde studies should be performed to localize the site and assess the severity of injury. With partial disruption, a guidewire may be passed from below to allow passage of a ureteral stent. If retrograde stent placement is not possible, antegrade stent placement through a percutaneous nephrostomy often is successful and results in control of the fistula. However, if a guidewire cannot be advanced to the bladder from above, percutaneous nephrostomy alone may not provide adequate drainage of an unobstructed system, increasing the likelihood of an open procedure. If the stent is successfully placed and subsequently removed after 4 to 6 weeks, it is mandatory that follow-up intravenous urography or ultrasonography be performed to rule out late stricture.

Successful reconstructive operative procedures rely on the anastomosis of well-vascularized tissues without tension in the absence of infection. Timing of the procedure is not as critical as with vesicovaginal fistula, because the repair is performed away from the area of injury. If the patient is otherwise in satisfactory condition, an open procedure may be performed as soon as the diagnosis is confirmed or conservative measures have failed.

A midline incision provides adequate exposure to the pelvic ureter and may be extended superiorly if a transureteroureterostomy is necessary or renal mobilization is required for maximal ureteral length. An extraperitoneal approach may be attempted, but often intraperitoneal identification is necessary, particularly if previous pelvic lymph node dissection has been performed. The ureter may be thick-walled and adherent secondary to chronic inflammation. The ureter can be identified as it courses over the iliac vessels, mobilized carefully with preservation of surrounding periadventitial tissue, and followed into the pelvis beneath the obliterated lateral umbilical ligament, which is divided. Vessels crossing the ureter distally may be sacrificed to gain additional length. The ureter should be divided as low as possible with preservation of blood supply.

If the bladder is normal and ureteral length is adequate, ureteroneocystostomy is the procedure of choice. The extravesical modified Lich technique, which is popular for renal transplantation, does not require a bladder incision or extensive mobilization. The bladder is distended with a No. 20 French Foley catheter until moderately tense. An oblique anterior bladder incision 4 to 5 cm long is made using cautery. Adventitial and detrusor muscle layers are divided and undermined with mucosa left intact. The ureter is spatulated posteriorly, and anchored proximally and distally to the mucosa with

5-0 chromic or 6-0 monofilament polyglyconate sutures. The mucosa is opened the length of the spatulation, and ureteral-to-bladder mucosa anastomosis is completed by running the proximal suture along one side and the distal suture back along the other, tying them at the ends. Bladder adventitia and muscle are then closed over the ureter in one layer with a running 3-0 chromic suture to create an antirefluxing tunnel. A Foley catheter remains in place for 3 to 5 days. The use of a double-J stent is optional. A suprapubic tube is not routinely used. A perivesical drain remains for several days.

Extravesical ureteroneocystostomy may be combined with a psoas hitch without opening the bladder. Mobilization of the contralateral wall of the bladder, with division of the superior vesical artery, may be required. The bladder is sutured to the psoas minor tendon lateral to the external iliac vessels with several 0 chromic sutures. The bladder should be secured to the psoas muscle before filling.

Alternatively, a transverse incision may be made across the anterior wall of the bladder, and two fingers inserted to retract the bladder laterally with fixation to the psoas tendon. A submucosal tunnel is fashioned for a distance of 3 cm. The ureter with stay suture attached is brought through the posterior wall and through the submucosal tunnel, and a new orifice created at the distal end of the tunnel. The ureter is spatulated anteriorly and anchored distally to muscle and mucosa with a 4-0 chromic suture placed deeply into the bladder wall. Interrupted ureteral-to-bladder mucosa sutures complete the anastomosis. The bladder is closed vertically in two layers. A double-J stent may be used. A suprapubic tube is optional but the Foley catheter remains in place for 1 to 2 weeks. The indwelling stent is removed endoscopically in 4 to 6 weeks.

Occasionally a Boari flap is required when a wider gap must be bridged. The bladder is mobilized as for the psoas hitch. Several centimeters of ureteral length can be gained by lateral dissection above the iliac vessels and mobilization of the kidney within Gerota's fascia if needed.

The required length of the flap should be measured with an umbilical tape before the bladder is cut. The flap should be based posteriorly and be 4 to 5 cm at the base and at least 3 cm at the apex, depending on the caliber of the ureter, to allow for adequate closure without constriction. Stay sutures are placed at the base and apex of the flap. A submucosal tunnel is created at the apex of the flap and directed toward the posterior wall of the bladder for 3 to 4 cm. A mucosal opening is created and the ureter brought through the tunnel. An anastomosis is performed as described above and the bladder wall is closed in layers over the ureteroneocystostomy.

In the presence of pelvic radiation, extensive inflammation, fibrosis, or a bladder unsuitable for use in reconstruction, options include transureteroureterostomy, permanent nephrostomy, or sacrifice of the affected renal unit by embolization or nephrectomy. For transureteroureterostomy, a midline incision provides optimal exposure; the ureters lie close together in the midline at the level of the sacral promontory. Maximal ureteral length is obtained and the ureter transected. The contralateral normal ureter is identified and mobilized above the iliac vessels for only a few centimeters. A passage that admits two fingers easily is bluntly created posterior to the left colonic mesentery and anterior to the great vessels. The tunnel may be created above or below the inferior mesenteric artery, depending on the extent of radiation. The ureter is transferred under the mesentery without tension or angulation and trimmed obliquely or spatulated to create an 8- to 12-mm opening. A matching length of ureteral wall is opened medially on the recipient ureter. The ends of the spatulation and recipient ureterotomy are approximated with 4-0 or 5-0 chromic suture. A continuous end-to-side anastomosis is performed. The back wall is closed with a running suture from the inside and tied to the lower suture. The front wall is closed from the outside and tied to the upper suture. The anastomosis is performed over a double-J stent catheter, which traverses the anastomosis to lie in the renal pelvis of the kidney on the side of the fistula. With a normal-caliber recipient ureter, a No. 6 or 7 Fr. stent will allow adequate drainage of both collecting systems. A retroperitoneal drain is placed. The stent is removed in 3 to 4 weeks.

If the functional ureteral length is very short or if the patient is elderly with underlying medical problems or advanced cancer, a permanent nephrostomy or sacrifice of the kidney is prudent. If a permanent nephrostomy is placed but does not control the fistula, open ureteral ligation may be required for effective urinary diversion. This may be performed through a small flank or left lower quadrant muscle splitting incision. In this instance, simple nephrectomy should be considered and is probably preferable to long-term nephrostomy drainage if the contralateral renal unit is normal. Alternatively, the ureter may be occluded percutaneously under fluoroscopic guidance or by injection of an occlusive polymer through a catheter from above.

The best approach to ureterovaginal fistula is prevention through careful pelvic dissection, identification of the ureters, and preservation of ureteral blood supply. Full intraoperative evaluation is warranted if injury is suspected. A high index of suspicion should be maintained postoperatively if vaginal drainage occurs. Fortunately, the urologist has an array of options for management of ureterovaginal fistula. A single well-planned and well-executed operation will solve the problem in most cases. There is no more grateful patient than one rendered dry. Selection of the best procedure depends on the judgment and experience of the surgeon and the condition of the patient.

SUGGESTED READING

Hedlund H, Lindstedt E. Urovaginal fistulas: 20 years of experience with 45 cases. J Urol 1987; 137:926.
Hinman F Jr. Atlas of urologic surgery. Philadelphia: WB Saunders, 1989:679.

POSTSURGICAL URETERAL STENOSIS

MAJID ESHGHI, M.D., F.A.C.S.
DAVID M. SCHWALB, M.D.

ETIOLOGY, PATHOGENESIS, AND DIAGNOSIS

A ureteral stricture is an area of narrowing caused primarily by some form of direct ureteral injury or vascular compromise (Table 1). Most strictures are diagnosed radiographically as a narrowed, poorly visualized ureteral segment with proximal hydroureteronephrosis and reduced renal function (Fig. 1), but some are identified incidentally, during ureteroscopy performed for other reasons, as a nondistensible area resistant to high-pressure irrigation or balloon dilatation. In a very small percentage of ureteral strictures there is no dilatation proximal, but the patient is symptomatic or forms stones.

Although most patients with ureteral stenosis present with symptomatic urinary tract infections, flank pain, or hematuria, 20 to 25 percent are asymptomatic, obstruction being discovered on imaging studies performed for routine follow-up or nonurologic purposes.

INDICATIONS FOR AND TIMING OF THERAPY

Treatment of ureteral stenosis is indicated in symptomatic patients (recurrent urinary tract infection, flank pain, or hematuria) and to prevent progressive renal insufficiency, and calculi caused by persistent obstruction. The stable, asymptomatic, minimally obstructing stricture that fails to produce deterioration in renal function can probably be left untreated in a reliable patient.

Thorough radiographic evaluation of the extent of ureteral stenosis is essential in preoperative planning because selection of a therapeutic option depends on the site, length, duration, and cause of the stricture. Knowledge of the functional status of the ipsilateral and contralateral kidney, the patient's medical condition, and the absence of concomitant ureteral involvement by ma-

Table 1 Common Causes of Ureteral Stricture*

Category	%	Common Examples	Pathogenesis
Urologic surgery	44	Ureteroileal anastomosis	Ischemia
		Ureterolithotomy	Recurrent malignancy
		Ureteroneocystotomy	
		Ureteroureterostomy	
General/vascular surgery	4	Aortobifemoral bypass	Surgical ligation, transection, or
		Abdominoperineal resection	clamping
		Colon resection	Ischemia
		Appendectomy	Periureteral inflammation
		Transplant ureter	
Gynecologic surgery	6.8	Hysterectomy (simple or radical)	Surgical ligation, transection, or
		Cesarean section	clamping
		Ovarian cystectomy	Ischemia
Endoscopic urologic procedure	20	Ureteroscopy — diagnostic and	Ureteral perforation or resection
		therapeutic	Ischemia and scarring
		Ureteral stone basketing	
		Percutaneous stone manipulation	
		Ureteral catheterization	
		Intraureteral lithotripsy	
		Electrocautery or laser	
		fulguration	
Stone passage	13.2		Ischemia
Miscellaneous	9	Retroperitoneal fibrosis	Infection
		Chronic urinary tract infection	Periureteral inflammation
		Pelvic radiation	
		Genitourinary TB	
		Recurrent pelvic carcinoma	
Unknown	3	No apparent cause	

*Review of eight large series of ureteral stenosis in 218 patients.

lignancy are important determinants of treatment recommendations.

Successful management of ureteral stenosis is defined as the absence of obstruction on contrast medium radiographic study, diuretic renography, or a Whitaker pressure perfusion study without an indwelling stent. Chronic indwelling ureteral stenting in patients with stenosis associated with recurrent pelvic malignancy is suboptimal therapy and is advised only for palliation of obstruction, owing to the high incidence of sepsis from urinary infection and obstruction.

Increased experience with retrograde and antegrade ureteral endoscopy, together with fluoroscopic techniques, has shifted the trend from open (Table 2) to endoscopic (Table 3) procedures for the definitive management of ureteral strictures.

ENDOSCOPIC THERAPY

Endoscopic management of ureteral stenosis (see Table 3) may be approached with simple ureteral catheterization, bougie dilatation, high-pressure transluminal balloon dilatation, or endoscopic and fluoroscopic cold- or hot-knife ureteral incision (endoureterotomy). Transluminal balloon ureteroplasty and visual hot- or cold-knife ureterotomy are the most commonly used noninvasive means of treating ureteral strictures, owing to their relatively high success rate, and the fact that they preclude the need for surgical repair and do not inter-

fere with subsequent successful operative reconstruction in failed cases. Endourologic correction of ureteral stricture is stressed, because over 85 percent of patients can be managed without open surgery and with a very short hospital stay and convalescence period.

URETEROVESICAL JUNCTION OBSTRUCTION

This condition is usually the result of endoscopic injury, reimplantation of the ureter, or prostate and bladder malignancy. The initial basic approach is cystoscopy and cannulation of the orifice, and possibly meatotomy or balloon dilatation, followed by insertion of an indwelling stent. If this fails, the patient requires a nephrostomy tube and antegrade placement of a guidewire with possible re-entry into the bladder, followed by antegrade balloon dilatation or retrograde endoureterotomy.

MECHANICAL DILATATION OF URETERAL STRICTURES

Mechanical dilatation of ureteral stenosis requires initial placement of an angiographic guidewire across the stenotic segment (usually a 0.035- or 0.038-inch Teflon-coated floppy tip or J-tip guidewire, although sometimes the more substantial Lunderquist torque or exchange wire is needed), followed by advancement of the dilating

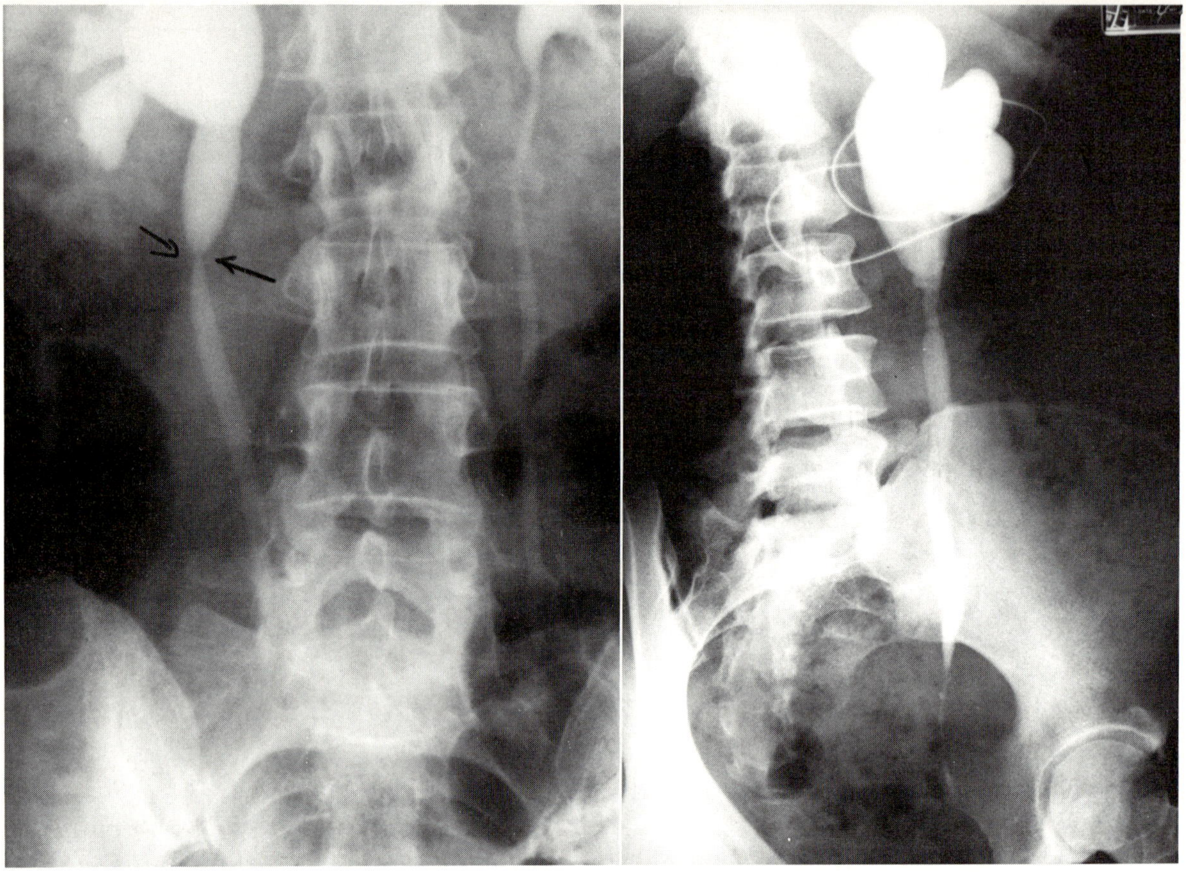

A **B**

Figure 1 *A,* Intravenous urogram in a patient with right upper ureteral stricture. Although the stricture is very short, it has caused dilatation of the proximal ureter and renal pelvis and blunting of the calices. *B,* Antegrade nephrostogram in a patient with a history of ureteral stone and ureterolithotomy. Note the distal ureteral obstruction as outlined by poor advancement of the dye in the distal segment.

instrument across the stenosis over the wire. A new generation of lubricated or slippery wires has made the initial negotiation through the stenotic area much easier and more successful. Unguided mechanical dilatation should never be performed because of the high incidence of ureteral perforation. At the completion of dilatation, the guidewire is left within the ureter to facilitate passage of a 6- to 8-Fr double-pigtail stent across the stenosis, which is left indwelling for 4 to 6 weeks. Ureteral catheters, flexible graduated, and bougie dilators are usually passed in a retrograde fashion, but angiographic Gruntzig-type balloon dilators can be negotiated across the stenosis antegrade via an existing nephrostomy tract or retrograde up the ureter through an endoscope, using fluoroscopic guidance. Catheter dilatation to 8 Fr and bougie dilation to 20 Fr of ureteral strictures, followed by stenting of variable intervals, has met some success, particularly with short strictures (Table 3). High-pressure balloon dilatation (12 to 16 atm) of a ureteral stricture, using a 6- or 7-Fr reinforced polyethylene Gruntzig-type angioplasty balloon with an inflated balloon diameter of 5 to 7 mm and balloon lengths of 4 to 10 cm, introduced over a wire and centered across the stricture, has fared

better, with shorter, membrane-like, more acute strictures (with success rates ranging from 48 to 74 percent) than with longer, fusiform, more chronic strictures (Table 3). With a pressure gauge connected between a mechanical hand injector and the balloon, the balloon is inflated slowly (0.5 ml per minute) using constant pressure with dilute contrast medium (30 percent hypaque) and left inflated for 1 to 5 minutes. Stricture dilatation is not complete until the waist or narrowing in the balloon at the stricture site is eliminated as seen fluoroscopically (Fig. 2). The ureter is stented with a 6- or 8-Fr double-pigtail stent for 1 to 6 weeks, depending on the length of the stricture. The major disadvantage of balloon dilatation is the high cost of the catheter, which is not reusable once inflated, owing to poor postinflation memory. The Olbert balloon, with good postinflation memory, can achieve high inflation pressures (12 to 16 atm) and can be reused, decreasing costs.

Potential complications of mechanical ureteral dilatation include ureteral perforation, especially with the bougie, if excessive shearing force is applied during passage, with development of a retroperitoneal urinoma and abscess and possible formation of recurrent or new

Table 2 Surgical Treatment of Ureteral Stricture

Type of Treatment	Author	No. of patients	Success Rate (%)	Comments
I. Stenosis from UPJ to iliac vessels				
A. Ureteroureterostomy and/or renal mobilization	Carlton (1971)	25	92	Used a watertight anastomosis
B. Davis intubated ureterotomy	Davis (1951)	NA	90	Stressed import of wrapping incision with fat to prevent adhesions
C. Bladder (Boari) flap	Thompson (1974)	23	100	100% had reflux, 87% with sterile urine; no restenosis
D. Ileal replacement	Boxer (1978)	89	81	Contraindicated when serum creatinine greater than 2.0
E. Renal autotransplantation	Bodie (1986)	23	87	Two kidneys removed postoperatively owing to bleeding
II. Pelvic ureteral stenosis				
A. Ureteroneocystostomy and/or psoas hitch	Ehrlich (1975)	52	95–100	Reflux: 2 cases; no restenosis
B. Bladder (Boari) flap	Flynn (1979)	41	95–100	
C. Transureteroureterostomy*	Udall (1973)	42	98	One failure required nephrectomy
III. All stenoses				
A. Ureterolysis and/or omental wrap	Baker (1988)	54	25–100	Success increased in presence of a functioning kidney and with addition of postoperative corticosteroids
B. Urinary diversion (cutaneous ureterostomy)	Faminella (1971)	70	Varied	1. Flush stoma: 95% stomal stenosis rate 2. Protruding stoma: 45–64% restenosis rate
C. Nephrostomy drainage (percutaneous or open)				Performed for temporary decompression of obstructed kidney in a septic patient For diagnostic evaluation of stricture extent
D. Nephrectomy				Definitive therapy in a completely nonfunctioning obstructed kidney (10% total renal function on renal scan)

*May occasionally be used for midureteral stenosis in the presence of severe ipsilateral pelvic adhesions or abscess.

ureteral strictures. Perinephric abscess and hematoma are potential hazards of antegrade ureteral manipulation through a percutaneous approach. Recently we demonstrated in animal studies that bougie, Teflon, and balloon ureteral dilatation of uninjured ureters causes universally a severe degree of mucosal damage, intramural hemorrhage, and macro- and microscopic perforation of the ureters. Scarring is rarely reported clinically after balloon ureteral dilatation and ureteroscopy, but in the minipig there was evidence of chronic scarring and muscle loss in 75 percent of unscarred ureters subjected to mechanical dilatation. These and previous studies by Oppenheimer, Hinman, and Davis on ureteral regeneration led us to consider simple ureteral incision the preferable means of managing ureteral stenosis.

URETEROSCOPIC ENDOURETEROTOMY

During the last 4 years at our institution, we have managed 61 ureteral strictures of various lengths via cold knife endoscopic ureterotomy using one of three techniques, with a stent-free success rate of 98 percent (see Table 3).

Instruments

The ureter is approached in a one-step procedure using hydraulic dilatation. As a result, there is no previous manipulation or instrumentation of the ureteral wall or mucosa, and ureteral strictures are clearly identified. Initially cold-knife ureteroscopic endoureterotomy was performed using an endoureterotomy scissors or catheter knife passed through the ureteroscope working channel to incise the stricture, but most recently we have incised strictures with one of three cold-knife ureterotomes. Our newest instrument is a 13-Fr cold-knife ureterotome specially designed for ureteral stricture. It has a tapered beak and a half-moon blade with a lumen that allows it to move back and forth over a guidewire to ensure that the cold knife at all times remains within the ureteral lumen (Fig. 3).

Table 3 Endourologic Management of Ureteral Stenosis

Type of Treatment	Author	Extent of Dilatation	No. of Strictures	Type of Stricture	Success Rate (%)	Comments
I. Mechanical dilatation						
A. Ureteral catheterization (Teflon)	Witherington (1980)	8 Fr	4	Short, postsurgical	100	50% required multiple redilatation before resolution
B. Bougie dilatation	Vliestra (1953)	Up to 20 Fr	37	NA	NA	Fair success
C. Balloon dilatation						
Antegrade	Banner (1984)	12 Fr	44	Varied length	48	Best response with short, membrane-like strictures
Retrograde	Eshghi (1988)	Up to 18 Fr	25	Varied length	74	
II. Endoscopic Incision						
A. Cold-knife	Eshghi (1989)	See text	61	Varied length	98	Failure in one patient with long stricture, treated successfully with ureteroureterostomy
B. Hot-knife	Thomas (1988)	Full-thickness incision, balloon dilated to 24 Fr, stented	14	NA	64	Strictures >1.5 cm failed

Cold-Knife Endoureterotomy

With two wires in place, the endoureterotome is advanced over a wire to the strictured segment, then withdrawn partially to give a wide view of the strictured area. From this position, the cold knife is advanced (Fig. 4) and can be directed into the narrow lumen of the strictured area to incise the stricture. In most cases, we insert the second wire at this stage from the back end of the endoureterotome, which exits through the shaft of the knife and is directed into the strictured area under vision. If two wires cannot pass through the narrow segment the procedure is done with one wire, but care must be taken not to kink the wire during the manipulation of the knife. If the lens is too close to the stricture, there will be no space for the cold knife to be seen and the ureteral wall may be perforated. A posterolateral incision of the ureter is recommended in all areas except over and near the crossing of the iliac vessels, where the incision should be made at the 12 to 2 o'clock position. In making the incision, one must be aware of the anatomic landmarks, paraureteral structures and surface anatomy, and vascular supply of the ureter in male and female patients (crossing of the uterine artery, ovarian vein, vas deferens, gonadal veins, iliac vessels, and medial blood supply of the ureter except in the very distal segment) (Fig. 5).

The main advantage of pressure-controlled hydraulic ureteral dilatation is that the flow of irrigant keeps the ureteral walls apart and prevents them from collapsing. As a result, the strictured segment is easily identified. After one or two arclike strokes along the stricture, the ureter slowly widens. This procedure should be continued until the lumen allows the scope to advance beyond the stricture. Incision into periureteral fat is not always required with simple and short strictures. With dense and recurrent strictures, incisions may be required in more than one location for maximal spreading of the stricture. In almost all the long and dense strictures that require multiple incisions, one encounters the periureteral fat that indicates the limits of the incision.

Bleeding is rarely a problem and fulguration is almost never needed and is in fact contraindicated, since electrocoagulation may result in thermal injury and, together with a scarred area with compromised blood supply, may lead to recurrent stricture. In our series over a 4-year period, there has been no need for fulguration and no patient has required transfusion.

At the completion of the procedure, a retrograde ureteropyelogram can be performed to check the efficacy of the incision and the lumen, but this is seldom needed or informative because of an incision into periureteral fat and contrast extravasation, which might

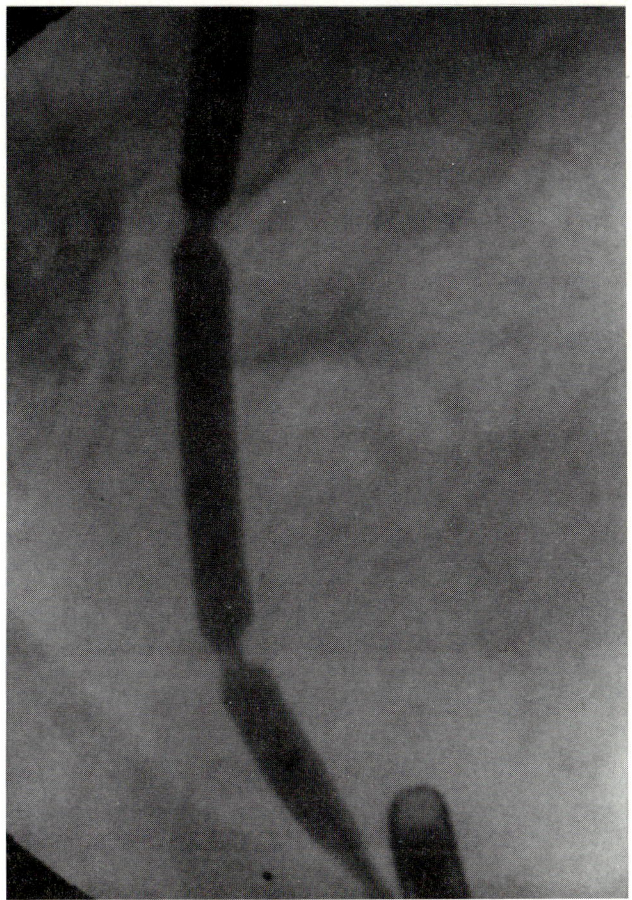

Figure 2 Balloon dilatation of the distal ureter in a male with renal stones. There are two areas of narrowing in the right ureter: one approximately 1 cm above the ureterovesical junction and the second at the lower margin of the sacroiliac joint. After completion of the dilatation, these areas of wasting should disappear, and the balloon must look fully inflated in its entirety.

interfere with fluoroscopic positioning of the ureteral stent. If there is any doubt as to the adequacy of the incision, a "balloon test" can be performed by inserting a low-pressure balloon catheter across the incised area, applying less than 20 PSI of pressure to the catheter. This will demonstrate clearly if any wasting still exists after the incision. Visual evaluation and easy excursion of the endoureterotome in the strictured area are usually adequate indicators of a successful incision.

Relative contraindications to endoureterotomy include abnormal coagulation parameters, the presence of retroperitoneal vascular grafts, previously operated ureters with abnormal positions (making wire and instrument passage difficult), and severe urinary tract infection. All efforts should be made to ensure sterile urine before the endoscopic incision.

Postoperative Stenting

An 8-, 10-, or 12-Fr double-pigtail or endoureterotomy stent is left in place for 4 weeks when one is stenting

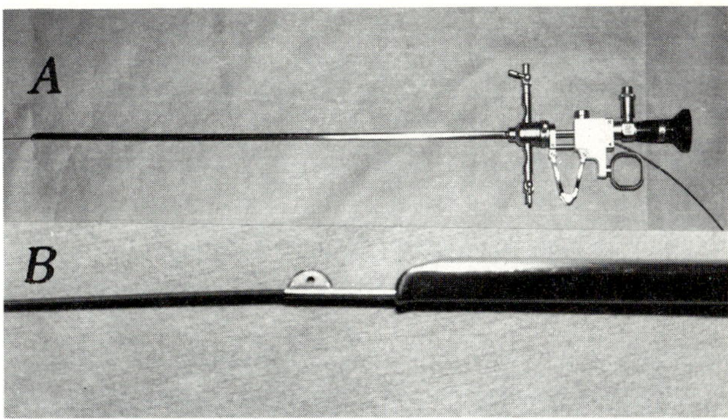

Figure 3 *A*, Assembled cold-knife endoureterotome with a guidewire inside the cutting element (Olympus, Lake Success, NY). *B*, Close-up of the tip of the instrument with the cold knife extending out of the sheath over the guidewire.

small, short strictures; 6 to 8 weeks are required for long and dense strictures that need extensive endoureterotomies. Stenting length is based on experimental work demonstrating that ureteral mucosa regenerates in 6 days and ureteral muscularis by 6 to 8 weeks.

In the absence of a full-thickness incision with visible periureteral fat, a special endouretotomy stent with side grooves and no internal lumen is used to allow for hydrostatic dilatation of the ureteral wall by the passing urine, which may improve patency and prevent stricture recurrence. With extensive incisions and visible fat this stent may be contraindicated, as it may lead to more urinary extravasation and produce delayed healing. Another option is a 6- to 8-Fr catheter with a 4-cm long 12-Fr diameter sleeve that can be repositioned along the shaft to correspond to the area of incision for mucosal regeneration around a maximal diameter. A 1- or 2-day period of Foley drainage is recommended to prevent vesicoureteral reflux. Perioperative intravenous antibiotics are administered followed by oral antibiotics until stent removal. After removal, follow-up consists of intravenous pyelography (IVP) at 3 months and diuretic renal scan and/or sonogram every 4 to 6 months.

Using this technique in 61 strictures, we had an initial success of 93 percent, which improved to 98 percent after a second incision in three patients who experienced recurrence 3 to 5 months after stent removal. Two patients have residual hydroureters with an open lumen because of long-standing stricture, but they are asymptomatic; if these two are considered failures, our overall success rate is 95 percent. One patient with a long upper ureteral stricture after ureterolithotomy failed balloon dilatation twice and endoscopic incision with scissors once, and underwent successful ureteroureterostomy (Fig. 6).

HOT-KNIFE ENDOURETEROTOMY

Although hot-knife endoureterotomy has been performed in a retrograde fashion with a 3-Fr electrode through the working channel of an endoscope for the treatment of ureteral stenosis (Table 3), the best results

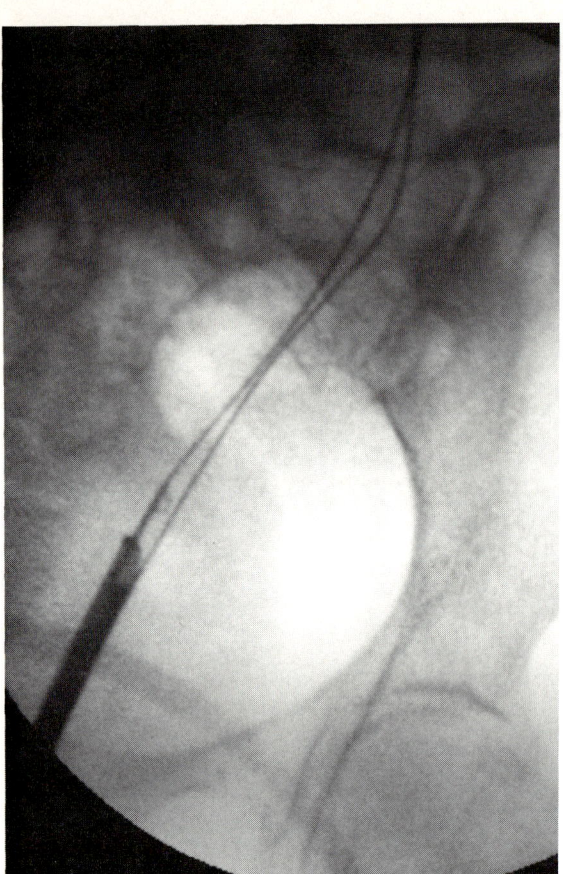

Figure 4 Fluoroscopic view of the incision of a left distal ureteral stricture with a cold-knife endoureterotome. The second guidewire is placed through the cold knife to maintain a constant intraluminal position of the blade.

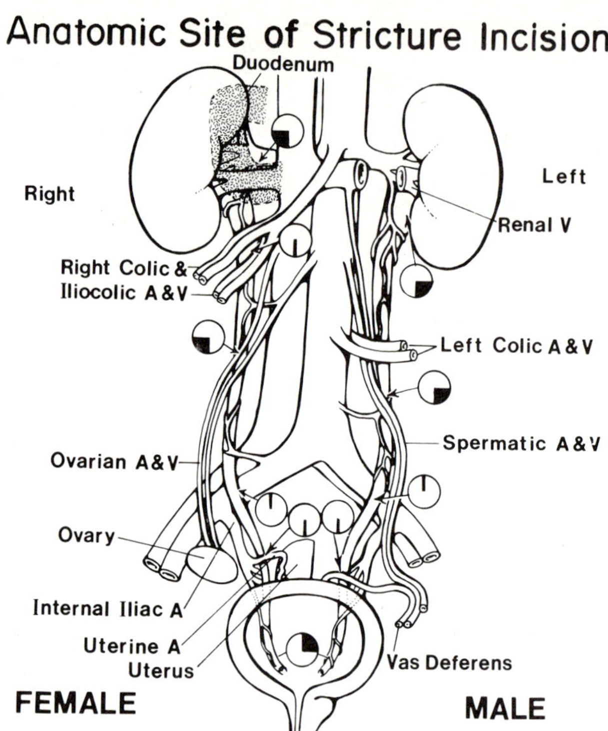

Figure 5 Recommended anatomic sites for incision of the ureteral strictures are based on the surface anatomy of the ureter and paraureteral structures. Observance of these sites will keep the incision away from the vital structures while at the same time preserving the blood supply of the ureter.

with this technique are described for antegrade incision in the management of ureterointestinal anastomotic strictures. Such strictures occur at variable intervals postoperatively, as a result of cancer recurrence, retroperitoneal metastasis, or benign disease (ischemia). Previously, standard surgical management included laparotomy with biopsy to rule out recurrence and reexcision of the anastomosis. Due to previous surgery and radiation this approach is associated with high rates of morbidity. As a result, the initial approach should always be the least invasive, regardless of cause.

Although antegrade high-pressure balloon dilatation followed by stenting of varying duration has met limited success (40 percent in 3 months and 16 percent in 1 year) in achieving stent-free cure in this difficult type of ureteral stricture, more encouraging results have been demonstrated with antegrade endoscopic hot-knife incision. Once a wire is negotiated across the stricture and into the bowel lumen, a flexible nephroscope is advanced antegrade to the point of obstruction. Under direct vision with a 3- or 5-Fr electrode passed through the working channel of the endoscope, the strictured area is incised until re-entry into the intestinal segment is achieved. It is advisable to have the intestinal segment filled with contrast media to assess stricture length and direction under fluoroscopy. After the stricture is recanalized, it is dilated further with a balloon and stented with a pigtail or custom-tailored catheter for the best drainage and patency of the anastomosis. The highest reported success rate (with 2.3-year follow up) with this technique is 58 percent; only one failure could have been considered for surgical recision (Table 4). This is not as high as the 89 percent success rate reported by the same group in nine strictures managed surgically, but for most patients this initial conservative approach is reasonable in view of its lower morbidity, the decreased cost, and the shorter hospital stay compared with open revision. For patients with advanced disease who fail endourologic management of an anastomotic stricture and are poor surgical risks, an indwelling ureteral stent, with frequent changes to prevent obstruction, is a reasonable alternative.

COLD-KNIFE URETEROSCOPIC ENDOPYELOTOMY AND INFUNDIBULOTOMY

During the last year we have extended the technique of cold-knife endoureterotomy to the ureteropelvic junction (UPJ) obstruction as well. With the cold-knife endoureterotome, the posterolateral aspect of the UPJ

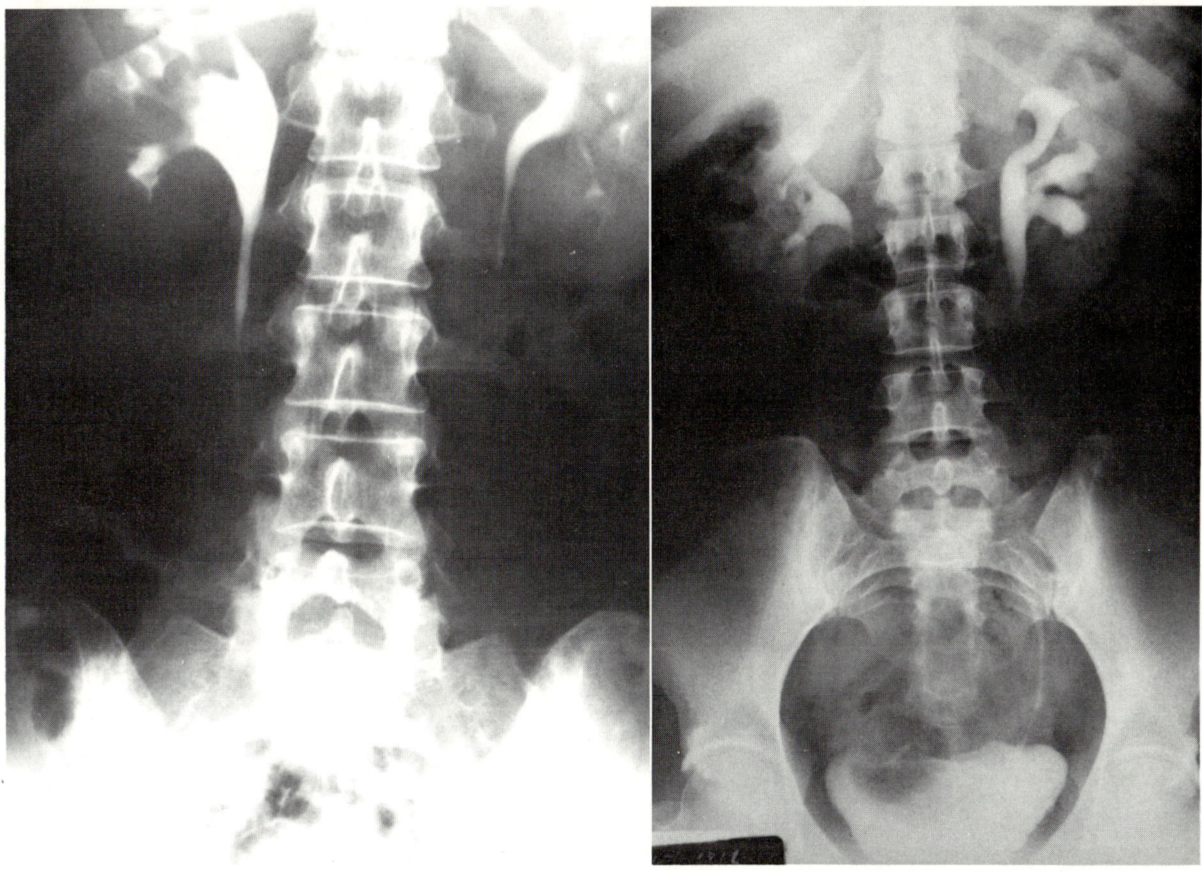

Figure 6 *A,* Postoperative intravenous urogram of the patient shown in Figure 1*A.* The patient underwent cold-knife endoureterotomy with 6 weeks of stenting. The blunting of the calices has almost disappeared and the dilatation of the renal pelvis and upper ureter has mostly subsided. *B,* Intravenous urogram of the patient shown in Figure 1*B.* Nine months after cold knife ureteroscopic endoureterotomy. Note that there is still a very mild fullness of the pelvis and the calices, which is probably due to long-term obstruction, but that the distal ureter is patent and the kidney drains well.

is incised full thickness into the fat. Postoperatively, a 10-Fr peripheral stent is placed for 6 weeks. Eight patients have undergone this procedure without failure. Three cases of ureterocalicostomy and infundibular stenosis have also been managed in this manner (Fig. 7).

SURGICAL TREATMENT OF URETERAL STENOSIS

Surgical repair for ureteral stenosis is indicated in the presence of an extremely long (>4 cm), dense stricture or a completely stenotic lumen (above the ureterovesical junction [UVJ]), or after multiple attempts at endourologic correction have failed.

Nonreconstructive procedures include surgical decompression of an obstructed kidney in a septic patient by nephrostomy drainage (percutaneous or open), or performed as a diagnostic procedure for antegrade evaluation of the extent of the stricture. Nephrectomy may be required in a nonfunctioning kidney that fails to function after decompression, in a severely infected kidney, in a very old patient with a normal contralateral

kidney, or in a situation in which failure of the primary ureteral repair may have fatal consequences (e.g., a urinary leak near a vascular graft).

Surgical reconstruction has been required in less than 6 percent of cases of ureteral stricture and obliteration at our institution over the last 5 years.

Ureteroureterostomy

Excision of the strictured ureteral segment with reanastomosis of the severed ends is indicated in the management of short fibrotic strictures more than 6 cm from the UVJ.

Absolute contraindications include inadequate length to achieve a tension-free anastomosis. Perianastomotic abscess, hematoma, or urinoma; previous surgical dissection or ureteral mobilization; previous injury, fibrosis, or radiation; and ureteral stenosis near a vascular graft or bypass are relative contraindications.

Surgical incision depends on the location of the ureteral stricture. In the absence of contraindications, successful repair is dependent on adequate debridement of the ureteral edges with preservation of blood supply,

Table 4 Endourologic Management of Ureterointestinal Anastomotic Stricture

Type of Treatment	Author	No. of Strictures	Balloon Size	Stent Size	Success Rate (%)	Comments
I. Ureteral stent	Smith (1979)	1	NA	9F	100	Stent remained indwelling
	Rose (1980)	3	NA	7.1–8.3 Fr	100	Stent remained indwelling
	Lange (1984)	17	NA	NA	58	Defined success as preserved renal function
II. High-pressure balloon dilatation (HPBD) and Stent	Shapiro (1988)	20	12 Fr	8–10Fr	16	1. Ureteroileostomy for cervical cancer or after pelvic RT resistant to HPBD 2. Ureteroileostomy for bladder pathology more amenable to dilatation
	Kramalowsky (1987)	4	15–36 Fr	5–18 Fr	0	
III. Hot-knife incision	Meretyk (1991)	19	30–36 Fr	16–22 Fr	57	See text

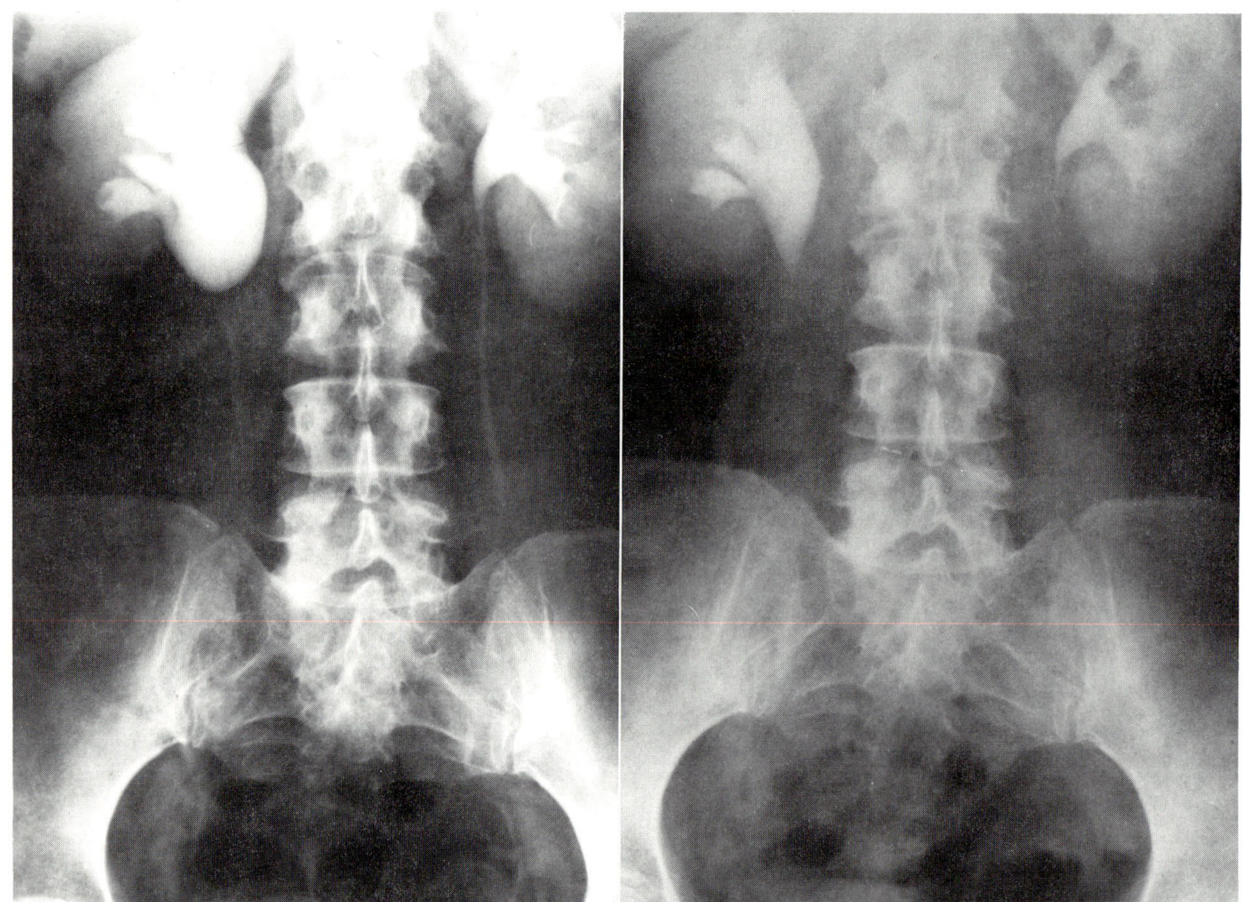

Figure 7 *A,* Preoperative intravenous urogram in a patient with right UPJ obstruction. Note the degree of dilatation of the renal pelvis and calices. *B,* Postoperative intravenous urogram in the same patient after cold-knife ureteroscopic endopyelotomy. Note that there has been a drastic decrease in the dilatation of the renal pelvis and the calices.

and a noncircular, spatulated, tension-free, watertight anastomosis performed with interrupted or continuous fine absorbable sutures (Fig. 8). Surgical adjuncts include wide renal mobilization with fixation to the retroperitoneum to gain 4 to 8 cm of proximal ureteral length, and the use of omentum or retroperitoneal fat to wrap the ureter, which may prevent restenosis. Stenting and proximal diversion with a nephrostomy are optional, but they will not prevent restenosis if a leaky, tense repair is performed. A Penrose or closed self-suction drain is placed near the anastomosis, since retroperitoneal collections are poorly resorbed.

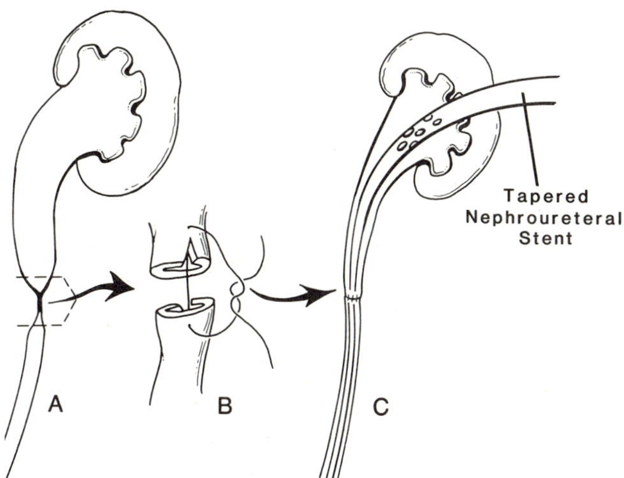

Figure 8 *A,* Technique of ureteroureterostomy. The stenotic segment is incised to obtain healthy tissue proximally and distally. *B,* The ureter is spatulated at opposite sides proximally and distally and reapproximated, and a watertight closure obtained. *C,* In very high strictures it may be worthwhile to use a tapered nephroureteral stent to provide proximal drainage as well as stenting of the anastomotic site.

Complications include prolonged urinary drainage with urinoma, possible ureterocutaneous fistula formation, and restenosis of the anastomotic site. If repair fails and restenosis occurs, secondary operations should be delayed after temporary nephrostomy diversion for 4 to 6 months.

Ureterolysis

When ureteral stenosis with associated renal obstruction is caused by periureteral fibrosis secondary to a benign or malignant retroperitoneal condition that is not reversible by drug ingestion (steroids) or drug withdrawal (methysergide), surgical correction is indicated. Through a transperitoneal midline incision, the ureters are exposed and bluntly dissected from the fibrotic process from the UPJ to below the iliac vessels, taking tissue for biopsy and frozen section to rule out malignancy and carefully avoiding vascular or ureteral injury. Once freed, the ureters are placed intraperitoneally or left retroperitoneally separated from the fibrotic process with fat or an omental wrap.

Complications include ureteral restenosis if the ureters are devascularized or if the fibrotic process recurs; urinary leak should injury occur; and if vascular injury occurs. Postoperatively, patients should be followed with periodic tests of serum creatinine levels and with intravenous pyelography (IVP) to rule out recurrence. Stenting is optional.

Davis Intubated Ureterotomy

Davis intubated ureterotomy can be performed for long ureteral strictures involving the upper ureter. Con-

traindications include the presence of periureteral inflammation, foreign bodies, or necrotic debris that may prevent unscarred healing. Like endoscopic ureterotomy, this procedure depends on uroepithelial regeneration at 4 to 7 days, followed by muscular regeneration of the defect from surrounding normal muscle by 6 to 8 weeks.

After full-thickness, longitudinal, external ureterotomy across the stenotic segment and into healthy ureter 1 cm proximal and distal, the entire ureter is stented with an internal pigtail stent and nephrostomy or a universal nephroureteral stent, and the incised area is surrounded with fat or omentum (Fig. 9). Penrose or closed-suction drains are placed near the affected area, and the stent is left in place for 6 to 8 weeks until the nephrostogram confirms proper healing.

Transureteroureterostomy

Transureteroureterostomy (TUU) is indicated for the treatment of middle third or pelvic ureteral strictures with accompanying ipsilateral pelvic infection, or inflammation in the latter case when ureteroneocystostomy is contraindicated. It can also be used as a secondary procedure when a previous ureteroureterostomy restenoses, always bearing in mind that technical errors jeopardize both collecting systems.

Contraindications include inadequate ureteral length to permit a tension-free anastomosis; previous ureteral injury or radiation; genitourinary tuberculosis; kidney stones; carcinoma; retroperitoneal fibrosis; and chronic infection, reflux, or obstruction of the recipient ureter.

Both ureters are approached transperitoneally. The donor ureter is mobilized proximal to the stricture, carefully preserving its blood supply. The ureter is then transected, tagged with a suture, and passed via a mesenteric tunnel anterior to the great vessels and cephalad to the inferior mesenteric artery to prevent its compression by the artery (Fig. 10). The anastomotic site of the recipient ureter is prepared with minimal dissection, a 1- to 2-cm longitudinal ureterotomy is made, and the donor ureter is anastomosed to the recipient after spatulation in a watertight, tension-free manner with fine absorbable sutures, wrapping the anastomosis with omentum. The area is drained extraperitoneally with a Penrose drain; stenting is optional. Proper patient selection prevents complications, with successful results in 95 to 97 percent of described cases.

Ureteroneocystostomy

Intra- or extravesical ureteral reimplantation into the bladder in an antirefluxing fashion is indicated in the treatment of ureteral stenosis within 6 cm of the UVJ, owing to the difficulty and higher failure rate of ureteroureterostomy of the pelvic ureter. The major contraindication to primary ureteroneocystostomy is excessive anastomotic tension. A vesicopsoas hitch or a Boari bladder flap allows primary vesical reimplantation of the

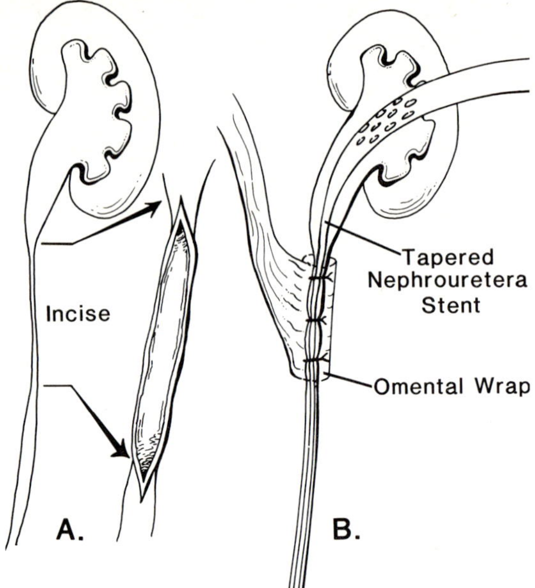

Figure 9 *A,* Davis intubated ureterotomy. The stenotic area is incised until the proximal and distal point of the incision show a wide lumen. *B,* A nephrostomy and a ureteral stent or a combination of a nephroureteral stent is used. The edges of the incised ureter can be partially reapproximated over the stent. It is helpful if a piece of omentum can be mobilized and wrapped around this segment to provide good blood supply for viability and regeneration of the ureter.

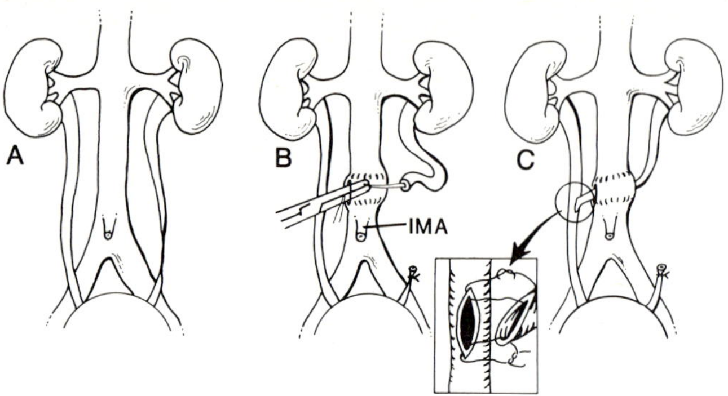

Figure 10 *A,* Technique of transureteroureterostomy. There is a long stricture in the left ureter that cannot be managed with ureteroureterostomy. *B,* Division of the ureter and retroperitoneal tunneling of the ureter in front of the aorta, above the level of the inferior mesenteric artery, to the contralateral side. *C,* End-to-side watertight anastomosis of the left ureter to the right ureter.

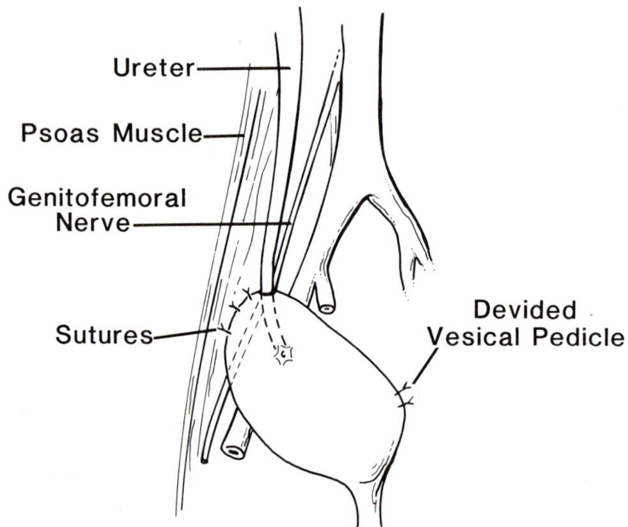

Figure 11 Completed psoas hitch. The right lateral superior aspect of the bladder is sutured to the psoas muscle. Sometimes, in order to achieve this degree of mobilization, the contralateral vesical pedicle needs to be divided. After the fixation of the bladder to the psoas muscle, the reimplantation of the ureter is performed.

ureter when there is a risk that tension on the anastomosis and excessive ureteral mobilization may result in restenosis and leakage.

The vesicopsoas hitch provides an additional 4 to 6 cm of length to reimplant the ureter into the bladder. It requires mobilization of the lateral bladder wall and stripping of the peritoneal reflection off the dome and posterior bladder wall. After a transverse anterolateral vesicotomy is made, two fingers placed within the bladder lumen displace the bladder over and above the iliac vessels, fixating the bladder to the medial aspect of the ileopsoas fascia with several heavy absorbable sutures without injuring the genitofemeral nerve or iliac vessels (Fig. 11). Sometimes, in order to obtain adequate mobility, the contralateral vesical arteries (lateral pedicle) must be divided. Antirefluxing reimplantation may then be performed by creating a long submucosal tunnel with minimal tension. The bladder is closed in two layers after suprapubic catheter placement, and a Penrose drain is placed near the anastomosis.

The Boari bladder flap provides 12 to 16 cm of extra distal ureteral length. This includes creating a pedicle tube bladder graft to bridge the long defect in cases of long (8- to 10-cm) lower ureteral strictures.

After complete lateral and posterior bladder mobilization, a flap is created from the posterior bladder wall 4 cm at the base and 3 cm at the apex, and may be spiraled anteriorly for more length (Fig. 12). The debrided, spatulated ureter is then reimplanted with a submucosal tunnel if possible, or to the end of the flap with inter-

rupted fine absorbable suture. The flap is closed in two layers, a suprapubic tube and Penrose drain are placed, and the anastomosis is usually left unstented.

Contraindications to the use of the psoas hitch and bladder flap are (1) a contracted, scarred, or irradiated bladder and (2) previous bladder surgery that could lead to vascular compromise and a greater risk of anastomotic leaks or restricture.

Ureteral Replacement with Bowel

Partial or complete intestinoplasty is indicated for the management of extensive ureteral stenosis that is not amenable to correction by any of the previously de-

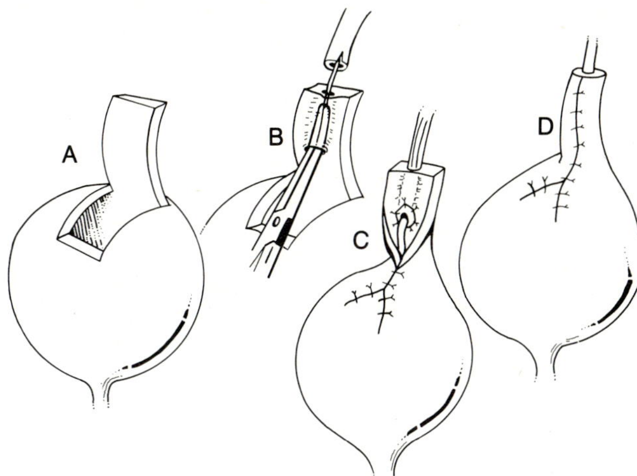

Figure 12 Technique of Boari flap with reimplantation of the ureter. *A,* development of the flap from the anteroposterior aspect of the bladder; *B,* development of the submucosal tunnel and advancement of the ureter; *C,* completion of the submucosal tunnel and fixation of the ureter; *D,* closure of the flap in a cylindrical fashion.

scribed methods. The most commonly used intestinal segment for ureteral replacement is ileum, but descending colon and appendix have been used with some success.

Contraindications to ileal ureter replacement include disorders of the intestinal tract such as Crohn's disease and diverticulitis, compromised renal function (creatinine > 2.0), and a functionally abnormal bladder.

After the integrity of the bladder and small bowel is assured, the patient is given a standard bowel preparation and antibiotics, and a long, midline, transperitoneal incision is made. The small bowel is mobilized and a segment of ileum 20 to 25 cm long with good vascular supply is isolated 15 cm proximal to the ileocecal valve. Bowel continuity is re-established with a stapled or sutured two-layer ileoileostomy. The bowel segment is passed through a mesocolic window into a retroperitoneal position, care being taken to ensure that the ileum is used in an isoperistaltic fashion. A pyeloileal, calicoileal, or ureteroileal anastomosis is performed proximally with a full-thickness single-layer absorbable suture. If the ileum is anastomosed to the renal pelvis, the ileal end is first spatulated. The ileovesical anastomosis is performed in one layer with fine absorbable suture. Use of a vesicopsoas hitch is advantageous to reduce the length of small intestine used, reduce its absorptive surface area, and eliminate a deep pelvic anastomosis. If a psoas hitch is not performed, the ileum is anastomosed to the bladder close to the trigone in a refluxing fashion with fine absorbable suture. The distal end can also be tapered and reimplanted with a tunnel or anastomosed to the bladder with a nipple valve.

For long ureteral strictures, one can use a 5- to 10-cm segment of ileum and taper it on the antimesenteric side over a Foley catheter. This tapered segment can then be interpositioned between the upper and

lower ureter, replacing the strictured area. The advantage of this technique is that it leaves the distal ureter intact and nonrefluxing.

The ileal ureteral anastomosis is protected proximally with a nephrostomy, and a suprapubic tube is placed in the bladder for irrigation of mucus with Penrose drains near each anastomosis. A nephrostogram performed at 10 days evaluates the anastomoses for leaks and determines the need for further stenting and drainage.

Complications include hyperchloremic, hyperkalemic metabolic acidosis (rarely seen in the presence of normal total renal function), reflux with potential upper tract deterioration (although the natural bowel peristalsis prevents high voiding pressures from being transmitted directly to the kidneys), mucous occlusion of the bowel segment or bladder, and anastomotic leak or stricture (which rarely occurs in the absence of tension and poor vascularity).

RENAL AUTOTRANSPLANTATION

Renal autotransplantation is indicated to treat long ureteral stenosis (1) in the absence of perirenal inflammation or underlying arteriosclerotic vascular disease, both of which may impair vascular perfusion and subsequent viability; (2) in the absence of severe renal parenchymal disease, which flushes poorly upon removal; and (3) when ureteral replacement by ileum is contraindicated or refused by the patient. It should also never be performed when equivalent results can be obtained by simpler measures, or as a desperate measure to save a poorly functioning kidney. The major advantage of autotransplantation over ileal ureter replacement is that it restores a healthy autologous excretory system without the associated complications of reflux and infection that affect the ileal ureter. Experience and technical competence in renal transplant are essential for a successful result.

After preoperative pelvic and renal arteriography to determine the number of renal arteries and evaluate the condition of the recipient vessels, a transperitoneal incision is made, the kidney is freed from all its attachments, and the renal vessels are identified and isolated with minimal manipulation to preserve ureteral blood supply. Intravenous mannitol and heparin are administered before dividing the renal artery and vein close to their junctions with the aorta and inferior vena cava. Renal viability is maintained with hypothermic pulsatile perfusion by means of one of various accepted mediums. After preparation of the pelvic vessels, the kidney is placed upside down in the ipsilateral iliac fossa and in a reverse anteroposterior position in the contralateral iliac fossa. A spatulated end-to-end anastomosis is performed between the renal and internal iliac arteries or end-to-side between the renal and external iliac arteries, and an end-to-side renal vein to external or common iliac vein anastomosis is performed with fine continuous cardiovascular Prolene suture.

After revascularization, urinary continuity is restored with ureteroureterostomy, pyeloureterostomy, ureteroneocystostomy, or pyelovesicostomy, depending on the state of the transplanted and native ureter. As an adjunct to pyelovesicostomy, which is performed with complete ureteral loss, a bladder flap may be created, as previously outlined, to increase ureteral length.

Complications include graft loss due to perihilar fibrosis with vascular thrombosis, renal hemorrhage, and urinary leak or ureteral restenosis.

Postoperative management consists of a renal scan on the first day to rule out vascular thrombosis and either a nephrostogram (if a nephrostomy is employed) at 10 days or IVP at 6 to 8 weeks in the absence of a nephrostomy.

URINARY DIVERSION

Although urinary diversion is rarely indicated in the elective operative repair of a ureteral stricture, rapidly performed cutaneous ureterostomy may be required in the face of an intraoperative anesthetic complication during a planned reconstructive procedure for ureteral stenosis.

The ureters are approached transperitoneally, mobilized cephalad to allow them to protrude over the skin by at least 2 cm, debrided to healthy tissue, spatulated, and tagged with a suture. A stoma site is selected, and a U skin incision is made down to fascia. A cruciate fascial incision is made straight into the abdominal cavity to admit an index finger. The U skin flap is sutured to the spatulated ureter with fine interrupted absorbable sutures and stented.

The most significant complication is stomal stenosis (50 to 60 percent) caused by the poor blood supply of the distal ureter. This is only a technique of last resort when the patient's condition precludes a lengthy attempt at reconstruction. A nephrostomy tube with ligation of the ureter may be a better alternative in patients who will undergo reconstruction later.

While the burgeoning increase in diagnostic and therapeutic endourological procedures on the ureter has reduced the need for surgical management and its associated higher morbidity and cost, aggressive ureteral dilation and ureteroscopy has contributed to an increase in the total absolute number and percentage of cases of ureteral strictures seen by urologists. As a result, urologists will be required to treat this condition more frequently than in the past.

Endourological treatment of stricture using high pressure balloon catheters and hot or cold knife incision should allow successful (50 to 98 percent) stent-free repair of most short strictures and should be considered as first-line treatment. In the presence of multiple failed endourological attempts at repair or extremely long strictures, operative repair is indicated, tailoring the procedure to the site and extent of the stenosis. Successful operative reconstruction depends on adequate ureteral debridement, preservation of ureteral blood supply, and performance of a tension-free, watertight anastomosis. Regardless of the technique utilized, the goals of management must be to restore ureteral continuity by removing obstruction, preserving renal function, and preventing morbidity and mortality by subjecting the patient to the minimum number of corrective procedures to obtain a satisfactory result.

SUGGESTED READING

Banner MP, Pollack HM. Dilation of ureteral stenosis. AJR 1984; 143:789.

Eshghi M. Dilatation of ureteral orifice for ureterorenoscopy. Urol Clin North Am 1988; 15:301.

Eshghi M. Endoscopic incisions of the ureter. Parts 1, 2, and 3. AUA Update Series, Volume 9, lessons 37–39, 1989.

Koontz WW, Klein FA, Vernon-Smith MJ. Surgery of the ureter. In: Walsh PC, Gittes RF, Perlmutter AD, Stamey TA, eds. Campbell's urology. 5th ed. Philadelphia: WB Saunders, 1986.

Merdyk S, Clayman RV, Kavoussi LR, Kramalowsky EV, Ricus DD: Endourological treatment of ureteroenteric anastomotic strictures: long-term follow up. J Urol 1991; 145:723.

Perlmutter AD, Stamey TA, eds. Campbell's Urology. 5th ed. Philadelphia: WB Saunders, 1986.

Silverstein JI, Libby C, Smith AD. Management of ureteroscopic injuries. Urol Clin North Am 1988; 15:515.

POSTIRRADIATION URETERAL STENOSIS

STEFAN A. LOENING, M.D., F.A.C.S.

Ureteral stenosis due to radiation injury is usually seen in the distal ureters and is related to radiotherapy of pelvic malignancies, most commonly cervical cancer treated by combined interstitial and external radiation therapy. Radiogenic ureteral injury can also occur after treatment of cancer of the bladder, prostate, and ovaries as well as other malignancies.

Radiogenic injury and subsequent stenosis is usually a bilateral process but in some cases is limited to one side. Unilateral radiogenic stenosis is especially common in patients treated with implanted radioactive seeds when misplacement or migration has occurred.

Ureteral stenosis from radiation injury usually develops slowly, but obstruction can occur as early as 6 months or as late as 20 years or more after the initial radiation treatment. Unless patients are followed closely with excretory urography or other diagnostic procedures, the stenosis may result in severe renal damage before being recognized.

In patients with known extraureteral primary malignancy, especially genitourinary cancer, it is necessary to differentiate thickening of the ureteral wall due to tumor metastases from that due to radiation, infection, or operative trauma, since treatment may vary greatly. Cancers of the genitourinary tract and colon are the most common neoplastic lesions involving ureters, accounting for 70 percent of the causes of extrinsic metastatic obstruction, but any other malignancy may extend to the retroperitoneum and lead to ureteral stricture. Unilateral obstruction is most often due to recurrent cancer.

PATIENT EVALUATION

Table 1 lists diagnostic procedures to evaluate and differentiate the causes of ureteral obstruction. The findings help in choosing the appropriate treatment. Radiographic studies, including excretory and retrograde urography, demonstrate the location and length of the ureteral stenosis, factors that are very important in choosing the proper treatment. By means of cystoscopy and retrograde studies, specimens can be obtained for cytologic study. The danger, however, of false-positive diagnosis in the presence of an inflammatory or reparative process or in previously irradiated tissue should be kept in mind by the cytopathologist, since most patients undergo irradiation, chemotherapy or surgery. The absence of nuclear chromatin abnormalities and a knowledge of the morphology of the primary cancer are the most important points in distinguishing this type of cellular reaction from malignancy. Spindle, stellate, and fibroblastic cells may simulate malignant cells.

Computed tomographic (CT) scans of the abdomen and pelvis may detect recurrent tumor, but malignant cells are rarely seen in patients with periureteral metastases or malignancies. Exploratory laparotomy with multiple direct biopsies would otherwise be the only other procedure to determine the cause of obstruction accurately unless a CT-guided biopsy can resolve the diagnostic problem.

Laboratory tests and retrograde studies may confirm bilateral obstruction resulting in renal insufficiency and the need for preliminary drainage procedures, such as percutaneous nephrostomy or retrograde stenting, before more definitive therapy is undertaken. Unilateral obstruction, on the other hand, often leads to fever, flank pain, or hypertension. Infection proximal to the ureteral obstruction may also indicate a preliminary drainage procedure before definitive surgical correction.

Voiding symptoms may suggest radiation damage in the bladder. These usually can be confirmed visually by cystoscopic examination, which shows typical damage of the bladder mucosa secondary to previous radiation therapy. Such radiation damage to the bladder may limit the choice of treatment. Bladder function can be further evaluated by urodynamic studies, but the history usually provides a good indication of the function and capacity

Table 1 Patient Evaluation

History and physical examination
Urine culture
Excretory urography
Cytoscopy
Retrograde urography and cytologies
Voiding cystourethrography
Computed tomography
DMSA DTPA renal scan
Urodynamic studies

of the bladder. Voiding cystourethrography may be considered as a further test for documentation purposes.

DMSA DTPA scan provides accurate and valuable information about total and differential renal function. The motility of the collecting system can likewise be assessed. The information on these two parameters again aids the choice of treatment.

THERAPEUTIC OPTIONS

Table 2 lists available treatment options in the management of patients with radiation damage. Observation, which may not be used enough, should be considered if the patient is asymptomatic and has a normally functioning contralateral kidney. Any surgical intervention in patients who have had previous radiation treatments carries a higher morbidity; this should be kept in mind especially in the case of patients who are otherwise asymptomatic.

Open surgical procedures available for palliative urinary diversion (formal nephrostomy, cutaneous ureterostomy, and ureterolysis) are generally contraindicated in advanced malignancies, since they are attended by significant morbidity and since only 40 to 50 percent of the treated patients survive more than 3 to 6 months, never leaving the hospital. Therefore, less aggressive therapy, such as plain percutaneous nephrostomy or endoscopic insertion of indwelling ureteral stents, may be more suitable in prolonging life without increasing morbidity and pain.

Balloon dilatation is a new technique, but it has not been shown to have consistent, long-lasting benefits in patients with the fibrotic reaction, as can be seen with radiation damage. The combination of balloon dilatation and incision can be considered if there is a short stenotic segment some distance from the pelvic vasculature.

Various self-retaining ureteral catheters, placed either retrograde or in a percutaneous antegrade fashion, can be used for stenting and draining of the collecting system. These can help in assessing the recovery of renal function and in treatment planning once an obstruction has been relieved. They also can be left in place for prolonged periods. Usually, the catheters need to be changed on a 2- to 3-month basis to prevent encrustation. Unfortunately, most patients also have symptoms of radiation cystitis and do not tolerate the indwelling ureteral catheters in spite of anticholinergic medications.

Table 2 Therapeutic Options

Observation
Balloon dilatation and incision
Ureteral stent (retrograde or percutaneous insertion)
Ureteral lysis
Ureteroneocystostomy
Transureteroureterostomy
Intestinal substitution of ureter
Supravesical diversion
   Ureterointestinal conduit
   Cutaneous ureterostomy
   Nephrostomy
Nephrectomy

Ureterolysis is rarely of benefit, but radiation may have caused obstruction by other means such as tubo-ovarian abscesses and lymphoceles. In such cases, ureterolysis is less likely to produce urinary fistulas than some other procedures, such as ureteroneocystostomy.

In patients with normal bladder function and no significant damage from radiation therapy to the bladder, ureteroneocystostomy is the most commonly performed corrective surgery. The bladder, however, needs to be assessed before this procedure to determine its distensibility, since a psoas hitch and/or a Boari flap may be needed to prevent any tension on the anastomosis.

In general, however, it is preferable to minimize mobilization of and surgery on the bladder to keep as much of the blood supply intact as possible. Tunneling of the ureter versus end-to-end anastomosis is not as important as a tension-free anastomosis and a good blood supply. The use of an indwelling double-J stent for a prolonged postoperative period is helpful because of the delayed wound healing in patients who have undergone previous radiation therapy.

Transureteroureterostomy (TUU) may be considered if the contralateral ureter has not been damaged by radiation therapy. This situation may arise owing to a misplaced seed or other processes (e.g., previous surgery, tubo-ovarian abscesses, lymphoceles). In this situation, a TUU is preferred to intestinal substitution because it is easier to perform and is associated with fewer complications.

Ileal substitution (ureteroileoneocystostomy) preserves renal function without the need for resorting to external diversion of urine. The effectiveness of this procedure is primarily due to the similarity between an isolated loop of small bowel and a segment of normal ureter. Small bowel is mobile with a rich blood supply and natural peristalsis. When distal ileum is damaged from irradiation, a more proximal segment or even jejunum can be used. Portions of small bowel (less than 25 cm in length) exhibit no prohibitive urinary electrolyte absorption. This procedure needs to be considered in patients with damage to the ureter extending above the pelvic brim.

Supravesical diversion becomes necessary when the bladder is so severely damaged that the above-mentioned procedures would not be of benefit. A ureterointestinal conduit is the preferred definitive supravesical diversion, especially in patients who have bilateral renal function. In patients with only one functioning renal unit, a nephrostomy has the advantage that it can be done percutaneously. As stated above, in regard to indwelling ureteral catheters, nephrostomy tubes must be changed at intervals of 3 to 4 months.

I prefer the transverse colon conduit urinary diversion in patients who have had pelvic radiation. It offers the following advantages:

1. This segment of bowel is less likely to be damaged by extensive pelvic irradiation; even the redundant transverse colon extending into the pelvis in many patients is mobile enough to receive less radiation than fixed pelvic structures.
2. A high ureteral or renal pelvic anastomosis can be achieved, thus using a segment of nonirradiated urinary tract.
3. Colon segments are less frequently complicated by stomal stenosis and related sequelae.
4. The effects of absorption of urine across the colon wall on renal function are minimized because of mass contraction emptying the segment and the resultant small residual volumes.
5. Other surgical procedures can be performed at the time of urinary diversion. Although proof of its superiority is still lacking, an antireflux colic anastomosis can be constructed optionally because of the thick wall colonic segment. In this group of patients, however, I have not performed antireflux anastomosis.

A simple nephrectomy is usually the last treatment option in patients who have failed previous corrective attempts or have not shown any substantial improvement in renal function after the placement of indwelling stents. It also may be indicated in patients with chronic renal infection and very poor renal function.

The many variables associated with radiogenic ureteral stenosis means that there is a range of therapeutic options to be considered. A detailed urologic evaluation allows the surgeon to choose the treatment option that is best suited to the patient's general condition and has the lowest likelihood of morbidity.

SUGGESTED READING

Dean RJ, Lytton B. Urologic complications of pelvic irradiation. J Urol 1978; 119:64.
Loening SA, Navarre RJ, Narayana AS, Culp DA. Transverse colon conduit urinary diversion. J Urol 1982; 127:37.
Perry CP, Massey FM, Moore TN, Erickson CA. Treatment of irradiation injury to the ureter by ileal substitution. Obstet Gynecol 1975; 46:517.

PRUNE-BELLY SYNDROME

RONALD RABINOWITZ, M.D., F.A.A.P., F.A.C.S.
WILLIAM C. HULBERT, Jr., M.D., F.A.A.P.

Prune-belly syndrome consists primarily of a triad of abnormalities: abdominal muscular deficiency, urinary tract abnormalities, and cryptorchidism. This is commonly referred to as the triad syndrome or the abdominal muscular deficiency syndrome. It has also been called the Eagle-Barrett syndrome. Prune-belly syndrome is seen almost exclusively in males and has an incidence of approximately one in 40,000 live births. In the complete syndrome there is marked deficiency of the abdominal muscles, allowing for easy palpation of abdominal viscera and visible intestinal peristalsis. The urinary collecting systems are bizarre and dysmorphic in appearance. The ureters are grossly dilated, tortuous, and commonly associated with massive vesicoureteral reflux. The urinary bladder is huge and often has a large urachal component. The proximal urethra has a classic appearance of a wide bladder neck and posteriorly dilated prostatic urethra, which tapers to a narrowed membranous urethra. The testes are intra-abdominal. Like other conditions, there is a spectrum of the severity of anomalies. There are many instances of incomplete forms of the syndrome, referred to as pseudo–prune-belly syndrome. These children may lack one or more of the major components of prune-belly syndrome, such as the abdominal laxity or cryptorchidism. The rare female with this condition usually has abdominal muscular deficiency as the major component, but she can have a severely affected urinary tract. In addition to the variability of involvement of the major components, there are often associated cardiac, orthopedic, and gastrointestinal abnormalities.

ETIOLOGY

Although the etiology of prune-belly syndrome remains unknown, many investigators now believe that prostatic hypoplasia is a critical element. This causes dilatation of the prostatic urethra and a functional obstruction leading to secondary dilatation of the urinary bladder and ureters, possibly with the formation of fetal ascites, resulting in abdominal distention. Perhaps the combination of massive bladder distention and abdominal muscular deficiency accounts for the cryptorchidism. Another theory of the etiology of prune-belly syndrome is an abnormal development of lateral plate mesoderm, which gives rise to the striated muscle of the abdominal wall and smooth muscle of the urinary tract. A third theory suggests that an abnormally large allantois, which is absorbed inside the abdomen, forming a large distended bladder and prostatic urethra, can also result in a distended prune-belly appearance of the abdomen. Chromosomal anomalies have also rarely been reported to be associated with this condition. There is an increased incidence of prune-belly syndrome in one member of monozygotic twin pregnancies.

Prune-belly syndrome has been diagnosed on prenatal ultrasound by observing the hugely dilated bladder and ureters and massively distended abdomen. In one reported instance, surgical construction of a fetal vesicostomy at 23 weeks' gestation resulted in marked improvement of the prune-belly appearance of the abdomen as well as the decompression of the urinary tract and resolution of the oligohydramnios.

EVALUATION

Infants with prune-belly syndrome must be evaluated for uropathology, pulmonary pathology, and associated anomalies.

Kidneys

When the newborn is found to have prune-belly syndrome, the urinary tract is initially evaluated with ultrasonography, renal function studies, and urine culture. The infant is then placed on antibiotic therapy and remains on long-term antibacterial prophylaxis. If renal function is satisfactory, the infant is evaluated electively with an intravenous urogram, voiding cystourethrogram (VCUG), and a functional upper tract study such as DMSA, DTPA, or MAG-3 renal scan. Some have gross renal failure secondary to renal dysplasia and may not survive the neonatal period. Others may have diminished renal function with severe hydronephrosis. Thus, the renal status can vary from normal to severe hydronephrosis and renal dysplasia.

Ureters

The ureters are initially evaluated with ultrasonography and intravenous urography. Since many reflux, VCUG also outlines the dilated ureters. Ultrasonography and fluoroscopy demonstrate that the distal ureters are progressively more dilated and less peristaltic than the proximal portions.

Urinary Bladder

The urinary bladder is huge and extends to the umbilicus, sometimes with a patent urachus. VCUG demonstrates the configuration of the dilated bladder, a dilated prostatic urethra with a somewhat narrowed membranous urethra that often meets the distal prostatic urethra at an abnormal angle, and often a urachal diverticulum.

Urethra

The proximal urethra, which is dilated in its prostatic portion, may be normal in its remainder. Often there is a narrowing of the membranous urethra, and this may even be atretic. Megalourethra is not uncommonly associated with prune-belly syndrome. Urethral abnormalities may make catheterization exceedingly difficult. VCUG can then be carried out by the percutaneous suprapubic route. Although posterior urethral valves have been reported in association with prune-belly syndrome, this is not a frequent association. Cystoscopy need not be employed if the VCUG demonstrates bladder and urethral anatomy well.

Testes

Classically, both testes in prune-belly syndrome are intra-abdominal, overlying the ureters at the level of the iliac vessels. However, some incomplete forms of the syndrome may have inguinal or even intrascrotal testes.

Abdominal Muscles

The abdominal wall defect in this syndrome responsible for the prune-belly appearance may be diffuse and severe or asymmetric and mild. Classically, the most affected areas are in the lower medial abdominal wall. The flanks bulge and the lower rib cage is flared. The abdominal organs are easily palpated through the thin, lax abdomen.

Lungs

Pulmonary status is extremely important in children with prune-belly syndrome. The pulmonary hypoplasia associated with oligohydramnios may result in neonatal death. Those who do not have pulmonary hypoplasia remain at significantly higher risk for pulmonary complications because of their decreased ability to clear pulmonary secretions as a result of their abdominal muscular deficiency. They have an increased risk for more severe pulmonary complications from upper respiratory tract infections. They are also at increased risk for anesthetic complications as well as postoperative atelectasis.

Associated Abnormalities

Prune-belly syndrome carries an increased risk of associated gastrointestinal, cardiac, and orthopedic deformities. These include imperforate anus, intestinal malrotation, ventricular septal defect, atrial septal defect, talipes equinovarus, and congenital dislocation of the hips.

MANAGEMENT

The urinary tract in children with prune-belly syndrome is generally managed nonoperatively, with close monitoring and follow-up and only selective surgical intervention in individualized cases. Renal function is evaluated from the newborn period onward. The degree of upper tract dilatation is monitored with ultrasonography and intravenous urography. Both studies are performed relatively early in the newborn as baseline studies. If renal function remains stable and the child remains free of infection while on antimicrobial prophylaxis, follow-up ultrasonography is performed at ages 4 to 8 months and an intravenous urogram is obtained at age 1 year. If the child continues to do well in terms of renal function, infection, and stable upper tract dilatation, ultrasonography is repeated at 6-month intervals until the age of 3 years, when an intravenous urogram is again performed. Thereafter, ultrasonography is performed yearly and intravenous urography every 3 to 4 years. Radioisotope renal scanning is performed in the infant and should be repeated periodically to assess individual renal function.

SURGICAL INTERVENTION

From a urologic standpoint, surgical intervention is carried out for the undescended testes and is considered for the ureters, bladder, urethra, and abdominal wall. Because of their relative importance, the surgical management of the ureters, bladder, and urethra will be discussed first. Although their surgical treatment may be considered separately, their management is intertwined. Abdominal wall plication may be performed in conjunction with any other reconstruction through a vertical midline incision that permits the abdominal wall fascia to be plicated transversely.

The entire dilated system is best decompressed, if necessary, by cutaneous vesicostomy. When there is progressive upper tract dilatation and/or deterioration of renal function in the absence of infection, temporary upper tract diversion may be considered.

Ureters

In the presence of marked vesicoureteral reflux, ureteral dilatation and tortuosity, and breakthrough urinary infections, improved urinary tract drainage is necessary. Extensive reconstruction can be employed, although alternative methods utilizing clean intermittent catheterization through the native urethra or a continent stoma may also be reasonable. Often, with urinary tract reconstruction, the ureteral dissection can be entirely transvesical. In addition, the lower ureters are much more deformed, dilated, and pathologic. The upper ureters may have near-normal caliber. A long length of excess ureter may be excised and the new ureteric orifice may have originally been in the middle to upper ureteral area. Reimplantation is performed by the Glenn-Anderson advancement technique with or without tailoring of the caliber of the ureteral segment to be reimplanted. This is combined with partial cystectomy, and each ureter is drained with a ureteral splint for 1 week. Because bladder function is generally poor and bladder emptying is impaired, postoperative evaluation with intravenous urography and/or renal scan may include postcatheterization studies.

Urinary Bladder

The huge bladder in prune-belly syndrome extends to the umbilicus, often as a urachal or pseudodiverticulum, and occasionally with a patent urachus. When temporary diversion is indicated, decompression of the bladder is the method of choice. The dome of the bladder or urachal component is brought through a fascial defect between the symphysis and umbilicus. If the urachal component is elongated and of tubular configuration, a portion may be excised. After a relatively small fascial segment is excised midway between the umbilicus and pubis, the muscularis of the bladder is sutured to rectus fascia and a skin flush stoma is created. In this condition, the stomal size should be rather generous, since stenosis is more of a problem than prolapse. With stabilization and/or improvement in renal function and upper tract dilatation, closure of the vesicostomy in conjunction with partial cystectomy should be considered. Unlike vesicostomy closure in other conditions in which the stoma is simply excised and a two-layered bladder closure carried out, I prefer to carry out closure of the vesicostomy in the prune-belly syndrome in conjunction with reduction cystoplasty. This may be performed through the same elliptical incision made to circumscribe the vesicostomy stoma at the time of closure. A lateral extension on each side of the ellipse is helpful for exposure. The dome of the bladder, which includes the entire urachal or pseudodiverticulum area, is excised as a wedge, and the bladder is closed. When ureteral reconstruction and/or reimplantation is undertaken, partial cystectomy or reduction cystoplasty is performed as part of the reconstruction.

Urethra

Although the urethra may be grossly deformed in prune-belly syndrome, active intervention is undertaken only in the presence of functional obstruction with associated urinary retention, infection, and/or progressive upper tract dilatation. Distal to the dilated prostatic urethra, folds of urethral wall may act as obstructing lesions. These may be endoscopically incised under direct vision using the Sachse optical urethrotomy blade. The membranous urethra may be quite stenotic. If a ureteral catheter can be passed through this stenotic segment, urethrotomy of this area may result in significantly improved emptying. This procedure may have to be performed on more than one occasion to achieve adequate caliber of the channel. When the penile urethra is grossly dilated (megalourethra), this may be associated with recurrent infections. Although a formal urethroplasty with excision of excess ventral urethra is often necessary, there are instances in which the redundant tissue may simply be plicated. The final result is similar, but there is a significantly lower incidence of complications such as fistula and infection, and postoperative urinary drainage is required for a significantly shorter time with the plication technique.

Testes

Orchidopexy may be the only surgical treatment necessary in some boys with prune-belly syndrome. Each testis may be approached through a high inguinal skin crease incision. If the testes can be operated on at approximately 6 months of age, a standard orchidopexy may be all that is necessary. If both testes are operated on simultaneously, a Pfaunenstiel incision may be used to improve intraperitoneal exposure. Often, the floor of the inguinal canal must be taken down to straighten and shorten the course of the spermatic vessels into the scrotum. This allows the cord structures to pass just lateral to the pubis on the way to the scrotum. The floor of the inguinal canal is then closed laterally, and the internal and external rings are superimposed on one another. In the older boy, the ability to bring the intra-abdominal testis down at one operation becomes more difficult unless one uses the Fowler-Stephens technique and divides the spermatic vessels. Because of an increased incidence of testicular atrophy when the testis is mobilized at the same time as spermatic vessel ligation, we prefer a staged Fowler-Stephens approach. The spermatic vessels are ligated and divided at the first operation, but the testis is left in situ. At a second operation 6 months later, the testis is mobilized, along with its vasal blood supply and new and increased collaterals, and moved into the scrotum.

When urinary tract intervention is necessary, testicular surgery may be combined with it. If the ureters are reimplanted, the testes may be mobilized with the distal ureters. In those instances when a vesicostomy was necessary, at the time of vesicostomy closure and partial cystectomy, a first-stage Fowler-Stephens procedure can be performed. When abdominal wall plication is carried out, the vertical midline approach can also be used for orchidopexy.

SUGGESTED READING

Greskovich FJ III, Nyberg LM Jr. The prune belly syndrome: a review of its etiology, defects, treatment and prognosis. J Urol 1988; 140:707–712.

Burbige KA, Amodio J, Berdon WE, et al. Prune belly syndrome: 35 years of experience. J Urol 1987; 137:86–90.

Woodard JR, Parrott TS. Orchidopexy in the prune belly syndrome. Br J Urol 1978; 50:348–351.

Orvis BR, Battles K, Kogan BA. Testicular histology in fetuses with the prune belly syndrome and posterior urethral valves. J Urol 1988; 139:335–337.

Snow BW, Duckett JW. The prune belly syndrome. In: Retik AB, Cukier J, eds. Pediatric urology. Baltimore: Williams & Wilkins, 1984:253–270.

CONGENITAL ADYNAMIC URETERAL SEGMENT WITH SECONDARY MEGAURETER

ANNE-MARIE HOULE, M.D., FRCSC
BERNARD M. CHURCHILL, M.D., FRCSC
GORDON A. McLORIE, M.D., FRCSC
ANTOINE E. KHOURY, M.D., FRCSC

The widespread use of pre- and postnatal ultrasonography has greatly increased the incidence of detection of asymptomatic ureteral dilatation in the pediatric population. This has given rise to what is probably the major debate in clinical pediatric urology today. This debate has continued whether ureteral dilatation indicates that obstruction is present in none, some, or all of the cases. This naturally has given rise to other clinical questions:

1. What is the risk of renal damage or destruction in the presence of asymptomatic ureteral dilatation?
2. Which cases require surgical correction?
3. If surgery is employed, which techniques are best?

To understand our philosophy of clinical management of this entity, it is essential to understand the underlying pathophysiology.

"Congenital adynamic ureteral segment" describes a lesion occurring in the distal 3 to 4 cm of the ureter. This segment is histologically and functionally abnormal. It is hypoplastic with an increased amount of collagen. The smooth muscle cell development is also imperfect, mainly in the regions where their plasma membranes are closely apposed. These areas, called nexi, represent a pathway for the transmission of impulses from one cell to another. These abnormalities result in inefficient urinary transport by the ureter in its terminal segment, and secondary dilatation of the proximal ureter as a compensatory mechanism to maintain low resting ureteral pressure. If the dilatation is significant, the term "secondary megaureter" is used to describe it. The degree of dilatation necessary to warrant the term "megaureter" is still a matter of debate. Previous publications from our unit have defined a megaureter as a minimal dilatation of more than 2 cm for more than half the length of the ureter as determined by imaging during appropriate physiologic circumstances. Recently, the increased use of ultrasonography as an imaging tool has changed our standard in the evaluation of ureterectasis. No standardized ultrasonographic criteria of what constitutes a megaureter have been defined thus far.

In 1976, an international pediatric urologic seminar held in Philadelphia proposed the following classification of the megaureter in three categories:

1. The refluxing megaureter:
   a. Primary: congenital primary reflux.
   b. Secondary: posterior urethral valves, neurogenic bladder dysfunction.
2. The obstructed megaureter:
   a. Primary: congenital adynamic segment.
   b. Secondary: extrinsic compression, posterior urethral valves, neurogenic bladder dysfunction.
3. The nonrefluxing, nonobstructed megaureter:
   a. Primary: idiopathic
   b. Secondary: polyuria, infection, residual dilatation after surgery.

Unfortunately, as with all classifications, this system has some pitfalls: (1) reflux and obstruction often coexist and (2) the megaureter of the prune-belly syndrome does not fit adequately into any of these categories. Although imperfect, the classification represents a useful tool in making the differential diagnosis of ureterectasis.

Historically, the dilated ureter was a very challenging problem to the general and pediatric urologist. Significant developments in antibiotics, anesthesia, imaging, physiologic studies, and surgical techniques have improved our understanding and clinical results of the treatment of megaureter. The studies of Hendren, Kalicinski and colleagues, Starr, and others have contributed significantly to current clinical success.

CLINICAL PRESENTATION

The history of the clinical presentation of this entity is divided into two periods: before and after the widespread use of ultrasonographic imaging. The incidental detection of asymptomatic ureteral dilatation has markedly changed in these two intervals. During the same period, most pediatric patients presented later in childhood suffering from recurrent urinary tract infection and occasionally flank pain and/or stones. Before the ultrasonographic era, only occasional asymptomatic patients were detected; these were undergoing cardiovascular imaging with radiopaque media that could subsequently be used at the same setting to visualize the urinary tract. The nature of ultrasonography markedly changed this situation in the following ways:

1. Ultrasound waves do not injure tissue and thus can be safely applied to mother and fetus. The clinical use of ultrasonography in clinical obstetrics has grown significantly, and in many areas virtually all pregnant women are surveyed in such a manner.
2. Ultrasonography can image soft tissues and specifically can detect dilatation of the urinary tract without the use of contrast material.

3. The clinical result of these two developments is that the number of asymptomatic ureteral dilatations detected in childhood has increased dramatically.
4. Patients are being detected at a much younger age, many antenatally.
5. The noninvasive nature of ultrasonography has been an attractive feature to referring pediatricians who frequently seek imaging of the urinary tract for various reasons; ultimately, detection of postnatal asymptomatic patients is significantly increased.

CLINICAL PHYSIOLOGY, PATHOPHYSIOLOGY, AND BIOHYDRAULICS

Our philosophy in the treatment of megaureter secondary to adynamic segment is based primarily on a fundamental understanding of the physiology, pathophysiology, and biohydraulics that are operative in the normal and abnormal ureter.

The principal function of the ureter is to transport urine from the kidney to the bladder. Since urine is a liquid, only compression and gravitational forces are effective in propelling the urine distally. In neonates, the ureter is short, approximately 10 to 12 cm in length, and thus gravity plays a limited role in urinary movement. Thus, urine is moved primarily by the force of compression. The fluid that does, or will, constitute urine is basically pressurized in three biologic compressors: the heart, the contracting ureteral bolus, and the contracting detrusor. The urine is thus propelled from these relatively high-pressure compressors to low-pressure receptor storage areas that include the renal pelvis and upper ureter, the storage detrusor, and the atmosphere (or amniotic sac). A simple hydraulic circuit consists of a compressor, a conduit, a receptor storage container, and a control mechanism (directional and/or intermittent). From a biohydraulic perspective, the urinary tract is made up of three such hydraulic circuits. These are named for the compressor and the low-pressure storage area and are attached in series; i.e., they are connected to one another consecutively: (1) the cardioureteral and pelvic system, (2) the ureteral-detrusor system, and (3) the detrusor-atmospheric system.

The law of conservation of mass applies in such conveyance systems. In simple terms, this law states that in a conveyance system matter must be conserved, and what goes into the system must come out. In more scientific terms, provided the flow rate is stable, the mass of fluid passing any particular point per unit time must be constant. A very significant practical application of this applies to the second circuit (the ureteral detrusor). When 1 g of urine leaves the ureter, 1 g of urine must be accommodated into the bladder. The law of conservation of energy is also applicable; this principle states that energy can neither be created or destroyed. It means that the energy present in the urine entering into a convey-ance system equals the energy present in the urine at the exit of the conveyance system plus the energy remaining in the conveyance system. Conversion of energy from one form to another is also important. Energy in each of the three hydraulic systems begins as chemical energy in the presence of adenosine triphosphate in the muscles of the biologic compressor. This energy allows the muscles to contract isometrically around entrapped liquid, converting the chemical energy into compression energy contained within the liquid. The valve system then allows the conversion of compression energy (which has no direction) to be converted into kinetic energy (which has assigned direction). When the urine enters into a reception storage container such as the bladder, it has velocity; thus, it has kinetic energy. There are three possible fates to such kinetic energy: (1) it can be taken up in the wall of the elastic container as potential energy of elastic force; (2) it can remain as compression energy in the urine within the container, such as the bladder; or (3) it can continue as kinetic energy. In a closed container, the distribution between compression energy and kinetic energy is governed by the law of Laplace, which states that

$$\text{Pressure} = \frac{\text{Potential Energy of Elastic Force}}{\Pi \times \text{Radius}^2}$$

The formation of the ureteral bolus in the ureter must also follow these same principles (Fig. 1). If urine is to accumulate in the ureter to form a low-pressure bolus, the wall of the ureter must be able to stretch and take up energy in the form of potential energy of elastic force. If this cannot occur, the ureteral bolus is not formed, and the urinary transport efficiency is impaired. Poiseuille's law governs the flow of liquid in hollow tubes. The law in its original form is applicable only to rigid tubes with constant geometry. It does not have a direct mathematical application to the urinary tract. Nevertheless, certain physical principles must be followed, including

1. The urinary flow is directly proportional to the pressure gradient. This gradient is the pressure in the ureter (pressure within the contracting ureteral bolus) minus the resting detrusor pressure.
2. Pressure in the ureteral bolus must be higher than the detrusor pressure for antegrade flow to occur.
3. Decreased ureteral contraction pressure and/or increased intravesical pressure can lead to inefficient urinary transportation and/or stasis.
4. The viscosity of urine in the biologic system is relatively constant.
5. As the radius of the conduit declines, but does not reach zero, the flow may be maintained by increasing the pressure gradient.
6. As flow rate increases significantly, the pressure gradient between the ureteral bolus and the resting detrusor must also increase.

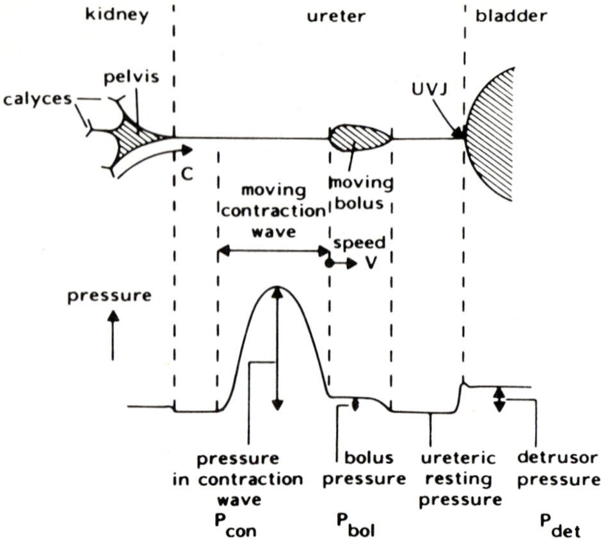

Figure 1 Schematic representation of a single bolus in the ureter moving from the renal pelvis to the bladder. Corresponding distribution of the pressure within the urinary tract is shown *(lower tracing)*. (Republished with permission by Griffiths DJ, Notschaele C. The mechanics of urine transport in the upper urinary tract: 1. The dynamics of the isolated bolus. Neurol Urodynam 1983; 2:155.)

Nature of Stasis

There has been significant controversy not only regarding the correlation between obstruction and dilatation, but also about the definition of obstruction. Everyone agrees that when the conduit radius is zero (e.g., occlusive ureteral ligature), the proximal biologic compressor is unable under any circumstances to overcome the significant distal resistance, and when urinary flow from the ureter or urethra falls to zero, obstruction clearly exists. Conduit problems are the primary types of urinary transport inefficiency that occur most commonly in adult clinical urology, but also in the experimental literature. The major adult urethral diseases consist primarily of benign prostatic hypoplasia (BPH), carcinoma of the prostate, and urethral stricture, and these are almost purely conduit problems. Similarly, in the ureter, ureteral calculus, ureteral ligature, and the occlusive effects of periureteral cancer are primarily pure conduit problems. Most of the models of hydronephrosis in the literature, beginning with Frank Hinman, Sr.'s original model involving ureteral ligation, are also purely conduit problems. In clinical pediatric urology, urinary transport inefficiency more often takes the form of an inefficient compressor, valve system, or storage container. Basically, four different approaches have been applied to a more definitive definition of incomplete obstruction. We prefer the terms "inefficient urinary transportation" or "urinary stasis." These methods include (1) evaluation of symptoms; (2) pressure flow studies; (3) time flow studies using a tagged solute, usually labeled with the radioactive technetium; and (4) proximal effects on the urinary collecting system, renal

structure, and function. Previous studies from our unit have clearly shown that there is no complete correlation between these methods of study. We believe, however, that the presence of proximal changes remains the best indicator in clinical pediatric ureteral problems. The other methods of study basically are never performed unless dilatation has been detected by ultrasonography or intravenous urography. Unfortunately, the proponents of pressure flow and time flow studies have been vigorously promoting these as the absolute "gold standard" to define stasis. We believe this type of article has shed more heat than light; we do not believe there is an absolute pat formula for demonstrating this.

We have found the following definition of urinary stasis clinically useful in analyzing ureteral detrusor system problems in children. We define stasis or inefficient urinary transportation as a state in which the proximal urinary system has undergone compensatory dilatation. We have previously published our belief that if stasis is defined as above, there are three causes that can affect any of the three biohydraulic systems:

1. Inefficiency of the biologic compressor generating compression energy and/or converting it to kinetic energy. Examples of this are the dilatation seen in the prune-belly syndrome and the problems in urinary transportation in grade V primary vesicoureteric reflux.
2. Excessive loss of kinetic energy in the urinary conduit, or inefficiency of converting kinetic energy to potential energy of elastic force in a urinary reservoir. Some examples of this include uncoordinated urethral control mechanism in the neurogenic bladder and low-compliance bladder as seen in posterior urethral valves or meningomyelocele.
3. Increase in urinary flow to such an extent that dilatation occurs.

By our definition, urinary transportation inefficiency exists when there is significant dilatation of any part of the urinary tract proximal to the affected area. We do not mean that every such inefficiency requires treatment, and in particular do not mean that any such inefficiency requires mechanical treatment or surgical intervention. We also acknowledge that, in very rare cases, calices have been abnormally formed in a large configuration in which no urinary transportation inefficiencies exists. This is the condition of so-called congenital megacalycosis. In these rare cases, there is usually significant enlargement of the calices but no significant dilatation of the pelvis or ureter. We thus find it an easy differential diagnosis on clinical and radiologic grounds.

In the adynamic segment, a ureter, because of its high collagen content, is unable to stretch and form a low-pressure ureteral bolus in the adynamic segment. The resulting inefficiency and the pumping action is very comparable with that which occurs in pericardial tamponade, when the heart is unable to pump efficiently because of lack of proper filling of the right ventricle. In addition, transmission of electrical impulses triggering the contraction in the adynamic segment is inefficient because of the abnormal nexi. Both of these mechanical and electrical physiologic factors contribute to inefficient urinary transportation in the segment. This results in proximal compensatory dilatation of the ureter. It is the nature and extent and severity of proximal changes that really determine the risk of renal injury.

Protective Compensatory and Destructive Decompensatory Mechanism

The body often reacts to pathologic inefficiency of liquid transportation by changes that are first compensatory and protective. If the compensatory changes are prolonged, persistent, and severe, they may in fact become decompensatory, which further aggravates the negative effect on the patient. The compensatory changes in a pragmatic fashion are usually designed to preserve the priority of function. An example of such compensatory changes are the circulatory changes that occur in hypovolemic shock. The circulation to the heart, brain, and lungs is determined to be the priority function. This is preserved by a compensatory mechanism that decreases the circulation to the kidneys, viscera, and limbs. If the pathologic insult is transient and not too severe, complete recovery from the compensatory changes can occur. In this example, the compensatory changes are protective. If the pathophysiologic changes are severe and persistent, significant changes may occur to the kidney, such as acute tubular necrosis, which becomes decompensatory and even lethal if not treated. The ureter has three functions: (1) low-pressure receptor and bolus formation storage to receive urine from the proximal urinary tract, and the pressure during this phase must be lower than the proximal biologic compressor that is delivering the urine to it; (2) contraction that acts as a biologic compressor with the coaptation of the ureteral wall to raise the pressure within the ureter; and (3) a simple urinary conduit.

The priority function of the three functions of the ureter is low-pressure storage so that proximal renal blood flow and glomerular filtration rate (GFR) can be sustained. If the degree of urinary transportation is mild or transient, these changes remain as compensatory protective changes. If the urinary transportation defect is persistent, pathologic, and severe, the proximal dilatation can be decompensatory change. Decompensation basically is due to inefficiency of the ureteral compressor. The ureteral compressor malfunction occurs through three mechanisms: (1) as the ureteral dilatation progressively occurs, it may reach the point where the ureter can no longer coapt, and thus can no longer entrap fluid and is unable to effectively compress it; (2) as the ureter dilates (as clearly shown in the recent studies), the area increases and thus the force per unit area or pressure that can generate it is decreased; and (3) Weiss and others have shown that as the ureter progressively dilates, it eventually becomes completely aperistaltic.

In severe cases, these three factors markedly interfere with the compressor biologic function of the ureter, and thus inefficiency of urinary transportation is further impaired. If these changes are severe and prolonged, the decompensatory change predisposes the kidney to injury. When urinary transportation inefficiency occurs, other compensatory mechanisms also occur to maintain a low pressure in the proximal collecting system so that renal blood flow and glomerular filtration can continue. These other mechanisms include a slow but progressive decline in GFR; postglomerular vasoconstriction to raise the GFR pressure; and reabsorption from the dilated collecting system.

Eventually, however, these changes become decompensatory. Hinman's original model, which was based on unilateral ligation of the ureter, showed that the decreases in renal function progressed from completely reversible to partially reversible to completely irreversible. This process of destruction was significantly accelerated by infection or inefficient circulation.

Significance of Dilatation

When ureteral dilatation is observed in pediatric patients, whether in utero or after birth, several questions need to be answered: (1) is the dilatation physiologic or pathologic?; (2) does it represent the extremely rare case of congenital megacalycosis?; (3) is it transient or persistent?; (4) if the dilatation represents a pathologic situation that is persistent, are the changes in the proximal urinary system mild and compensatory or severe and decompensatory?; and (5) is there a risk of renal damage or has renal damage or destruction already occurred?

As mentioned previously, these questions are answered by four techniques. Often we forget the simple use of clinical signs and symptoms. Proximal compensatory and decompensatory changes in the collecting system and kidney are still the best guide in determining the significance of urinary transportation inefficiency in a particular clinical setting. The following factors are clinically important in determining the significance of ureteral and proximal upper urinary tract dilatation in the pediatric population.

Whether Changes are Temporary or Persistent. There is little doubt that many ureteral dilatations in the fetus detected by ultrasonography are subsequently shown by postnatal imaging and other studies to be of no pathologic significance. Pathologic studies of aborted fetuses in which ureterectasis was detected by ultrasonography also showed that a significant percentage of them are normal. There seems little doubt that ureterectasis detected in such circumstances can be secondary to temporary transportation inefficiency or perhaps even a physiologic factor. The following factors are important in the physiologic explanation of this.

Polyuria. Poiseuille's law and extensive clinical experience indicate that a significant polyuria can result in ureteral dilatation. If the ureter is called on to deliver a progressively increased volume of urine, the contraction pressures rise and the frequency of peristalsis increases. If the volume is still further increased, the resting pressure gradually rises until ultimately a very high resting pressure and contraction pressure is maintained, and a continuous high-flow state is established. Imaging in patients with diabetes insipidus, for instance, clearly shows that their ureters are dilated. The fetus has a limited capacity to concentrate urine, and thus polyuria is almost certainly a physiologic factor in such cases.

Increased Bladder Pressure. Imaging, particularly in the fetus, may be done when the fetus is not voiding and bladder pressure is high. If subsequent imaging is done during the same sitting, the ureter may be considerably less dilated.

Infection. Boyarski showed some years ago that bacterial endotoxins directly interfere with ureteral smooth muscle activity and ureteral compressor capability. Thus, infection can be a cause of transient ureteral dilatation.

All these factors may be important in the neonate, and it is important to determine whether a ureteral dilatation is transient (and thus probably not of much pathologic significance) or persistent. If the changes are shown to be transient, we also suggest subsequent reimaging to confirm that they were temporary.

Site and Extent. Isolated dilatation occurring only in the distal ureter represents minimal compensatory change. Dilatation just proximal to the adynamic segment provides a low-pressure reservoir just above the site of inefficient urinary transportation (the adynamic segment). If the proximal ureter maintains a relatively normal caliber above the area of dilatation, the proximal ureter maintains good compressor capabilities. On the other hand, dilatation that involves the whole ureter, renal pelvis, and calices is much more likely to be significant. Unlike some authors, we attach much significance to the presence of caliectasis. This is particularly so when it is combined with pyelectasis and ureterectasis, thus essentially ruling out the rare case of megacalycosis. If the calix is dilated as a result of urinary transportation inefficiency, it was the last available site of compensatory protective changes before direct nephron involvement.

Degree of Dilatation. As discussed previously, dilatation of the ureter is initially protective and compensatory. If the dilatation is severe, however, the compressor function of the ureter is impaired and the changes become decompensatory.

Presence of Peristalsis. Previous radiologic studies and more recent ultrasonographic studies by Weiss and others clearly showed that the dilatation progresses toward a decompensatory degree that peristaltic activity decreases. They showed that the presence of an aperistaltic dilated ureter correlates well with a decompensated ureter and a high risk of renal injury. On the other hand, a peristaltic dilated ureter is still compensatory and there is less risk of renal injury.

Ureteral Tortuosity. We have noted a good clinical correlation between a dilated tortuous ureter and parenchymal injury. All of these really indicate the degree of upper tract dilatation. McLorie and colleagues evolved a scoring system to evaluate more objectively the degree of upper tract dilatation. This was originally elaborated to evaluate the dilatation occurring secondary to lower urinary tract effects of neurogenic bladder. There is an excellent statistical correlation between the degree of dilatation of the upper collecting system and the renal injury as evidenced by parenchymal thinning in the neurogenic bladder. We believe that the scoring system is equally applicable to other types of urinary transport inefficiency. The point scoring system evaluates four characteristics: caliectasis, pyelectasis, ureterectasis, and tortuosity. The scoring system was 0 for absent changes, 1 for mild, 2 for moderate, and 3 for severe. Thus, a very severe degree of hydroureteronephrosis would have a maximal score of 12, whereas a score of 1 would indicate very minor changes and a score of 0 normality.

Renal Injury. In children, this occurs by three mechanisms. First, experimental models have clearly shown that dysplasia and hypoplasia can be produced by experimental in utero inefficient urinary transportation. Second, Hinman showed that progressive hydronephrosis eventually leads to renal destruction even in the absence of infection, although infection clearly accelerates the process. Third, Hodson showed that a reflux nephropathy type of injury can lead to segmental scars.

Thus, we believe that the presence of any renal injury associated with urinary transportation inefficiency in a child is a valid reason for careful consideration of surgical treatment. Other authors do not advocate surgery for pediatric hydronephrosis until 40 to 60 percent of renal function has already been lost. It is important to realize that, under most circumstances, this function is irreversibly lost. We believe that this loss can be prevented in many such cases, and that is particularly important to avoid such irreversible loss of renal function in a child.

Pressure Flow Studies. The use of pressure flow studies to study upper urinary tract transportation problems in children has been advocated and popularized by Whitaker. It is important in these studies to recognize several limitations, as described by Toguri and others. These tests are often prone to technical error, and the Whitaker test uses an exogenous supplemental compressor unit composed of a Harvard pump and syringe. Thus, the procedure basically tests the conduit capabilities of the ureter, rather than its ability as a biologic compressor. We believe that pressure flow studies using such extracorporeal auxiliary compressors must be clearly differentiated from pressure flow studies that study the relationship between the efficiency of the patient's own biologic compressor and the resultant ureteral or urethral flow. We believe that our previous and current studies clearly show that although Whitaker-type studies or more recent innovations of Mitchell are helpful, they should not be interpreted as an absolute.

Time Flow Studies. There is also a growing, dangerous tendency to rely absolutely on time flow studies, particularly furosemide (Lasix) or various types of furosemide renography. These studies all involve the use of tagged radioactive solute with a diuretic effect induced by furosemide. Again, these studies have a significant deficiency. The pressure gradient necessary to cause the flow has two significant deficiencies: the pressure gradient is not simultaneously measured and the test is semiquantitative at best.

Again, we find the test useful, but warn against using it as an absolute definition of the presence or absence of significant urinary transportation inefficiency or obstruction. Particular caution has to be applied to the adynamic segment, where often the test just measures the movement of solute from upper to lower ureter. Measurements must be taken not only at the upper and lower ureter, but also in the bladder. The methods used in such studies must be constructively and critically analyzed by the urologist responsible for the management of a particular child. Again, this is not to suggest that such tests are not useful.

ANTENATAL MANAGEMENT OF URETERECTASIS

Beyond doubt, maternal ultrasonographic examination has changed the clinical presentation of many urologic disorders. Hydronephrosis and ureterectasis are probably the best examples. It has also left the pediatric urologist with new dilemmas, challenges, and unanswered questions. Indeed, the exact natural history of ureteral dilatation remains unknown. Reports describing spontaneous postnatal resolution of prenatally diagnosed upper urinary tract dilatations are even more confusing. In addition, the accuracy with which the antenatal diagnosis is confirmed postnatally is far from perfect. All these factors pose a new dilemma in the management of prenatally diagnosed ureterectasis.

The adynamic segment with secondary megaureter, unlike posterior urethral valves and bilateral ureteropelvic junction (UPJ) obstruction, rarely causes oligohydramnios. Bilateral disease is rare and the potential for end-stage renal disease low. However, since the accuracy of ultrasonographic antenatal diagnosis is only 66 percent, it is mandatory to have a well-planned scheme when a pregnant woman is referred for evaluation and treatment of antenatally diagnosed ureterectasis in the fetus. An algorithm of the decision process we have been following in such situations is depicted in Figure 2.

Many factors should be considered when dealing with an antenatal diagnosis of ureterectasis. First, as mentioned earlier, the accuracy of ultrasonographic antenatal diagnosis is mediocre, and up to 34 percent of such antenatal diagnoses are wrong. This makes a supposedly appropriate antenatal intervention potentially hazardous in one third of the cases. Second, even today, attempts to assess fetal renal function during normal and abnormal pregnancy have been unsuccessful. Although fetal urinary electrolytes were thought to be a clue in the evaluation of fetal renal function, more recent reports by Elder and colleagues failed to confirm

Table 1 Significance of the Lecithin/Sphingomyelin (L/S) Ratio

Value of L/S Ratio	*Probability of Respiratory Distress Syndrome*
>2:1	Minimal risk
1.5–1.9	Possibility of mild to moderate respiratory distress syndrome
1.0–1.49	Relative immaturity: moderate to severe respiratory distress syndrome
<1.0	Death

their reliability. The amount of amniotic fluid remains the most reliable guide to date. Third, with the current means of antenatal investigation, the identification of a fetal kidney is not usually possible before the 16th week of pregnancy. Until recently, a kidney could be identified in 90 percent of fetuses by the 17 to 20th weeks, and in 95 percent by the 22nd week. The intrarenal architecture can be defined with some detail only by the 20th week of gestation. The contribution of urine to the amniotic fluid is not significant before the 15th week of life. Proximal airway branching of the lungs has been completed by the 16th week. It is therefore unlikely that any intrauterine surgical manipulation would affect the pulmonary hypoplasia when it is caused by failure of airway branching, because the oligohydramnios would be detected too late. On the other hand, oligohydramnios presenting later during pregnancy will interfere with the alveolar development. This type of pulmonary hypoplasia might be alleviated by antenatal intervention. Maturation of the lungs may be accelerated by administration of corticosteroids. The lecithin/sphingomyelin ratio serves as a tool to assess pulmonary maturity and its progression under treatment. Table 1 summarizes its significance. Other information from the amniotic fluid and the urine electrolytes of the fetus should be taken into account when a decision for antenatal intervention is contemplated. Chromosomal and other major organ abnormalities that are known to be frequently associated with renal malformation should be ruled out.

Fourth, reports describing spontaneous resolution of prenatal diagnosed ureterectasis are becoming more frequent. Many newborns diagnosed as having uni- or bilateral ureterectasis were managed conservatively for up to 28 months of follow-up in one series by Keating and colleagues. This might be explained by the high urine outflow state that fetuses have: their urine output is as high as four to six times the urine output of a newborn.

Premature delivery after artificial maturation of the lungs is not without risk and the renal damage is usually already irreversible. Antenatal diversion, either percutaneously or in an open procedure, is also putting both fetus and mother at significant risk; hemorrhage, sepsis, abortion, premature labor, and maternal or fetal death are not uncommon after these procedures. The most worrisome problem remains the possibility that neither the pulmonary complication nor the renal damages can be prevented by this risky intervention.

Taking all this into account, antenatal intervention

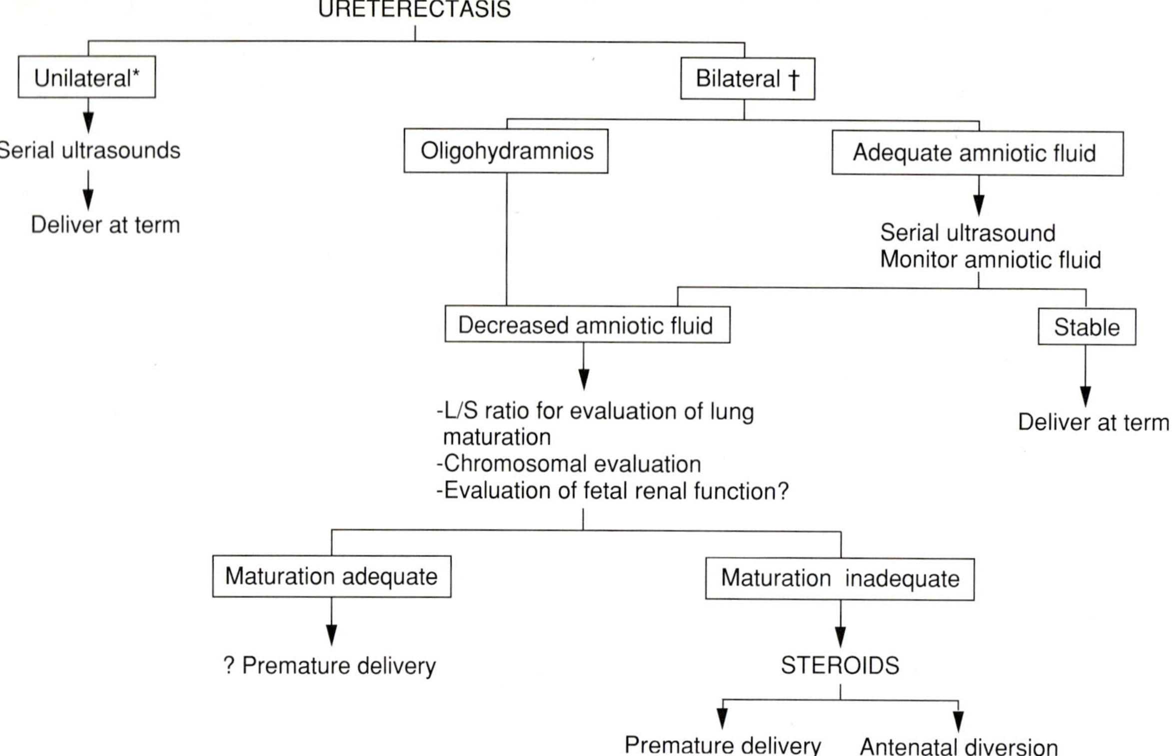

Figure 2 Antenatal management of ureterectasis. L/S ratio, lecithine/sphingomyelin ratio; * normal contralateral kidney; † or disease in a solitary kidney.

or premature delivery should be reserved for extreme cases such as severe and progressive oligohydramnios and dilatation in which end-stage renal disease is a probability, but may be reversible, and in which the pulmonary function is adequate. This decision process should be left to highly qualified individuals in specialized centers, where the risks and benefits of such intervention can be meticulously weighed.

POSTNATAL INVESTIGATION

The first step in postnatal investigation is usually an ultrasonographic examination, to identify and confirm ureteral dilatation. This also assesses the residual ipsilateral parenchyma, evaluates the contralateral kidney, and rules out the possibility of an intra-abdominal mass with extrinsic compression. More recently, with newer forms of ultrasonography and more sophisticated probes, it has also become possible to evaluate the peristaltic activity of the dilated ureter. As mentioned earlier, it seems that the peristaltic activity correlates with the degree of renal injury. This of course is only preliminary information, which must be supported by more definitive evaluation.

Voiding cystourethrography (VCUG) should be the second step and is the cornerstone of differential diagnosis, by separating a refluxing megaureter from a nonrefluxing one. It is also useful when a bladder outlet obstruction or neurogenic bladder dysfunction is sus-

pected. Intravenous pyelography (IVP) is also helpful: it gives a better definition of the anatomy of the collecting system and can identify associated anomalies such as duplication with or without ureterocele, and UPJ obstruction that could have been missed otherwise. Also, it is IVP that reveals the severity of the dilatation and/or tortuosity. For those of us with a surgical inclination, precise imaging of the collecting system continues to be important. Determination of the exact number, site, and extent of sections in the urinary tract where urinary transport is inefficient is essential to the elaboration of a surgical management plan. Thus, IVP remains a valuable tool. The timing of this examination is also controversial in the neonate. Usually, it is not recommended that an IVP be performed before 44 weeks of gestational age because of defective concentrating ability of the neonatal kidney.

The next step in the evaluation of a megaureter is a diethylenetriaminepentaacetic acid (DTPA) renal scan. Determination of total and differential renal function either by GFR measurements or by extraction factor measurements are of special interest. The DTPA renal scan with furosemide injection may be useful to confirm obstruction, but in our experience is not very reliable for distal ureteral transport problems. When a secondary megaureter is suspected, urodynamic studies are helpful in defining the contractile and storage properties of the bladder. If the diagnosis remains doubtful, cystoscopy and retrograde pyelography may be the only way to

Table 2 Postnatal Investigation of Ureterectasis

Examination	Purpose
Ultrasonography	Identification of ureterctasis
	Assessment of ipsilateral and contra-lateral parenchyma
	Assessment of ureteral peristaltis
	R/O intra-abdominal mass
VCUG	Identify refluxing megaureter
	R/O bladder outlet obstruction or neurogenic bladder dysfunction
IVP	Anatomic definition
	Assessment of dilatation and tortuosity
	Identification of other anomalies
	duplication of and/or ureterocele
	UPJ obstruction
	Megacalycosis
	Extrinsic compression
	Estimation of function
	Parenchymal thickness and/or scarring
DTPA renal scan	Assessment of renal function
	GFR
	Extraction factor
Lasix washout renal scan	Evaluation of obstruction
Urodynamic studies	Assessment of bladder function (when necessary)
Cytoscopy: retrograde pyelogram	R/O bladder outlet obstruction
	Assessment of neurogenic bladder dysfunction
	Better anatomic definition of UV junction

confirm it. Table 2 represents a summary for the investigation of a postnatally diagnosed megaureter.

POSTNATAL DIFFERENTIAL DIAGNOSIS AND MANAGEMENT OF AN ADYNAMIC SEGMENT

After this tailored investigation, the entire working urinary tract is understood and a precise pathophysiologic process resulting in a dilated ureter can be identified. It can be secondary to either infection, polyuria, high intravesical pressures, vesicoureteral reflux, or urinary transport inefficiency within the ureter itself. Next, three crucial questions need to be answered: (1) is the patient's life in jeopardy?, (2) is the total renal function in jeopardy?, and (3) is a renal unit in jeopardy? To answer these as they pertain to an adynamic segment, three important factors must be evaluated: (1) the degree and severity of decompensation of the dilated ureter, (2) the presence and/or severity of renal injury, and (3) bi- or unilateral disease in a solitary system.

Once all these are studied and understood, the way to treat an adynamic segment becomes clear. Figure 3 represents a simplified algorithm of our approach to such management. It is important to realize that the real difference between the management of uni- and bilateral disease is our degree of conviction. Also, the advent of aminoglycosides has changed our ability to treat infection in the face of urinary transport inefficiency, and temporary proximal diversion is rarely needed.

PROS AND CONS OF OBSERVATION VERSUS SURGERY

Two schools of thought have emerged regarding the significance and resultant management of this entity: the "wait and see" or "observation school," and the more aggressive "surgical school." It is more important to realize that the distinction between the two schools of thought is not absolute. The strongest advocates of the "wait and see" approach are operating on severe cases, particularly patients who have already undergone significant renal injury (loss of 40 to 60 percent of ipsilateral renal function). On the other hand, even the most aggressive surgeons acknowledge that some of these cases, particularly when detected in utero, have little mechanical significance and do not warrant surgical correction. There are also other points of agreement between the two schools, regarding the importance of infection and the danger of renal injury in this congenital uropathy compared with other congenital uropathies. These schools of thought clearly acknowledge, as Hinman showed in the early 1920s, that infection accelerates renal injury when combined with urinary transport inefficiency. There is little doubt that antibiotic prophylaxis is extremely important in the prevention of renal injury. Continuous prophylaxis is usually more effective than intermittent prophylaxis. It is also well accepted that once infections occur, the longer the delay in the establishment of antibiotic treatment, the greater is the degree of renal damage. Thus, aggressive treatment of pyelonephritis, especially in the context of urinary transport inefficiency, is clearly advocated by both schools. There is also overall agreement that this entity is less dangerous in terms of significant renal injury and the incidence of end-stage renal disease than other congenital uropathies. Clearly, diseases such as posterior urethral valves, meningomyelocele, bilateral UPJ obstruction, ectopic ureterocele, congenital uropathies associated with significant anorectal problems, and even grade V primary vesicoureteral reflux all pose a greater risk of end-stage renal disease than does this entity. However, despite the similarities, we must not minimize the differences between these two schools of thought.

There is a significant difference of opinion over where to draw the line of separation between cases that definitely require corrective surgery and those that are best served by observational therapy. The "wait and see" school advocate that surgery in pediatric hydronephrosis is not indicated until there is clear, objective demonstrable evidence from nuclear medicine studies that significant renal damage, possibly as high as 40 to 60 percent, has already occurred. Conversely, the "surgical school" advocate that surgery is indicated once decompensatory changes are clearly demonstrated in the ureter. This school believes that in such cases, the likelihood of irreversible renal damage is high and that surgery should be performed. We subscribe to the latter school of thought.

In light of the above discussion, we believe that it is important to outline the pros and cons of observation

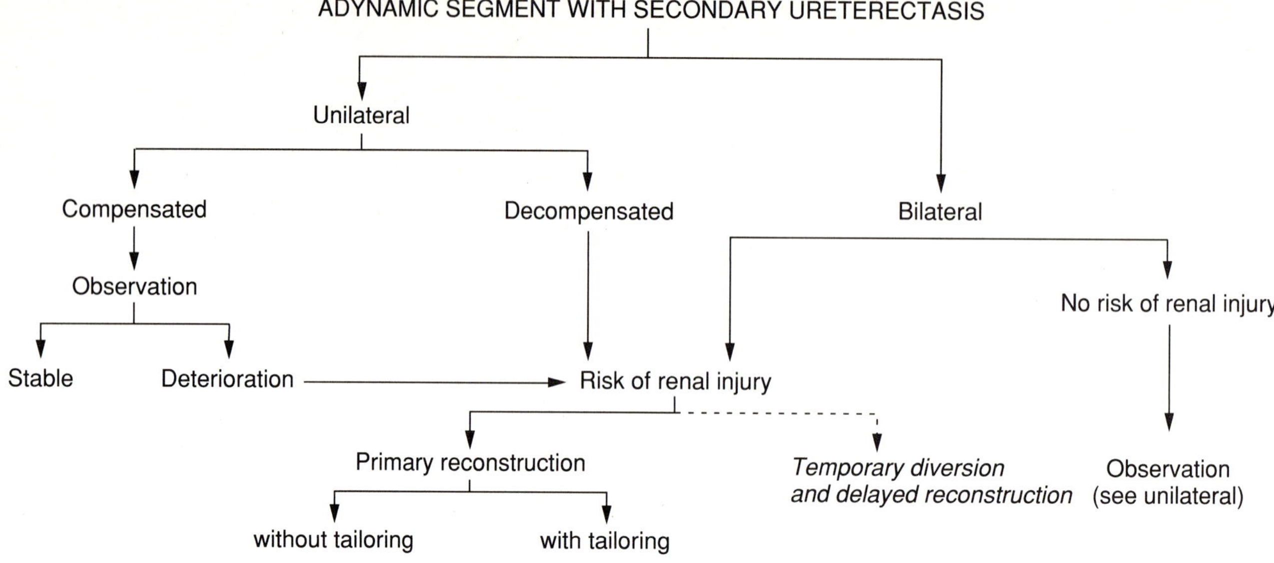

Figure 3 Postnatal management of an adynamic segment with secondary megaureter.

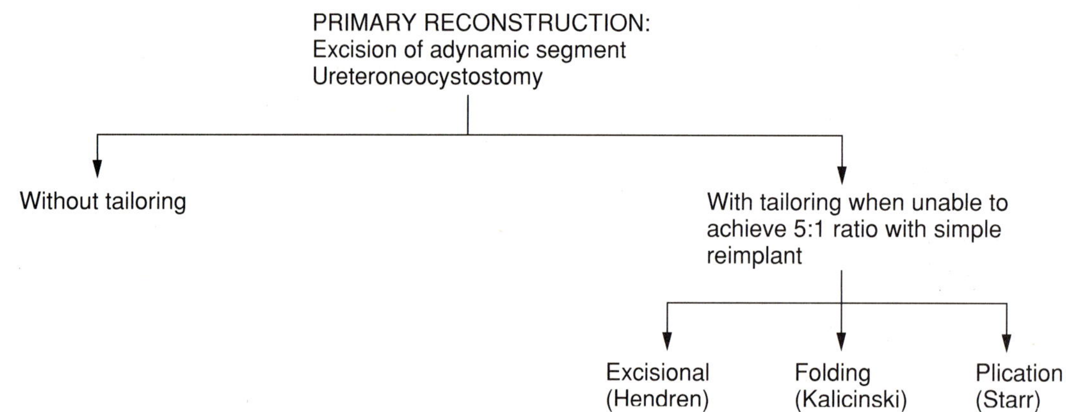

Figure 4 Preferred surgical treatment.

and surgery, so that readers can make up their own minds in this continuing debate.

The first advantage of observation is that it can be temporary, whereas surgical is definitive. If clinical and imaging studies indicate that the situation is deteriorating, a child on observation therapy can subsequently undergo surgery. The period of observation, whether used as a definitive method of management or as a temporary measure, allows one to determine whether the ureterectasis is transient or persistent, and whether the upper tract changes are progressive, stable, or improving. Observation also allows further maturation of the child and resolution of other problems that might predispose the child to undue risk associated with anesthesia and surgery.

The dangers of observation therapy are more subtle. This is usually a unilateral disease. In our extensive experience of pediatric renal transplant, it is an extremely rare cause of end-stage renal disease. Thus, catastrophic problems arising from observation therapy are extremely unusual. It is important to remember that although renal scanning is a convenient way of evaluating overall renal function and differential renal function, it is far from foolproof. DTPA renal scan may overestimate the GFR by as much as 20 percent, and becomes even less accurate as the age of the child and renal function decrease. Thus, renal damage, even irreversible damage, may be occurring during this period of observation. The second problem with observation therapy is more subtle. It is what we call the "politician's dilemma." If one projects to the parents that a particular case of urinary transport inefficiency associated with an adynamic segment is severe and probably will require surgery at some stage, and then proposes a period of observational therapy, the astute parent will almost automatically detect the indecision, and ask the pertinent question: "If you firmly believe the child's renal function is in danger, why don't you correct it earlier?" There is definite room for an intermediate school of management involving observation and possible or

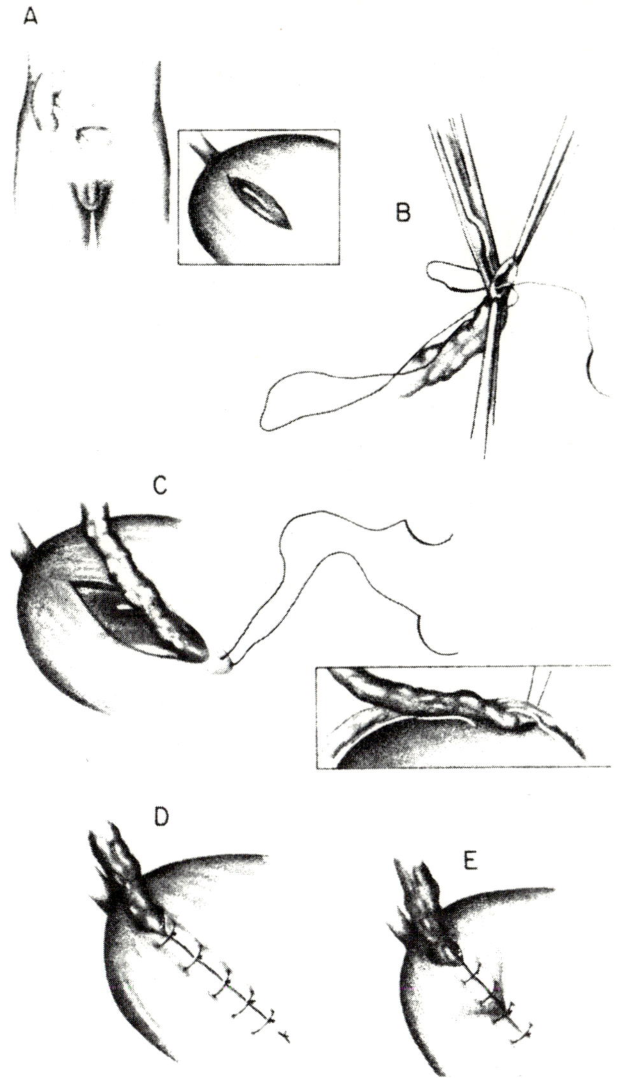

Figure 5 *A,* Insert shows incision in the anterior wall of the bladder through the muscularis and submucosa, with the mucosa bulging owing to antibiotic solution in the bladder. *B,* Double-armed 3-0 polyglycolic acid suture to evert the spatulated tip of the ureter. *C,* Needles of polyglycolic acid suture being passed from inside out through the bladder wall through a small opening in the mucosa. Inset shows a sectional view of the ureter lying outside the mucosa with the tip inside the bladder lumen. *D,* Approximation of bladder muscle over the ureter to construct a tunnel. *E,* Second layer of sutures to provide added strength to the tunnel. (Republished with permission by Wasnick RJ, Butt KMH, Laungani G, et al. Evaluation of anterior extravesical ureteroneocystostomy in kidney transplantation. J Urol 1981; 126:306–307.)

probable surgery. Historically, even in patients with very definite grounds for surgery, an observation period of 6 to 12 months is seldom detrimental provided meticulous prevention of infection is achieved. This waiting period allows the parents to have the child at home in order to achieve early psychological bonding. It also allows the child to grow and mature. Stevens advocated that one wait until the child's weight reaches approximately 10kg before attempting surgical intervention if the anomaly to be corrected is not life-threatening. Although such a guideline is very pragmatic, we have found it extremely useful. This period allows one to confirm that the changes are persistent and pathological and perhaps progressive.

We are quite comfortable in managing patients with normal proximal ureteral compression capability (see guidelines for detection above) and those in whom serial studies clearly show progressive significant improvement.

SURGICAL OPTIONS

Our indications for surgery for this entity are as follows:

1. The presence and/or progression of irreversible renal damage to the ipsilateral renal unit secondary to urinary transport inefficiency in a child on antibiotic prophylaxis. However, if the renal damage is the result of medical or parental delay in the initial institution of antibiotic therapy, especially in the face of two minor urinary transportation problems, the observation period would still be allowed.
2. Demonstration of proximal (i.e., caliceal, pelvic, or ureteral) changes that are becoming decompensatory. These pathophysiologic changes have been extensively discussed above (see the section "Clinical Physiology, Pathophysiology, and Biohydraulics").

If these factors are present, the urologist can decide for temporary urinary diversion with either delayed or primary reconstruction.

Temporary diversion, either percutaneous or open with delayed reconstruction, is not our preferred method of treatment. The efficacy with which aminoglycosides can control infection in urinary transport inefficiency has caused this option to be rarely chosen at our institution. No open temporary diversion has been performed for this condition over the past 15 years.

A percutaneous diversion (percutaneous insertion of a nephrostomy tube) may still be required in life-threatening situations such as a septic newborn with renal failure and severe ureterectasis and tortuosity. This procedure would accelerate the extermination of the infection and the recovery of renal function, preserve the residual functioning renal mass, and help in the metabolic stabilization of the infant until a definitive correction can be dispensed.

The usual surgical option chosen at the Hospital for Sick Children in Toronto is primary reconstruction, which includes excision of the atretic adynamic segment and ureteroneocystostomy, with or without tapering of the ureter (Fig. 4).

Another area of uncertainty is the timing of surgical correction. As mentioned above, an observation period of 6 to 12 months is seldom detrimental if antibiotic

Table 3 Pros and Cons of Different Tapering Techniques

Tailoring Techniques	Pros	Cons
Folding (Kalicinski, Ehrlich)	Preservation of blood supply No need for stenting Lower risk of leakage Shorter hospital stay	Bulk of tissue Tortuous ureter
Plication (Starr)	Simpler technique Lower risk of leakage Stenting period shorter Shorter hospital stay	Reduction only up to 50–60% Tortuous ureter Bulky to reimplant
Excisional (Hendren)	Ideal for massively dilated and/or tortuous ureter Better tailoring	May jeopardize blood supply Longer period of stenting Longer hospital stay Higher risk of leakage

prophylaxis is provided and infection prevented. This time frame usually corresponds to the relatively long waiting lists in the Canadian health care system. Thus, most newborns with this congenital abnormality, even when there is a definite surgical indication, are observed on prophylactic antibiotics for that period. During that time, the child can grow and reach approximately 10kg, develop psychological bonding with the parents, and have a chance to either improve or spontaneously resolve the urinary transport problem.

PROS AND CONS OF DIFFERENT SURGICAL TECHNIQUES OF RECONSTRUCTION

Many areas of discussion still persist over the surgical correction of an adynamic segment. Every urologist would agree that the distal, nondilated atretic segment of ureter should be excised. A variety of surgical techniques are available for reimplantation. The reader is referred to the multiple description of the Politano-Leadbetter, Paquin, and Cohen and the combined extra-

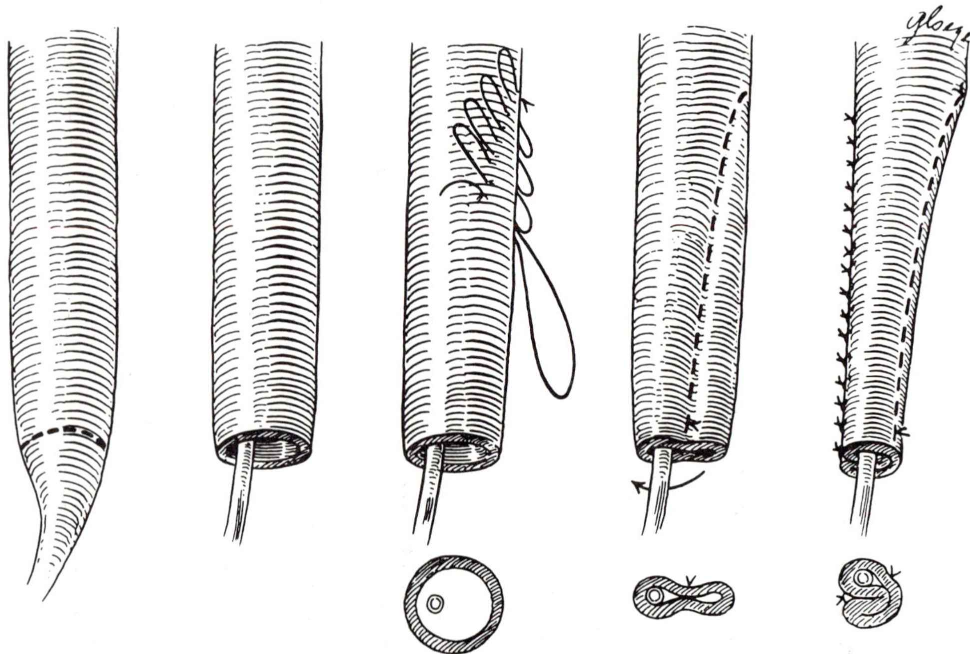

Figure 6 The atretic distal segment is excised. A horizontal mattress suture is applied to the lateral surface, and the ureter is folded under. (Republished with permission by Ehrlich RM. The ureteral folding technique for megaureter surgery. J Urol 1985; 134:668. © by Williams & Wilkins.)

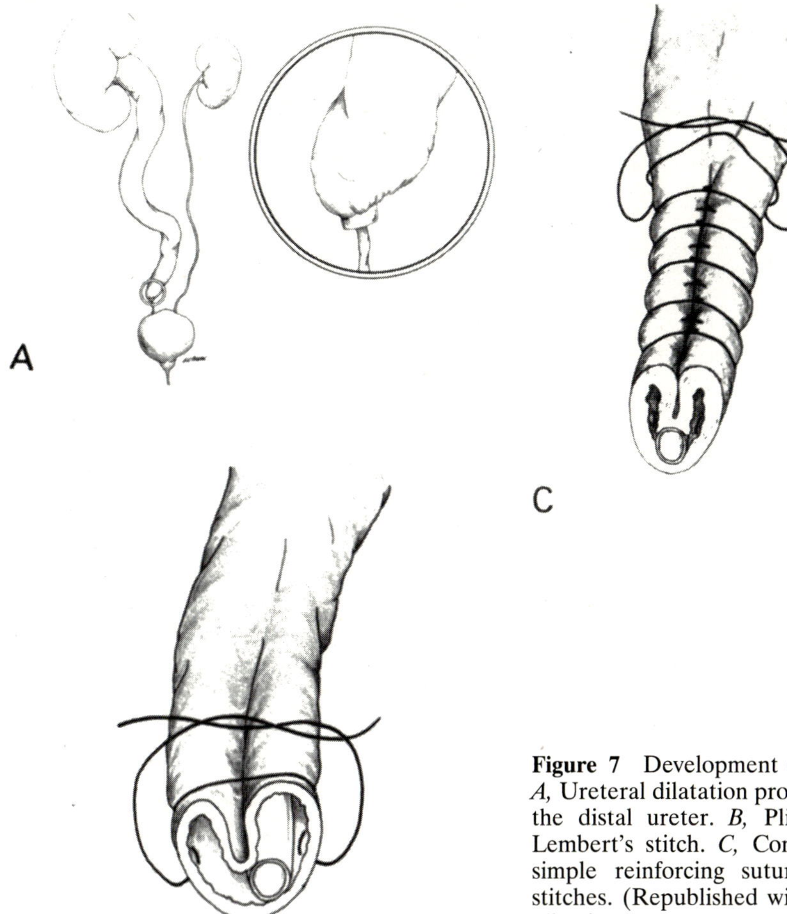

Figure 7 Development of the ureteral plication procedure. *A,* Ureteral dilatation produced by an aluminum band around the distal ureter. *B,* Plication of the dilated ureter with Lembert's stitch. *C,* Completion of ureteral plication with simple reinforcing sutures placed between the Lembert stitches. (Republished with permission by Starr A. Ureteral plication. A new concept in ureteral tailoring for megaureter. Invest Urol 1979; 17:153 © by Williams & Wilkins.)

and intravesical techniques of ureteroneocystomies, all of which have passed the test of time and are highly successful. The Lich-Gregoir technique is also simple and fast and allows tailoring of the ureter if necessary, and so far seems to achieve results comparable with those of more classical techniques of reimplantation. This technique must be differentiated from the extravesical reimplantation described by Zaontz, in which the ureter is *not* disconnected from the bladder. In the case of an adynamic segment, the ureter has to be disconnected, the distal atretic segment excised, and the ureter reimplanted extravesically as in a kidney transplant (Fig. 5).

In the decision to taper or not to taper, the following guidelines have proved reliable and allowed a high success rate:

1. If it is not possible to achieve a 5:1 ratio between the length of the tunnel and the diameter of the ureter by other means (bladder mobilization, ureteral mobilization), we taper. In our hands, extensive bladder mobilization by dividing the urachus and the obliterated umbilical artery, and mobilizing the peritoneum off the bladder dome usually provides the mobility to bring the bladder up to the ureter, and the length to create an adequate tunnel. This avoids the need to taper the ureter.
2. If, after the adynamic segment is excised, the ureteral peristalsis is disorganized and/or inefficient, we taper.
3. If, after the adynamic segment is excised, the ureteral diameter in diastole is more than 2.5 cm, we taper.

At least three different tailoring techniques have been described, each with its advantages and disadvantages. Table 3 summarizes the pros and cons and Figures 6 to 10 are representations of these techniques. For some years we have used the classical excisional Hendren technique. With strict adherence to simple surgical techniques, this technique has been very successful so far. Gentle handling, minimal manipulation of the ureter, optical magnification, and meticulous dissection of the ureter, preserving the "mesoureter," allow precise identification of the vascularization of the ureter and its preservation (Figs. 11 and 12). This technique is our first choice for all remodeling and should be used whenever

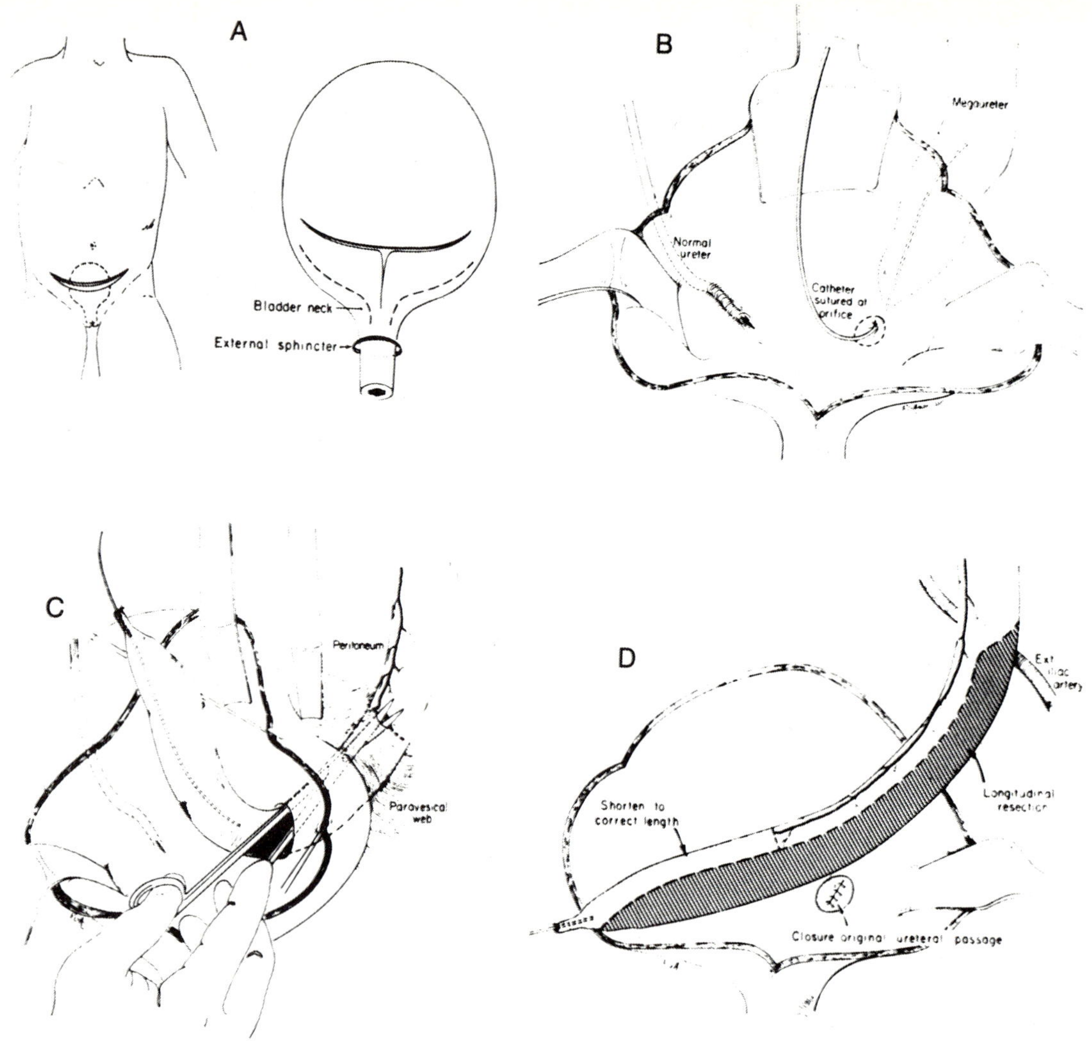

Figure 8 Classic excisional Hendren tapering technique. *A,* Incision on the bladder. *B,* Placement of the ureteral stent. *C,* Intravesical dissection of the megaureter. *D,* Shaded area: segment to be excised. (Republished with permission by Hendren WH. Operative repair of megaureter in children. J Urol 1969; 101:493.)

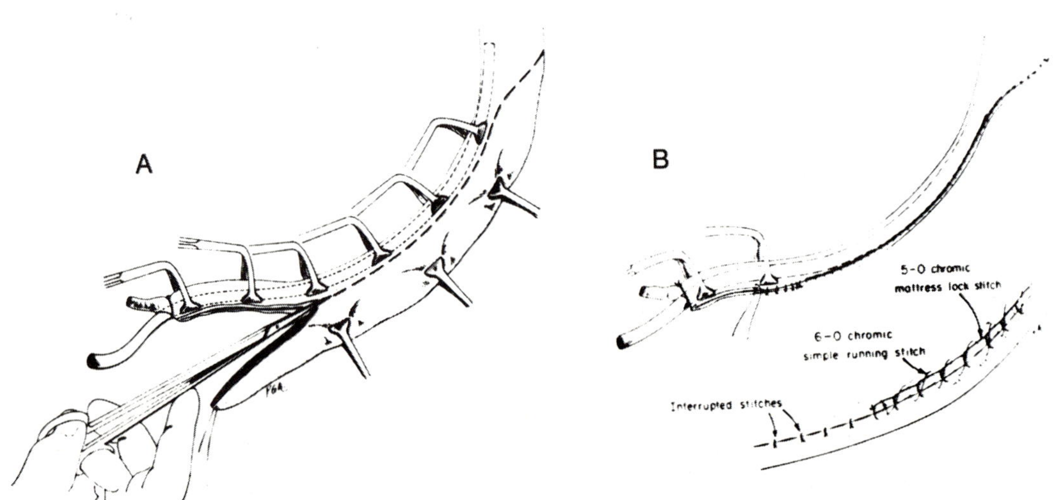

Figure 9 Classic excisional Hendren tapering technique. *A,* Placement of the clamps on the segment to be kept. *B,* Sutured ureter.

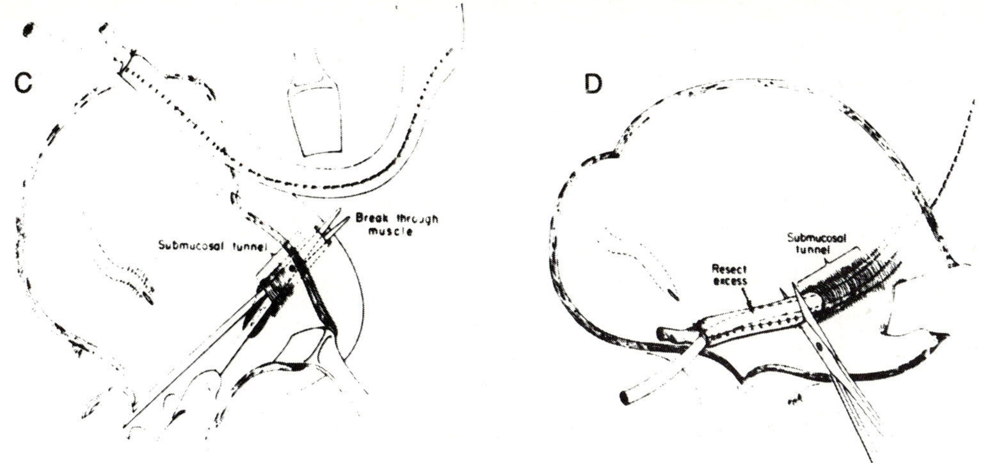

Figure 9, cont'd. *C,* Politano-Leadbetter reimplantation. *D,* Excision of a redundant length of ureter. (Republished with permission by Hendren WH. Operative repair of megaureter in children. J Urol 1969; 101:494.)

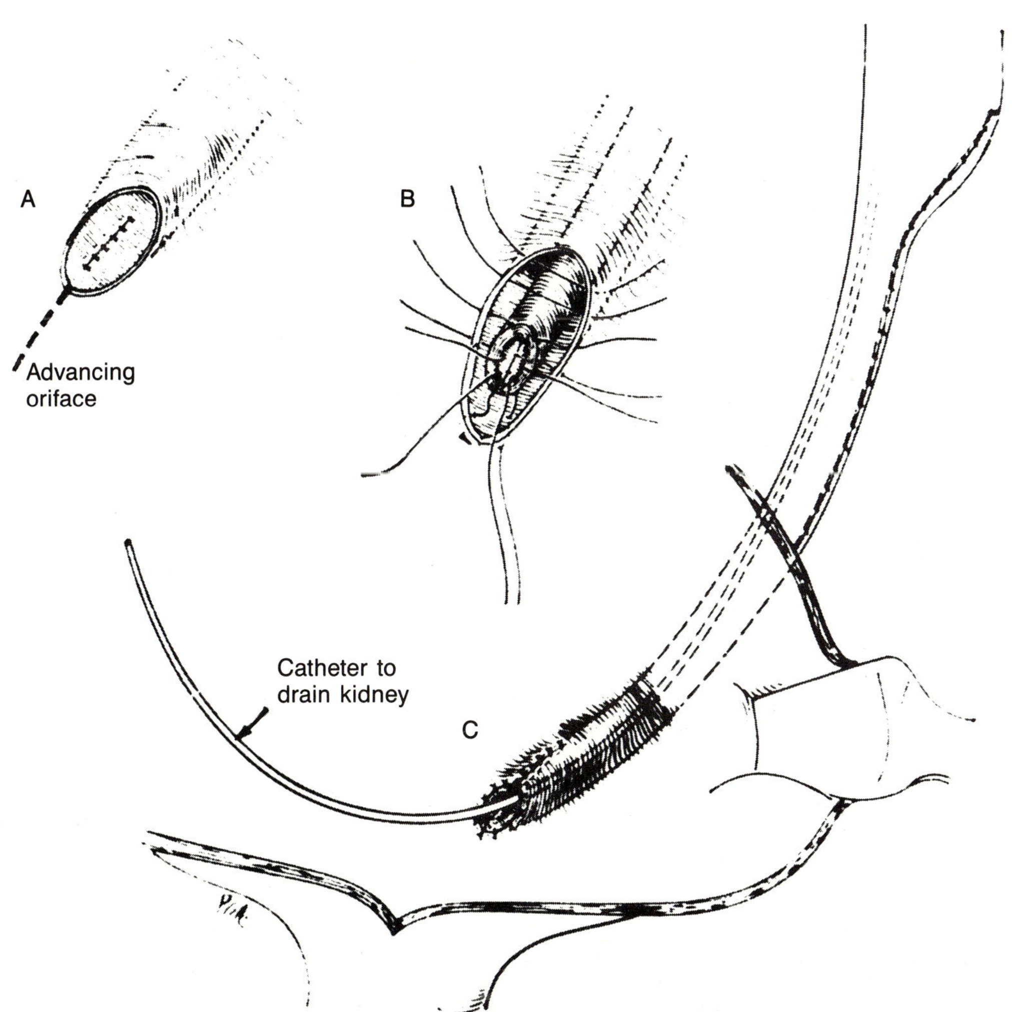

Figure 10 Classic excisional Hendren tapering technique. *A,* New orifice. *B,* Suturing the new orifice. *C,* Indwelling ureteral stent. (Republished with permission by Hendren WH. Operative repair of megaureter in children. J Urol 1969; 101:495.)

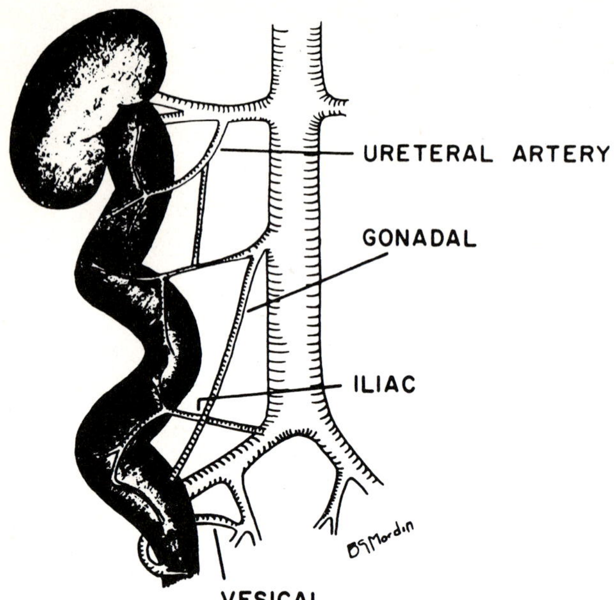

Figure 11 Blood supply of the megaureter and different patterns of final distribution. (Republished with permission by Hanna MK. Megaureter. In: King LR, ed. Urologic surgery in neonates and young infants. Philadelphia: WB Saunders, 1988:189.)

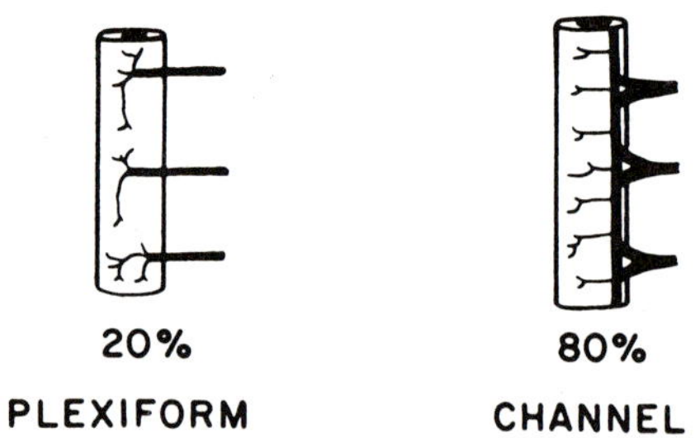

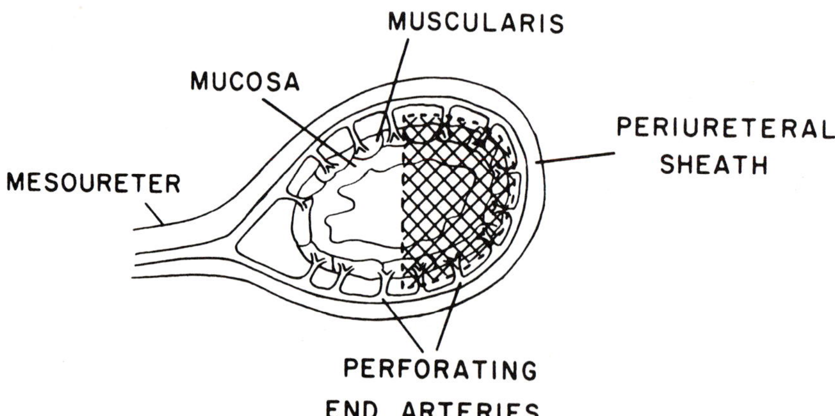

Figure 12 Final distribution of perforating "end arteries" from juxtaureteral vessels within the ureteral adventia. The shaded area represents part of the ureteral wall that should be excised. (Republished with permission by Hanna MK. Megaureter. In: King LR, ed. Urologic surgery in neonates and young infants. Philadelphia: WB Saunders, 1988:190.)

the ureter is massively dilated and tortuous: it allows for better tailoring. Hendren himself has modified his technique (Hendren II) and no longer uses his special noncrushing clamps. He now tapers the ureter "free-handed." In Hendren II, the ureter is dissected on its blood supply (mesoureter). The adventitia is meticulously reflected off the muscularis, beginning at a point in the circumference of the ureter 180 degrees opposite the blood supply. The ureter is then detubularized longitudinally on its antimesenteric border. The redundant muscularis and mucosa are then excised in equal amounts on both sides of the mesoureter, and the ureter is retubularized by a locking running suture over the mucosa reinforced by an adventitial layer. The critical point in Hendren I technique is the placement of the clamps on the segment of the ureter that will be kept, leaving the segment to be excised outside the clamps (see Fig. 9). The main disadvantage of this technique is the possibility of jeopardizing the blood supply of the ureter. Other inconveniences are a longer stenting time, the potential risk of urinary leakage, and a longer hospital stay. With the two other techniques, the folding (Kalicinski) (see Fig. 6) and the plication (Starr) (see Fig. 7), there is no suture line leakage, and either stents are not required or the stenting period is shorter; theoretically, these should preserve lower blood supply to the ureter. We have some reservations about these techniques. First, a significant amount of redundant tissue is folded over and placed into the tunnel, and this probably interferes with urinary transportation and/or prevention of reflux. More important, when the ureter is tortuous, we do not believe that these techniques are as good as the classical or modified Hendren technique.

The question of stenting versus nonstenting arises. Rabinowitz and colleagues reported a series of patients who underwent unilateral or bilateral ureteroneocystostomies with tapering (Kalicinski technique) in which no stent, and in some cases no urethral catheter, was used. Although it appears highly cost effective, in his small series of 19 patients, one underwent bilateral surgery and the other had surgery on his solitary system. Both of these patients had some degree of postoperative acute renal failure requiring prolonged hospitalization, and one had percutaneous nephrostomy. This suggests that patients undergoing unilateral surgery also have renal function impairment ipsilaterally, but that because of the normal contralateral unit, this is not clinically detected. The question to be decided is the severity of the renal injury, transient or permanent, that this postoperative complication involves. We recommend that this uncertainty be alleviated by stenting these kind of repairs. Nowadays, with the smaller scopes and instruments, double-J stents can be placed and removed with minimal risk, and burdensome external stents are no longer required.

SUGGESTED READING

Hanna MK. Megaureter. In: King LR, ed. Urologic surgery in neonates and young infants. Philadelphia: WB Saunders, 1988:160.

Hendren WH. Operative repair of megaureter in children. J Urol 1969; 101:491.

Kalicinski ZH, Kansy J, Kotarbinska B, Joszt W. Surgery of megaureters—modification of Hendren's operation. J Pediatr Surg 1977; 12:183–188.

Starr A. Ureteral plication. A new concept in ureteral tailoring for megaureter. Invest Urol 1979; 17:153.

Weiss RM, Coolsaet BLRA. The ureter. In: Gillenwater JY, Grayhack JT, Howards SS, Duckett JW, eds. Adult and pediatric urology. Chicago: Year Book, 1987:777.

VESICOURETERAL REFLUX

PHILLIP F. NASRALLAH, M.D.

It has been almost 40 years since Hutch's treatise on vesicoureteral reflux (VUR). Since that time, several thousand articles have been published on this subject, answering many clinical and pathophysiologic questions concerning VUR. It is now apparent that spontaneous resolution of reflux occurs in approximately 60 percent of patients who present with this problem. Lower grades of reflux are more likely to resolve spontaneously. The mechanism of resolution appears to be improvement in bladder function and dynamics, and not a change in ureteral anatomic configuration. During the conservative management of reflux, one can reliably prevent renal scarring by prophylaxis against infection. Conversely, renal scarring seems to occur only in association with breakthrough urinary tract infection (UTI). Sterile reflux in the presence of normal bladder dynamics is not injurious to the kidney. Intrarenal reflux due to incompetence at the renal papilla is an important factor in the pathogenesis of renal scarring.

However, many questions about VUR remain unclear. Management of the female adolescent with mild reflux who has been treated conservatively for years remains a controversial problem. Since reflux can be diagnosed antenatally, appropriate management of newborns with significant VUR is still uncertain. In adults with vesicoureteric reflux, factors other than infection may lead to eventual renal demise once renal scarring has occurred. There is also doubt whether endoscopic reflux management will, for the most part, replace surgical management in the future.

This chapter addresses the management of children with VUR. Although the main focus is on primary VUR, one important form of secondary VUR, reflux in association with non-neurogenic dysfunctional voiding, is discussed in detail.

DIAGNOSIS

The diagnosis of VUR is made in four specific clinical situations. Children presenting with UTI are the most common population found to have VUR. Second, prenatal ultrasonography is providing another population of patients with reflux. Third, many patients with dysfunctional voiding are found to have VUR. Lastly, approximately 30 percent of siblings of refluxing patients are found also to have reflux.

There does not seem to be any argument that radiologic imaging should be performed in all children with proved UTI. If the ultimate goal in management of children with infection is to prevent renal scarring, documentation of those conditions that increase the risk of scarring is essential if that goal is to be achieved. With today's imaging techniques, it makes little sense to subject children to repeated UTI before radiographic screening. The one exception to this rule is a girl whose first UTI occurs after attempts at toilet training and whose symptoms are completely confined to the lower tract (dysuria, urgency, incontinence). In this subset of patients, it is acceptable to wait until recurrence of infection before proceeding with radiographic screening. In all other patients with documented UTI, radiologic screening is mandatory.

Appropriate imaging for the upper tracts in a patient with UTI is renal ultrasonography in both males and females. Ultrasonography is a proved method of accurate upper tract evaluation in children with UTI and has several advantages in the pediatric age group. There is no need for bowel preparation, injections are avoided, and there is no radiation exposure. Lower tract evaluation can be either with voiding cystourethrography (VCUG) or nuclear cystography. Males require VCUG, because definition of bladder neck and urethral anatomy is essential. In females, I routinely order a nuclear cystogram as a screening test because it has the advantage of very low radiation exposure as well as very high sensitivity to the presence of reflux. In most pediatric centers, however, a standard radiographic VCUG remains the initial evaluation of the lower tract. This test, although higher in radiation, defines bladder anatomy better and allows the practitioner to grade reflux accurately under the international grading system. In most instances it is prudent to wait until after UTI has been treated in order to obtain a cystogram of either the conventional or the nuclear variety. However, in patients with recurring pyelonephritis in whom a previous cystogram has been negative, a repeat cystogram during the period of infection may reveal a patient in whom reflux only occurs in the presence of UTI. Infection can alter vesicoureteral dynamics and allow reflux to occur in an orifice that is otherwise competent. It is important to document such cases because prevention of infection is essential in this population lest the upper tracts be repeatedly exposed to bacteria.

VUR can be a cause of prenatally detected hydronephrosis. Serial fetal ultrasonography may show variability in the degree of hydronephrosis caused by reflux. An ultrasonographic examination after birth may also be normal. Since the infant kidney is more susceptible to renal scarring from infection, it is my practice to follow all patients who have had prenatally diagnosed hydronephrosis with VCUG (Fig. 1). VUR is treated with antibiotic prophylaxis unless a precipitating cause (posterior urethral valves, neurogenic bladder) can be found.

In patients with dysfunctional voiding, with or without UTI, VUR can be a part of the clinical picture. In these patients, a standard radiographic voiding cystogram is the best method of lower tract evaluation. Figure 2 is a perfect example of reflux secondary to bladder dysfunction. Note the other subtle signs that indicate to the practitioner that reflux is one of many sequelae to abnormal bladder dynamics. The dilated urethra and the serrated, irregular bladder and small

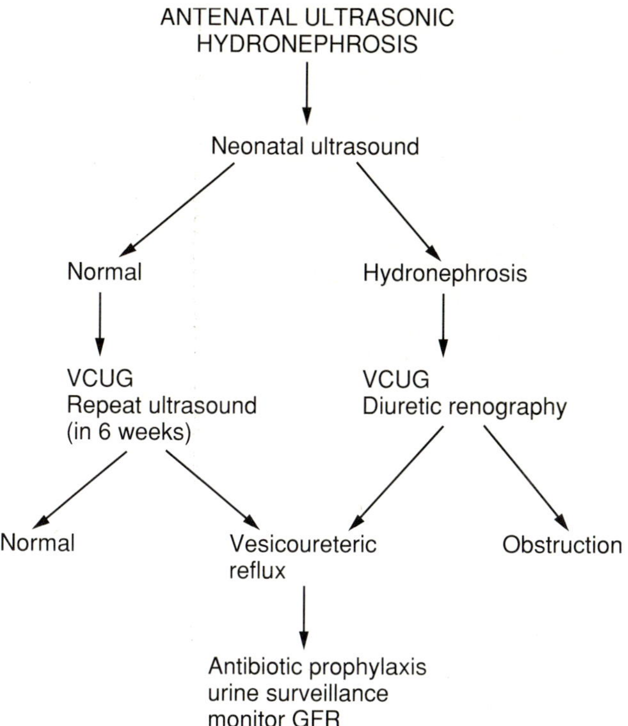

Figure 1 Algorithm for the detection and management of VUR in newborns.

diverticulum also indicate increased bladder pressure. Reflux in this clinical setting is secondary to abnormal bladder dynamics, not a primary anatomic problem. Urodynamic evaluation is essential in such children, and patience and persistence in conservative management is the key. Koff and associates have reported resolution of reflux in these patients with improvement in bladder dynamics.

Finally, Jerkin's series of refluxing probands with associated sibling reflux in 30 percent of cases has emphasized the need for sibling evaluation. It has been my experience that when patients' reflux is secondary to bladder dysfunction and of a mild degree, there is no significant incidence of reflux in their siblings. The evaluation of siblings varies with the aggressiveness of the practitioner. Some recommend both upper and lower tract evaluation with renal ultrasonography and nuclear cystography to limit radiation exposure to asymptomatic patients. My own recommendation is simple ultrasonographic screening as long as the sibling does not have a history of UTI.

CONSERVATIVE AND NONOPERATIVE TREATMENT

King and others have shown that in large series of refluxing patients treated initially with nonoperative management, approximately 65 percent can be expected to resolve the reflux spontaneously. As a general rule, the lower the grade of reflux, the greater is the chance

of spontaneous resolution. It is also clear from the work of Smellie and colleagues that the prevention of renal scarring is intimately tied with the ability to prevent breakthrough infection during this period of spontaneous resolution. After the initial diagnosis of VUR, a trial of nonoperative therapy is reasonable for every patient, even those with severe grades of reflux. This initial trial of medical management serves to establish parental rapport. Parental confidence cannot be minimized in the present litigious climate. Prophylaxis consists of either co-trimoxazole or nitrofurantoin at a dosage of one fourth the therapeutic amount given at bedtime. In newborns with reflux, a more prudent choice for prophylaxis is amoxicillin drops, again at the same dosage once daily. After several months, the infant can be switched to another form of prophylaxis once liver enzymes have been established. Office follow-up is done every 3 months to make sure that the urine remains infection free. Repeat imaging is done on a yearly basis. Renal growth and parenchymal thickness can be followed very accurately with ultrasonography. If there is question about renal scarring, a 2, 3-dimercaprol succinic acid (DMSA) radionuclide renal scan can more accurately define cortical injury. Follow-up cystography should be done with a nuclear cystogram, since this decreases the gonadal radiation exposure by at least 100-fold. The greater sensitivity to reflux of this test makes it ideal as a follow-up imaging study.

Most patients entered into such a conservative arm of treatment can be expected to show spontaneous resolution of VUR. However, several complex clinical problems can occur during conservative therapy and warrant further discussion. Reflux in the face of dysfunctional voiding requires great patience and perseverance during conservative therapy. The aim should be prevention of pyelonephritis and improvement in bladder dynamics. To this end, anticholinergic medication is often necessary in conjunction with antibiotic prophylaxis. These children may have more frequent episodes of breakthrough infection than their continent counterparts, but as long as these are of an afebrile, nonpyelonephritic nature, surgery is not necessary. Bouts of upper tract infection mandate surgery. Every effort must be made to allow the child to achieve a coordinated voiding pattern in the hope that reflux will resolve. Reimplantation in a dysfunctional bladder is more difficult, and the failure rate of such surgery is higher than in children with normal bladder dynamics.

A female patient approaching puberty who has had a benign clinical course but continues to reflux poses a specific dilemma. These patients are more susceptible to pyelonephritic episodes during pregnancy, but it seems that antireflux surgery does not protect this population against the development of pyelonephritis. Patients who have undergone successful antireflux procedures still carry a significant risk of pyelonephritis with pregnancy. Many surgeons choose to operate on this group, eliminating reflux as the patient enters adult life. It has been my practice to follow these patients expectantly and operate only on those who demonstrate recurring UTI

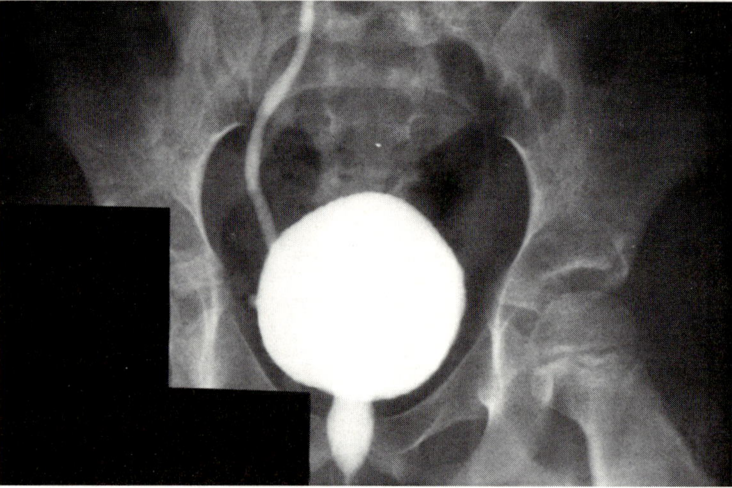

Figure 2 Grade II VUR seen in conjunction with detrusor hyperactivity. The patient is having difficulty with toilet training. Note the dilated urethra and small diverticulum.

once antimicrobial prophylaxis has ceased. It is this group of patients who may benefit the most from endoscopic reflux control, since this is an effective and safe procedure with minimal risk and morbidity.

The newborn patient with significant reflux poses another dilemma. If one accepts the "big bang" theory of renal injury, early infection is to be avoided at all costs lest the delicate kidney be subjected to bacterial insult. Cystoscopy plays an important role in such infants with high-grade reflux, since it can help define grossly abnormal vesicoureteral anatomy. Evaluation of these infants must be thorough so that precipitating causes of reflux such as neurogenic bladder or bladder outlet obstruction can also be eliminated. Primary VUR in these infants should be treated aggressively but nonoperatively, because reimplantation of a dilated ureter in an infant bladder is not an easy task. Even significant reflux in such infants can be seen to improve or resolve (Fig. 3).

Of patients with VUR and ureteral duplication, nonoperative therapy can be successful in approximately 50 percent. Kaplan demonstrated spontaneous cessation of reflux in five of 23 patients and improvement in six others. Reflux into the lower pole is the rule. When reflux is into an upper pole system alone, endoscopy is indicated and usually discloses an orifice at the bladder neck.

CYSTOSCOPY

The practitioner should be ready to use cystoscopy in a variety of clinical situations to define better optimum treatment. In patients followed conservatively for several years without resolution of reflux, cystoscopy may shed valuable light on the potential for spontaneous resolution. I also routinely perform cystoscopy in patients with ureteral duplication and reflux. Patients at

the two extremes of age—i.e., infants with high-grade reflux and teenage girls—can benefit from endoscopic evaluation of the orifice. The cystoscopic findings are valuable in the management of this controversial group of patients. Finally, any patient whose clinical course during nonoperative therapy is stormy (recurring episodes of breakthrough infection or worsening of the grade of reflux) deserves the more complete evaluation that cystoscopy provides.

Parental education and cooperation is essential if nonoperative therapy is to be successful. The parents' role in administering antibiotic prophylaxis, in recognizing breakthrough infection, and in complying with imaging schedules cannot be minimized. In this regard, patient education pamphlets explaining the condition of VUR, the consequences of untreated infection, and the plan for follow-up imaging studies and urinalysis are of great help to the practitioner.

OPERATIVE TREATMENT

Breakthrough UTI despite prophylactic antibiotics remains the most common indication for surgical correction of reflux. Severe grades of reflux (III to V, international classification) that do not improve with such conservative therapy also are best treated surgically. Other indications for surgery continue to be parental preference or frustration, cystoscopic findings that militate against spontaneous resolution, upper tract changes during conservative therapy, or an itinerant family. Preoperative evaluation of the patient should include recent imaging studies. I prefer that a recent nuclear cystogram be part of the preoperative work-up, to help define patients who initially were shown to have unilateral reflux but who subsequently have developed reflux on both sides. In this situation, both ureters should be reimplanted at the time of surgery. Although cystos-

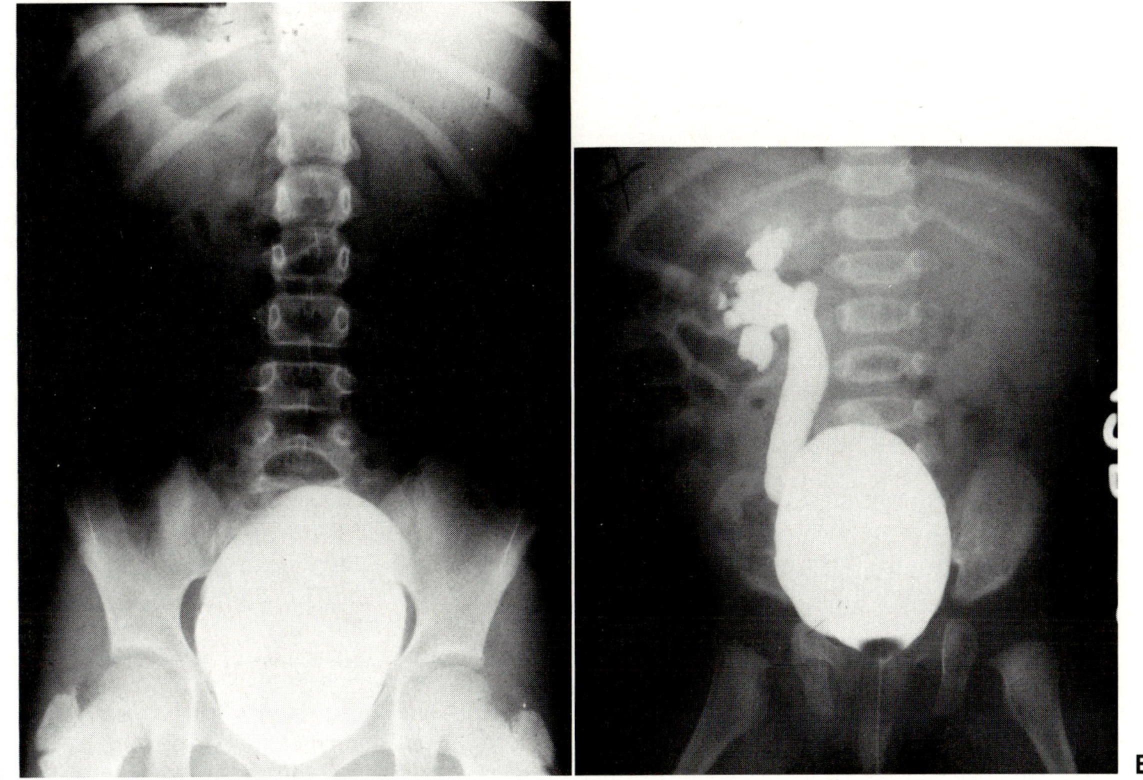

Figure 3 Severe VUR seen in a newborn *(A)* that resolves spontaneously in 2 years *(B)*.

copy in patients with unilateral reflux may reveal an unexpectedly abnormal-appearing contralateral orifice, it has not been my practice to reimplant such a ureter if it cannot be shown to reflux with nuclear cystography preoperatively. The practitioner must be sure that normal bladder dynamics exist and that the reflux is not the result of dysfunctional voiding. Urodynamics are valuable in this setting if there is any doubt about the patient's bladder coordination. In patients with renal scarring, it is best to document renal function and blood pressure accurately preoperatively to provide a baseline for future follow-up.

Antireflux surgery can be a same-day surgical procedure, with admission after the operation. In most patients, it is not necessary to have blood typed and cross-matched, since blood loss in antireflux procedure should be minimal. The urine should be sterile before ureteral reimplantation. For this reason, I routinely check the urine 1 week preoperatively and begin appropriate antibiotic therapy if an unexpected infection is encountered.

Choice of Surgical Procedure

There are many ways to approach the refluxing ureter surgically. The Leadbetter-Politano ureteral reimplantation enjoyed popularity for a number of years, but most such reimplantations can now be done by either a modified ureteral advancement or cross-trigonal reimplantation. These procedures essentially preserve the ureteral hiatus and have all but eliminated the obstructive complications that were occasionally seen with the Leadbetter-Politano procedure. They are also less bloody and easy to perform. Although the Cohen reimplantation has been shown to be effective and complication free, consideration of future ureteral access for stone disease or other diagnostic testing has made a modified Glenn-Anderson ureteral reimplantation more attractive for most cases of VUR. If the trigone is not expansive and if ureteral advancement alone will not result in a sufficient length of tunnel, the ureteral hiatus can be moved superiorly by incising the bladder mucosa and muscle in the course of the ureter. By moving the ureter 1 or 2 cm in upward direction and closing the incised muscle beneath the new ureteral hiatus, one can achieve an adequate tunnel length without risk of angulation. Routine stenting is not performed unless the ureters have been tailored or other significant anatomic problems exist, such as ureterocele or ureteral duplication. A Foley catheter is left in place for 1 week to promote bladder healing. The patient is often sent home with catheter drainage, because postoperative hospitalization is required for only 2 to 3 days.

If adequate ureteral length cannot be achieved through purely intravesical dissection, an extravesical dissection can be performed. The dissection should be carried out well above the obliterated umbilical artery, and this artery can be divided between ligatures to ensure that angulation to the ureter does not occur. An appropriate tunnel length to ureteral width should be in the ratio of 4:1. For larger ureters, tapering may be necessary. Again, intravesical dissection is possible in most of these patients, and the ureteral tailoring can be performed with Hendren clamps. It is necessary to tailor only that portion of the ureter that will be reimplanted, so the tailoring can be confined to the distal 6 to 7 cm of ureter. My personal choice is to resect the lateral aspect of the ureter and close this ureter in two layers over a ureteral stent, using the Hendren clamps. The ureteral folding technique has some appeal because there is no risk of urinary leak and little risk of interrupting the blood supply of the ureter when folding is performed. However, the technical problem of dealing with the large amount of tissue in submucosal tunnel still makes conventional ureteral tapering appealing to me.

POSTOPERATIVE CARE

Postoperative care includes intravenous fluids for at least 24 hours. Administration of D5 and Ringer's lactate at a rate of 25 percent over maintenance ensures a good urinary output. Since this is a same-day surgical procedure, patients are often dehydrated from having nothing by mouth for extensive periods. Bladder spasms tend to be the most immediate problem in the postoperative period. These can be handled by prophylactic oxybutynin, 2.5 to 5.0 mg three times a day as well as B & O suppositories at an appropriate dose. Caudal anesthesia can be performed with bupivacaine after reimplantation, but there is a risk of systemic absorption of the anesthetic agent. The side effects of this can be seizure or cardiopulmonary collapse. For this reason, I simply use postoperative analgesia and bladder spasm control without caudal anesthesia. The largest Foley catheter that the urethra will allow is left in place for 7 days. Small males usually require a suprapubic tube, ureteral stents being brought out through a separate stab wound in the abdomen. The patient remains on intravenous therapy until fluids can be taken orally. Once the diet has returned to normal and bladder spasms are at a minimum, such a patient may be discharged home. I keep the patient on antimicrobial therapy until cystography documents a successful reimplantation. This means that the patient is discharged on therapeutic doses of antibiotics and then returns to the normal preventive dosage of medication after catheter removal.

The biggest concern postoperative is ureteral obstruction. Despite the virtual elimination of this complication by the techniques discussed, it is still necessary to ensure that the reimplanted ureter is draining well. For this reason, I perform renal ultrasonography 1 month postoperatively to make sure there is no hydronephrosis. Edema at the orifice may take several weeks to subside. Suspected ureteral obstruction can be evaluated by diuretic renal scan, antegrade pyelography, or cystoscopy and retrograde pyelography. Approximately 6 months postoperatively, nuclear cystography is performed to evaluate the success of the antireflux procedure. If no reflux is seen, the antimicrobial prophylaxis

is discontinued. If reflux continues, the patient is maintained on prophylaxis for another year and repeat studies are done at this time. Usually, persistent reflux is of a low grade and spontaneous resolution is probable. The same approach is taken for low grades of contralateral reflux that appear after successful reimplantation on the opposite side. In my experience, this is of low grade and resolves spontaneously. This possibility should have been discussed with the parents so that surprises are kept to a minimum. A final repeat renal ultrasound examination is done 1 year postoperatively to ensure that occult hydronephrosis is not occurring secondary to distal ureteral obstruction.

Long-term follow-up is important, especially for children who have shown any degree of renal scarring. Patients whose kidneys are unscarred are probably not at risk for any future problems. However, those who have shown any degree of scarring may fall into the group of patients at risk for focal glomerulosclerosis under the hyperfiltration theory of Brenner. For this reason, yearly urinalysis to check for proteinuria and blood pressure determinations are necessary in these and all children who have demonstrated any amount of cortical loss.

In the rare patient who develops postoperative obstruction, repeat surgery is best postponed for several months. Temporization can be done through the use of a percutaneous nephrostomy tube or placement of a double-J ureteral catheter if possible. In the reoperated cases of obstruction, both intra- and extravesical dissection of the ureter is necessary to make sure that the ureter has an unkinked course. Elimination of tension on the ureteral vesical anastomosis may dictate a psoas hitch. A transureteroureterostomy is an attractive alternative to repeat ureteral reimplantation, but this does risk injury to a nondiseased ureter.

Parents must be aware of the risk of surgical complications such as obstruction (1 percent) or persistent reflux (3 to 5 percent). Up to 20 percent of contralateral ureters may reflux postoperatively. Although this is usually transient, parental concern can be minimized by proper preoperative education. The same is true for postoperative urinary infection. It is surprising how many parents expect ureteral reimplantation to eliminate infection, rather than prevent renal exposure to infected urine.

ENDOSCOPY

As we enter the 1990s, no review of VUR is complete without discussing endoscopic management of this disease. O'Donnell has shown high success with low complications in the management of primary VUR by subureteric injection of Teflon particles. This initial enthusiasm has been dampened by experimental evidence showing migration of these particles. The clinical significance of this microscopic migration into lymph nodes, liver, brain, and other tissues is still uncertain. Work with bovine collagen is continuing and encouraging results are being reported. However, long-term follow-up is lacking. The hope of endoscopic management is exciting, especially for certain clinical subgroups such as adolescent females with mild to moderate reflux in whom an open surgical procedure is not appealing. The technique is simple and involves the placement of either a collagen or Teflon deposit immediately under the submucosal ureter. This effectively buttresses the ureter and can be done on an outpatient basis in a matter of minutes. The morbidity and complication rate is negligible, and O'Donnell has shown a success rate in excess of 80 percent with this technique. With the development of newer materials, this may be the procedure of choice for a large percentage of patients with VUR.

ADULT VESICOURETERAL REFLUX

There are special considerations for adults with VUR. Reimplantation is indicated if they are experiencing recurring episodes of pyelonephritis. Surgery is more difficult in adults because the bladder occupies a position deeper in the pelvis. It is rare to see the development of new scars in adult VUR. Malek and colleagues showed that 93 percent of 67 adults became free of pyelonephritis after successful reimplantation, but in patients with renal scarring, proteinuria, or hypertension, correction of reflux had no effect on the progression of renal damage. Since focal glomulosclerosis is often seen in these kidneys, hyperfiltration injury may play a part in renal damage.

SUGGESTED READING

Hutch JA. Vesicoureteral reflux in the paraplegic: cause and correction. J Urol 1952; 68:457.
Jerkins GF, Noe HN. Familial vesicoureteral reflux: a prospective study. J Urol 1982; 128:774.
Kaplan WE, Nasrallah PF, King LR. Reflux in complete duplication in children. J Urol 1978; 120:220.
King LR, Zami SO, Belman AB. Natural history of vesicoureteral reflux: outcome of a trial of non-operative therapy. Urol Clin North Am 1974; 1:441.
Koff SA, Lapides J, Piazza DH. Association of urinary tract infection and reflux with uninhibited bladder contraction and voluntary sphincteric obstruction. J Urol 1979; 122:373.
Malek RS, Svensson J, Neves RJ, Torres VE. Vesicoureteral reflux in the adult. III. Surgical correction: risks and benefits. J Urol 1983; 130:882.
Malek RS, Svensson J, Torres VE. Vesicoureteral reflux in the adult. I. Factors in pathogenesis. J Urol 1983; 130:37.
O'Donnell B, Puri P. Treatment of vesicoureteric reflux by endoscopic injection of Teflon. Brit Med J 1984; 289:7–9.
Smellie JM, Edwards D, Normand ICS, Prescod N. Effect of VUR on renal growth in children with UTI. Arch Dis Child 1981; 56:593.

ECTOPIC URETEROCELE

RONALD R. PFISTER, M.D., F.A.A.P., F.A.C.S.
MARTIN A. KOYLE, M.D., F.A.A.P., F.A.C.S.

Ectopic ureterocele can be defined as a cystic dilatation of the terminal end of a ureter in which the terminal ureter lies in a position other than the orthotopic site; usually these sites include the distal trigone, bladder neck, or urethra. Although there have been many classifications, the one that comes closest to general acceptance is that put forth by F. Douglas Stephens:

1. Stenotic. Orifice is inside the bladder and is the presumed site of obstruction.
2. Sphincteric. Orifice of the ureterocele may be normal, even patulous, but lies in the floor of the urethra so that the ureter leading to it is obstructed by the internal sphincteric mechanism.
3. Sphincterostenotic. (Combination of I and II).
4. Cecoureterocele. Ureterocele that extends beneath the mucosa of the trigone and the urethra.
5. Blind ureterocele. Ureterocele with no orifice or kidney above the proximal extension of its ureter.
6. Nonobstructed ureterocele.

Ectopic ureteroceles usually subtend the upper moiety of a duplex system and most often occur in white girls. The detection of a ureterocele is increasingly made in the antenatal period with the advent of the widespread use of ultrasonography (Fig. 1). Renal and bladder ultrasonography accompanying a voiding cystourethrogram is also widely accepted as a first-line investigation of urinary tract infections in children, and ureteroceles may often be picked up by these routine imaging methods as well. In general, ultrasonography is the best definitive study since a voiding cystourethrogram, and to a lesser degree the intravenous pyelogram (IVP), may obscure and "white out" the ureterocele by the contrast medium density. A diethylenetriaminepenta-acetic acid (DTPA) scan may also suggest a ureterocele by demonstrating a nonfunctioning or poorly functioning upper pole with or without ureteral distention. Ureteroceles are also detected clinically when they prolapse externally through the urethra (Fig. 2) or as a result of investigation for urinary retention. The prolapsed ureterocele, the obstructing ureterocele, or a ureterocele causing recurrent urinary tract infection mandates early surgical correc-

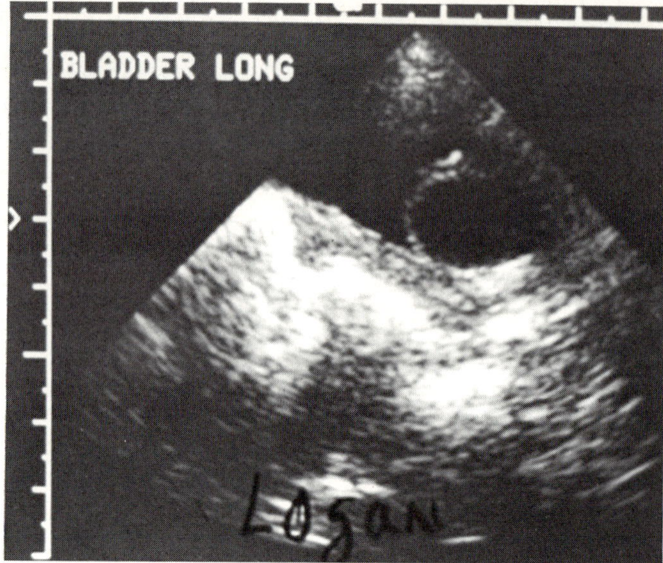

Figure 1 Ultrasonogram of the bladder and ureterocele.

tion. In asymptomatic newborns, however, urgent intervention is not necessarily a pressing issue. Management is therefore an individual matter. In the case of a sick child or infant, management of the infection is of primary importance. Most often antibiotics (e.g., aminoglycosides and ampicillin or a third-generation cephalosporin) can control the infection and temporize the situation to prepare for elective intervention, but occasionally decompression of the obstructed system is necessary. In such instances, acute decompression can be accomplished best by one or both of two methods. In the case of a duplex system, the upper segment can be large and amenable to percutaneous catheter drainage. This is especially pertinent in a septic neonate who is a poor anesthetic risk. Should this route prove not to be feasible, transurethral decompression is a possibility. The niceties of performing a low transurethral incision of the ureterocele may not be simple, however, since some are huge and orientation can be difficult endoscopically, particularly if there are bilateral ureteroceles. In such cases, a simple puncture of the ureterocele is appropriate, secondary repair at a later date possibly being necessary from reflux resulting from such unroofing. It must also be borne in mind that transurethral drainage may not be sufficient and a percutaneous nephrostomy may be necessary in addition. Other forms of drainage—e.g., cutaneous pyelostomy or ureterostomy—are not without their difficulties and require secondary closure later on. In the case of a loop ureterostomy, the ureter can be significantly shortened, and thus later reimplantation compromised. Pyelostomy is easy only if the pelvis is large and therefore conveniently brought to the skin; otherwise the risks of injuring the ureteropelvic junction are considerable, thus compounding the problem. In a duplex system, there is no pelvis in the upper pole, and an upper pole ureterostomy puts the lower pole ureter at risk. It therefore seems prudent to perform percutaneous nephrostomy preferentially if adequate drainage is not obtainable endoscopically.

PREFERRED APPROACH

The conventional management of ureteroceles depends on whether the system involved is single or duplex. In the single system, conventionally the ureterocele is resected, the bladder wall reinforced, and the ureter reimplanted. This may sound straightforward, but the surgery is lengthy and not easy, especially in an infant. The ureterocele may be so large, however, that no other route is feasible. We would resort to this approach only if the ureterocele was such that orientation was difficult endoscopically, but an ectopic ureterocele usually connotes a duplex system, and this entails several approaches. Our own approach is described below.

PATIENT SELECTION

Almost all ureteroceles that we currently encounter are in neonates or infants, having been discovered incidentally by antenatal ultrasound or as the result of a work-up for urinary tract infection. In our experience, the number of prolapsed ureteroceles presenting as such have been very few and have been easily reduced. If possible, we prefer to manage the ureterocele endoscopically irrespective of the patient's age or presentation.

TIMING OF SURGERY

Infection, if present, must be brought under control by either oral or intravenous antibiotics, with adjuvant drainage if necessary. After approximately 2 weeks,

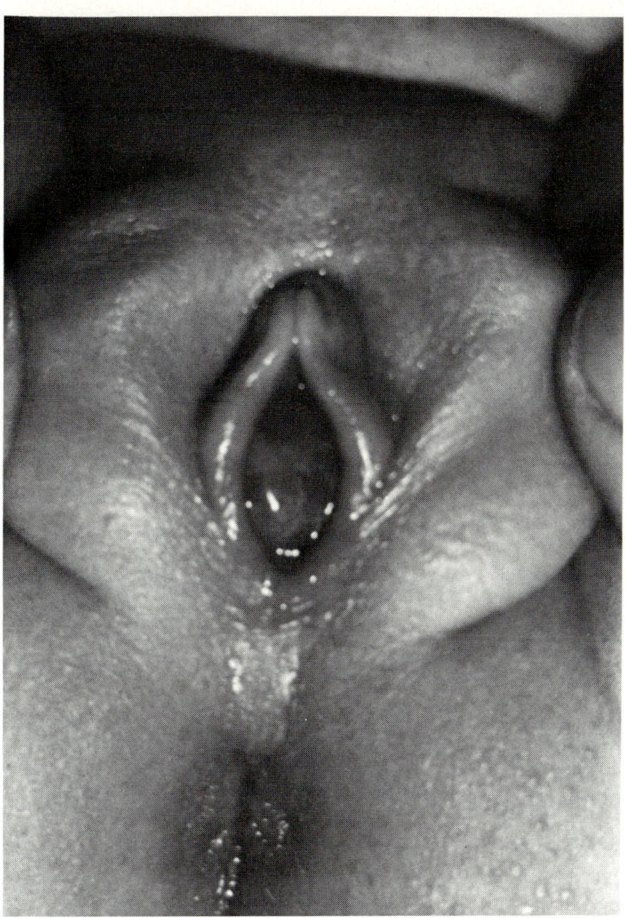

Figure 2 Prolapsed ureterocele.

cystoscopy and transurethral incision of the ureterocele are attempted. If the patient is asymptomatic, the procedure can be more electively scheduled. In the case of a neonate, it is important to allow bonding between the mother and child for a month or so before surgery.

PREOPERATIVE PREPARATION

Much has been made of the need to evaluate the function of the kidney with particular reference to that portion of the kidney subtended by the ureterocele. This has been important in determining whether a resection of the upper pole with its attendant ureter should be done. Tank has shown in a series of 40 cases following endoscopic incision of the ureterocele that only six required urgent intervention, and 20 (50 percent) improved in renal function after decompression. It becomes moot, therefore, whether renal function is initially demonstrated in the upper pole of the duplex system, since demonstrated function is not a determinant as to the choice of procedure: incision of the ureterocele or upper pole nephrectomy and ureterectomy. However, it is important to determine the function of the upper pole or the kidney itself in overall monitoring, however, and

this should be part of the preoperative work-up. The DMSA scan has been particularly helpful compared with the intravenous urogram and/or DTPA scan in quantitating the function of the affected segment.

CHOICE OF PROCEDURE

In the case of either single or duplex systems, our first approach is a low transurethral incision of the ureterocele on the medial distal aspect. Tank suggested the incision be proximal and lateral, but we have taken an opposite tack in order to prevent ureteral reflux if possible (Fig. 3). In boys, the urethra often restricts the use of a resectoscope, necessitating a small 7.5- to 10-Fr cystoscope, the ureterocele being incised by either a Bugbee electrode or a ureteral catheter through which a wire stylet is threaded. The end of the ureteral catheter containing small perforating eyes must be removed when using such a stylet to prevent arcing of the current through the eyes, thus injuring the urethra. It is easier to make the incision with the resectoscope, using the small single-wire electrode, than with the Bugbee or the ureteral catheter with the stylet, however. The incision should be made at the base of the ureterocele medially and transversely as small as possible to achieve decompression. The thickness of the ureterocele is often much greater than expected, and the incision may be thwarted by the collapse of the ureterocele. In such cases, abdominal or flank pressure can fill the ureterocele. The ureterocele may be difficult to see and demonstrate. A ureterocele collapsed by intravesical pressure can be filled by inserting a small ureteral needle into the base of the bladder and distending it with contrast material. In one of our patients, we could not penetrate the ureterocele, but the problem was ultimately solved by partial nephrectomy and ureterectomy. So far we have treated five patients—four girls and one boy—with ages ranging from newborn to 4 years old. All patients are currently free of infection or symptoms. Two still minimally reflux into the lower pole system; one required a partial nephrectomy and ureterectomy, as stated above. As to the question of function, it seems to have had no impact so far. As long as the system drains and no longer refluxes, or refluxes minimally, there appears to be no indication for future intervention. We would not advocate a partial nephrectomy and ureterectomy merely because of nonfunction. As for the reflux into the lower pole system, our inclination is to wait for spontaneous resolution. So far we have not been forced to resort to ureteral reimplantation, and in one patient, reflux into the ureterocele resolved spontaneously.

Recently we have attempted to correct the lower pole reflux by subureteric injection of Teflon (i.e., the STING). We have insufficient data to comment on the efficacy of this procedure in such a duplex system, but theoretically it seems possible. Should transurethral incision of a ureterocele prove unsatisfactory, an open surgical approach is necessary. There is general agreement that upper pole nephrectomy and removal of its

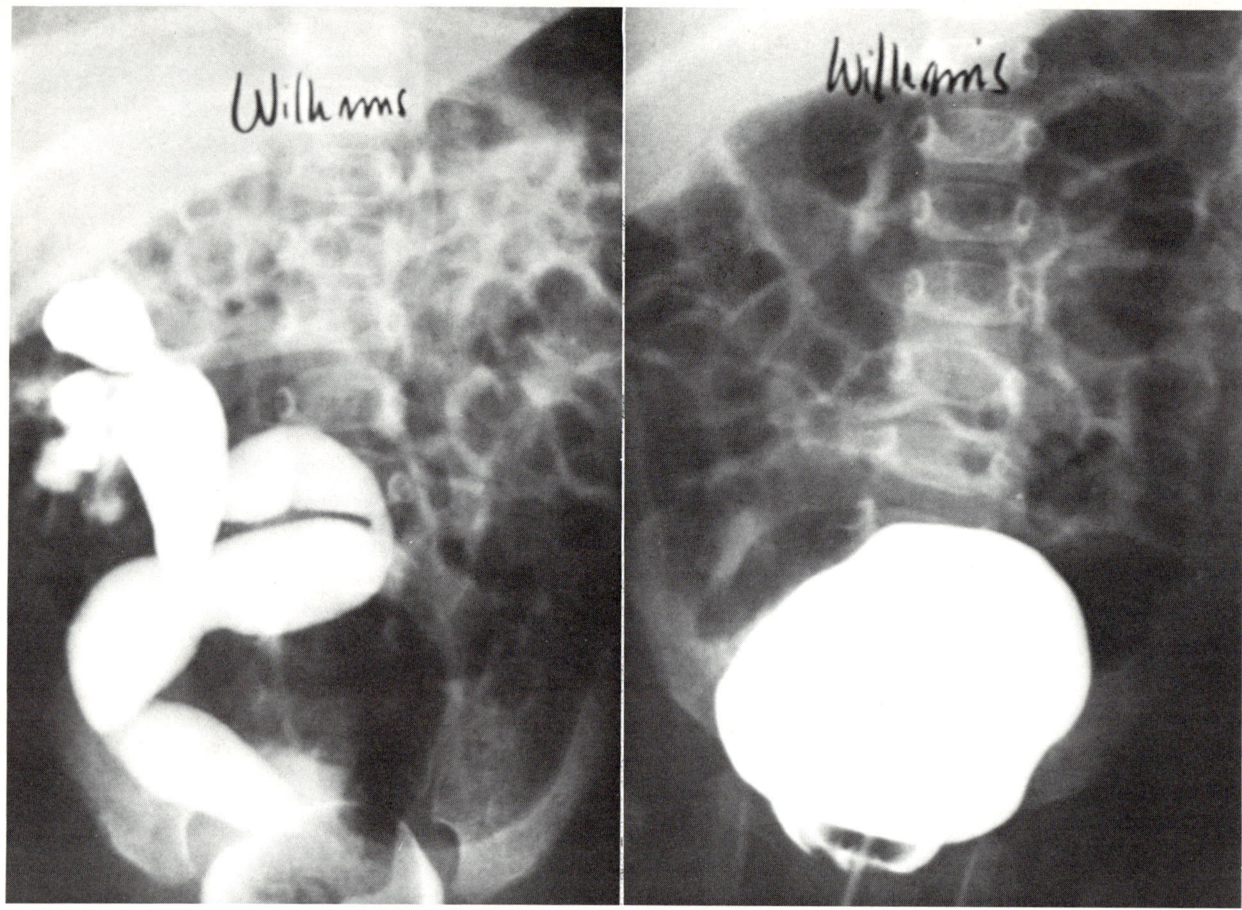

Figure 3 Transurethral incision into a ureterocele. *A,* Preoperative view, with reflux into the lower pole system. *B,* Postoperative view, no reflux.

attendant ureter as far as possible is appropriate if the upper pole is seen to be nonfunctional on DMSA scan. It has been reported that 30 to 60 percent of patients treated in this manner will require a second procedure to remove the residual upper pole ureteral stump and reimplant the lower pole ureter. This problem has prompted reports advocating one-stage intravesical resection of the ureterocele and total reconstruction. Conversely, 50 to 70 percent needed only an upper pole nephrectomy and upper pole ureterectomy without the need for ureteral implantation and ureterocele resection. In the case of a small infant, the additional surgery is a matter for concern. Even large ureteroceles can flatten out and become asymptomatic when they are completely decompressed. After upper pole nephrectomy, we have chosen to excise the upper pole ureter only as far distally as possible through a single incision. The walls of the upper pole and the lower pole ureter become virtually confluent and share a common blood supply in the distal aspect of both ureters. This can lead to inadequate resection of the upper pole ureter, with a resultant diverticulum-like stump. The upper pole ureter in its distal segment is lateral to the lower pole ureter; it passes around and under the lower pole ureter in its

most distal segment. If a ureteral catheter is in place in the orthotopic lower pole ureter, it is possible to remove the lateral wall of the ectopic ureter without injuring the orthotopic one. The filleted ureter can be left open if closure seems hazardous. Bladder drainage plus local drainage are sufficient to seal the open ureter. As for partial nephrectomy itself, little has been mentioned in most reports of the surgical procedure itself. It is important to recognize that the upper pole ureter is medial to the lower pole ureter and passes under the renal vessels. Occasionally the ureter is encased in inflammatory tissue and is difficult to separate from the vessels. In removing the upper pole cap of the kidney, it is sometimes helpful to open the dilated upper pole ureter, place a finger into the collecting system, and with a Bovie resect the cap against one's finger. It is not essential to peel back the capsule, which may be difficult, since the upper pole may have an irregular surface and scarring. On rare occasions, the upper pole may show reasonable function, in which case two choices present themselves: (1) upper pole ureteral anastomosis to the pelvis of the lower pole or (2) dual ureteral reimplantation as a single unit into the bladder.

MANAGEMENT OF THE DISTAL URETER

If reflux is a continuing problem after upper pole resection and ureterectomy, reimplantation and resection of the ureterocele will be necessary. In a single system, only the top half of the ureterocele is resected, leaving enough bladder mucosa to close the hiatus once the ureter has been reimplanted. The bladder wall also may be weak in the area of the ureterocele and should be plicated to prevent a subsequent paraureteral diverticulum. If the ureterocele subtends the upper pole of the duplex system, reimplantation becomes more complex. The orthotopic lower pole should be catheterized and most of the ureterocele resected, leaving enough to close the mucosa over the repair site. Occasionally, the ureterocele extends well into the urethra. Care must be taken to avoid injury of the urethra, and one must leave a little of the distal lip of the ureterocele to act as a urethral valve. A residual stump can be removed from the orthotopic ureter, leaving the common wall intact, or if the length of the common wall is short, the entire section involving both ureters can be removed, leaving the single orthotopic ureter to be reimplanted. Occasionally the common wall is lengthy, and resection of the two ureters high enough to obtain separate walls would leave too short a ureter for tension-free reimplantation. In such cases, only the lateral wall of the ectopic ureteral stump is removed, leaving the blood supply and the common wall intact.

In our opinion, resection of the ureterocele and reimplantation in the neonate should not be attempted by any other than the most experienced of surgeons. There is no urgency to complete everything in the first effort. It has generally been conceded that ureteral reimplantation and tapering in the neonate is unnecessary and hazardous, and the same appears true for a single-stage surgical correction of a ureterocele. A transurethral incision, in the manner described, appears to circumvent many problems and can save much surgical effort.

SUGGESTED READING

Gonzales ET Jr, Decter R. Management of ureteroceles in the newborn. Urologic surgery in neonates and young infants. Philadelphia: WB Saunders, 1988:204.

Kaplan GW, Brock WA, Kroovand KL, Tank ES. Management of ureterocele. Controversies in urology. Chicago: Year Book, 1989.

Rich MA, Keating MA, Snyder HM, Duckett JW. Low transureteral incision of single system intravesical ureteroceles in children. J Urol 1990; 44:120.

VESICOVAGINAL FISTULA: POSTSURGICAL

BERNARD LYTTON, M.B., F.R.C.S.

The diagnosis of a urinary vaginal fistula should always be considered in a woman who complains of incontinence after pelvic surgery. Vesicovaginal fistula accounts for 85 to 90 percent of cases and ureteral vaginal fistula for 10 to 15 percent. Occasionally, both may be present or fistulas may be multiple. The urinary incontinence usually takes the form of a continual leakage but may mimic true stress incontinence, especially in younger women in whom the urine may collect in the vagina; if the patient has a tight introitus, urine will be voided only on coughing or straining, or even at the time of normal urination when patients usually complain of double voiding. The diagnosis may be established by visualization of the fistula on cystoscopy or vaginoscopy, or by putting methylene blue into the bladder and seeing it leak into the vagina. Vaginal leakage may be visualized directly with a well-lighted speculum or by carefully placing a sponge into the vaginal vault and watching for staining of the proximal end. The most useful imaging studies are intravenous pyelography (IVP) to demonstrate any ureteral abnormality that may be indicative of a ureterovaginal fistula, or vaginography in which contrast material is injected through a Foley catheter placed in the vagina with the balloon inflated to occlude it. Often, the diagnosis can be re-established by seeing a small amount of contrast appear in the bladder or ureter. A vaginogram may be particularly helpful for fistulas that are difficult to define.

The patient may complain of postoperative leakage almost immediately or this may be delayed for several days or even weeks, depending on whether it is caused by direct injury or follows a vaginal cuff infection with perforation into the bladder.

Patients with vesicovaginal fistulas are generally unhappy. They have just suffered through one major procedure, they are wet, and there is no effective method for diverting or collecting the leaking urine. The urologist needs to be sympathetic but firm and exercise good judgment as to the best treatment and optimal time to recommend surgical repair. The patient needs support and reassurance that the problem will be successfully resolved. Careful records need to be kept in case of future litigation.

TREATMENT

The following outline for management applies only to fistulas in women who have not received any pelvic irradiation. Initially the fistula may be treated by placement of a urethral catheter, and sometimes this provides sufficient drainage to allow the fistula to close spontaneously. Once the tract becomes epithelialized, it is very unlikely to heal spontaneously.

When the fistula is only pinhole-sized, fulguration of the fistulous tract with a No. 3 Fr Bugbee electrode has been curative on a few occasions. Electrodes are inserted into the fistula through a cystoscope. The approach may be transvesical, transvaginal, or a combination of both. It is important to use only sufficient current to destroy the epithelial lining. Excessive fulguration may result in initial closure due to edema, but a recurrence of the fistula when the burned tissue sloughs. This procedure has the advantage that it can usually be performed in the office under local anesthesia together with a little sedation. An indwelling Foley catheter should be worn for 2 weeks. The patient should be warned that this procedure is not always successful.

Timing of Surgical Repair

It has traditionally been advocated that repair should not be undertaken for at least 3 months after the initial injury, to allow all the inflammatory action in the tissues to subside. Because of the discomfort and distress that frequently accompanies the waiting period, many surgeons now advocate immediate repair and have had satisfactory results. An immediate repair gives the patient a reasonable chance of early relief from incontinence, and even if the operation is unsuccessful, little time will have been lost if the secondary repair is performed after an interval of 2 to 3 months. Our own practice has been to undertake repair of the fistula as soon as most of the surrounding edema and inflammatory action have subsided, which may be much sooner than 3 months. In the presence of a great deal of inflammation, an operative repair would be difficult and very likely fail. In some cases repair can be carried out immediately as there is very little inflammatory action; in others an interval of 3 to 6 weeks may be required. Badenoch and colleagues reported 19 patients with vesicovaginal fistulas, seven of which were operated on in less than 6 weeks and 12 in more than 6 weeks after injury. Repair was by the abdominal route and all were successful.

Preoperative Preparation

It is preferable to remove the catheter a few days before surgery and administer an antibacterial agent to ensure sterile urine. Postmenopausal women should receive systemic estrogens or apply an estrogen cream vaginally for about 1 week preoperatively to improve the vascularity and thickness of the vaginal tissues.

Administration of steroids preoperatively to diminish the inflammatory response has been advocated by Collins and colleagues to facilitate early operative repair, but this does not appear to be necessary in most cases.

Fistulas can be repaired by either a transvaginal or a transabdominal approach. The transvaginal approach, although less familiar to urologists, is preferred when the conditions are suitable, because it obviates the need for another abdominal incision and what is often a tedious dissection to free the bladder from the adherent rectus muscles and overlying peritoneum. The advantage of the vaginal approach may be compared with those of a transurethral resection of the prostate versus transvesical prostatectomy. Most simple fistulas can be repaired transvaginally, but the transabdominal approach is recommended when the vaginal vault is deep and fixed, when there are multiple fistulas, when the fistula cannot be catheterized, or when the defect is very large (>2 to 3 cm).

Transvaginal Repair

When there have been several unsuccessful attempts at vaginal repair, a transabdominal repair is probably advisable in most cases. Successful closure of the fistula is achieved in 75 to 95 percent with both the vaginal and abdominal routes. Most failures are related to previous pelvic radiation or some unusual anatomic or technical problem such as loss of vaginal wall, involvement of the proximal urethra, postoperative bowel complications, or extensive scarring from multiple previous operations.

The patient is placed in an exaggerated lithotomy position with the buttocks well over the edge of the table so that a weighted vaginal speculum of appropriate size can be placed in the vagina to expose the vault. Some surgeons prefer to place the patient in the prone position. The lower abdomen should be left exposed to enable a suprapubic tube to be inserted into the bladder through a small incision under direct vision. The labia are sutured to the medial aspect of the thighs to provide good exposure of the introitus, and a weighted speculum is placed in the vagina to expose the fistula and scarred vault. The anterior vaginal wall is retracted with a narrow, straight Deaver retractor. A small Foley catheter should be passed through the fistula into the bladder and the balloon inflated. Traction on the catheter will pull the fistulous opening down toward the introitus and makes it easier to excise. When the fistula track is too small to accept a catheter, a guide wire or a No. 4 or 5 Fr ureteral catheter is passed first. This can be done through the cystoscope to pass the guide through either the bladder or the vaginal opening. A No. 6 Fr or No. 8 Fr Foley catheter is then tied to the end of the ureteral catheter and railroaded through the fistula into the bladder. When the fistula cannot be catheterized owing to its length or tortuosity, it is probably best to repair it via a transvesical approach, as this allows for better visualization of the anatomy to ensure complete excision of the fistula. Vaginal exposure may be improved by performing a posterolateral episiotomy. The ureters should then be catheterized with No. 5 Fr ureteral stents so that their position can be readily identified during the dissection and repair.

The vaginal mucosa should be circumcised about 2 to 3 mm from the edge of the fistula with sharp dissecting scissors. The vaginal incision may be extended longitudinally both anteriorly and posteriorly to provide better access to the bladder (Fig. 1*A*). The incision is deepened until a plane between the vagina and bladder is established. This is usually recognizable in one or more areas where the vagina is not adherent to the bladder, and separates fairly easily. The plane is developed from these areas into the adherent scar tissue, enabling the vaginal flaps to be completely separated from the bladder for a distance of at least 1 to 2 cm from the site of the fistula in order to completely free the bladder from the vagina. The peritoneal reflection may be seen or entered under the posterior part of the vaginal flaps. The peritoneum usually can be easily dissected off the bladder and vagina to allow it to be closed or used as a flap to interpose between the vesical and vaginal repairs. Care must be taken to avoid any injury to, or inclusion of, any adherent bowel.

The bladder portion of the fistula is now excised together with any surrounding scar tissue. A small incision should be made first so as to identify the ureteral catheters and ureteral orifices before completing the excision of the fistula, as these are often in close proximity. The bladder is closed transversely. A 000 plain catgut suture is placed at each end of the defect, and should include both the mucosa and underlying muscle. Each suture is run to the middle of the defect and tied to the other (Fig. 1*B*). This allows the mucosa at the ends of the defects to be closed under vision to ensure a watertight closure. The bladder suture line is then embrocated using interrupted 00 chromic catgut sutures to reinforce the repair. Hemostasis is secured by light fulguration or by oversewing the bleeding vessels with

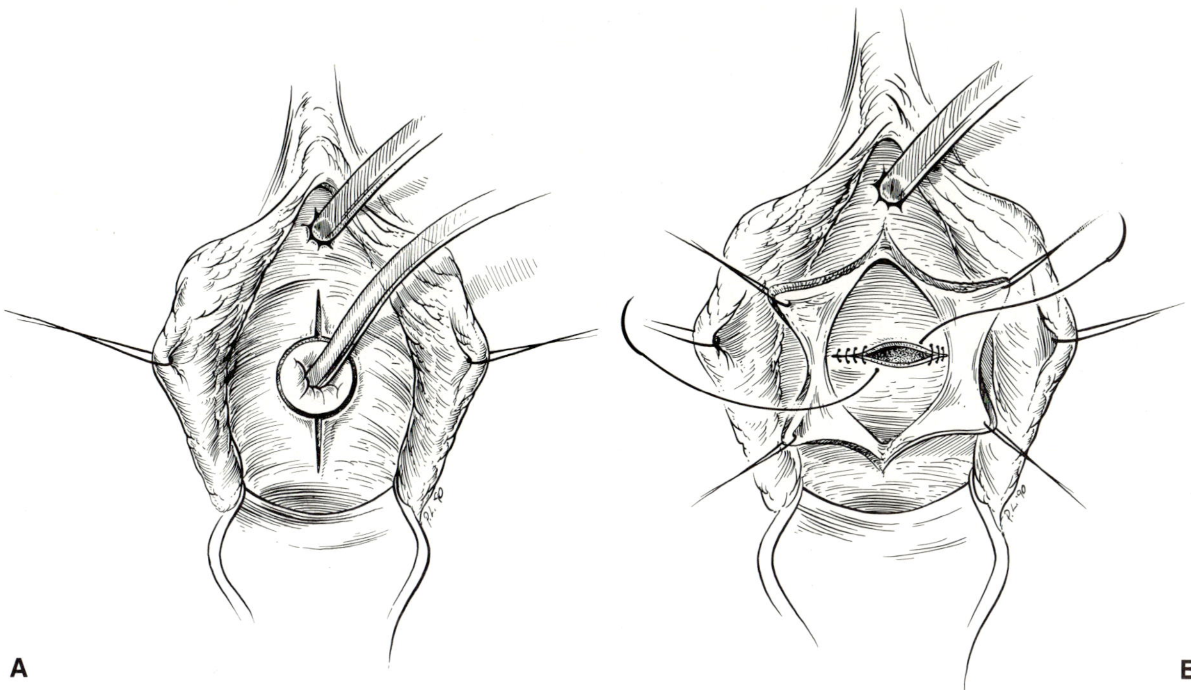

Figure 1 Vaginal approach. *A,* Small Foley catheter in fistula and vaginal incision around it. *B,* Mobilization of vaginal flaps complete. Bladder opening being closed transversely from each end with running 000 chromic catgut sutures.

000 chromic sutures. The suture line may be covered with fascia or a flap of peritoneum for extra protection. Once the bladder closure is completed, if the bladder has been adequately freed from the vagina, it will retract away from the vaginal incision. The vagina is sutured with interrupted 00 polyglycolic sutures. No drains are inserted, but the vagina is packed with 2-inch-wide gauze impregnated with either iodoform or Betadine to control oozing. The packing is placed fairly tight with the speculum in position, so that on removal of the speculum the packing assumes the correct tension. A No. 26 Fr Malecot catheter is placed suprapubically through a small midline incision. It is better that this not be a percutaneous stab, in order to avoid injury to the peritoneum, which often is adherent to the anterior surface of the bladder after an abdominal operation. No urethral catheter is inserted to obviate any pressure on the repair. The ureteral stents are taped to the thigh and attached to drainage bags. The vaginal pack and ureteral stents are removed after 24 hours. An antibacterial, usually a cephalosporin, is given preoperatively and for 24 hours postoperatively. The patient is usually sent home after 1 week with a suprapubic tube in place. Cystography is performed 2 weeks after surgery, and if there is no leakage the tube is removed. If there is concern for the viability of the tissues or if it is a secondary or tertiary repair, a Martius graft can be placed over the vesical repair to reinforce it. The graft is prepared by mobilizing the labial fat pad together with the corpus cavernosum muscle on its vascular pedicle. A tunnel is created with the finger under the lateral vaginal flap to the root of the graft, which is then brought through and sutured over the bladder repair.

A partial culpocysis or Latzko procedure is an alternative vaginal operation that does not require such an extensive dissection. The mucosa of the vagina is denuded around the fistulous opening for about 1 cm. The bladder is then embrocated over the fistula tract with two layers of interrupted 00 chromic sutures, and the vaginal mucosa is approximated with interrupted 00 polyglycolic sutures. This procedure, while simpler, tends to carry a higher recurrence rate and results in some shortening of the vagina (see Fig. 2).

Transabdominal Repair

There are basically two transabdominal approaches. One is transperitoneal with a racket incision in the bladder that circumscribes the fistula, and the other is transvesical and extraperitoneal. The latter, the one I prefer, is performed when vaginal access is difficult, when the fistula and vaginal vault are relatively immobile owing to extensive scarring, and when the fistula cannot be cannulated preoperatively owing to the length and tortuosity of the tract. Furthermore, inability to catheterize the fistula makes it more difficult to ensure complete excision, and consequently there is a greater risk of recurrence.

The patient is placed supine on the operating table, after both ureters are catheterized and the vagina prepared with Betadine. The bladder is filled with 200 to 300 ml of saline to facilitate the dissection. A transverse

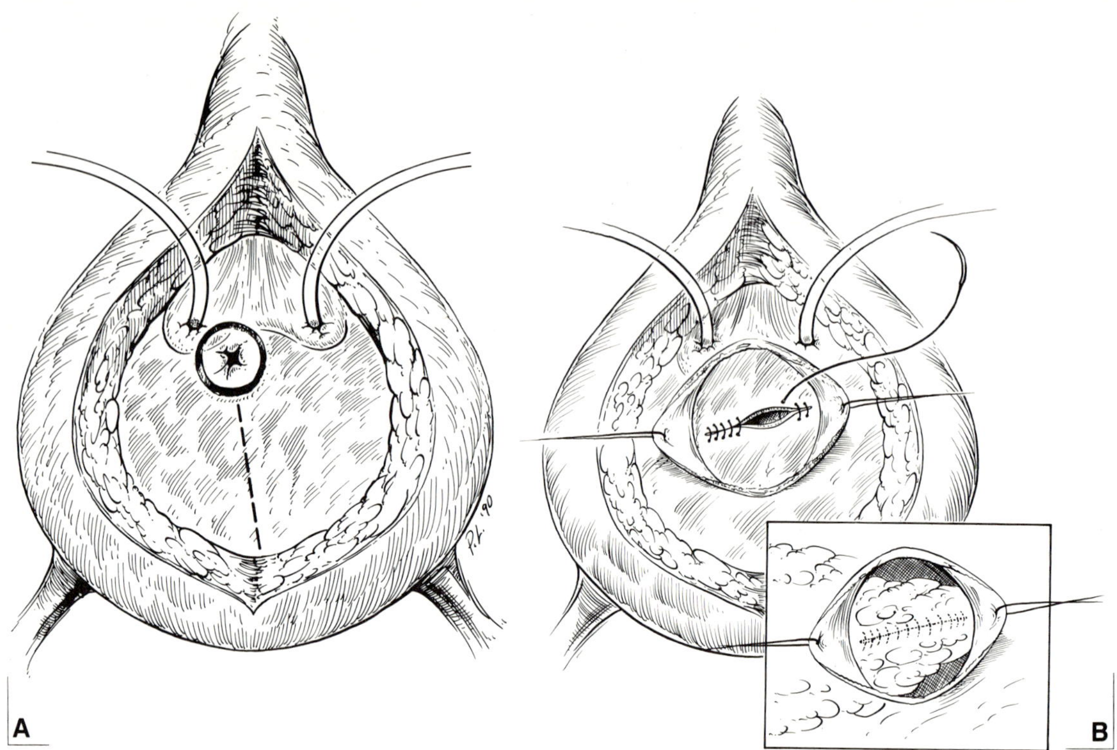

Figure 2 Transvesical approach. *A,* Circumcision of bladder fistula. Dotted line shows alternative racquet incision. Note catheters in ureters. *B,* Closure of vaginal defect. Inset shows interposition of properitoneal fat or appendix epiloica.

or longitudinal incision is made in the lower abdomen, usually through the previous scar. The rectus muscles are divided in the midline just above the symphysis to avoid opening the peritoneum inadvertently. The rectus muscles are separated off the underlying bladder and peritoneum. This usually needs to be done by sharp dissection, because these structures are often adherent from the previous surgery. The peritoneum is reflected off the anterior surface of the bladder.

Transvesical Approach

The anterior bladder wall is incised longitudinally and a self-retaining bladder retractor inserted. The posterior wall is retracted with a middle blade on the self-retaining retractor or a medium-size Deaver to expose the trigone and fistula site. The fistula site and surrounding scarred area are then circumcised with a small long-handled knife or sharp dissecting scissors (Fig. 2 *A*). The incision is deepened through the muscle until the plane between the bladder wall and the vagina is entered. The bladder muscle is dissected off the vagina circumferentially until the bladder is entirely free. Again, the peritoneal reflection will be seen under the proximal or cephalad flap and can be dissected off to facilitate the bladder closure. The fistulous track and scar tissue are excised from the vagina, and the defect in the vagina is closed with a running polyglycolic suture, embrocated with a few interrupted sutures of the same

material. The suture line may be covered with a flap of peritoneum or, if necessary, an epiploic appendix from the sigmoid brought through a small opening in the peritoneal pouch behind the bladder (Fig. 2*B*). The defect in the bladder muscle is closed transversely with a running 00 chromic catgut suture, and the overlying mucosal layer is closed with a 000 plain catgut suture. A No. 26 or 28 Fr Malecot catheter is then placed through a separate stab incision in the bladder and secured to the bladder wall with 2-0 chromic catgut suture. The anterior incision in the bladder is closed in two layers with catgut sutures, a running 000 plain for the mucosa and interrupted 00 chromic for the muscle layer. It is preferable to put the suprapubic tube through a separate stab incision in the skin so as to avoid contamination of the abdominal incision with urine that sometimes leaks around the catheter. The tube should be secured to the skin with a nylon suture. The ureteral catheters are brought out through the suprapubic stab incision together with the tube, and are removed after 24 hours. The vagina is packed with impregnated gauze, which is removed after 24 hours.

Transperitoneal Approach

The anterior incision in the bladder is carried upward through the lower peritoneal reflection. Care must be taken to avoid any adherent bowel loops, which must be dissected off the peritoneal surface of the bladder. The edge of the bladder is grasped with Allis forceps, and the incision is carried over the dome and down the posterior wall to its point of adherence to the vagina and then continued around the fistula to complete the racket incision. The lateral edge of the bladder is dissected free from the vagina. The fistula and scar tissue are excised en bloc and the vaginal defect is closed as previously described. An epiploic appendix, a peritoneal flap, or a portion of the greater omentum may be used to cover the vaginal closure. The omentum can be mobilized if too short to reach by first separating it from the transverse colon, and then dividing the short gastric vessels along the greater curvature of the stomach to allow the omentum to drop down on a vascular pedicle derived from the right gastroepiploic artery. The bladder is then closed in two layers as described. A suprapubic tube is placed in the bladder through a separate stab incision.

Repair of Vesicovaginal Fistula After Pelvic Irradiation

This type of fistula poses a special problem, because the tissues are poorly vascularized, and viability and healing is impaired by the radiation. These fistulas often develop spontaneously many years after the original surgery and radiation.

The essential feature in the repair is the interposition of a well-vascularized, nonirradiated graft. It is preferable to perform the repair vaginally if possible, since the tissues of the lower abdominal wall and pelvis have been irradiated and bowel loops are often adherent in the pelvis. When the approach has to be from above, omentum is probably the best graft to interpose between the bladder and vagina.

When a vaginal approach repair is performed, a vascularized musculocutaneous graft of gracilis muscle and overlying skin is transposed to the perineum on its neurovascular pedicle. It is advisable to have the collaboration of a plastic surgeon familiar with the preparation of this type of graft. The vesicovaginal fistula is dissected out as previously described, and the bladder is separated from the vagina by sharp dissection. A tunnel is then created under the vaginal flap into the medial aspect of the thigh where the graft has been raised. The graft is brought through the tunnel, the muscular surface is used to close or reinforce the bladder defect, and the cutaneous portion is sewn to the edges of the vaginal defect. It is

Table 1 Repair of Vesicovaginal Fistula (17 Patients, 1980–1990)

	Vaginal Repair	*Transvesical Repair*
Posthysterectomy	12 patients (12 closed) 1 had 3 previous repairs 2 had 1 previous repair	2 patients (2 closed) 1 had previous repair
Postradiation	3 patients 1 Martinus graft (1 failed 4 weeks postoperatively) 2 gracilis myocutaneous flaps (2 closed)	

helpful to divert the urine away, using large, single-J ureteral stents, which are exteriorized with the suprapubic tube and left in position for 7 to 10 days. It is probably advisable to leave the suprapubic tube in place for at least 3 weeks and to perform cystography before removal of the tube to ensure that closure is sound.

When the vagina and bladder cannot be separated, a colpocleisis may be the only way to close the defect. In severe cases in which the tissues become too indurated to enable a formal repair to be performed or in which the defect is too large, a suprapubic diversion using an ileal conduit or continent pouch is the only alternative.

SUGGESTED READING

Badenoch DF, Tiptaft RC, Thakar DR, et al. Early repair of accidental injury to the ureter or bladder following gynaecological surgery. Br J Urol 1987; 59:516–518.

Barnes R, Hadley H, Johnston O. Transvaginal repair of vesicovaginal fistulas. In: Whitehead ED, Leiter E, eds. Current operative urology. Part 31: Surgery of urinary fistula. Philadelphia: Harper & Row, 1984:973.

Eisen M, Jurkovic K, Altwein J-E, et al. Management of vesicovaginal fistulas with peritoneal flap interposition. In: Whitehead ED, Leiter E, eds. Current operative urology. Part 31: Surgery of urinary fistula. Philadelphia: Harper & Row, 1984:977.

Keettel WC, Schring FG, DeProsse CA, et al. Surgical management of urethrovaginal and vesicovaginal fistulas. Am J Obstet Gynecol 1978; 131:425.

VESICOVAGINAL FISTULA: POST RADIATION THERAPY

ELROY D. KURSH, M.D.

Vesicovaginal fistulas that develop after radiation therapy are particularly vexing management problems. Most of these occur following radiation therapy for carcinoma of the cervix, which was the predominant treatment for this condition in the 1940s. Radiation therapy continues to be widely used and apparently is as effective as surgical treatment, despite the fact that the cervix is not particularly radiosensitive. This is because the cervix and vagina tolerate radiation well, allowing large doses to be administered with relatively good results and cure rates, and the cervix is particularly well suited to local radium implantation. Unfortunately, the large radiation dose may lead to injury to adjacent organs such as the bladder, rectum, and small bowel.

Most complications of radiation therapy appear relatively soon after the treatment is completed, often within 6 to 12 months. However, there is evidence that urinary and rectosigmoid complications are increasing in incidence 5 years after treatment and may be noted even 30 years later. Not only does the radiation therapy cause significant tissue injury, but tissue necrosis may be enhanced by progressive arteriosclerotic vascular disease that frequently occurs with aging.

Patients present with varying degrees of urinary incontinence that develop months or years after completion of radiation therapy. A history of large doses of radiation therapy to the pelvis suggests that the incontinence may be related.

Associated radiation-induced genitourinary complaints may include intermittent hematuria and marked irritative bladder symptoms such as frequency and urgency related to radiation cystitis or bladder fibrosis. Patients may also complain of symptoms related to radiation proctitis such as bloody stools, diarrhea, or painful bowel movements.

EVALUATION

The diagnosis of a vesicovaginal fistula is suspected on the basis of the history and is usually relatively easy to establish. Urine may be noted to be exiting from the vagina, and the fistula may be visualized on vaginal speculum examination. A bladder-filling test confirms the diagnosis by noting drainage of fluid from the fistula in the vagina as it is inserted into the bladder via a catheter or cystoscope. Similarly, various dye solutions such as methylene blue or indigo carmine may be used to fill the bladder as the potential fistula site in the vagina is observed.

A patient who develops a vesicovaginal fistula after radiation therapy should be considered to have recurrent cancer until it is proved otherwise. Evaluation is made in conjunction with the primary physician who delivered the radiation therapy, e.g., a gynecologist. A computed tomographic scan of the pelvis is obtained to assess evidence of recurrent cancer or a possible pelvic mass. A pelvic examination is performed, preferably with the patient under anesthesia, and the edge of the fistula is biopsied.

Evaluation of the status of the bladder is particularly important because it has significant impact on the choice and outcome of therapy.

Cystoscopy is performed to confirm the diagnosis of a vesicovaginal fistula and assess bladder status. The size, location, and degree of associated inflammation, and other pathologic conditions such as radiation cystitis and/or bladder fibrosis that may complicate a vesicovaginal fistula are noted. The urologist should try to obtain some idea of bladder compliance, although this may be difficult if the fistula is large, owing to inability to fill the bladder. Likewise, urodynamic testing may be impossible in a patient with a large fistula. Video urodynamic evaluation may be helpful in assessing urethral sphincter function.

TREATMENT

Repair of a radiation-induced vesicovaginal fistula presents a particularly challenging surgical problem. Obviously, it is not considered if the patient has recurrent cancer. An accurate preoperative assessment of bladder function is imperative, since the patient must have a reasonably compliant functional bladder, capable of maintaining continence, for surgical correction to be contemplated. The ultimate solution to an insufficient storage capacity is augmentation cystoplasty, but this is not always feasible owing to associated radiation-injured small or large bowel and the fibrotic condition of the bladder. Therefore, some form of supravesical urinary diversion may be the only reasonable alternative.

If the urologist concludes that surgical correction of a radiation-induced vesicovaginal fistula is appropriate, it is important to time the repair to maximize the likelihood of a successful outcome. When the fistula develops acutely, shortly after the cessation of radiation therapy, it is necessary to await resolution of the acute radiation injury. Repeat speculum examinations of the vagina are performed to estimate the degree of necrosis and inflammation, and cystoscopy is repeated. Generally, a period of 6 months or more is required to allow the acute necrosis and inflammation to subside before undertaking surgical repair. On the other hand, a fistula that develops years after the radiation insult has a more rigid, indurated, fixed appearance and may have little associated necrosis or acute inflammation. In this instance, it may be possible to avoid a long delay when timing the surgical procedure.

Once the surgery is undertaken, a standard repair is fraught with the risk of failure, since radiation-damaged tissue heals poorly. Not only is the radiation-damaged tissue fibrotic, but associated vasculitis minimizes blood supply and impairs normal healing. In order to strengthen the repair and increase the likelihood of success, it is necessary to interpose nonradiated, well-vascularized tissue between the bladder and vagina.

One possibility is to use the bulbocavernosus muscle and fat pad in a procedure also known as the Martius operation. A variety of vaginal incisions can be employed, although a flap that can be advanced later is preferred. The irradiated, fixed, fibrotic fistula edge is excised and the vaginal mucosa dissected off the bladder. After closing the bladder side of the fistula, a separate labial incision is made on either side. The bulbocavernosus muscle and fat pad, which are usually based posteriorly, are rotated under a subcutaneous tunnel and the vaginal mucosa to cover the bladder closure. Closure of the vaginal mucosa by a variety of techniques completes this procedure.

I prefer to avoid the vaginal approach to repair a postirradiation vesicovaginal fistula for several reasons: (1) it is generally difficult to dissect the fibrotic radiation-damaged vaginal mucosa off the fistula and bladder; (2) excision of the edges of the bladder side of the fistula is often avoided using the vaginal technique, which may be necessary to attempt to close better vascularized tissue; and (3) the bulbocavernosus fat pad may have been injured by its proximity to the radiation field.

I prefer to use a suprapubic, transvesical, transperitoneal approach to correct a postirradiation vesicovaginal fistula. Preoperative preparation includes mechanical and antibiotic bowel preparation, since it may be necessary to lyse a significant number of adhesions to gain access to the pelvis. Care is taken to ensure sterile urine, and broad-spectrum parenteral antibiotic coverage is started preoperatively. A povidone-iodine (Betadine) douche is administered the night before surgery.

After anesthesia is induced, the patient is placed in the lithotomy position with the lower extremities in strapped foot restraints so that the surgeon has access to both the abdomen and vagina. I employ the Allen stirrups for this purpose because of their ease of manipulation. The vagina, the perivaginal area, the entire abdomen, and the upper portion of both lower extremities to below the knees are prepared with Betadine, and the patient is draped to allow access to the suprapubic area, the vagina, and the medial aspect of each thigh.

A lower abdominal midline incision is made. A transverse incision should be avoided, since it may be necessary to extend this incision to gain adequate access to the upper abdomen in order to mobilize the omentum later in the procedure. The small bowel is mobilized and packed out of the way, and adhesions are frequently incised to gain access to the pelvis.

The bladder is opened in the midline longitudinally. A No. 5 or 6 Fr ureteral catheter is passed to 25 cm bilaterally. A plane is established between the vagina and bladder without attempting to separate the perito-

neal reflection from the bladder wall. It is helpful for the surgeon to keep either the index and long fingers of his free hand or the hand of an assistant in the vagina when establishing this plane in order to ascertain the exact location in the vagina. Another option is to pack the vagina with a Betadine-impregnated vaginal pack to help define the location of the vagina. To determine the exact location of the fistula, it is often helpful to insert a small Foley or Fogarty catheter through the fistula from the opened bladder. Bivalving the bladder down to the fistula site is usually avoided in order to obviate the need for a large posterior bladder closure later in the procedure, especially in a bladder that is already compromised secondary to radiation injury. After an adequate plane is established between the vagina and the bladder with the use of a Metzenbaum scissors, the diseased tissue from the bladder and vaginal edges of the fistula is sharply excised. The serosa and muscularis of the bladder is closed longitudinally with interrupted 2-0 absorbable suture material, and the mucosa is closed with a running 4-0 chromic catgut suture. The vagina is closed in an opposite transverse direction using interrupted 2-0 absorbable sutures. If the vagina is pliable enough, it may be feasible to invert the initial layer of closed vagina with a second layer using interrupted Lempert-type sutures of absorbable suture material, although this is the exception for a radiation-induced fistula.

A decision is made regarding the degree of radiation-induced injury, the viability and strength of the tissue supporting the sutures, and the satisfaction with the repair that has already been completed. If there is any concern about the adequacy of repair or the risk of recurrence, which is usual, I do not hesitate to use a well-vascularized gracilis muscle flap or rectus flap interposed between the bladder and vagina. Otherwise, an omental pedicle graft is employed.

Depending on the anatomy of the omentum, a variety of omental flaps can be mobilized to gain adequate access to the pelvis. The omental blood supply comes from the right gastroepiploic artery, which is a branch of the gastroduodenal artery, and the left gastroepiploic artery, which is a branch of the splenic artery. The right and left omental arteries extend down each side of the omentum, and there is a variable middle omental artery. If the omentum is long enough, an L-shaped incision can be made in the omentum close to the transverse colon, basing the omental flap on either the right or left omental arteries. If the omentum is short, it is necessary to mobilize the omentum from the transverse colon and make the inverted L-shaped incision close to the stomach in order to gain sufficient length of omentum to reach the pelvis. This often requires extending the abdominal incision. When designing an omental flap, it is usually relatively easy to locate the omental blood supply by palpation.

If the surgeon chooses to use a gracilis muscle flap, dissection between the bladder and vagina proceeds caudal to the fistula under the contralateral ureter in the direction of the thigh of the donor gracilis muscle. Again, it is helpful for the examiner to keep the examining fingers on his free hand in the vagina in order to discern its anterior edge. The dissection terminates near the bladder neck in a plane beneath the endopelvic fascia in the prevesical space. An incision is made in the endopelvic fascia anteriorly on the side of the donor thigh, extending for several centimeters, which is large enough to admit the belly of the gracilis muscle. This incision in the endopelvic fascia connects to the already established plane between the bladder and the vagina where the gracilis muscle flap will sit.

Either the same surgical team or a second team, possibly headed by a plastic surgeon, prepares the gracilis muscle flap. This may be done while the initial team is operating in the pelvis. Either a long skin incision is made extending over the course of the muscle on the medial thigh, or three smaller skin incisions are made along the same course, to permit mobilization and rotation of the muscle into the pelvis. The gracilis muscle is a relatively small adductor originating on the pubic arch and inserting into the proximal tibia. Rotation of the distal portion of the muscle into the pelvis does not compromise ambulation in any way. The distal tendinous insertion of the muscle is incised but is usually discarded later once the distal muscle belly is properly positioned and fixed in place. Usually, there are two branches of the deep femoral artery supplying the muscle from a lateral position in the proximal third of the muscle. Doppler ultrasonography can be used to assist in their localization. It may be necessary to sacrifice the distal branch of the artery to gain additional length, which can usually be done without altering viability of the flap. The origin of the muscle on the pubic arch is not disturbed. Using blunt and sharp dissection from both the thigh and the pelvis, a tunnel is created between the upper thigh and the urogenital diaphragm medial to the inferior pubic ramus. The distal muscle is rotated medially to enter this space. If necessary, additional length may be gained by adducting the leg. The muscle is brought through the openings in the urogenital diaphragm and the endopelvic fascia to enter the space posterior to the bladder. Another option is to bring the gracilis muscle through a perforation in the obturator fossa. After the muscle is properly positioned, it is affixed in place to the adjacent endopelvic fascia with a few interrupted 2-0 chromic catgut sutures. The distal end of the muscle is usually sutured in place on the bladder to buttress the previously closed bladder side of the fistula. Alternatively, it can be sutured onto the vagina over the previously closed vaginal side of the fistula. For a particularly difficult fistula, I do not hesitate to use both a gracilis muscle flap and omentum interposed between the bladder and vagina, or even gracilis muscle flaps from each thigh. Omentum has the added advantage of helping absorb adjacent fluid collections that might accumulate, to enhance the possibility of a successful outcome.

A rectus flap is another option in interposing well-vascularized tissue between the bladder and vagina. Either rectus can be mobilized from the upper abdomen to fit easily in the pelvis without tension. Use of the rectus flap has the advantages of avoiding an incision and dissection in the thigh and the need for the inferior dissection between the bladder and vagina, which is usually a difficult part of the procedure when a gracilis flap from the abdominal incision is employed. The rectus flap is an appealing choice if the fistula is not located too inferior on the bladder base, making it difficult to fix the flap in place well below the fistula site in the bladder. On the other hand, it is relatively easy to suture a gracilis flap in place to cover an inferiorly positioned bladder defect easily.

After the fistula repair is completed, the ureteral stents are removed. A large Foley catheter is employed as a cystostomy tube brought through a separate stab incision, and a large urethral Foley catheter is also inserted. A Jackson-Pratt drain is placed in the space of Retzius and brought through a separate stab incision. Closed suction drainage is also used to drain the medial thigh.

For several days postoperatively, the lower extremity of the donor gracilis muscle is kept relatively adducted, and the bed is adjusted so that the lower extremities are elevated with the hips flexed. The patient is allowed to ambulate, but sitting in the chair is avoided to minimize the risk of venous stasis and subsequent venous thrombosis. The drains are left in place until drainage is minimal. The suprapubic cystotomy tube is usually removed approximately 1 week postoperatively, and the urethral catheter is removed a few days later when the suprapubic drainage has ceased.

If in the urologist's judgment bladder compliance is inadequate to permit satisfactory storage and continence, it is preferable to perform a urinary diversion unless an augmentation cystoplasty is feasible. Many factors must be considered in deciding which form of urinary diversion to use, such as the age of the patient, her motivation for undergoing a continent urinary reservoir, and the condition of the bowel, which may also have associated radiation injury.

Since radiation-induced vesicovaginal fistulas are relatively rare, most urologists do not encounter them often enough to gain experience or proficiency in repairing them. Whatever approach the surgeon chooses when undertaking surgical correction of such fistulas, careful attention to detail and proper surgical technique is mandatory. The planes between the bladder and vagina must be carefully dissected and defined and the blood supply to the individual structures maintained as well as is feasible. If possible, apposition of suture lines should be avoided. The repair described in this chapter has the distinct advantage of excellent visualization of both the bladder and vaginal edges of the fistula, allowing for satisfactory closure and the interposition of well-vascularized, nonirradiated tissue between the vagina and bladder. Also, most urologists are more familiar with the suprapubic transperitoneal, transvesical exposure of a vesicovaginal fistula, which makes this type of repair an attractive option.

SUGGESTED READING

Fleischmann J, Picha G. Abdominal approach for gracilis muscle interposition and repair of recurrent vesicovaginal fistulas. J Urol 1988; 140:552.

Obrink A, Bunne G. Gracilis interposition in fistulas following radiotherapy for cervical cancer: a retrospective study. Urol Int 1978; 33:370.

Ryan JA Jr, Gibbons RP, Correa RJ Jr. Urologic use of gracilis muscle flap for nonhealing perineal wounds and fistulas. Urology 1985; 23:456.

Zoubek J, McGuire EJ, Noll F, DeLancey JOL. The late occurrence of urinary tract damage in patients successfully treated by radiotherapy for cervical carcinoma. J Urol 1989; 141:1347.

ENTEROVESICAL FISTULA

HUGH A. G. FISHER, M.D., F.A.C.S.

Enterovesical fistula has a wide spectrum of etiology, presentation, and management. Diagnosis may be reliably made in most cases, provided that clinical suspicion is high and available tests are systematically utilized. Treatment of the underlying cause, complete excision of diseased bowel, drainage of abscesses, and adequate bladder closure are the cornerstones of successful management.

An enterovesical fistula is an abnormal communication between the intestinal tract (including small bowel, appendix, or large bowel) and the urinary bladder. Congenital fistulas to the bladder are rare and are associated with imperforate anus of the supralevator type. These fistulas more commonly communicate with the prostatic urethra in the male or with the vagina in the female. Most enterovesical fistulas are acquired and are secondary to primary bowel pathology of inflammatory or neoplastic etiology (Table 1). Primary bladder cancer accounts for approximately 5 percent of fistulas. There is a male preponderance of 2:1 to 3:1, owing to the relative incidence of related diseases in each sex, and the protective positioning of the uterus and vagina between bowel and bladder in the female. In patients without primary bowel or bladder pathology, factors predisposing to the formation of an enterovesical fistula include previous urologic, gynecologic, or colorectal surgery; active pelvic malignancy; and previous radiation therapy, all of which compromise protective natural anatomic barriers. Three types of enterovesical fistulas are recognized: (1) ileovesical, most commonly caused by regional ileitis (Crohn's disease) and less commonly by malignant tumors of the ileum, foreign bodies, trauma, tuberculosis, or schistosomiasis; (2) appendicovesical, secondary to ruptured appendicitis with abscess formation; and (3) colovesical or rectovesical, associated with diverticulitis, granulomatous colitis, carcinoma of the sigmoid colon and upper rectum, or primary bladder carcinoma. Fistulas rarely occur spontaneously in the lower two thirds of the rectal vault because of the thick

Table 1 Etiology of Acquired Enterovesical Fistula

Inflammatory
    Regional ileitis (Crohn's disease)
    Granulomatous colitis
    Diverticulitis
    Appendiceal abscess
Neoplastic
    Small bowel
    Colorectal
    Bladder
    Prostate
    Ovary
    Cervix
    Endometrium
    Vagina
Traumatic
    Pelvic surgery
    Radiation
    Foreign body
Infectious
    Tuberculosis
    Schistosomiasis

double layer of Denonvilliers' fascia in men anteriorly and the interposition of the vagina in women.

The clinical presentation of enterovesical fistula ranges widely from a completely asymptomatic patient to one who is acutely ill. Presenting symptoms predominantly involve the urinary tract. Most patients have a urinary tract infection. Two thirds of patients have pneumaturia, although air in the urinary tract may also be caused by gas-producing organisms or fermentation of glucose by diabetic urine or be introduced during urinary tract instrumentation. Fecaluria, on the other hand, is pathognomonic of enterovesical fistula, but occurs in less than 50 percent of patients. Abdominal pain or dysuria is present in more than 50 percent of patients, while fever, urinary frequency, gross hematuria, urine passage per rectum, diarrhea, or testicular pain occur in 5 to 30 percent. Significantly, particularly in patients with colovesical fistula secondary to diverticulitis, there may be no history of abdominal pain or previous bowel complaints, with very mild or absent urinary symptoms. In this setting, the diagnosis of fistula is typically delayed for months or even years until more alarming symptoms occur. Often, failure to cure a urinary tract infection with appropriate antimicrobial therapy, particularly in a male, is the only clue that a fistula is present.

On physical examination, a palpable abdominal mass is the most frequent finding, being present in one-third of cases. Fever, abdominal tenderness, cutaneous fistula, or unilateral epididymo-orchitis may be associated findings.

Urinalysis usually reveals pyuria and microscopic hematuria. Undigested food fibers may be present. Contrary to expectation, a single aerobic organism is usually isolated from the urine, with *Escherichia coli, Streptococcus faecalis, Klebsiella, Proteus,* or *Pseudomonas* most frequently cultured. Polymicrobial infections occur in only 20 to 30 percent of cases. Rarely, anaerobic organisms may predominate, requiring specific cultures if clinical suspicion of fistula is high.

Documentation of the presence of an enterovesical fistula and its localization may be difficult. Orally administered charcoal appearing in the urine confirms the presence of a fistula, but this test is not very sensitive and does not define the fistula's location. Radionuclide ingestion techniques are more sensitive but are not widely used. Methylene blue dye administered orally or injected per rectum is not recommended because systemic absorption and excretion of the dye make interpretation of the test meaningless.

Conventional radiologic studies, including intravenous urography, cystography, and upper and lower gastrointestinal series, reveal the communication in less than 35 percent of cases. Recovery of barium by centrifugation of an aliquot of urine and radiography following barium enema has improved diagnostic accuracy in colovesical fistula and may detect as little as 0.001 ml of barium. Computed tomography (CT) may demonstrate air or orally administered contrast material in the bladder, a mass effect, or bladder or bowel wall thickening.

Cystoscopy remains the best single procedure for diagnosis, and enables direct visualization of the fistulous tract or demonstrates an edematous "herald" patch of mucosa on the posterior wall, lateral walls, or dome in 80 percent of patients. This endoscopic appearance may be confused with primary bladder cancer, particularly in a patient with no abdominal symptoms or history of bowel disease. Sigmoidoscopy or colonoscopy rarely allows visualization of the fistulous communication but is essential to define underlying bowel pathology.

The systematic application of available diagnostic tests should permit accurate preoperative diagnosis of the etiology and location of the fistula. However, not infrequently, the fistula is suspected preoperatively but found only at the time of exploratory laparotomy, or sometimes not at all. Fortunately, correction of the precipitating bowel pathology, particularly if inflammatory, usually results in spontaneous closure of a very small fistula.

Although the urologist is often called on to diagnose an enterovesical fistula, management relies on the coordinated efforts of the urologist, the general surgeon, and often a nutritionist. The approach to management is dependent on the etiology, manner of presentation, and location of the fistula and on the nutritional status and general medical condition of the patient. Patients may be acutely ill or asymptomatic, elderly or young, well nourished or malnourished, and harboring advanced carcinoma or benign disease. This spectrum of presentation demands individualization of treatment, with considerable judgment and flexibility regarding the timing of surgical intervention and choice of procedure.

INFLAMMATORY FISTULA

Sixty to 80 percent of enterovesical fistulas are secondary to inflammatory bowel disease. Treatment is primarily surgical, the timing and extent of which is dependent on the severity of the underlying bowel condition rather than on the presence of the fistula. Long-term, nonoperative management is often indicated in Crohn's disease to improve nutritional status and to allow inflammatory bowel disease to become quiescent. Through the use of oral antibiotics, steroids, and elemental diets, gastrointestinal and urinary symptoms are considerably improved, but spontaneous fistula closure rarely occurs. In the asymptomatic elderly patient with colovesical fistula who is not a candidate for surgery because of underlying medical problems, spontaneous closure cannot be expected to occur, yet the patient may remain remarkably free of complications for years. Indeed, fistula formation permits initial drainage of an intra-abdominal abscess and is partially therapeutic.

Initial management of the critically ill patient includes intravenous administration of broad-spectrum antibiotics with aerobic and anaerobic coverage, hydration, bowel decompression, and nutritional supplementation if needed. Urinary retention may aggravate sepsis and should be relieved by catheter drainage. Urinary tract sepsis is usually promptly controlled with antimicrobials alone, whereas intra-abdominal abscess or bowel obstruction requires prompt surgical intervention.

In the patient with controlled sepsis or one not requiring immediate exploration, full diagnostic studies should be performed before definitive surgical management. It is imperative that broad-spectrum antibiotics be administered before urinary tract diagnostic instrumentation for prevention of sepsis. A full bowel preparation should be initiated using cathartics, oral antibiotics, and cleansing enemas whenever possible. However, in Crohn's disease, cathartics should be used with caution, and bowel preparation with 5 to 7 days of a liquid and elemental diet is preferred.

Just as the manner of presentation of enterovesical fistula varies greatly, so do the operative findings. With ileovesical fistula, an inflammatory phlegmonous mass is commonly encountered encompassing the ileum, cecum and bladder dome; in colovesical fistula, the inflammatory mass encompasses the sigmoid colon and dome or left lateral bladder wall. Abscesses may be present within the inflammatory mass and may be extensive. Bowel obstruction may be present. In regional ileitis, internal fistulas are often encountered, most commonly ileosigmoid in location. Right ureterolysis may be necessary, and careful inspection for unsuspected ileoureteral fistula must be made. The fistulous tract may vary from being nonvisible to being several centimeters in length. Conversely, chronic fistulas from either small or large bowel may be associated with minimal perivesical inflammation, no abscess, and a well-epithelialized fistulous tract.

Excision of all diseased bowel and the fistulous tract is the key to successful management. When exploratory laparotomy is performed as an emergency procedure for obstruction or abscess with poorly prepared bowel, a staged approach with proximal fecal diversion, with or without bowel resection, should be employed. Bowel diversion alone may not resolve sepsis, and abscesses should be drained thoroughly. Whenever possible, excision of all diseased bowel and proximal ileostomy or colostomy with Hartmann pouch creation is preferable to a bypass procedure or simple diversion alone. Re-establishment of bowel continuity is then made at a later date under more ideal conditions.

In a patient with adequately prepared bowel, no abscess, controlled sepsis, and adequate nutrition, a one-stage procedure with resection of diseased bowel, primary anastomosis, and closure of fistula is preferred. Management of concomitant internal fistulas—for example, between ileum and sigmoid colon—may involve complete local resection of both involved bowel segments or resection of the diseased segment, fistula excision, and primary closure of the sigmoid colon, with or without proximal diverting colostomy, depending on the appearance of the bowel. The presence of an enterovesical fistula in this setting has little influence on the management of the bowel condition.

Opinions differ regarding the extent of vesical resection that is necessary before bladder closure. Both simple "pinching off" of the fistulous tract and closure with one or two sutures or more extensive excision of inflamed tissue produce satisfactory healing, provided that abscesses are adequately drained and all diseased bowel is excised. My personal preference is to excise bulky inflammatory tissue that may harbor microabscesses and obtain a clear margin for meticulous bladder closure.

Bladder closure should be in layers. Again, opinions vary regarding the use of absorbable or nonabsorbable sutures, favorable results being obtained with each. I use an inner layer of running absorbable suture on the bladder mucosa, a second running muscular layer as needed, and an outer nonabsorbable layer in interrupted fashion.

Suprapubic tube placement is rarely indicated for enterovesical fistula. The urethral catheter remains in place for 5 to 7 days, and a cystogram is performed before catheter removal in patients with extensive bladder resection, neoplasm, or previous irradiation. Fistula persistence or recurrence after appropriate surgical management of the underlying inflammatory bowel condition is uncommon and is most often due to inadequate resection of unrecognized diseased bowel or flare-up of bowel disease, particularly in Crohn's disease, which can involve large and small bowel.

NEOPLASTIC FISTULA

Management of cancer-related enterovesical fistulas depends on whether the fistula is present at the time of initial diagnosis or occurs secondarily after definitive cancer therapy. These fistulas are most commonly associated with neoplasms of the colon or rectum, bladder, cervix, ovary, endometrium, or prostate.

Resectable adenocarcinoma of the colon or rectum with fistulization to the bladder may be managed by en bloc excision of the bowel, fistulous tract, and portion of the bladder wall when feasible. Alternatively, when posterior wall, trigone, or bladder neck is involved, a total pelvic exenteration may be required. In this situation, the left colon may be used for urinary diversion to avoid a bowel anastomosis and save operating time. The prognosis depends more on the presence or absence of positive nodes than on the presence of a fistula, and long-term disease-free survival is possible. For the patient with an unresectable fistula who is undergoing proximal colostomy, palliative urinary diversion should be considered if ureteral obstruction is present, no distant metastases can be demonstrated, and life expectancy is more than 1 year.

Enterovesical fistula formation associated with gynecologic malignancies or bladder or prostate carcinoma usually occurs after initial treatment by surgery, irradiation, or both and is often associated with recurrent tumor. These fistulas may be multiple and involve both small and large bowel, with concomitant enterovaginal or vesicovaginal fistulas in women. Considerable judgment and individualization regarding the extent of operative intervention must be exercised. If recurrent or persistent disease is locally confined and resectable, aggressive resection with pelvic exenteration is sometimes warranted, particularly if further effective treatment exists, such as chemotherapy for ovarian or bladder cancer. The presence of synchronous bilateral ureteral obstruction or vesicovaginal fistula is an additional indication for supravesical diversion in selected patients. Unfortunately, development of these fistulas after extensive pelvic surgery and irradiation is most often associated with extensive local recurrence or distant metastases with poor long-term survival. Bowel diversion above the level of the fistula and bladder drainage by means of an indwelling catheter may provide significant palliation.

RADIATION-INDUCED FISTULA

Enterovesical fistula occurring after definitive irradiation for pelvic malignancy must be approached with caution. Recurrent tumor should be ruled out by appropriate radiologic studies and biopsies. Radiation damage is often extensive, all diseased bowel cannot be excised, and potentially poorly healing bladder and bowel tissue must be used in the repair. Fibrosis may be extensive, but inflammatory reaction and abscess formation are not commonly encountered. Following excision of involved bowel, fistulous tracts, and a small portion of bladder, meticulous closure of both bowel and bladder in layers is paramount. Also, a well-vascularized pedicle of omentum should be interposed between the bladder and bowel suture line to help prevent recurrence. The catheter is left indwelling for 4 to 6 weeks, and a cystogram is performed before its removal.

SUGGESTED READING

Amendala MA, Agha FP, Dent TL, et al. Detection of occult colovesical fistula by the Bourne test. AJR 1984; 142:715–718.
Carson CC, Malek RS, Remine WH. Urologic aspects of vesicoenteric fistulas. J Urol 1978; 119:744–746.
McConnell DB, Sasaki MT, Vetto RM. Experience with colovesical fistula. Am J Surg 1980; 140:80–84.
Schraut HW, Block GE. Enterovesical fistula complicating Crohn's ileocolitis. Am J Gastroenterol 1984; 79(3):186–190.

EXSTROPHY OF THE BLADDER

MARK C. ADAMS, M.D.
ALAN B. RETIK, M.D.

Exstrophy of the bladder, which occurs in one per 30,000 live births, is a severe malformation that represents one of the most difficult challenges to the urologic surgeon. Classic exstrophy is the most common form of the exstrophy-epispadias complex, occurring more than twice as frequently as isolated epispadias. Cloacal exstrophy and split symphysis variants account for less than 10 percent of patients within this complex. Males are affected more commonly than females, with a ratio of 2.3:1. The risk of recurrence within a given family appears to be approximately one in 100.

Theoretically, exstrophy results from failure of caudal migration of the cloacal membrane secondary to impaired mesodermal ingrowth. Breakdown of the abnormally located membrane then results in an absent anterior wall and exposed posterior bladder. Variations in the degree of failure of migration and the timing of breakdown account for the different forms of the complex.

Prenatal diagnosis of bladder exstrophy can occasionally be made by the inability to visualize a distended bladder on sonography. At birth the diagnosis generally is immediately apparent. These are usually healthy babies with rare anomalies unrelated to the genitourinary and musculoskeletal defects. The exposed bladder is variable in size and generally has soft, pliable mucosa at birth. The upper urinary tract is almost always normal. The umbilicus is low set and located just above the bladder. The rectus muscles diverge at the umbilicus to insert on the widely separated pubic rami. Males have a short, stubby penis with severe dorsal chordee. Undescended or retractile testes and inguinal hernias are not uncommon findings. In females, the clitoris is bifid and the vagina is often short with a stenotic, anteriorly displaced orifice. Duplication of the female genital system is occasionally present. The perineum is short in both sexes, and the rectum is usually drawn anteriorly.

The surgical treatment of bladder exstrophy is complex and constantly evolving. Goals of therapy include a cosmetically acceptable appearance of the abdominal wall and genitalia, preservation of renal and sexual function, and urinary continence. Optimal treatment of children with exstrophy requires immediate care by a surgeon with expertise and interest in the malformation. Our bias in the treatment of exstrophy is toward primary bladder closure and staged reconstruction. We reserve urinary diversion, whether continent or not, for patients who fail such reconstruction.

PRIMARY BLADDER CLOSURE

Medical assessment of the child with exstrophy, with emphasis on the cardiopulmonary system, should be made as soon as possible after birth. The bladder should be covered with plastic wrap to avoid trauma to the delicate mucosa. We obtain renal ultrasonography to evaluate the upper urinary tracts. Males with a very small, dystrophic phallus may be considered for sex reassignment, but this is rarely indicated with classic exstrophy. Much time must be spent with the parents of these children early on so that they begin to understand the implications of the malformation and the complexity of surgical reconstruction. This is the beginning of a lifelong commitment to these patients and their parents.

Primary exstrophy closure should be performed in the first 48 hours of life if at all possible. Within this time frame, the bony pelvis is pliable and edematous, fibrotic changes in the bladder mucosa have not yet occurred, and the bladder and abdominal wall can usually be closed without iliac osteotomies. Closure after that time generally requires iliac osteotomies for approximation of the pelvic ring. We have occasionally seen newborns with bladder plaques so small that they could not be inverted at all with digital manipulation. We have been able to close the bladder of several of these children secondarily after several years of growth.

Bladder closure begins with an incision along the

mucocutaneous border of the bladder, taking care to avoid rolling skin within the bladder. We identify the ureteral orifices at the onset and place stents. The bladder muscle is then separated from the umbilicus superiorly and the peritoneum swept off the bladder. This allows extraperitoneal dissection behind the lateral edges of the bladder before separation of the bladder from the recti muscles. The dissection is carried on to the periosteum of the inferior ramus of the pubis on either side, freeing up the lateral aspect of the urogenital diaphragm tissue. The mucocutaneous incision is continued on either side of the posterior urethra, leaving a plate approximately 2 cm wide. This incision is deepened to dissect the urethral plate away from the medial aspect of the urogenital diaphragm in order to allow the bladder neck and urethra to fall back. The urethral plate can be continued out to the introitus in females. In males, we generally cut across the urethral plate just distal to the verumontanum. This plane is developed down to the divergent corpora, which are then dissected proximally away from the ischiopubic rami. Care must be taken to avoid injury to the lateral neurovascular bundles. The freed corpora give additional length to the penis and can then be approximated in the midline. The penile length gained results in an equivalent urethral defect between the posterior and anterior urethra. This defect can be covered with paraexstrophy skin flaps as described by Johnston and Duckett. These flaps of thin, mucosa-like skin lateral to the posterior urethra are based on the distal urethra and rotated distally and medially. The flaps can be approximated to the posterior urethra proximally and to each other in the posterior and anterior midline to create a tubularized neourethra. Care must be taken, however, that these flaps are well vascularized and of adequate width, or a stricture and bladder outlet obstruction will result. The mucosa and muscle of the bladder, bladder neck and posterior urethra can then be closed in the midline anteriorly. The urogenital diaphragm tissue likewise can be approximated over the bladder neck and urethra anteriorly as a separate layer. We leave ureteral stents and a Malecot suprapubic catheter in place for urinary drainage. No tubes are left in the urethra. The pubic symphysis is approximated in the midline by horizontal mattress sutures of 2-0 nylon. Good approximation is facilitated by simultaneous inward rotation of the greater trochanters. The knots of these sutures should be placed anteriorly to avoid erosion into the urethra. The rectus muscles and remainder of the abdominal wall can be closed in the midline. We place these patients in modified Bryant traction using adhesive skin traction to immobilize the pelvis.

The patient is left in traction for 3 weeks during healing. The ureteral stents are left in place as long as they divert urine away from the bladder, generally about 2 weeks. Once the patient is out of traction, the suprapubic tube is clamped and residuals are checked to ensure good bladder emptying. If emptying is not complete, we proceed with cystoscopy and urethral calibration. If poor emptying causes hydronephrosis, urethral dilatation and, on occasion, intermittent catheterization are necessary. These children, now converted to a complete epispadias with incontinence, should undergo intravenous pyelography or renal ultrasonography every 6 months for upper tract surveillance. They are continued on daily antibiotics, since almost all have reflux. Upper tract dilatation secondary to retained urine, reflux, and infection occasionally necessitate ureteral reimplantation at an early age.

Bladder capacity, as determined by voiding cystography or cystoscopy, usually increases as the child grows. If, by age 2 to 3 years, capacity is not increasing appropriately, we proceed with epispadias repair so that additional resistance created by the neourethra may help increase bladder capacity. Otherwise, at 3 to 4 years of age when bladder capacity reaches approximately 60 ml, we proceed with ureteral reimplantation and bladder neck reconstruction to achieve urinary continence.

BLADDER NECK RECONSTRUCTION

We prefer a modified Young-Dees-Leadbetter procedure for bladder neck reconstruction and often split the intrasymphyseal band as described by Peters and Hendren, to maximize exposure to the posterior urethra and bladder neck. Splitting the symphysis also allows for narrowing of a greater length of urethra, bladder neck, and bladder and eventually a longer area of functional resistance. To accomplish this, the bladder and bladder neck are mobilized widely. The bladder is opened in the midline and a sound or catheter passed through the urethra. This facilitates the sometimes difficult dissection of urethra from symphysis. After the urethra is safely away, the intrasymphyseal band is divided, exposing the entire female urethra and the male urethra well proximal to the prostate.

The ureters are reimplanted well up on the fixed posterior bladder, leaving the old trigone for tubularization. The ureters can be tunneled across the bladder or in a cephalad direction from their hiatus. We then mark and incise a posterior strip of mucosa 15 to 18 mm wide and 45 to 50 mm long extending up to the upper trigone. The triangles of muscle lateral to this strip are denuded of mucosa. Deep lateral dissection on either side of the bladder neck and urethra provides adequate mobilization for tension-free tubularization. We tubularize the mucosa, submucosa, and superficial muscle using a single layer of interrupted suture. The denuded muscle flaps are then wrapped over the mucosal tube in a tight, but not strangulating, manner. We overlap these flaps in a pants-over-vest fashion using horizontal mattress sutures. The bladder is then closed and the pubis reapproximated. To increase resistance and prevent kinking, we suspend the urethra and bladder neck from the pubis and rectus sheath in the manner of Marshall, Marchetti, and Krantz. We have not found intraoperative manometry to be useful. Ureteral stents help divert urine, and the bladder is drained with a suprapubic cystostomy tube and a small silicone catheter through the urethra. The pelvis is kept immobilized by wrapping the thighs in a position of adduction and mild internal rotation for 2 weeks. After 2 to 3 weeks the urethral catheter is removed and the suprapubic tube clamped. Residuals are checked, using the suprapubic tube to ensure adequate bladder emptying. We avoid urethral instrumentation for at least 4 weeks after surgery. At that point, cystoscopy, urethral calibration, and dilatation as appropriate are performed if bladder emptying is poor. The patient and family must be prepared to begin intermittent catheterization at this point in some cases. The dry interval between voiding or catheterization may initially be short, but should increase with time as the patient learns how to void and bladder capacity increases; this process, however, may take up to several years.

GENITAL RECONSTRUCTION

Genital reconstruction in the male is performed about 1 year after the incontinence operation, unless necessary earlier. If the phallus is dependent and there is adequate penile skin, the dorsal urethral plate may be tubularized from the pubis through the glans. Much more commonly, in our experience, the urethral plate is tethered and must be divided. Usually we find that, to achieve a dependent phallus of maximal length, extensive proximal dissection and mobilization of the corpora is again necessary, followed by corporal rotation and, at times, placement of dorsal dermal grafts to the corpora. Aggressive penile lengthening in this manner generally leaves a sizable defect between the ends of the divided urethral plate. If there is adequate penile skin, we use a vascularized interposition graft of ventral preputial skin to bridge such a defect. Preservation of adequate skin coverage for the penis is imperative, however, to avoid shortening or burying the phallus, and free grafts of nongenital skin or bladder mucosa are sometimes necessary for the urethroplasty.

RESULTS OF STAGED RECONSTRUCTION

Initial bladder closure without osteotomies during the first 48 hours, or with osteotomies later, should be achieved with a very low rate of dehiscence. These patients generally are born with good renal function and delicate upper tracts. With close follow-up and appropriate treatment, upper tract deterioration should be rare. Ultimate urinary continence after reconstruction has been reported in 45 to 86 percent of patients, the best results being achieved by Jeffs.

If incontinence persists after initial bladder reconstruction, we consider that urodynamic evaluation is important to determine whether there is a problem with outflow resistance, bladder compliance, or both. For inadequate outflow resistance, we initially favor reoperative bladder neck tubularization, although some patients eventually may require artificial sphincter placement. Bladder augmentation is necessary for some patients to achieve an adequate functional bladder capacity. After multiple operations, fibrosis of the bladder outlet may prevent urinary continence. In such patients, continent urinary diversion may eventually be considered.

Fistula formation, even in experienced hands, occurs in up to 40 percent of cases after epispadias repair. This fistula rate is apparently independent of the sequence of genital and bladder neck repair. In up to 80 percent of male patients, the penis eventually has a horizontal or downward angulation when flaccid, and most are able to have satisfactory sexual intercourse. Fertility in males may be impaired owing to injury to the verumontanum or to retrograde ejaculation, but 50 percent of married men with exstrophy in the Mayo Clinic series fathered children. Fertility in females is probably not affected, although cesarean section should be performed for delivery to prevent injury to the reconstructed pelvic diaphragm. Uterine prolapse during pregnancy is common.

The risk of developing adenocarcinoma in the exstrophied bladder has been noted to be 400 times greater than in the normal population. However, the malignant potential of the exstrophic bladder closed at an early age is unknown. Long-term surveillance of these patients for tumor development is prudent.

CLOACAL EXSTROPHY

Cloacal exstrophy, occurring in one per 200,000 live births, results from failure of caudal migration of the cloacal membrane and separation of the cloaca by the urorectal septum. Two exstrophied hemibladders are divided by a fissure of hindgut or cecum. The ileum is often prolapsed, and the terminal hindgut is short and blind ending. The musculoskeletal anomalies of exstrophy are present; other anomalies such as omphalocele and meningocele are common. Unlike classic exstrophy, upper urinary tract abnormalities are frequent.

This devastating anomaly was once almost universally fatal; now over 80 percent of infants with this condition survive. Immediate surgical care should include repair of the omphalocele, separation of the hindgut from the hemibladders, closure of the hindgut fissure, and end colostomy. The functionalized hindgut generally grows remarkably, and the shortgut syndrome is eventually avoided in most patients in whom all bowel is preserved. In many patients, the hemibladders may be approximated and closed at the same initial procedure, although bladder closure may be staged if the infant is ill or if the abdominal wall is insufficient. In nearly all males, the phallus is inadequate and gender reassignment is necessary. In such cases, orchiectomy should also be performed during the newborn period. Spinal anomalies should be diagnosed and treated at an early age to minimize neurologic deficits.

Urinary continence can be achieved in some of these patients with staged reconstruction similar to that described for classic exstrophy. The prognosis, however, is not nearly equal to that of classic exstrophy, and many more of these patients will need urinary diversion. Most will require bladder augmentation to achieve an adequate bladder capacity, and when necessary, the stomach should be used to avoid decreasing the absorptive intestinal surface. In some patients there will not be adequate urethral, bladder neck, and urogenital diaphragm musculature to achieve good outflow resistance. Concurrent neurogenic dysfunction may also contribute to the poorer prognosis for urinary continence. In terms of the gastrointestinal tract, a permanent end colostomy is appropriate for many patients, although some may be candidates for a continent fecal stoma, and a few may achieve continence with a perineal pull-through procedure.

SUGGESTED READING

Johnston JH. The genital aspects of exstrophy. J Urol 1975; 113:701.

Lepor H, Jeffs RD. Primary bladder closure and bladder neck reconstruction in classical bladder exstrophy. J Urol 1983; 130:1142.

Lowe FC, Jeffs RD. Wound dehiscence in bladder exstrophy: an examination of the etiologies and factors for initial failure and subsequent closure. J Urol 1983; 130:312.

Peters CA, Hendren WH. Splitting the pubis for exposure in difficult reconstructions for incontinence. J Urol 1989; 142:527.

Young HH. Exstrophy of the bladder: the first case in which a normal bladder and urinary control have been obtained by plastic operation. Surg Gynecol Obstet 1942; 74:729.

CONGENITAL BLADDER DIVERTICULA

R. DIXON WALKER, M.D.

Bladder diverticula are protrusions of bladder mucosa through the bundles of detrusor muscle and may be primary or secondary. Primary bladder diverticula are not associated with urethral obstruction, whereas secondary diverticula occur with increased intravesical pressure, either from urethral obstruction in males or from neurogenic bladder in either sex. Bladder diverticula must be distinguished from other abnormalities that may appear to be diverticula on initial studies. Bladder "ears" are lateral herniations of the entire bladder wall that occur in infants and small children and which usually resolve spontaneously. Urachal diverticula occur as part of the prune-belly syndrome and represent a urachal compartmentalization of the bladder that may allow for poor emptying. An hourglass-shaped bladder is an acquired abnormality most often seen with neurogenic bladder or the Hinman-Allen syndrome (urethral dyssynergia). Rarely, bladder duplication may present in such a way as to initially appear to be a bladder diverticulum.

Congenital bladder diverticula are of two types. Those that are associated with vesical ureteral reflux (Hutch's diverticula) occur because of a weakening in the suprahiatal musculature. They may occur equally between sexes. Most often they are small or of moderate size, with most being 1 cm in diameter or less and 2 to 3 cm being the extreme. Reflux often resolves with small diverticula, particularly if the orifice does not enter the diverticulum itself. There is some question as to whether these small diverticula are primary or secondary, since some authors consider that they occur as a result of the reflux.

Primary congenital bladder diverticula occur more often in boys and the ostium is not suprahiatal. The ostium may be close enough to the ureteral orifice, however, that the gradual enlargement of the diverticulum incorporates the orifice and causes reflux. These are not common. In 20 years of pediatric urologic practice in which more than 300 major cases per year have been treated, I have operated on five primary congenital bladder diverticula, four of which occurred in males and none of which were associated with reflux. All occurred at the base of the bladder and several were in close proximity to the ureteral orifice. Whereas the periureteral diverticulum is usually small, primary congenital bladder diverticula are often large; in two such personal cases, the diverticulum was as capacious as the bladder. Large bladder diverticula in males may cause bladder outlet obstruction because they fail to empty and distort the bladder neck.

It has been reported that congenital bladder diverticula are found in association with several syndromes, including multisystemic disease. Syndromes in which bladder diverticula are known to occur include Menkes', Williams', and Ehlers-Danlos. Hofmann and colleagues presented evidence of the hereditary nature of some cases, seven patients in one family having congenital bladder diverticula.

The pathology of congenital bladder diverticula traditionally has been that they are associated with a mucosal outpouching covered by serosa, but this is not true. Most diverticula have varied amounts of muscle, inversely proportional to the size of the diverticulum. A diverticulum cannot be distinguished by etiology on the basis of its pathologic appearance. Concern has been raised about the histology of the transitional epithelium in long-standing diverticula. Some studies have shown chronic inflammation in 80 percent of diverticula removed, but other studies such as that of Hofmann and colleagues indicated that the transitional epithelium was normal in most cases. Because chronic inflammation is reported in many patients, concern has been raised about the unknown risk of transitional cell carcinoma. It has been suggested that up to 10 percent of adults with a diverticulum will develop a transitional cell tumor. The prognosis of a transitional cell tumor arising in a diverticulum may be worsened by two factors: a delay in establishing the diagnosis because the tumor is not readily accessible, and early invasion of adventitia because of attenuated muscle within the diverticulum.

DIAGNOSIS

The diagnosis of a bladder diverticulum is most often made with intravenous urography or voiding cystourethrography. This is usually done as part of an evaluation for urinary tract infection or for symptoms of abnormal voiding. Intravenous urography is being done less commonly in children than previously and large diverticula may be seen on abdominal ultrasonography. Whereas cystoscopy may be important for diagnosis in adults, it is most often performed in children at the time of surgery to define the relationship of the diverticulum to the ureteral orifice.

THERAPEUTIC ALTERNATIVES

The management of periureteral diverticula associated with reflux is primarily dependent on the management of the reflux itself. The presence of such a diverticulum does not preclude spontaneous resolution of the reflux unless the ureter enters the diverticulum. Surgical management of reflux associated with a diverticulum should include excision of the diverticulum as part of the procedure. The question of management should be addressed to those diverticula that persist after nonsurgical resolution of the reflux. Most of these are small and do not require surgery, and it is doubtful whether they place the patient at a greater risk for transitional cell cancer. Those that are large or that retain urine should be managed surgically.

Congenital bladder diverticula unassociated with reflux are most often managed surgically. The clearest indications for surgical management are in patients with recurrent urinary tract infection or voiding difficulties. In the asymptomatic or minimally symptomatic patient, observation may be satisfactory for small diverticula. The dividing line is strictly arbitrary, but I would draw it at a diameter of about 1 to 2 cm. It must be recognized that observation will often be interpreted by the patient as meaning that the diverticulum is unimportant; therefore, noncompliance in long-term follow-up will be a problem.

Congenital diverticula that may require surgery include those that are larger than 2 cm; those that drain poorly; those whose location and size has incorporated the ureteral orifice, causing vesical ureteral reflux; and those associated with recurrent urinary tract infections, voiding abnormalities, or stone. The presence of multiple diverticula is suggestive of a secondary problem, and these patients should be investigated for neurogenic bladder or urethral obstruction.

Diverticula diagnosed during the newborn period should be given 6 to 12 months to see if they will improve spontaneously. Large diverticula in newborns, particularly those associated with hydronephrosis or causing bladder outlet obstruction, may be managed initially with cutaneous vesicostomy and delayed diverticulum repair. Even in neonates, however, large diverticula can be excised if care is used during the surgical procedure. In older children, all but the largest diverticula are followed for several months to see whether there is any initial improvement. However, my experience is that diverticula rarely become smaller, and most eventually require surgery. These patients are usually maintained on prophylactic antibacterial therapy and it is imperative that the urine be sterile before the surgical procedure is performed.

OPERATIVE PROCEDURE

The surgery should be performed on an inpatient basis with a postoperative admission for 3 to 7 days. After the patient is given a general anesthetic, cystoscopy is performed to identify the ureteral orifice in relationship to the diverticulum. Cystoscopy is performed with a No. 8 to 10 Fr instrument using a 0- and 30-degree lens. I use a video camera so that the pathology can be recorded and all participants in the room can see. In younger children and infants, the endoscopy is performed with the child's legs in frog-leg position and the buttocks on two towels. Older children and adolescents are placed in stirrups. In males, one should visualize the urethra to rule out urethral obstruction. Viewing the interior of the bladder, the operator should investigate the proximity of the ureteral orifice to the mouth of the diverticulum. It may be necessary to catheterize the ureteral orifice to assess this. Indications of a very irritated bladder, particularly one that appears to be acutely infected, should be cause for terminating the procedure, with repeat surgery after the inflammatory process is resolved. In those in whom the bladder wall is not inflamed, one may proceed with the open procedure.

The patient is reprepped and draped so that the surgeon has access to the lower abdomen and the urethra. A Pfannenstiel incision is made and carried down to the rectus fascia, which is divided in the line of the incision, and the underlying rectus muscle is split in the midline to expose the bladder. The perivesical space is developed lateral to the bladder so that the Dennis-Browne retractor with two scoop blades can be placed. Two traction sutures are placed in the bladder dome, and the bladder is opened with the Bovie. No suction should be applied to the bladder mucosa lest it be made edematous; rather, the assistant should place suction on a moist gauze sponge. Both ureteral orifices should be identified and catheterized with a No. 3.5 or 5 Fr feeding tube even though they appear not to be associated with the diverticulum. On the basis of previous radiologic studies and visualization at the time of surgery, the size of the diverticulum is determined. Small or moderate-sized diverticula can be managed intravesically; larger diverticula are likely to require extravesical dissection.

Small-to-moderate diverticula (up to 2 cm) may be managed intravesically. The mouth of the diverticulum, including a 2-mm rim of mucosa, is incised with a needlepoint Bovie. A four-quadrant, figure-of-eight suture of the incised mouth is placed and tagged as a holding suture. If the diverticulum is small, a Fogarty catheter may be placed in the diverticulum; if larger, a 5-ml Foley balloon may be used. This facilitates dissection. In both instances the catheter is incorporated with the figure-of-eight suture so that appropriate traction may be applied. The diverticulum is then dissected from the underlying muscle and adventitia much as an intramural ureter is freed before reimplantation. A combination of blunt and sharp dissection is performed with Metzenbaum or DeMartel scissors and a Kitner dissector. Bleeding points should be electrocoagulated. Once the diverticulum is dissected free and excised, the mucosa at the edges of the incision is gently freed by sharp dissection from the underlying muscle for a distance of several millimeters. The muscle is then reapproximated with interrupted, absorbable suture and the mucosa closed with a fine running absorbable suture. If the ureter is intimately attached to the diverticulum, it should be dissected free and a crosstrigonal reimplant performed at the cephalad end of the incision, treating the diverticular recess as a large ureteral vesical hiatus. Some surgeons have described grasping the base of the diverticulum with Allis clamps and inverting the mucosa. Although in many instances this may permit easy dissection, it has the distinct potential of incorporating other important structures, such as the rectum, into the clamps and thus causing a severe injury.

Large diverticula are approached with a combined intra- and extravesical approach. After inspection of the inside of the diverticulum and catheterization of the ureteral orifice, the diverticulum is packed with a moist gauze. In order to prevent a ureteral injury, the urethra should be identified outside the bladder, by first identifying and ligating the obliterated hypogastric artery on the ipsilateral side. By tracing the proximal end of the obliterated artery to its base, one can identify the ureter retroperitoneally. It should be freed up and isolated with a vessel loop. Then, working in the perivesical space, one can identify the diverticulum packed with moist gauze, and free it from the bladder and ureter by a combination of blunt and sharp dissection. Most of the diverticulum can be dissected down to a small neck, which can be divided with the Bovie. The mucosa is then closed from the outside with a fine running absorbable suture and the muscle with interrupted absorbable suture. If the diverticulum is intimately attached to the ureter or if there is ureteral injury, a Paquin or crosstrigonal reimplantation may be done.

Occasionally, a diverticulum will enter close to the bladder neck. In such instances a reimplantation of the ureter is probably required, and great care must be given to the reapproximation of the bladder neck muscle to avoid incontinence.

The bladder can be drained with a suprapubic tube or Foley catheter; I prefer the latter because the period of hospitalization is shortened. Ureters, even if reimplanted, usually do not require stents. The bladder is closed in two to three layers with absorbable sutures. A Penrose or Jackson-Pratt drain is placed anteriorly if the procedure was entirely intravesical, or in the perivesical space if an extravesical approach was used.

Drains are removed when drainage ceases, and the bladder catheters are removed in 5 to 7 days. The patient is maintained on anticholinergic therapy while the catheter is in place, and on antibacterial therapy for 4 to 6 weeks postoperatively. An ultrasonogram of the kidney is obtained 6 to 8 weeks after surgery to confirm that it has not damaged the ureters, and voiding cystourethrography is performed 3 to 6 months postoperatively to confirm that the bladder is now normal. Long-term follow-up and repeated cystograms should not be necessary. I usually follow the patient for any recurrence of urinary tract infection and obtain one long-term ultrasonogram 1 to 2 years postoperatively to check whether the kidneys are still normal.

ADVANTAGES AND DISADVANTAGES

A critic of this approach may suggest that bladder diverticula are much more common than those that present to the urologist and that the morbidity is overstated. This is because patients who present do so because they have problems, and thus any assessment of the incidence of disease within a diverticulum is not accurate unless normal asymptomatic patients are also investigated. Despite this distraction, the urologist can only work with the facts presented. In the case of a congenital bladder diverticulum in a child, the long-term sequelae, including the potential risk of transitional cell cancer, represent a strong argument for repair.

SUGGESTED READING

Hofmann R, Hegemann M, Mauermayer W, et al. Hereditary autosomal dominant form of bladder diverticula in male patients. J Urol 1984; 131:338.

Jarow J, Brendler CB. Urinary retention caused by a large bladder diverticulum: a simple method of diverticulectomy. J Urol 1988; 139:1260.

Peterson LJ, Paulson DF, Glenn JF. The histopathology of vesical diverticula. J Urol 1973; 110:62.

Verghese M, Belman B. Urinary retention secondary to congenital bladder diverticula in infants. J Urol 1984; 132:1186.

ACQUIRED BLADDER DIVERTICULA

NEHEMIA HAMPEL, M.D., F.A.C.S.

Diverticulum of the bladder represents protrusion of the vesical mucosa through the bladder wall. Usually its wall contains little or no continuous layer of bladder muscle. Bladder diverticula are classified in two groups: congenital, occurring mostly in children, and acquired, occurring mostly in adults. The latter are by far the most common. Acquired bladder diverticula are encountered in association with bladder outlet obstruction. The condition can be anatomic, as in benign prostatic hyperplasia, and bladder neck obstruction, or neurogenic, as in spinal cord injury. Bladder saccules have the same etiology as acquired bladder diverticula and, for practical purposes, protrusions that do not bulge out of the bladder wall should be called saccules; protrusions larger than 2 cm are considered diverticula. Most diverticula arise anterolateral to the ureteral orifices or on the trigone; only a few arise from the fundus of the bladder. The cause of acquired bladder diverticula is widely recognized as obstruction. The factors permitting diverticula formation in some bladders are less certain, as are the reasons for their formation at a given part of the bladder. Causes of bladder outflow obstruction and diverticula formation include benign prostatic hyperplasia, carcinoma of the prostate, bladder neck obstruction, urethral strictures, and detrusor sphincter dyssynergia in patients with neurogenic bladder disorders.

Most bladder diverticula are diagnosed by cystoscopy and some are incidentally identified during excretory urography. The best radiologic identification of bladder diverticula can be made by cystography with anteroposterior, oblique, and drainage static x-ray films, or by fluoroscopy. The latter is seldom used for primary diagnosis of diverticula but can be helpful in the assessment of location, size, and drainage. The most important evaluation of bladder diverticula is the endoscopic examination. Care should be taken to perform a complete inspection of every diverticulum. If standard rigid cystoscopy is not adequate, flexible cystoscopes are readily available and usually permit complete inspection of all diverticula. Diverticula should be evaluated in regard to their location in the bladder, the size of the opening, the size of the diverticula, and how well they drain after micturition.

Most bladder diverticula are of small size, and up to 35 percent of patients have multiple diverticula. Symptoms related to bladder diverticula alone are difficult to distinguish from complaints of the associated bladder outlet obstruction. Diverticula occur in 1.4 to 13 percent of these patients. Larger diverticula have a greater potential of causing complications that may eventually require surgical correction. Excluded are symptoms related to carcinoma in bladder diverticula.

Complications and the most significant clinical relevance of bladder diverticula include incomplete emptying, recurrent urinary tract infections, stone formation (up to 16 percent), and tumor formation (2.9 to 6.7 percent). Less common occurrences include peridiverticulitis, spontaneous rupture, upper urinary tract obstruction, and (rarely) urinary retention secondary to bladder neck compression (Table 1).

TREATMENT

Except in cases of malignancy, primary treatment should be directed toward relief of bladder outlet obstruction and removal of diverticular stones, if present. In the past, diverticulectomy was probably more commonly performed than today. During the treatment of bladder outlet obstruction, when stones are present, they can be either disintegrated in the diverticula or displaced into the bladder and treated there. Electrohydraulic lithotripsy is much safer than mechanical stone crushers. It is an unusual impacted large stone that fails endoscopic treatment and requires open surgery. In most cases, symptoms are alleviated, because diverticula are seldom the principal cause of the urinary difficulty. Persistent or recurrent symptoms after initial resolution may be directly attributable to bladder diverticula.

Vesical diverticulectomy was first described by Czerny in 1897. Since that time, numerous techniques to treat bladder diverticula have been described; the most common are listed in Table 2.

The indications for surgical treatment of bladder diverticula are persistent urinary tract infections caused by poor drainage, ineffective bladder emptying secondary to filling of the diverticulum during voiding, large calculi, interference with ureteral drainage, and bladder outlet obstruction. A separate indication is the presence of neoplasm within the diverticulum.

Before surgery is contemplated, urine should be sterilized, and the absence of bladder outlet obstruction should be demonstrated by pressure flow studies, cystourethroscopy, or voiding cystourethrography. Fluoroscopy can identify significant enlargement of diverticula during voiding. Bladder catheterization will not distinguish residual urine in the bladder from residual limited to the diverticulum. Once the indication for surgical treatment has been established, a choice has to

Table 1   Complications of Bladder Diverticula

Recurrent urinary tract infection
Stones
Malignant tumors
Large diverticula that fail to empty
Spontaneous rupture
Ureteral obstruction
Urinary retention
Peridiverticulitis
Spontaneous rupture

Table 2 Surgical Treatment of Bladder Diverticula

Endoscopic Surgery
    Fulguration of mucosa
    Incision of diverticular neck
    Resection of diverticular neck
    Combination of incision/resection and fulguration

Open Surgery
    Excision
        Intravesical
        Extravesical (extra- or transperitoneal)
        Combined intra- and extravesical
    Marsupialization
    Drainage with mucosal abolishment

be made between endoscopic and open procedures. As a general concept, larger diverticula are probably best treated by open excision; smaller ones are more suitable for endoscopic treatment. Decreased morbidity, major complications, convalescence time, hospital stay, and cost are reported advantages of endoscopic surgery. In spite of the reported success of endoscopy, the chief controversy regards its effectiveness in cases of larger diverticula. An endoscopic approach may not be effective in eliminating large diverticula, may fail to manage stones, and can be followed by significant peridiverticular inflammatory reaction. This can be caused by urinary extravasation or as a result of extensive fulguration of the diverticular mucosa. Subsequent open surgery may become more difficult should endoscopic treatment be unsuccessful.

Several approaches have been advocated for endoscopic treatment of bladder diverticula. To be successful, it has to address two problems: relieving obstruction at the neck of the diverticulum and decreasing or eliminating most of it. Obstruction of the neck can be treated with single inferior or multiple incisions that can be made through the resectoscope with a roller electrode or Collings electrode (diverticulotomy). An alternative method is to use a resection loop and to cut carefully the inferior lip of the orifice. Small cuts are then made around the entire circumference of the orifice until an adequate opening is created. Although the orifice of the diverticulum usually consists of a thick muscular ring, there is a danger of perforation, and care must be taken to perform incisions or resection carefully and with small bites. If perforation is encountered, the procedure should be terminated and the bladder drained. Bleeding points at the diverticular neck can usually be controlled without difficulty by coagulation. The inside of the diverticulum should be fulgurated with a roller electrode. Fulguration should begin at the dome and gradually advance toward the opening. All the mucosa is carefully treated. When transurethral prostatectomy is done in conjunction with diverticular surgery, it may be easier to address the diverticulum first. During transurethral prostatectomy, care must be taken not to overdistend the bladder. A continuous-flow resectoscope can be advantageous in maintaining low intravesical pressure during endoscopy. Postoperatively, if needed, the blad-

der may be maintained on continuous low-pressure irrigation to prevent blood clot retention. Foley catheter drainage is maintained for 4 to 5 days. Before the catheter is removed, a cystogram is obtained to demonstrate lack of extravasation. Reported results of endoscopic treatment of bladder diverticula indicate that successful eradication occurs in 60 percent of patients; another 30 percent exhibit about 80 percent reduction in size.

Open diverticulectomy is preferred for removal of large diverticula. The surgeon should be familiar with the various intra- and extravesical approaches. Before surgery, endoscopy of the bladder and diverticula is mandatory to rule out tumor in a diverticulum. Inability to visualize all the wall may warrant diverticulectomy. If the diverticulum is near the ureteral orifice or if the diverticula are very large, placement of ureteral catheters is warranted. During exploration, identification of the ureter can be greatly facilitated by palpation for the ureteral catheter, thus preventing inadvertent ureteral injury. The bladder is exposed through a midline extraperitoneal or a Pfannenstiel incision. The peritoneum has to be dissected free from the abdominal pelvis. Of the open surgical procedures described, I initially try an extraperitoneal extravesical approach. A Foley catheter placed in the bladder during the surgery is used to distend the diverticulum and assists in the identification and dissection of the diverticulum. If surrounding tissue adherence prevents safe dissection, the diverticulum may be opened or a combined intra- and extravesical approach can be continued. When the bladder is opened, the dissection is facilitated by packing the diverticulum with gauze, placing a large balloon Foley catheter, or inserting a finger into the diverticulum. The diverticulum is divided at the bladder and completely excised. In rare cases when ureteral insertion is into the diverticulum or close to it, it may become necessary to perform ureteroneocystostomy of the ipsilateral ureter. To prevent a later risk of development of carcinoma, the mucosa should be completely removed.

The opening in the bladder is closed in several layers with absorbable sutures. The mucosa is closed with running suture and the muscle with interrupted figures of eight. A large tubular drain is left in the perivesical space and brought out through a separate incision. Suprapubic cystostomy Malecot catheter is placed and can usually be removed after 7 to 10 days. It is recommended that cystography be performed and that a trial of voiding with the cystostomy catheter blocked be made before one removes it. Marsupialization and drainage without diverticulectomy clearly should be used only as a last resort for patients with acute infection or abscess formation, or in whom the diverticula are impossible to dissect.

The incidence in bladder diverticula of neoplasms, most of which are transitional cell carcinomas, is between 1.5 and 13.5 percent, which indicates that a relationship exists between the two. An attractive explanation for the high incidence is that activation of carcinogens in urine is enhanced by the prolonged stasis of urine in the poor-emptying diverticula. This is similar to the contributing factor in the development of urothelial tumors within the bladder. When diverticular mucosa is examined, chronic inflammatory and premalignant changes are found in approximately 80 percent of all diverticula. These data suggest that carcinoma is more likely to occur in bladder diverticula, and some have even suggested the need for prophylactic diverticulectomy. Most reports express a dismal prognosis for bladder neoplasms originating in diverticula. In an alarming series from the Mayo Clinic, only 16 percent of the patients survived 1 year after onset of symptoms. The thinness of the diverticular wall (which has a scanty layer of muscles, if any at all) and the occult location are responsible for the poor prognosis. Thus, at presentation, most neoplasms are of high grade and advanced stage. These conditions preclude treatment at early and potentially curable stages.

No clear evidence is available comparing prognosis and result of treatment when same-grade and same-stage neoplasms in tumors in the normal bladder wall and tumors in the diverticular wall are compared. The grave prognosis of diverticular neoplasms is most probably related to anatomic factors leading to the local spread and early dissemination. Patient prognosis is linked to the extent of spread at the time of presentation. Therefore, the importance of surveying bladder diverticula for neoplasms cannot be overemphasized. Endoscopic examination of the diverticular mucosa should include all of the surfaces, and a flexible cystoscope should be used whenever necessary. If the slightest suspicion exists, cytology and mucosal biopsies should be obtained.

Neoplasms in bladder diverticula should probably not be treated endoscopically, with the exception of very small, low-grade papillary neoplasms. I do not believe that a correct assessment of the depth of penetration can be made in the thin wall of bladder diverticula. Use of a resectoscope is likely to cause perforation, with the risk of dissemination. The high incidence of premalignant changes in the diverticular mucosa support this opinion. Prophylactic diverticulectomy in patients with superficial tumors elsewhere in the bladder mucosa should be performed if it is difficult to survey the diverticulum or if premalignant changes are demonstrated on biopsy.

With the rising popularity of organ-preserving local excision for bladder neoplasms, a comparison between diverticulectomy and total cystectomy is appropriate. There are no objective reports comparing diverticulectomy (partial cystectomy) with radical cystectomy for invasive neoplasm in bladder diverticula. When it is anatomically possible, I recommend partial cystectomy with extensive local excision and bilateral pelvic lymphadenectomy. When adequate removal is in doubt, radical cystectomy with bilateral pelvic lymphadenectomy should be performed when the patient is an acceptable surgical risk. When invasive disease is present, adjuvant multidrug chemotherapy can be considered as well as local radiation therapy. The benefits of both forms of treatment in neoplasms of bladder diverticula are not yet established.

SUGGESTED READING

Clayman RV, Shahin S, Reddy P, Fraley EE. Transurethral treatment of bladder diverticula. Urology 1984; 23:573.

Kelalis PP, McLean P. The treatment of diverticulum of the bladder. J Urol 1967; 98:349.

Lowe FC, Goldman SM, Oesterling JE. Computerized tomography in evaluation of transitional cell carcinoma in bladder diverticula. Urology 1989; 34:390.

Melekos MD, Asbach HW, Barbalias GA. Vesical diverticula: etiology, diagnosis, tumorigenesis, and treatment. Urology 1987; 30:453.

URACHAL CYSTS AND ANOMALIES

KENDALL A. ITOKU, M.D.
ANTHONY A. CALDAMONE, M.D., F.A.C.S., F.A.A.P.

DESCRIPTION

The urachus is a fibrous cord extending from the anterior bladder wall to the umbilicus, traveling between the peritoneum and the transversalis fascia. Early in embryonic life, the urachus is the connection between the allantoic stalk and the anterior cloaca (urogenital sinus), or future bladder. During the fourth to fifth months of gestation, as the bladder descends into the pelvis, the urachus becomes a thin-caliber tube, and at approximately the time of birth, it becomes a vestigial fibrous cord. The urachus is composed of three histologic tissue types: an inner transitional epithelium, a submucosal connective tissue layer, and an outer smooth muscle layer. In addition, the urachus is enveloped in two layers of umbilicovesical fascia, which can limit the spread of infection.

Urachal cysts and anomalies are rare clinical entities. In the largest review of these cases, Blichert-Toft and Nielson collected only 315 cases from the world literature covering a period of more than 400 years. Disorders of the urachus are generally classified into four groups (Fig. 1): (1) patent urachus, (2) urachal sinus, (3) urachal diverticulum, and (4) urachal cyst.

Failure of closure of the urachal lumen results in free communication between the bladder and umbilicus, or congenital patent urachus. The disorder typically presents soon after birth with urine draining from the

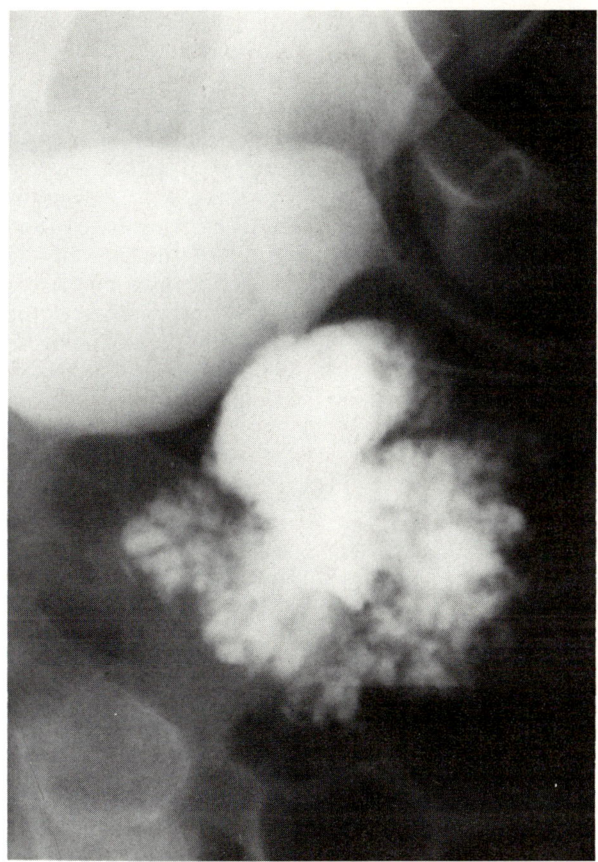

Figure 1 The four anatomic variations of urachal anomalies. (Modified from Bauer and Retik. Urachal anomalies and related umbilical disorders. Urol Clin North Am 1978; 5:195.)

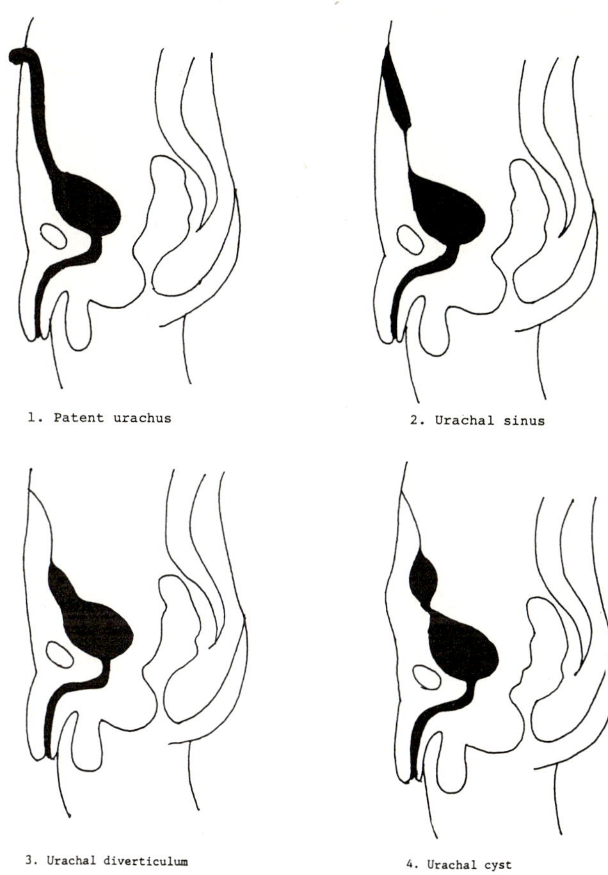

Figure 2 An infected urachal cyst in a 17-year-old boy: percutaneous sinogram with a concomitant cystogram.

umbilicus. Often, the umbilicus has a tumor-like appearance. An acquired form of patent urachus has been described in adults, usually associated with outlet obstruction. A fistulogram confirms the diagnosis, defines the anatomic conditions, and rules out a patent omphalomesenteric duct. Patent urachus can be associated with bladder outlet obstruction in neonates and adults, and a voiding cystourethrogram should be performed to rule out this possibility. Patent urachus has been associated with other genitourinary anomalies, including vesicoureteral reflux, solitary kidney, ureteropelvic junction (UPJ) obstruction, and hydronephrosis, although cause and effect is not always apparent. It may also be seen with prune-belly syndrome. A screening intravenous pyelogram is recommended to rule out an associated anomaly. Early treatment of the patent urachus is essential to avoid potential urinary infection and sepsis. The best treatment is complete excision of the urachus down to the level of the bladder through an extraperitoneal approach. Simple ligation or cauterization of the lumen involves a high likelihood of recurrence. Excision of a cuff of bladder has been recommended to eliminate the risk of adenocarcinoma arising in the urachal remnant, of which there have been several reported cases. If bladder outlet obstruction is detected, it should be repaired either concomitantly with or before the definitive treatment of the patent urachus.

A urachal sinus is a blind external sinus opening at the umbilicus, usually the result of a small urachal cyst that becomes infected and opens to the umbilicus. In rare cases it may drain into the bladder as well, creating the syndrome of an alternating sinus. Sinography should be performed to define the extent of the sinus. Simple drainage or cauterization is inadequate because recurrences are common. The most definitive treatment again is excision of the entire tract along with the umbilicus. A cuff of bladder should be included in the resection if patency to the bladder is demonstrated. Most series report good results with complete excision of the tract without bladder excision, and this is probably adequate, especially if the sinus ends well away from the apex of the bladder.

A diverticulum at the apex of the bladder can be of urachal origin. This anomaly has been associated with prune-belly syndrome and occasionally with urethral or vesical neck obstruction. If the diverticulum is narrow mouthed, stones may form within it. Usually this condition is asymptomatic and detected only incidentally, often during a work-up for urinary tract infection. The recommended treatment is complete excision of the diverticulum, but only if it is symptomatic. Obviously, if urethral or vesical neck obstruction is detected, it should be corrected.

Incomplete obliteration of the urachal lumen allows formation of a urachal cyst. These cysts provide the greatest challenges in diagnosis and management among the urachal anomalies. They are often silent and usually go undetected until they become infected. The symptoms caused by an infected urachal cyst are variable and can mimic a variety of abdominal and pelvic disorders, including severe cystitis, pelvic inflammatory disease, appendicitis, and acute abdomen. Common signs and symptoms include fever, lower abdominal mass, lower abdominal tenderness, and voiding complaints. The infection is usually contained within the planes of the umbilicovesical fascia, but several cases of rupture into the peritoneal cavity have been reported. Diagnosis can be made best with ultrasonography or computed tomography (CT), revealing a cavity adjacent to the dome of the bladder. Often, however, the diagnosis is made incidentally on exploration for appendicitis or suspected acute abdomen. If the diagnosis of urachal cyst is known, the patient should be screened for other genitourinary anomalies, because a significant association has been noted.

Treatment of an infected urachal cyst includes systemic antibiotics followed by one of three surgical options: (1) incision and drainage, (2) primary excision, or (3) initial incision and drainage (or percutaneous drainage) followed by excision of the remnant as an interval procedure. Drainage alone is inadequate therapy, carrying recurrence rates of approximately 30 percent. Primary complete excision may be performed when the infection is limited. Total removal of the cyst wall is essential, since adenocarcinoma can develop in the remnant. Percutaneous aspiration with indwelling catheter placement provides drainage of the abscess, and allows radiographic determination of the size of the cavity and any communications with abdominal viscera (Fig. 2). Initial drainage also allows for resolution of the inflammatory process, making subsequent definitive surgery easier with less risk of bladder injury. Excellent results with minimal complications have been demonstrated in all series reviewed.

SUGGESTED READING

Bauer SB, Retik AB. Urachal anomalies and related umbilical disorders. Urol Clin North Am 1978; 5:195.

Blichert-Toft M, Nielson OV. Congenital patent urachus and acquired variants. Diagnosis and treatment. Review of the literature and report of five cases. Acta Chir Scand 1971; 137:807.

Goldman IL, Caldamone AA, Gauderer M, et al. Infected urachal cysts: a review of 10 cases. J Urol 1988; 140:375.

Jeffs RD, Lepor H. Management of the exstrophy-epispadias complex and urachal anomalies. In: Walsh PC, Gittes RF, Perlmutter AD, Stamey TA, eds. Campbell's urology. 5th ed. Philadelphia: WB Saunders, 1986:1915.

Rich RH, Hardy BE, Filler RM. Surgery for anomalies of the urachus. J Pediatr Surg 1983; 18:370.

BLADDER AND URETHRAL FOREIGN BODIES

ANTON J. BUESCHEN, M.D.

Foreign bodies in the bladder and urethra have been seen by all urologists, but no urologist will encounter the long list of objects reported to have been found in the lower urinary tract. Some objects found in the bladder have produced much amusement and amazement. It is alleged that a urologist inserted a cystoscope into the bladder and found a snake looking at him. The imagination of those placing unusual foreign bodies in the bladder and urethra is not to be exceeded by the ingenuity of urologists in deciding how to remove the objects.

ETIOLOGY

A complete list of objects found in the bladder and urethra is not provided here, since it is almost endless. The most common means of entrance of lower urinary tract foreign bodies are (1) penetrating injuries with bullets or explosive devices; (2) introduction of objects by patients or sexual partners; (3) iatrogenic insertion of objects such as catheters or fragments of catheters, pieces of instruments, nonabsorbable sutures, metallic clips, or surgical sponges; and (4) migration of objects from the gastrointestinal tract, pelvic organs (IUDs), and surgically repaired hip joints.

CLINICAL PRESENTATION

Occasionally patients present with a history of having inserted a foreign body into the lower urinary tract. Often, however, they do not provide such a helpful history because they are unaware that a foreign body is present or deny it owing to embarrassment or a psychological illness.

Foreign bodies usually cause persistent pyuria, bacteriuria, and hematuria. Urethral obstructive symptoms may be present. Occasionally a perforation of the urinary tract by the foreign body causes a clinical picture of urinary extravasation and sepsis with associated abscess, fistula, or severe hemorrhage. A bladder stone may contain a foreign body.

EVALUATION AND DIAGNOSIS

Persistent dysuria, pyuria, bacteriuria, or hematuria should lead to evaluation that will identify the foreign body. Intravenous urography and cystoscopy are performed in most situations. The plain film reveals radiopaque foreign bodies, but many are not radiopaque and the intravenous urogram is normal. Retrograde urethrography is helpful in patients with symptoms suggesting urethral obstruction, and cystography is performed in those presenting with a clinical picture of bladder rupture.

TREATMENT

Patient Selection

All foreign bodies should be removed, since urinary tract infections and stones develop eventually in all cases and urinary obstruction in some.

Timing of Surgery

The foreign body should be removed fairly soon after it has been recognized. However, it should be removed urgently if it has caused complications resulting in fever or sepsis.

Preoperative Preparation

Since infection occurs commonly with foreign bodies, all patients should have a urine culture and be treated with broad-spectrum bactericidal antibiotics.

Choice of Procedure

The size, shape, location, and composition of the foreign body should be considered in choosing the surgical method of removal. Most foreign bodies in the urethra and bladder can be removed endoscopically. However, this requires the urologist to have a surgical repertoire that includes all endoscopic instruments and occasionally some innovative planning.

Most small objects in the bladder can be grasped and removed with a flexible alligator forceps, cup biopsy forceps, or the three-pronged grasping forceps. A direct vision lithotrite can be used to fragment a larger object or one with an attached stone. An ultrasonic or electrohydraulic lithotripsy probe can be used to fragment a foreign body that has calcified. Nonabsorbable sutures can be cut with cystoscopic scissors and removed with grasping forceps. A resectoscope sheath and an Ellik evacuator can remove some small foreign bodies, or larger ones that have been fragmented.

Urethral foreign bodies can also be removed with a grasping forceps. Small objects in the urethra can be engaged and removed with a stone basket. If the sharp end of an object is pointing toward the urethral meatus, it may be better to push the object into the bladder; it can then be grasped by the blunt end and removed endoscopically.

An open surgical procedure is sometimes necessary when the foreign body is too large to remove endoscopically or when the patient has a bladder rupture, a pelvic abscess, or perforation of adjacent organs. An open removal of a foreign body in the bladder is usually quite easy. Postoperative temporary bladder drainage is accomplished with a suprapubic cystostomy tube in males or a urethral Foley catheter in females.

COMPLICATIONS

Postoperative complications are rare. The persistent dysuria, pyuria, hematuria, and bacteriuria resolve quickly after the foreign body has been removed. Psychological disorders should be considered and treated in patients who have inserted the foreign bodies.

SUGGESTED READING

Grumet GW. Pathologic masturbation with drastic consequences: case report. J Clin Psychiatry 1985; 46:537–539.

Kenney RD. Adolescent males who insert genitourinary foreign bodies: is psychiatric referral required? Urology 1988; 32:127–129.

Wheeler JS, Babayan RK, Austen G Jr, Krane RJ. Urologic complications of hip arthroplasty. Urology 1983; 22:499–503.

VAGINAL PROLAPSE

JERRY G. BLAIVAS, M.D.

Vaginal prolapse is one of the most common afflictions of women. It is a generic term that denotes a weakness of the musculofascial structures that support the bladder, urethra, uterus, cul-de-sac, and rectum. The resultant abnormalities include cystocele, urethrocele, uterine prolapse, enterocele, and rectocele, respectively. Predisposing factors include advancing age, childbirth, previous pelvic surgery, and chronic constipation. Treatment is usually elective, depending on the nature and severity of symptoms, but in rare instances ureteral obstruction or urinary retention demands prompt intervention. For milder degrees of prolapse, conservative therapy consists of pelvic floor exercises, biofeedback, or electrical stimulation. For more overt prolapse, insertion of a vaginal pessary is acceptable to many patients.

Surgical repair of prolapse may be accomplished by any of a number of techniques designed to reconstruct the weakened pelvic floor and perineum.

ANATOMY

The pelvic floor is formed primarily by the levator ani muscle, which forms a diaphragm-like plate of musculofascial tissue that attaches to the pubis, the side walls of the pelvis, and the coccyx and sacrum. On the anterior surface of the levator there is a condensation of endopelvic fascia known as the arcus tendineus that runs parallel to the pelvic side walls. I believe that it is important to incorporate this fascial condensation into the surgical repair of stress incontinence. The vagina is a muscular tube lined with stratified squamous epithelium that extends from the cervix to the vulva. The urethral meatus opens into the anterior vaginal wall behind and posterior to the clitoris. The bladder base lies just above the anterior vaginal wall, from which it is separated and supported by the musculofascial tissue of the levator ani. The cervix lies behind and above the bladder, and its os opens into the proximal portion of the vagina. Support for the cervix is derived from the levator complex and from the strong cardinal and uterosacral ligaments. The upper and posterior portion of the vagina lies adjacent to the cul-de-sac, which extends lower than the apex of the vagina in over 90 percent of women. The posterior wall of the vagina covers the rectum and cul-de-sac.

The distal urethra is attached to the undersurface of the pubis by dense collagenous tissue and is fixed at this point, so that even patients with massive cystourethrocele simply rotate posteriorly about this fixed point. The strength and integrity of the "pubourethral ligaments" is the subject of considerable controversy. Some authors believe that these structures are primarily responsible for anchoring the vesical neck and proximal urethra to the undersurface of the pubis; others, including myself, believe that the pubourethral ligament is at best a flimsy structure that adds little to overall support.

The cardinal and uterosacral ligaments are the primary supporting structures of the uterus and cervix. These ligaments are derived from extension and condensation of the levator complex. They are essential components in the surgical repair of enterocele. The rectum is supported posteriorly by a strong muscular sling composed of puborectal and pubococcygeal muscle. Anteriorly, these muscles decussate between the posterior vaginal wall and rectum to provide further support.

The urogenital diaphragm is composed of the skeletal muscle and fascia that lie in the triangular area formed by the ischial tuberosities and the inferior ramus of the pubis. There are two fascial layers: a superficial and a deep layer. The superficial fascia encloses the superficial transverse perineal muscles, the bulbocavernous muscle, and the ishiocavernous muscle. The deep layer encloses the deep transverse perineal muscles, fat, and loose connective tissue. The perineal body is an important anatomic landmark. It lies between the rectum and vagina and consists of the common insertion of the superficial and deep transverse perineal muscles, the bulbocavernous muscle, the external anal sphincter, and the levator.

CYSTOURETHROCELE

Cystocele is prolapse of the bladder into the vagina; urethrocele is prolapse of the urethra. In most instances the two conditions coexist as a cystourethrocele. They may be defined both radiographically and clinically. Radiographically, cystocele is best diagnosed by a lateral or oblique projection at the time of cystography. It is defined as a prolapse of the bladder base below the inferior ramus of the symphysis pubis. This is most apparent when the patient is coughing or straining. A urethrocele is defined as rotational descent of the proximal urethra. On clinical examination, cystourethrocele is apparent as a bulging of the bladder base and proximal urethra into the vagina. The degree of cystourethrocele may be subjectively graded. In the most overt cases, the prolapse extends beyond the introitus.

Cystourethrocele causes symptoms either by inducing stress incontinence, by causing difficulty in voiding, or by causing discomfort due to the anatomic distortion of the pelvic floor. The usual symptoms of cystocele are those of a pressure sensation in the vagina that is often described as a gnawing, aching discomfort. Some patients complain that it is difficult to sit or walk because they feel the mass effect of the prolapse. In more severe cases the vaginal wall becomes ulcerated and inflamed from the local pressure. In some patients the anatomy of the cystocele is such that during increases in intra-abdominal pressure it protrudes below the vesical neck and actually causes an incomplete obstruction, thereby preventing stress incontinence. In others the cystocele appears to make voiding much more difficult, particularly when the patient pushes or strains. This is probably caused by the cystocele acting as a vent for intravesical pressure.

Stress incontinence is very common among women with cystourethrocele. It is thought to be due to an unequal transmission of pressure during stress when the vesical neck descends into the vagina and outside the influence of abdominal pressure. It therefore follows that surgical correction of this type of incontinence is directed toward preventing the abnormal descent of the neck and proximal urethra that occurs during sudden increases in intra-abdominal pressure.

At least 10 percent of patients who undergo primary cystocele repair subsequently develop stress urinary incontinence unless a urethropexy type of operation is simultaneously performed. For this reason, a careful examination for the possibility of latent stress incontinence should be made in every patient in whom cystocele repair is contemplated. A practical way to test for the possibility of stress incontinence is to examine the patient with a full bladder and a pessary in place. Lateral upright cystography or videourodynamics may disclose subtle degrees of stress incontinence that are not apparent clinically. In my opinion, even the slightest degree of stress incontinence or vesical neck weakness should be corrected at the same time that the cystocele is repaired.

UTERINE PROLAPSE

Uterine prolapse is most often seen as a manifestation of a generalized pelvic floor weakness. Many women with uterine prolapse are asymptomatic and require no treatment. When treatment is elected, a vaginal pessary often offers symptomatic relief. The most effective surgical treatment is hysterectomy performed at the same time and through the same approach as the pelvic floor repair.

ENTEROCELE

An enterocele is a herniation of the cul-de-sac between the rectum and vagina. It usually contains small bowel but may contain large bowel, omentum, or ovary. As a clinical entity it is most often seen after hysterectomy and is known as a "pulsion" enterocele. A "traction" enterocele, caused by uterine descent, is uncommon. Symptoms of enterocele are generally due to the mass effect of the prolapse and include a pressure or bearing-down sensation, pain, or ulceration of the vaginal mass. Treatment is elective except in rare instances of bowel obstruction.

RECTOCELE

Rectocele is a bulging of the rectum into the posterior vaginal wall. In addition to generalized symptoms due to the mass effect, patients often describe difficulty in moving the bowels. Many patients note that the bowel difficulties are improved by exerting manual pressure over the posterior vaginal wall during defecation. Most patients with rectocele also have a weakness of the urogenital diaphragm that, if surgical treatment is chosen, should be repaired at the same time (perineorraphy).

Surgical Treatment

Treatment is elective and based on symptoms. For a small cystourethrocele, virtually all the "urethropexy" operations seem to be equally efficacious. The choice of surgery has more to do with the preference of the individual surgeon than with inherent differences between the operations. Nevertheless, certain general guidelines should be borne in mind when selecting the procedure. Operations performed primarily through the vagina, such as the Raz and Stamey urethropexy, clearly carry less patient morbidity and can be effectively accomplished even in very obese women. Abdominal urethropexy operations such as the Marshall-Marchetti-

Krantz or Burch may be much more difficult and carry much more morbidity in obese patients. On the other hand, the abdominal urethropexy operations have mostly withstood the test of time. Long-term success rates with these operations are 70 to 80 percent. The vaginal urethropexy operations have simply not been performed long enough to evaluate the long-term success rates.

In my opinion, the general principle underlying all urethropexy operations is not to "suspend the vesical neck," but rather to prevent its abnormal descent during increases in intra-abdominal pressure. Although this may sound like semantics, I believe that the distinction is important. The goal of surgery is simply to strengthen the musculofascial tissue that surrounds the vesical neck and urethra. This requires restoring the functional anatomy of the endopelvic fascia and levator complex as a strong support. To this end it is important that the tissue being used for the repair be subjectively tested at the time of surgery to make sure it is strong enough to provide the necessary support. This is best accomplished by exposing the tissue and, under direct vision, grasping it with a forceps or suture and feeling for its strength.

When sutures are placed for the purpose of providing support, another general principle must be borne in mind. If the sutures are placed too close to the urethra, when one pulls up there is a tendency to compress the urethra; when sutures are placed too far away from the urethra, lateral attachments of the endopelvic fascia prevent any meaningful change in support when the sutures are tied. To ensure that this does not happen, when a vaginal approach is used it is important to sever the lateral attachments of the endopelvic fascia from the pubis and ischium. This is automatically accomplished when one perforates the endopelvic fascia with either blunt finger dissection or a scissor. In abdominal urethropexy operations, it may not be necessary to sever these lateral attachments because the sutures are placed completely under direct vision.

For larger cystoceles, I prefer a standard anterior colporrhaphy. If there is a significant uterine prolapse, vaginal hysterectomy is generally the treatment of choice. If a urethropexy operation for stress incontinence is necessary at the time of anterior colporrhaphy, I prefer the Raz modification of the Peyrera. The endopelvic fascia alongside the vesical neck is perforated at its junction with the ischium, and the retropubic space is entered. The lateral edge of the endopelvic fascia, including the arcus tendineus of the levator, is grasped with a long Allis clamp and gently brought into the wound under direct vision. A No. 2 Prolene suture on a curved Mayo needle is passed through this tissue in three or four bites of running suture with both ends left long. The procedure is repeated on the other side. A small transverse incision is made several centimeters above the symphysis pubis, and an index finger is placed in the vaginal wound into the retropubic space. The vaginal finger is palpated just beneath the rectus muscle, and a Stamey needle is passed to the lateral edge of the vaginal finger, care being taken at all times to keep the finger between the needle and the bladder and urethra. The needle is then passed through the vaginal wound, both ends of the suture are threaded through the needle, and the suture is transferred to the abdominal incision. This is repeated on the other side, but the suture is not tied until the pelvic floor reconstruction is completed.

For anterior colporrhaphy a vertical incision is made on the anterior vaginal wall from the vesical neck to the cervix if the uterus is still present, or to the vaginal vault if it has been removed. Lateral flaps of vaginal epithelium are dissected all the way to the side walls of the pelvis. This dissection proceeds immediately beneath the vaginal epithelium in the "bloodless plane" identified by the glistening white surface of the tissue. The "bloodless plane" is not always so bloodless.

The cystocele is reduced with a narrow Deaver retractor or a sponge stick. The endopelvic fascia overlying the lateral aspect of the vaginal portion of the bladder is approximated with interrupted figure-of-eight sutures of 0 chromic catgut.

Next, cystourethroscopy is performed to make sure there has been no injury to the bladder urethra or ureters by the sutures. Accurate placement of the vesical neck sutures is ensured by visual inspection. A percutaneous suprapubic tube is placed and the position checked cystoscopically.

Excess vaginal epithelium is excised and the anterior vaginal wall closed with interrupted sutures of 2:0 chromic catgut. The long Raz sutures are tied in the abdominal wound with just enough tension to prevent descent of the vesical neck. No attempt is made to pull up on these sutures. This completes the cystocele repair.

If rectocele, enterocele, and vaginal outlet laxity are present they are repaired as follows. An Allis clamp is placed at the lower border of each labia minora, positioned so that when these are approximated in the midline, the resulting vaginal width comfortably admits three fingers. An incision is made by excising a thin strip of tissue between the clamps with a Metzenbaum scissor. The vaginal epithelium is mobilized off the rectum to the vaginal apex. The pararectal fascia is dissected as far laterally as possible and the edge of the levators is identified. If an enterocele is present, the peritoneum is identified and incised. The hernia contents are reduced, excess peritoneum is excised, and high ligation of the sac is accomplished with pursestring sutures of 0 chromic catgut. The cardinal and uterosacral ligaments are approximated with 0 chromic catgut. This completes the enterocele repair.

The rectocele repair is begun by approximating the pararectal fascia in the midline with figure-of-eight sutures of 0 chromic catgut. In the lower portion of the repair it is usually possible to approximate the levators

in the midline, but as one approaches the apex of the vagina, only the pararectal fascia is mobile enough to use in the repair. If the dissection is difficult, digital examination of the rectum can easily be performed to aid in identification of its walls. Once the rectocele has been repaired, excess vaginal epithelium excised, and approximated in the midline with 2:0 chromic catgut sutures.

The perineal muscles and levators in the perineal portion of the wound are approximated in the midline and the vaginal wall is closed. Care is taken to ensure that the introitus and vaginal canal comfortably admit three fingers. If the outlet is too small, offending sutures are removed. A vaginal pack saturated with aqueous lubricating jelly is placed in the vagina.

Complications

The most distressing complications of pelvic floor reconstruction are vesicovaginal fistula, ureterovaginal fistula, ureteral injury, and dyspareunia due to a scarred and narrowed vagina. Adherence to meticulous surgical technique is the best means of avoiding these untoward occurrences. Of particular importance is the avoidance of blind suture ligation of bleeding within the depths of the vaginal wound. Suture ligatures are rarely necessary, but when they are used they should be applied only under direct vision. Most bleeding may be controlled by applying pressure, completing the operation in a reasonable time, and applying a vaginal pack. When laceration of the bladder is suspected, it should be confirmed by cystoscopic examination and repaired as if it were a fistula. If sutures from the incontinence procedure were inadvertently placed through the bladder, they may simply be removed. If ureteral injury is suspected, retrograde ureterography should be performed; if the injury is confirmed, it should be repaired by appropriate technique with a ureteral catheter left indwelling.

Urinary retention is another complication. It may be managed with prolonged suprapubic drainage until the vaginal wound has healed. If it persists for more than 1 month, the patient is begun on intermittent self-catheterization and urodynamic studies are performed. Impaired or absent detrusor contractility is treated with continued intermittent self-catheterization. If urethral obstruction is found and persists, consideration is given to urethrolysis.

SUGGESTED READING

Blaivas JG, Vaughan ED. Urinary incontinence. Semin Urol 1989; 7:59–138.
Mattingly RF, Thompson JD. TeLinde's operative gynecology. Philadelphia: JB Lippincott, 1985.

SEMINAL VESICLE CYSTS

JONATHAN P. JAROW, M.D.

Seminal vesicle cysts are a rare and challenging urologic problem. Disorders of and surgery upon the seminal vesicles were more common earlier in the century, owing to the high prevalence of inflammatory lesions of the lower urinary tract. Since malignancy of the seminal vesicles is extremely rare and most inflammatory lesions can now be treated with antibiotics, cysts have become the most common reason to operate on the seminal vesicles. The term "seminal vesicle cyst" is a misnomer because most of these lesions are due to either ejaculatory duct obstruction or ectopic ureter. However, the radiographic appearance of these lesions, particularly on ultrasonography, is cystic.

Owing to the relative inaccessibility of the seminal vesicles, located deep in the pelvis between the bladder, prostate, and rectum, pathologic processes are not well understood and not easily detected. Cysts of the seminal vesicles can remain asymptomatic for many years unless complicated by infection or hemorrhage. They are usually congenital but may also be acquired through obstruction of the ejaculatory duct. Congenital lesions are frequently associated with anomalies of the upper urinary tract.

The ureter and seminal vesicle share a common origin from the mesonephric duct with the vas deferens, the ejaculatory duct, and part of the epididymis. The mesonephric duct drains the mesonephros into the urogenital sinus when the fetal cloaca divides at 5 weeks. At this time, a ureteric bud grows cranially from the mesonephric duct to meet with the metanephrogenic blastema. Proper timing and positioning of this juncture is necessary for normal development of the adult kidney. The seminal vesicle separates from the mesonephric duct much later in fetal development, at 13 weeks. Abnormal timing in the development of the ureteric bud can result in an ectopic ureter draining into the seminal vesicle. In addition, abnormalities of the mesonephric duct may result in delay or complete failure of ureteric bud formation, and subsequently a dysplastic or absent kidney.

Acquired causes of seminal vesicle cysts are usually inflammatory in origin. Infections of the genitourinary tract as well as trauma may be associated with ejaculatory duct obstruction. These lesions present in a similar manner to seminal vesicle cysts but are not associated with upper tract anomalies.

The management of patients suspected to have seminal vesicle cysts should be based on the clinical presentation. Specifically, patients complaining of infertility should be managed differently from those with a symptomatic pelvic mass.

EVALUATION

The differential diagnosis of a male pelvic cyst includes seminal vesicle cyst, müllerian duct cyst, prostatic retention cyst, and ejaculatory duct diverticulum in descending order of frequency. Other lesions that may present in a similar fashion include tumors of the bladder or rectum and a pelvic abscess (Table 1). Presenting symptoms may include hematospermia, perineal pain, urinary retention, dysuria, or infertility. Semen analysis findings consistent with seminal vesicle disease include reduced ejaculate volume (less than 1.5 ml), hematospermia, and, with bilateral disease, low sperm count. The age at the time of presentation has been reported to range from in utero detection by maternal ultrasonography to the eighth decade. However, most patients present between the third and fourth decades. The position of the seminal vesicles high in the pelvis makes all but large cysts difficult to palpate by rectal examination. Cystoscopic evaluation will reveal nonspecific findings, including elevation of the trigone and potentially a hemitrigone. Therefore, the diagnosis is invariably based on clinical suspicion and some form of radiologic imaging.

Table 1   Differential Diagnosis of a Male Pelvic Mass

Seminal vesicle cyst
Müllerian duct cyst
Prostatic retention cyst
Ejaculatory duct diverticulum
Bladder tumor
Rectal carcinoma
Pelvic abscess

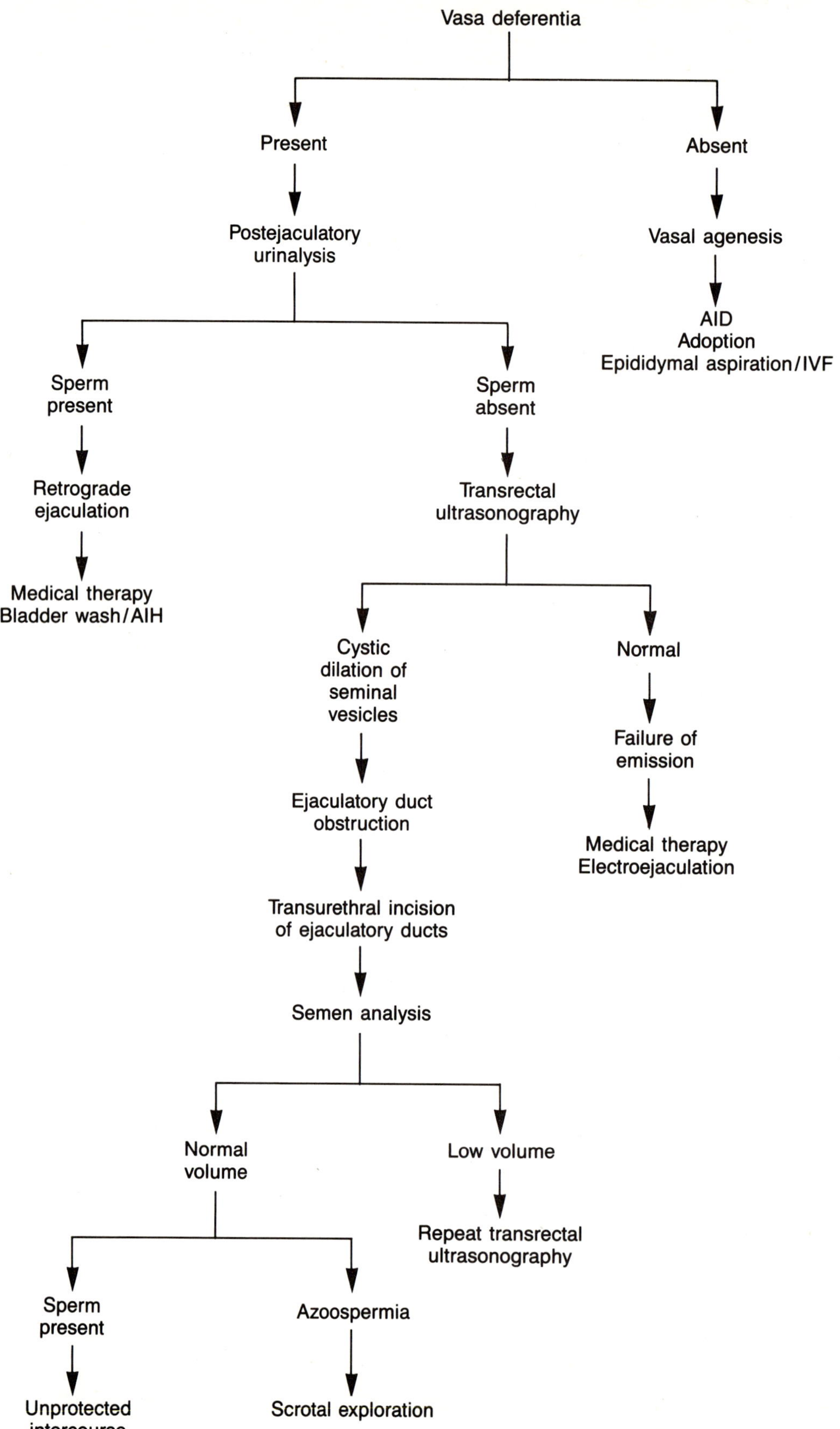

Figure 1 Algorithm for the evaluation and treatment of the infertile patient with decreased ejaculate volume with or without azoospermia.

Table 2 Male Pelvic Cysts

Cyst	Position	Sperm	Size	Upper Tract Anomalies
Seminal vesicle cyst	Cranial/lateral	+	+ + +	Yes
Müllerian duct cyst	Midline	−	+ +/+ + +	Rare
Ejaculatory duct cyst	Lateral	+	+ +	No
Prostatic retention cyst	Peripheral prostate	−	+	No

The size, location, and presence of sperm within a cyst (Table 2) are the factors used to determine the organ of origin. A variety of radiologic imaging tools have been employed to evaluate pelvic cysts, including computed tomography (CT), magnetic resonance imaging (MRI), vasoseminal vesiculography, and direct cyst puncture with cystography. Both CT and MRI can identify cystic lesions within the pelvis, but their resolution is sometimes insufficient for a more specific diagnosis. Both vasography and direct cyst puncture are better at establishing the organ of origin of the cyst. Cyst puncture has the advantages of providing fluid for microscopic examination of sperm, and may be therapeutic. However, these tests are invasive and have associated risks. Transrectal ultrasonography is supplanting other radiologic imaging techniques in the management of these patients. High-resolution probes placed in close proximity to the lesion can provide much more information than either CT, or MRI. In addition, with the same methodology used for prostatic biopsy, transrectal ultrasonography can provide guidance for transperineal needle aspiration of these lesions.

Patients presenting with symptoms referable to a mass lesion of the seminal vesicles should undergo transrectal ultrasonography initially. Seminal vesicle cysts appear as echo-free cavities located laterally outside the prostate gland and beneath the bladder. However, if this does not provide a definitive diagnosis, ultrasonography-guided needle aspiration with cystography can be performed next. Aspirated fluid should be analyzed for sperm and a cytology test obtained to rule out the rare malignancy. A final diagnosis should be made on the basis of these findings using the criteria listed in Table 2. In addition to the evaluation of the pelvis, patients with seminal vesicle cysts should undergo imaging of the upper tracts because of the frequent association of renal anomalies.

In contrast, the approach to infertile patients suspected of having a seminal vesicle cyst (low ejaculate volume) should use a different algorithm (Fig. 1). The differential diagnosis includes vasal agenesis, ejaculatory duct obstruction, and ejaculatory dysfunction (retrograde ejaculation or failure of emission). These disorders can be diagnosed by physical examination of the vas deferens and a postejaculatory urinalysis. After other causes are ruled out, transrectal ultrasonography should be performed to differentiate between failure of emission and ejaculatory duct obstruction. Failure of emission can usually be suspected on the basis of history,

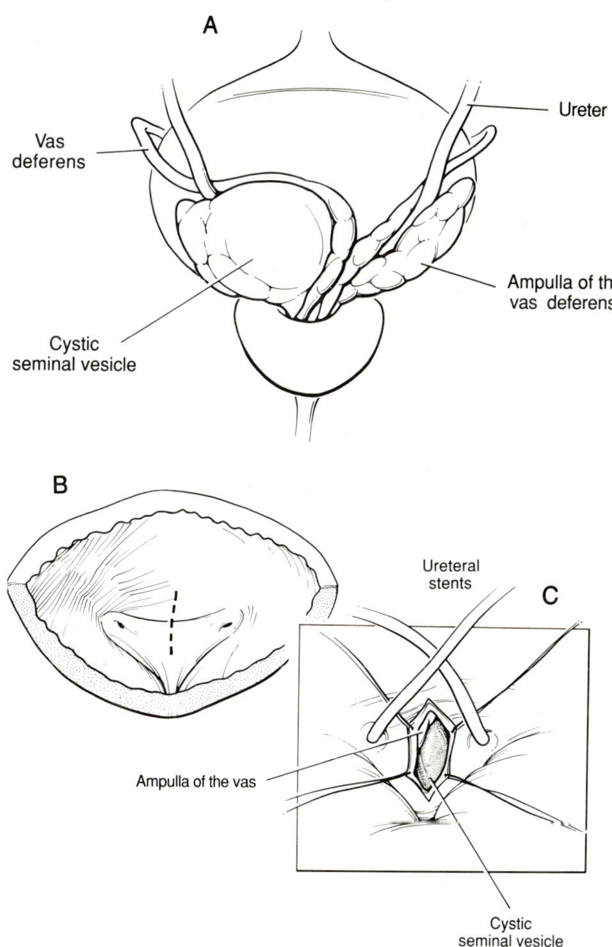

Figure 2 Transvesical approach to excision or marsupialization. *A,* Posterior view of the pelvis with a large seminal vesicle cyst. *B,* Longitudinal incision through the trigone between ureteral orifices. This approach allows removal of the entire seminal vesicle under direct vision, avoiding injury to the rectum and ureters *(C)*.

whereas ejaculatory duct obstruction having no typical presentation can be easily identified by the cystic dilatation of the seminal vesicles seen on ultrasound images.

TREATMENT

In a patient with a symptomatic seminal vesicle cyst, initial treatment should be aspiration: many of these

Table 3 Treatment Options

Observation

Aspiration

Transurethral incision in ejaculatory ducts

Excision
    Transperitoneal
    Extraperitoneal
    Transvesical
    Perineal
    Posterior

Marsupialization into bladder
    Transurethral
    Transvesical

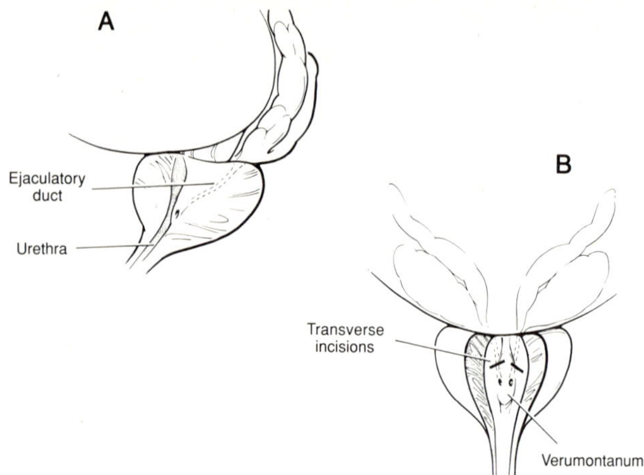

Figure 3 *A, B,* Transurethral incision is the preferred treatment of infertile patients with cystic dilatation of the seminal vesicles due to ejaculatory duct obstruction. Incisions are made perpendicular to the path of the ejaculatory ducts, just cranial and lateral to the verumontanum, using cutting current.

lesions remain asymptomatic for many years after a single aspiration. Cytology tests should be obtained to rule out a rare but possible malignancy. Asymptomatic lesions detected incidentally can be followed with periodic transrectal ultrasonography. Failure of aspiration or the development of recurrent symptoms after aspiration are an indication for surgical treatment in patients in whom infertility is not the primary complaint. Surgical approach will vary, depending on the size and location of the cyst (Table 3). For smaller cysts located adjacent to the bladder, a transurethral unroofing procedure similar to that used for müllerian duct cysts is very effective. The end result will be similar to that of an open marsupialization procedure. Care should be taken to identify and avoid resection of the ureters.

Open surgical procedures are best reserved for very large symptomatic cysts, since the increased size makes the operation easier. Several approaches have been described: perineal, posterior, transperitoneal, extraperitoneal, and transvesical. The transvesical approach is preferable because of the decreased risk of injury to the ureters and rectum. The perineal approach may be just as good for surgeons familiar with this technique. However, when an ectopic ureter is suspected, an abdominal approach is necessary to search for and remove any associated renal tissue.

Transvesical excision or marsupialization of a seminal vesicle cyst is performed through a lower abdominal incision. The bladder is opened and retraction maintained with a self-retaining retractor (Balfour with a bladder blade or ring retractor). The ureteral orifices should be identified and cannulated. A longitudinal incision is then made in the trigone between the orifices (Fig. 2). In a case with ipsilateral renal agenesis, the trigonal incision can be biased toward that side and an ectopic ureter identified if present. Dissection behind the bladder will reveal the ampullae of the vasa and the seminal vesicles. Placement of stents within the ureters will help prevent inadvertent injury. The abnormal seminal vesicle can now be excised or marsupialized into the trigone. The bladder should be closed in multiple

layers with absorbable suture. Both an extravesical drain and an indwelling catheter should be used.

Infertile patients with ejaculatory duct obstruction should undergo transurethral incision of the ejaculatory ducts rather than an initial aspiration. This is performed with the Collings knife using cutting current. Bilateral incisions should be made lateral and cranial to the verumontanum over the path of the ejaculatory ducts (Fig. 3). Simultaneous massage of the seminal vesicles and prostate transrectally will reveal a cloudy effluent when the ducts have been opened adequately. Unfortunately, some patients with ejaculatory duct obstruction develop a secondary, more proximal obstruction of the excretory ducts of the testis owing to an epididymal blow-out. If a follow-up semen analysis reveals normal ejaculate volume and azoospermia, scrotal exploration should be performed to rule out epididymal obstruction (see Fig. 1). One should be prepared to perform an epididymovasostomy at this time.

Scrotal exploration in a patient with persistent azoospermia after incision of the ejaculatory ducts should be performed as follows. The testes and vasa are delivered through bilateral scrotal incisions. A partial-thickness transverse incision is made through the vasa, and vasal fluid collected. Examination of this fluid for sperm determines proximal patency. Vasography is then performed to confirm distal patency. If sperm are present within the vas, the vasotomy should be closed using microsurgical technique and the transurethral incision of the ejaculatory ducts repeated on the basis of vasographic findings. If intravasal azoospermia is detected, the transverse incision should be completed and an end-to-side microsurgical anastomosis performed proximal to the level of epididymal obstruction.

SUGGESTED READING

Arey LP. Developmental anatomy. Philadelphia: WB Saunders, 1974.

Jarow JP. Transrectal ultrasonography in the evaluation of male infertility. In: Resnick MI, ed. Prostatic ultrasonography. Philadelphia: BC Decker, 1990.

Littrup PJ, Lee F, McLeary RD, et al. Transrectal ultrasound of the seminal vesicles and ejaculatory ducts: clinical correlation. Radiology 1988; 168:625–628.

Shabsigh R, Lerner S, Fishman IJ, Kadmon D. The role of transrectal ultrasonography in the diagnosis and management of prostatic and seminal vesicle cysts. J Urol 1989; 141:1206–1209.

URETHRAL DUPLICATION

MARK F. BELLINGER, M.D.

Duplication of the urethra is uncommon. Most occur in the male and are midline in location (sagittal duplications), but anatomic findings vary greatly (Fig. 1). Collateral duplications (side by side) are usually associated with duplications of the lower genitourinary tract and disordered external genitalia. Although many systems of classification have been proposed, the scheme of Effman and colleagues is most complete in describing duplications in the male (Table 1). To this scheme must be added female urethral duplications. Type IA duplications are the most common, while type IIB are the most rare. An appreciation of the potential anatomic spectrum of urethral duplication and a systematic approach to the patient are important, since incomplete evaluation or ill-planned surgical intervention may cause irreparable harm to the dominant urethra or to continence mechanisms.

CLINICAL PRESENTATION

Many patients with urethral duplication are asymptomatic. Duplication may be evident on examination of the genitalia in infants or adults. Dorsal duplications may appear as a double meatus, a dorsal glanular groove or cleft, an elongated mucosal strip on the dorsum of the penile shaft, or a penopubic sinus; they are commonly associated with dorsal chordee. Ventral duplications are usually less striking on examination and are not associ-

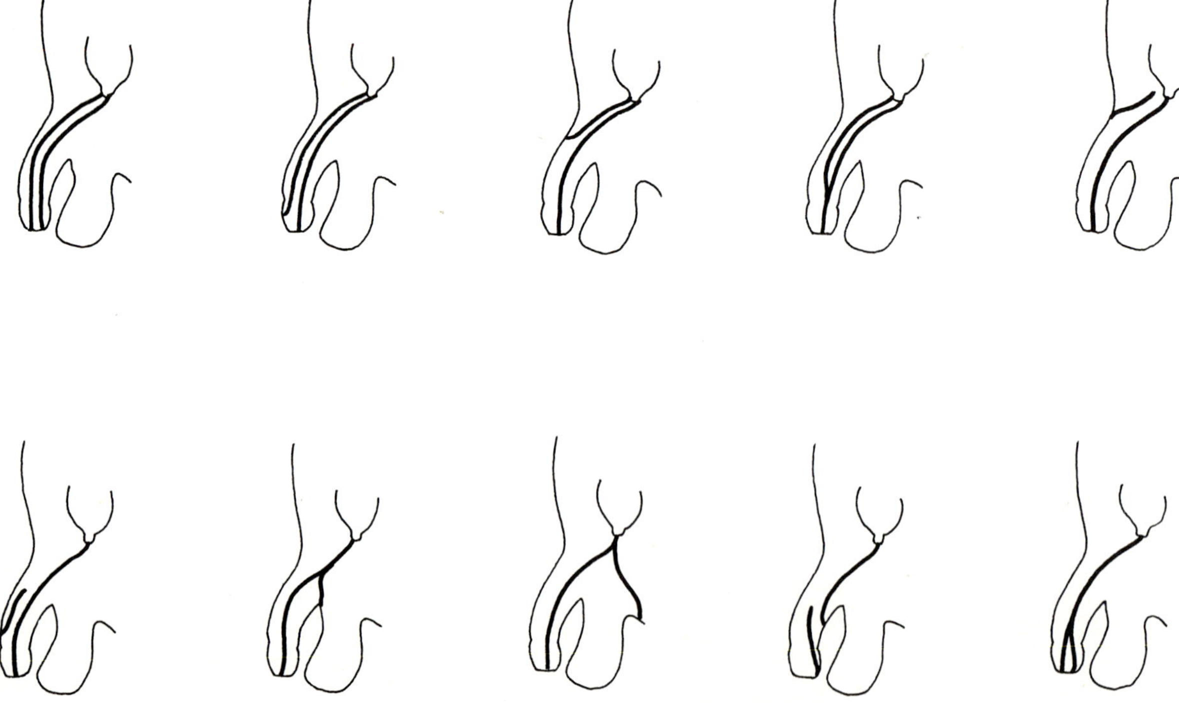

Figure 1 Variations of urethral duplication.

ated with chordee. Two urinary streams may be evident on micturition. Incontinence is rare even in complete duplications (type II), because both urethras usually exit through a common bladder neck. However, incontinence may result when the accessory urethra exits the bladder from a more eccentric location. When present, incontinence is usually mild and stress related rather than a continuous dribbling. Urinary tract infection is uncommon, but nonspecific or sexually related urethritis, especially of the accessory urethra, is a frequent complaint. The accessory urethra may be more susceptible to infection because of a thinner wall and lack of normal wash-out during voiding. Symptoms of vesical outlet obstruction may occur if the proximal accessory urethra is wide but narrows distally, allowing the proximal channel to balloon and compress the primary bladder outlet during micturition. Infants with variations of caudal regression and anomalous perineal and genital anatomy may be found to have urethral duplication when aberrant micturition from a perineal meatus is discovered.

EVALUATION

Evaluation of the patient with suspected urethral duplication should begin with a complete examination of the genitalia and perineum. Suspected blind-ending duplications can be gently probed and any discharge cultured. The sacral area should be inspected for abnormal folds or dimples, especially in patients with

Table 1 Classification of Urethral Duplication

Type I	Blind incomplete urethral duplication (accessory urethra) A. *Distal:* opens on dorsal or ventral surface of penis but does not communicate with bladder or urethra. B. *Proximal:* opens from urethral channel and ends blindly in periurethral tissue; may be difficult to differentiate from urethral diverticula or Cowper's ducts

Type II	Complete patent urethral duplication
	A. *Two meati*
	  1. Two noncommunicating urethras arising independently from bladder
	  2. Second channel arises from first and courses independently into second meatus.
	B. *One meatus*
	  Two urethras arise from bladder or posterior urethra and unite into a common channel distally (spindle duplication)

Type III	Urethral duplication as component of partial or complete caudal duplication (male or female)
Type IV	Accessory phallic urethra in females
Type V	Congenital prepubic sinus in females

Modified from Effman EL, Lebowitz RL, Colodny AH. Duplication of the urethra. Radiology 1976; 119:179.

anomalous or ambiguous genitalia. When possible, the voided urinary stream should be observed to determine which urethra is dominant. A Valsalva maneuver may produce a discharge from the accessory meatus. Upper tract anatomy should be evaluated by screening ultrasonography in all cases. If abnormal findings are noted, further radiographic studies are warranted. The most important part of the evaluation is complete radiologic assessment of both urethral channels. This usually necessitates both retrograde urethrography and voiding cystourethrography (Fig. 2), both of which should include anteroposterior, lateral, and oblique views. It should be noted that a widened intersymphyseal distance (> 1 cm) is found in most patients with dorsal epispadiac urethral duplication. Endoscopy may be carried out as a preliminary investigation or coincident with surgical repair. The location of a verumontanum and normal sphincteric mechanisms should be noted. Frequently, one or both urethras may be too small to allow endoscopy, even with small pediatric instruments. Large instruments should not be forced, or stricture may result and considerably worsen potential reconstructive efforts for the dominant urethra. Urodynamic studies may be performed but are not usually as helpful as radiography.

NONSURGICAL TREATMENT

Not all patients with urethral duplication require surgical treatment. Asymptomatic blind-ending duplications, for example, may cause no symptoms. If urethritis is a presenting complaint, cultures should be taken and appropriate antibiotic therapy administered. Cultures for gonorrhea and chlamydia should be included.

SURGICAL TREATMENT

Considerations in Surgical Repair

Surgical therapy for urethral duplication may be performed because of chordee, incontinence, infection, or abnormal urinary stream, for cosmetic reasons, or for a combination of the above. When one is considering surgical treatment for urethral duplication, it is always important to evaluate both urethras completely. The basic tenet of reconstruction is that in the vast majority of patients the ventral urethra is dominant and more normal in terms of both structure and function. The use of optical magnification or microsurgical technique is important in most urethral reconstructive procedures in order to maximize functional and cosmetic results. In all cases of penile surgery, adjunctive local or caudal anesthesia combined with the use of intraurethral anesthetic jelly smooths the postoperative course.

Dorsal Duplications

Dorsal urethral duplications may be complete or incomplete, and radiographic and endoscopic findings

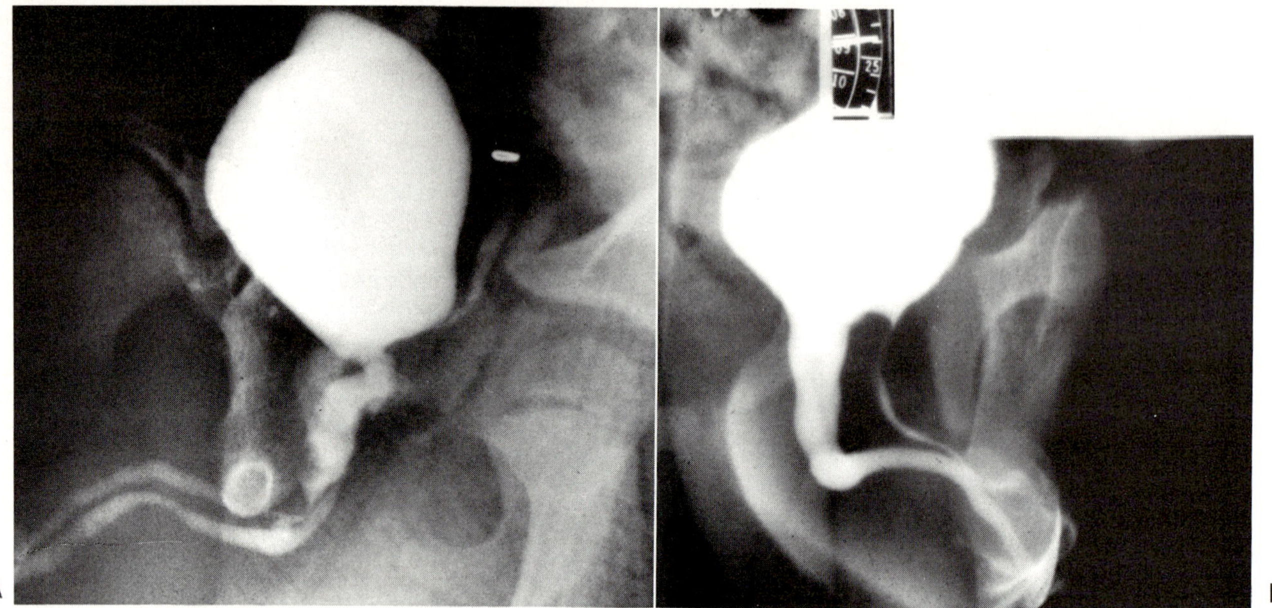

Figure 2 Voiding cystourethrography *A,* in a boy with imperforate anus and type IIA2 urethral duplication and *B,* in a boy with isolated diphallus.

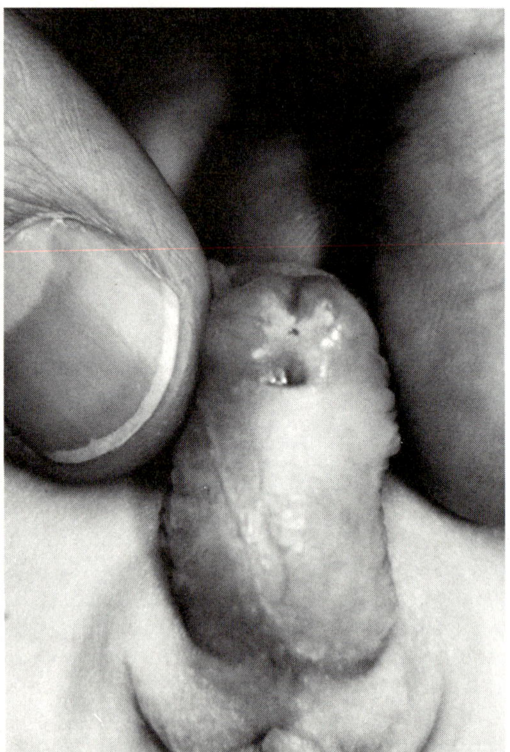

Figure 3 Coronal hypospadias. The pinpoint opening proximal to the glanular cleft was a dorsal blind-ending duplication 1 cm in length.

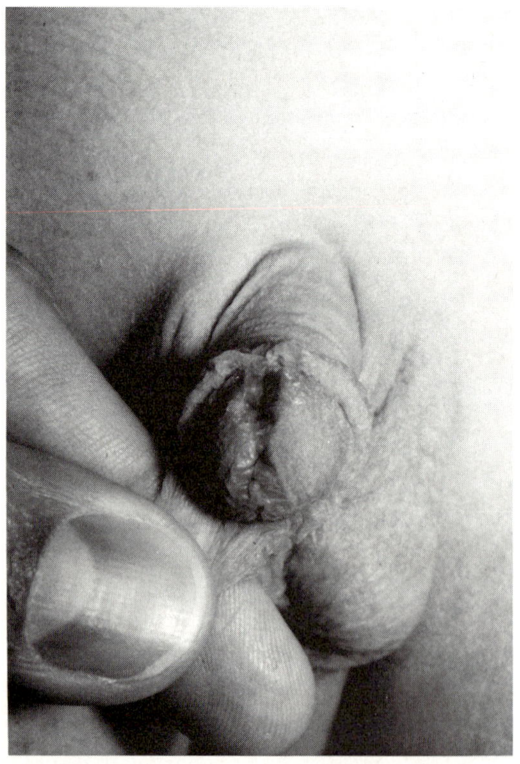

Figure 4 Glanular meatus of a dorsal duplication that ended blindly in the infrapubic space.

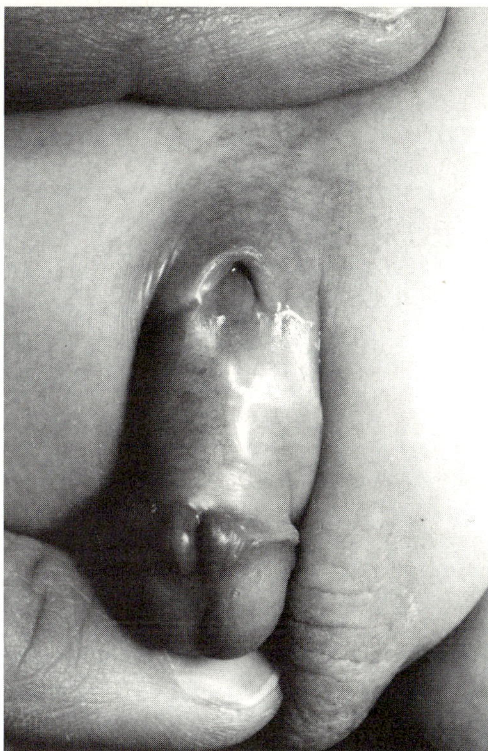

Figure 5 Penopubic urethral duplication associated with a dorsal glanular groove.

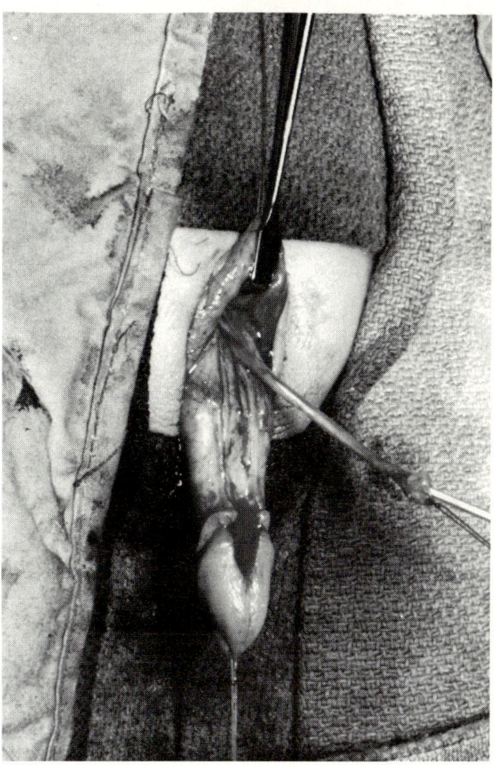

Figure 6 Excision of the urethral duplication seen in Figure 5.

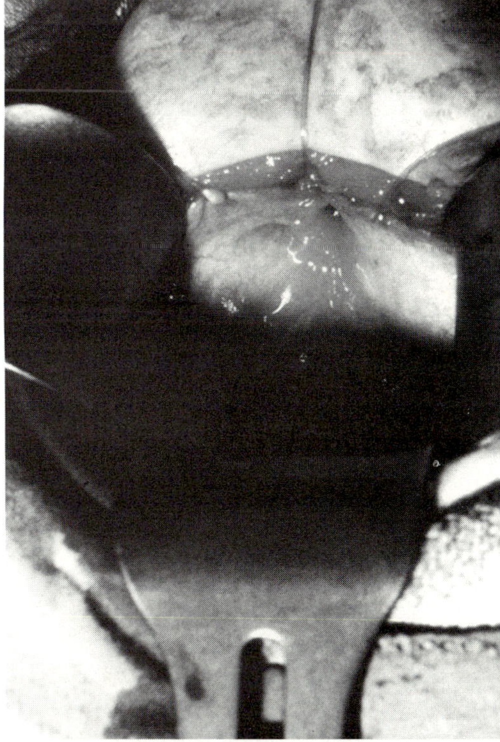

Figure 7 Duplicate bladder neck at cystostomy. There was a common musculature and no incontinence. The patient voided through both urethras.

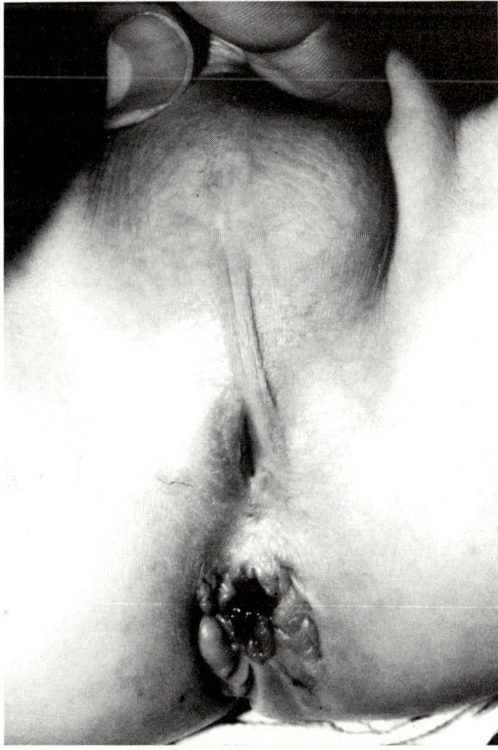

Figure 8 Midline ventral urethral duplication in a boy with imperforate anus. The dorsal urethra was dominant.

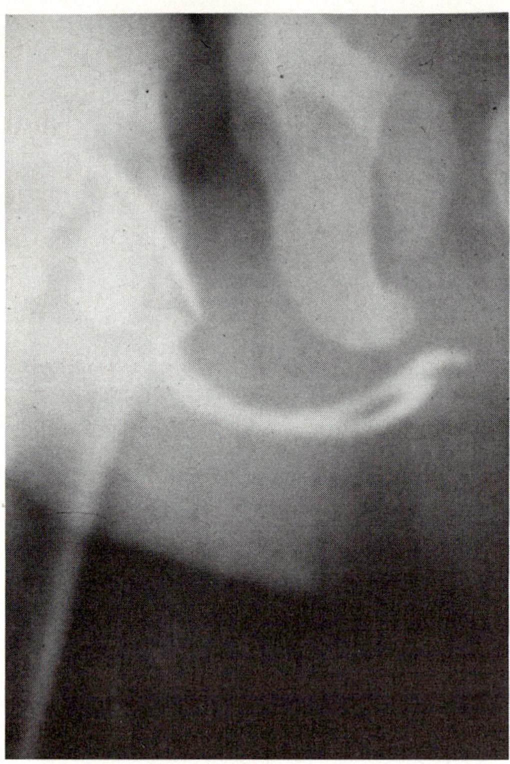

Figure 9 Type IIB (spindle) duplication.

will dictate the most appropriate surgical approach. Type II duplications associated with incontinence require complete excision. All patients with dorsal duplication should undergo assessment by artificial erection at the start of the procedure, since the presence of chordee may greatly influence the surgical approach. Before surgery, it is imperative to be certain that the dorsal urethra is not dominant.

Glanular Urethral Duplications

Type IA duplications are most commonly seen in association with hypospadias (Fig. 3). These blind-ending accessory pits in the distal urethral plate are usually short and cause no problems. They should be examined with a lacrimal duct probe at the time of urethroplasty, however, and if they are deep (>3 mm), should be marsupialized into the urethral plate by simple midline incision of the septum between the duplication and the urethral plate. This ensures that the duplication will not become a diverticulum after urethroplasty and act as either a source of infection or a blind passage that will interfere with subsequent urethral catheterization.

A duplicate meatus in close juxtaposition to the normal meati may be representative of either a complete (type II) or an incomplete (type IA) duplication. If there is incontinence, complete excision of the accessory urethra will be required (see below). If there is no

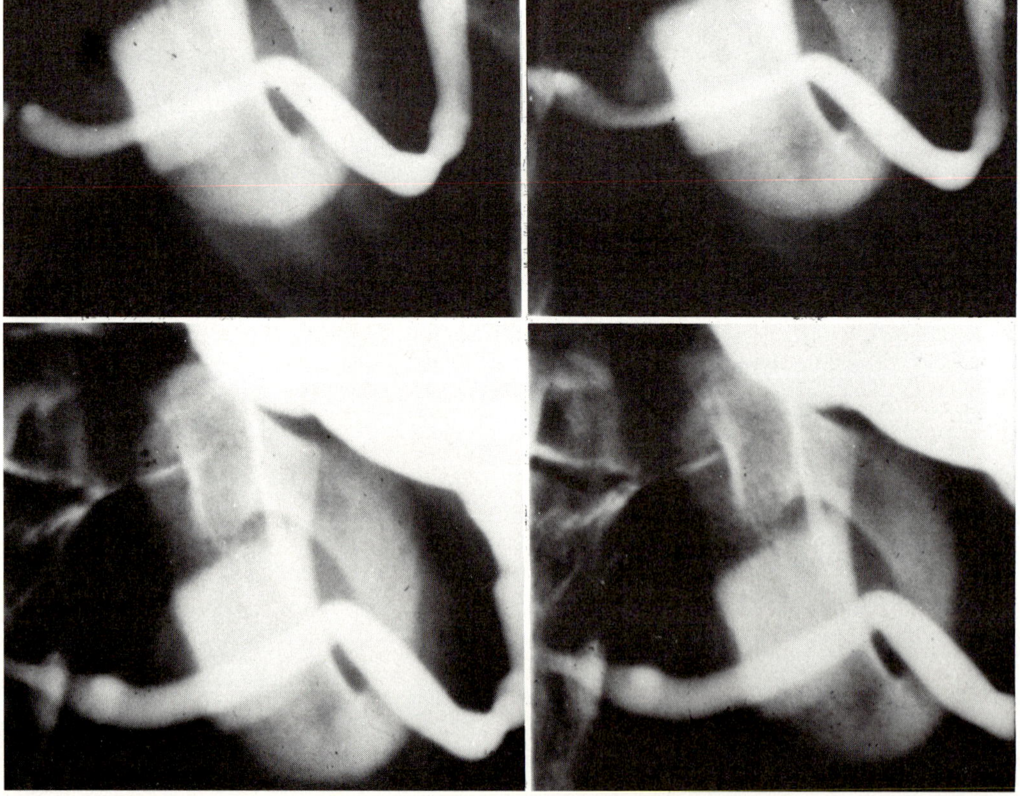

Figure 10 Lacuna magna as seen on a voiding cystourethrogram in a boy with bloody spotting. The small dot of contrast near the meatus is the duplication.

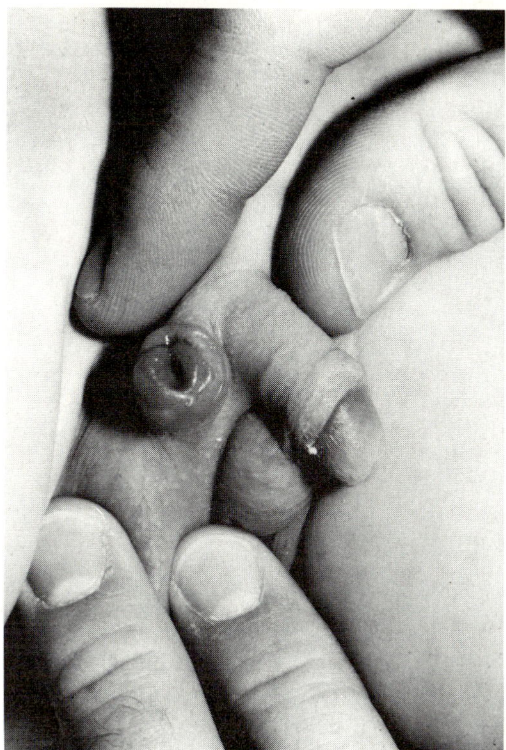

Figure 11 Urethral duplication in association with isolated diphallus.

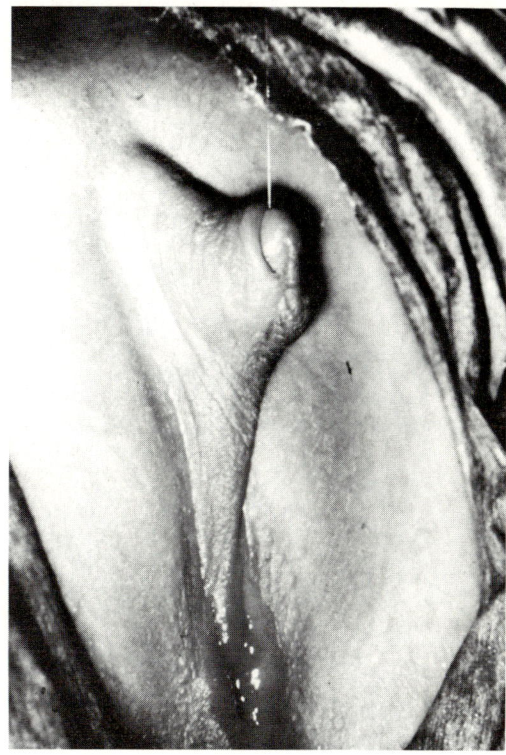

Figure 12 Accessory phallic urethra in a female. A stream of urine exits the glanular urethra.

incontinence, this cosmetic situation is usually best handled by division of the distal septum separating the two meatus, using optical magnification and fine instruments. In most cases, no suture is required unless the septum is thick, in which case one or two fine (6-0 or 7-0) absorbable sutures may be placed to control bleeding. No catheter is required, and intraurethral anesthetic jelly will decrease postoperative dysuria.

The proximal glans penis may be the site of a duplicate urethral meatus (Fig. 4) or the glans may be grooved with a mucosal surface in association with a proximal penile meatus (Fig. 5). In the latter situation, the mucosal groove appears to represent the urethral plate of the accessory urethra. In both cases, an artificial erection should be performed using a tourniquet at the base of the penis, a small (25-gauge) needle, and parenterally compatible saline. The blind-ending duplication should be excised completely, inserting a small lacrimal duct probe, intravenous catheter, or feeding tube to better define the tract. Careful instillation of methylene blue into the accessory urethra may help to define its path, but this is usually messy. If the tract is short and there is no chordee, a simple circumferential incision around the meatus extended up the midline over the duplication serves well (Fig. 6). The glanular groove should be de-epithelialized and trimmed. Skin closure must be precise, approximating the glanular edge and coronal margins perfectly to create optimal cosmesis.

Penile or Penopubic Urethral Duplications

Penile or penopubic urethral duplications (see Fig. 5) are commonly associated with dorsal chordee. Artificial erection may be helpful before, during, and after dissection of the accessory urethra. Under optical magnification the meatus is circumscribed. Penile meatal dissection is accomplished by a circumferential subcoronal incision and degloving of the dorsum of the penis or its entire shaft, depending on the degree of exposure necessary. Dorsal neurovascular structures must be preserved, and dissection should follow the midline, close upon the surface of the urethra, guided by a small catheter or lacrimal duct probe (Fig. 6). When the duplication extends into the infrapubic space, the dorsal penile skin may be divided in the midline and this incision carried up over the pubic symphysis in the midline or as a "T" to gain exposure to the symphysis. Since the intersymphyseal distance is usually abnormally wide, the intersymphyseal band may be divided to achieve better exposure. If the duplication extends into the dominant urethra, a catheter or sound will help define normal structures to avoid an incomplete dissection leaving a urethral diverticulum, or an overzealous dissection potentiating urethral narrowing and stricture. Complete duplications that enter the bladder or bladder neck (type IIA or IIB) require an additional Pfannenstiel incision and cystostomy in order to completely excise the proximal urethra. Since most duplicate urethras share a common bladder neck when both are continent, bladder

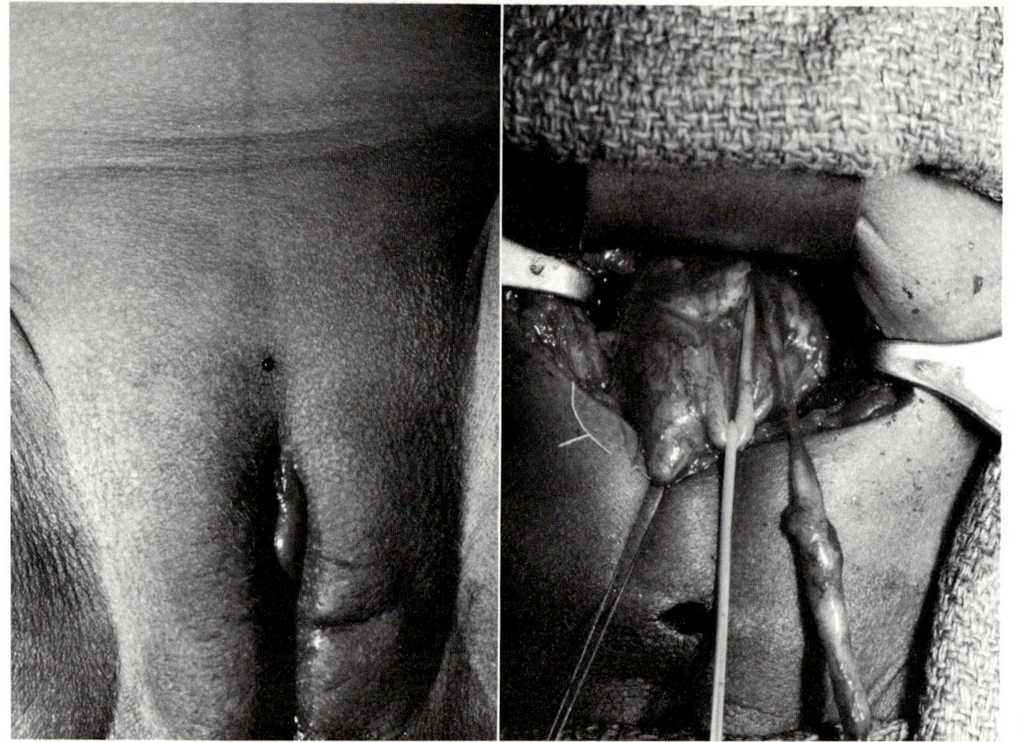

Figure 13 *A,* Congenital prepubic sinus in a female. A small dot of methylene blue in the midline marks the sinus. *B,* The sinus has been dissected to its blind-ending termination at the anterior bladder wall near the urachal remnant.

neck musculature should be carefully preserved (Fig. 7). This is best accomplished by circumscription of the accessory bladder neck with dissection of the mucosal channel distally to join the dissection previously carried out from the meatus. Once the urethral mucosa has been excised, the muscular defect is simply approximated and the bladder mucosa closed. After the duplication has been excised, artificial erection should be repeated. Persistent dorsal curvature is usually remedied by careful excision of midline fibrous tissue, again avoiding neurovascular structures. When modest chordee persists, ventrolateral plicating sutures may help to straighten the penis. Severe chordee, however, uncommonly necessitates isolation and preservation of dorsal neurovascular structures and excision or incision of the dysgenetic tunica albuginea with replacement by dermal graft or tunica vaginalis. Postoperative urinary diversion is not necessary in most cases. If the urethra or bladder has been opened, diversion may be advisable for 3 to 10 days, depending on the age of the patient and the complexity of the repair. Most infants are best managed by a small Silastic stent with several extra side holes cut, passed 1 to 2 cm beyond the bladder neck and sewn through the glans penis using a nonabsorbable suture to transfix both glans and catheter. The catheter is allowed to drain into the outer layer of a double diaper and removed later in the office. Bladder spasms and catheter-related problems are minimal with this technique. Foley catheter or suprapubic drainage may be appropriate in older patients.

Ventral Duplications

Ventral urethral duplications (Fig. 8) may present more problems in management than dorsal duplications, since the dorsal urethra (which lies in a more normal position and has a more orthotopic meatus) is usually hypoplastic. The ventral channel thus requires a more complex reconstructive effort. Artificial erection should be performed intraoperatively, although chordee is less of a problem than with dorsal duplications. In many instances, the ventral urethra opens very low on the perineum or in the perianal area. In these patients, the possibility of using any portion of the duplication as part of the reconstructed urethra should be examined carefully before any portion of it is excised. Rectal or anal ectopia of the dominant ventral urethra may be associated with severe upper tract changes and renal failure, necessitating temporary cutaneous vesicostomy drainage to allow upper tract decompression before urethral reconstruction. Urethroplasty of the ventral channel may be accomplished by single- or multiple-stage repairs using standard hypospadias techniques, with excision of the dorsal duplication if the distance to be bridged is not excessive. Bladder mucosal grafts or free grafts of preputial skin may be used. A determined effort should be made to avoid both hair-bearing and extragenital skin in reconstruction. Use of the dorsal urethra in certain instances can be accomplished by division of the urethrourethral septum, using the dorsal marsupialized urethra as a portion of the reconstruction. In limited instances, very slow, chronic dilatation of an atretic dorsal urethra with graduated, indwelling Silastic catheters may produce a urethra of satisfactory caliber. This may then be used as a primary urethra when anastomosed to the proximal ventral channel or after the ventral limb of a Y-type duplication is excised. Postoperative urinary diversion is managed as in cases of dorsal urethral duplication.

Miscellaneous Urethral Duplications in Males

Type IIB (spindle) duplications are rare and may be asymptomatic (Fig. 9). They may be difficult to differentiate from false passages caused by traumatic instrumentation. Although reports of endoscopic division of the intervening septum have appeared, symptomatic spindle duplications rarely require treatment. An open surgical approach may be needed if symptoms occur.

Type III duplications are associated in most cases with severely disordered perineal and genital anatomy and upper tract anomalies, and frequently with spinal dysraphism. Treatment must be highly individualized.

The lacuna magna is a distal dorsal urethral diverticulum (essentially a type IB duplication) that may cause bloody urethral spotting in boys (Fig. 10). No treatment is necessary in most cases, but transmeatal excision of the valve leaflet (the valve of Guérin) may relieve symptoms in severe cases.

Collateral urethral duplication in males is uncommon except in association with diphallus (Fig. 11).

Urethral Duplication in Females

Female urethral duplications are uncommon unless associated with cloacal anomalies or syndromes of

caudal regression, but two isolated types have been reported with some regularity.

Accessory phallic urethra in females (Fig. 12) is associated with disordered perineal anatomy: a prominent clitoris lacking its usual "chordee," a posteriorly placed urogenital sinus, and deficient perineal anatomy (absent or hypoplastic labial structures). Feminizing genitoplasty may be indicated. The accessory urethra is usually so small that excision is not necessary. The ventral urethra, as in males, is predominant and commonly hypospadiac.

Congenital prepubic sinuses in female infants occasionally become symptomatic because of bloody or purulent discharge (Fig. 13*A*). These sinuses end blindly in the anterior bladder wall or perivesical fat and appear to represent a form of dorsal urethral duplication. Local excision of the entire tract is indicated for symptomatic relief. This may entail a circumferential excision of the tract, guided by placement of a small lacrimal duct probe. A Pfannenstiel counterincision may be necessary to accomplish complete excision (Fig. 13*B*).

SUGGESTED READING

Effman EL, Lebowitz RL, Colodny AH. Duplication of the urethra. Radiology 1976; 119:179.

Psihramis KE, Colodny AH, Lebowitz RL, et al. Complete patent duplication of the urethra. J Urol 1986; 136:63.

Gross RE, Moore TC. Duplication of the urethra. Arch Surg 1950; 60:749.

Woodhouse CRJ, Williams DI. Duplications of the lower urinary tract in children. Br J Urol 1979; 51:481.

Campbell J, Beasley S, McMullin N, et al. Congenital prepubic sinus. Possible variant of dorsal urethral duplication (Stephens type 2). J Urol 1987; 137:505.

CONGENITAL URETHRAL STRICTURE

DAVID A. BLOOM, M.D.
JOHN C. NORBECK, M.D.

Urethral stricture is one of the index diseases of urology and one of the first that had appropriate operative treatment. These strictures occur almost exclusively in males and most have a definable cause. It

may be difficult to distinguish a congenital urethral stricture from other restrictive lower tract lesions or from an acquired stricture. Semantics further confuse the issue: in a sense, meatal stenosis is a distal urethral stricture just as bladder neck obstruction is arguably a proximal stricture. Urethral atresia is another distinct lesion, consisting of a long segment of hypoplastic and narrow urethra.

In this chapter, we define congenital urethral stricture as a short luminal restriction within the course of the urethra and exclude postoperative strictures, posterior urethral valves, bladder neck obstruction, and meatal lesions. Barring an obvious history of urethritis, trauma, or instrumentation, it may be impossible to prove that a stricture is not acquired. Some authors question the existence of congenital strictures and suggest that they be described as of unknown origin. It is likely that some reported cases of congenital stricture were related to occult injuries or inflammations.

We believe congenital stricture does exist but is rare. Kaplan and Brock found that congenital strictures accounted for one in seven pediatric urethral strictures. Only eight cases of presumed congenital stricture had been published before 1961, and it is unusual for more than one or two bona fide congenital strictures to present to a busy pediatric urologic service in the course of a year. Cobb and colleagues' report of 26 congenital strictures in boys over a 3-year period failed to exclude previous instrumentation or trauma. The claim of embryologic origin of stricture was based on a lack of previous infection and on the predictable location of the lesions in the proximal bulb. A mild straddle injury or a long forgotten kick can leave its mark in a child's urethra just as a long-forgotten and denied episode of gonococcal urethritis leaves a scar years later in an adult. Reports of identical urethral strictures in fathers and sons or in siblings support the congenital origin of some strictures. Abnormal urethral canalization during the first trimester and incomplete rupture of the cloacal membrane are possible causes of congenital stricture. One might assume that a true congenital stricture would be a stable restriction and a secondary stricture would be progressive, but this is not always the case. Congenital strictures may begin as soft mucosal rings (Fig. 1), although fibrosis may occur over time. The usual location is in the bulbous or penile urethra.

SYMPTOMS AND DIAGNOSIS

A stricture has a lumen smaller than that of the urethral meatus. Even a narrow stricture may be asymptomatic, particularly in a young patient who has never realized a normal urinary stream. Once the degree of blockage becomes significant, symptoms develop in addition to morphologic and functional changes of the bladder and upper urinary tracts. The typical presentations of urethral stricture include decreased force and caliber of the urinary stream, stranguria, prolonged voiding times, dribbling, hematuria, urinary retention, and failure to thrive. Audible stream insufficiency is an occasional diagnostic complaint. Diagnosis may be made by stream observation, hand-timed urine volumes (home uroflowmetry), instrumental uroflowmetry, voiding cystourethrography, retrograde urethrography, cystourethroscopy, and urethral sounding. The urethral pressure profile may show a high gradient at the site of stricture. Ultrasonography of the urethra may demonstrate a stricture. In most patients, we have found voiding cystourethrography alone to be adequate to rule out a urethral stricture (Fig. 2), although concomitant retrograde imaging offers the most complete study. Urinalysis should accompany any stricture evaluation, and ultrasonography can readily prove that the upper urinary tracts are normal.

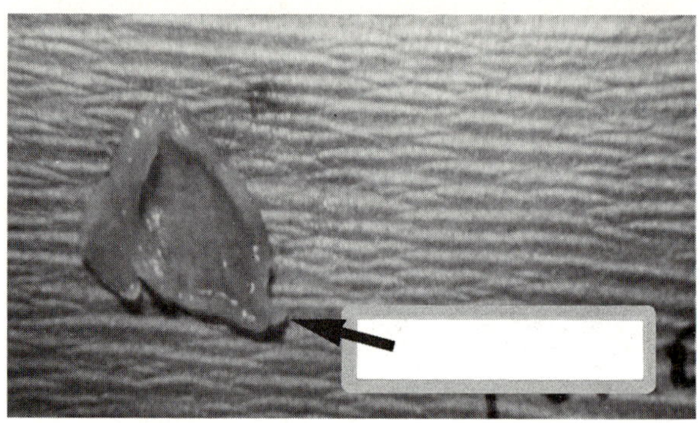

Figure 1 Excised congenital stricture in a 15-year-old boy with gradual awareness of dysuria, decreased force and caliber of stream, and intermittent terminal hematuria. Voiding cystourethrogram (see Fig. 2) demonstrated a bulbar stricture. Uroflowmetry demonstrated a peak flow rate of 12 ml per second with a volume of 350 ml. At cystourethroscopy, this fold was found in the bulbous urethra and removed.

Symptoms disappeared postoperatively and peak flow rate exceeded 45 ml per second with a volume of 450 ml. One year later, bloody spotting recurred and the stream became weak. Peak flow rate was 10 ml per second with a volume of 550 ml. Cystoscopy revealed a diaphragmatic stricture in the bulbous urethra. Internal urethrotomy resolved the symptoms and improved the flow rate. Two years later, symptoms recurred and a recurrent stricture was found and cut. He has been well now for 2 years with daily catheterization.

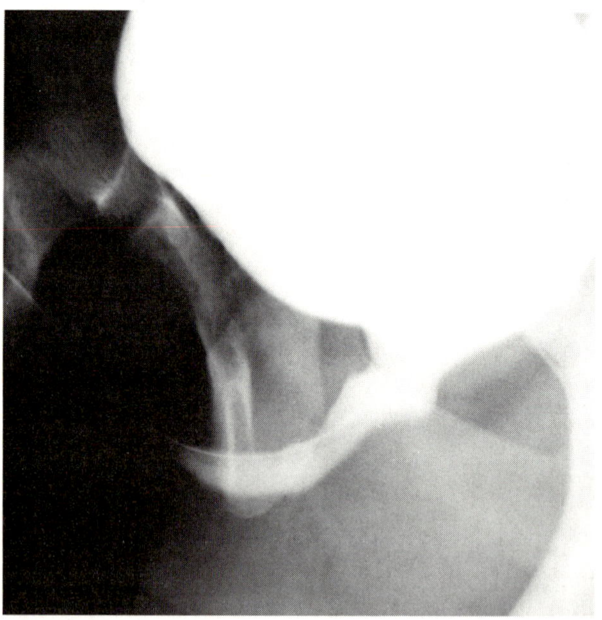

Figure 2 Voiding cystourethrogram in the patient described in Figure 1.

TREATMENT

The preferred treatment is endoscopic with perioperative antibiotics. Urethral dilatation, the standard treatment of centuries, may be effective for a filmy stricture or a very discrete diaphragmatic stricture that, once ruptured, may be unlikely to recur. However, dilatation carries the disadvantage of producing a circumferential urethral injury that may heal by further cicatricial formation. Success rates with dilatation alone range from 20 to 60 percent. Balloon dilatation has the advantage of directing the distention to the specific area of the stricture. This minimizes the longitudinal urethral damage but still creates a short circumferential injury. For a more substantial stricture that involves a longer segment of urethral wall, we utilize internal urethrotomy with sharp cold-knife incisions at the 5, 7, and 12 o'clock positions. Urethrotomy should extend to a point proximal and distal to the breadth of the stricture. To prevent periurethral fluid extravasation, a lubricated Silastic Foley catheter must be passed immediately after the urethrotomy and cystoscope removal. Unless the procedure is unusually difficult and bloody, the catheter is left in place for 48 hours and oral antibiotics are continued for 5 days. To eliminate the risk of recurrence, the urethra is sounded in the clinic at 2 weeks, 1 month, 2 months, 4 months, 8 months and 1 year. Alternatively, older boys can be monitored by uroflowmetry.

RECURRENT STRICTURES

A first recurrence is treated by repeat internal urethrotomy. Percutaneous or endoscopic steroid injection into the strictured area with a fine needle at the time of repeat urethrotomy may prevent restricture. If recurrences persist, daily intermittent urethral catheterization prevents contraction of the damaged lumen during wound healing until the lumen is stable. In young boys, however, daily calibration may be unwelcome. For a very short segment of recurrent stricture, resection and end-to-end urethral anastomosis may solve the problem. One must be certain that the urethral edges anastomosed are healthy. In occasional situations, temporary proximal diversion and two-stage Johanson urethroplasty is necessary. In the first stage, healthy urethra proximal to the stricture is identified and marsupialized to the skin. The incision is carried distally through the stricture, which is also marsupialized. After an interval in excess of 6 months, the urethra is reconstructed by means of simple closure or substitution urethroplasty.

FOLLOW-UP

The success of any treatment for urethral stricture cannot be ascertained in a few months of follow-up. The patients must be followed through childhood, although we do not believe follow-up urethrography to be necessary unless coexistent vesicoureteral reflux is under surveillance. Young children should undergo periodic urethral calibration and older children may be monitored by uroflowmetry. Renewed symptoms, urinary infection, or hematuria should prompt re-evaluation. Urethrography, either antegrade or retrograde, will document recurrence of the lesion. In a child with a history of stricture and recurrent symptoms, direct cystourethroscopy with provision for internal urethrotomy is a reasonable approach, obviating repetitive and unpleasant diagnostic interventions and radiation.

Acknowledgement. The authors thank Dr. Michael L. Ritchey for his help with this manuscript.

SUGGESTED READING

Bloom DA, Foster WD, McLeod DG, et al. Cost-effective uroflowmetry in men. J Urol 1985; 133:421–424.

Cobb BG, Wolf JA Jr, Ansell JS. Congenital stricture of the proximal urethral bulb. J Urol 1968; 99:629–631.

Currarino G, Stephens FD. An uncommon type of bulbar stricture, sometimes familial, of unknown cause: congenital versus acquired. J Urol 1981; 126:658–662.

English PJ, Pyror JP. Congenital bulbar urethral stricture occurring in a father and a son. Br J Urol 1986; 58:732.

Gibbons DM, Koontz WW, Smith MJ. Urethral strictures in boys. J Urol 1979; 121:217–220.

Harshman MW, Cromie WJ, Wein AJ, Duckett JW. Urethral stricture disease in children. J Urol 1981; 126:650–654.

Jones DJ. Congenital bulbar urethral stricture. Br J Urol 1987; 60:186.

Kaplan GW, Brock WA. Urethral strictures in children. J Urol 1983; 129:1200–1203.

Netto NRJ, Martucci RC, Goncalves ES, Freire JC. Congenital stricture of male urethra. Int Urol Nephrol 1976; 8:55–61.

Redman JF, Fraser CP. Apparent congenital anterior urethral stricture in brothers. J Urol 1979; 122:707–708.

POSTERIOR URETHRAL VALVES

PATRICK C. CARTWRIGHT, M.D.
JOHN W. DUCKETT, M.D.

Posterior urethral valves represent the most common cause of lower urinary tract obstruction in boys. It occurs in approximately one of every 5,000 male births and may result from abnormal persistence of the distal portion of the Wolffian system. Typical valves (type I) are membranous leaflets of varying thickness extending distally from the verumontanum onto the lateral urethral walls and fusing anteriorly proximal to the external sphincter.

All portions of the urinary tract proximal to the obstructing valves may be abnormal. The abnormality ranges in severity from prostatic urethral dilatation with only mild trabeculation of the bladder to the more common picture of severe bladder trabeculation, vesicoureteral reflux, tremendous hydroureteronephrosis, and varying degrees of renal insufficiency. Management of valves remains a fascinating and complex problem. During a career, every urologist will see boys with posterior urethral valves, and a solid knowledge of basic management principles is mandatory. This chapter details the practical aspects of our approach to such patients (Fig. 1).

INITIAL MANAGEMENT

Prenatal

A presumptive ultrasonographic diagnosis of posterior urethral valves may be made in a fetus with a consistently distended, thickened bladder associated with unilateral or bilateral hydroureteronephrosis. Attempts to decompress the urinary tract of the fetus with posterior urethral valves have been made either with a vesicoamniotic shunt or with surgical diversion of the urinary tract to the skin.

We consider fetal intervention for presumptive posterior urethral valves to be experimental and not applicable in the standard clinical situation. There are several reasons for this belief: (1) substantial risk to mother and fetus, (2) diagnostic error of up to 20 percent, (3) the rarity of true oligohydramnios in these patients, and (4) unproven benefit. It must be realized that the severely affected fetus with oligohydramnios will not be detected before midpregnancy; at this point, there generally is severe renal dysplasia, which is not likely to respond to bladder decompression. When the pros and cons are weighed, fetal intervention for valves is not our management choice at this time.

Ideally, a baby with suspected posterior urethral valves should be delivered in or very near a facility ready to provide care, thus avoiding a long journey for a potentially ill neonate. There is no reason to consider early delivery of a fetus with suspected posterior urethral valves.

Neonatal

Most of these patients are seen as neonates, many with prenatal diagnoses. Owing to the homeostatic effect of the placenta, these newborns are generally metabolically stable at birth. Significant renal insufficiency, present in 10 to 20 percent, may result in rapid deterioration after birth, and daily tests of electrolytes and creatinine values are necessary. An occasional boy with posterior valves has severe renal dysplasia associated with pulmonary hypoplasia and may die rapidly from respiratory failure. The neonate with posterior urethral valves not diagnosed prenatally may present with a palpable bladder, palpable hydronephrotic kidneys, a dribbling stream, a urinary tract infection or sepsis, failure to thrive, or ascites.

Bladder drainage is established in boys suspected of having posterior urethral valves. We use a No. 6 or 8 French feeding tube taped (using benzoin) to the penis and suprapubic area. A Foley catheter should be avoided, since the balloon may cause intense bladder spasm with resultant complete ureteral obstruction. Catheterization may sometimes be difficult owing to the dilated prostatic urethra and hypertrophied bladder neck deflecting the catheter posteriorly. If this is a problem, a finger in the rectum will push the posterior wall of the prostatic fossa anteriorly while passing the catheter. If this is still unsuccessful, a stylet can be fashioned out of a piece of 22-gauge surgical stainless steel wire and placed into the lumen of the feeding tube with a coudé bend at the tip. With the tip directed anteriorly, the bladder neck can often be negotiated. The catheter should never be forced if not passing easily. Alternatively, percutaneous suprapubic tube drainage can be established.

Through the bladder catheter a voiding cystourethrogram (VCU) is obtained. This shows the dilated prostatic urethra, trabeculated bladder, and prominent bladder neck and any associated vesicoureteral reflux (50 percent) (Fig. 2). Retrograde urethrography does not suffice for diagnosis. Renal ultrasonography is used to assess the degree of hydroureteronephrosis, the amount of renal parenchyma present, and its echogenicity and differentiation.

Newborns presenting with or developing significant renal insufficiency require meticulous metabolic care to minimize acidosis, hyperkalemia, and disorders of hydration. Bladder drainage may result in rapid postobstructive diuresis in an azotemic patient, requiring salt and water replacement intravenously. A persistent diuresis associated with escalating hypernatremia suggests obstruction-induced renal tubular insensitivity to antidiuretic hormone. These children must receive free water replacement and be followed closely with frequent weighing, since losses greater than 5 to 10 percent of body weight may cause hypovolemic shock.

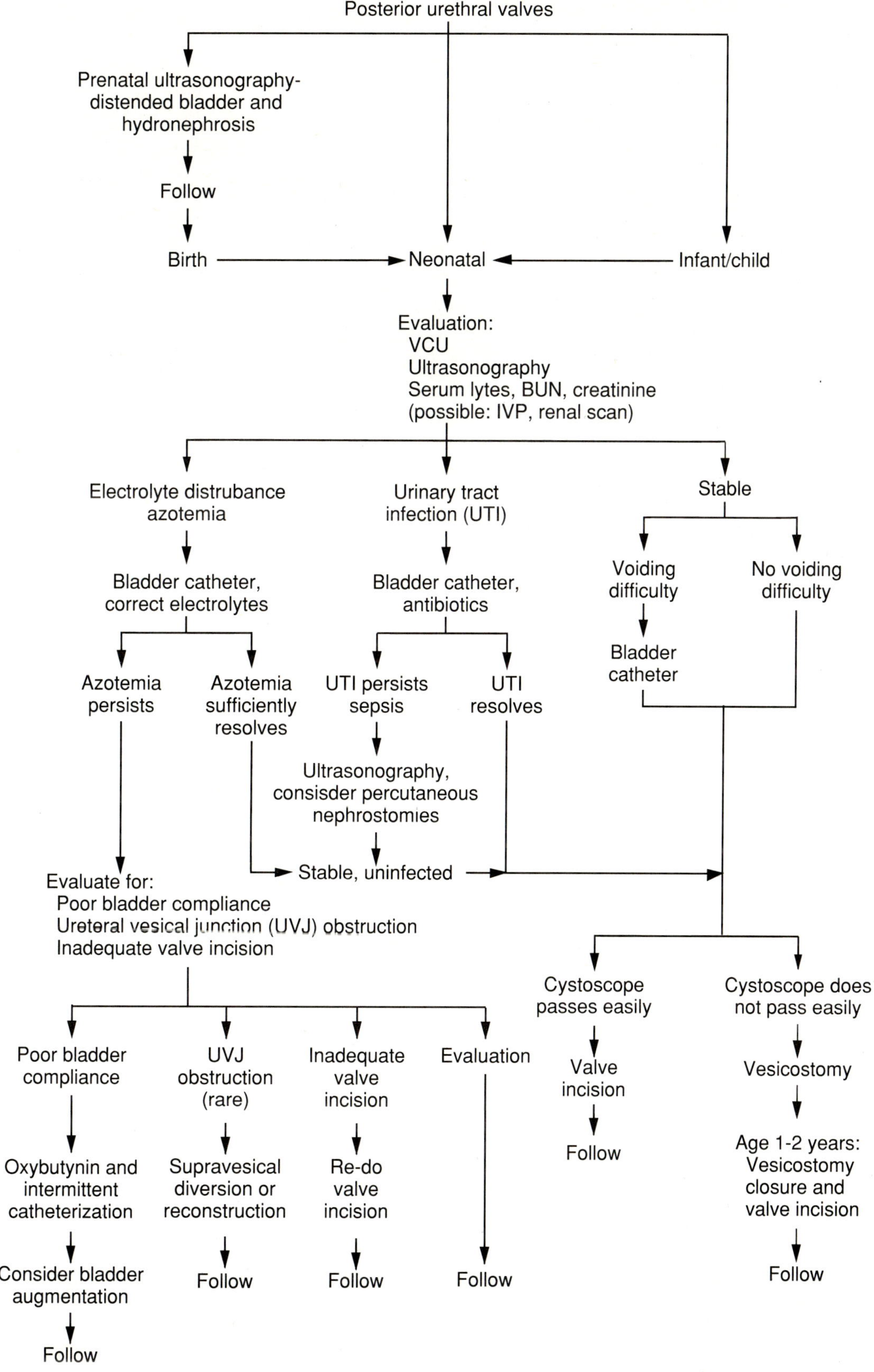

Figure 1 Treatment algorithm for posterior urethral valves.

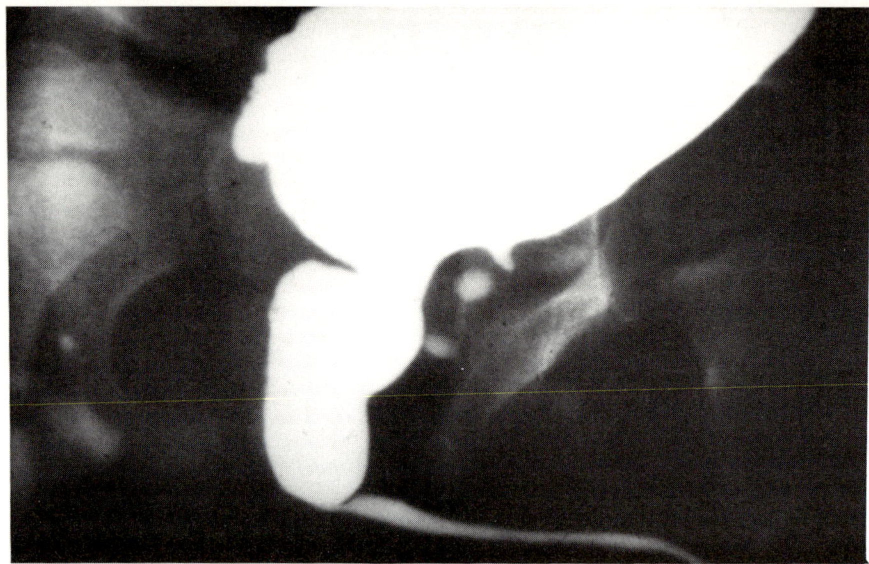

Figure 2 Voiding cystourethrogram in a patient with posterior urethral valves. Note the distended prostatic urethra with a normal-caliber urethra distally.

Boys presenting with urinary infection should be started on gentamicin and ampicillin to cover gram-negative organisms as well as enterococcus. This regimen may be used in neonates with renal insufficiency if gentamicin is redosed on the basis of serum levels. Purulent debris in the dilated upper tracts of a septic child may occasionally require percutaneous nephrostomy drainage for a good response. Those presenting without clinical infection should be started on penicillin VK prophylaxis at 15,000 U per kilogram once daily. Those older than 6 weeks at diagnosis can start on sulfamethoxasole-trimethoprim (SMX-TMP), 0.25 ml per kilogram once daily, or nitrofurantoin, 1.5 mg per kilogram once daily.

After stabilization of the child, the primary surgical therapy should be directed toward relief of the urethral valvular obstruction without regard to the severity of upper tract dilatation. Neonatal endoscopes as small as 7.5 to 8 Fr with a 3 Fr working channel make safe endoscopic valve incision possible in most neonates. No dilatation of the urethra should be performed if these small instruments do not pass readily. The cystoscope is passed and the valve cusps are evaluated. These may be very translucent and filmy or at times thickened with substantial tissue. There is fusion anteriorly, which is the primary portion of the valve that must be incised. Others have advocated destruction of the valve cusps at the 5 and 7 o'clock positions as well. If the urethra allows passage of an infant resectoscope (11 Fr or larger), a resecting loop bent together into a hook shape is very suitable for assessing and incising the valves (as described in the following section).

In most newborn males, the urethra does not accept the infant resectoscope; the smaller neonatal scope with a 3 Fr Bugbee electrode through the working channel can be used in these cases. The valve is best incised by placing the instrument at the external sphincter and advancing the Bugbee electrode a few millimeters beyond so that the cutting tip can be well seen. The cautery is set on a "pure cut" mode. The valve can then be ablated in the midline anteriorly in small bites, advancing the electrode and cystoscope as one unit toward the bladder neck. This allows for controlled division of the valve without pulling the cutting electrode toward the external sphincter. The valve incision should be carried down to where the apex is flush with the anterior urethral wall. The electrode can be pulled gently along the anterior urethra to see whether there is still any irregularity or bump indicating incomplete valve incision. Deeper incision into the urethral wall will predispose to stricture. Once the valve appears incised, suprapubic bladder compression should yield a strong urinary stream. It is optional to leave a catheter in place overnight or use no bladder drainage at all.

Occasionally, in premature or small neonates, the urethra will not readily accept any cystoscope. In the past, a perineal urethrotomy was performed through which the cystoscope could be placed. We prefer instead not to risk any injury to the urethra, but to divert the urinary tract by means of a vesicostomy. This can be done through a small transverse lower abdominal incision midway between the umbilicus and pubis. The bladder dome is mobilized and matured to the fascia and skin as a vesicostomy. It is crucial to bring out the dome and not the anterior bladder wall so that prolapse of the vesicostomy does not occur. Identifying the urachus is valuable in ensuring that the dome is brought out. Comparison studies have shown a similar clinical course between patients diverted with a vesicostomy and those undergoing primary valve incision. We prefer valve incision when possible, but vesicostomy remains an adequate temporizing procedure in children with a small-caliber urethra. Vesicostomy is also an appropriate procedure for the surgeon who is unfamiliar with urethral valve resection or is without proper cystoscopic equipment.

When the patient is approximately 1 year of age, the vesicostomy can be closed at the same time the valves are incised. It is not appropriate, however, to concomitantly create a vesicostomy and incise the valves. This commonly results in stricturing in the area of the valve resection. Antegrade valve resection by going through the vesicostomy with a cystoscope has been reported but is not generally applicable.

Postoperatively, patients are observed for the presence of a continually distended bladder or any difficulty with voiding. In addition, some patients need to be maintained on bicarbonate replacement owing to their renal insufficiency. These boys are continued on prophylactic doses of antibiotics to maintain sterile urine. In general, cystography is performed at 6 weeks after valve incision to assess the urethra and the degree of reflux, and also ultrasonography to evaluate the upper tract dilatation.

Infants and Children

Boys whose condition is not detected during the neonatal period will present later with clinical signs of urinary tract infection, failure to thrive, daytime wetting, straining to void, weak stream, signs of renal failure, or a suprapubic mass. Endoscopic incision of the valves is virtually always possible since the urethra is of adequate caliber. The initial assessment and management is otherwise much like that for younger patients.

The infant resectoscope is positioned just proximal to the external urethral sphincter, and the resectoscope loop (bent into a hook) is passed through the opening in the valve and then drawn back distally, engaging the valve cusp in the anterior midline. With the cautery set on a "pure cut" mode, the foot pedal is tapped until the loop resects through the valve tissue. This is done in small bites until the apex of the incision is flush with the anterior wall of the urethra. With an adequate destruction, the hooked loop should draw back toward the scope without catching on any lip of tissue.

Once valves are incised in a boy, the relationship between the urologist and the patient has just begun. Proper follow-up is vital as many complications of posterior urethral valves may occur over time.

PROBLEMS ASSOCIATED WITH POSTERIOR URETHRAL VALVES

Inadequate Valve Incision

It can be difficult to judge the adequacy of valve resection in the operating room. An "on-the-table" postoperative compression cystourethrogram should generally show a decompressed prostatic urethra with a distended anterior urethra distal to the valves if valve incision is adequate. Complete bladder emptying and resolution of the marked hydroureteronephrosis as shown by ultrasonography support adequate valve incision, as does a drop in the creatinine level. Resolution of reflux (25 percent) may take longer to become evident, and chemoprophylaxis should continue.

Findings that arouse suspicion for inadequate valve incision include persistently distended bladder, recurring urinary tract infection, and persistent hydronephrosis or elevated creatinine.

It is usually best not to rush back to the operating room too quickly unless the clinical picture clearly points to a problem. A few months of observation generally will allow the patient to declare whether urethral obstruction still exists.

Persistent Hydronephrosis

The vast majority of patients with posterior valves start with severe hydroureteronephrosis. Although obstruction may be relieved shortly after birth, most valve ureters remain somewhat atonic and dilated. However, it is a rare ureter that is truly obstructed and in need of surgical intervention.

As described before, our first intervention without regard to the degree of hydronephrosis is valve incision or vesicostomy to divert the lower tract. A few patients (<10 percent) with persistent hydronephrosis associated with recurring infection or elevated creatinine levels benefit from a higher urinary diversion. This generally consists of bilateral pyelostomies or high-loop cutaneous ureterostomies. In patients coming to high diversion, we have generally found the prognosis to be poor, with renal biopsies at the time of high diversion confirming significant dysplasia or renal damage.

When the decision is difficult, a renal scan with Lasix wash-out can be helpful in assessing the degree of obstruction. It is crucial to remember that the full bladder in a valve patient can functionally obstruct the outflow from the ureter. Placement of a catheter to drain the bladder at the time of the study is important. A pressure perfusion study is often misleading in this situation.

Reflux

Fifty percent of these patients at diagnosis have reflux, either unilateral or bilateral. After valve incision, 25 percent of these have spontaneous resolution. The VURD syndrome occurs in about 20 percent of patients: a combination of posterior urethral *v*alves, *u*nilateral *r*eflux, and renal *d*ysplasia on the refluxing side. The left kidney is involved in 80 percent of cases and is often nonfunctioning. A nephroureterectomy at some point to improve voiding dynamics and to remove a reservoir for recurrent infections is appropriate. The VURD syndrome appears to be a protective phenomenon. The uninvolved kidney is often minimally hydronephrotic and functions very well owing to the "pop off" protection from intravesical pressure offered by the enormous refluxing system on one side.

Patients with reflux into functioning kidneys are maintained on prophylactic antibiotics, and many of these resolve over time. If recurrent infections are present, reimplantation is usually recommended. Reimplantation of a dilated ureter that may require tapering into a trabeculated, thickened valve bladder carries a lower success rate (70 to 80 percent) than a reimplant into a normal bladder.

Recurrent Urinary Tract Infection

Recurrent urinary tract infections may reflect persistent obstruction at some level. Incomplete bladder emptying with persistent ureteral obstruction is usually the problem. Recurrent infections therefore elicit a urodynamic work-up to assess possible obstruction, along with a diuretic renal scan and a VCU.

Incontinence

Transient incontinence is fairly common after valve incision. It has been shown that with careful technique there is rarely injury to the external sphincter. Persistent incontinence may be related to poor sensation of bladder fullness or myotonic failure with resultant overflow incontinence. In addition, uninhibited bladder contraction may be present with resultant urge incontinence. Urodynamic assessment of the bladder is important in patients with incontinence, as discussed below.

Bladder Dysfunction

About 10 percent of patients with posterior urethral valves eventually have significant bladder dysfunction. This should be suspected in patients with persistent incontinence, urinary frequency or urgency, poor stream, increasing hydronephrosis, worsening renal function, or recurrent bladder infections. The pattern of incontinence may be stress, urge, or constant dribbling. These patients need urodynamic evaluation to evaluate the storage capacities of the bladder and assess for hyperreflexia, myotonic failure, and poor compliance. Those with hyperreflexia can often be treated successfully with oxybutynin. Intermittent catheterization is appropriate in patients with myotonic failure. Those with poor compliance may develop what is described as the "full valve bladder" syndrome with resultant hydroureteronephrosis due to persistently elevated intravesical pressures. Oxybutynin and intermittent catheterization may be adequate in some patients, but others will require bladder augmentation to ensure low-pressure storage of an adequate urine volume.

Urethral Stricture

Urethral stricture after valve incision has become less common with the use of smaller cystoscopes, and occurs in very few patients. In the past, strictures were noted in the distal or bulbous urethra as a result of dilatation or trauma in passing the scope or a catheter. Stricture may occur at the site of valve resection if a deep coagulating current is used or if the valve is incised before establishing urine flow with a vesicostomy or ureterostomy.

Postoperative strictures can be diagnosed by retrograde urethrography. These strictures are treated like other traumatic strictures: visual internal urethrotomy is the first step, followed by open procedures if needed.

Renal Insufficiency and Failure

Up to 30 percent of patients with posterior valves develop renal insufficiency or failure. A few patients with severe renal insufficiency die shortly after birth from the associated pulmonary hypoplasia. A second group of patients have reasonable pulmonary function but severe renal insufficiency, which is evident during the first few weeks of life. These patients must be followed closely, along with the pediatric nephrologist, using dietary manipulations and appropriate medications to control their hyperkalemia and acidosis. Adequate dependable urinary tract decompression is essential, and these are some of the few patients whom we consider for upper tract diversion. These children may progress toward renal failure within the first month or years of life and require dialysis or transplantation. The third group of patients are those who have moderate renal insufficiency during their first years of life, but good urinary tract drainage overall. As they progress through puberty and acquire more body mass, they often suffer progressive renal insufficiency, and they may need transplantation or dialysis toward the end of puberty or early in adulthood. Unfortunately, a slightly poorer graft survival is reported in posterior valve patients undergoing renal transplantation than in the other transplant groups, perhaps because of poor bladder function.

Despite the renal insufficiency present in up to 30 percent of these patients, it should be remembered that the other 70 percent maintain adequate or borderline renal function throughout their lifetime with avoidance of urinary infections and proper overall management. Some dietary restriction of protein is probably advisable for the future in light of the popular hyperfiltration theory of renal stress.

SUGGESTED READING

Duckett JW, Snow BW. Disorders of the urethra and penis. In: Campbell's urology. 5th ed. Philadelphia: WB Saunders, 1986.

Glassberg K. Current issues regarding posterior urethral valves. Urol Clin North Am 1985; 12.

Peters C, et al. The urodynamic consequences of posterior urethral valves. J Urol 1990; 144:122.

Rittenberg MH, et al. Protective factors in posterior urethral valves. J Urol 1988; 140:993.

Warshaw BL, et al. Prognostic features in infants with obstructive uropathy due to posterior urethral valves. J Urol 1985; 133:240.

ANTERIOR URETHRAL VALVES

R. LAWRENCE KROOVAND, M.D.

The congenital anterior urethral valve is an uncommon cause of infravesical urinary obstruction in boys. The differentiation between the anterior urethral valve and the anterior urethral diverticulum appears one of semantics, although the anterior urethral valve in the fossa navicularis may be embryologically different from that in the penile or bulbous urethra. For the purpose of this discussion, the terms "anterior urethral valve" and "anterior urethral diverticulum" are synonymous. Forty percent of anterior urethral valves occur in the bulbous urethra, 30 percent at the penoscrotal junction, and 30 percent in the penile urethra; they are uncommon in the fossa navicularis.

The anterior urethral valve in the fossa navicularis appears the result of failure of the invaginating ectoderm of the glanular urethra to merge perfectly with the distal advancing urethral plate; urethral canalization may then produce a flap or diaphragm that could obstruct the urinary stream. The etiology of the anterior urethral valve in the penile or bulbous urethra is also uncertain, but may be accounted for if an anterior urethral diverticulum undermines the distal penile urethra, creating a "valvelike" distal lip that may obstruct the urinary stream. Anterior urethral diverticula may develop when there is a defect in development of the corpus spongiosum because of incomplete migration and midline fusion of the spongious tissue from the inner genital folds, resulting in an abnormal support to penile urethra and corpus spongiosum and the potential for outpouching and diverticulum formation.

DIAGNOSIS

Most important in management of the anterior urethral valve is a timely and accurate diagnosis. A minimally obstructive valve may produce few if any symptoms and is generally discovered in childhood during evaluation for voiding dysfunction. Other anterior urethral valves may cause severe urinary outlet obstruction and upper tract deterioration and be complicated by urosepsis. Such anterior urethral valves are most often diagnosed during the neonatal period or in infancy.

It is the signs and symptoms of urinary outlet obstruction that most often prompt urologic investigation. Penile or perineal swelling during voiding, a poor urinary stream, postvoid dribbling, failure to thrive, or recurrent urinary tract infection may also indicate a need for urologic investigation and lead to the diagnosis of an anterior urethral valve. In my experience, the voiding cystourethrogram with oblique voiding films has proved the most accurate and reliable uroradiographic study to identify the anterior urethral valve. Anterior urethral valves are often missed during examination of the urethra, which may appear normal unless the entire urethra, from the membranous portion to the external urethral meatus, is included in all uroradiographic studies. Unfortunately it is a common error to omit this portion of the male urethra from voiding uroradiographic studies. Voiding cystourethrography also defines the status of the bladder and any vesicoureteral reflux present. Retrograde urethrography frequently does not define the anterior urethral valve, because the retrograde introduction of contrast material tends to flatten out the valve lip against the urethral mucosa, making identification of the valve difficult if not impossible. Similarly, cystourethroscopy may fail to demonstrate the presence of an anterior urethral valve, as the valve lip tends to flatten out against the urethral mucosa during examination. If the working port of the cystourethroscope is left in the open position, expression of the distended bladder while the cystourethroscope is withdrawn from the urethra permits antegrade flow of irrigant down the urethra, potentially elevating the valve lip and permitting identification of the anterior urethral valve. In addition to voiding cystourethrography and cystourethroscopy, an evaluation of the upper urinary tract by intravenous pyelography (IVP), isotope renography, or renal ultrasonography should be made.

TREATMENT

Management of boys with an anterior urethral valve requires surgical ablation of the valve and possibly also the associated diverticulum, especially if it is large or traps urine. The method of and urgency for management of the anterior urethral valve differ, depending on the age and clinical situation of the child at the time of diagnosis. For the minimally symptomatic older child with an anterior urethral valve in the fossa navicularis, management is either by endoscopic cauterization (incision) or by sharp excision. Endoscopic incision or ablation of the anterior urethral valve in the distal urethra or fossa navicularis may be difficult owing to the anatomic location of the valve. The infant resectoscope with a fulgurating electrode is used to stroke the urethral surface gently and engage the valve lip. Incision of the valve lip with cutting current electrocoagulation will disrupt the tissue and relieve any obstruction present. Since stricture formation is a considerable risk after any fulguration procedure in the anterior urethra, the same care and finesse required for treatment of posterior urethral valves is mandatory when the anterior urethral valve is endoscopically ablated. The proper-size cystourethroscope or resectoscope must be used to prevent iatrogenic urethral injury. The cutting current used should be the minimal current necessary to incise the valve lip. Incision into the wall of the corpus spongiosum or glanular tissue must be avoided to prevent excessive bleeding or extravasation of urine and the potential for stricture formation. In some situations, a crochet hook may be used to engage the valve lip and prolapse it through the urethral meatus, permitting sharp excision.

For infants or neonates with moderate-to-severe urinary outlet obstruction and/or urosepsis, urinary diversion in the form of temporary transurethral catheter drainage and metabolic stabilization is generally prudent, delaying surgical management until they are clinically and metabolically stable and reconstructive surgery is more appropriate. After a period of transurethral drainage, the degree of decompression of the urinary upper tract may be determined with ultrasonography. When the upper tract is well decompressed after initial catheter drainage and the anterior urethral valve is associated with a large diverticulum, simple marsupialization of the diverticulum (cutaneous urethrostomy) provides prolonged nonintubated relief of outlet obstruction and reduces the risk of serious urosepsis, while permitting growth and development before definitive management. Some infants do not maintain appropriate upper tract decompression after cutaneous urethrostomy or may develop recurrent urosepsis, but may progress satisfactorily after a cutaneous vesicostomy. For cutaneous vesicostomy I prefer the Blocksom technique, which is simple and easy to perform. This technique does not produce significant surgical change in the bladder and is easy to reverse. Cutaneous vesicostomy should be performed only if preliminary transurethral catheter drainage improves upper tract drainage. If the upper urinary tract remains dilated after a period of transurethral drainage, or if cutaneous vesicostomy is unsuccessful in eliminat-

ing urinary infection or upper track dilatation, high urinary diversion (cutaneous pyelostomy) should be considered.

An alternative management approach in the minimally symptomatic infant with an anterior valve and a large anterior urethral diverticulum is a primary one-stage reconstruction excising the obstructing valve lip combined with reduction urethroplasty, resecting all redundant urethral tissue.

Once the diverted child is medically stable and a period of growth and development has been achieved, urinary tract reconstruction and surgical management of the anterior urethral valve and any problematic anterior urethral diverticulum is appropriate. Before closure of a cutaneous pyelostomy, an antegrade pyelogram should be obtained to evaluate ureteral peristalsis and ureteral obstruction and the appropriateness of urinary undiversion. Voiding cystourethrography should also be performed so that any persistent vesicoureteral reflux can be corrected simultaneously with other reconstructive procedures. I advocate a one-stage reconstruction: reversal of the upper tract diversion (vesicostomy, pyelostomies), correction of any ureteral obstruction or vesicoureteral reflux present, and urethroplasty with excision of the valve lip and resection of the "associated" anterior urethral diverticulum and urethral reconstruction. Postoperative urinary diversion is generally transurethral, employing a C-splint and urethral catheter, although suprapubic urinary diversion is also a viable option. The transurethral bladder catheter is removed 3 to 4 days after surgery and the urethral C-splint after 7 to 10 days. The advantage of the C-splint is that it

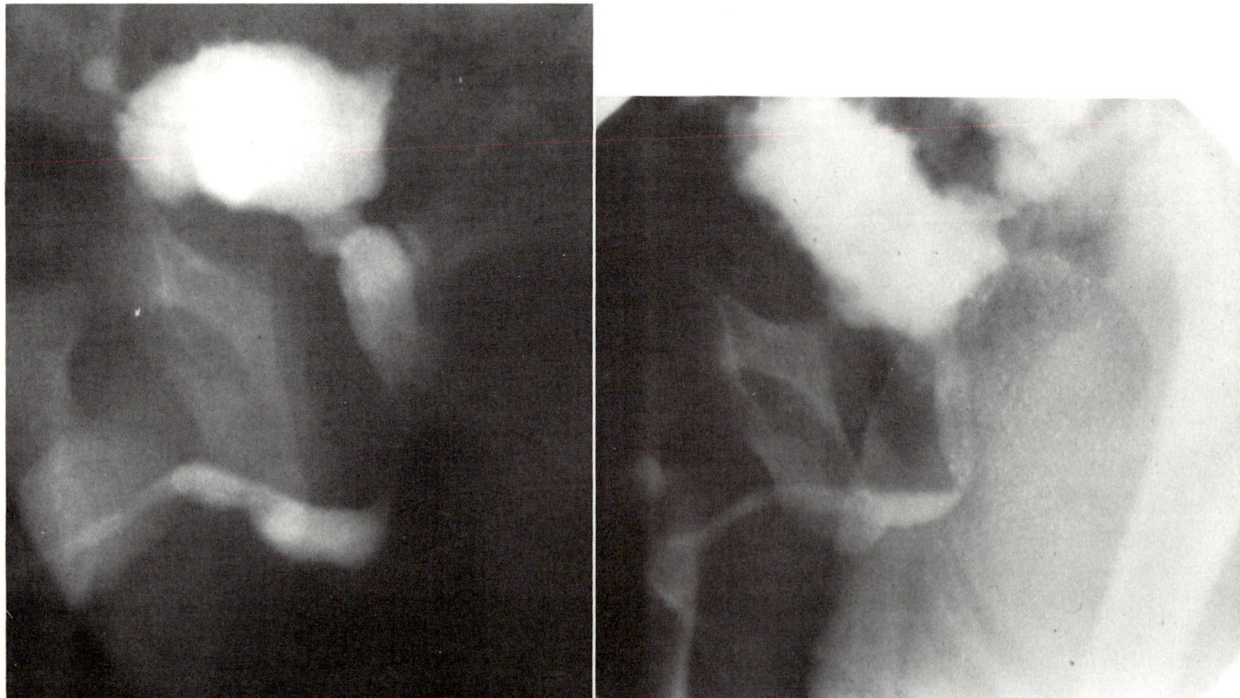

Figure 1 Case 1. *A*, Uroradiograph demonstrating the anterior urethral valve. *B*, Results of endoscopic resection.

provides for prolonged urethral intubation, but because it does not extend into the bladder, urinary tract infection and bladder spasm are infrequent complications. After any major upper tract reconstruction (ureteral tapering, pyeloplasty), the use of pediatric double-pigtail indwelling ureteral stents should be considered. The stents are removed endoscopically 4 to 6 weeks after surgery, when they are no longer necessary.

CASE STUDIES

A high index of suspicion and appropriate uroradiographic investigation should make the diagnosis of the anterior urethral valve a simple task. As outlined, the management of the anterior urethral valve must be individualized and flexible, but is most often straightforward and governed by the basic principles of reconstructive pediatric urology. The following three cases demonstrate individual application of the principles discussed above.

Case 1

A 10-year-old boy presented with dysuria and hesitancy. Physical examination was unremarkable. A microscopic urine sample contained an occasional white cell. A urine culture was negative. Uroradiographic evaluation demonstrated an anterior urethral valve with mild bulbous urethral dilatation (Fig. 1A) and minimal bladder trabeculation. Endoscopic resection of the valve lip produced resolution of the voiding symptoms and the urethral uroradiographic findings, although mild bladder trabeculation persisted. Long-term follow-up has been satisfactory (Fig. 1B).

Case 2

Pediatric urologic consultation was requested to evaluate a newborn male born with imperforate anus and an abnormal-appearing penis. On physical examination, in addition to the imperforate anus, the child had a large saccular dilatation of the urethra, dorsal glanular chordee, and a bifid scrotum (Fig. 2A). Renal ultrasonography demonstrated absence of the right kidney and a normal-appearing left kidney without evidence of hydronephrosis or ureteral dilatation. Voiding cystourethrography demonstrated a normal bladder without evidence of vesicoureteral reflux. Urethral films demonstrated an anterior urethral valve associated with a large anterior urethral diverticulum (Fig. 2B).

Transurethral catheter drainage provided initial urinary drainage, but because of intercurrent medical problems initial management was by marsupialization of the anterior urethral diverticulum (cutaneous urethrostomy) and subsequently by open excision of the valve lip and excess urethra tissue, with urethral reconstruction and sleeve reapproximation of the penile shaft skin. Long-term follow-up has been satisfactory.

Case 3

This premature infant was hospitalized in the neonatal intensive care unit for management of respiratory distress and sepsis. The urethra was noted to bulge on voiding with only a dribbling urinary stream. On examination, a bulge was noted on the ventral surface of the penis (Fig. 3A). Plain abdominal films demonstrated evidence of a resolving right-sided adrenal hemorrhage. Voiding cystourethrography demonstrated bilateral and vesicoureteral reflux (Fig. 3B). Voiding films demon-

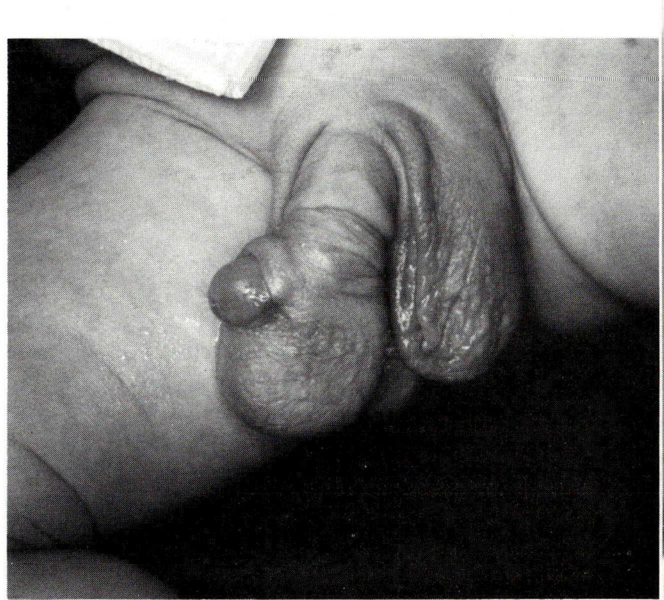
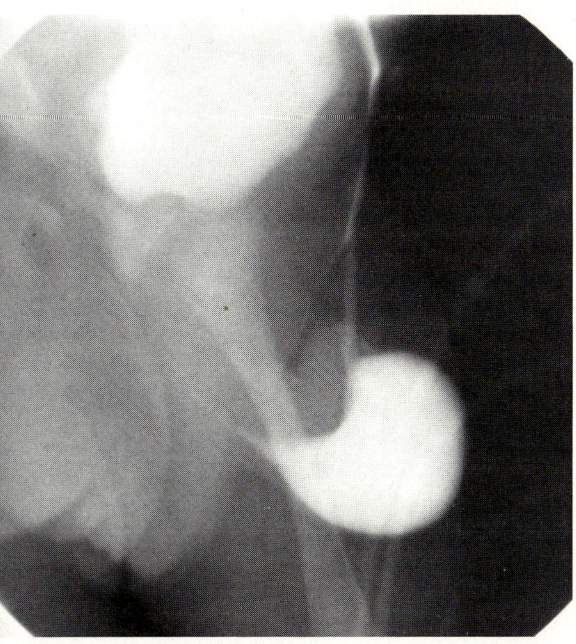

Figure 2   Case 2. *A,* Newborn infant with saccular dilatation of the urethra, dorsal glanular chordee, and bifid scrotum. *B,* Anterior urethral valve and diverticulum in the same infant.

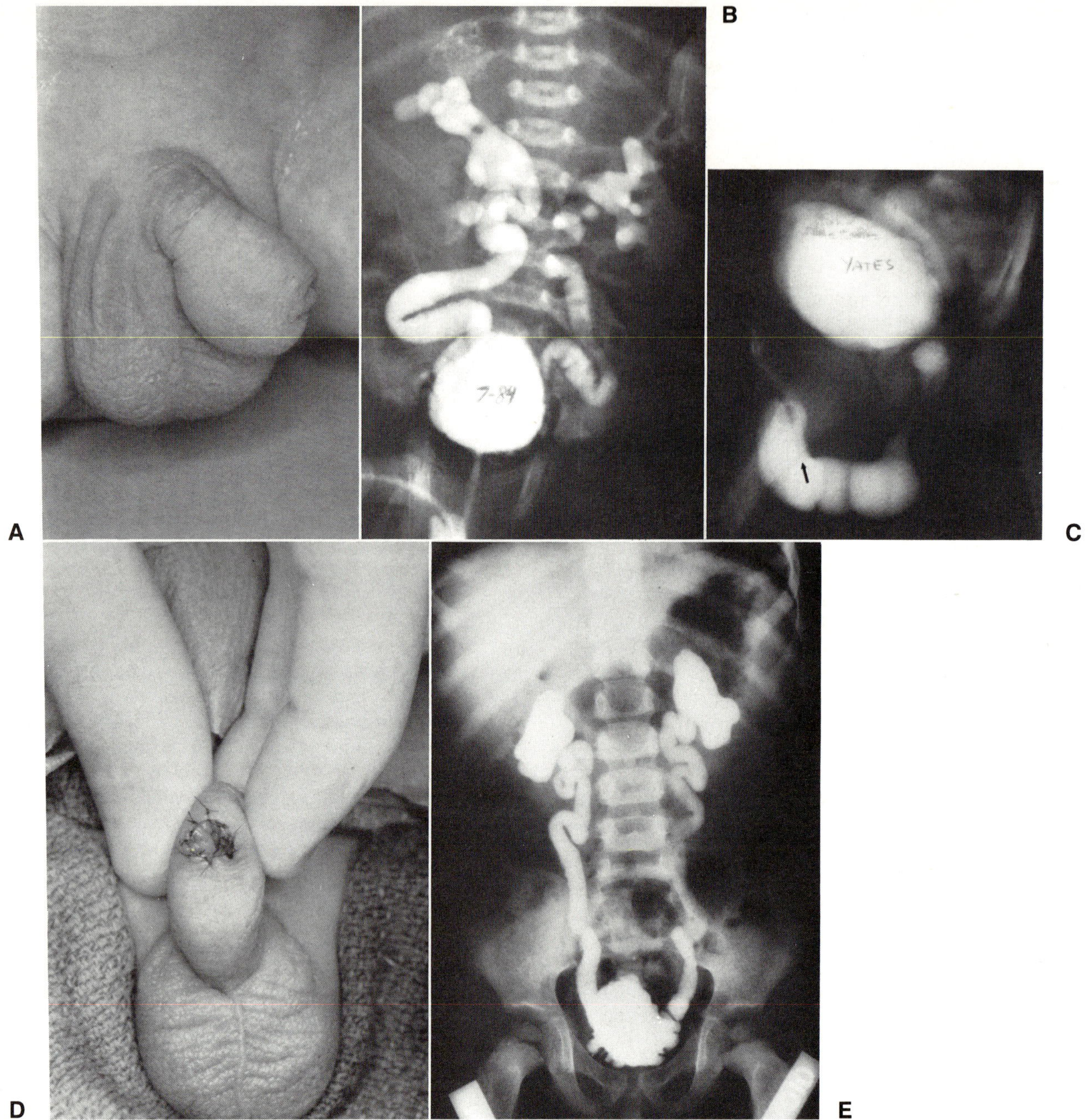

Figure 3 Case 3. *A,* Bulge on the ventral surface of the penis in a premature infant. *B,* Bilateral, vesicoureteral reflux demonstrated by voiding cystourethrography. *C,* Anterior urethral diverticulum as seen on voiding films. *D,* Cutaneous urethrostomy. *E,* Lessening of vesicoureteral reflux after urethrostomy.

strated a large anterior urethral diverticulum undermining the distal urethra (Fig. 3*C*). The valve lip is identified by the arrow. Isotope renography demonstrated nonfunction of the right kidney with excellent function of the left kidney.

After initial transurethral catheter drainage and upper tract decompression, the diverticulum was marsupialized (cutaneous urethrostomy) (Fig. 3*D*). Follow-up uroradiographic studies demonstrated a lessening but persistence of the vesicoureteral reflux (Fig. 3*E*). Because of recurrent urosepsis, the child underwent a right nephroureterectomy and a cutaneous vesicostomy. The recurrent urosepsis resolved and the upper tract changes on the left improved. Subsequently a left ureteral reimplantation, open excision of the valve lip, and a reduction urethroplasty (to manage the large, poorly draining anterior urethral diverticulum) produced a satisfactory long-term outcome.

SUGGESTED READING

Chaviano AH, Firlit CF. Anterior urethral valves. In: Resnick MI, Kursh E, eds. Current therapy in genitourinary surgery. Philadelphia: BC Decker, 1987:261.

Lewis E, Palmer J. Anterior urethral valves. Urology 1981; 18:494.
Scherz HC, Kaplan GW, Packer MG. Anterior urethral valves in the fossa navicularis in children. J Urol 1987; 138:1211.
Tank ES. Anterior urethral valves resulting from congenital urethral diverticula. Urology 1987; 30:467.

URETHRAL DIVERTICULA IN FEMALES

ELROY D. KURSH, M.D.

The incidence of urethral diverticula in women may be higher than suspected, but the true incidence is unknown. They usually present in the third or fourth decades of life and may be single or multiple. Their size varies from 0.5 to 6 cm; most are 2 to 3 cm. The ostia are almost always located posteriorly in the urethra. Finger-like projections may dissect around the urethra or under the base of the bladder, which may complicate the surgical excision. The contents of the sac consist of urine, pus, stones, or debris.

CLINICAL PRESENTATION AND PATIENT SELECTION

The most characteristic symptoms of urethral diverticula are postmicturition dribbling and the expression of pus or urine from the urethral meatus when pressure is placed on the suburethral mass, such as during intercourse. In fact, few patients present with these symptoms and most complain of nonspecific urologic problems, the most common being dysuria and frequency. Other commonly reported symptoms are refractory cystitis, urgency, dyspareunia, hematuria, urethral pain, and the patient's observation of an anterior vaginal wall mass. The association of stress urinary incontinence is generally reported to vary between 12 and 30 percent of cases, but has been noted to be as high as 70 percent. One recent series emphasized that a surprising number of patients presented with urinary incontinence as the only complaint. Hematuria deserves special attention, since it is observed more frequently in patients with carcinoma arising in a urethral diverticulum.

By far the most important factor in establishing a diagnosis of urethral diverticulum is awareness of the entity. The urethra should be examined routinely, especially in patients with rapidly recurring urinary tract infections. The most common finding is induration or palpation of a mass beneath or lateral to the urethra. The urethra and anterior vaginal wall are stripped with the examining finger while the urethral meatus is observed for discharge consisting of pus, blood, or urine. Unfortunately, the expression of discharge from a urethral diverticulum is not noted nearly as often as most urologists anticipate, despite the fact that they expect this finding to be characteristic or necessary to establish a diagnosis.

In my experience, the most productive diagnostic tool when a urethral diverticulum is suspected is a voiding cystourethrogram (VCU) performed in the standing position under fluoroscopic control. It may also be helpful to occlude the meatus transiently during voiding in an attempt to fill the diverticulum with contrast media. A postvoid film is also particularly helpful in identifying diverticula that may not be seen on other x-ray films during the VCU. Positive-pressure urethrography using either a Davis-TeLinde or a Trattner double-balloon catheter has been thought to be the most reliable radiologic means of establishing the diagnosis of a urethral diverticulum. Realistically, positive-pressure urethrography is somewhat cumbersome to perform and rarely reveals diverticula that are not demonstrable by a standard VCU.

I do not advocate the preoperative urodynamic testing recommended by some authors. It has been suggested that urethral profilometry is a useful screening tool for patients with a urethral diverticulum, since it reveals a typical bicornuate curve. However, this bicornuate curve has been variably noted, and the study cannot be used to confirm with reliability the diagnosis of a urethral diverticulum. I also do not consider urodynamics helpful in discerning which patients may benefit from a concomitant urethropexy, preferring to rely on the history and physical findings. It has been demonstrated that the distributional overlap in urethral pressure profile parameters comparing normal females with those who have stress urinary incontinence is too great to make the UPP diagnostically useful. In my opinion, urodynamics and, more specifically, urethral profilometry are useful only in selected patients with urethral diverticula, primarily those with incontinence or symptoms of bladder instability.

TREATMENT

An incidentally discovered diverticulum in an asymptomatic patient requires no treatment, but surgical excision is appropriate in symptomatic women. Although a variety of surgical techniques have been described, I do not believe there is one surgical technique that is suitable for every type of urethral diverticulum. Fibrosis and scarring may make this supposedly simple procedure more difficult than anticipated, and bleeding may be encountered that may be significant at times.

Whichever surgical treatment is chosen, it is important to sterilize the urine preoperatively. Preoperative antibiotics should be administered according to previous culture data; if none are available, broad-spectrum antibiotics are started well before surgery.

Rarely, endoscopic means have been employed to treat urethral diverticula. The basis for endoscopic treatment rests on the creation of a wide-mouthed diverticular cavity to provide free drainage and clearance of infection. This technique is rarely appropriate except to treat a diverticulum in an awkward position such as in the roof of the urethra, particularly if it contains calcifications.

Marsupialization of the sac has been reported; the urethral floor is incised through the level of the urethral diverticulum and the epithelial margins of the urethra and vagina are approximated with a running absorbable suture. In essence, this technique represents a generous distal meatotomy through the diverticulum sac and can be employed only for a distal diverticulum in order to avoid damage to the sphincter mechanism. I prefer to avoid this procedure, since it may result in sphincter damage or lead to urethral shortening, which contributes to the development of stress urinary incontinence, not an infrequent association in these patients. The marsupialization procedure also results in a patulous type of hypospadiac urethral meatus, which can cause spraying of the urinary stream or pseudoincontinence secondary to vaginal filling.

The most popular surgical procedure has been transvaginal excision of the sac. A longitudinal vaginal incision is made and the urethral diverticulum is excised after being carefully dissected from the adjacent tissues. The urethra is closed with fine absorbable suture over an indwelling urethral catheter. A second layer of closure is achieved by approximating the urethrovaginal fascia, and the vaginal mucosa is closed last. This relatively simple technique is perfectly adequate for most urethral diverticula if the sac is not large or if the ostium appears to be located distally.

If the diverticulum is large or if the ostium is in the proximal urethra, a variety of modifications help to achieve a multilayer closure and increase the likelihood of a satisfactory outcome. An inverted, U-shaped anterior vaginal wall incision is made. After the posterior-based anterior vaginal wall flap is mobilized, a transverse incision is made in the periurethral fascia. A plane is established between the periurethral fascia and the diverticulum both superiorly and inferiorly. This plane may sometimes be difficult to establish because of the degree of associated inflammation. The exposed urethral diverticulum is excised, and its communication with the urethra often establishes a relatively large urethral defect. The urethra is closed longitudinally with 3-0 absorbable suture over a No. 14 French Foley catheter. The periurethral fascia is closed transversely

with interrupted 2-0 absorbable sutures, and the vaginal flap is closed last with a running 2-0 absorbable suture. An advantage of this technique is the avoidance of apposing suture lines. If the urethral defect is large, and especially if there is considerable inflammation in adjacent tissues, a bulbocavernosus fat pad graft is sutured over the urethral closure as an intervening layer. This so-called Martius flap employs a posteriorly based bulbocavernosus muscle and fat pad, which is mobilized through a separate labial incision and rotated under the skin of the labia and anterior vaginal mucosa to cover the urethral closure.

An alternative approach is worth mentioning, since it may be valuable in dealing with very large proximal diverticula associated with considerable inflammation. The hazards of extensive subtrigonal dissection are alleviated by leaving a portion of the diverticular wall intact and marsupializing it to the vaginal mucosa.

If patients exhibit stress urinary incontinence preoperatively, a concomitant endoscopic urethropexy is advisable. Experience has shown that the procedure can be safely performed without risk of infection if precautions are taken. It is emphasized that the decision to perform a urethropexy is not based on preoperative urodynamic findings, but on the patient's symptoms and documentation of stress urinary incontinence. A urethropexy should also be considered, even in the absence of preoperative stress urinary incontinence, if a large proximal diverticulum is excised leading to apparent loss of support of the proximal urethral segment. If a urethropexy is required, it should be done by placing a helical suture of No. 2 Prolene through the pubocervical fascia and anterior vaginal wall, as described by Raz, and avoiding the use of Dacron bolsters or other foreign materials, which are much more likely to become infected in the face of an infected urethral diverticulum. The supporting urethropexy sutures are placed before mobilization and excision of the suburethral diverticulum in order to minimize the risk of pus extruding from the diverticulum and contaminating the retropubic space. The supporting urethropexy sutures are not tied until the diverticulum excision and repair are completed.

POSTOPERATIVE COURSE

For most straightforward urethral diverticula repairs, a No. 14 French indwelling urethral catheter is left in place for 7 to 10 days. Patients are usually admitted to the hospital for 1 to 2 days, although the procedure has been done on an ambulatory basis. Parenteral antibiotics are administered during the hospital stay, and oral agents are continued until after the catheter is removed.

If there is any concern about the integrity of the urethral closure because of weakness of the tissues due to associated infection, the large size of the ostium, or the proximal location of the diverticulum, a punch suprapubic cystostomy catheter is placed at surgery. In this event, a VCU is often performed 7 to 14 days postoperatively to assess the urethral reconstruction site before removal of the catheters. A cystostomy tube is also used if a concomitant urethropexy is performed, and is not removed until the patient is voiding reasonably well and postvoid residuals are less than 75 to 100 ml. Intermittent catheterization is avoided in order to prevent disruption or injury of the operative site in the reconstructed urethra.

COMPLICATIONS

The most commonly employed procedure is the transvaginal diverticulectomy. A combined review in seven different reports of over 400 patients in whom this approach has primarily been employed revealed a significant complication rate of 17 percent. Recurrent urinary tract infection was the most common complication, occurring in 5 percent. Urethrovaginal fistula formation was noted in 4 percent, but some were asymptomatic and did not require surgery, depending on their size and location. An additional 4 percent of

patients developed recurrent or persistent diverticula. Other complications included urinary incontinence, urethral stricture, bladder injury, and persistent urinary symptoms.

Approximately 2 percent of patients develop postoperative stress urinary incontinence. This undoubtedly results from loss of urethral support, particularly in the vicinity of the proximal urethral segment and bladder neck, suggesting that a concomitant urethropexy is advisable in some patients even when stress incontinence is not present preoperatively.

SUGGESTED READING

Downs RA. Urethral diverticulum in females. Urology 1987; 29:201.

Ginsburg DS, Genadry R. Suburethral diverticulum in the female. Obstet Gynecol Surv 1984; 39:1.

Leach GE, Bavendam TG. Female urethral diverticula. Urology 1987; 30:407.

Leach GE, Schmidbauer CP, Hadley HR, et al. Surgical treatment of female urethral diverticulum. Semin Urol 1986; 4:33.

URETHRAL DIVERTICULA IN MALES

BARRY A. KOGAN, M.D.

Diverticula of the male urethra are most often asymptomatic and undiagnosed. Those associated with significant urologic pathology are uncommon, with only about 250 reported in the literature. Diverticula are generally classified as either congenital or acquired, the latter accounting for more than 90 percent.

ETIOLOGY

Congenital diverticula of the posterior urethra are the result of associated conditions, including the stump of an ectopic ureter, an enlarged prostatic utricle as a result of an intersex condition, or the residual of a rectourethral fistula consequent upon repair of a high and imperforate anus. A large "diverticular" posterior urethra is also seen in the prune-belly syndrome and is presumed to be caused by hypoplasia of the prostate.

Congenital anterior urethral diverticula are also commonly called anterior urethral valves. They are nearly always ventral and probably result from a failure of development of the corpus spongiosum. The ostium can be small to moderate; with voiding, the diverticulum distends, pushing the distal lip dorsally, thereby ob-

structing the urethra and forcing more urine into the diverticulum, which in turn causes further urethral obstruction (Fig. 1). Occasionally, dilated Cowper's ducts can also act as diverticula. Although the theory is somewhat controversial, a distal, dorsal diverticulum (called the lacuna magna or valve of Guérin) is thought to cause clinical problems. This small diverticulum, probably formed when the distal urethral plug does not meet exactly with the proximal urethra formed by the fusion of the labioscrotal folds, may account for dysuria or bloody urethral spotting in boys.

Acquired urethral diverticula, when posterior, are most often secondary to urethral instrumentation, repair of traumatic urethral disruption, or prostatic abscess. Anterior urethral diverticula are the most common. They are generally asymptomatic and result from previous urologic intervention. The majority, commonly known as false passages, are usually the result of a difficult attempt at catheterization and rarely cause problems until future attempts are made. Similarly, diverticula are common after hypospadias surgery; however, with the exception of minimal postvoid dribbling or difficulty with urethral catheterization, these rarely cause problems. When noted, a distal obstruction should be sought, because high voiding pressures may lead to dilatation of the proximal repair, which is unsupported by corpus spongiosum.

Symptomatic diverticula are most often the result of urinary incontinence, primarily neurogenic incontinence. They are generally in the anterior urethra and usually result from attempts to gain continence with penile clamps or condom catheters placed too tightly and too long in the same position (partly as a result of

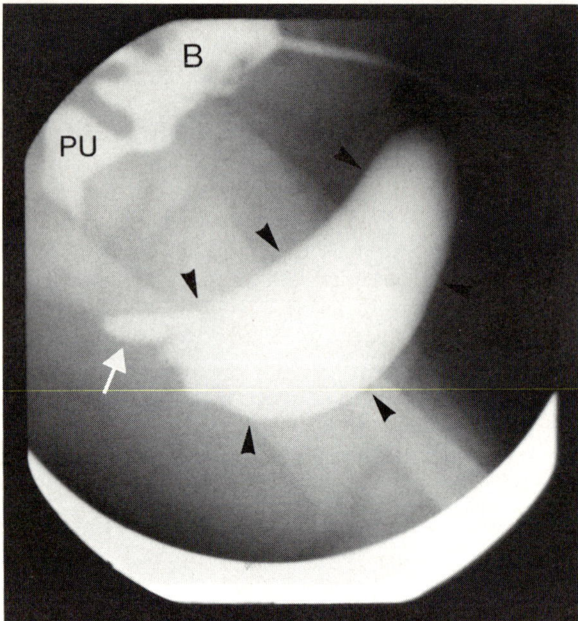

Figure 1 Voiding cystometrography performed via a suprapubic cystostomy in a 1-week-old boy with massive bilateral hydroureteronephrosis. The bladder (B) is small and trabeculated, the prostatic urethra (PU) dilated, and the deep bulbous urethra (*white arrow*) normal. The enormous anterior urethral diverticulum (*black arrowheads*) is severely obstructive.

decreased penile sensation in these patients). Another cause is chronic urethral catheter drainage, which prevents normal drainage of urethral secretions, resulting in urethritis, urethral abscess formation, and eventually a diverticulum (as well as urethral fistulas in severe cases). Occasionally, gonorrhea, tuberculosis, or bilharzial infections also lead to urethral abscesses and diverticulum formation.

SYMPTOMS

The symptoms of urethral diverticula depend on their location. Those in the posterior urethra are generally noted only with recurrent urinary infections (the pocket of urine acting as a reservoir makes eradicating the infection very difficult). If these remain uninfected, however, they are likely to be asymptomatic and rarely require treatment.

By contrast, major anterior urethral diverticula, even when uninfected, can cause symptoms. Most common is postvoid urinary dribbling, which can be troublesome enough to require treatment. As noted above, congenital anterior diverticula often present with significant outflow obstruction and nearly always require repair.

DIAGNOSIS

On physical examination, a posterior urethral diverticulum may go unnoticed. Often, however, it will be found as a boggy (and, if inflamed, extremely tender) lesion in the region of the prostate on rectal examination. Anterior diverticula are noted as a fullness on the ventral surface of the penis, particularly when the patient is examined immediately after voiding. Further, urine may be expressed during the examination. In severe cases, a urinary fistula may also be seen.

Urinalysis and culture are essential. For posterior urethral diverticula, an examination of expressed "prostatic" secretions or collection of a urine sample after rectal examination may be extremely helpful. When there is no clear-cut cause, cultures for gonorrhea and tuberculosis should be obtained. Careful radiographic evaluation is essential. A good plain film that includes the entire penis is important, because the combination of a diverticulum and stasis can lead to a urethral calculus. Retrograde urethrography is extremely important for both diagnosis and treatment (Fig. 2). In most instances, voiding cystourethrography should also be performed. This will delineate the anatomy more physiologically and may be the only way to demonstrate posterior urethral or extremely distal diverticula (extra attention should be paid to visualizing the entire distal urethra). In some patients, catheterization is difficult and voiding cystourethrography is not feasible.

TREATMENT

Most diverticula are asymptomatic and never require treatment, and neither do those with relatively mild symptoms. For instance, boys with postvoid urinary dribbling after hypospadias surgery may be taught to express the trapped urine after each void. Similarly, many patients and families may only need reassurance that the lacuna magna is the cause of the bloody spotting and is benign. In most cases, investigation and intervention are unnecessary.

Nonetheless, patients with significant infection, calculus formation, marked postvoid dribbling, or urethral abscess require surgical intervention. Just as radiographic evaluation is essential before treatment, endoscopy is extremely helpful at the time of repair, both in accurately assessing the lesion and the tissues around it and in calibrating the distal urethra to ensure that no obstruction exists. Knowledge of the size of the ostium is very important, and this may not be apparent from radiographic studies alone. Similarly, after previous urethroplasty, the presence of hair in the urethra or diverticulum may not be apparent until endoscopy. In most instances, treatment must be planned to eliminate this portion, as the hair will lead to chronic infection, calculus formation, or both.

For some patients, endoscopic treatment alone may suffice. A posterior urethral diverticulum from a residual of an ectopic ureter can often be treated by electrocautery, which will contract the lesion to the point where it is functionally insignificant. Other narrow-mouthed, shallow diverticula can be treated by endoscopic incision of the meatus, allowing better drainage. Similarly, when dysuria or urethral spotting is significant enough to

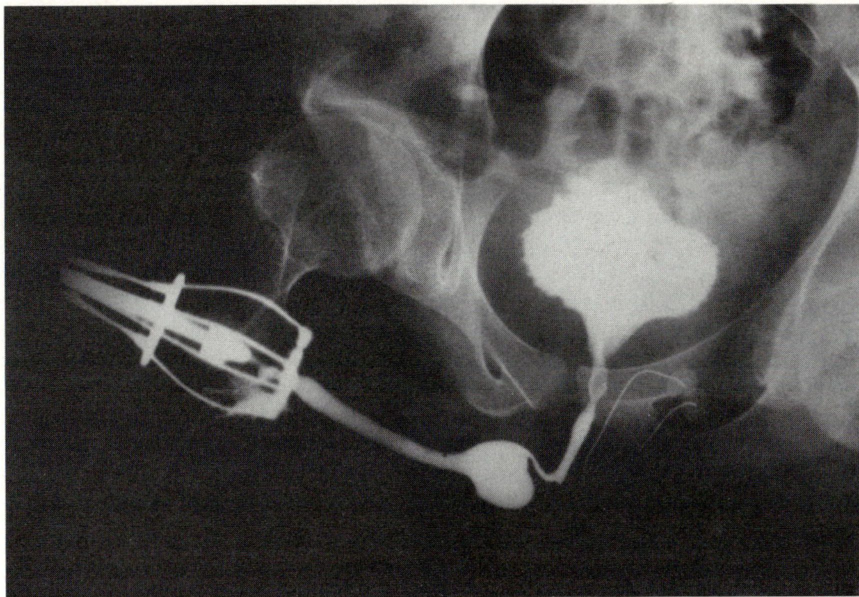

Figure 2 Retrograde urethrogram in a 15-year-old boy awaiting urinary undiversion. The anterior urethral diverticulum is the result of chronic urethral catheter drainage and resultant urethritis and urethral abscess.

warrant intervention, lesions of the lacuna magna can usually be treated by endoscopic or "open" transmeatal unroofing.

When open urethroplasty is necessary, the incision and dissection should be planned so that suture lines do not overlap. Traditionally, this is done by degloving the penis with a circumcising incision; however, operative trauma is often less with an incision lateral to the diverticulum and dissection of a ventral skin flap with its random blood supply based on the contralateral side. In addition, when previous operations have been performed (e.g., hypospadias surgery), it is best to avoid crossing previous suture lines or vascular pedicles. Delineating the exact location of the diverticulum at the start of the dissection is important. Although this can often be done either blindly by passing a bougie or endoscopically by passing a Fogarty balloon into the diverticulum and inflating it there, it is often preferable to observe the diverticulum directly by distending the entire anterior urethra with fluid. This is best done by passing the appropriate-size feeding tube or catheter to the midpoint of the urethra and injecting methylene blue while compressing the perineal urethra and simultaneously obstructing the meatus. This technique defines a diverticulum, clearly delineates any fistula, and stains the urethra (particularly any abnormal, irregular, and unhealthy tissue). It makes premature entry into the urethra during dissection obvious and it can easily be repeated.

The incision in the diverticulum must also be planned to avoid overlying suture lines. Although much of the diverticular lining will be removed, the position of the incision is important in order to allow later tissue coverage over the repair. The amount excised is assessed by passing an appropriate-size sound or catheter past the diverticulum; in general, a slight excess is preferable to avoid urethral stricture formation. The full thickness of the diverticulum is not excised; rather, the lining is removed, leaving the outer tissue (without its epithelium) for coverage to prevent a leak. The urethra itself is closed with a running 7-0 blue chromic suture, inverting the edges to prevent fistula formation. Again, previous staining of the urethral mucosa with methylene blue is helpful. The previously de-epithelialized outer layer of the diverticulum is then positioned with another running layer of 7-0 blue chromic in such a way as to cover the previous suture line completely. The skin coverage, previously designed to avoid overlying suture lines, is sewn in place with interrupted 6-0 blue chromic. In general, a drain is not left, but a Silastic urethral stent is. A suprapubic cystostomy is optional; it is highly recommended in patients with previous urethritis or surgery. Urinary diversion is maintained for 7 to 21 days, depending on the surgeon's preference (a shorter time is advisable when tissue viability is good). Optical magnification ($3\times$ to $7\times$) is helpful throughout. In very young infants with anterior urethral valves, in elderly patients, or in those with severe inflammation, it may be more appropriate to perform a first-stage Johansen urethroplasty initially (i.e., an external urethrotomy), which allows for urinary drainage and treatment of infection. Closure can then be performed as appropriate, at least 6 months later.

Posterior urethral diverticula are a special group. Fortunately, they rarely require treatment. When it is necessary and endoscopic treatment either fails or is not feasible, the best approach is transabdominal (the perineal approach is possible but is generally more difficult and dangerous). Although approaching the diverticulum from above is also technically demanding and exposure is generally achieved by opening the base of the bladder in the midline of the trigone, it provides excellent visualization of the anatomy. Postoperative care is typical of any bladder surgery.

Complications resulting from these repairs should be minimal. Fistulas and strictures are possible, but should be rare with careful attention to dissection and closure. The most common complication is recurrence, which can result from a failure to diagnose and treat a distal stricture or from insufficient excision of the original diverticulum. Both causes are preventable. In general, operative repair of this unusual lesion should yield excellent results.

SUGGESTED READING

Firlit CF, King LR. Anterior urethral valves in children. J Urol 1970; 108:972–975.

Marya SKS, Kumar S, Singh S. Acquired male urethral diverticulum. J Urol 1977; 118:765–766.

Mohan V, Gupta SK, Cherian J, et al. Urethral diverticulum in male subjects: Report of 5 cases. J Urol 1980; 123:592–594.

Ortlip SA, Gonzalez R, Williams RD. Diverticula of the male urethra. J Urol 1980; 124:350–355.

Tank ES. Anterior urethral valves resulting from congenital urethral diverticula. Urology 1987; 30:467–469.

MEGALOURETHRA

R. DIXON WALKER, M.D.

Megalourethra is defined as a congenital enlargement of the anterior urethra and must be distinguished from similar congenital and acquired abnormalities. Megalourethra is caused by an insufficiency of erectile tissue and occurs in two forms. Fusiform megalourethra results from a deficiency of erectile tissue of both corpus spongiosum and corpus cavernosum, and may occur in a spectrum of severity. These children are incapable of having an erection. With our present state of knowledge this aspect of the abnormality is uncorrectable. About half of these cases are associated with prune-belly syndrome, and many of these children have defects that are incompatible with life. Scaphoid megalourethra, although more common than the fusiform variety, is still rare and also frequently associated with prune-belly syndrome. This entity is characterized by a deficiency only in the corpus spongiosum. Thus, these children can have satisfactory erections, albeit with a characteristic dorsal curvature that does not seem to impede them as adults in having intercourse. The other characteristic feature of their disease is the ballooning or "frog's throat" of the ventral urethra as they void. In some instances they may retain significant amounts of urine in this patulous urethra and appear incontinent. I have described a more common variant of scaphoid megalourethra that occurs in association with hypospadias. These patients are characterized by having dorsal curvature with erection and a very large hypospadiac meatus.

Congenital megalourethra must be distinguished from other congenital and acquired diseases that appear similar. Congenital urethral diverticulum with or without anterior urethral valves has a similar clinical appearance but usually can be distinguished by voiding cystourethrography. A urethral diverticulum secondary to hypospadias repair is remarkably similar to megalourethra in its appearance, clinical symptomatology, and treatment.

THERAPEUTIC ALTERNATIVES

For the patient with fusiform megalourethra, early recognition of the abnormality is important because an excellent option is to change the child's sex. This remains largely a theoretical option because the disease is so rare and the children so ill. In two cases of fusiform megalourethra that I have seen, one infant died at several months of age and the parents of the other refused to consider gender reassignment. This latter child is currently 13 years old and has never had an erection. In my opinion this parental decision may be more difficult than that concerning children with micropenis. Since many of these patients have either life-threatening problems or a poor prognosis, sexual options are of low priority. Nevertheless, in those few patients in whom there is a good prognosis, early decision making is important.

The child with scaphoid megalourethra with or without hypospadias should have renal imaging, since there is a reasonably high incidence of other congenital abnormalities. Urine should be cultured and infections appropriately treated. Surgical repair depends on the size of the megalourethra and how much it bothers the patient. Minimal postvoiding incontinence can be managed by learning to massage and empty the urethra after voiding.

PREFERRED APPROACH

Patient Selection

Patients with fusiform megalourethra are candidates for genitoplasty and sex conversion only if their other abnormalities are not life threatening and there is a reasonable prognosis.

Patients with scaphoid megalourethra should have surgical correction if the megalourethra is associated with a hypospadias, if there are recurrent infections, if the capacity of the urethra is so large that it is difficult to empty, or if the size is a cosmetic problem for the patient.

Timing of Surgery

Surgical correction of fusiform megalourethra should be delayed until the prognosis of the child is determined and all underlying medical problems resolved. Once a decision is made about whether the child should be raised as a boy or a girl, genitoplasty can be accomplished at any time in the first year of life.

Surgical correction of scaphoid megalourethra with or without hypospadias is best done when the child is about 1 year of age or when the indication presents itself. Recommendations for genital surgery with hypospadias, which indicate that surgery can safely be done in the 6- to 12-month age group, are probably applicable to this more unusual abnormality.

Preoperative Preparation

Patients with fusiform megalourethra first require resolution of problems in other organ systems that may make them surgical risks. In infants being considered for gender reassignment this should be thoroughly discussed with the parents, and psychological assistance should be available if necessary.

Patients with scaphoid megalourethra require preparation the day before surgery. This includes a thorough history and physical examination, hemogram, urinalysis and urine culture, renal profile, and blood typing. Black patients require documentation of whether they have sickle cell trait or disease.

After general anesthesia has been initiated, I prefer preoperative antibiotics, usually cephazolin in a dose of 25 mg per kilogram of body weight. I follow this postoperatively with cephazolin in four intravenous divided doses, with a total daily dose of 50 mg per kilogram of body weight. After the patient is receiving oral feedings, I switch to oral cephalexin, given at a daily dose of 50 mg per kilogram of body weight and divided into four doses.

Choice of Procedure

The procedure of choice for fusiform megalourethra is gender reassignment surgery. Almost all male gender reassignment surgery is done with microphallus, and thus there is not a problem in dealing with a bulky penis. The experience in gender reassignment in this disease process remains theoretical and anecdotal. Goals of the surgery are to develop labia majora from the scrotal skin, remove gonadal tissue, and reduce penile bulk to clitoral size. The latter may be impossible, and total resection of the penis may be required. Shaft skin inversion with preservation of the glans penis, as is done in creating a vagina for adult male transvestitates, is probably not practical in this group.

Patients with scaphoid megalourethra without hypospadias are probably best served by an operation that mobilizes all shaft skin as in a hypospadias repair and then reduces the diameter of the urethra to a normal size by excising the redundant urethra and reapproximating around a stent. The suture should be absorbable and suture lines watertight and inverted with a running fine suture (5-0 or 6-0 polyglycolic acid). Diversion can be with the stent or suprapubically. There is no reason not to manage these operations like hypospadias repairs, doing the procedure on an outpatient or short-stay admission basis and letting the stent drain into the diaper or a drainage bag for 4 to 7 days.

The patient who presents with the combination of hypospadias and scaphoid megalourethra almost always has the enlarged meatus midshaft or distal. Since the associated chordee is dorsal and does not require correction, the only consideration is reducing the size of the urethra and constructing a tube to the end of the penis. I think this is best done with a meatal-based flap, either Horton-Devine flip flap or a Mustardé. The latter procedure particularly lends itself to this diagnosis, since it is easier to reduce the caliber of the urethra by excising a wedge of tissue on the side of the urethra closest to the corpus cavernosum. Drikett and Keating have described the pyramid procedure for such cases with equally good results. As in other hypospadias repairs of this magnitude, the procedure can be done on an outpatient or short inpatient basis and diversion can be into a drainage bag or a diaper. My preferred method of stenting is similar to that of Mitchell. A No. 10 Fr Silastic tube is precut to be 15 cm. To use it as a stent, I cut out a 1-mm strip of the back wall, bevel the end, and pass it into the bladder. The end of the stent is then spatulated and sewn to the meatus with a 5-0 nylon suture. The stent can be irrigated with a 6-ml syringe and small angiocatheter if necessary.

POSTOPERATIVE COURSE

The patient is given cephalexin for 7 to 10 days postoperatively. I prefer to wrap the penis with a 2-inch Kling soaked in saline. The child is placed in diapers and the stent allowed to drain into the dressing and the diaper. The diapers are changed every 3 or 4 hours except at night; at each change, the dressing is irrigated with sterile normal saline by the parent. If this dressing comes off it is replaced by a loose 4 × 4 dressing and irrigated by the parent. The stent is usually left in for 4 to 7 days and removed, along with the dressing, in the outpatient clinic, using loops to identify the nylon suture easily and to cut it.

The child is examined 6 weeks postoperatively and again at 1 year to note any complications.

COMPLICATIONS AND SEQUELAE

The general complications of this procedure are no different from those of any genital procedure: loss of tissue from compromised circulation, infection, and hematoma. Specific complications include fistula formation and recurrence of the divertulum. Fistulas should be repaired by any of the multitude of acceptable outpatient procedures 4 to 6 months after the original procedure. Recurrence of the diverticulum is a more difficult problem, and repeated correction should be done only if it is large and troublesome. Sometimes urethral meatotomy may be necessary to decrease distal urethral resistance.

There is no medical treatment for patients with megalourethra. The treatment choice is whether or not to perform surgery. The indications for surgery have been previously discussed. In my experience, most parents choose surgical treatment for any genital abnormality, since their expectations are that the penis should be as normal as possible.

SUGGESTED READING

Dorairajan T. Defects of spongy tissue and congenital diverticula of the penile urethra. Aust N Z J Surg 1963; 32:209.
Mortensen PHG, Johnson HW, Coleman GU, et al. Megalourethra. J Urol 1985; 134:358.
Wilson JA, Walker RD. Megalourethra and hypospadias. J Urol 1982; 129:556.
Drikett JW, Keating MA. Technical challenge of the megameatus intact prepuce hypospadias variant: the pyramid procedure. J Urol 1989; 141:1407.

HYPOSPADIAS AND CHORDEE

A. BARRY BELMAN, M.D., M.S. (Urology)

Hypospadias is one of the most common congenital genitourinary problems seen in boys. Its incidence approaches five to seven per 1,000 male births. It is an abnormality virtually independent of other genitourinary pathologic conditions, although the incidence of undescended testes, hernia, and an enlarged utriculus masculinus is reportedly increased in these children. Therefore, evaluation of the urinary tract is not indicated in boys with isolated hypospadias.

Treatment of hypospadias remains purely a surgical endeavor. With improved techniques, virtually every boy with hypospadias is a candidate for surgical intervention. Most now agree that surgery is best carried out as early as possible, but certainly before the second birthday. Aside from ancillary support in terms of proper anesthesia, nursing, and the general health of the child, the only limiting factor is penile size. In most instances, technical considerations do not limit planning correction at 6 months for the full-term infant. Correction can be carried out even earlier if timed with another, more pressing problem (hernia). Occasionally, hormonal stimulation may be necessary in infants with a small glans or limited preputial skin in whom that skin is an essential ingredient in completing the repair. Two injections of testosterone can be given either intramuscularly (testosterone enanthate, 25 mg) or applied daily (10 percent

testosterone proprionate cream). Treatment should be initiated about 6 weeks before the planned surgical correction.

Chordee is an associated condition occurring in about 35 percent of boys with hypospadias. The severity of chordee relates directly to that of the hypospadias. Often, meatal position is not entirely indicative of the degree of pathology, because some with severe chordee may appear to have the meatus at the coronal sulcus. However, close inspection will clarify the extent of the pathology. Upon release of chordee, the meatus in this circumstance may well be found at the penoscrotal junction.

A few patients present with chordee despite a more or less normally placed urethral meatus. The first clue to an abnormal penis is the recognition of absent ventral foreskin. Release of chordee generally requires either urethral transection or dorsal plication (the Nesbit procedure). In most patients, however, the urethra is abnormal, and either complete urethral release or urethral transection with an interpositional graft becomes necessary to achieve a straight penis.

Dorsal chordee has also been reported both in conjunction with and independent of hypospadias. Delay in surgical therapy is advised for those with dorsal chordee alone, since the extent of this problem and its clinical ramifications may not be clear until after puberty and full penile development.

Release of Chordee. Release of chordee before urethroplasty is the mandatory first step for proper care of the hypospadiac penis. To correct chordee, excision or incision of the thickened ventral bands that may be the rudimentary spongiosum of the uncanalized urethral groove is necessary. These fibers or bands may even extend proximal to what appears to be the normal urethra. In fact, dissection of the normal, proximal urethra from the corpora for a short distance is part of a routine hypospadias repair to ensure correction of chordee. With more severe forms of hypospadias, chordee may persist even after both extensive ventral dissection and proximal urethral mobilization. The use of fine transverse incisions to filet Buck's fascia, as well as a midline incision between the corporeal bodies, may be required to release chordee completely. Others have advocated a deep transverse fascial incision across the midline to include both corporeal bodies for complete release of chordee, the resultant defect being covered with a free dermal or tunica vaginalis graft. I have never had to apply the latter principle and have instead achieved penile straightening with multiple small transverse incisions. The neourethra, which is formed at the same time, is then used to cover the fascial defects and may serve the same purpose as a free tunica vaginalis graft.

Technical Considerations. The use of fine, nonreactive suture material, made possible by the routine application of optical magnification, has played a significant role in improving the results of hypospadias repair. Although some authors advocate use of an operating microscope, most "hypospadiologists" are satisfied with 2.5 to 3.5 × optical magnification. Although some continue to use fine chromic catgut for formation of the urethra and/or skin closure, I prefer to use 6-0 and 7-0 polyglactin (Vicryl) exclusively. Admittedly, the suture material may remain for several weeks and in some children can result in troublesome "suture tracks" (epithelial bridges).

Prevention of Complications. Ensuring flap viability and avoiding crossing suture lines are the two most important steps in the prevention of complications. The use of a well-vascularized pedicle flap to create the urethra with widely spatulated anastomoses has resulted in a marked reduction in complications of hypospadias repair, and made success with a single-stage procedure possible in virtually every circumstance. In addition, the application of a complete layer covering the neourethra, applying either a de-epithelialized skin flap or a pedicle of tunica vaginalis, has reduced the incidence of urethrocutaneous fistulas to close to zero. A de-epithelialized flap can generally be created from residual split hooded prepuce even after creation of the urethra from a transverse preputial island flap. Skin is removed from the residual preputial flap and swung over the neourethra into the glans, if possible (Fig. 1). When, in the most severe forms of hypospadias, there is inadequate skin for creation of a de-epithelialized cover, tunica vaginalis based on a pedicle from the spermatic cord can be harvested and swung distally over the entire neourethra into the glans. Either of these methods will allow the new urethra to be completely covered, avoiding the crossing of suture lines.

Cosmesis. An additional goal in hypospadias repair beyond achieving a straight penis with a meatus in a functional position is to normalize its appearance. This means creating the urethral meatus at the tip of the glans and excising excessive skin to leave the patient with the appearance of a normally circumcised phallus. Leaving a collar, as described by Firlit, helps to achieve this goal. A normal midline raphe can also be achieved in most instances by using a midline closure rather than interdigitating flaps.

Postoperative Management. This has also undergone tremendous changes in recent years. The use of a suprapubic tube is reserved for the most severe scrotal or perineal abnormalities. Patients with glanular hypospadias or coronal hypospadias without chordee can be sent

A   B

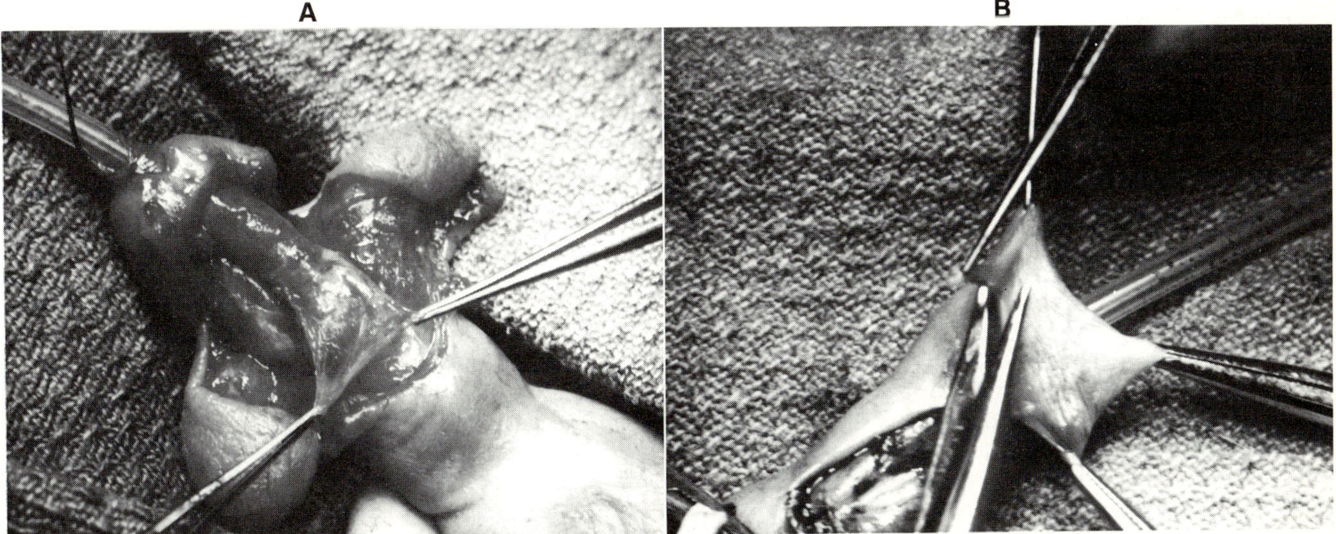

Figure 1 *A,* Transverse preputial island flap neourethra funneled through the glans. Fine forceps are holding up redundant subcutaneous tissue from the pedicle flap, which is used to cover the proximal anastomosis. *B,* Right half of the split prepuce being de-epithelialized to cover the new urethra.

home, voiding through the repairs. The remainder do well with an intravesical stent draining into a diaper. A No. 5 or 8 feeding tube, tied to the glans and allowed to drain into the outer of two diapers, offers a safe and reliable means of postoperative management.

In addition, bulky compression dressings have been replaced by a double layer of Tegoderm, which remains in place for 3 to 4 days. A bulky dressing is used for severe proximal repairs, allowing scrotoperineal compression for 48 hours.

Anesthesiologists have been helpful in providing postoperative pain relief in this group of patients. A caudal block of 0.25 to 0.5 percent bupivacaine can give sustained pain relief for 4 to 6 hours. This allows the patient to awaken peacefully immediately after surgery, avoiding straining with possible disruption of the dressing and increased venous pressure that might lead to hematoma formation.

SURGICAL PROCEDURES

Glanular Hypospadias

The introduction of the MAGPI broke a barrier leading to more lenient criteria for surgical candidates. Extension of the use of this operative procedure to those with hypospadias proximal to the coronal sulcus has led to dissatisfaction with its results by some. However, for realistic candidates with glanular hypospadias, the MAGPI procedure continues to offer an opportunity to normalize penile appearance.

An alternative to the MAGPI for those with a wide glanular groove is the GAP procedure. This is performed by de-epithelializing skin at the lateral margin of the glanular groove, carrying that de-epithelialization proximal to the meatus. The urethra is then lengthened by approximating the two resultant skin edges, the inner edge with running subcuticular 7-0 Vicryl to create the urethra, and the outer or glanular edge with mattressed 6-0 or 7-0 Vicryl. Redundant skin is then excised and the edges are approximated with interrupted 6-0 Vicryl suture. A double layer of Tegoderm is applied as a postoperative dressing and the patient is discharged the day of surgery, voiding through the new repair.

Distal Hypospadias Without Chordee

A megameatal variant of distal hypospadias exists that is generally unrecognized at birth, since the foreskin in this condition may be complete. The distal urethra and meatus is patulous and the glans flattened and widely grooved. Repair often requires tailoring of the urethra proximal to the wide meatus. The glanular portion is fashioned by tubularizing the ventral glanular tissue and then closing the glans over the extended urethra, in a manner similar to that of the GAP procedure or as originally described by King. In this situation, redundant ventral skin proximal to the meatus may be de-epithelialized and extended over the initial suture line that was used to create the distal urethra and

interposed between it and the glans closure. This will markedly reduce the risk of fistula.

Meatus-based Flaps

The Mathieu procedure offers a highly successful means of dealing with coronal and subcoronal hypospadias. By creating a vascularized flap proximal to the meatus, which is then flipped distally and anastomosed to a strip of glanular tissue distal to the glans, one can normalize the penis with minimal risk of complications. It is important to leave sufficient subcutaneous tissue both to vascularize this meatus-based flap and to provide for a second layer over the lateral suture lines. Running 7-0 subcuticular Vicryl sutures are used to close the urethra, which should be about 1 cm in width. The incisions in the glans to create the strip must be carried down to Buck's fascia to allow sufficient mobility of lateral glanular tissue to close over the new urethra without tension. After the lateral closures are completed, subcutaneous tissue from the pedicle is sutured on each side to the depths of the glanular incision with three or four interrupted 7-0 Vicryl suture. Finally, to protect the repair further and add both vascularity and another layer, the hooded prepuce is split and one of the wings de-epithelialized and laid into the glans, completely covering the new urethra. This tissue is also sutured to the depths of the glanular incisions with interrupted 7-0 Vicryl, and the most terminal portion is sutured to the urethral meatus. The glans is closed with interrupted, mattressed 6-0 Vicryl suture. To create a normal-appearing penis, the original circumferential subcoronal incision had been carried out sufficiently proximal to the coronal sulcus to prevent suturing shaft skin directly to the glans. Excessive skin is removed and skin edges approximated with 6-0 Vicryl suture. A double layer of Tegoderm is applied and the patient discharged the day of surgery, voiding through the repair. The Tegoderm is removed after three or four days.

Onlay Island Flap Repair

An onlay island repair is advised if the penis is straight and the meatus too proximal, or if there is inadequate ventral skin, to allow a meatus-based flap. The length of tissue required to cover the urethral defect is measured and marked out on the undersurface of the dorsal prepuce. The prepuce is then split at this level and the portion intended for the urethroplasty swung ventrally. The dorsal surface is partially de-epithelialized, creating an island of foreskin (undersurface) on a well-vascularized pedicle. Parallel incisions are made from the meatus distally into the glans, isolating the urethral groove, similar to the Mathieu repair. The urethra is created using running 7-0 Vicryl to anastomose the foreskin island to the strip outlined distal to the meatus. On the side ipsilateral to the pedicle the suture is run on the inside of the urethra, whereas on the opposite side, a running inverting subcuticular suture is employed on the outer edge. The remaining, opposite portion of the hooded prepuce is de-epithelialized and swung into the glans to cover the new urethra, suturing it to the depths of the glans with 7-0 interrupted Vicryl. The glans is then closed with mattressed 6-0 Vicryl suture and excessive skin excised to create a normal circumcised appearance to the penis. In this circumstance, an intravesical stent is used to drain the bladder for 3 to 7 days. A No. 8 feeding tube, tied in place by the 3-0 vertical glanular traction suture routinely used in hypospadias repairs, is allowed to drain directly into the outer of two diapers. The child is placed on oxybutynin hydrochloride (Ditropan) and trimethoprim-sulfamethoxazole (Bactrim) while the tube is in place.

Hypospadias with Chordee

Release of chordee by dissection distal to the hypospadiac meatus, as described earlier, is mandatory before creation of the new urethra is considered. Chordee release will result in retraction of the meatus and necessitate the creation of a neourethra from this point to the tip of the glans. It has always been my preference to use a pedicle flap rather than a free graft to create the urethra. In virtually every virginal circumstance this can be achieved, although hormonal pretreatment may occasionally be required as previously noted. The transverse preputial island pedicle is ideal for this, and after release of chordee, the undersurface of the foreskin should be dissected from the remainder of the dorsal skin on a long vascular pedicle. It is not uncommon, when this procedure is initially attempted, that the dorsal skin that is to remain to cover the penis is devascularized as an uninitiated surgeon attempts to create an excessively well-vascularized pedicle. In fact, the amount of tissue necessary to maintain viability of the pedicle is minimal. However, to prevent penile torque, the dissection of the vascular pedicle should be carried to the penile base. It is my preference to then swing the island flap ventrally and create the anastomosis between the hypospadiac meatus and the pedicle before its tubularization. This is carried out in a widely spatulated fashion with interrupted 7-0 Vicryl over the feeding tube that will be used for drainage. The urethra is created by tubularizing the island flap with a running 7-0 subcuticular Vicryl suture over the feeding tube. A neourethra of adequate length to reach the tip of the glans is thus formed. The glans is split and lateral dissection carried out to prevent tension following closure. The meatus is created with interrupted 7-0 Vicryl suture, and a de-epithelialized flap of remaining skin is brought over the entire repair. If there is inadequate skin remaining for de-epithelialization, tunica vaginalis is harvested by delivering one testis, opening the tunica vaginalis inferiorly and freeing a wide strip based on the spermatic cord. Care must be taken to fulgurate the edges of the tunica vaginalis to prevent hematoma formation. This tissue is then sutured both to the glans and laterally to cover the neourethra. Needless to say, this suture should not encroach on the pedicle to

the island flap. Skin edges are then approximated with mattressed 6-0 Vicryl on the ventral midline and interrupted 6-0 Vicryl subcoronally. The intravesical feeding tube is tied in place with the previously placed 3-0 silk glanular traction suture and a double layer of Tegoderm is applied. The patient is discharged the same day on Bactrim and Ditropan, the double diaper drainage technique described previously employed.

For the majority of those with severe, more proximal hypospadias, a single-stage repair can also be applied. Generally, shiny parameatal skin exists in the midline from the meatus to the penoscrotal junction. This skin can be isolated and rolled into a tube in the manner described by Thiersch, thus creating a penoscrotal hypospadias. The repair from this point is similar to that just described. The patient is not discharged the day of surgery, but a compression dressing is applied to the scrotoperineal region for 24 to 48 hours. This is done over the double layer of Tegoderm, which is removed as an outpatient on the fourth day. The intravesical stent is kept indwelling for 10 days.

Complicated Repeat Hypospadias

The usual methods are often not appropriate for patients who have undergone previous attempts at repair and who have a meatus in an abnormal location and/or persistent chordee. It is infrequent that adequate skin persists to allow both urethroplasty and penile skin coverage. Thus, nonpenile tissue may be necessary to create the urethra. Endoscopy may be helpful to determine whether any part of the previously constructed urethra can be applied to the repair. In many instances, however, the entire urethra or most of it must be excised because of scars, stenoses, and hair growth. To release chordee, the entire urethra, including that which is reusable, must be dissected from the shaft, and residual scar and tissue causing persistent chordee excised. This may often require aggressive dissection accompanied by significant bleeding. However, urethroplasty cannot be entertained until one is assured that the penis is straight. In this situation, dorsal plication may occasionally be used in the older patient to achieve a straight penis, but in most cases, aggressive ventral dissection is successful. If adequate penile skin does not exist to create the urethra, a free graft of bladder epithelium is harvested through a suprapubic incision. About 50 percent more width and length than that measured should be obtained to allow for anticipated contracture of the free graft. The bladder is closed with a suprapubic tube left in place. The epithelial graft is then tubularized with running, locked 6-0 or 7-0 Vicryl suture, and a wide spatulated anastomosis is created proximally. Bladder epithelium tends to pout at the meatus, leaving a wet, irritated surface. To avoid this, a pedicle flap of hairless distal shaft skin can almost always be fashioned to create the glanular urethra to which the free bladder graft is anastomosed in a widely spatulated fashion. Multiple layers are used to cover the free graft to hold it firmly in place while ingrowth of blood vessels occurs. A silicone stent is left in the urethra, extending from the bulb distally just beyond the meatus, and secured with two sutures at the glans. Tegoderm is applied, and the patient kept at bed rest for 4 days and hospitalized for 6 days. He is discharged postoperatively with both stent and suprapubic tube in situ after removal of the Tegoderm dressing. This diversion is maintained for 2 weeks with the suprapubic tube clamped after removal of the stent. After confirmation that the patient is voiding without difficulty, the suprapubic tube is removed.

Results of Hypospadias Surgery

With the above techniques the incidence of complications has been reduced to an absolute minimum. For patients with distal hypospadias without chordee, including candidates for the MAGPI, GAP, or meatus-based flap procedures, complications should be close to zero. The fistula rate for those requiring a transverse island flap is less than 3 percent, including those with scrotal and perineal hypospadias. Patients with complicated repeat hypospadias repairs requiring free grafts have a complication rate of about 20 percent. With improvement in techniques and the results currently being obtained at major pediatric medical centers, it is apparent that additional training in hypospadias repair and an opportunity to carry out these procedures on a regular basis are essential for maintenance of these skills.

SUGGESTED READING

Belman AB. Anomalies of the urinary tract: urethra. In: Kelalis PP, King LR, Belman AB, eds. Clinical pediatric urology. Philadelphia: WB Saunders, 1985.

Belman AB. Deepithelialized skin flap coverage in hypospadias repair. J Urol 1988; 140:1273.

Belman AB, Kass EJ. Hypospadias repair in children under one year of age. J Urol 1982; 128:1273.

Duckett JW. Hypospadias. In: Gillenwater JY, Grayhack JT, Howards SS, Duckett JW, eds. Adult and pediatric urology. Chicago: Year Book, 1987.

Hendren WH, Horton JE Jr. Experience with one-stage repair of hypospadias and chordee using free grafts of prepuce. J Urol 1988; 140:1259.

Oesterling JE, Gearhart JP, Jeffs RD. Urinary diversion in hypospadias surgery. Urology 1987; 29:513.

Zaontz MR. The GAP (glans approximation procedure) for glanular/coronal hypospadias. J Urol 1989; 141:359.

EPISPADIAS

MICHAEL J. LEMMERS, M.D.
EDWARD S. TANK, M.D.

The embryologic defect resulting in epispadias occurs early in development. Aberrant mesodermal accumulation in the cloacal ridges can bridge the cloacal membrane and establish precursors of the genital tubercle which are displaced caudally relative to the urogenital diaphragm. Subsequent differential growth and regression of these disordered anlagen produce a urethral groove situated dorsally relative to phallic or clitoral tissue. Abnormal cephalad extension of the cloacal membrane contributes to the occurrence of vesical exstrophy in association with epispadias. Because the developmental error occurs so early in these conditions, the most severe anomaly, exstrophy, is observed more frequently than isolated epispadias. The comparatively rare condition of epispadias affects roughly four times as many male infants as females, and is associated with variable degrees of compromised genitourinary function and structural deformity.

CLINICAL ISSUES

The principal clinical problems arising from epispadias include compromised sexual function, especially in male patients, and urinary incontinence. As in hypospadias, individual cases of male epispadias may be designated distal (glanular), middle (penile), or proximal (penopubic), depending on the position of the urethral meatus. Unlike hypospadias, however, the more proximal forms of epispadias occur more frequently than the distal forms: proximal epispadias accounts for about 60 percent of cases, whereas distal forms occur in only about 15 percent. As one would expect, the severity of the malformation influences the continence rate; virtually all patients with distal epispadias are continent, but over 90 percent of those with proximal epispadias are not. The anatomic features of epispadias, depending on degree, include flattening and dorsal separation of the glans, a dorsal urethral groove, variable dorsal chordee with foreshortening of the phallus, divergence of the symphysis pubis associated with lateral displacement of the proximal corpora cavernosa and with malformation of the external urinary sphincter, and bladder neck incompetence.

In female epispadias, the clitoris is bifid, and the

severity of superior labial separation and flattening of mons pubis is determined by the magnitude of the symphyseal diastasis. The relative degrees of female epispadias are gauged, as in the male, by the extent of urethral and bladder neck deformity, varying from a patulous meatus to complete dorsal urethral split with incompetent sphincter mechanisms.

The continuum of epispadiac deformities, from distal epispadias to complete vesical exstrophy, may be divided conveniently (albeit somewhat artificially) by the position of the urethral plate and bladder neck relative to the fibrous band bridging the symphyseal gap. In this discussion, only epispadiac anomalies in which the urethra and bladder neck are located posterior to the intersymphyseal band will be considered. When these structures are situated anteriorly, the principles and techniques of exstrophy management are appropriate. Before deciding on a surgical approach, the urologist should remember that as the degree of epispadias increases, the probability of vesical and ureterovesical dysfunction also increases. Diminished bladder capacity and vesicoureteral reflux must be recognized preoperatively and addressed directly in the plan of management.

RECONSTRUCTIVE APPROACH

Any surgical approach to epispadias must correct both the functional and cosmetic abnormalities. Therapeutic objectives include the establishment of urinary continence and urethral repair without compromising upper tract or renal function, and the construction of functionally and cosmetically adequate external genitalia. The initial assessment of epispadiac children should include careful physical examination to ascertain the degree of epispadias and to confirm that the deformity is in fact limited to epispadias. Special attention should be given to the magnitude of symphyseal separation and to the position of the urethra relative to the intersymphyseal band. The physician and parents should reach agreement regarding the presence or absence of urinary continence. Voiding cystourethrography should be performed to assess bladder capacity, bladder neck anatomy, and ureterovesical function. If there is any question of possible renal compromise, differential baseline renal function should be determined, perhaps most conveniently by radionuclide renography.

In preparation for surgery, the urologist should counsel parents thoroughly about the complex nature of the deformity, the potential requirement for a staged repair, the possibility of numerous complications, and the uncertainty of the final cosmetic and functional result. By about 1 year of age, the genital tissues have reached a point beyond which their relative growth rate is markedly slowed until puberty. Therefore, little if any advantage is gained by delaying surgery until later in infancy. Some authorities report helpful enlargement of the male genitalia after preoperative administration of testosterone enanthate (2 mg per kilogram intramuscularly 5 and 2 weeks before surgery). The urologist's role

is also facilitated by the use of optical magnification (loupes or an operating microscope), delicate instruments (such as ophthalmologic tools), and fine suture. Preoperative and postoperative antibiotics are recommended to maintain sterile urine and to avoid infection around fresh flaps or grafts.

Continent children with epispadias usually have adequate bladder capacity and no vesicoureteral reflux. In these patients, one may plan a single-stage repair consisting of urethroplasty and genitoplasty. Male patients with distal epispadias and no chordee may be managed by advancement or flap urethroplasty and dorsal closure of the glans. With middle epispadias, artificial erection will help ensure adequate resection of chordee. After recessing the meatus and releasing chordee, it may be desirable to lengthen the phallus by dissecting the crura of the corpora cavernosa partially off the pubic rami, taking care to avoid vascular insufficiency. Once the corpora are approximated in the midline, one must decide whether to perform dorsal or ventral urethroplasty. If the native urethra is short, the distance to the tip of the phallus can become quite long. In this situation, the proximal urethra and bladder neck may be redirected between the corpora toward the perineum, effectively converting the problem into proximal hypospadias, which can be addressed by tubularized flap or graft urethroplasty during the same operation or during a second-stage procedure delayed at least 6 months. When minimal chordee release or phallic lengthening are necessary for middle epispadias, the urethral meatus may remain quite close to the tip of the glans penis. Again, techniques from hypospadias surgery may be borrowed and inverted to complete the urethra dorsally and to close the glans. As in hypospadias surgery, cautious surgical judgment is essential, since a failed primary urethroplasty will almost always make secondary attempts technically much more difficult.

Continent female patients with epispadias generally have adequate local tissues that permit a single-stage repair. Periurethral mucosa can be elevated and sutured in the midline to accomplish at least partial urethral closure. If necessary, the remnant urethra can be mobilized and redirected inferiorly, using a tubularized graft or flap to bridge the gap between the urethral margin and the target meatus. This approach carries the risk of compromising bladder neck function and rendering the patient incontinent. Clitoral components can be mobilized and approximated in the midline. Wide labial and pubic flaps may be rotated medially to allow juxtaposition of the labia superiorly and construction of a satisfactory mons. Attention must be directed to the symmetric use of future hair-bearing skin.

Incontinent children with epispadias require much more extensive procedures. We recommend a two-stage repair for incontinent male epispadiacs who have adequate bladder capacity (>60 ml). During the first stage, bladder neck reconstruction and genitoplasty are performed, while the urethroplasty is deferred at least 6 months. After the urethral plate is elevated, dorsal chordee tissue is resected completely, penile lengthening is accomplished as described above, and the glans penis is closed. Lateral penile skin can usually be mobilized to achieve shaft coverage; the surgeon should reserve preputial skin for future urethroplasty whenever possible. Intersymphyseal tissue may be interrupted in the midline, and the bladder neck dissected anteriorly and laterally. Bladder neck reconstruction is accomplished by urethrovesical tubularization, employing the method of Young-Dees-Leadbetter (YDL) or the transverse modified YDL technique as practiced at the Indiana University Medical Center. One may also employ an anteriorly based detrusor flap as described by Tanagho. This latter technique is particularly useful when trying to redirect the bladder neck toward the perineum between the corpora cavernosa. Ureteroneocystostomy may be necessary for the correction of vesicoureteral reflux or to recess the ureteral orifices from the new bladder neck. The surgeon may choose any of several intravesical or extravesical techniques, depending on specific bladder neck and ureteral anatomy as well as surgical exposure. We prefer to bring ureteral stents out through the anterior wall of the bladder and abdomen. To conclude the first stage, intersymphyseal tissue should be reapproximated over the reconstructed bladder neck; osteotomy and closure of the diastasis is unnecessary. Excessive mobility of the reconstructed bladder neck posterior to the intersymphyseal band should be reduced by suspension sutures through the perivesical or periurethral tissues in the vicinity of the new bladder neck. Dead spaces should be drained appropriately. The catheter draining the bladder doubles as an appropriate stent for 7 to 10 days, exiting through the neomeatus located dorsally at the base of the phallus or on the perineum, depending on the method of bladder neck reconstruction.

At least 6 months after completion of the first stage, urethroplasty is performed. We prefer to avoid reusing tissues that have been mobilized and repositioned previously because of technical difficulties in elevating scarred tissues and unreliable revascularization. Instead, we tend to select tubularized flaps or grafts, usually constructed from preputial skin. Tunneling on the dorsal aspect of the phallus can be challenging, especially in the face of dense, contracted scar tissue. If the neomeatus has been directed toward the perineum, one has the advantage of applying a tubularized flap or graft to the unoperated ventral aspect of the corpora. If there is insufficient penile and preputial skin to fashion the neourethra and to cover the repair, it becomes necessary to harvest and tubularize distant full-thickness grafts from the medial arm, far-lateral abdomen, or bladder mucosa.

For the incontinent female epispadiac with adequate bladder capacity, reconstruction of the bladder neck is performed as described above, with ureteroneocystostomy when necessary. In the process, the neourethral meatus is directed to an appropriate site and the intersymphyseal and fascial tissues are closed over the repair. The extensive vulvoplasty outlined earlier is then employed in the closure of the subcutaneous and cutaneous layers.

The addition of inadequate bladder capacity to incontinence in male epispadiacs can compromise upper tract function and the outcome of bladder neck reconstruction. In this situation, the first stage of the repair should include genitoplasty and urethroplasty. The fractional increase in urethral resistance sometimes raises intravesical pressure enough to cause gradual expansion of the bladder volume. If reflux is not corrected during this first stage, the urologist should place the child on suppressive antibiotics to ensure sterile urine until the second stage can be accomplished. Bladder neck reconstruction and ureteroneocystostomy (if necessary) are performed when the bladder enlarges to an acceptable capacity for age. Failure of the bladder to expand is thought by some authorities to be an indication for augmentation cystoplasty at the time of bladder neck reconstruction. In female epispadiacs with low bladder capacity, the decision to augment the bladder can be deferred until the outcome of the complete first-stage operation is known. Parents should be warned of the risks of high intravesical pressures or low-pressure, incompletely drained bladders, as the clinical situation warrants.

The postoperative care of these patients at any stage of repair rests on familiar surgical principles. After bladder neck reconstruction, we usually divert urine away from the repair with a tension-free indwelling catheter or a suprapubic cystostomy tube in combination with a flexible Silastic bladder neck stent. These are removed after 7 to 10 days. Following urethroplasty, we recommend the Mitchell "splent" technique; about one quarter of the circumference of a flexible Silastic tube is removed longitudinally, providing a urethral stent that responds to intraluminal pressure and thus minimizes the risk of superficial pressure necrosis. Dressings should be nonocclusive and nonconstricting. Antibiotic ointments are frequently helpful in minimizing the adherence of dressings or clothing to fresh wounds. Small drains are sometimes necessary to prevent undesirable accumulation of serous fluid or blood in the vicinity of fresh flaps or grafts. We recognize that systemic antibiotics cannot overcome technical errors, but we continue to recommend their use in the postoperative period because even minimal, localized infections around marginally vascularized tissues undoubtedly contribute to the occurrence of fistulas and strictures.

COMPLICATIONS AND OUTCOME

Like the operative management of hypospadias and exstrophy, the surgical repair of epispadias ranks among the most challenging of urologic endeavors. Even with sound technique and judgment, the surgeon, patient, and parents should expect a high rate of complications. Urethrocutaneous fistulas occur in 15 to 30 percent of patients after urethroplasty, depending on the extent of the procedure. Sometimes, small fistulas without distal obstruction can be dissected and closed edge to edge, with care being taken to cover the repair with well-vascularized subcutaneous tissue and skin. Other fistulas may require debridement and closure with an island flap or a patch graft. Strictures may occur anywhere along the neourethra but are most common at the proximal and distal anastamoses. Preventive measures include the avoidance of circular anastamoses, constricting tunnels, or injury to the vascular supply of tubularized flaps. Another complication of urethroplasty is the formation of pseudodiverticula, with or without distal obstruction, sometimes requiring careful dissection and reduction urethroplasty.

The genital component of epispadias repair in the male can provide increased phallic length, but overzealous dissection of the crura may result in corporeal necrosis and impotence. Inadequate resection of dorsal chordee may leave the patient with a functionally significant deviation of the erect penis. However, subcutaneous fibrosis after skin mobilization ("skin chordee") can also cause shaft irregularities and must be distinguished from true chordee at the time of revision. Undue tension on reapproximated glanular flaps may cause edge necrosis and lead to failure of the glanuloplasty and perhaps also the distal urethroplasty. Remodeling of the female external genitalia is sometimes necessary for cosmetic reasons as the tissues fill out and mature during puberty.

The outcome of bladder neck reconstruction is less than optimal, even with meticulous technique. We advise parents of a 60 to 75 percent chance of success in achieving urinary continence with current methods. Revision of bladder neck repairs is not only difficult but often unsatisfying. If total continence is not accomplished on the first attempt, the contributory factors should be reviewed. A careful assessment of bladder capacity and intravesical pressure should be repeated, and the urethral pressure profile of a quiet patient may give the surgeon an idea of the magnitude of the urethral resistance deficit. Males who have persistent incontinence after complete repair but a continuous, unobstructed conduit from bladder to glans and some degree of bladder neck resistance, may be candidates for observation only; prostatic enlargement through puberty may resolve incontinence in this instance. Aside from formal revision of the bladder neck repair, delayed intervention for persistent incontinence may require an obstructing procedure such as a bladder neck sling or an artificial urinary sphincter. We do not advise placement of an artificial sphincter distal to the bladder neck around a neourethra. When the postoperative outlet resistance is too high, clinical problems stemming from elevated intravesical pressure or high postvoid residual urine may appear. Depending on the anticipated difficulty in achieving reduced urethral resistance, bladder neck revision, stricture repair, or augmentation cystoplasty may be necessary. High-pressure bladders must be studied for persistent or recurrent vesicoureteral reflux, which should be managed appropriately if present.

SUGGESTED READING

Kropp KA. Bladder neck reconstructive surgery in children. AUA Update Series 1989; 8:314–319.

Monfort G, Morisson-Lacombe G, Guys JM, Coquet M. Transverse island flap and double flap procedure in the treatment of congenital epispadias in 32 patients. J Urol 1987; 138:1069–1071.

Peters CA, Gearhart JP, Jeffs RD. Epispadias and incontinence: the challenge of the small bladder. J Urol 1988; 140:1199–1201.

URETHRAL PROLAPSE

ELLEN SHAPIRO, M.D.

Prolapse of the female urethra is a circumferential eversion of the distal urethra through the urethral meatus. Urethral prolapse appears as a rosette- or donut-shaped collar of hemorrhagic, friable, edematous tissue with the urethral meatus in the center (Fig. 1). This is an uncommon entity, occurring in approximately one in 3,000 children. It is seen in both prepubertal and postmenopausal females. Urethral prolapse has been observed in children as young as 5 days old, but the average age is 5 years. In older women, the average age of presentation is 57 years. In most series, more than 90 percent of children with urethral prolapse are black, whereas most of the adults reported with this benign condition are Caucasian.

ETIOLOGY

The exact etiologic factors leading to urethral prolapse are unknown. Despite the reported occurrence of urethral prolapse in a set of identical twins and the increased incidence in black children, the changing racial distribution pattern makes it difficult to propose either a genetic or a racial predisposition for this condition. Various theories have been proposed to explain both the congenital and the acquired forms of this condition. The congenital theories include weak pelvic floor structures, inadequate pelvic attachments to the urethra, excessive urethral mobilization, excessive redundancy of the mucosa, and an abnormally patulous urethra. Lowe and colleagues performed an en bloc

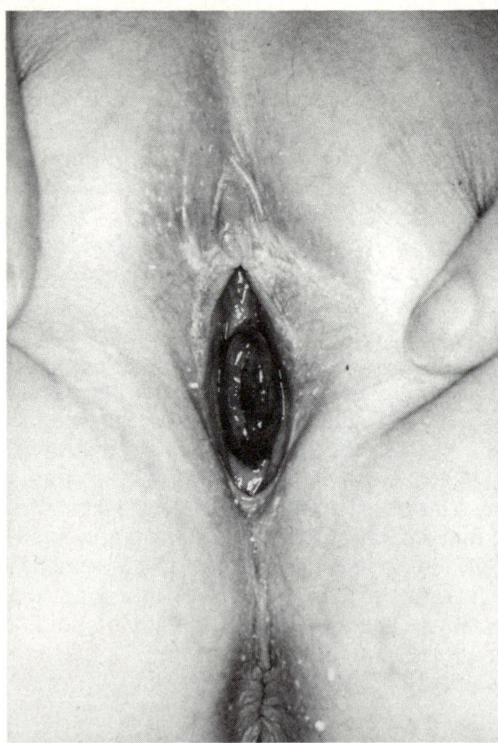

Figure 1 Urethral prolapse presenting with a donut-shaped collar of hemorrhagic edematous tissue with the urethral meatus in the center.

dissection and serial sectioning of the normal and prolapsed prepubertal female urethra. The normal urethral mucosa is surrounded by a plexus of vascular channels and intermixed longitudinal smooth muscle bundles. This resembles erectile tissue and has been termed corpus spongiosum urethrae muliebris. Surrounding this corpus spongiosum is a thick layer of smooth muscle arranged in a circular-oblique pattern. The outermost layer is skeletal muscle, concentrated primarily at the trigone and meatal regions. Lowe and colleagues proposed that urethral prolapse results from poor attachments between the longitudinal and circular-oblique smooth muscle of the urethra subjected to repeated episodes of increased intra-abdominal pressure.

Acquired causes of this disorder include trauma from childbirth, all forms of increased abdominal pressure, urethral coitus, malnutrition, and neuromuscular deficiency. Although sexual abuse is a possible cause, this is more likely to result in meatal contusion than in prolapse. Estrogen deficiency has been implicated, since there is a bimodal distribution of urethral prolapse among female population on both sides of the hormonal peak.

PRESENTATION

Most children with urethral prolapse present with blood spotting in their underclothes. Others complain of micturitional disturbances, including dysuria and urinary frequency. Although mucosal ulceration may cause introital pain, the mass of a prolapsed urethra can be asymptomatic and can be detected incidentally on routine examinations. Voiding complaints, including dysuria, urinary frequency, stranguria, a decrease in the force of the urinary stream, gross hematuria, and tenesmus, are more common in older patients.

The diagnosis of urethral prolapse is usually made on inspection of the introitus. The finding of a complete circular prolapse of mucosa with a centrally located urethral opening is pathognomonic for urethral prolapse. If there is any doubt of the diagnosis, the abnormal appearance of the introitus must be differentiated from urethral polyps, papilloma, condyloma, sarcoma botryoides, prolapsed ectopic ureterocele, hydrometrocolpos, paraurethral cysts, and periurethral abscess. If there is partial or eccentric prolapse of one wall, the diagnosis of ectopic ureterocele should be considered. An intravenous pyelogram or ultrasonogram will demonstrate a prolapsed ectopic ureterocele. In older females, urethral caruncle presents as a reddened tender swelling arising from the lower half of the urethral meatus. Other unusual differential diagnoses include cervical prolapse, hemangioma, malacoplakia, and carcinoma. Cystoscopy is rarely necessary to diagnose urethral prolapse definitively, but it is helpful as a means to further define micturitional complaints or gross hematuria in older females.

THERAPEUTIC ALTERNATIVES

When a patient is first diagnosed with urethral prolapse, conservative measures may be initiated until elective surgery is possible. Sitz baths and bed rest may help the vascular congestion. Estrogen creams may be employed in addition to antibiotic therapy, since the normal defense barriers to bacteria may be altered. Reduction of the prolapse by placement of a catheter has also been advocated. These nonoperative methods have had long-term success, justifying an initial conservative approach to the management of urethral prolapse. Although some improvement may be seen, a persistent, bleeding prolapsed urethra should be surgically excised. Numerous procedures have been proposed for the treatment of urethral prolapse, including suprapubic urethropexy, cautery excision, surgical ligation, and cryosurgery. More aggressive therapy is rarely needed. These alternative methods of excision are of historical interest and involve greater morbidity and potential for urethral stricture. After surgical excision, the outer epithelial and inner mucosal layers are circumferentially approximated with fine interrupted absorbable sutures. Short-term catheterization is recommended to avoid postoperative urinary retention.

Lowe and colleagues recommend the surgical reduction technique for the prolapsed urethra. This entails incising the constricting meatal ring if there is no evidence of thrombosis or necrosis of the prolapsed mucosa. The vascular congestion is relieved, permitting reduction of the prolapsed mucosa. Sutures are placed through the mucosa and urethral wall and into the periurethral vestibule to obliterate the plane between the smooth muscle layers.

COMPLICATIONS

The most common complication following treatment of urethral prolapse is its persistence or recurrence. Etiologic factors should be investigated. After surgical excision the recurrence rate is less than 5 percent. If no contributing factors can be implicated, a suprapubic urethropexy may be indicated. Overzealous excision of the urethra may result in a hypospadiac deformity with excessive vaginal voiding and incontinence. Meatal stenosis is uncommon after excision of the urethral prolapse if performed properly.

SUGGESTED READING

Belman AB. Anomalies of the urinary tract: urethra. In: Kelalis PP, King LR, Belman AB, eds. Clinical pediatric urology. Philadelphia: WB Saunders, 1985:786.

Lowe FC, Hill GS, Jeffs RD, Brendler CB. Urethral prolapse in children: insights into etiology and management. J Urol 1986; 135:100–103.

MICROPENIS

CLAUDE C. SCHULMAN, M.D., Ph.D.
A. M. SASSINE, M.D.

A micropenis is defined as a normally formed but diminutive male organ that has a stretched length less than 2 to 2.5 standard deviations below the mean (Fig. 1). At 12 weeks of gestation the penis is completely developed, measures 3.5 mm, and increases in size (0.7 mm per week), measuring 35 mm at term. The newborn has a penis 35 ± 4 mm in length and 11 ± 1 mm in diameter. In boys 1 to 12 years old, the norms are 40 to 65 mm in length and 11 to 17 mm in diameter; after 12 years, there is progressive pubertal development of the penis until the adult norms are reached.

Neonatal identification of the condition allows for the greatest flexibility in management and the best outcome.

PATHOPHYSIOLOGY

Under hormonal control, the external genitalia and perineum undergo morphogenesis between 6 and 12 weeks of gestation. By the 12th week of gestation, male and female perineal and external genital organs are completely differentiated. The transformation of the genital tubercle into a penis is influenced by dihydrotestosterone, the product of fetal testosterone, and by 5-α-reductase, which is produced in the fibroblast of the perineum.

A hormonal defect occurring before 12 weeks of gestation is influenced by maternal stimulation of the fetal testosterone system and will result in a penis with varied ambiguity. A defect occurring after 12 weeks is related to the fetal endocrine system and will result in a normally developed but small penis.

ETIOLOGY AND DIAGNOSIS

Associated clinical syndromes should be suspected in a boy presenting with a micropenis (Table 1). The

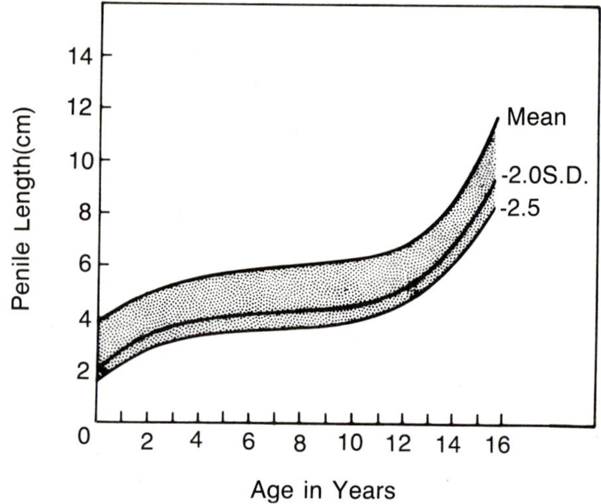

Figure 1 Stretched penile length. Micropenis is defined as a length less than 2.0 to 2.5 standard deviations (S.D.) from the norm at a specific age. (Republished with permission by Joseph DB, Bauer SB. Micropenis. In: Resnick MI, Kursh E, eds. Current therapy in genitourinary surgery. Toronto: BC Decker, 1987.)

clinical examination and biologic explorations lead to diagnosis in 75 to 80 percent of cases. The penis is stretched and measured after depressing the preputial fat. A karyotype study is indicated to ascertain chromosomal sex. Fifty percent of boys with micropenis have congenital hypothalamic pituitary abnormalities. Micropenis is exceptional within Klinefelter's syndrome with a 47XX karyotype. Testicular deficiencies are less common. The rudimentary testis often leads to male pseudohermaphroditism with sometimes a micropenis. Curiously, the micropenis is less common with anorchia. More frequent are the polymalformative syndrome with or without karyotype abnormalities. One of the easiest to diagnose is the Prader-Willi syndrome.

For neonatal identification of micropenis and in order to diagnose the congenital deficiency in gonadotropins, the serum levels of luteinizing hormone (LH) and testosterone should be obtained between the first and second month of age. If micropenis is diagnosed in a young boy, an hCG stimulation test should be performed to differentiate between a central or a testicular abnormality in the production of androgens. If there is a central abnormality and no appreciable growth of the

Table 1 Causes of Micropenis

Hypothalamic-pituitary abnormalities
  Kleinfelter's syndrome
  Björeson's syndrome
  Anorchia
  Rudimentary testes

Testicular disorders
  Kallmann's syndrome
  Prader-Willi syndrome
  Robinow's syndrome
  Anencephaly
  Hypopituitarism

End-organ failure

Idiopathic

penis with hCG therapy, end-organ responsiveness should be evaluated by measuring 5-α-reductase and receptor site activity.

TREATMENT

Management of micropenis should be directed toward early evaluation, diagnosis, and treatment. Neonatal identification allows for the greatest flexibility in management and the best treatment outcome. These infants respond best to androgen stimulation or replacement. Sex reassignment is most appropriate for newborns who do not respond to hormonal manipulation. In these, such a phallus will never develop into a sexually or cosmetically effective organ. A team approach combining the pediatric urologist, endocrinologist, and psychologist must discuss this issue openly with the family, explaining that poor sexual identity related to an inadequate penis can have profound psychological repercussions.

If it is agreed that the child is to be raised as a female, orchiectomy and external genitoplasty are required as soon as feasible before the age of 6 months.

Prepubertal boys with a primary testicular abnormality will benefit from androgen therapy. Parenteral administration is preferable to topical administration of testosterone, which requires daily and adequate manipulation of the genitals. A dosage of 2 mg per kilogram is administered intramuscularly every 3 weeks for 3 months. During the prepubertal and pubertal periods, other courses of therapy are needed. Postpubertal or adult males require a penile lengthening procedure or a penile prosthesis to provide adequate penile length and enable them to achieve satisfactory sexual intercourse. In all cases psychological support is needed.

AMBIGUOUS GENITALIA

ANTHONY A. CALDAMONE, M.D., F.A.C.S.,
F.A.A.P.

Ambiguous genitalia in the newborn presents as an urgent condition requiring a well-formulated diagnostic protocol and prompt assimilation of information to arrive at a propitious recommendation regarding the sex of rearing. The major difficulty in dealing with this problem is that many conditions have genital ambiguity as their presentation. The atmosphere for the parents is one of confusion, anger, guilt, and anxiety. This situation must be explained to the parents in such a way as to best allay their anxiety and to allow a short time to arrive at a definitive recommendation before the infant's discharge from the hospital. We rely on a team approach consisting of a pediatric endocrinologist, geneticist, pediatric urologist or surgeon, and primary pediatrician. Generally a decision should be arrived at within the first week of life.

The evaluation and management, both medical and surgical, of the newborn presenting with ambiguous genitalia is emphasized here. A brief review of normal sexual differentiation is provided as background for evaluation and management, followed by a general classification of intersex conditions.

NORMAL SEXUAL DIFFERENTIATION

Before the sixth week of gestation the human fetus is sexually undifferentiated, since the gonad cannot be distinguished as an ovary or testis. Sexual differentiation is a sequential process that can be divided into three stages, each subsequent stage depending on the preceding one. The chromosomal sex, which is determined at fertilization, dictates the differentiation of the gonad (gonadal sex), which in turn dictates differentiation of the internal ductal system and external genitalia (phenotypic sex).

Chromosomal sex is determined at the moment of conception and is based on the sex chromosome complement of the fertilizing sperm. This concept, however, is rather simplistic, since at least 19 genes on both the sex and autosomal chromosomes have been identified that are involved in the determination of fetal sex. A recent work has identified a sequence of genes located on the distal portion of the short arm of the Y chromosome within 1A. In addition, there are many common sequences of this genetic material located on the X chromosome.

The gonadal sex is established by the seventh week of gestation. At this stage, the fetus contains two internal ductal systems, wolffian and müllerian, and undifferentiated external genital primordia recognized as protuberances anterolateral to the cloacal membrane. Both internal ductal systems are derived from the mesonephric renal system. That portion of the urogenital sinus distal to the termination of these ducts contributes to external genital development, whereas the proximal portion develops into the bladder, trigone, and posterior urethra.

Phenotypic sexual differentiation is predicated on the establishment of gonadal sex. If an ovary is developed, the wolffian duct involutes, persisting only in its terminal portion as Gartner's ducts in the females. The müllerian ducts develop into the proximal vagina, uterus, and fallopian tubes. The exact role that ovarian development and secretion plays in female phenotypic differentiation is uncertain. Since ovarian development lags behind genital development to some degree, and since, in cases of agenesis of the gonads, female phenotypic development occurs regardless of the chromosomal complement, it is thought that the ovaries do not play a determining role in the early stages of female differentiation. It is possible that this process occurs under the influence of the high estrogen milieu from the placenta and maternal circulation.

Male phenotypic differentiation is predicated on the elaboration by the testis of two distinct hormonal substances: testosterone and müllerian inhibitory substance (MIF). These are produced and secreted by the 8-week stage of development. MIF causes the involution of the müllerian ducts and is produced by the fetal Sertoli cells.

Immediately following müllerian duct regression, the wolffian ducts develop under the influence of testosterone secreted by the fetal Leydig cells. The wolffian ducts evolve into the epididymis, vas deferens, and seminal vesicles. This process occurs as a direct action of testosterone on the ductal structures. By the twelfth week of gestation, differentiation of the wolffian ducts is completed. External virilization, however, relies on the ability of the tissues involved to convert testosterone into a more potent androgen, dihydrotestosterone. The cytoplasm of the target cells possesses the enzyme 5-alpha-reductase, which is necessary for this conversion. Once dihydrotestosterone is formed, a cytoplasmic receptor binds to the hormone and transports it to the nucleus, where it acts on DNA to direct the formation of various proteins necessary for virilization of the external genitalia.

DISORDERS OF SEXUAL DIFFERENTIATION

On the basis of the embryologic events described, disorders of sexual differentiation can be better understood and appreciated. Intersexuality can be thought of as resulting from overandrogenization of the female or underandrogenization of the male. In turn, these can occur from events occurring at the chromosomal, gonadal, or phenotypic stages of development. Not all intersex states lead to ambiguous genitalia. Those states in which chromosomal, gonadal, or internal phenotypic disorders do not influence external phenotypic expression may have normal-appearing external genitalia. There are also some disorders in which, in spite of normal external genitalia, the internal ductal system either is poorly developed or develops along lines inconsistent with external genital sexual differentiation. These cases may present with infertility, delayed puberty, primary amenorrhea, inguinal hernia with müllerian contents in a phenotypic male, or inguinal hernia with a gonad in a phenotypic female. A classification of various intersex states based on a chromosomal, gonadal, or phenotypic etiology is presented in Table 1.

EVALUATION OF THE NEWBORN WITH AMBIGUOUS GENITALIA

History

A careful history should include questioning regarding maternal ingestion of androgens, progestational agents, or other drugs during pregnancy. Some of these agents, which can affect virilization of the female genital system, may have been prescribed to prevent spontaneous abortion. A history of virilization of the mother

Table 1 Classification of Intersex

Disorders of chromosomal sex
  True hermaphroditism
    (46 XX or 46 XY or mosaic)
  Mixed gonadal dysgenesis
    (46 XY/45 XO)
  Klinefelter's syndrome
    (47 XXY)
  Sex reversal syndrome
    (46 XX male)
  Turner's syndrome
    (46 XO)

Disorders of gonadal sex
  46 XY gonadal dysgenesis
  46 XX gonadal dysgenesis
  Gonadal agenesis (regression)

Disorders of phenotypic sex
  Female pseudohermaphroditism (46 XX)
    Congenital adrenal hyperplasia
    Exogenous virilization
    Virilizing tumor (maternal)

Male pseudohermaphroditism (46 XY)
  Deficiency of müllerian inhibitory substance
  Deficient androgen synthesis
  Androgen insensitivity
  5-Alpha-reductase deficiency
  Dysgenetic gonads

during pregnancy may signal a maternal virilizing tumor (arrhenoblastoma, luteoma).

Many intersex conditions are inheritable; consequently, a thorough family history should be obtained. A history of similar problems in other family members should be sought. One should also ask if there are family members with a history of unexplained death in infancy, delayed puberty, amenorrhea, hirsutism, infertility, and salt craving. Androgen insensitivity syndromes are inherited in an X-linked recessive trait; therefore, a similar disorder may be present in a maternal aunt, uncle, cousin, or sibling. Congenital adrenal hyperplasia (CAH, adrenogenital syndrome) is transmitted as an autosomal recessive disorder, and consequently other siblings may be affected.

Physical Examination

The most important finding on physical examination is the presence or absence of palpable gonads. Although ovaries may present in the inguinal region, they rarely descend to the distal canal, labioscrotal folds, or scrotum. The presence of palpable gonads excludes the diagnostic category of female pseudohermaphroditism, which is the most frequent cause of neonatal genital ambiguity. If both gonads are descended and normal to palpation, male pseudohermaphroditism is most likely. Various degrees of hypoplastic or undescended gonads occur in a variety of intersex conditions.

The size of the phallus (stretch length and diameter) along with the location of the urethral meatus should be carefully determined. Most cases of ambiguous genitalia have a single urogenital sinus; however, patients with the more severe forms of androgen insensitivity syndrome and 5-alpha-reductase deficiency may have separate urethral and vaginal openings.

Hyperpigmentation of the labioscrotal folds and the areola is commonly seen in CAH owing to excess circulating adrenocorticotropic hormone. Rectal examination should be performed to assess the presence of müllerian structures. Specifically the uterus may be palpable as a midline structure on rectal examination in the newborn. Physical signs of dehydration and salt wasting should be observed, since these symptoms commonly present with CAH (most commonly, 21-hydroxylase deficiency). Blood pressure should be checked because patients with certain types of CAH (11-beta-hydroxylase deficiency) have hypertension caused by retention of sodium. Other congenital anomalies may also be present with certain cases of intersex.

Laboratory Evaluation

The evaluation of the newborn with ambiguous genitalia is divided into chromosomal, biochemical, and radiographic/endoscopic/surgical examination. Chromosomes may be evaluated by buccal smear or culture of peripheral blood leukocytes. The buccal smear technique relies on the presence of clumped nuclear chromatin along the nuclear membrane, thereby repre-

senting the inactivated X chromosome of an XX complement. Depending on the familiarity of the laboratory, Barr body interpretation should be viewed with caution, since only 20 percent or more of nuclei of normal female cells and up to 2 percent of normal male cells contain Barr bodies. Additionally, Barr body counts in the normal female may be low in the first few days of life. More recently, the Y chromosome has been identified on buccal smear by fluorescence microscopy after staining with quinacrine. Owing to inherent difficulties in the interpretation of the presence or absence of Barr bodies by buccal smear, it is probably more prudent to base the sex of rearing on formal chromosomal analysis, which requires a 3-day period of incubation.

The chromosomal complement is extremely helpful in determining the etiology of the ambiguous genitalia, although by no means singularly diagnostic. An XY karyotype most often indicates one of the various causes of male pseudohermaphroditism, although in a smaller percentage of cases it may indicate true hermaphroditism or 46 XY gonadal dysgenesis. An XX pattern most often indicates female pseudohermaphroditism except in those rare cases in which it is associated with true hermaphroditism or 46 XX gonadal dysgenesis. An XO or XO mosaic pattern indicates gonadal dysgenesis (Turner's syndrome) or mixed gonadal dysgenesis, respectively.

Biochemical evaluation is most helpful in CAH. Elevated urinary levels of 17-ketosteroids and pregnanetriol are very suggestive of a deficiency of 21-hydroxylase or 11-hydroxylase. Serum levels of 17-hydroxyprogesterone are significantly elevated in 21-hydroxylase deficiency, which is the most common enzymatic defect in CAH. Other plasma cortisol precursors may also be measured to document rarer forms of CAH enzymatic deficiencies. Electrolytes should also be obtained, since many patients with CAH are significant salt losers.

Serum testosterone is normally elevated above prepubertal levels within the first 6 to 8 weeks of life owing to an unexplained LH surge in the perinatal period. Measurements of serum testosterone and dihydrotestosterone are helpful in determining the causes of male pseudohermaphroditism. An additional way to test androgen production is by administration of human chorionic gonadotropin (hCG). No response in serum testosterone level after 3 consecutive days of hCG therapy indicates either the lack of androgen-producing tissue (gonadal dysgenesis, gonadal agenesis) or deficient androgen production. The latter possibility can be diagnosed by measuring plasma or urinary levels of testosterone precursors. If there is an effective rise in testosterone, either androgen insensitivity or 5-alpha-reductase deficiency is likely. Androgen insensitivity is characterized by a normal ratio of testosterone to dihydrotestosterone with elevated serum testosterone and dihydrotestosterone to varying degrees, while in 5-alpha-reductase deficiency the ratio is greater than 30:1.

The radiographic evaluation of genital ambiguity in

the newborn includes abdominal and pelvic ultrasonography and contrast genitography. The purpose of radiography is to determine the status of the internal ductal system. Ultrasonography may nicely demonstrate a uterus and vagina in the newborn; however, these structures may not be readily apparent to the novice observer (Fig. 1). The ability of ultrasonography to demonstrate conclusively the presence or absence of ovaries in the infant is limited. The purpose of contrast genitography is to show the common urogenital sinus, urethra, and vagina, if present. In addition, an indentation on the dome of the vagina represents a uterine cervical impression, indicative of internal müllerian structures (Fig. 2). Retrograde contrast genitography is preferable to voiding cystourethrography, since the latter may not reflux contrast medium into a vaginal pouch. Documentation of internal müllerian structures excludes most causes of male pseudohermaphroditism except those due to dysgenetic gonads in which there is a deficiency of MIF.

If genitography is equivocal, endoscopy of the urogenital sinus, urethra, and vagina can be performed to further elucidate the anatomy. Exploratory laparotomy and gonadal biopsy should be done early only in cases in which a definitive diagnosis cannot be established by chromosomal, biochemical, and radiographic evaluation, and only if findings will influence the sex of rearing. Laparoscopy may also be helpful in these cases.

ASSIGNMENT OF SEX OF REARING

Sex assignment should be made only after all the significantly contributory information is available. This should be done in concert with a geneticist, endocrinologist, and surgeon. The female pseudohermaphrodite should be raised as a female regardless of the degree of virilization. Since all these patients have normal ovaries, fallopian tubes, uterus, and vagina, fertility is possible.

The male pseudohermaphrodite presents a complex problem. It is difficult to predict whether virilization with adequate phallic growth will occur at puberty. Neonatal response to testosterone in androgen synthesis deficiency, partial androgen insensitivity, or mild forms of 5-alpha-reductase deficiency may be reassuring as to later virilization; however, this is only speculative. The sex of rearing is primarily based on the degree of virilization and adequacy of the phallus at birth. A child with a significantly short penile stretch length that does not respond to exogenous hCG or testosterone should be reared as a female without regard to diagnostic testing results. If these children are raised as males, the result is psychologically devastating because they are often inadequately virilized. Children are thought to reach a level of well-differentiated psychosexual identity by 1½ to 2 years of age; therefore, gender reassignment beyond that age is unwise.

When the diagnosis of mixed gonadal dysgenesis is made (46 XY/XO), there are several factors that favor female sex assignment. Although infantile even after puberty, a uterus and vagina are present. These patients are commonly of rather short stature. Finally, the testes are usually infertile and carry an increased potential for malignancy.

The true hermaphrodite with an adequate phallus should be raised according to the degree of external virilization. If there is a normal testis that can be placed in the scrotum, a male assignment should be made. Female assignment should be made if there is an inadequate phallus, or if normal müllerian duct struc-

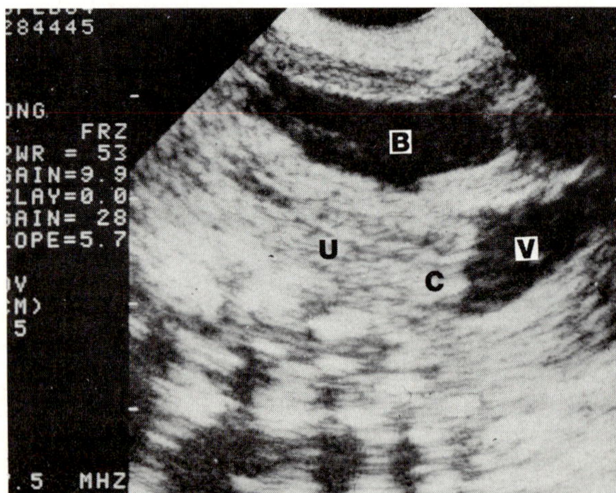

Figure 1 Ultrasonogram of a newborn with ambiguous genitalia and a common urogenital sinus, demonstrating bladder (B), vagina (V), cervix (C), and uterus (U). The diagnosis was congenital adrenal hyperplasia.

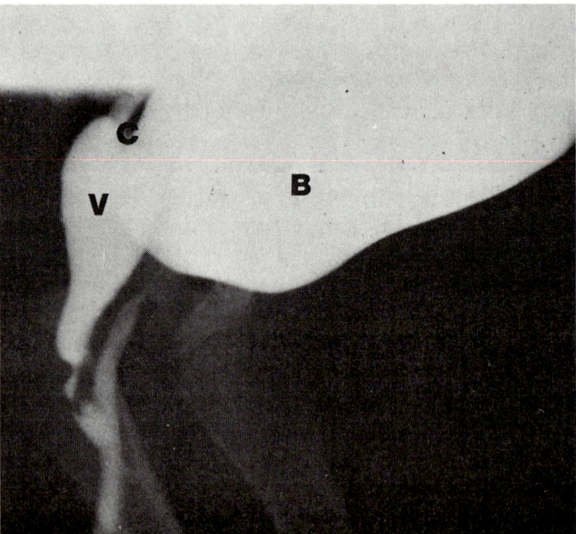

Figure 2 Contrast genitogram in a newborn with a common urogenital sinus. The vagina (V) is nicely demonstrated with cervical (C) impression on the dome. B represents the bladder.

tures exist with a normal ovary on one side and either a testis or an ovotestis on the other side.

SURGICAL MANAGEMENT OF INTERSEX STATES

Surgical intervention in intersex conditions has three purposes: (1) diagnostic-exploratory laparotomy and gonadal biopsy, (2) gonadectomy for dysgenetic gonads or gonads inconsistent with the sex of rearing, and (3) external genital reconstruction.

The indications for exploratory laparotomy and gonadal biopsy have dwindled over recent years owing to significant improvement in our diagnostic capabilities. However, if following chromosomal, biochemical, and radiographic evaluation a definitive sex assignment cannot be made, a detailed or laparoscopic surgical exploration of the internal ductal system along with biopsy of each of the gonads is indicated. The gonadal biopsy must be performed in such a way as to sample all representative areas of the gonad. This is particularly important in the ovotestis in which the separate portions occur at the poles of the combined gonad.

There are basically two indications for gonadectomy: (1) gonads that are inconsistent with the sex of rearing and (2) gonads that have malignant potential. The first indication arises in cases of androgen-insensitivity patients raised as females, severe cases of defective androgen synthesis and 5-alpha-reductase deficiency, true hermaphroditism, and mixed gonadal dysgenesis. The second indication arises in 46 XY gonadal dysgenesis (Swyer's syndrome) and mixed gonadal dysgenesis. There have been cases of Swyer's syndrome in which a gonadoblastoma had been present as early as 15 months of age; therefore, gonadectomy should be undertaken at the time of diagnosis.

Reconstructive surgery falls into two categories: (1) repair of hypospadias, chordee, bifid scrotum, penoscrotal transposition, and/or orchidopexy; and (2) feminizing genitoplasty—clitoral reduction and vaginoplasty. The first category will not be discussed here, since it follows the general tenets of each individual procedure and is not specific for the intersex condition.

Congenital adrenal hyperplasia is the most common condition for which a feminizing genitoplasty is indicated. The surgical correction of the virilized external genitalia is both cosmetic and functional. There are two schools of thought as to the timing of this reconstruction. Some believe that this reconstruction should be done immediately after the child is stabilized on glucocorticoid and mineralocorticoid therapy. Their rationale is that taking a child home who appears normal significantly reduces parental anxiety and guilt. Others, however, reserve this procedure as an elective operation to be done within the first year of life. With this approach, the longer time on corticosteroid therapy often results in clitoral shrinkage. Also, complete correction in the neonatal period can be a technically difficult procedure. If parental acceptance is judged to be satisfactory, it is probably best to delay correction until 6 to 9 months of age. When the clitoris is severely masculinized, however, clitoroplasty prior to initial discharge from the hospital is appropriate.

Clitoroplasty and vaginoplasty can usually be performed together. In such situations vaginoplasty is best performed first, because this permits a better anatomic arrangement in creating the labia. It may be necessary to delay vaginoplasty in certain cases in which there is a very high outpouching of the vagina (long common urogenital sinus). In this setting it is advisable to perform the clitoroplasty early in infancy for cosmetic effect, reserving the vaginoplasty until 2 to 4 years of age when the structures are somewhat larger, thus reducing technical complications.

Several methods are available to improve the appearance of a virilized clitoris, including simple recession, reduction, and amputation. The choice of procedure depends primarily on the size of the phallus and the surgeon's preference. Several factors should be taken into account, however. The clitoris is a localized focus for sexual stimulation in the female, and it is therefore preferable to preserve at least part of this focus for later sexual activity. It has been noted that adolescent girls who had undergone total clitorectomy in early childhood reported inhibition of sexual arousal. Simple concealment or recession of a large clitoris may result in a conspicuous and at times painful erection on sexual arousal. The goal, therefore, is to obtain a well-concealed clitoris that maintains erectile activity on sexual stimulation without causing pain or embarrassment.

I prefer a procedure in which the erectile tissue is shelled out of Buck's fascia after proximal individual ligation of the corporeal bodies. This not only reduces the erectile tissue but also preserves the glans with its dorsal neurovascular bundle. If the glans is conspicuously large, however, a glans wedge resection may be performed. Similarly, the corporeal tissue and surrounding fascia may be plicated to achieve shortening of the clitoral shaft. The clitoris is then recessed by suturing it to the periosteum of the undersurface of the pubis.

It is important to preserve all the overlying skin of the clitoris: the foreskin, if you will. This skin can be split in the midline and fashioned into labial minora.

Vaginoplasty involves exteriorizing the vagina to the perineal skin, thus creating separate urethral and vaginal orifices and eliminating the common urogenital sinus. For the very mild degrees of virilization a simple cut-back procedure by a Heineke-Mikulicz rearrangement suffices. For moderate virilization with a moderate-length urogenital sinus, a perineal flap vaginoplasty provides a well-vascularized skin flap, which is anastomosed to the posterior wall of the vagina, thus creating a perineal vaginal opening. This is an inverted U-shaped flap with its apex at the posterior lip of the urogenital sinus opening. Dissection is on the posterior wall of the urogenital sinus until the posterior vaginal wall is isolated. The posterior wall is then incised in the midline to allow for its anastomosis to the skin flap.

It is anticipated that the most common complication of vaginoplasty will be stenosis of the vaginal outlet. I do not advocate postoperative vaginal introital dilatation in this very young age group. Unless problems develop related to urinary reflux or entrapped secretions, revision should be delayed until after puberty.

In those conditions of severe virilization in which there is a very high vaginal take-off from the urethra, vaginoplasty should be delayed until later in childhood or even after puberty.

ANORCHIA

GLEN S. GERBER, M.D.
CASIMIR F. FIRLIT, M.D., Ph.D.

Congenital anorchia is a rare condition manifested as bilaterally absent testes in an otherwise phenotypically normal male. The disorder is characterized by a normal 46XY karyotype as well as the absence of müllerian structures. These findings help to distinguish anorchia from gonadal dysgenesis, Klinefelter's syndrome, extreme forms of hypogonadotropic hypogonadism, and male and female pseudohermaphroditism. However, the differentiation that is most important is between anorchia and bilateral cryptorchidism. It is estimated that no gonadal tissue will be found upon surgical exploration in 0.5 percent of boys with bilaterally undescended testes. Therefore, the incidence of true congenital anorchia is approximately one in 10,000 to 20,000 male infants.

The etiology of anorchia has not been determined. Since the male external genitalia develop under the influence of fetal testosterone during the 6th to 13th weeks of gestation, it is apparent that functioning testicular tissue was present during this interval. For this reason, the most widely supported theory holds that vascular occlusion, most likely secondary to intrauterine torsion, occurred during testicular descent. The frequent operative finding of a small nubbin of fibrotic tissue at the end of the vas deferens also supports a vascular etiology.

DIAGNOSTIC EVALUATION

When confronted wth a male child with nonpalpable testes, it is important to examine carefully the external genitalia. The presence of hypospadias in this setting raises concern over sexual ambiguity. As mentioned above, true congenital anorchia implies that the genitalia are normal except for the absence of testes. It is also necessary to perform a digital rectal examination to check for internal müllerian structures. Important points in the history include familial disorders of sexual development as well as possible maternal disease or exposures during pregnancy. In addition, karyotyping of the patient is needed when neither testis can be palpated.

The efficacy of several radiographic imaging techniques in localizing nonpalpable testes has been investigated. The results from invasive modalities such as spermatic arteriography and gonadal venography have been very inconsistent. Therefore, the potential morbidity associated with these methods makes their use unjustifiable. Less invasive techniques such as computed tomography (CT), ultrasonography, and radionuclide scanning may sometimes help to localize a nonpalpable gonad. However, a negative result does not rule out the presence of a testis, and surgical exploration may still be necessary. Recently, several reports of the use of magnetic resonance imaging (MRI) to localize nonpalpable testes have been published. As is true for the older radiographic modalities discussed above, MRI may be helpful in some instances, but failure to locate gonadal tissue does not rule out the need for more definitive exploration. In addition, the expense of MRI further limits its value in localizing nonpalpable testes. For these reasons, radiographic evaluation of nonpalpable testes is of limited utility.

ENDOCRINOLOGIC EVALUATION

The endocrinologic evaluation of boys with bilateral nonpalpable testes plays an important but controversial role in the differentiation between anorchia and cryptorchidism. Classically, anorchism is characterized by elevated basal levels of gonadotropins, especially follicle-stimulating hormone (FSH), and a low level of testosterone that fails to respond to an appropriate human chorionic gonadotropin (hCG) stimulation test. Some authors have stated that when there is no testosterone response to hCG, the diagnosis of anorchia is assured and surgical exploration is unnecessary. However, we have reported two cases that contradict this view, both being well-differentiated males with normal 46XY karyotypes. Each child had normal basal gonadotropin levels and no testosterone response to hCG. At surgical exploration, testes were noted bilaterally, with few Leydig cells seen on histologic evaluation. These cases demonstrate that the lack of a testosterone response to hCG stimulation does not rule out the presence of testes. Rather, the unresponsiveness to hCG may be evidence of dysfunctional or nonexistent Leydig cells. In addition, anorchid males may have normal gonadotropin levels. Recent studies suggest that the latter finding may in part be age dependent. During the first 3 to 4 years of life, serum levels of gonadotropins are elevated in anorchid boys, but these subsequently decrease to normal until the ninth year of life, when they again rise. It is postulated that the normal gonadotropin levels seen in middle childhood are due to a steroid-independent, central nervous system inhibition of pulsatile luteinizing hormone–releasing hormone (LHRH) secretion.

Present recommendations for hormonal evaluation when congenital anorchism is suspected are as follows (Fig. 1). Regardless of the age at presentation, gonadotropin levels and an hCG, testicular tissue is present and exploration is indicated. When gonadotropin levels are elevated and there is no response to hCG tests, anorchism is assured and no further search for the testes is necessary. However, when FSH and LH levels are normal, a negative hCG stimulation test does not rule out the presence of testicular tissue. Further evaluation is therefore warranted.

SURGICAL EVALUATION

The search for nonpalpable testes can be performed by laparoscopy, surgical exploration, or both. Regardless of which method is chosen, the absence of the testis is not assured unless a blind-ending spermatic vessel is seen. The mere presence of the vas deferens without an adjacent gonad does not prove that the testis is absent, since gonadal structures may be separate from the epididymis and vas deferens.

Laparoscopy is often preferred to laparotomy as the initial means of exploration for nonpalpable testes, for several reasons. Both methods require general anesthesia, but laparoscopy is less invasive and can be performed through a much smaller incision. In addition, if the testes are seen, this information can be very helpful in planning the surgical approach during the same period of anesthesia. Alternatively, if blind-ending spermatic vessels are visualized bilaterally, there is no need for formal surgical exploration. Some surgeons do not feel comfortable with this approach, however, and may choose to perform surgical exploration regardless of the findings at laparoscopy. This decision must be individualized and is often predicated on the surgeon's level of experience with laparoscopy.

Laparoscopy is performed after first emptying the urinary bladder by catheterization. A small incision is made inferior to the umbilicus and deepened to the level of the midline fascia. A small insufflation needle is passed into the peritoneal cavity as the anterior abdominal wall is lifted. One to 3 L of carbon dioxide are then instilled until adequate distention of the peritoneal cavity is achieved. After the patient is placed in the Trendelenburg position, the needle is removed and the laparoscope introduced. The area between the renal fossa and internal ring can then easily be inspected bilaterally.

Formal surgical exploration is best performed through a modified Gibson incision that allows for adequate intraperitoneal and retroperitoneal inspection. As mentioned above, it is essential that blind-ending spermatic vessels be visualized before it is concluded that the testes are absent.

TREATMENT

Once it has been established that the testes are absent, it is advisable to insert testicular prostheses.

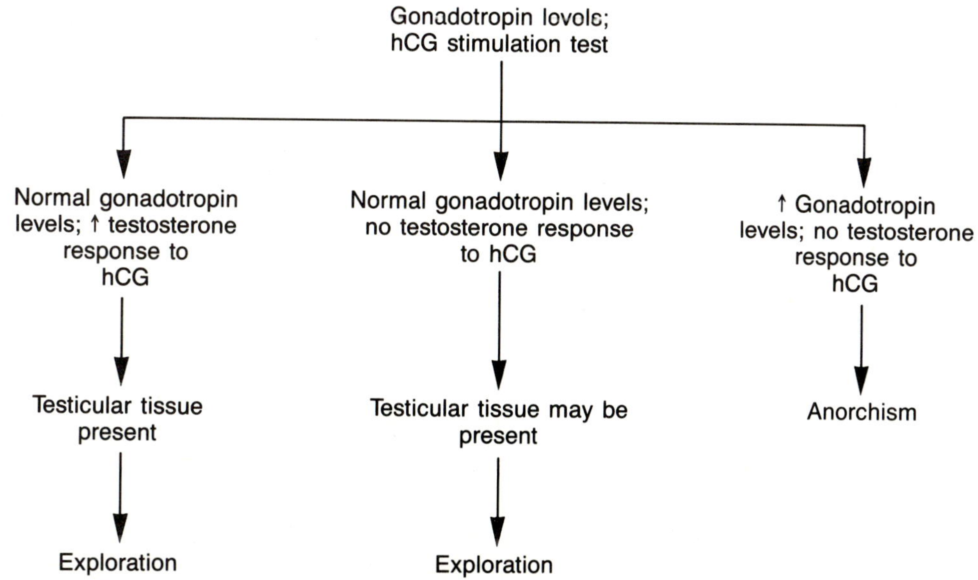

Figure 1 Algorithm for endocrinologic evaluation of boys with suspected congenital anorchism.

These may be important to the patient and parents for psychosocial reasons. If placed in infancy, the prostheses may be exchanged for larger ones at puberty if requested. The prostheses can be implanted at the time of surgical exploration for the absent testes, or at any time thereafter via an inguinal incision. The inguinal approach is preferred because of reports of prosthesis extrusion through the scrotal wound. A vaginal speculum may facilitate prosthesis placement during the inguinal approach. After a subcutaneous plane is developed from the inguinal region down into the scrotum, the speculum is inserted into this plane and spread until a canal is created into the most dependent portion of the hemiscrotum. An appropriately sized testicular prosthesis is inserted and is pushed into the scrotum. A pursestring suture is then placed through the dartos layer superior to the prosthesis to keep it secured in the dependent scrotum.

Hormone replacement is also necessary in anorchid boys. Before puberty, growth will be normal and supplemental androgenous steroids are unnecessary. However, exogenous testosterone is needed to achieve a normal pubertal growth spurt. Testosterone can be supplied either in monthly injections of long-acting testosterone enanthate or in daily oral doses of testosterone undecenote. Generally, monthly injections are preferred. Testosterone replacement therapy should be continued after puberty for psychosocial reasons.

SUGGESTED READING

Bartone FF, Huseman CA, Maizels M, Firlit DF. Pitfalls in using human chorionic gonadotropin stimulation test to diagnose anorchia. J Urol 1984; 132:563–567.

Bloom DA, Ayers JW, McGuire EJ. The role of laparoscopy in management of nonpalpable testes. J Urol (Paris) 1988; 94:465–470.

Jarow JP, Berkovitz GD, Migeon CJ, et al. Elevation of serum gonadotropins establishes the diagnosis of anorchism in prepubertal boys with bilateral cryptorchidism. J Urol 1986; 136:277–279.

Kier R, McCarthy S, Rosenfield AT, et al. Nonpalpable testes in young boys: evaluation with MR imaging. J Radiol 1988; 169:429–433.

Lustig RH, Conte FA, Kogan BA, Grumbach MM. Ontogeny of gonadotropin secretion in congenital anorchism: sexual dimorphism versus syndrome of gonadal dysgenesis and diagnostic considerations. J Urol 1987; 138:587–591.

UNILATERAL CRYPTORCHIDISM IN CHILDREN

GEORGE W. KAPLAN, M.D., M.S.

The unilateral undescended testis is one of the most common problems encountered in children with urologic disorders. There is considerable controversy surrounding both diagnosis and management, largely because there is a lack of precise definition of terms. The normal testis in children or adults resides in a dependent position at the base of the scrotum; any variation may represent cryptorchidism. Some authors limit the term "cryptorchidism" to the intra-abdominal testis, but I believe this is too stringent a definition. Others consider that any testis that has reached even the upper extent of the scrotum is fully descended; I view this as too liberal a definition. It is known that some testes that are not in the scrotum at birth will descend spontaneously during the first few months of life. If descent has not occurred by 6 to 9 months of age, however, it is not likely to do so. There is evidence, based on electron microscopy, that histologic development of the testis begins to lag after roughly 2 years. Thus, according to current thought there is an interval between 9 months and 2 years of age during which cryptorchidism is optimally treated.

One factor that makes therapeutic decisions difficult is testicular retractility. In my opinion, testicular retractility is nothing more than an exaggeration of the normal cremasteric reflex. Many children, because they are bashful, ticklish, frightened, or cold, exhibit testicular retractility during examination. If there is a well-documented history that the testis has been in the scrotum in infancy, testicular retractility becomes a very tenable possibility. Similarly, if the scrotum is normally developed on the affected side, it is more likely that the testis has been scrotally located in the past (i.e., that testicular retractility is present).

EVALUATION

Initial evaluation in the office provides an opportunity to examine the child for the purpose of diagnosis, but, more important, provides an opportunity to educate the parents about the problem at hand and to explore the therapeutic options. I tend to obtain the history from the parents before undressing or examining the child, to allow the child a brief period to become comfortable with my presence. Important elements of the history include associated disorders, a family history of cryptorchidism, a history of hernia, any scrotal abnormalities noted during infancy, and any previous comments on the child's genitalia by physicians.

After taking a complete history, I examine the child; he does not undress completely but merely drops his trousers and raises his shirt. I place the child in a "frog leg" position supine on the table and observe the scrotum for a few seconds. One must specifically note whether the hemiscrotum is hypoplastic and whether a testis appears to be visible in the scrotum. If it is visible, I attempt to trap the testis between the scrotum and the pubis by placing my index finger and thumb over the left and right scrotal inlets, respectively. I then can palpate the hemiscrotum with my other hand to determine whether what I have identified visually is indeed the testis. If no testis is palpable in the scrotum, I gently palpate in the inguinal canal, using the flat portion of my fingertips. If no testis is palpable in the groin, the perineum is carefully examined for evidence of perineal ectopia.

If testicular retractility is suspected on the basis of a history of scrotal placement, a well-developed ipsilateral hemiscrotum, or a contralaterally exaggerated cremasteric reflex, I often recommend a trial of chorionic gonadotropin: 50 IU per kilogram of body weight intramuscularly every 5 days for a total of five doses. If the testis has not descended within 1 week of the final dose, I accept this as evidence of true cryptorchidism and recommend surgery. However, if the testis descends, hormonal therapy can be discontinued. This establishes a diagnosis of testicular retractility, and even if the testis ascends in the future, it may be expected to redescend spontaneously at or before puberty. Most available evidence seems to indicate that retractile testes develop normally.

Although the testis seems retractile, if a hernia or communicating hydrocele is uncovered on the affected side, I consider that orchiopexy is warranted at the time of hernia repair, because many apparent instances of iatrogenic cryptorchidism have been produced after such repair in children with retractile testes. Similarly, if an infant has an undescended testis and a symptomatic hernia on the affected side, I believe that orchiopexy should be accomplished at the time of the hernia repair rather than as a separate procedure, because secondary orchiopexy after hernia repair is more difficult and results in testicular injury more often than does a primary procedure.

Imaging studies are thought inappropriate for children with undescended testes, especially if unilateral. If the testis is palpable, imaging studies are unnecessary for confirmation. If the testis is not palpable, imaging studies may show a testis in the inguinal canal but often fail to demonstrate a testis intra-abdominally. For this reason, imaging studies cannot be relied on to establish conclusively that no testis is present.

If the testis is not palpable, either in the office or with the patient under anesthesia at the time of surgical repair, laparoscopy is of definite assistance in therapy. A small incision is made at the lower edge of the umbilicus with a No. 11 blade. A Veres needle is introduced into the abdominal cavity and the abdomen is filled with carbon dioxide to a pressure of approximately 20 mm Hg (which corresponds to a distended, tympanitic abdomen). A short laparoscopy trocar is introduced through the same incision. The posterior peritoneum is then inspected with the patient in the Trendelenburg position. The vas deferens has a characteristic appearance and can easily be identified as it emerges from behind the bladder and courses toward the internal ring. Similarly, the spermatic vessels can be identified coursing in the retroperitoneum as they approach the vas deferens. If a testis is located intra-abdominally, it can easily be identified. If the vas and vessels are seen to course into the inguinal canal, it then is apparent that any testicular structures must be within the canal. If the vas and vessels end blindly before reaching the internal ring, it can be presumed that a vascular accident resulted in atrophy and subsequent disappearance of the testis.

The management of an intra-abdominal testis, especially if this is unilateral, is controversial. Some authors feel that these are best removed because there is a normal testis on the contralateral side and because of a high likelihood that germ cells will be absent or of poor quality. The eventual functional utility of the testis remains in question. If one is rather less nihilistic regarding the functional prognosis of intra-abdominal testes, it must be recognized that moving a testis from an intra-abdominal location to the scrotum can be difficult. It is partly for this reason that I consider localization of the testis with laparoscopy to be helpful. If the testis resides near the internal ring and has an apparently lengthy vascular pedicle, it can be anticipated that standard maneuvers will result in scrotal placement of the testis. Conversely, if the testis is near or above the iliac vessels and if the spermatic vessels are not at all redundant, it can be expected that no amount of dissection alone will result in scrotal placement.

Transection of the spermatic vessels to achieve sufficient length to reach the scrotum has been practiced since Bevan first described orchiopexy in the late 19th century. This maneuver has reportedly produced variable results. About 30 years ago, Fowler and Stephens demonstrated in experimental animals that collateral circulation exists for the testis and that in many instances the spermatic vessels can be transected if the collateral circulation is not disturbed. After transecting the spermatic vessels, some authors have reported success rates of 70 to 90 percent. My personal series produces results far less satisfactory and has consistently achieved less than 50 percent success.

It was for this reason that a prospective attempt at microvascular anastomosis of the spermatic vessels to the inferida epigastric vessels was used to achieve orchiopexy for intra-abdominal testes. I have worked in conjunction with an experienced microvascular surgeon who is accustomed to anastomosing very small vessels. Using this kind of talent, I have been able to achieve satisfactory scrotal position in all instances and testicular survival in 90 percent of cases in children 1 to 2 years old. However, whether any functional benefit is produced by this endeavor remains to be seen.

The timing of operations for undescended testes has changed in recent years. Since it is unlikely that the testis will descend spontaneously after 6 to 9 months of age and it is thought that histologic development does not progress if the testis is not scrotally placed by 2 years of age, I prefer to operate when the child is roughly 1 year old. This offers some other benefits. The anesthetic risk is the same at this age as at any subsequent time during childhood. The children seem to tolerate these operations better psychologically and tend to recuperate much more quickly at younger ages. Lastly (and most subjectively), the operations appear to be easier in younger children. They are usually performed on an outpatient basis and the children are at the hospital for approximately 5 to 6 hours, including the time in the operating room.

The child is placed supine on the operating table and general anesthesia is induced. If the testis was previously nonpalpable, repeat palpation of the groin under anesthesia is performed. After skin preparation with antiseptic, the abdomen is draped appropriately: if the testis is not palpable, the abdomen is draped so that a higher incision can be used; if it is palpable, a standard groin incision is used. An inguinal incision is made in a skin crease roughly at the midpoint of the inguinal canal. The skin landmarks used to place the incision are the pubic tubercle and the anterior superior iliac spine. The internal ring lies roughly two thirds of the distance along that line, closer to the anterior superior spine than to the pubic tubercle. The incision is usually 3 to 4 cm in length, depending on the size of the child.

After Scarpa's fascia has been incised, the processus vaginalis may be identified emerging from the external inguinal ring. If so, the tunica vaginalis is grasped with a hemostat and the gubernacular attachments are transected. Dissection is continued outside the processus vaginalis up to the external ring. The inguinal canal is then opened in the direction of the fibers of the external oblique aponeurosis. Care is taken to avoid transecting the ilioinguinal nerve. Dissection is carried up to the internal ring, removing all cremaster fibers but not yet opening the processus vaginalis (and presumably the internal spermatic fascia).

When the testis, processus vaginalis, and cord structures have been dissected free to the internal ring, an assistant places caudal traction on the testis, and the anterior wall of the processus vaginalis is grasped and opened. The posterior wall is held taut so that the spermatic vessels and vas deferens can be visualized. Using a fine-pointed scissors (such as Joseph dissecting scissors), the posterior aspect of the processus vaginalis is dissected free from the spermatic vessels and the vas deferens. I do not infiltrate this area with saline, because in my experience this causes more problems than it solves. After the processus vaginalis has been completely transected, it is gently teased from the cord until a retractor can be placed between the posterior aspect of the processus vaginalis and the cord structures.

At this point, dissection is carried further cephalad, and the lateral aspect of the transversalis fascia (the so-called lateral spermatic fascia) is incised parallel to the direction of the spermatic vessels. This tends to allow the vessels to move medially and produces some increase in spermatic cord length. When enough length has been achieved so that the testis easily reaches the scrotum, the processus vaginalis is twisted and transfixed with a permanent suture.

In the rare event that sufficient length cannot be

achieved by this maneuver, the floor of the inguinal canal can be opened by incising the transversalis fascia, and dissection is carried under the inferior epigastric vessels. The testis can then be passed under the inferior epigastric vessels to emerge from a point that would normally correspond to the external ring. This maneuver was originally described by Prentiss and was used routinely by many surgeons. However, its use is now reserved for unusual situations in which the testis cannot be easily brought all the way to the scrotum.

The scrotum is then dilated by passing an index finger through the inguinal wound into the scrotum. A scrotal counterincision is made through the scrotal skin over the finger, and the skin is dissected from the underlying dartos muscle to create a pouch between the skin and the dartos muscle in which the testis will eventually reside. The distal extent of the processus vaginalis is incised to expose the tunica albuginea. The testis is then passed into the subdartos pouch that has previously been created. Small sutures are placed between the dartos and the tunica albuginea. It has previously been shown that these sutures are of temporary benefit only and that the major fixation occurs because the tunica albuginea lies in contact with the dartos muscle. This fixation should prevent testicular torsion in the future and, it is hoped, ensure permanent scrotal placement of the undescended testis. The scrotal skin is then closed with an absorbable suture. Bupivacaine is infiltrated into the area around the ilioinguinal nerve and into the subcutaneous tissues, unless the anesthesiologist has administered a caudal anesthetic for postoperative pain relief. The external oblique aponeurosis is closed with permanent suture, Scarpa's fascia is usually reapproximated with interrupted suture, and the skin is closed with a subcuticular absorbable suture. Although I have used staged orchiopexy in the past, it seems inappropriate to resort to staged orchiopexy if there is a contralaterally normal testis.

In instances when the testis reaches the scrotum but does not achieve a truly dependent position, I prefer to hold the testis in place during the postoperative period by passing a nylon suture through the testis and out through the scrotal wall, tying that over a small cotton bolster. Although rubber band traction has been used in the past, as has the Torek procedure, it is my belief that neither of these maneuvers is necessary in modern surgical practice, and the Torek procedure is probably best relegated to history.

COMPLICATIONS

Complications are not very frequent with the above operative procedure, but they may include injury to a looping vas through inadvertently transecting it before recognizing its presence. I therefore confine dissection to the area outside the processus vaginalis, because in reality this means confining it to the area outside the internal spermatic fascia. The vas deferens traverses a space between the internal spermatic fascia and the processus vaginalis, and if dissection has not entered that plane, it is unlikely that the vas will be injured inadvertently.

Occasionally the ilioinguinal nerve is injured or transected, as in any inguinal wound. To prevent this, one should try to identify the nerve early in the procedure and be aware of its position throughout.

In my experience of repeat surgery, the most common reason for failure has been the first surgeon's failure to transect the processus vaginalis. I feel strongly that orchiopexy should never be performed without dissection up to the internal ring and transection of a processus vaginalis.

The vas deferens can also be injured in the course of dissecting the processus vaginalis from the cord. If it is transected, it is my opinion that it should be immediately repaired at the same time, using either magnifying loupes or a microscope.

Inadequate dissection to allow for easy scrotal placement will probably result in retraction of the testis; one must therefore be relatively vigorous in dissection. However, too vigorous dissection of the spermatic vessels may result in their attenuation and occasionally their avulsion during high dissection in the retroperitoneum. Bladder injuries theoretically could occur with medial dissection along the hernia sac, but in my experience this is more common with hernia repair than with orchiopexy.

If laparoscopy has not been performed, it is insufficient to explore the groin and, on finding no testis, abandon the procedure. In this instance, I feel strongly that the peritoneum must be opened and that both vas and vessels must be identified and traced to their termination before one can diagnose with assurance absence of the testis.

SUGGESTED READING

Forest MG, David M, LeCoy A, et al. Kinetics of the hCG induced steroidogenic response of the human testes. III. Studies in children of the plasma levels of testosterone and hCG, a rationale for testicular stimulation test. Pediatr Res 1980; 14:819.

Fowler R and Stephens FD. The adle of testicular vascular anatomy in the salvage of high undescended testes. Aust New Zealand J Surg 1959; 29:92.

Hadziselimovic CF. Cryptorchidism, management and implications. New York: Springer-Verlag, 1983.

Harrison CB, Kaplan GW, Scherz HC, et al. Microvascular autotransplantation of the intra-abdominal testis. J Urol 1990; 144:507.

Lowe DH, Brock WA, Kaplan GW. Laparoscopy for localization of nonpalpable testes. J Urol 1984; 131:728.

Prentiss RJ, Weickgenant CJ, Moses JJ, and Frazier DB. Undescended testis: surgical anatomy of spermatic vessels, spermatic surgical triangles and lateral spermatic ligaments. J Urol 1960; 83:686.

Scorer GC, Farrington GH. Congenital deformities of the testis and epididymis. London: Butterworths, 1971.

UNILATERAL CRYPTORCHIDISM IN ADULTS

PAUL E. ANDREWS, M.D.
REZA S. MALEK, M.D., M.S., FRCSC, F.A.C.S.

In the pediatric urologic practice, cryptorchidism is the most common surgical problem, with an incidence of 30 percent in premature infants. The incidence decreases to 3 percent in term infants, and at 1 year of age, only 0.8 percent remain cryptorchid. Despite widespread knowledge of the benefits of early orchiopexy in preserving spermatogenic potential, diminishing or preventing malignant degeneration in the undescended testis, and helping in early detection of testicular cancer, some children remain untreated and eventually present for evaluation in adulthood.

Approximately 10 percent of patients with germ cell cancer of the testis have a history of undescended testis. The risk of malignancy is 30 to 40 times greater in an undescended testis than in a normally descended testis. The peak incidence is in the third and fourth decades of life; approximately 70 percent of all germ cell tumors of the testis are seen in patients between 15 and 35 years of age. The location of the undescended testis does not affect the age at which patients present with a malignancy. In the past, there was a general belief that an abdominal testis was more prone to malignant degeneration. To date, there has been no study corroborating this assertion. Therefore, it is thought that the risk of tumor development is not related to the natural location of the undescended testis. Carcinogenesis is neither altered nor diminished by continued observation. Another important aspect of cryptorchidism is its effect on fertility. Cryptorchid testes that remain undescended have very few, if any, germ cells. The tubules have a decreased diameter and their basement membranes are thickened. Therefore, spermatogenesis usually is severely impaired and the contribution, if any, of such a testis to the overall production of spermatozoa is minimal.

In order to assess the therapeutic alternatives, it is necessary to consider risk of malignancy, spermatogenic potential, location of the testis, risk of the surgical therapy itself, available imaging techniques, and the patient's concerns.

THERAPEUTIC ALTERNATIVES

Management of the undescended testis in adults requires locating the impalpable gonad, decreasing the risk of malignancy, and clarifying the prognosis with regard to fertility. Surgical alternatives are orchiectomy and orchiopexy. Orchiopexy is not practical, however, because it does not decrease the risk of malignancy but still carries the risk of surgery; the only benefit it offers is easy physical examination. Orchiectomy eliminates the risk of cancer in the undescended testis but does not decrease the risk of malignancy in the contralateral, normally descended testis, which was reported by Batata et al. in 1982 to be as high as 14 percent. Therefore, the only two practical therapeutic alternatives in adults are removal of the undescended testis followed by observation of the normally descended testis, or simply observation of both testes.

An analytic approach to the management of cryptorchidism after puberty was first described by Martin and Menck in 1975. They advocated removal of the undescended testis in patients with unilateral cryptorchidism who were younger than 50 years of age and in all patients with abdominal cryptorchidism, regardless of age. From another analysis in 1985, Farrer and associates concluded that cryptorchid patients younger than 32 years of age should undergo orchiectomy and that those older than 32 years of age should be observed. This conclusion is based on the point where the two relative risk curves cross (Fig. 1). The two studies differ, the most important difference being that the later study takes into account diagnostic and therapeutic advances that have dramatically improved survival rates.

Spermatogenesis is usually severely impaired in the testis that remains undescended beyond early childhood. The contribution of this testis to reproduction is therefore minimal and there can be little justification for preserving it on this basis. However, the androgenic potential in these testes is usually preserved. The Leydig cells appear relatively hyperplastic and marked interstitial fibrosis is often present. Leydig cell atrophy with impaired testosterone production has been described. However, the testosterone production in these testes usually is adequate to sustain puberty and sexual function, even in bilateral cryptorchidism.

Observation of both the cryptorchid and the normally descended contralateral testis is the other practical alternative in adults. This implies that the patient must be followed because there is a risk of a germ cell tumor developing in the undescended testis. The patient must be compliant and willing to undertake a lifetime of follow-up examinations. Imaging technology must be available to permit adequate assessment of the undescended testis. Even if the patient undergoes orchiectomy, he must be followed because of the increased risk of malignancy in the normally descended contralateral testis.

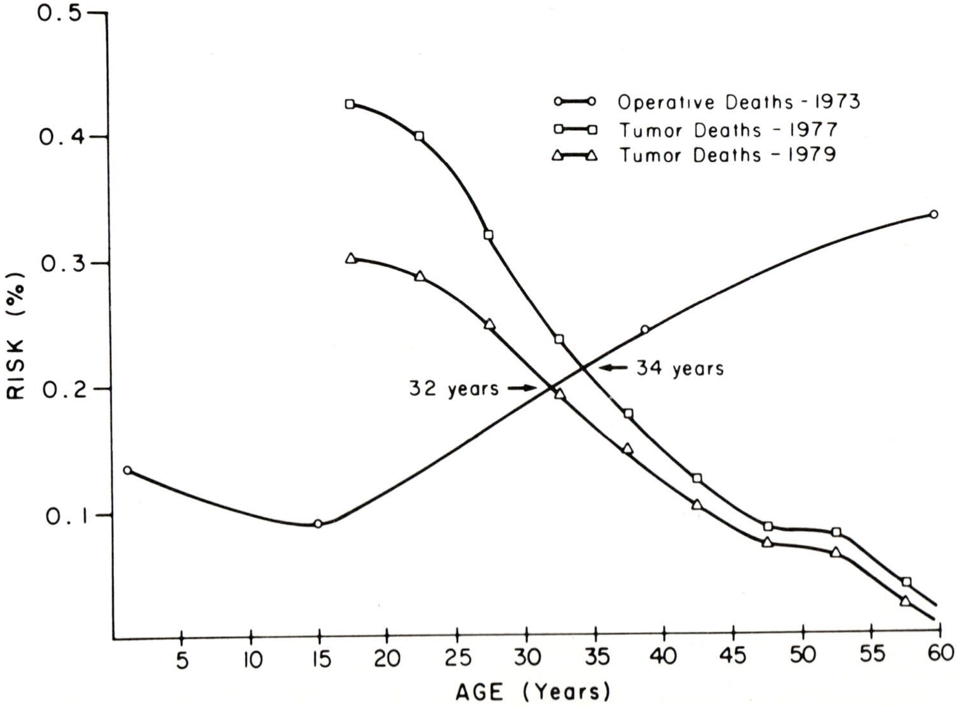

Figure 1 Lifetime risk of death from testicular tumors for white male patients with cryptorchidism (1977 and 1979) compared with the risk of death from surgery (age- and ASA class–specific). (Republished with permission by Farrer JH, Walker AH, Rajfer J. Management of the postpubertal cryptorchid testis: a statistical review. J Urol 1985; 134:1071–1076. By permission of Williams & Wilkins.)

PREFERRED APPROACHES

The approach to the postpubertal patient with cryptorchidism is based on (1) whether the testis is palpable or impalpable, (2) the symptoms, and (3) the age of the patient with regard to the risk of malignancy as opposed to the risk of surgery. Other important variables are the condition of the patient, the state of the contralateral testis, and the cosmetic results.

In general, any patient who presents with symptoms thought to be secondary to an undescended testis should undergo exploration and orchiectomy. An abdominal testis that presents with acute abdominal pain has a greater than 60 percent chance of containing a malignancy. An adult with an inguinal hernia and an undescended testis should undergo orchiectomy at the time of inguinal hernia repair. Similarly, a postpubertal patient who presents with an inguinal testis and a history of recent irritation of that testis secondary to work-related or athletic activity should undergo orchiectomy.

Palpable Undescended Testis

In 80 percent of patients with unilaterally undescended testis, the undescended gonad is palpable in the inguinal region. The approach to this group of patients is based on analytic data presented by Farrer and associates that assess the relative lifetime risk of death secondary to testicular cancer and the risk of death from surgery. Patients under 32 years old are better served by

orchiectomy. However, patients over 32 should simply be observed, because in these, the risk of surgery is greater than that of testicular cancer.

For a palpable undescended inguinal testis, orchiectomy should be performed through an inguinal incision. The testis usually is in the superficial inguinal pouch of Douglas. The removed testis should be thoroughly examined by the pathologist, who should look specifically for carcinoma in situ, defined as seminiferous tubules containing Sertoli cells and atypical germ cells. The atypical germ cells are large and the DNA content is highly aneuploid. Carcinoma in situ has been identified as a premalignant change in the testicular tubular epithelium. Approximately 30 percent of patients with carcinoma in situ of the testis have a history of cryptorchidism. The risk of invasive tumor growth developing in a postpubertal undescended testis with carcinoma in situ is 50 percent at 5 years after diagnosis.

Patients with germinal testicular cancer are at increased risk of cancer developing in the contralateral testis. Furthermore, carcinoma in situ has been found in the normally descended testis in 20 percent of patients who have had carcinoma in the contralateral cryptorchid testis.

Patients older than 32 years of age with a palpable unilateral undescended testis who are managed by observation should undergo a baseline ultrasonographic examination. Follow-up should be semiannual to annual, and a complete physical examination should be per-

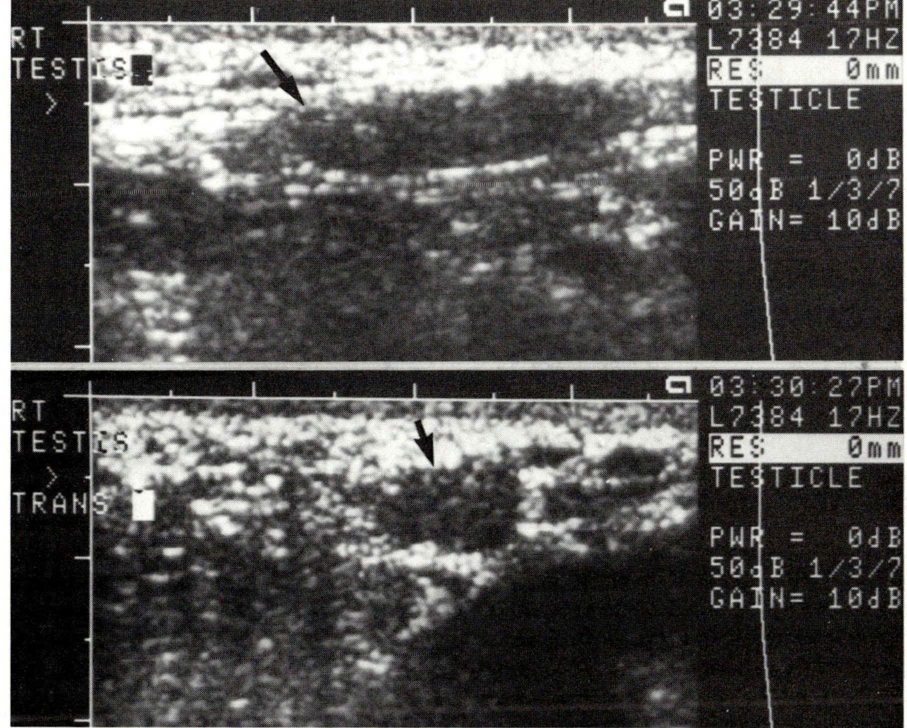

Figure 2 Ultrasonogram of right inguinal testis (*arrow*) in a 37-year-old man. *Upper,* Longitudinal view, showing atrophic testis in right inguinal canal. *Lower,* Transverse view.

formed. If follow-up is impossible for the patient or if he is noncompliant, orchiectomy is recommended.

Impalpable Undescended Testis

In approximately 20 percent of the cryptorchid population, the testis is impalpable because it is intra-abdominal, intracanalicular, or atrophic or absent. The impalpable testis constitutes a diagnostic challenge. The location or absence of the testis must be verified.

Various diagnostic modalities, including ultrasonography, computed tomography (CT), magnetic resonance imaging (MRI), gonadal venography, and laparoscopy, may be used to identify the impalpable undescended testis. Ultrasonography is the least invasive and therefore is the initial test used to identify the undescended testis (Fig. 2). However, this method is limited in the evaluation of an intra-abdominal testis and in differentiating lymph nodes from the undescended testis. When the ultrasonographic examination is inadequate technically or if no testis is visualized, CT or MRI is used. Both are useful in identifying an intra-abdominal or intracanalicular testis. Intraoperative search for an impalpable undescended testis can be time-consuming, and preoperative localization allows for a planned surgical approach.

CT is the preferred imaging tool for localization of an intra-abdominal testis. It also permits differentiation between the spermatic cord and enlarged lymph nodes.

The main advantage of CT over MRI is the use of gastrointestinal contrast medium to help differentiate nonopacified bowel loops from the undescended testis.

Like CT, MRI is a sensitive modality for localizing the undescended testis, and it provides excellent tissue characterization. An additional advantage is the capability of obtaining multiplanar images, which are helpful in depicting an undescended testis in the inguinal canal (Fig. 3).

Selective gonadal venography and laparoscopy are invasive diagnostic modalities. Venography is useful in locating an impalpable undescended testis, and it is possible to predict testicular agenesis by visualizing a blind-ending gonadal vein. This technique requires a skillful angiographer experienced in selective catheterization of the gonadal vein. Laparoscopy also has been useful for locating an intra-abdominal testis accurately and for inspecting the spermatic vessels and vas deferens entering the internal inguinal ring. Laparoscopy also can demonstrate blind-ending spermatic vessels or vas deferens within the abdomen.

The review by Farrer and associates indicated that treatment of the impalpable testis should be the same as that of the palpable testis. There are no data to indicate that an abdominal testis poses a greater risk of malignancy than an inguinal testis. Furthermore, the most important factor in survival when there is a germ cell tumor in the undescended testis is tumor stage, and this is independent of the location of the undescended testis.

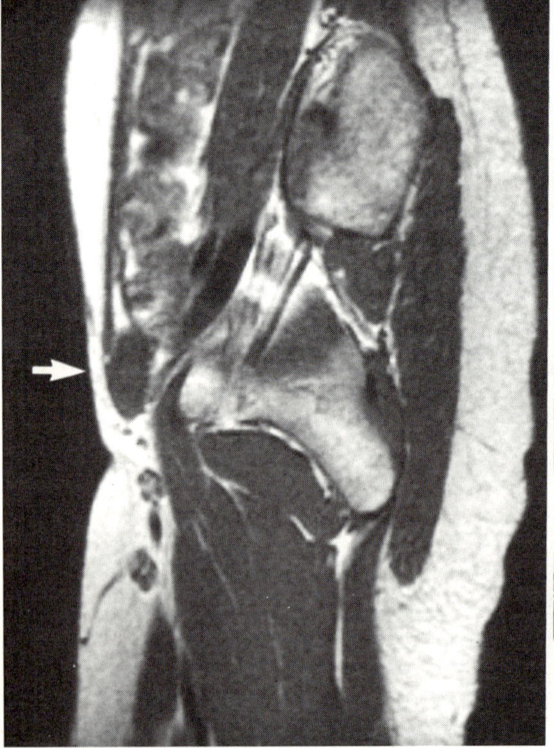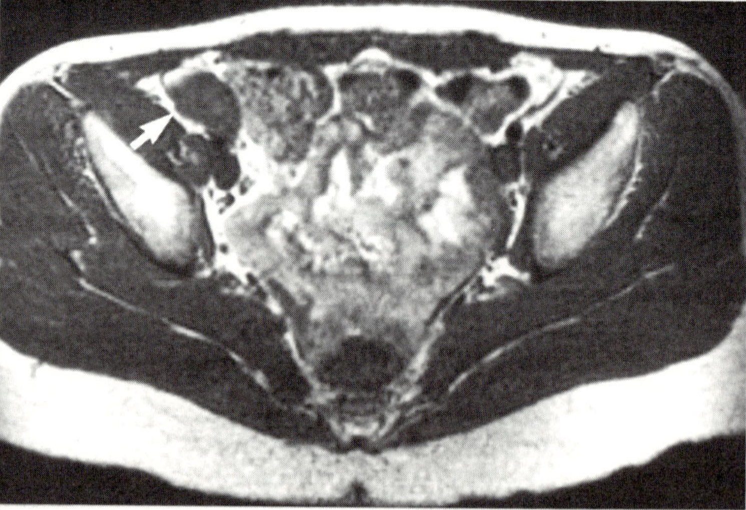

Figure 3 Magnetic resonance image in a 27-year-old man demonstrates a right inguinal testis (*arrow*). *Left,* Sagittal view. *Right,* Transverse view.

Many authors recommend exploration of all impalpable testes, regardless of the patient's age.

Observation requires a lifetime of follow-up visits and the use of ultrasonography or other imaging techniques. The major obstacles to observation are cost effectiveness and the need for excellent patient compliance. However, the risk of a germ cell tumor developing in a patient older than 50 years of age is extremely small. Our recommendation is therefore to explore in healthy patients younger than 50 years of age who have an impalpable undescended testis not visualized by ultrasonography or other imaging techniques. Laparoscopy before surgical exploration may help locate such a testis. Patients younger than 50 years of age with an impalpable undescended testis visualized by one of the imaging techniques may be observed with periodic imaging. Patients older than 50 years of age who have an impalpable undescended testis can be observed with very little risk of development of a germ cell tumor.

Method of Exploration

Most impalpable undescended testes (80 percent) are within the inguinal canal; the remaining 20 percent are intra-abdominal. A unilateral impalpable testis is approached through an inguinal incision. Most such testes are found in the inguinal canal or just inside the internal inguinal ring. Preoperative imaging can be helpful in choosing the correct incision and directing the intraoperative search. If no testis is found on opening the inguinal canal, the incision should be extended superolaterally to explore the retroperitoneum. The finding of only the vas does not justify the conclusion that the testis is absent. However, the finding of blind-ending spermatic vessels is proof that the testis is absent. If the testis

or spermatic vessels are not identified retroperitoneally, the peritoneum must be opened. When a testis or spermatic vessels are not found, monorchia exists. Unilateral testicular absence occurs in approximately 4 percent of cases of impalpable testis.

MANAGEMENT

In the past, orchiectomy was the accepted treatment for unilateral undescended testis in the adult because of the increased risk of testicular germ cell cancer. However, analysis of the relative risks of surgery and observation and recent advances in the treatment of testicular cancer have made other options available (Fig. 4).

In the postpubertal patient with an undescended testis, orchiopexy is not a rational therapeutic option. Orchiectomy is the recommended treatment if the patient is less than 32 years old and has a palpable undescended testis or if he is less than 50 years old, is healthy, and has an impalpable undescended testis not visualized by any imaging techniques. Furthermore, any patient who presents with symptoms secondary to an undescended testis should undergo orchiectomy.

Observation is the recommended treatment if the patient is more than 32 years old and the undescended testis is palpable or is impalpable but can be visualized by imaging techniques. All patients more than 50 years of age may be observed, regardless of whether the testis is palpable or is located by available imaging techniques. Observation requires semiannual to annual physical examination and imaging of the undescended gonad, good patient compliance, and absence of symptoms.

Ultrasonography, computed tomography, and mag-

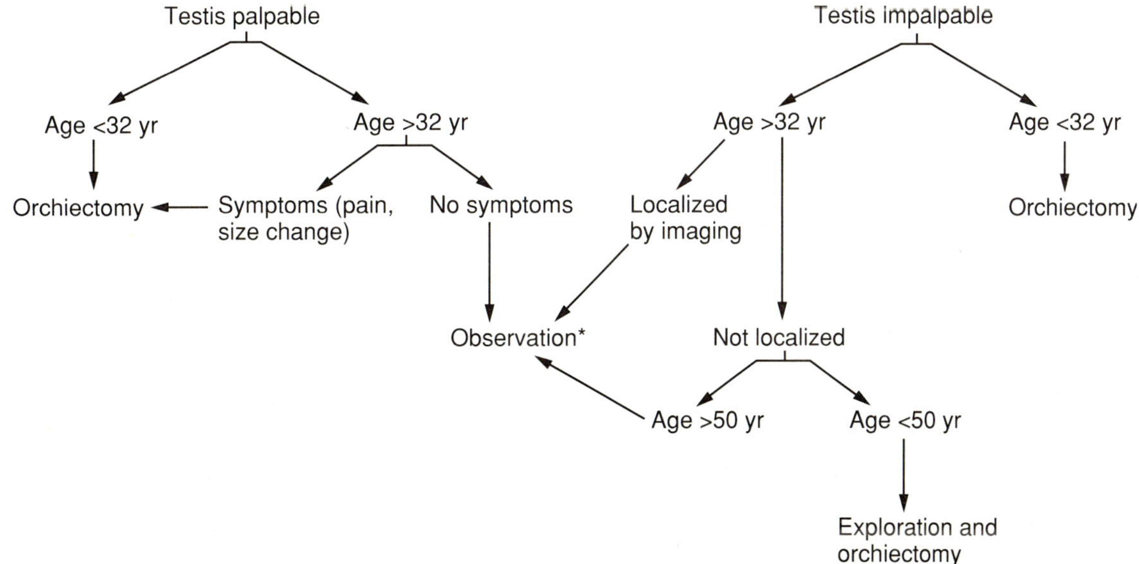

Figure 4 Plan for management of unilateral undescended testis in adults. *With routine physical examination and ultrasonography.

netic resonance imaging are useful for localizing an impalpable testis. Ultrasonography has been particularly useful in the follow-up examination when the testis is impalpable. Any patient to be observed should undergo baseline ultrasonography of both testes. Finally, each patient must be treated individually, with attention paid both to the patient's concerns and to the risk/benefit ratios of available treatment options.

Copyright 1990 Mayo Foundation.

SUGGESTED READING

Batata MA, Chu FCH, Hilaris BS, et al. Testicular cancer in cryptorchids. Cancer 1982; 49:1023–1030.
Farrer JH, Walker AH, Rajfer J. Management of the postpubertal cryptorchid testis: a statistical review. J Urol 1985; 134:1071–1076.
Giwercman A, Müller J, Skakkebaeck NE. Carcinoma in situ of the undescended testis. Semin Urol 1988; 6:110–119.
Martin DC, Menck HR. The undescended testis: management after puberty. J Urol 1975; 114:77–79.
Whitaker RH. Neoplasia in cryptorchid men. Semin Urol 1988; 6:107–109.

BILATERAL CRYPTORCHIDISM

DAVID B. JOSEPH, M.D.
STUART B. BAUER, M.D.

Bilaterally undescended testes have been reported in 10 to 30 percent of boys who present with a cryptorchid abnormality. Cryptorchidism occurs in approximately 3 percent of full-term infants weighing over 2,500 g. Of those testes that will descend, approximately 60 percent do so by the first 2 months of life. It is rare for a testicle to descend after an infant is 1 year of age. The incidence of cryptorchidism at this time is 0.8 percent and it remains as such throughout puberty and early adulthood.

The occurrence of an undescended testis is also related to prematurity and birthweight. Cryptorchidism occurs in approximately 21 percent of premature infants weighing 1,500 to 2,500 g and 60 to 70 percent of male infants under 1,500 g.

Unfortunately, there is no universally accepted terminology to define the undescended testis in character or location. The lack of standardization in describing testicular position is probably one reason for the extreme variability of results from treatment options reported by different investigators. In this chapter, we have attempted to define our approach to bilaterally undescended testes in a systematic and standardized fashion.

DIAGNOSIS

First, an undescended testis is defined as palpable or nonpalpable. Of the palpable testes, it is essential to differentiate the retractile from the truly undescended testis. A retractile testis is one that can be brought into the scrotum and will stay there on repeated examination.

An undescended testis may or may not be manipulated into the scrotum, but if it is, on its release it returns to either its original position or to one just above the scrotal sac. Therefore, the undescended testis is characterized according to its resting location: intracanicular, between the internal and external ring; pubic, at the level of the external ring or overlying the pubic tubercle; or ectopic, in the superficial superior thigh or perineum.

PHYSICAL EXAMINATION AND IMAGING

To determine the true position of a testicle, an appropriate examination is required in a cooperative child. A compassionate, unhurried examination is mandatory. The examiner's hands should be similar to the child's body temperature while the ambient temperature needs to be warm. These conditions are important in order to prevent the cremasteric muscle from tethering a retractile testicle and mimicking an undescended organ. Getting the child to relax after he undresses is paramount. A glance at his scrotum as he does this can provide a clue to where the testicle resides under normal conditions. Allowing the child to relax on the examination table for a few moments, distracting his attention, and then slowly moving one's hands to the genital area is another way to reduce anxiety, which may cause the testicle to retract. Sometimes it is helpful if the child assumes a cross-legged or squatting (baseball catcher's) position to allow for cremasteric relaxation and descent of a retractile testis. Often, we have resorted to teaching parents how to examine their child while he is asleep or being bathed. Despite these maneuvers, it may still be difficult in a few children to differentiate between a retractile and a truly undescended testis.

It has been documented that testes previously categorized as retractile may become trapped and truly undescended at a later age. Because of this, we recommend a yearly follow-up in any child diagnosed with a retractile testis until that testis is well seated in the scrotum.

In our experience, diagnostic imaging for the non-palpable testis is of limited value. Nonpalpable testes have been identified by computed tomography (CT) and magnetic resonance imaging (MRI), but we do not consider either test sensitive or specific enough in localizing the testis to change our therapeutic plan. We do not believe that the need to sedate the child, the added expense, and the additional radiation are justified. Inguinal and pelvic ultrasonography, although inexpensive and atraumatic, has limited reliability and should be reserved for boys with an associated hypospadias who require urinary tract assessment, and for infants with bilaterally nonpalpable gonads who are evaluated for an intersex abnormality.

TREATMENT

The treatment of bilaterally undescended testes depends on several variables: the age at which the child presents, the ability to palpate one or both testes, and the location of any palpable testis. Ideally, we prefer to initiate treatment before 1 year of age, after which time spontaneous descent is unlikely. Early intervention may prevent mitochondrial degeneration, decreased germ cell production, and increased collagen deposition surrounding both spermatogenic and Leydig cells. These changes begin in undescended testes as early as 18 months of age and are progressive with time.

Hormonal manipulation for testicular descent remains controversial and has met with limited success. Parenteral hCG testing has had inconsistent results for inducing testicular descent. It is possible that testes reported to respond to hCG were in fact retractile and did not require surgical treatment in the first place. Recently, gonadotropin-releasing hormone (GnRH) has been used for inducing testicular descent. Both Cryptocur (GnRH produced by Hoechst) and Buserelin (GnRH analog produced by Hoechst) have been used experimentally in the United States and abroad, again with controversial and inconsistent results in inducing testicular descent. There is evidence that the combined use of GnRH and hCG may have a synergistic effect in improving the rate of testicular descent. In addition, Buserelin may prove beneficial in stimulating germ cell proliferation, which is depressed in cryptorchidism. At this time, the GnRH analogs are not available for use in the United States. Further investigation is needed to determine their efficacy.

At the present time, we limit the use of preoperative hormonal manipulation to children with bilaterally nonpalpable testes as part of the evaluation of anorchia. In children with bilaterally nonpalpable testes, pretreatment levels of testosterone, luteinizing hormone (LH), and follicular-stimulating hormone (FSH) are obtained. We then proceed with an hCG stimulation test, administering 1,000 IU of hCG intramuscularly every other day for a total of three doses. Forty-eight hours after the last injection, a testosterone level is obtained. A 20-fold increase in testosterone over baseline is considered positive and suggests the presence of at least one testicle. If there is no significant elevation of testosterone and the baseline level of LH is elevated, anorchia is presumed to be present and further evaluation and treatment are based on that diagnosis.

We are not enthusiastic about the use of hCG for initiating descent of the cryptorchid testis, but it may induce descent of the retractile testis and can be of benefit in differentiating these two entities. The use of hCG also stimulates an increase in vascularization to the testis with elongation of cord structures and enlargement of the scrotum. An investigation is currently under way to determine whether this is indeed occurring. If so, the preoperative use of hCG may prove effective in otherwise difficult cases.

Our surgical approach to the child with bilaterally undescended testes is based on the presence and location of a palpable testis. If both undescended testes are palpable, we limit our surgical exposure to the region of each respective inguinal canal. In most cases, both testes can be brought down during the same period of anesthesia, using a standard dartos pouch technique. If one side is technically difficult or if there is a doubt of testicular viability, we suggest deferring contralateral orchiopexy until the outcome of the surgically treated side has been assessed. Although this necessitates a second anesthetic, the delay allows for re-evaluation of surgical options based on the results of the initial procedure. Testicular viability in these cases is best assessed by physically palpating the gonad for consistency and measuring its growth with an orchidometer. If there is concern about testicular atrophy, a technetium-99m pertechnetate testicular scan or color Doppler ultrasonography can be performed to assess blood flow.

In children with one or two nonpalpable testes, we perform laparoscopy immediately before the planned orchidopexy. Laparoscopy is easily and quickly performed with minimal morbidity. It is helpful in diagnosing the vanishing testis, which has been reported in 20 to 88 percent of nonpalpable testes. The surgeon should not rely solely on a blind-ending vas, but must identify blind-ending gonadal vessels to make the diagnosis. In the older, chubby child, laparoscopy has helped to localize a difficult-to-palpate inguinal testis; both the vasal and testicular arteries can be seen exiting through the internal ring. In such instances, a limited surgical exploration over the respective inguinal canal is all that is required. Some surgeons now believe that no exploration is necessary if blind-ending vessels are noted intra-abdominally.

When one undescended testis is palpable and the contralateral testis has been identified at laparoscopy as intra-abdominal, we begin with a standard dartos pouch orchidopexy on the palpable testis. Once that side has been placed in the scrotum successfully, we proceed with a Fowler-Stephens orchidopexy on the contralateral side, either during the same period of anesthesia or at a later date. In this circumstance, we do not advise percutaneously ligating the testicular artery at the time of initial laparoscopy, because this would have to precede the standard dartos pouch orchidopexy. If the viability of the testis operated on were in question, both testes could potentially be in jeopardy.

When both testes are located intra-abdominally, we stage our repair by concentrating on one testicle at a time in order to confirm its viability before proceeding with contralateral orchidopexy. The initial approach to the intra-abdominal testis can be either a Fowler-Stephens orchidopexy undertaken immediately after laparoscopy, or a staged procedure after percutaneously occluding the testicular artery through the laparoscope followed by an open Fowler-Stephens operation 6 to 8 weeks later.

When performing the Fowler-Stephens operation, a low Pfannenstiel intra-abdominal incision can be made, which allows excellent access to the retroperitoneum and easy ligation of the proximal testicular artery. We routinely use Doppler ultrasonography to ascertain testicular blood flow after temporary occlusion of the testicular artery by a bulldog clamp before transecting the vessel. If adequate blood flow is not identified on intraoperative Doppler monitoring or if brisk bleeding is not encountered after incising the tunica albuginea, we do not proceed with the Fowler-Stephens repair but consider testicular autotransplantation. If adequate blood flow is confirmed by either Doppler ultrasonography or brisk bleeding, the artery is transected as proximally as possible. A wide segment of posterior peritoneum is then mobilized between the distal artery and vas in order not to disrupt the distal anastomotic arcade between the vasal and testicular arteries. If testicular size and viability are noted to be good on postoperative assessment, a Fowler-Stephens approach is undertaken on the contralateral testis 3 to 6 months later. If testicular viability has not been maintained, options are discussed with the family to place the remaining testicle either into the scrotum with autotransplantation or to a location where it can be easily palpated with minimal manipulation of its blood supply.

The approach to bilateral cryptorchidism in older, prepubertal, and pubertal children needs to be individualized. We rarely suggest orchiectomy, even in pubertal males. Although the incidence of testicular tumor is greater in an undescended testis, we do not believe it is great enough to consider removal in those testes that can be brought down easily into the scrotum. We do advocate testicular biopsy in any pubertal child undergoing orchidopexy in the evaluation of carcinoma in situ. We also perform testicular biopsy on all intra-abdominal testes. In pubertal children, if one of the intra-abdominal testes can be easily placed in the scrotum but the contralateral testis cannot, it may be best to remove that gonad. However, we try to place the testis in a superficial inguinal position for easy examination only if its absence would threaten future testosterone availability. Fortunately, this is rare.

In children with multiple congenital abnormalities, including mental deficiencies producing conditions in which fertility may not appear to be an important future consideration, we believe orchidopexy is still appropriate. It is essential that these boys have their gonads placed in a position that is easily accessible for self-examination or assessment by their caretaker or physician. If the testes cannot be placed in a readily palpable position, they should be removed.

In treating children with a nonpalpable testis, there is a possibility of anorchia. Under such circumstances, we routinely advise families of the availability of a testicular prosthesis, believing these to be appropriate in infants or young children. Inserting an infant-sized prosthesis at this time does not necessitate replacement with a larger size unless the boy wants it. The prosthesis can be exchanged for one of adult size after puberty. Otherwise, the infant size becomes small and inconspicuous in relation to the native testis. We believe that the early formative years are most important for developing an appropriate self-image. In some children, delay in placing a testicular prosthesis may result in feelings of inadequacy during adolescence. This is especially true for boys with bilateral anorchia.

SUGGESTED READING

Cendron M, Keating MA, Huff DS, et al. Cryptorchidism—orchidopexy and infertility: a critical long-term retrospective analysis. J Urol 1989; 142:559–561.

Colodny AH. Undescended testis—is surgery necessary? N Engl J Med 1986; 314:510–511.

Hadziselimovic F, Herzog B, Buzer M. Development of cryptorchid testes. Eur J Pediatr 1987; 146(suppl 2):8–12.

Kogan SJ, Tennenbaum S, Gill B, et al. Efficacy of orchidopexy by patient age one year for cryptorchidism. J Urol 1990; 144:508–509.

Rajfer J, Handelsman DJ, Swerdloff RS, et al. Hormonal therapy of cryptorchidism: a randomized, double-blind study comparing human chorionic gonadotrophin and gonadotrophin-releasing hormone. N Engl J Med 1986; 314:466–470.

HYDROCELE IN CHILDREN

WILLIAM A. BROCK, M.D., F.A.C.S., F.A.A.P.

The pathophysiology of hydroceles in children differs from that in adults. Hydroceles may occur in children secondary to local inflammatory conditions within the scrotum, such as torsion of a testicular appendage, but the vast majority are congenital in nature, being due to communication between the scrotum and the peritoneal cavity through a persistently patent processus vaginalis. The processus vaginalis is an outpouching or extension of the peritoneal lining through the internal inguinal ring that forms during the third month of gestation and normally persists only within the scrotum. The processus vaginalis resembles the open finger of a glove that enters the groin through the internal inguinal ring and extends into the scrotum beside the spermatic cord and testis. The exact developmental reason for this projection of peritoneum is unknown, but it is thought to be important in descent of the testis. Failure of the inguinal portion of the processus vaginalis to obliterate may lead to a communicating hydrocele, a hydrocele of the cord, or an indirect inguinal hernia.

The processus vaginalis is patent at birth in 94 percent of boys. By 1 year of age, the incidence of patency has decreased to 57 percent, and by adulthood, autopsy studies reveal an incidence of 20 percent. Since clinical hernias and hydroceles occur much less frequently, the presence of a patent processus vaginalis does not always lead to development of a hydrocele or hernia, and most never become clinically apparent.

The only difference between a congenital hydrocele and a congenital inguinal hernia is the diameter of the patent processus and the contents of the sac. If the processus is large enough to permit bowel, omentum, or other abdominal viscera to pass through the internal inguinal ring, a clinical indirect inguinal hernia results. If the opening in the processus is only large enough to allow peritoneal fluid to pass to the scrotum, a communicating hydrocele results. A hydrocele of the spermatic cord occurs when partial, distal obliteration of the processus causes localized loculation of fluid within the spermatic cord above the testis.

Most congenital hydroceles are clinically apparent at birth and present as an asymptomatic scrotal swelling that tends to vary in size from day to day. Increases in intra-abdominal pressure during daytime activity cause more fluid to enter the hydrocele, enlarging it. During sleep the fluid is reabsorbed or re-enters the peritoneal cavity, causing the hydrocele to appear smaller and softer in the morning. Some infant hydroceles may attain a very large size, causing the penis to retract and appear hidden in the prepubic fat. On occasion, a congenital communicating hydrocele first presents later in infancy or childhood. The lack of symptoms, the presence of a normal underlying testis, and the absence of other signs of inflammation confirm the diagnosis of a simple hydrocele. Delayed appearance or persistence of a communicating hydrocele are seen with increased frequency in children with ascites or ventriculoperitoneal shunts or in those on peritoneal dialysis.

DIAGNOSIS

On examination, the hydrocele is smooth and nontender and readily transilluminates. The overlying skin is neither thickened nor inflamed and often displays a bluish tint. The hydrocele sac can extend variable distances up and down the spermatic cord, and usually surrounds and hides the testis, which is palpable within the posterior aspect of the hydrocele or may be visible on transillumination. Occasionally, the sac terminates proximal to the testis and presents as a supratesticular mass. Manual compression of the hydrocele may cause partial emptying, confirming its communicating nature. A flap valve mechanism along the inguinal portion of the processus or loculations within the scrotum may prevent emptying of the hydrocele by manual compression, but all hydroceles in children should be considered to be communicating in nature when treatment is planned. If a hydrocele empties rapidly and completely as soon as compression is attempted, it is considered the equivalent of an inguinal hernia, since the processus is large enough to admit bowel and is at risk for development of an incarceration.

It is sometimes difficult to determine whether scrotal swelling in an infant contains bowel or merely fluid, since both transilluminate. Digital rectal examination may reveal irregularity and swelling in the area of the ipsilateral internal ring if viscera are indeed present within the sac, whereas a simple communicating hydrocele will be associated with a very smooth internal ring and pelvic side wall.

A hydrocele of the cord presents as a fusiform, translucent mass along the course of the spermatic cord in the groin or upper scrotum. These are usually somewhat mobile, nontender, and tense and are not freely compressible. The spermatic cord can usually be traced proximally and distally from the mass, confirming its origin within the cord. If a question exists regarding differentiation from a paratesticular neoplasm, ultrasonography will confirm the fluid-filled nature of a hydrocele of the cord.

Other causes of scrotal swelling in children are relatively easy to differentiate from hydroceles and hernias. Acute inflammatory conditions, such as torsion of a testicular appendage, may be associated with a hydrocele; these should be suspected if there is associated pain, tenderness, and inflammation. Testicular neoplasms may also be associated with hydroceles and are usually apparent on careful palpation or transillumination. If there is a possibility of a neoplasm, scrotal ultrasonography will clarify an inconclusive physical examination.

TREATMENT

The decision to repair a communicating hydrocele surgically is based on several factors. Most hydroceles resolve spontaneously during the first 18 months of life and therefore do not require surgical intervention until this age. In addition, those hydroceles that do persist beyond this age rarely progress to a clinical hernia and are thus repaired primarily for cosmetic reasons. Inguinal hernias, on the other hand, never resolve and are associated with an inordinately high risk of incarceration in infants. Sixty-nine percent of all incarcerations occur in children younger than 1 year of age, most often during the first 3 months of life. Thus, an inguinal hernia in an infant is repaired soon after diagnosis if the child is otherwise medically stable. In contrast to the older child, a communicating hydrocele in an infant younger than 1 year of age may progress to a frank inguinal hernia and, in my experience, is more often complicated by incarceration when it does progress. Parents of infants with hydroceles should therefore be advised of the signs and symptoms of this complication, and early repair should be undertaken if a frank hernia develops.

Because of the difference in pathogenic mechanisms, hydroceles in children are treated differently from those in adults. Nonsurgical management by percutaneous drainage or sclerotherapy is ineffective in children. The surgical approach is directed primarily at the internal inguinal ring and ligation of the patent processus vaginalis, rather than at the tunica vaginalis within the scrotum. The internal ring is located approximately one third of the way *up* from the pubic tubercle toward the anterior superior iliac spine and an equal distance *medial* to the inguinal ligament. Since the skin in a young child can easily be moved back and forth over the external oblique aponeurosis to expose the deeper tissues, the incision can be placed cosmetically in a nearby lower abdominal skin crease. Scarpa's fascia is divided and the external oblique aponeurosis identified and cleaned. It is helpful to identify the inguinal ligament laterally and follow this distally to the spermatic cord as it exits the external inguinal ring in order to establish localizing landmarks.

If the hydrocele is not large and loculated, it is not necessary to divide the external oblique through the external ring, because it will not be necessary to deliver the testis. In this case, a small incision is made in the direction of the fibers of the external oblique aponeurosis, and the slips of the cremaster muscle are identified as they surround the spermatic cord. The muscle fibers are bluntly separated to reveal the internal spermatic fascia, which is gently grasped to lift the cord from between the cremaster fibers, which are brushed inferiorly.

Once the cord has been elevated, the processus vaginalis is identified along the anteromedial aspect of the cord within the flimsy enveloping layer of internal spermatic fascia. Blunt forceps are used to open the internal spermatic fascia longitudinally, and the processus is lifted away from the adherent vas and vessels and divided between clamps. The vas and vessels are very susceptible to permanent occlusion by crush injury and should never be directly grasped or clamped. The proximal portion of the processus is then lifted and bluntly teased up from within the confines of the internal spermatic fascia, back to the level of the internal inguinal ring, where it is ligated and divided. Care must be taken to avoid injury to the vas deferens, which may become entrapped within the ligature placed on the peritoneum at the internal ring. If the processus cannot be identified within the spermatic cord, it is helpful to trace the cord proximally to the internal inguinal ring, where the peritoneum can be identified as it tents up and points to the processus vaginalis.

If the hydrocele can be emptied easily through the distal stump of the processus, it is not necessary to deliver the testis into the operative field. However, some hydroceles are loculated and require drainage to avoid what appears to the parents to be a failed intervention, either by creation of a wide window in the tunica vaginalis or by formal eversion of the hydrocele sac. In these latter instances, it may be necessary to divide the external inguinal ring to allow delivery of the testis and scrotal portion of the hydrocele. Care must be taken to ensure that the testis has been properly replaced within the scrotum to avoid the development of iatrogenic cryptorchidism. Peritoneal fluid should not reaccumulate after division of the processus, but a local inflammatory hydrocele sometimes occurs after delivery of the testis. This usually resolves over 3 to 4 months.

It usually is not necessary to reconstruct the internal inguinal ring or repair the floor of the inguinal canal. The cord is simply replaced in its anatomic position and the wound closed with interrupted or running absorbable sutures in the external oblique aponeurosis and Scarpa's fascia, and interrupted subcuticular sutures in the skin.

In contrast to the debate surrounding the young child with an indirect inguinal hernia, I feel that contralateral exploration is unnecessary in the child with an apparently unilateral hydrocele who is older than 18 months of age, since asynchronous appearance of a contralateral clinical hydrocele is unusual after this age. If a contralateral communicating hydrocele is suspected but not obvious, it may be possible to prove its presence by insufflating the peritoneal cavity with carbon dioxide (pneumoperitoneum) through the clinically apparent processus. This is performed by first intubating the processus with a No. 5 or 8 Fr catheter, securing the tube and sealing the processus with an encircling silk suture. Carbon dioxide is then insufflated until the abdomen is tense, at which time the contralateral groin is palpated. The presence of subcutaneous crepitus or a mass in the contralateral groin or scrotum proves the existence of a patent processus. Although absence of crepitus does not absolutely rule out an occult patent processus, the number of false-negative studies is low. Pneumoperitoneum is not necessary as a routine procedure in most patients, because a clinical hydrocele infrequently occurs at a later date in children with a silent patent processus at the time of initial surgery. The procedure should be reserved for children in whom a contralateral communication is clinically suspected but not proved.

Unilateral or bilateral hydrocele repair is performed on an outpatient basis in otherwise healthy children, who are then seen once on follow-up approximately 2 weeks after surgery.

COMPLICATIONS AND RECURRENCE

The complications associated with hydrocele repair are similar to those associated with repair of an inguinal hernia. These include accidental division or crush injury of the vas deferens or spermatic vessels in approximately 1 percent of patients. If the processus that has been excised is examined pathologically and it appears that a segment of vas deferens has been inadvertently removed, it is useful to examine the diameter of the segment in question, since it is known that small embryonal remnants that are normally present within the spermatic cord may microscopically resemble the vas.

Recurrence of a communicating hydrocele is rare.

SUGGESTED READING

Harrison CB, Kaplan GW, Scherz HC, Packer MG. Diagnostic pneumoperitoneum for detection of the clinically occult contralateral hernia in children. J Urol 1990; 144:510–511.
Popek EJ. Embryonal remnants in inguinal hernia sacs. Hum Pathol 1990; 21:339–349.
Powell RW. Intraoperative diagnostic pneumoperitoneum in pediatric patients with unilateral inguinal hernias: the Goldstein test. J Pediatr Surg 1985; 20:418–421.
Tolete-Velcek F, Leddomado E, Hansbrough F, Thelmo WL. Alleged resection of the vas deferens: medicolegal implications. J Pediatr Surg 1988; 23:21–23.

HYDROCELE IN ADULTS

J. PATRICK SPIRNAK, M.D.

A hydrocele is a collection of serous fluid between the two layers of the tunica vaginalis, which normally surrounds the testis. It is the most common benign cause of scrotal swelling and has been estimated to occur in up to 1 percent of the adult population. A hydrocele is thought to be due to an imbalance between the production and reabsorption of serous fluid secreted by the tunica vaginalis. A primary or idiopathic hydrocele is one in which no underlying urologic abnormality is identified and there is no history of scrotal or groin surgery. Secondary hydroceles occur as a result of any process that acts either to stimulate increased production of fluid by the tunica (e.g., trauma, tumor, inflammation) or to decrease the resorption of this fluid (e.g., inguinal surgery). About 10 percent of testicular tumors are associated with a hydrocele. In patients between the ages of 18 and 35 years in whom a hydrocele appears suddenly, a malignancy must be ruled out.

An accurate diagnosis can usually be made on physical examination. A smooth, cystic-feeling mass completely surrounding the testis and not involving the spermatic cord is characteristic of a hydrocele. When transilluminated light is readily transmitted. On occasion, the hydrocele may be so large or tense that palpation of the underlying testis is impossible. In such cases, scrotal ultrasonography is diagnostic and rules out any underlying testicular abnormalities. Adult hydroceles do not communicate with the peritoneal cavity and thus should not diminish in size as the patient changes position from upright to supine.

Small asymptomatic hydroceles require no treatment other than reassurance of the patient. Indications for intervention include scrotal discomfort or disfigurement due to the sheer size of the mass. Treatment options include needle aspiration, aspiration with injection of a sclerosing agent, and surgical excision. Simple needle aspiration is seldom therapeutic, because the cause of the problem is not addressed and the fluid typically reaccumulates. Excellent results are possible with either surgical excision or needle aspiration combined with injection of a sclerosing agent. Several sclerosing agents have been used successfully, including tetracycline, phenol, and tetradecyl sulfate. Success rates ranging from 33 to 100 percent have been reported, but multiple treatments may be required to achieve these results.

When intervention is indicated, I recommend surgical excision as the most effective form of treatment. A number of surgical procedures have been described, including evagination of the hydrocele sac or "bottle" procedure, excision of the hydrocele sac with oversewing of the cut edges, or plication of the hydrocele sac (the Lord procedure). Although all three of these are effective forms of treatment and may be safely performed on an outpatient basis with the patient under local anesthesia, I believe that the Lord procedure is associated with less scrotal dissection, and therefore less postoperative swelling and fewer complications.

The Lord procedure is performed routinely with the patient under local anesthesia. After the ipsilateral groin and scrotum are shaved, a cord block is performed using a 25-gauge needle. Typically, 7 to 10 ml of 0.5 percent bupivacaine hydrochloride (Marcaine) is injected. An additional 5 to 10 ml of a 50 percent mixture of 1 percent lidocaine and 0.5 percent bupivacaine is injected directly into the skin and subcutaneous tissue directly over the site of the planned transverse scrotal incision. A 4- to 5-cm incision is made through the skin and subcutaneous tissue. The anterior wall of the hydrocele is identified and incised the length of the incision. The testis is delivered through the incision. The hydrocele sac is plicated using 3-0 chromic suture; typically, eight to ten of these plicating sutures are required to obliterate the sac. The testis is returned to the scrotum and the incision is closed. A drain is not generally used.

The major complication of hydrocele surgery is excessive scrotal swelling, which may exceed the mass effect produced by the hydrocele. The degree of swelling is related to the extent of the scrotal dissection. The Lord procedure eliminates the need for excessive mobilization of the hydrocele sac, thus minimizing postoperative morbidity and recovery time. Most patients are able to return to work 7 days after surgery. No recurrences have been reported.

SUGGESTED READING

Kaye KW, Clayman RV, Lange PH. Outpatient hydrocele and spermatocele repair under local anesthesia. J Urol 1983; 130: 269–271.

Savion M, Wolloch Y, Savir A. Phenol sclerotherapy for hydrocele: a study in 55 patients. J Urol 1989; 142:1500–1501.

Spirnak JP, Resnick MI. Hydrocele repair: the Lord procedure. Contemp Urol 1989; 55–57.

SPERMATOCELE

DONALD R. BODNER, M.D.

Spermatoceles are epididymal cysts so named because of the frequent finding of sperm in the cyst fluid. They are the most common cystic condition encountered within the scrotum. Spermatoceles are usually found at the head of the epididymis, adjacent or posterior to the superior pole of the testicle. Spermatoceles vary in size from several millimeters to many centimeters in diameter, and may be single or multiple, unilateral or bilateral. They typically present as incidental scrotal masses found on routine physical examination. They may be discovered by an individual during self-inspection of his scrotum and testicles, or when large, by palpation by his partner. Spermatoceles are usually asymptomatic except when quite large, and then may be associated with testicular discomfort.

The etiology of spermatoceles remains controversial. It is believed they may originate as a diverticulum from the tubules found in the head of the epididymis. With spermatogenesis over time, the diverticulum increases in size, ultimately producing a spermatocele. Spermatoceles are also believed to form as a result of infection (epididymitis) or trauma. If any portion of the epididymis becomes obstructed by scar formation, a spermatocele can form.

DIFFERENTIAL DIAGNOSIS

The differential diagnosis of a painless scrotal mass includes spermatocele, hydrocele, hernia, varicocele, tuberculosis of the epididymis, and tumors of the testicle or epididymis. Acute inflammatory processes involving the epididymis or testicle, such as epididymitis, orchitis, or testicular torsion, are associated with a high degree of pain and should not be confused with spermatocele.

Diagnosis of a spermatocele is best made on physical examination. The finding of a cystic, painless mass at the head of the epididymis that transilluminates and can be definitely differentiated from the testicle is generally sufficient to confirm the diagnosis. Spermatoceles often feel cystic to palpation, but may be firm in consistency when chronic and simulate a solid epididymal or testicular mass. It is important to ensure that the mass is in fact in the epididymis and not in the testicle. Masses in the testicle are testicular tumors until histologically proved otherwise. If uncertainty exists, ultrasonography of the scrotum will confirm the diagnosis.

Hydroceles are common and can be confused with a spermatocele. Hydroceles are a collection of fluid in the tunica vaginalis and either are anterior to the testicle or completely surround the testicle. It is often difficult to palpate the testicle in the presence of a hydrocele, but hydroceles characteristically transilluminate and, if aspirated, yield clear, straw-colored fluid. Varicoceles are a common finding in young men and represent a dilatation of the pampiniform plexus above the testicle. Diagnosis is made by examining the patient in the standing position and confirming the presence of the tortuous veins along the spermatic cord above and posterior to the testicle. When tuberculosis involves the epididymis, a nontender epididymal mass associated with sterile pyuria and beading of the vas deferens is found.

PATIENT SELECTION

Small cysts of the epididymis are best left alone, as are larger cysts when asymptomatic. Only when the cysts are associated with discomfort and are enlarging in size, or when the patient wants the spermatocele removed, should surgical intervention be considered. The patient should be made aware that spermatocelectomy will not improve fertility and should not be performed for this reason. It is also possible that pain may persist after spermatocele removal.

SPERMATOCELECTOMY

Once it has been decided to proceed with spermatocelectomy, the procedure can be performed on an outpatient basis. The technique is performed easily under local or general anesthesia. A transverse scrotal incision is made , ensuring adequate hemostasis. The testicle is delivered from the scrotum, and both the testicle and epididymis are carefully inspected after the tunica vaginalis is opened. The incision is extended to the wall of the cyst of the epididymis. The cyst is often adherent to the underlying epididymis and spermatic cord structures. Sharp and blunt dissection can be used to separate the spermatocele from the testicle and epididymis. The origin of the cyst from the epididymis is isolated, clamped, and ligated with an absorbable suture.

Care is taken not to injure the blood supply to the testicle and not to disturb the continuity of the vas deferens or epididymis. Often the cyst can be removed intact. If the cyst is opened, murky fluid containing spermatozoa is found. Multilocular cysts of the epididymis can be excised in the same manner.

Hemostasis must be ascertained before returning the testicle to the scrotum. The scrotum is then closed in two layers with an absorbable suture. A drain is generally not required. Fluffs and a scrotal support are applied. The patient is advised to apply ice to the scrotum for 24 hours and change the dressing in 1 to 2 days. Complications are infrequent and include scrotal hematomas, testicular atrophy if the blood supply to the testicle is injured, and occasionally infertility if the epididymis is transected.

SUGGESTED READING

Hinman F Jr. Atlas of urologic surgery. Philadelphia: WB Saunders, 1989:311.

Howards SS. Surgery of the scrotum and its contents. In: Walsh PC, Gittes RF, Perlmutter AD, Stamey TA, eds. Campbell's urology. 5th ed. Philadelphia: WB Saunders, 1986.

VARICOCELE IN ADULTS

FLOYD A. FRIED, M.D.

Although the presence of varicosities of the pampiniform plexus of veins had been known for centuries, it was not until 1885 that Barwell described the atrophy associated with this entity. In 1952, Tulloch reported the improved semen quality in an infertile male after the correction of bilateral varicoceles, and subsequent fathering of a child. Today, growing evidence suggests that a varicocele may impair normal testicular function. These arguments are difficult to resolve in the absence of a randomized trial, since not all men with varicoceles are infertile, and even in a population of infertile couples receiving no therapy there exists a baseline pregnancy rate approaching 20 percent.

The incidence of varicoceles is about 15 percent in the general population of adult males. Interestingly, the incidence of varicoceles in men seen in infertility clinics ranges from 21 to 41 percent. The marked prevalence for the left side (78 to 93 percent) is commonly attributed to the differences in venous anatomy, the left spermatic vein being almost 10 cm longer than the right. Furthermore, there is thought to be some element of increased venous pressure in the left renal vein (and hence the left spermatic vein) because of its retroaortic position as it courses to join the vena cava. Bilateral varicoceles occur in 2 to 20 percent and right-sided lesions in 1 to 7 percent of patients.

Varicoceles are probably acquired, because only sporadic cases are noted in children and by age 19 the incidence is 16.2 percent, which is similar to that in the adult population.

Several studies have been performed to determine whether varicoceles are harmful to spermatogenesis, and have demonstrated differences in the histologic appearance of testes associated with varicoceles. Pathologic examination reveals thickening of the tubules, maturation arrest, and decreased spermatogenesis. Changes in the Leydig cells are also described. The presence of Leydig cell hyperplasia is said to be associated with poor results after surgical repair, whereas patients with Leydig cell atrophy have a better prognosis after varicocele repair.

Further evidence of the adverse effects of varicoceles on testicular function is implied by reports describing an exaggerated pattern of response of luteinizing hormone (LH) and follicle-stimulating hormone (FSH) after stimulation with luteinizing hormone–releasing hormone (LHRH). In patients observed after varicocele repair, there was a return to normal of their response to LHRH. Numerous investigators have described histologic changes in the contralateral testis of varicocele patients, although the mechanism remains unclear. Finally, Rhesus monkey models of varicocele have produced similar histologic changes in the ipsilateral testis that eventually begin to involve the contralateral testis. The changes observed include increased testicular temperatures (bilaterally), decreased sperm count, increased blood flow (bilaterally), and disorganized spermatogenesis seen histologically (bilaterally). On the basis of these observations, there is growing reason to believe that varicoceles somehow damage the sperm-producing capacity of testes.

DIAGNOSIS

A simple grading system for varicoceles has been devised based on the size of the lesion: grade I, clinically inapparent; grade II, palpable and moderate in size; and grade III, large lesions that are visible. The diagnosis of grades II and III lesions is generally straightforward, being based on physical findings of a dilated pampiniform plexus with the patient in the standing position that collapses in the supine position. Detection of smaller varicoceles and assessment of the contralateral testis pose some problems. A variety of diagnostic measures have been used. Thermography using heat-sensitive materials that detect increased temperatures has received some attention, but I have not found this to be necessary. Venography should not be used routinely but only in certain situations such as a failed varicocele repair, or in a person who has had previous surgery in the inguinal or scrotal area in whom the examination is confused by scarring. Some have found the radionuclide scan to be helpful, but I have no experience with this and rely on auscultation with the Doppler stethoscope. I would emphasize the following points for its successful use:

1. Examine a number of patients with obvious varicoceles before using it to assess the less obvious. The examination should always be carried out with the patient standing with his back against an immovable object such as a wall or the end of the examining table.
2. Use ample amounts of contact gel.
3. Listen for the easily heard pulsation of the spermatic artery, which can be distinguished from scrotal vessels by compressing the cord structures as they pass over the pubic tubercle (this is why the patient should be up against an immovable object). If you are listening to the spermatic vessel, its pulsation will diminish and can be obliterated by this maneuver.
4. The spermatic veins are close to the artery. If you have listened to obvious varicoceles, you will easily recognize the low-pitched continuous hum heard throughout the cardiac cycle: it sounds like wind blowing through trees and may intensify during inspiration. I believe this should be

present before the diagnosis of a varicocele is made.
5. If the diagnostic finding of a varicocele is not heard, have the patient slowly perform a Valsalva maneuver. In most patients, there will be a rush of blood into the pampiniform plexuses. This probably does not represent a true varicocele, but rather reflects the increased venous pressure and engorgement. This finding can also be obliterated by pressure on the spermatic cord as it passes over the pubic tubercle during the Valsalva maneuver.
6. If there are Doppler findings consistent with a varicocele, the Doppler stethoscope can be used to determine whether there are collateral veins communicating with it. In the presence of collateral veins, compression of the cord over the pubic tubercle will not obliterate the auscultatory findings of the venous hum heard throughout the cardiac cycle. If there are no significantly sized collateral veins, pubic tubercle pressure will definitely obliterate the venous hum.

INDICATIONS FOR SURGICAL REPAIR

What constitutes the indications for surgical repair is a controversial subject. I use the following criteria:

1. Results of several semen analyses that are consistent and demonstrate a low count, low motility, and an increased number of abnormal forms. This has been described as a "stress pattern."
2. A couple who have had timed sexual exposures for at least 18 months without a pregnancy.
3. A woman who has undergone an infertility evaluation, including documentation of ovulation, usually by basal body temperature charts; documentation of the adequacy of the luteal phase of the cycle; and a postcoital (Huhner) test showing decreased numbers of spermatozoa.
4. A decrease in testicular volume if pronounced or progressive. I suspect that at this point the changes are likely to be irreversible.
5. Adolescents who have had an LHRH stimulation test with an exaggerated response; this is defined as an LH value greater than 45 μIU per milliliter and an FSH value greater than 15 μIU per milliliter within 1 hour after stimulation with 100 μg of LHRH.

Some authors advocate an aggressive attitude toward varicocele repair in children, arguing that the procedure is safe and may prevent infertility in later years. This has not yet been proved.

I do not advocate varicocele repair for a patient with (1) an abnormal hormonal profile (i.e., elevation of FSH and/or LH—this is usually associated with testicular failure); or (2) azoospermia in the presence of unobstructed vasa and epididymides.

THERAPEUTIC OPTIONS

In recent years transvenous embolization has been reported to be effective for the obliteration of a varicocele. The procedure may require up to 3 hours to perform and cannot be completed in about 15 percent of cases. Patients are also worried about the radiation exposure required to accomplish this. The long-term results indicate a failure rate similar to that of surgical repair, and there is always the potential for migration of the veno-occlusive device and perforation of the spermatic vein. This procedure is worth considering in a patient in whom surgery has failed.

My current preference is for surgical repair of varicoceles. In most cases, it takes less than 1 hour to perform, is an outpatient procedure, has minimal morbidity, and costs about the same as the transvenous embolization procedure. There are two surgical approaches. The first is the retroperitoneal (Palomo) procedure, which is performed through a small transverse lateral incision just above the internal inguinal ring. The main advantage of this technique is that there are fewer branches of the spermatic vein at this level, and the consequences of accidental ligation of the internal spermatic artery are said to be of less significance. The major disadvantage is that there is a real possibility of missing collateral vessels distal to the point of ligation. The second approach is the inguinal procedure (Ivanissevich), described below.

INGUINAL APPROACH

Although this procedure can be performed with local infiltration and cord block, I would caution against this, because it has been shown that local infiltration of the spermatic cord can result in vascular injuries. General or regional anesthesia is preferred. A 5- to 6-cm incision is made just as for an inguinal herniorrhaphy. The incision is extended to the fascia of the external oblique, which is carefully opened in the direction of its fibers, care being taken to avoid injury to the underlying ilioinguinal nerve. The spermatic cord structures are elevated by sweeping an index finger from lateral to medial against the pubic tubercle, and a Penrose drain is placed beneath the cord. At this point, the patient is placed in reverse Trendelenburg position to distend the veins. The cremasteric fascia is opened and the obvious veins are dissected free from the surrounding structures. This should be done with the aid of magnification, because the spermatic artery is frequently included in this dissection. A few drops of papaverine over the vessels usually dilate the artery and assist in its identification. Small lymphatics can also be seen and should be left undisturbed in order to

minimize the possibility of hydrocele formation postoperatively. Before the main veins are clamped and divided, the patient should be placed in the Trendelenburg position to empty the varicocele before it is tied off. The main vessel is ligated with 00 or 000 ligature at two sites about 1 to 2 cm apart, and an intervening segment of the vein is excised and submitted to the pathology department. The cord should be thoroughly examined for small veins, and any found should be ligated. Next, with the previously placed Penrose drain, the cord is elevated and the floor of the inguinal canal examined. Often small or moderate-sized veins are seen passing into the floor or coursing medially to the contralateral side. These vessels can easily be missed if this maneuver is omitted; if additional veins are found, they are ligated without taking a segment.

COMPLICATIONS

Hydrocele formation has been reported to occur after internal spermatic vein ligation. It is thought to be due to the injury to the lymphatics as they course within the cord structures. This is best avoided by the use of magnification to permit identification of these structures. Ligation of the spermatic artery may also occur and is also best prevented by the use of magnification and topical papaverine to aid the dissection. Injury to the ilioinguinal nerve, resulting in sensory loss or scrotal pain, is recognized as a complication of the inguinal incision. Awareness of the nerve's location, not only while incising the external oblique fascia but also during the closure, usually prevents this problem.

POSTOPERATIVE CARE

Patients can usually be discharged on the day of surgery. Progressive return to full physical activities over a 2- to 3-week period is advised. In view of the approximately 80-day transit time of spermatozoa through the reproductive tract, I obtain a semen analysis 12 weeks after the procedure. If several such analyses fail to demonstrate improvement, I use a course of human chorionic gonadotropin (hCG), 5,000 U per intramuscular injection, as shown in Table 1.

Table 1 Administration of Human Chorionic Gonadotropin After Surgery for Varicocele

Week	Number of Injections
1	3
2	2
3	2
4	1
5	1
6	1

SUGGESTED READING

Hadziselimovic F, Herzog B, Liebundgut B, et al. Testicular and vascular changes in children and adults with varicocele. J Urol 1989; 142:583.

Vermeulen A, Vandeweghe M. Improved fertility after varicocele correction: fact or fiction? Fertil Steril 1984; 42:249.

Yarborough MA, Burns JR, Keller FS. Incidence and clinical significance of subclinical scrotal-varicoceles. J Urol 1989; 141:1372.

VARICOCELE IN CHILDREN

IHOR S. SAWCZUK, M.D.
TERRY W. HENSLE, M.D.

A varicocele, by definition, is an abnormal dilatation of the veins of the pampiniform plexis. Although varicoceles are predominantly found on the left side, bilaterality does occur. Varicoceles seem to affect fertility in that approximately 13 percent of adult males in the United States with varicoceles are infertile. This rate of varicocele-associated infertility in adults is remarkably close to the incidence of varicoceles found in adolescents. The question is, are the infertile adults with varicoceles the same patients who developed varicoceles as adolescents? For this reason, it is important to know whether varicocele correction in the adolescent will affect fertility in the adult. It is well known, from both clinical studies and animal models, that a unilateral varicocele can cause bilateral histologic testicular changes that generally consist of epithelial degeneration in the germinal centers, interstitial fibrosis, and spermatogenic impairment. If these changes occur during puberty (the critical growth period), irreversible testicular damage may occur and subsequent varicocele correction in adulthood may not improve fertility.

Varicoceles are rare in the prepubertal child, but with the onset of puberty the incidence increases dramatically. This increased incidence is most probably related to the physiologic changes that occur during puberty and that affect the internal spermatic vein. Testicular mass increases tremendously with the onset of puberty, along with an associated increased intratesticular blood flow. Because of this excessive perfusion, a functional overload of the internal spermatic vein may occur and collateral vessels can develop. This excess perfusion alone does not cause varicocele formation. Various anatomic features of the left spermatic vein also must occur, including the sharp entry angle of the vein into the left renal vein, the long length of the left spermatic vein compared with the right, and the possible "nutcracker" phenomenon created by the aorta and superior mesenteric artery, compressing the left renal vein and subsequently increasing pressure within the left spermatic vein.

Clinically a varicocele presents as a peritesticular mass classically described as a "bag of worms." Physical examination with the patient in both the supine and upright positions, with and without the Valsalva maneuver, is the diagnostic method of choice. Varicoceles are classified according to grade as shown in Table 1. Since varicoceles may cause a loss of testicular volume, both the affected and contralateral testis must be measured, preferably with an orchidometer. In children, the presence or absence of secondary sex characteristics must also be noted. In the pubertal group, if a discrepancy is detected in testicular size and a varicocele is not palpated. Doppler ultrasonography may aid in detecting a subclinical varicocele. Other modalities that have been used in the diagnosis of a varicocele include conventional and contact scrotal thermography and radionuclide scans, neither of which is particularly useful in the adolescent, and sperm analysis, which is not practical for use in the adolescent. Remember the other causes of scrotal swelling in a child, such as hernia, hydrocele, and testicular torsion or tumor.

INDICATIONS FOR SURGERY

The ultimate goal of varicocele correction in the adult is an improvement in spermatogenesis and fertility potential. It appears that the histologic changes seen in the testes of patients with varicoceles are progressive and more severe with larger varicoceles. With the recognition that early surgical correction of varicoceles may normalize testicular volumes, there has been an increased tendency to correct varicoceles earlier, particularly in the adolescent. Currently, our indications for the surgical correction of an adolescent varicocele include (1) large varicoceles (grade III), (2) symptomatic lesions, (3) marked testicular volume discrepancies, and (4) bilateral lesions.

Varicoceles are rare in prepubertal males; therefore, such a diagnosis in a prepubertal child should be suspect. Occasionally we see patients with a difference in

Table 1 Varicocele Grading

Grade I: Small, detected only by Valsalva
Grade II: Moderate, detected without Valsalva
Grade III: Large, visible before palpation

From Dubin L, and Amelar RD. Varicocele size and results of varicocelectomy in selected subfertile men with varicocele. Fertil Steril 1970; 21:607.

testicular volumes but no clinical varicocele. Since there are no clear data concerning testicular size in this group, testicular volume discrepancy alone is not an indication for surgical correction of a clinical or subclinical varicocele. We recommend that these children be re-examined at puberty with testicular volume determinations to see if a varicocele develops on the affected side. Serum levels of follicle-stimulating hormone, luteinizing hormone, and testosterone are usually normal in adolescents with varicoceles, and for this reason we do not obtain them.

THERAPEUTIC ALTERNATIVES

Percutaneous embolization of the internal spermatic vein with a balloon, coil, or sclerosing agents has been advocated as a nonsurgical form of varicocele ablation in adults. In the adolescent, however, because of the size of the vessels, the percutaneous technique poses more risks than does conventional surgical therapy. We do not use any percutaneous technique as a form of primary varicocele therapy in the adolescent. The use of laparoscopy has increased dramatically, and outpatient laparoscopic varicocele ligation may develop into an attractive alternative to traditional operative varicocele ligation techniques in appropriate patients.

SURGICAL TECHNIQUE

Several different surgical approaches to varicocele correction have been described. The scrotal approach rarely permits identification and ligation of all the collateral vessels and should not be used. Both the inguinal and retroperitoneal approaches can be used. We prefer the inguinal approach, using a transverse skin incision to localize the spermatic cord at the internal ring. The dilated spermatic vein and collaterals are easily identified and ligated at this location. Extreme care should be taken to identify and preserve both the vas deferens and the testicular artery. We have found the use of optical magnification a great help in doing the procedure accurately. Varicocele surgery in the adolescent may be performed on an outpatient basis.

Postoperative complications include hydrocele formation, which is due to excessive lymphatic ligation, and varicocele recurrence, which is due to not interrupting all the collaterals. With proper care and attention, damage to the vas deferens should not occur. If the testicular artery is inadvertently ligated, collateral testicular blood supply through the vasal artery should prevent testicular atrophy. Postoperative evaluation should include scrotal examination for varicocele persistence and measurement of the testis to determine whether the size discrepancy has been arrested or whether testicular size or volume has increased.

SUGGESTED READING

Buch J, Cromie W. Evaluation and treatment of preadolescent varicocele. Urol Clin North Am 12:177–186.

Denver D, Ginsburg M, Millet D, Feinstein M, Cockett A. Nutcracker phenomenon. 1986; 27:541.

Fisch H. The surety of surgical repair of varicoceles. Contemp Urol 1991:68–74.

Reitelman C, Burbige K, Sawczuk I, Hensle T. Diagnosis and surgical correction of the pediatric varicocele. 1987; 138:1038–1040.

VASOVASOSTOMY

ARNOLD M. BELKER, M.D.

As time has elapsed since bilateral vasectomy became popularized in the United States in the 1960s and 1970s, increasing divorce rates have led more men in second marriages to consider a vasectomy reversal procedure. My personal approach to vasectomy reversal reflects my bias that microsurgical anastomotic methods yield better results than do nonmicrosurgical methods. I routinely perform vasectomy reversals on an outpatient basis.

PATIENT SELECTION

Virtually any man who requests a vasectomy reversal is a candidate for the procedure. Patients should understand that chances for a fertile postoperative result decrease as the obstructive interval, which is the time from vasectomy to its reversal, lengthens. Systemic antisperm antibodies, which are present in 50 to 70 percent of vasectomized men, seem to impair fertility after a reversal procedure in a small percentage of men. Unfortunately, there is no test for sperm antibodies that has prognostic significance regarding fertility after a reversal when the test is performed before the reversal. We know that men who have higher levels of serum or seminal plasma sperm antibodies are more likely to have impaired fertility than men who have low levels or no sperm antibodies. However, routine sperm antibody tests before vasectomy reversals are unreliable indicators of postoperative fertility. In 130 of my patients who underwent preoperative and serial postoperative tests for serum sperm agglutinating and immobilizing antibodies, the one patient with the highest levels achieved a conception.

Before a patient actually undergoes a vasovasostomy procedure, I strongly recommend that his wife undergo a gynecologic evaluation. This evaluation does not need to consist of anything more than elicitation of a history and an office pelvic examination. Its purpose is to ensure that the wife does not have any abnormality that might prevent her from becoming pregnant. It is embarrassing to discover for the first time 12 to 18 months after a successful vasovasostomy that the wife has irremediable infertility.

ANESTHESIA

Almost all reversals can be performed with the patient under local anesthesia. For this purpose, I use a mixture of equal parts of 1 percent plain lidocaine to accomplish the immediate onset of anesthesia and 0.5 percent plain bupivacaine for a longer duration of anesthesia. After infiltrating and incising the scrotal skin, I infiltrate perivasal tissue above the level of the vasectomy with the local anesthetic mixture. This is sufficient anesthesia for vasovasostomy. If testicular manipulation or epididymal surgery is required, a more complete spermatic cord block may be necessary. If the obstructive interval spans more than 7 to 8 years, when the need for vasoepididymostomy becomes more likely, I prefer continuous epidural anesthesia. The longer amount of time required for vasoepididymostomy compared with vasovasostomy often leads to restlessness during the critical microsurgical anastomotic suturing when local anesthesia is used. I prefer not to be diverted from the operative procedure by the need to control the patient's restlessness with intravenous sedatives. Therefore, epidural anesthesia is used and sedation is controlled by the anesthesiologist in such circumstances. I also prefer epidural anesthesia when performing repeat vasovasostomy after failure of an initial vasovasostomy procedure, because reoperative procedures require more dissection than the first procedures.

OPERATIVE PROCEDURE

Placement of Incision

Vasovasostomy is performed routinely through short, vertical, anterior scrotal incisions. When the vasectomy has been performed at a very high level or when an unusually long length of the vas has been resected, I prefer an infrapubic incision. This allows easy access to the ends of the vas when the vasectomy site is at a high scrotal level. It also enables mobilization of a sufficient length of the abdominal end of the vas to bridge any length of gap between the ends of the vas, and thus avoid anastomotic tension when a long gap exists. If vasoepididymostomy is required, the scrotal contents may easily be displaced upward through the infrapubic incision.

Dissection of Vas Ends

If vasovasostomy and not vasoepididymostomy is required, one needs to exteriorize only the ends of the vas and not the entire scrotal contents. When the ends of the vas are isolated, the blood supply to the vas is preserved by taking care not to strip the perivasal tissue away from the transected ends of the vas. The vascular leash in the perivasal tissue should be ligated and divided at the level of transection of the vas. When the old scarred ends of the vas are resected, the surgeon must be certain that all scarred portions have been resected and that the ends of the vas that are to be joined appear normal. If scarred ends are joined, the anastomosis is doomed to failure. To minimize the chance of scarring, only bipolar cautery should be used to control bleeding on the adventitia of the vas, and the surface of the transected end of the vas should never be cauterized.

The ends of the vas must be mobilized sufficiently to avoid tension on the anastomosis. As a further measure to prevent such tension, I approximate the perivasal tissue along the base of each isolated end of the vas with interrupted polyglycolic acid sutures (Fig. 1).

If the vasectomy has been performed in the convoluted portion of the vas, the lumen of the testicular end of the vas may be eccentrically situated or extremely elongated. In such instances, sequential resection at 1-mm intervals of the testicular end will quickly result in a centrally situated, relatively small, testicular end lumen.

Preparation for Anastomosis

I prefer to sit rather than stand while performing microsurgical procedures. Because the pedestal of the ordinary operating room table interferes with placement of the surgeon's and assistant's legs, a plain wooden table (22.5 inches wide × 78.5 inches long × 32 inches tall) has been constructed and is used routinely for microsurgical genital procedures. The tabletop is covered with foam rubber pads enclosed in conductive rubber. Use of this table allows ample room under it for the legs of both surgeon and assistant and thus enables them to be comfortably seated during the entire microsurgical procedure.

I always perform the anastomosis while situated on the left side of the patient. This is done so that the sutures that are placed from outside to inside of the mucosal layer of the narrow abdominal end lumen will be placed through the anterior aspect of the mucosal layer on the abdominal end. Other surgeons may find that suturing of the mucosal layer of the abdominal end

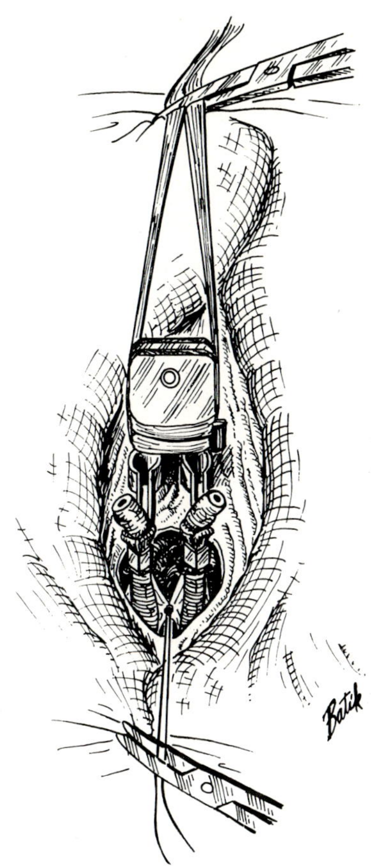

Figure 1 Before the approximating clamp is applied, the suture used to approximate spermatic fascia is left long and is tagged to drapes on the surgeon's side (*bottom*). After the approximating clamp has been applied and folded, a double wrap of umbilical tape around the hinge post of the clamp is tagged to drapes on the assistant's side (*top*). Thus, the anastomosis is stabilized bilaterally. (Republished with permission by Belker AM. Microsurgical repair of obstructive causes of male infertility. Semin Urol 1984; 2:91.)

of the vas is easier if performed from the right side of the patient.

Intraoperative Examination of Vas Fluid

As soon as the scarred testicular end of the vas has been resected, the fluid from that end is examined microscopically for sperm content. If sperm or sperm heads (without tails) are present, vasovasostomy is performed. If sperm are absent and the vas fluid is watery (clear, colorless, and transparent), vasovasostomy is performed. If the vas fluid does not contain sperm and appears thick and creamy, vasovasostomy will result in low postoperative patency (sperm in semen) and pregnancy rates, and vasoepididymostomy therefore is performed. If sperm are not present in cloudy vas fluid, the results of vasovasostomy are sufficiently good for only vasovasostomy to be necessary. However, I recommend that vasoepididymostomy be performed when

sperm are absent and the vas fluid appears cloudy if the obstructive interval is longer than 8 years.

Anastomotic Method

Before anastomotic suturing is performed, patency of the abdominal end of the vas is verified by observing the free flow of Ringer's solution instilled through a 24-gauge blunt tip needle. After the testicular end vas fluid has been sampled for sperm content and the patency of the abdominal end of the vas has been verified, the perivasal fascial approximating suture is tagged to the drapes on the surgeon's side. A hinged, folding, vas-approximating clamp is then applied from the assistant's side, secured to the drapes with a double wrap of umbilical tape, and folded. This results in bilateral stability of the vas ends (see Fig. 1). The approximating clamp is placed onto the vas ends from the assistant's side so that the hinge post of the clamp will not interfere with motion of the tips of the surgeon's instruments during the anastomotic suturing. I prefer the two-layer microsurgical anastomotic method of vasovasostomy (Fig. 2). Modified single-layer microsurgical vasovasostomies (Fig. 3) do have patency and pregnancy rates comparable with those of two-layer microsurgical anastomoses. However, I routinely perform two-layer vasovasostomy to maintain the microsurgical skills that are required to perform vasoepididymostomy when that procedure is necessary.

When the entire anastomosis is performed with the vas-approximating clamp folded, the surgeon is able to see clearly where each suture is placed. During placement of the anterior inner mucosal layer sutures from outside to inside the lumen, the surgeon must verify that the sutures indeed pass into the lumen so that they include the mucosa itself, and also so that they do not penetrate so deeply that they include the mucosa of the opposite posterior wall. All mucosal layer sutures are tied after they are placed until space remains for only the last three anterior sutures. Then, all three remaining mucosal layer sutures are placed before any of them are tied. This method avoids difficulty in placement of the last mucosal layer suture when all previous sutures have been tied. The mucosal 10-0 nylon sutures should include about one fourth of the thickness of the muscular wall of the vas, and the outer muscular layer 9-0 nylon sutures should include the outer one third to one half of the muscular wall. Generally, five to eight mucosal layer sutures and seven to nine muscular layer sutures are used.

After the anastomotic suturing has been completed, the vas-approximating clamp is removed carefully and the anastomosis is returned into the scrotum. Wound closure is performed in a routine fashion. The entire procedure is performed skin to skin first on one side and then on the other. This avoids loss of the local anesthetic effect before skin closure on each side. Drains are not needed after microsurgical vasovasostomy owing to the meticulous hemostasis required for microsurgical procedures.

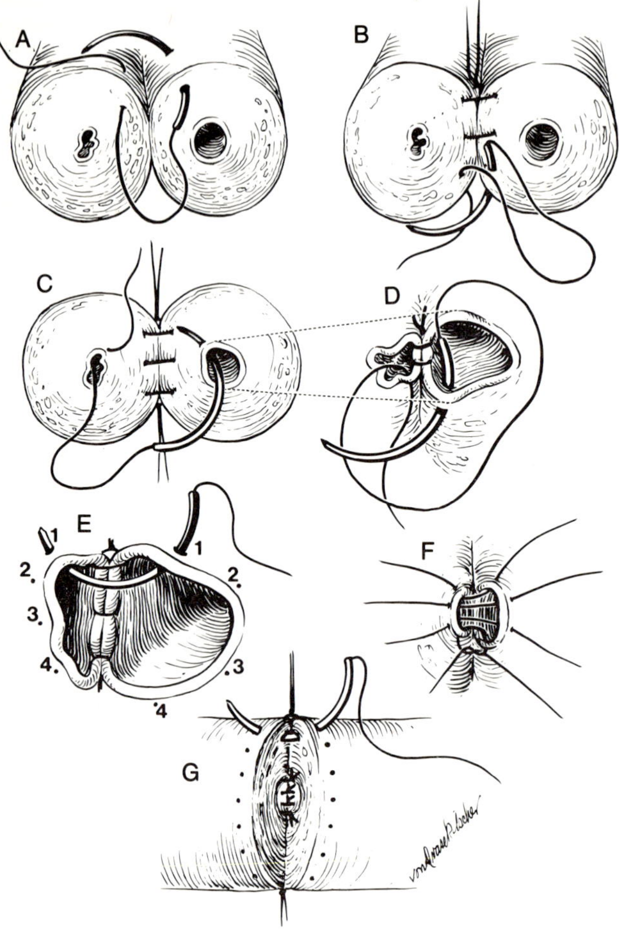

Figure 2 The two-layer microsurgical anastomotic method of vasovasostomy. Note the discrepancy in luminal diameters. *A, B,* Three posterior row muscular layer sutures are placed so that the knots are outside. Only 90 degrees of circumference is approximated, leaving full access to the mucosa. End sutures are left long and tagged. *C, D,* Note the change in magnification indicated by broken lines. Three (sometimes two) posterior row mucosal sutures are placed with knots extraluminal. Successive sutures are placed from the assistant's side toward the surgeon's side. *E,* Four (sometimes three) anterior row mucosal sutures are placed in the order indicated by the numbers. *F,* Sutures are cut long and left untied until all anterior row mucosal sutures are placed. Sutures are then tied in reverse order of placement. *G,* Anterior 270 degrees (diagram depicts only 180 degrees) of muscular layer sutures are placed, using two tagged end posterior muscular layer sutures for traction to aid placement of anterior muscular layer sutures. (Republished with permission by Belker AM. Microsurgical two-layer vasovasostomy: simplified technique using hinged, folding-approximating clamp. Urology 1980; 16:376. © by Williams & Wilkins)

POSTOPERATIVE CARE

I do not use either antibiotics or steroids. Patients are requested to remain at home for 1 week postoperatively and to avoid heavy physical activity and use a scrotal support for 1 month. The rather long limitation of heavy physical activity and use of a scrotal support is based on my observations of disrupted anastomoses when performing repeat vasovasostomy in patients who had been allowed to resume any activity that was comfortable as soon as they desired after the initial procedure. I also request patients to avoid ejaculation for 2 weeks after the procedure. This advice is based on histologic observations by Stanwood S. Schmidt of the rate of healing of canine vas anastomoses some years ago. Semen analyses are obtained starting 2 months postoperatively and then every 2 months subsequently either until normal sperm concentration and motility have been reached and maintained for several times, or until a pregnancy occurs.

COMPLICATIONS

Scrotal hematoma and infection are rare. I estimate that each occurs in less than 2 percent of patients who undergo vasovasostomy. After bilateral microsurgical vasovasostomy was performed in most of the 500 patients who underwent vasectomy reversal procedures, testicular atrophy occurred unilaterally in three, presumably as a result of compromised blood supply. One other patient developed bilateral inflammatory hydrohematoceles, which required surgical repair 2 weeks postoperatively. Several other patients developed small scrotal hematomas that responded to simple symptomatic treatment and did not require surgical intervention.

RESULTS

The Vasovasostomy Study Group of five surgeons recently reported results of 1,247 first-time microsurgical vasectomy reversals. There was no statistically significant difference in patency or pregnancy rates postoperatively between patients who underwent modified one-layer and those who had two-layer microsurgical anastomoses. Patients who had a histologically proved sperm granuloma at the vasectomy site bilaterally did not have statistically significant different patency or pregnancy rates than patients who had histologically proved absence of a vasectomy site sperm granuloma bilaterally. Among the five surgeons, overall patency rates ranged only from 85 to 87 percent and overall pregnancy rates from 48 to 54 percent. The average overall patency and pregnancy rates were 86 and 52 percent, respectively.

New guidelines were developed to give patients seeking vasectomy reversals prognostic information based on the length of the obstructive interval. If this was less than 3 years, patency occurred in 97 percent of the patients and pregnancy in 76 percent of their wives. Patency and pregnancy rates, respectively, for longer obstructive intervals were 88 and 53 percent for 3 to 8 years, 79 and 44 percent for 9 to 14 years, and 71 and 30 percent for 15 years or longer.

Among patients who underwent first-time reversals, the average time until conception postoperatively was 12

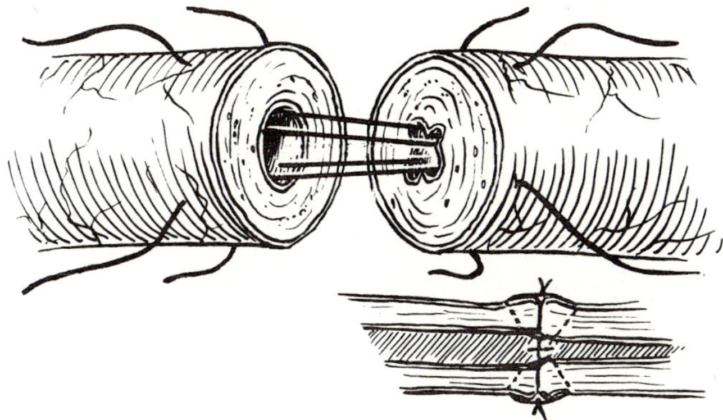

Figure 3 The method of vasovasostomy used by most surgeons who do not use optical magnification, and by some surgeons who use optical loupes or the operating microscope for magnification, is shown. Inset shows side view of the anastomosis. Full-thickness sutures are placed and tied, and then more superficial outer muscular layer sutures are placed and tied. (Republished with permission by Belker AM. Vasovasostomy. In: Resnick MI, ed. Current trends in urology. Vol. 1. Baltimore: Williams & Wilkins, 1981:20. Copyright by Williams & Wilkins.)

months, the spontaneous abortion rate was 20 percent, and the male-to-female ratio of children (1.0252:1) was no different from that in the general population. Congenital anomalies occurred in 1 percent of the children, compared with 3 percent in the general population of newborns.

Among 76 repeat vasectomy reversals that I have performed, 69 were second reversals and seven were third reversals. Of 55 patients who underwent repeat reversal and in whom postoperative semen analyses were performed, 18 (33 percent) were azoospermic postoperatively. This is a considerably higher rate of postoperative azoospermia than the rate of 14 percent that occurs after first reversals. Sixteen (44 percent) of my 36 repeat reversal patients who were eligible for pregnancy rate calculations achieved a pregnancy. Among 222 patients who underwent repeat vasectomy reversal by the Vasovasostomy Study Group, 25 percent were azoospermic postoperatively and 43 percent achieved a pregnancy postoperatively. Patients who request repeat vasovasostomy should understand that patency and pregnancy rates are lower after repeat than after first-time reversal procedures.

SUGGESTED READING

Belker AM. Vasovasostomy. In: Resnick MI, ed. Current trends in urology. Vol. 1. Baltimore: Williams & Wilkins, 1981:20.

Belker AM. Vasovasostomy and vasoepididymostomy. AUA Update Series. Vol. 1. lesson 2. Houston: American Urological Association, Office of Education, 1981.

Belker AM. Microscopic vasovasostomy. Videotape for Urology Today series, Male infertility. 8th ed. Vol. 4. No. 1. Norwich, NY: Norwich Eaton Television Network, Norwich Eaton Pharmaceuticals, 1984.

Belker AM. Microsurgical vasectomy reversal. In: Lytton B, Catalona WJ, Lipshultz LI, McGuire EJ, eds. Advances in urology. Vol. 1. Chicago: Yearbook, 1988:193.

Belker AM, Thomas AJ Jr, Fuchs EF, et al. Results of 1,469 microsurgical vasectomy reversals by the Vasovasostomy Study Group. J Urol 1991; 145:505.

VASOEPIDIDYMOSTOMY

ANTHONY J. THOMAS, Jr., M.D.

Complete obstruction of the epididymis can have a variety of causes. Among the more common are a previous inflammatory event; a congenital disjunction between the vasa and the epididymides; or a more distal obstruction somewhere along the course of the vas deferens, which can cause the delicate and highly convoluted tubule to rupture from pressure-induced changes within its lumen.

PREOPERATIVE EVALUATION

Azoospermic men should be carefully evaluated for the presence of a surgically correctable lesion. When there is complete epididymal blockage, the testes are normal in size (>20 cm^3) and the vasa are readily palpable without evidence of induration. The epididymis may feel full and firm, although in some this fullness is subtle. The volume of semen is normal (>1.5 ml). It has an alkaline pH, and fructose is present in the seminal plasma in a quantity greater than 150 mg per deciliter. The serum follicle-stimulating hormone (FSH) level is normal if active spermatogenesis is present in both testes, but can be mild-to-moderately elevated in men who have a normal testis on one side and a smaller, more poorly functioning contralateral testis.

The patient should have at least two semen analyses that reveal no sperm. A postejaculatory urine sample is examined to rule out the possibility of retrograde ejaculation, particularly when the semen volume is marginal.

If there is a strong suspicion of a correctable obstruction, the testis biopsy, vasogram, and vasoepididymal anastomoses can be carried out during the same operative event. If there is any doubt of the presence or absence of active spermatogenesis, the patient may be brought to the operating room fully prepared for microsurgical reconstruction and the testis biopsy may be performed using local anesthesia combined with a mild intravenous sedative. If the testes are of equal and normal size, only one side need be biopsied. If spermatogenesis is not found or if its adequacy cannot be determined, the small scrotal incision is closed and the patient sent home pending further examination of the biopsy material. When a frozen section is properly cut and fixed, it is not difficult to evaluate it for the presence of active spermatogenesis. As a quick, adjunctive test, a "touch preparation" of the tissue sample can easily be prepared and examined for the presence of long-tailed sperm. After the biopsy sample is sharply cut from the testis, it is dabbed on a sterile glass slide five or six times and the slide immediately fixed by putting it into absolute ethyl alcohol or spraying it with an appropriate fixative.* The slide is then treated with Wright's stain, rinsed, and examined.

OPERATIVE TECHNIQUE

Once the biopsy has been read and spermatogenesis determined to be adequate, the patient is anesthetized and the appropriate procedures are carried out. The testes are exposed through two separate scrotal incisions. An x-ray film of the pelvis, including the scrotum, is taken. The straight portion of one vas deferens is isolated on the medial side of the cord structures, care being taken not to injure its closely adherent artery and vein. A 2-cm segment of the vas deferens is freed up and held taut between two towel clips. A 30-gauge lymphangiogram needle,† its tubing attached to a 3-ml syringe

filled with saline, is inserted into the vas lumen, and 1 to 2 ml of saline is injected. If there is no resistance and no extravasation with the saline injection, the syringe is exchanged for one containing a 1:1 mixture of Renografin 60 and saline. Approximately 1.5 to 2 ml is injected and another radiograph taken. If there is no distal obstruction, the vas lumen is visualized as a fine white line, traversing the inguinal canal, dipping behind the bladder, merging with the seminal vesicle and ending in the ejaculatory duct. If more contrast material is injected and another radiograph taken, the contrast will be readily apparent in the bladder, indicating patency of the ejaculatory duct. The contralateral vas is isolated and cannulated in a similar fashion. Unless there is a specific history of inflammation or previous surgery on that side, only saline need be injected and no further radiographs need be taken. If 5 to 8 ml of fluid can easily be pushed through the lumen of the vas deferens, it is unlikely that there is a distal obstruction.

Once patency of the vasa is confirmed, each epididymis is carefully examined for signs of obstruction. At times this can be identified by an area of blue-brown discoloration beneath the epididymal tunic (Fig. 1). This most likely represents a point of sperm extravasation, the coloration being caused by lipofuchsin granules, a breakdown product of the epididymal cells. In some instances, when the point of obstruction is not readily apparent, it will be necessary to explore the epididymis

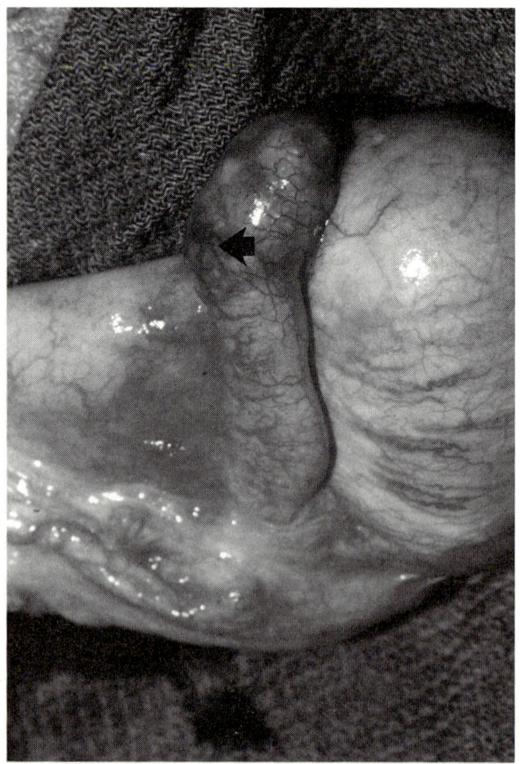

Figure 1   Dilated caput epididymidis with an area of discoloration (*arrow*) indicating the point of obstruction.

---

*Spray-cyte, Clay Adams, div. of Becton Dickinson Co, Rutherford, NJ or Surgipath Cytology Fixative, Surgipath Medical Industries, Inc, Grayslake, IL.

†No. 6657, Becton-Dickinson Co.

from the tail, cephalad until normal-appearing motile or nonmotile sperm are identified.

After the epididymis is examined and before the tubule is opened, the proximal portion of the vas deferens is freed up on the medial side of the testis. The vasal vessels are individually ligated with 6-0 nylon sutures, and the vas deferens along with its artery and vein is transected and freed from the surrounding, loose areolar tissue for a distance of approximately 6 to 8 cm, long enough to bring the cut end to the epididymal tubule without tension.

The operating microscope is necessary to explore the epididymal tubule properly. When no obvious point of obstruction is apparent, the tunic overlying the cauda is incised with a small, round-tipped scalpel, care being taken not to open the tubule below. With a round-tip microscissors, a small window of tunic is removed. Thumb and forefinger are used to compress gently the sides of the epididymis, causing the convoluted tubule to

protrude through the window of the tunic. Using the round-tip microscissors again, a single loop is carefully freed from the surrounding tissues, and once isolated is unroofed (Fig. 2*A* and *B*).

The fluid exuding from the opened lumen is placed on a sterile glass slide and a drop of saline added, which dilutes the fluid and allows for easier identification of sperm, if present. I prefer to have a light microscope in the operating room so that I can examine the slides immediately, rather than spending the time and the added cost of sending them to the pathologist.

If no sperm are found in the portion of the tubule opened, the epididymal tunic is incised 0.5 cm more cephalad, and another loop of tubule is isolated and unroofed. This procedure is repeated until long-tailed sperm are found. With experience, the surgeon can sometimes identify the site of obstruction early in the exploration and incise the tubule just above that level.

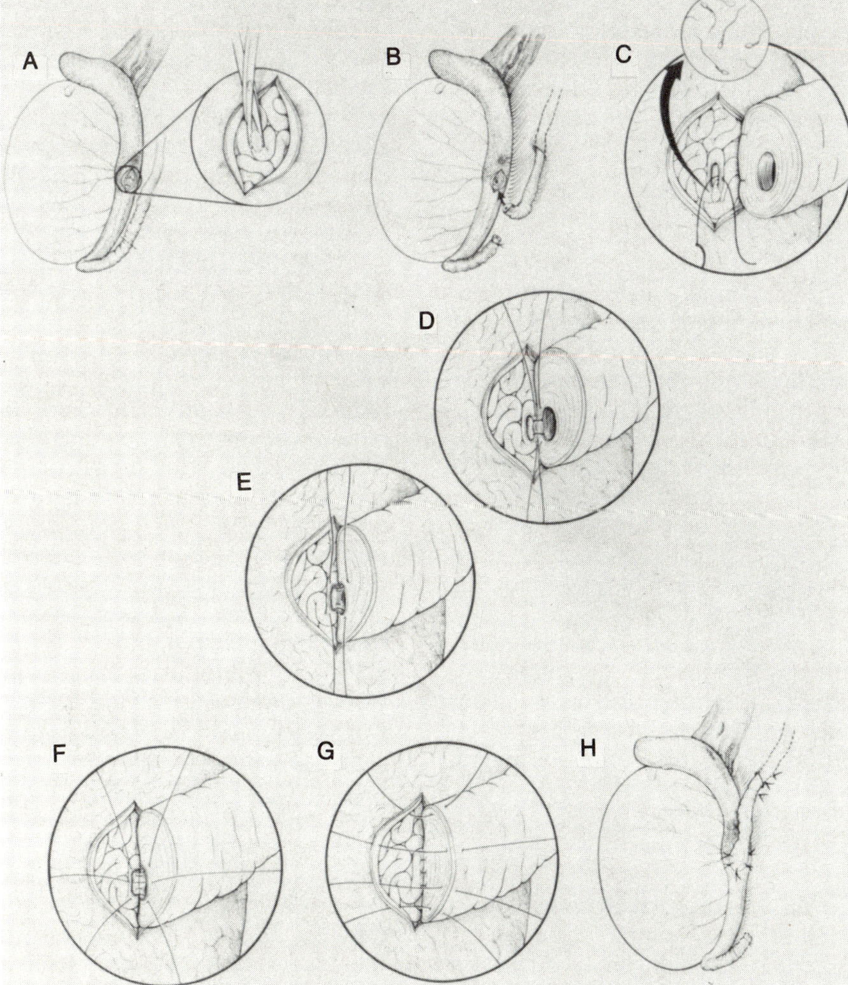

Figure 2 *A* to *H,* Method of end-to-side microsurgical vasoepididymostomy. Republished with permission by Howards S, Thomas A. Surgical treatment of infertility. In: Lipshultz L, Howards S, eds. Infertility in the male. Chicago: Mosby-Year Book, 2nd ed., 1991:366.

Until that experience is gained, it is best to begin in the distal, cauda epididymidis and move proximal, as required.

When the proper level is found and the portion of the tubule exuding sperm opened, a 10-0 suture is passed from the outside into the lumen. This suture is helpful in later identification of the lumen, which tends to collapse as fluid drains out from it. The cut end of the convoluted vas is brought beneath the cord structures to the lateral side of the epididymis where the tunic had been opened (see Fig. 2*B*). Two 9-0 sutures are passed through the adventitia and muscularis of the vas, securing it to the edge of the epididymal tunic at the level of the opened tubule (Fig. 2*C*). The mucosa of the vas lumen is then sutured to the opened tubule with four to six individual 10-0 sutures incorporating the "identification suture" within the circumferential approximation of the two lumens (Fig. 2*D* to *F*). After the placement of these sutures, the muscularis and adventitia of the vas are secured to the epididymal tunic with 9-0 nylon sutures, equally spaced about the end of the vas deferens (Fig. 2*G*). Three or four 9-0 nylon sutures are placed along the length of the vas, attaching it along the inner surface of the tunica vaginalis (Fig. 2*H*). These sutures serve to keep tension off the anastomosis as the testis is manipulated back into the scrotum, as well as during the initial healing phase.

POSTOPERATIVE CARE

Acetaminophen with codeine is given for the discomfort experienced after vasoepididymostomy. In most instances it need be taken only for a day or two. Patients are requested not to participate in any strenuous work or exercise for 2 weeks, and intercourse is prohibited for 3 weeks. With these restrictions, most men are able to return to work within days after surgery. The patient is seen and a semen sample examined during the fourth postoperative week. Many men have no sperm in their semen at this time. It may take 3 to 12 months before sperm are evident in the semen and even longer for motility to increase to levels at which one might anticipate a pregnancy capable of being established. If the anastomosis is performed in the more proximal level of the epididymis (caput), sperm motility may remain low, and the chance of a pregnancy occurring is less than in patients with anastomoses to the corpus or cauda.

COMPLICATIONS

Scrupulous attention to detail will minimize morbidity from this procedure.

Patients who present with epididymal obstruction are generally healthy, young, and highly motivated to do whatever they can to make their surgery successful. There are rarely specific medical or anatomic problems to prevent either general or regional anesthesia from being offered. If regional anesthesia is selected, I prefer epidural to spinal anesthesia because it offers the ability to tailor the anesthetic's time of effectiveness while minimizing the possibility of the often severe headache that can occur after spinal anesthesia. Since some of these procedures can take as long as 4 to 5 hours, I routinely place sheepskin pads beneath the patient's buttocks and heels to minimize the postoperative soreness that sometimes occurs after prolonged procedures in anesthetized, immobile patients.

Meticulous hemostasis during dissection and closure will prevent most large hematomas from forming, although most men undergoing vasoepididymostomy can expect some ecchymoses and mild scrotal swelling after the surgery. An ice bag placed over the scrotum immediately after and for the first 24 hours following the surgery minimizes swelling and adds to the patient's comfort and ease of convalescence.

When there is extensive scarring from previous surgery or infection, care must be taken in dissecting the vas deferens away from the other cord structures, as it is possible to injure the arterial blood supply inadvertently and cause atrophy of the testis. Optical loops and the operating microscope are sometimes needed to isolate the vas safely, maintaining the vascular integrity of it and the testis.

Although postoperative antibiotics are not essential, I have made it a practice to give each patient a 7-day course of doxycycline, 100 mg twice a day.

VASOEPIDIDYMOSTOMY FOLLOWING VASECTOMY OR FAILED VASOVASOSTOMY

As mentioned earlier, a distal vasal obstruction can cause a more proximal blockage through a pressure induced "blow-out" anywhere along the epididymal tubule. The problem the surgeon faces is when to explore the epididymis in the course of performing a vasectomy reversal. The absence of sperm in the fluid from the proximal (testicular) end of the vas deferens is not in itself reason to perform a vasoepididymostomy. A recent review by members of the Vasovasostomy Study Group of more than 1,400 men who underwent vasectomy reversal pointed out that of 83 patients who had bilateral absence of sperm from the proximal vas and underwent vasovasostomy only, 50 (60 percent) developed sperm in their semen, and 20 of 65 (31 percent) men went on to establish a pregnancy with their spouses. There is an increased incidence of sperm absence in the vas fluid along with an increased duration of obstruction. All surgeons must develop their own approach to the postvasectomy patient with regard to when to explore the epididymis. In the absence of sperm, when there is clear or opaque fluid coming from the proximal vas, there is a much higher probability of sperm return to the semen than when there is thick, creamy fluid and a long obstructive interval (>10 years). In some men, there may be no fluid seen in the vas, and in those with a longer obstructive interval, I expose and carefully explore the epididymis. There is no hard and fast rule that covers for

Table 1 Results of Vasoepididymostomy

Author(s)	No. of Patients	No. with Sperm	No. Pregnant
Fogdestam et al.	41	35 (85.3%)	15 (36.6%)
Silber	190	146 (77%)	94 (49%)
Thomas	69*	57 (82%)	26† (44%)

*Patients followed a minimum of 3 months.
†Based on 59 men followed for a minimum of 6 months.

all circumstances. One must be comfortable in performing either a vasovasostomy or vasoepididymal anastomosis and have the patient prepared for either procedure, depending on the intraoperative findings.

RESULTS

The proper use of the operating microscope has led to almost a doubling of the patency and pregnancy rates compared with men undergoing vasoepididymostomy without magnification. In my patients and those of other experienced microsurgeons, patency rates range between 75 and 85 percent, with pregnancies occurring in 35 to 50 percent of the spouses (Table 1).

SUGGESTED READING

Belker AM, Thomas AJ, Fuchs EF, et al. Results of 1469 microsurgical vasectomy reversals by the Vasovasostomy Study Group. J Urol 1991; 145:505–511.

Fogdestam I, Fall M, Nilsson S. Microsurgical epididymovasostomy in the treatment of occlusive azoospermia. Fertil Steril 1986; 46: 925–929.

Silber SJ. Results of microsurgical vasoepididymostomy: role of epididymis in sperm maturation. Human Reprod 1989; 4:298–303.

Thomas AJ. Vasoepididymostomy. In: Rajfer J, ed. Common problems in infertility and impotence. Chicago: Year Book, 1990:217.

Thomas AJ. Vasoepididymostomy. Urol Clin North Am 1987; 14: 527–538.

XANTHOGRANULOMATOUS PYELONEPHRITIS

ROBERT B. SMITH, M.D.

Xanthogranulomatous pyelonephritis is a rare form of pathologic change that accompanies chronic renal infection. It represents an unusual response to chronic infection, in which there is migration of fat-laden histiocytes (xanthoma cells) that cause a replacement lipomatosis. It is found in less than 1 percent of patients with a history of renal infection who undergo pathologic examination. Clinically, it is often confused with renal cell carcinoma, hydronephrosis, or perinephritis. Only rarely is it diagnosed preoperatively.

CLINICAL FEATURES AND DIAGNOSIS

Xanthogranulomatous pyelonephritis is more often seen in females in midlife, but it has been reported in children. Up to 60 percent of the patients present with a palpable kidney. This is usually associated with multiple symptoms, including flank pain, fever, chills, malaise, anorexia, weight loss, and anemia, and is accompanied by persistent urinary tract infection, often despite prolonged antibiotic therapy. *Escherichia coli* and *Proteus mirabilis* are by far the most prevalent organisms involved. Anaerobic organisms have been reported as additional causative agents. One third of these patients have a history of urinary tract calculi. Patients often, but not invariably, have pyuria and microscopic hematuria. Up to 50 percent have a hepatic dysfunction syndrome with an elevated alpha$_2$-globulin level, an abnormal prothrombin time, and an elevated alkaline phosphatase level. This hepatic dysfunction syndrome is not dissimilar to that seen in cases of renal cell carcinoma, and therefore these two diagnostic entities can often be confused. It is especially common for these patients to be misdiagnosed as having renal cell carcinoma because of the presence of flank mass, pain, and systemic symptoms, which are indicative of an advanced malignancy.

The radiographic appearance of xanthogranulomatous pyelonephritis is varied, having little in the way of characteristic findings. A mass lesion is often appreciated on intravenous pyelography with rather ill-defined renal margins. In cases of diffuse lesions, the kidney often does not function. The presence of calcifications in the area of the kidney should alert one to the possible diagnosis of xanthogranulomatous pyelonephritis. In a few cases this disease is focal. Caliceal distortion can be seen on intravenous pyelography in addition to dilatation of the collecting system from previous or current stones or infection. Renal ultrasonography may confirm the presence of a

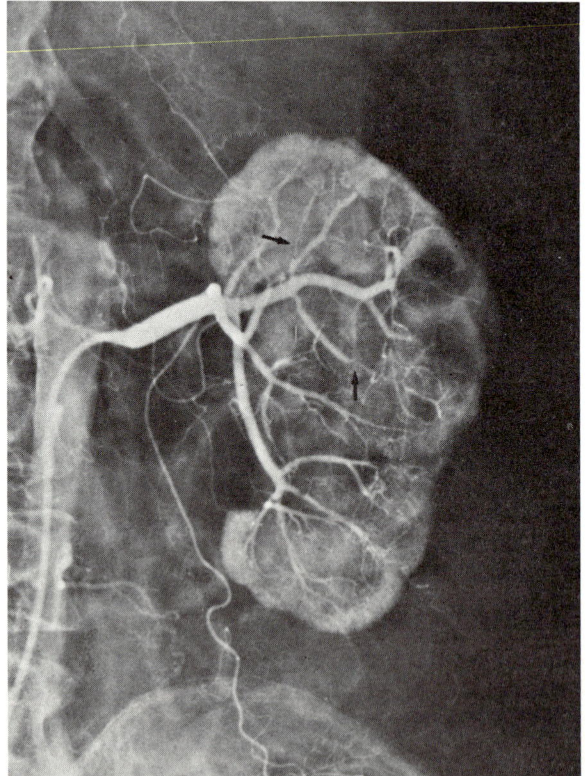

Figure 1 Renal angiogram of pathologically proved xanthogranulomatous pyelonephritis. Note the encasement of arterioles with mass effect, with splaying of arterioles. Also note the irregular and narrowed arteries (*arrows*) with near-occlusion.

364

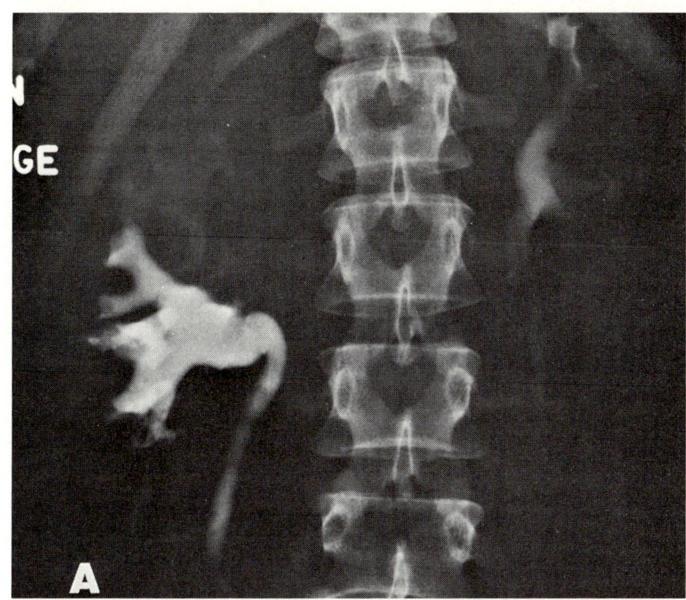

Figure 2 A 19-year-old female with a 7-day history of fatigue, anorexia, and right upper quadrant pain. Urine culture and sensitivity was positive for *Enterobacter*. The patient was also noted to have elevated bilirubin and alkaline phosphatase levels. Urine culture and sensitivity for tuberculosis was negative. *A,* Intravenous pyelogram demonstrates an obstructed upper pole infundibulum with secondary hydrocalices proximal to this infundibulum. *(Continued on next page)*

stone in the diffusely enlarged kidney. The dilated collecting system is noted as well as a possible mass effect in those early cases that are localized. In diffuse cases it is difficult to differentiate pyelonephritis from simple hydronephrosis secondary to a pelvic stone (peripheral anechoic pattern and central echogenic areas). On computed tomography (CT), the enlarged kidney or mass effect is noted, the parenchyma being replaced with relative low-density areas with rims that may enhance with the administration of contrast medium. Stones that may be present and noted would help to confirm the diagnosis of xanthogranulomatous pyelonephritis. Renal angiography should differentiate this lesion from renal cell carcinoma, since the arteriographic appearance of xanthogranulomatous pyelonephritis is less varied than that seen on intravenous pyelography (Fig. 1). The typical neovascularity and tumor blushes seen in renal cell carcinoma are not present in xanthogranulomatous pyelonephritis; however, not all renal cell carcinomas are hypervascular, hence the confusion. In addition, the segmental arteries in xanthogranulomatous pyelonephritis are often irregular and narrowed or occluded and may be stretched around masses in the replaced parenchyma. They are often fewer in number than normal. The main renal artery itself can also be narrowed and attenuated. Defects in the parenchyma are often noted on the nephrogram phase of the arteriogram, correlating with areas of parenchymal replacement by fat and with dilated hydrocalices. Both on the CT scan and angiogram there can be evidence of this lesion extending through the renal capsule and producing a significant perinephric mass, causing even more confusion with renal cell carcinoma.

The disease process is rarely bilateral. Most cases diffusely involve one kidney. Up to 20 percent are focal. This is usually the type of disease noted in children and young adults (Fig. 2). Xanthogranulomatous pyelone-

phritis can be classified in regard to the extent of extrarenal extension. It can (1) involve only the kidney in either a local or diffuse manner, (2) involve the perinephric fat, or (3) present as a diffuse infiltrating process in the retroperitoneum. Xanthoma cells (fat-laden histiocytes) may be sloughed in the urine and would be a valuable diagnostic test preoperatively in distinguishing this entity for renal cell carcinoma. The absence of these cells, however, does not exclude the diagnosis of xanthogranulomatous pyelonephritis. Increased use of urine cytology in a search for xanthoma cells, and improved scanning techniques with ultrasonography, CT, and magnetic resonance imaging in the future may help differentiate this lesion from renal cell carcinoma preoperatively.

Treatment

Most patients are treated surgically because of concern over missing a neoplastic lesion or because of the systemic symptoms that this lesion causes. When there is legitimate confusion with renal cell carcinoma, "radical nephrectomy" is generally the treatment of choice. Also, in cases of diffuse involvement of kidney, this is probably appropriate therapy even if the diagnosis of xanthogranulomatous pyelonephritis is made preoperatively. Since most of the kidneys with diffuse disease contribute little if anything to overall renal function, they are probably best removed because of the symptoms related to the lesion and because they represent a long-term focus of urinary tract infection or sepsis. "Radical nephrectomy" should be done in an expeditious manner, and proper preoperative preparation, including systemic antibiotic therapy and bowel preparation, should be performed. In cases of diffuse retroperitoneal involvement, the risk of bowel injury is significant. Such patients should have preoperative

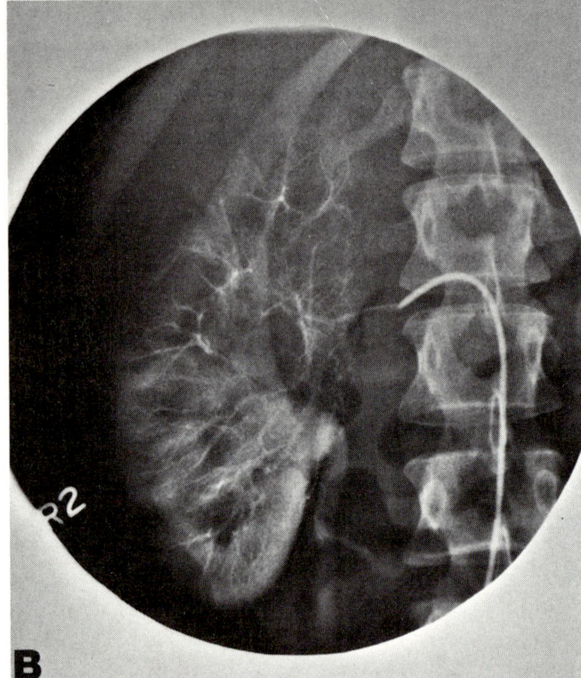

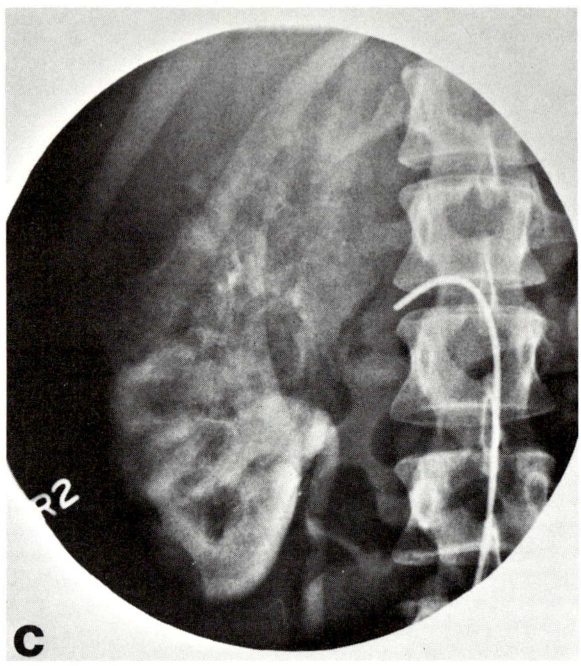

Figure 2 *(Continued)*   *B* and *C,* Delayed renal angiogram and nephrogram demonstrating a poor-quality nephrogram in the upper pole with attenuated upper polar arterioles. The patient underwent right upper pole nephrectomy. The peritoneum was noted to be densely adherent to the upper pole. Pathologic examination revealed multiple areas of abscess and fibrosis within the parenchyma in addition to the hydrocalices. There were multiple areas microscopically, demonstrating large foamy histiocytes and multinucleated giant cells in a granulomatous arrangement. Acid-fast stain was negative. The final diagnosis was infundibular obstruction with secondary hydrocalix (acute) and chronic xanthogranulomatous pyelonephritis with abscess formation.

preparation in the form of mechanical cleansing of the bowel with neomycin and erythromycin. In cases of diffuse retroperitoneal involvement, the operative risk may be significant. This process can involve the great vessels, liver, diaphragm, and bowel mesentery and represents the same surgical challenge as an extensive renal cell carcinoma. Thus, in such cases, the indications for surgery (i.e., symptoms) must justify these increased risks. Surgical exposure in such cases should be excellent, as for a large renal cell carcinoma. The incision of choice is a large 11th interspace flank incision in an attempt to remove all Gerota's fascia and perinephric fat intact. One should carefully avoid entry into the chest in these patients because of the possibility of contaminating the chest with bacteria. However, in our experience, when this has occurred we have not had sequelae. The

complications and sequelae of this procedure are no different from those in any cases involving a difficult nephrectomy. A Penrose drain should be left in the renal fossa postoperatively because of the infectious nature of the lesion, and systemic antibiotics should be continued for 7 days, directed by the urine culture and renal tissue culture results.

In cases of focal disease, medical therapy may suffice. In other cases with localized disease, partial nephrectomy is performed if the diagnosis is made preoperatively (see Fig. 2). This is especially indicated in the pediatric population with localized disease. In cases of partial nephrectomy, the collecting system should be closed in a meticulous manner. It is my preference to leave an internal double-J stent in position for the initial postoperative period.

RENAL AND PERIRENAL ABSCESS

KEVIN PRANIKOFF, M.D.

Flank abscesses can be broken down into three categories depending on the space that they occupy. A renal abscess refers to a process entirely confined to the renal parenchyma, usually in the cortex. A perirenal abscess is one that also involves the perinephric fat but is confined within Gerota's fascia. If the infectious process extends through Gerota's fascia to the retroperitoneum or is isolated in the retroperitoneum external to Gerota's fascia, it is termed a pararenal abscess. Treatment is initiated based on location and size and altered based on patient response (Fig. 1).

RENAL ABSCESS

The etiology of renal abscesses began to change significantly about 30 years ago with the advent of broad-spectrum antibiotics. Before that time, the most common organism seen was *Staphylococcus* and the route of infection was by hematogenous spread. More recently, gram-negative organisms have become most common, and most abscesses have been a result of the extension of a pyelonephritic process. A staphylococcal abscess should be suspected in patients who clinically appear to have pyelonephritis but have a negative urine culture with no history of urinary tract infections. These patients often have a history of a skin infection in the previous few months. More commonly, patients present with a positive urine culture but do not respond appropriately to antibiotic therapy. These abscesses often present in a less specific manner, with patients being admitted with a fever of unknown origin.

Diagnosis

The diagnosis of renal abscess has been revolutionized over the past 15 years, primarily because of newer imaging modalities. The primary contributions have been from computed tomography (CT) and advances in ultrasonography, which have permitted more accurate imaging of the area and, when necessary, have also allowed for needle aspiration. There is a more limited role for gallium-67 scanning and indium-111–labeled leukocyte scanning. It is often difficult to differentiate between an intrarenal mass and an inflammatory process. Focal renal inflammation may present in a spectrum ranging from lobar nephronia or focal pyelonephritis to a frank abscess with central liquefaction and a thick fibrotic wall. Ultrasonography and CT may show a homogeneous center, or it may be inhomogeneous with internal echoes due to cellular debris or loculations within the abscess cavity. The differential diagnosis apart from renal abscess must include a renal tumor with

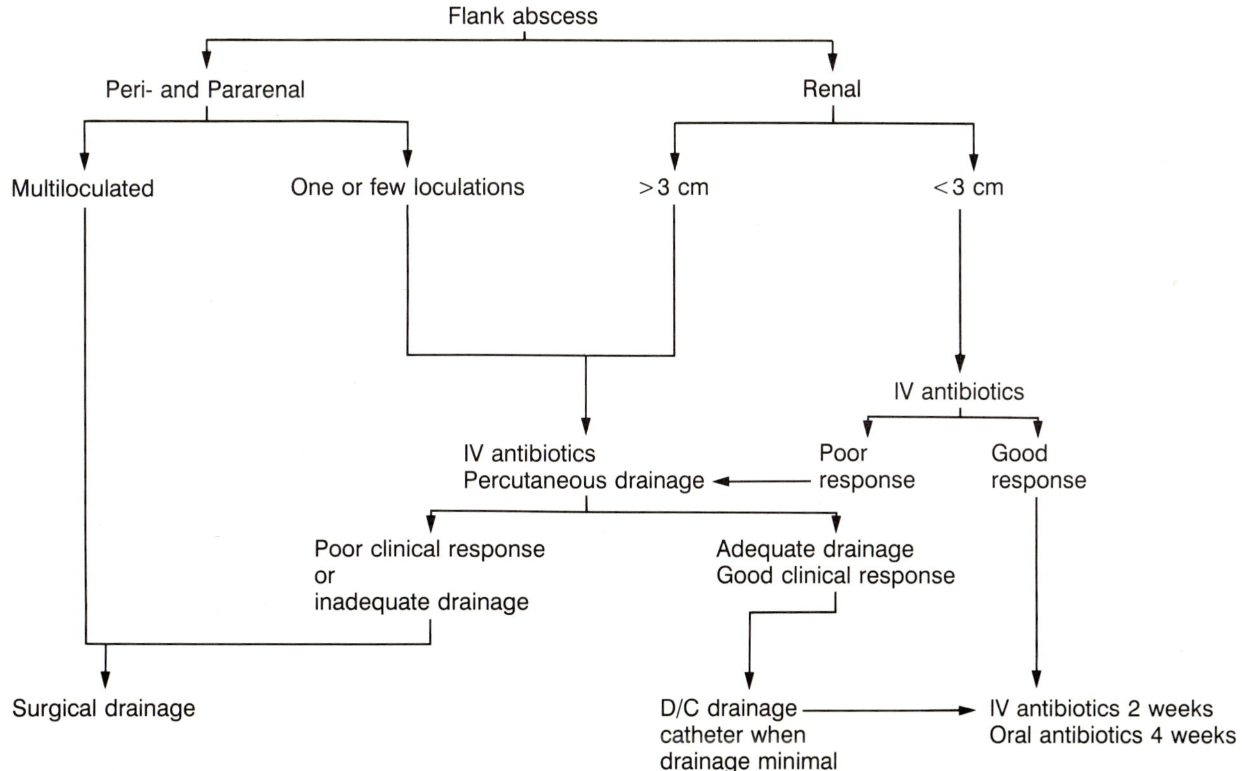

Figure 1 Treatment of flank abscess.

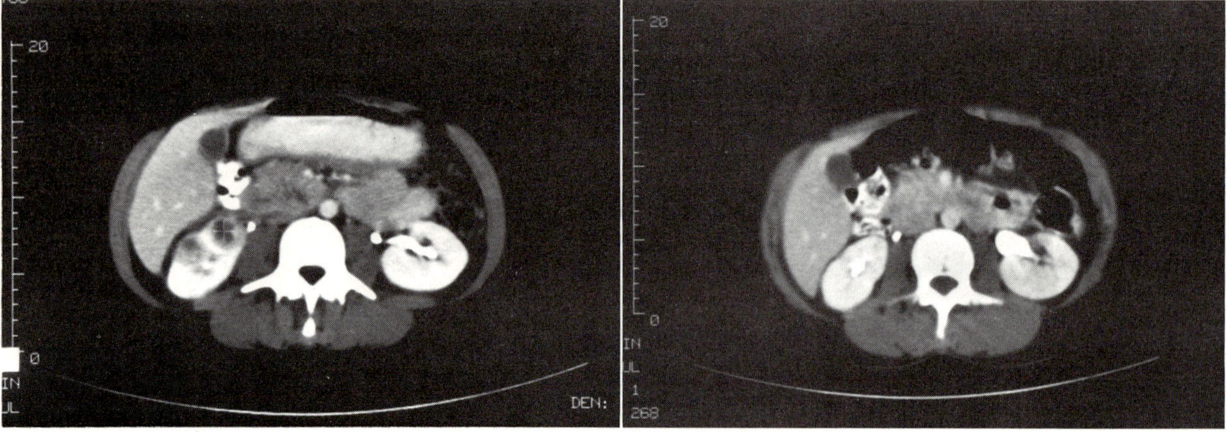

Figure 2 *A,* Renal abscess in a 38-year-old woman treated by antibiotics alone. *B,* Two-month follow-up demonstrating resolution.

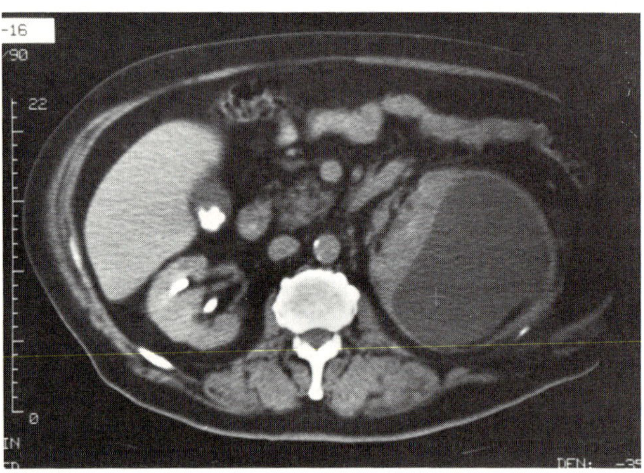

Figure 3 This large renal abscess in a 72-year-old man was successfully treated by percutaneous drainage.

necrosis or xanthogranulomatous pyelonephritis. Rarer still in the differential are vascular lesions, adult Wilms' tumor, and multiloculated cystic nephroma.

Treatment

Imaging has revolutionized not only diagnosis, but also our ability to treat these lesions more conservatively and follow their course more accurately. Traditional open surgical drainage may now be obviated in many instances. Because these lesions are relatively rare, there is no randomized prospective trial comparing various forms of treatment in matched lesions. In view of their wide clinical spectrum, such a study would be difficult to perform. This is an area in which clinical judgment and close follow-up of the patient's course are of primary importance.

It has become obvious that antibiotics alone are capable of curing lobar nephronia and small renal abscesses. It is my preference to use only antibiotics and close follow-up in abscesses that are 3 cm or less in diameter (Fig. 2). The patient is followed with serial imaging studies to watch the resolution of the process. Intravenous antibiotics are continued for 10 days to 2 weeks. Oral antibiotics are continued after this for at least 4 weeks. If the generalized fever and malaise are not beginning to resolve over 3 to 4 days, this treatment should be reconsidered.

If the abscess is greater than 3 cm in size, or if there is poor clinical response to antibiotics alone, the abscess is aspirated (Fig. 3). Aspiration for culture is also indicated if urine cultures are negative. If aspiration is necessary, I prefer to leave a small drainage tube in place if technically possible. An alternative is to aspirate all the contents. The drainage tube is left in place until minimal drainage is noted. Antibiotics are given as described above. These tubes may require irrigation to keep open, and some authors prefer to instill antibiotics directly into the cavity. If the patient's course does not respond appropriately or if the abscess cavity cannot be adequately drained owing to loculations or for technical reasons, open surgical drainage is indicated. When a patient is clinically stable but loculations militate against complete percutaneous drainage, surgical drainage without nephrectomy can generally be accomplished. If the patient is toxic and not responding to more conservative measures, a nephrectomy is occasionally required to stabilize the situation. This scenario is most often seen in diabetics or otherwise compromised patients.

If a complex abscess is to be treated initially by open drainage, antibiotics are always started preoperatively. Broad-spectrum antibiotics appropriate for the urinary tract are used until cultures become available. In the face of a negative urinalysis, adequate staphylococcal coverage must also be instituted.

PERIRENAL ABSCESS

Perirenal abscesses result from the direct extension of an intrarenal process. Antibiotics alone are not adequate treatment in these instances. If the patient is stable and the abscess appears well localized, an attempt at percutaneous aspiration and drainage may be undertaken. Follow-up is as described for an intrarenal abscess. If inadequate drainage is effected or a poor clinical response noted, open surgical drainage is indicated.

PARARENAL ABSCESS

Pararenal abscesses may be of renal origin with the continuation of a perirenal process, or may result from the spread of an unrelated extrarenal process in the retroperitoneum or subdiaphragmatic areas. Treatment is as described for a perirenal abscess.

RENAL TUBERCULOSIS

NICHOLAS A. ROMAS, M.D.

In the United States, as in other developed countries, tuberculosis decreased during the last half of this century. In recent years, however, its incidence has increased. The acquired immunodeficiency syndrome (AIDS) and other factors such as immigration have been cited as an explanation for this resurgence. The World Health Organization has estimated that throughout the world there are 10 million new cases of all forms of tuberculosis, mostly in Third World countries. These worldwide figures become very important when a massive immigration occurs. For example, in the late 1970s large numbers of "boat people" from Indochina, Haiti, and Cuba entered the United States. During the 1980s we witnessed the emergence of AIDS with a concomitant increase in tuberculosis. After 5 to 8 years, approximately 8 to 10 percent of patients with pulmonary tuberculosis develop genitourinary disease. If new treatment for AIDS extends the life span of this group of patients, we may see an increase in the number of cases of genitourinary tuberculosis. Renal tuberculosis may not become a forgotten disease in areas that have immigrants from emerging nations and a high incidence of AIDS.

PATHOGENESIS

Mycobacterium tuberculosis and *M. bovis* are the two members of the *Mycobacterium* genus most likely to cause renal tuberculosis. In any country where steps have been taken to eliminate tuberculosis from cattle and to pasteurize milk, disease due to the bovine bacillus is uncommon. Atypical organisms can cause disease that is indistinguishable clinically, radiologically, and histologically from that caused by *M. tuberculosis* or *M. bovis*. This diagnosis should not be based on a single isolation, and usually the patient has had previous treatment with steroids, or immunosuppressive drugs or has AIDS. Renal tuberculosis is the result of the dissemination of tubercle bacilli via the bloodstream, usually from the lungs, but the site can be other parts of the body such as the gastrointestinal tract. There will be foci of infection in both kidneys even though clinical disease is usually manifested unilaterally. The primary lesion is usually in the glomerulus and it may heal rapidly or progress. Subsequent granuloma formation and giant cells may lead to caseous necrosis through the wall of the calix, forming the first radiologically visible lesion. Further spread occurs along the mucosal surfaces of the renal pelvis and calices and down the ureter to the bladder. Healing is characterized by fibrosis and later calcification. This process causes distortion of the renal pelvis, leading to partial or complete autonephrectomy (putty kidney). Fibrosis affects the ureter, and strictures may occur at the ureterovesicular junction, at the ureteropelvic junction, at the midureter, or (in females) where the ureter passes under the broad ligament. An early stricture of the ureter may lead to a nonfunctioning kidney in several weeks. The bladder also heals by fibrosis, and a severely contracted bladder may occur. This process may cause obstruction of the ureter on the apparently normal side. Renal blood supply may be impaired, and the fibrosis occurring in the healing process results in hypertension. Tuberculous prostatitis and epididymitis usually is secondary to renal tuberculosis, but may be blood-borne.

SUGGESTED READING

Finn DJ, Palestrant AM, DeWolf WC. Successful percutaneous management of renal abscess. J Urol 1982; 127:425–426.

Hoverman IV, Layne OG, Jones DW, Guerriero WG. Intrarenal abscess. Arch Intern Med 1980; 140:914–916.

Levin R, Burbige KA, Abramson S, et al. The diagnosis and management of renal inflammatory processes in children. J Urol 1984; 132:718–721.

Richie JP, Kachel TA, Eichhorn JH. In: Scully RE, Mash EJ, McNeely WF, McNeely BV, eds. Case Records of the Massachusetts General Hospital. N Engl J Med 1989; 321:813–823.

Thorley JD, Jones SR, Sanford JP. Perinephric abscess. Medicine 1974; 53:441–451.

CLINICAL PRESENTATION

Tuberculosis of the genitourinary tract has no classic clinical presentation. The vast majority of patients have been born abroad and the most common symptoms are frequency, nocturia, and dysuria. The next most common complaint is a tender epididymis, which may at times form draining sinuses. Symptoms may be few or absent even in the presence of advanced disease. With the slow progression of the disease, affected kidneys may be severely damaged without apparent symptoms. The physical examination may be unremarkable but may show chronic draining epididymal sinuses; a beaded, indurated vas deferens; and a shrunken, irregular, hard nodular prostate.

DIAGNOSIS

Skin testing and a chest x-ray examination (including an apical lordotic film) are important initial studies in a patient suspected of having genitourinary tuberculosis. If the skin test is negative in the absence of anergy with a normal chest film, further testing should not be terminated. Urinary test results may vary considerably, but sterile acid pyuria is the classic finding. Secondary infections are often observed, and after treatment, sterile pyuria will persist. All patients suspected of having genitourinary tuberculosis should have a minimum of three clean-catch, fresh-voided, morning urinary specimens. These should be cultured and stained for acid-fast bacilli. An intravenous pyelogram (IVP) may be revelatory. The plain film of the abdomen may show punctate calcification or large areas of renal calcification. After injection of contrast media, the range of findings may include delayed visualization and excretion, "moth-eaten" calices, exclusion of one or more calices, parenchymal cavitation and scarring, ureteral strictures with hydroureteronephrosis, and bladder wall thickening and contraction. Computed tomography (CT) is often the initial modality to suggest the inflammatory nature of a mass seen on IVP and to suggest that tuberculosis may be the causative disease. Cystoscopy may reveal the "pepper-and-salt" pattern around one or both ureteral orifices. Retrograde pyelography may be necessary if the kidneys are poorly functioning.

MEDICAL TREATMENT

The basic principles in the medical treatment of genitourinary tuberculosis are as follows:

1. Multidrug therapy is required.
2. Treatment should be continued for 6 months or longer if necessary.
3. Patient compliance is of the utmost importance in following this prolonged medical regimen.

For years the standard accepted treatment for genitourinary tuberculosis consisted of triple-drug che-

motherapy administered daily for a minimum of 2 years. The agents most often given (depending on sensitivity) included streptomycin, kanamycin, isoniazid, cycloserine, ethambutol, rifampin, and para-aminosalicylic acid (PAS). Since 1970, there has been a change in thinking with regard to duration of treatment, drug selection, and drug dosage. The important experiment that ushered in short-course chemotherapy was performed in the late 1960s at the Pasteur Institute. Infected mice were treated with a combination of isoniazid and rifampin and showed negative cultures after only 4 months of therapy. This result had not been duplicated previously with other antituberculous drugs. The important contribution of the rifampin-isoniazid combination to shortening of therapy soon became clinically evident.

Tubercle bacilli exist in two populations, one large and rapidly dividing, and one smaller, persistent, and more slowly dividing. Both rifampin and pyrazinamide have been found to have excellent sterilizing activity and also the capability of destroying persistent bacilli. Early drug resistance to either drug is uncommon. Pyrazinamide has been found to eliminate the slowly dividing bacilli, and it has its major impact during the first 2 months of therapy. Pyrazinamide has been available for years but had fallen into disrepute because of hepatotoxicity during long-term therapy. This toxicity was dose related (2 g per day), but with the use of 1 g per day in short-course trials there has been much less toxicity.

Ethambutol, PAS, and cycloserine are all bacteriostatic drugs and their role in short-course chemotherapy is diminishing, as they do not add anything to the bactericidal activity of the regimen. Rifampin is highly bactericidal but requires at least 4 months of therapy, and isoniazid sterilizes to a somewhat lesser degree. Gow and colleagues from Great Britain initially indicated that a 9-month intensive multidrug therapy was satisfactory, and then in the mid-1980s reported an effective 4-month program. The treatment consists of a 2-month daily course of rifampin, isoniazid, and pyrazinamide followed by isoniazid and rifampin three times per week for 2 months. Skutil and colleagues from Czechoslovakia confirmed the British report that short-term chemotherapy was effective for urogenital tuberculosis. Daily administration of rifampin (600 mg), isoniazid (300 mg), and pyrazinamide (1,000 mg) in the hospital for 2 months was followed by daily administration at home of 600 mg rifampin and 300 mg isoniazid for 4 months. The urinary reversion rate was less than 1 percent.

Our standard chemotherapy for genitourinary tuberculosis is isoniazid, 300 mg per day; rifampin, 600 mg per day; and pyrazinamide, 1000 mg per day. Pyridoxine (vitamin B_6), 25 mg per day, should be added to the medication to prevent the unusual occurrence of peripheral neuropathy seen with isoniazid. This regimen is continued for 2 months or until susceptibility tests are returned. If no unusual findings are reported from these tests, isoniazid and rifampin are continued for 4 months. A recent study demonstrates a high frequency of drug resistance, especially to isoniazid and rifampin, among homeless patients. In this group of patients, careful susceptibility tests should be performed and various combinations of drugs used, with prolonged therapy. During medical therapy, cultures are performed every 2 months and then every 6 months for 3 years. Renal scans and ultrasonography are performed on a 2-month basis to determine the degree of renal function as well as the development of hydronephrosis. After treatment, ultrasonography is performed every year for 3 years.

Drug Toxicity

The most important side effect of isoniazid, rifampin, and pyrazinamide is hepatic toxicity. Patients may present with a wide range of clinical findings including jaundice, malaise, fever, anorexia, nausea, and vomiting. Often an asymptomatic transient rise in transaminase and alkaline phosphatase levels may occur during the first 3 months of therapy; this has no clinical significance. Isoniazid is especially prone to cause serum glutamic-oxaloacetic transaminase (SGOT) elevation.

Additional rare side effects associated with rifampin are a flulike syndrome and thrombocytopenia, often associated with the development of antibodies to this agent. Rifampin may stimulate the drug-metabolizing enzyme system of the liver. As a result, the serum concentration of the following agents may be reduced when given along with rifampin: cardiac glycosides, oral contraceptives, anticoagulants, oral antidiabetics, corticosteroids, narcotics, and analgesics.

Sensitization rashes occur with all the antituberculous drugs. An alternative drug may be used or the patient may be desensitized by giving a small dose and gradually increasing it. Another approach is to continue the normal dosage with concomitant use of steroids.

SURGICAL TREATMENT

Nephrectomy

The role of nephrectomy in the treatment of tuberculosis remains controversial. In the United States, the approach is conservative. Nephrectomy is performed in patients with intractable pain, uncontrollable fever, persistent hematuria, bacterial resistance, or uncontrollable hypertension caused by a poorly functioning kidney and who are not responsive to antihypertensive medication. The British approach is to proceed with nephrectomy whenever the kidney appears nonfunctioning or indicates irreversible damage.

There is clinical evidence to support the conservative approach of not performing nephrectomy until indicated. The combination of rifampin and isoniazid has been found to have a potent sterilizing effect. Besides the animal studies, a human pathologic investigation of nephrectomy specimens after various chemotherapeutic regimens noted that rapid tissue sterilization occurred in patients who received rifampin and isoniazid for 6 to 8 months. There is no doubt that the role of nephrectomy in the treatment of renal tuberculosis remains controversial.

If nephrectomy is contemplated, the patient should have received at least 3 weeks of antituberculous therapy. The kidney should be approached through an extraperitoneal flank incision. Dissection may be difficult and the kidney is often adherent to adjacent organs. The artery and vein may be poorly defined and individual ligation impossible, and therefore a pedicle ligation of heavy absorbable suture may be used. As much of the ureter should be removed as is technically feasible, and there is no need to bring the ureter to the skin, as has been advocated in the past.

URETERAL STRICTURE

In genitourinary tuberculosis, the lower ureter is most commonly involved with stricture disease. In the past, the more conservative approach was to perform ureteral calibration and dilatation routinely. With today's new endoscopic procedures, we use balloon dilatation and insertion of a double-J indwelling stent, which can be left in place for 3 to 6 weeks. If this fails, ureteroneocystostomy is performed. These distal ureteral strictures are usually short, and therefore after excision of the diseased segment, reimplantation is generally successful. If adequate ureteral length is not obtained, a psoas hitch or Boari flap should be used.

Strictures in other parts of the ureter are rare but may be managed by balloon dilatation and insertion of a double-J indwelling stent. Ureteropelvic junction strictures secondary to tuberculosis are also rare and are best handled by a dismembered pyeloplasty. The anastomosis should be stented and a nephrostomy tube left in place for 3 weeks. None of the above operative procedures should be performed until a minimum of 3 weeks of antituberculous drug therapy has been given.

TUBERCULOUS CYSTITIS: AUGMENTATION CYSTOPLASTY

In a few patients with genitourinary tuberculosis, extensive fibrosis of the urinary bladder may occur during the healing process. The bladder has a markedly reduced capacity and may develop ureteral obstruction or vesicoureteral reflux. Bladder augmentation may be performed with the cecum or sigmoid colon. If ureteral reimplantation is necessary, the cecal segment is preferred with reimplantation of the ureters into the segment of ileum. There may also be an associated bladder-neck or urethral contracture, which may be treated via an endoscopic incision.

TUBERCULOUS EPIDIDYMITIS AND PROSTATITIS

Epididymitis may commonly be the first manifestation of genitourinary tuberculosis. The patient may present with a painful swelling of the epididymis or with fistula formation. The clinician should have a high degree of suspicion and, in addition to routine cultures, should obtain stains and cultures for acid-fast bacilli. Patients should be given standard antituberculous therapy; some may require epididymectomy. Tuberculous epididymitis and prostatitis may both be hematogenous but may be caused by infected urine from the kidneys. Tuberculous prostatitis is often confused with carcinoma of the prostate. After an appropriate course of chemotherapy, residual induration can be biopsied percutaneously. Occasionally, tuberculosis is found by the pathologist after subtotal prostatectomy for benign disease. For miliary disease, which has been reported to occur during the postoperative period, antituberculous therapy should be instituted.

The incidence of pulmonary tuberculosis has recently increased in the United States because of growing numbers of AIDS patients. No increase in genitourinary tuberculosis has been reported, because this condition occurs 5 to 7 years after pulmonary tuberculosis, and AIDS patients currently are dying before this time. AIDS patients may be expected to contact genitourinary tuberculosis at a shorter time interval because of their poor immunologic status.

The initial therapy for genitourinary tuberculosis is chemotherapy, and surgery is required only in special clinical settings. The disease is rare and the diagnosis is often made late in the clinical course.

Acknowledgment. The author would like to thank Mrs. Marilyn Carlin for technical assistance on this manuscript.

SUGGESTED READING

Gow JG, Barbosa S. Genitourinary tuberculosis: a study of 1,117 cases over a period of 34 years. Br J Urol 1984; 56:449–455.

Laidlaw M. Renal tuberculosis. In: Scientific foundations of urology. Chicago: Year Book, 1990.

Pablos-Mendez A, Raviglione MC, Battan R, Ramos-Zuniga R. Drug resistant tuberculosis among the homeless in New York City. N.Y. State J 1990: 351–355.

Skutil V, Varsa J, Obstinik M. Six-month chemotherapy for urogenital tuberculosis. Eur Urol 1985; 11:170–176.

IDIOPATHIC RETROPERITONEAL FIBROSIS

ROBERT P. GIBBONS, M.D., F.A.C.S.

Idiopathic retroperitoneal fibrosis is a nonspecific inflammatory process of uncertain etiology that appears as a dense fibrotic, hard, gray-white mass of varying thickness most frequently encountered from the fourth lumbar to the first sacral vertebrae. The fibrosis envelopes, but rarely invades, the aorta, vena cava, and ureters and may extend from the midbony pelvis to the renal pedicle. All identifiable causes of fibrosis must be excluded, and deep biopsy specimens must be confirmatory before establishing the diagnosis of "idiopathic."

The symptoms of idiopathic retroperitoneal fibrosis are caused by encasement of the ureters, arteries, veins, and nerves. Initially, there is a cellular phase believed to be related to vasculitis, hypersensitive states, autoimmune reactions, or generalized collagen disease foilowed by the development of an extensive fibrotic plaque. A few patients give a history of taking the ergot derivatives methysergide (Sansert) or lysergic acid di ethylamide (LSD) or methyldopa (Aldomet), amphetamines, or phenacetin. Many patients are asymptomatic, but an insidious, dull, noncolicky pain in the lower flank radiating into the lower abdominal quadrant is the most frequent symptom, followed by nonspecific gastrointestinal symptoms, anorexia, weight loss, and fever. An elevated erythrocyte sedimentation rate (ESR) (greater than 30 mm in 1 hour) is found in most patients. Anemia, if present, is usually proportional to the degree of azotemia.

The diagnosis is suggested in most patients by the intravenous pyelogram, which typically demonstrates medial deviation of the middle third of the ureters with extrinsic compression and proximal ureteral obstruction, tortuosity, and hydronephrosis. A bulb retrograde ureterogram confirms the distant extent of the process. A No. 5 or 6 Fr olive-tipped or Flexi-tipped ureteral catheter can usually be readily passed through the area of ureteral narrowing. Computed tomography confirms the presence and extent of the fibrotic process. Renal ultrasonography is most helpful in determining the resolution or return of hydronephrosis in follow-up. Radioisotope renal function and/or flow studies are reserved for patients with bilateral disease when there is a question regarding renal function.

THERAPEUTIC ALTERNATIVES

In the majority of cases, ureterolysis is the procedure of choice to establish the diagnosis and relieve the ureteral obstruction. Patients should discontinue taking any implicated drugs. In the presence of minimal obstruction, relief of the hydronephrosis within a few weeks is sometimes seen after the drug is discontinued.

Corticosteroids (prednisone, 40 mg per day) are sometimes used in patients with mild degrees of obstruction who have also been ingesting one of the possible incriminated drugs. Some investigators believe that surgery should be avoided until a trial of corticosteroid therapy is given to all patients with a history and laboratory and radiographic evidence of idiopathic retroperitoneal fibrosis. Patients with an early (cellular) stage of disease can be expected to respond more favorably to corticosteroids than those with advanced and extensive fibrosis. The obvious risk in treating without a tissue diagnosis is delaying treatment of a possibly more serious underlying malignant condition. The primary objective of therapy should be to establish the diagnosis by retroperitoneal biopsy and to preserve renal function by relieving ureteral obstruction.

Patients with azotemia secondary to ureteral obstruction can have indwelling double-J ureteral stents placed to decompress the upper urinary tracts. After dilatation of the ureter to the size of the stent, these stents can generally be passed to the renal pelvis. This allows the patient to be brought into the best possible metabolic and nutritional status before surgery.

PREFERRED APPROACH

Most patients are found to have bilateral involvement of the ureters even though hydronephrosis may appear to be unilateral on the roentgenogram. Accordingly, it is imperative that transabdominal exploration of both ureters be performed. Before surgery, double-J ureteral stents should be placed into both ureters. These aid in later identification of the ureters and in the blunt dissection of the ureter from the surrounding fibrosis and provide "internal" drainage in the event of inadvertent ureterotomy. They also tend to hold the ureters in their new location and allow the surgeon to identify any potential area of kinking. A long midline incision is used to expose the retroperitoneum from the level of the renal pedicle to the bladder. The retroperitoneum can be opened in the midline with flaps undermined laterally to expose the ureters, or incisions can be made lateral to the ascending and descending colon to reflect these structures medially to expose the ureters. Deep biopsies in the midline below the bifurcation of the great vessels are taken to establish the diagnosis. The ureters should be identified where they are not involved, i.e., at the level of the kidney or bladder, and followed into the area of fibrosis. Blunt dissection between the ureteral adventitia and the fibrotic process with a finger or a right-angled clamp is usually possible. If there is invasion of ureteral wall, a malignant process is usually present. The resultant ureteral wall is thickened, and the dissection is aided by the presence of the previously placed stent. A dissection of the ureteral musculature to expose the mucosa is not necessary and can result in ureterotomy, which should be avoided. Any adhesive bands in the proximal tortuous ureter should be sharply divided to ensure ureteral straightening up to the renal pelvis. Both ureters are freed from the renal pelvis to the bladder.

After mobilization, several techniques are available to keep each ureter away from the area of fibrosis. The ureter can be (1) transposed laterally and anteriorly with retroperitoneal fat placed between it and the pathologic process; (2) transposed laterally and this location maintained by suturing a "sling" of unopened peritoneum to the underlying psoas muscle; (3) transposed to an intraperitoneal position; or (4) wrapped in a sleeve of omentum. This is accomplished by first mobilizing the omentum from the transverse colon and then the greater curvature of the stomach by ligating and dividing the short gastric branches. The right and left gastroepiploic arteries are left intact, and the mobilized omental apron is vertically divided to the right of the middle omental artery, thereby creating two pedicle flaps of approximately the same size. These omental pedicle grafts are then brought around the hepatic and splenic flexures, which, if mobilized completely, usually allow the omental pedicle to reach the distal normal ureter. The omental pedicle graft is then wrapped around both ureters from the renal pelvis to the bladder. It is important that kinking of the ureter be avoided during any of these transposition techniques. A drain is placed only if a ureterotomy has been made or if there is concern regarding the vascular status of the ureter.

FOLLOW-UP

I recommend that systemic corticosteroids (prednisone, 20 mg per day for 5 months and then a tapering dose for 1 month) be given after surgery in all patients except those few with a minimal degree of obstruction. The ESR generally falls to normal. The ureteral stents are removed in 6 to 12 weeks. Recurrence after completion of corticosteroid therapy is not unusual, and follow-up should include determination of ESR and creatinine values and renal ultrasonography at 3-month intervals for the first year, 6-month intervals for the second year, and then annually thereafter, with the patient returning sooner upon any return of symptoms. The degree of renal recovery is dependent on the length and degree of obstruction present before treatment. If the obstruction has been chronic, persistent hydronephrosis can be expected but should not progress.

If recurrent ureteral obstruction occurs, it is often associated with an elevation of the ESR, and once again corticosteroid therapy should be instituted. If there is no improvement, re-exploration is necessary. Repeat ureterolysis can be difficult in this situation unless the ureters have been wrapped in omentum. If a short segment of a ureter is fibrotic, primary resection with reanastomosis can be performed. If insufficient viable ureteral length results from re-exploration, ureteral replacement with small bowel, autotransplantation, or urinary diversion is an option. Nephrectomy is reserved for patients with symptomatic kidneys that alone would not support life.

RETROPERITONEAL FIBROSIS OF KNOWN ETIOLOGY

THOMAS J. ROHNER, Jr., M.D.

Retroperitoneal fibrosis (RF) is an inflammatory fibrotic disorder, most commonly occurring in the L5–S1 region, resulting in encasement and constriction of the great vessels, nerves, and ureters. It was first described by Albarran in 1905 but did not receive specific recognition as a distinct entity until Ormond reported two patients in 1948, the second of whom underwent ureterolysis with successful long-term relief of ureteral obstruction. The cause of RF remained obscure until 1966, when this disorder was described in 27 patients taking methysergide for headache. Approximately two thirds of reported cases are considered to be of idiopathic origin (i.e., no inciting agent or associated disease could be identified); the other one third have been associated with or due to drugs or medical conditions listed in Table 1.

PATHOLOGY

The gross appearance of RF is that of a whitish-gray hard mass that can range from several millimeters to several centimeters in thickness. Microscopically, a spectrum of findings may be seen, ranging from a nonspecific, subacute inflammatory infiltration of lymphocytes, plasma cells, eosinophils, and polymorphonuclear leukocytes to relatively acellular dense collagenous tissue with few chronic inflammatory cells. In patients with aneurysmal dilatation of the aorta and autoimmune disease, vasculitis and perivasculitis evidenced by lymphocytic and plasma cell infiltration is prominent. It has been suggested that the more prominent cellular infiltration characterizes the active early phase of RF and that the relatively acellular collagenous tissue is typical of disease of longer duration. In one large series, retroperitoneal malignancy was found in 8 percent of patients.

ETIOLOGY

Although the resulting retroperitoneal fibrotic process may behave and appear histologically similar, the causes or associations listed in Table 1 may have several different etiologic mechanisms.

Both localized and metastatic carcinoid tumors have been associated with RF, presumably through secretion of serotonin (5-hydroxytryptamine) known to cause fibrosis of the lungs, cardiac valves, endocardium, and vascular intima. Methylsergide, LSD, and ergot derivatives have serotonin receptor blocking activity and are

Table 1 Recognized Association With Retroperitoneal Fibrosis

Drugs:
- Methysergide maleate
- Methyldopa
- Beta-blockers
- LSD (lysergic acid diethylamide)
- Reserpine
- Phenacetin
- Amphetamines
- Ergotamine alkaloids
- Haloperidol
- Hydralazine

Retroperitoneal tumors
- Hodgkin's disease
- Metastatic carcinoma (breast, carcinoid, colon, lungs, pancreas, stomach, kidney)
- Lymphoma, sarcoma

Iatrogenic chemicals
- Avitene
- Talcum powder
- Methyl methacrylate

Infection
- Tuberculosis
- Gonorrhea
- Syphilis

Inflammatory disease
- Ascending lymphangitis
- Chronic inflammatory bowel disease
- Ruptured diverticulitis
- Sarcoidosis
- Systemic lupus erythematosus
- Sclerosing cholangitis
- Ankylosing spondylitis
- Fibrous thyroiditis (Riedel's)

Hemorrhage
- Previous abdominal and pelvic surgery
- Henoch-Schönlein purpura with hemorrhage

Periarteritis
- Aortic or iliac artery aneurysm with atherosclerosis (chronic periaortitis)
- Collagen vascular disease

Radiation therapy

Other

thought to produce fibrosis by increasing local concentrations of serotonin, although this has not been proved and the mechanism whereby serotonin leads to fibrosis is not clearly known. Another possibility is that these drugs and others listed may act as a hapten, the resultant vasculitis and fibrosis being a manifestation of an autoimmune response.

RF secondary to inflammatory bowel disease or perforation probably represents an extension of that primary disease but may involve a unique patient response to inflammation.

Recent studies have suggested that the RF in patients with aortic aneurysms or severe atherosclerosis with attenuation of the media is a result of a plasma cell IgG-mediated hypersensitivity response to ceroid, an insoluble polymer of oxidized lipid and protein components of atheromatous plaque, with inflammation of the adventitia and surrounding tissue and subsequent fibrosis.

CLINICAL PRESENTATION

RF occurs most frequently (50 percent) in patients between the ages of 40 and 60 years, but has been described in all age groups including pediatric patients. Most clinical series show a 2:1 male predominance.

The most common presenting symptoms are shown in Table 2, as described by Koep and Zuidema in their review of 481 cases. The great majority of patients experienced back or flank pain for several months before the diagnosis was finally made. Physical findings are remarkably few and do not often help with diagnosis, except in patients presenting with lower extremity edema.

DIAGNOSIS

The diagnosis of RF of both idiopathic and known etiology is aided by a careful history and knowledge of the drugs and entities associated with the condition but is fundamentally dependent on awareness or suspicion of the disease and appropriate radiologic and laboratory studies.

There are no specific laboratory tests for RF, but anemia and azotemia may be present if the disease has been of sufficient duration to cause significant ureteral obstruction. An elevated erythrocyte sedimentation rate (ESR) is found in over 90 percent of patients and may be useful to monitor the activity of the inflammatory process postoperatively. Eosinophilia and leukocytosis have also been described.

In most older clinical reports, intravenous pyelography (IVP) has been the most frequently abnormal and characteristic radiologic study. Typical findings on excretory urography include bilateral hydronephrosis with dilated tortuous upper ureters, with medial deviation of the ureters at the sacral promontory. It should be recognized that only unilateral obstruction may occur; medial deviation of the ureters may occur as a normal variant and is not necessarily an indication of RF. IVP provides only indirect evidence of RF and is dependent on ureteral obstruction to suggest the diagnosis. For this reason, early RF may not be detected by excretory urography.

More recently, ultrasonography, computed tomography (CT), and magnetic resonance imaging (MRI) have been of more diagnostic help in evaluating patients with suspected RF. Ultrasonography as a screening study to detect hydronephrosis is appropriate, but because of body habitus and bowel gas may not detect the actual retroperitoneal mass. CT will show a retroperitoneal fibrotic mass of homogeneous density that envelops but does not displace the aorta and vena cava, and may extend laterally to involve the ureters. Subsequent studies report additional advantages of MRI, including coronal and sagittal views to determine more accurately the cephalad and caudal extent of involvement, and elimination of the need for intravenous contrast agents in patients with renal impairment. An

Table 2   The Most Common Symptoms of Patients with Retroperitoneal Fibrosis

Symptom	Percentage
Backache	34
Flank pain	34
Abdominal pain	24
Weight loss	13
Nausea, vomiting	4
Edema	3
Malaise	2.5
Gastrointestinal bleeding	3
Unilateral swollen leg	2

important finding in both CT and MRI scanning is that RF causes envelopment of the aorta and vena cava anteriorly with lateral extension to involve the ureters, while retroperitoneal malignancy including lymphomas tends to involve lymph nodes posterior to the great vessels causing anterior displacement. The improved diagnostic information afforded by these two modalities should improve the ability to discriminate between RF and retroperitoneal malignancy.

TREATMENT

The objective of treatment is to provide relief of ureteral obstruction with restoration or preservation of renal function. In a lesser number of patients, fibrotic compression of the aorta, iliac vessels, and vena cava causes significant morbidity and requires therapeutic consideration.

Cystoscopy and bilateral ureteropyelograms are indicated early for both diagnosis and therapeutic benefit. The retrograde studies should reveal a normal distal ureter without intraluminal filling defects and a tapering dilated ureter above the level of obstruction. Despite the obstruction to urinary flow caused by fibrosis interfering with ureteral peristalsis, it is generally possible to pass a No. 5 or 6 Fr ureteral catheter up the ureter with relief of obstruction. A double-J indwelling ureteral stent should be placed to relieve obstruction and improve renal function. If it is not possible to pass a ureteral catheter, percutaneous nephrostomy should be performed to provide drainage. Renal function should be permitted to improve or stabilize, which may take a few weeks; if it does not improve after ureteral stenting, it should be recognized that stents do not always provide adequate renal drainage. A cystogram showing reflux to the upper tracts and subsequent emptying of the upper tracts on a drainage film should be taken if renal function does not improve as expected. Percutaneous nephrostomy should be carried out if drainage provided by ureteral stents is not satisfactory.

If the patient is taking a drug suspected of causing RF, it should be discontinued. Spontaneous resolution or improvement of RF after drug cessation has been reported but is not likely. It should be noted that only 1 percent or at most 3 percent of patients taking methysergide, and even fewer patients taking other drugs, will develop RF. The possibility of other causes, including occult retroperitoneal malignancy, must always be borne in mind.

CT or MRI scans of the abdomen and chest will provide important diagnostic information, including the extent of the retroperitoneal mass and the presence or absence of abdominal aortic aneurysm, and should be of significant help in determining whether occult or retroperitoneal malignancy is present and the amount of renal cortex remaining.

Surgical intervention with bilateral ureterolysis, multiple deep biopsies of surrounding fibrosis, and omental wrapping appears to provide the best long-term results. This approach allows histologic confirmation of RF and has been shown to produce a successful outcome in 60 to 90 percent of patients; for these reasons, it is my recommended treatment. Elderly patients with long-standing obstruction and poor residual renal function have a worse prognosis. The procedure is carried out through a midline transabdominal incision extending from xiphoid to pubis. Inspection and palpation of intraperitoneal structures is done to exclude unsuspected malignancy or perforation. The ureters are identified and freed by mobilizing the right colon and left colon, including the hepatic and splenic flexures; identifying the ureters at a point where they are free of surrounding fibrosis; and following them distally to their involved portion. A right-angled clamp placed anterior to the ureter with sharp incision of the overlying fibrosis generally permits easy blunt finger mobilization of the ureter. Actual invasion of the ureteral wall is unusual with true RF, but is common with surrounding malignancy.

After mobilization of the ureter, several biopsies of the surrounding fibrosis should be sent for both frozen and permanent sections, to provide adequate sampling to exclude malignancy with desmoplastic response. The ureters should be mobilized from the renal pelvis to the deep pelvis. The mobilized ureter should be surrounded by peritoneum in one of two ways. The posterior peritoneum medial to the ascending and descending colon can be incised with the ureter brought medially and the peritoneum closed posterior to the internalized ureter with sutures. If this is technically difficult, the ureter can be placed lateral to the colon with peritoneum brought beneath it and sutures placed to maintain the ureter with peritoneum behind it. Omental wrapping of both ureters is recommended and appears helpful in preventing obstruction from recurrent fibrosis. This is done by freeing the omentum from the transverse colon, ligating and dividing the short gastric vessels to the midomentum, and splitting the omentum longitudinally, with blood supply to the right omental segment provided by the gastroepiploic branch of the pancreaticoduodenal artery and to the left omental segment by the left gastroepiploic artery. The omental segments can either be brought behind the splenic and hepatic flexures and sutured loosely around the ureter as a sleeve, or if the ureters have been brought medially and placed in-

traperitoneally, the divided omental segments can be brought directly down and sutured about the ureters. Even though only one ureter may be obstructed, we recommend bilateral ureterolysis and omental wrapping, since the later contralateral recurrence rate may be as high as 20 to 58 percent, with ipsilateral recurrence of 10 percent. Steroids have been used successfully most often for later contralateral recurrence, but it is preferable to minimize that possibility by mobilizing and wrapping both ureters at the time of initial surgery.

There is some evidence that postoperative adjunctive steroid therapy for 6 to 8 weeks improves results, and it seems especially indicated in patients with associated vascular compromise. The dosage and duration of adjuvant steroid therapy has not been clearly established, but prednisone or prednisolone at an initial dose of 30 to 60 mg daily for 10 days, with tapering over a 2-month period, has been used successfully.

Late recurrences of RF have been reported as long as 9 years after initial therapy. Thus, long-term follow-up is essential and should consist of a complete blood count, tests of BUN and creatinine levels and ESR, and ultrasonographic examination of the kidneys at least annually.

Alternative Treatment: Urinary Drainage and Steroid Therapy

The major advantages of surgical exploration and ureterolysis include the opportunity to obtain tissue confirmation excluding malignancy and to provide more predictable relief of ureteral obstruction. Although no clinical trials have been done, anecdotal reports suggest that an alternative to surgical exploration is steroid therapy in conjunction with renal drainage by ureteral stents or percutaneous nephrostomy.

The availability of CT should improve diagnostic discrimination between RF and retroperitoneal malignancy and may make steroid therapy a reasonable option in patients who have RF associated with drugs, periaortitis associated with aortic aneurysms of nonsurgical size, and collagen or autoimmune disease. Contrast enhancement of the retroperitoneal mass has been described and may indicate the early active phase of RF, which appears to be most responsive to resolution by steroid therapy. Steroid therapy has been reported to result in regression of ureteral obstruction within a few days and actual resolution of the retroperitoneal mass within 6 to 8 weeks.

CT-guided needle aspiration biopsies cannot exclude malignancy with certainty, but since the treatment of extensive retroperitoneal malignancy is so unsatisfactory, a delay of several weeks for a trial of steroid therapy is not of harmful consequence. In the past, steroid therapy was reserved for patients in poor medical condition, those experiencing recurrence of ureteral obstruction after ureterolysis, those with obstruction of the contralateral ureter after unilateral ureterolysis and biopsy-proven RF, and those with poor renal function. Evidence of steroid efficacy was largely provided by improvement in renal drainage as seen by IVP and decreased ESR. The dosage and duration of successful steroid therapies vary considerably: all employ high initial doses in the range of 30 to 60 mg of prednisone or prednisolone intravenously daily for 10 days, followed by tapering over 6 to 8 weeks. Continued treatment with low-dose prednisone (5 to 10 mg daily) for up to several years has been recommended. The cessation or tapering of steroids has been associated with recurrent ureteral obstruction and elevation of the ESR. Thus, the major disadvantages of steroid therapy include the unpredictable response rate, which may be as low as 30 percent, and the need for long-term steroid therapy. RF of long duration and histologically composed of hyalinized collagen may not respond to steroids to the same degree as the active early more cellular phase. Azathioprine, 150 mg per day for 6 weeks, has also been used successfully in treating RF.

The side effects of long-term steroid therapy, including increased susceptibility to infection, osteoporosis with compression fractures, peptic ulcer disease, myopathy, and psychiatric disturbances, have been well described and favor short-term courses of treatment.

COMPLICATIONS

The ureters are generally lysed easily from the underlying fibrosis, but a ureter may be inadvertently injured during lysis, or because of significant adherence it may be necessary to resect a short segment. Ureteroureterostomy should be performed over an indwelling stent and a drain left. Ureterolysis should be done carefully and efforts made to avoid injury to the adventitia. Late complications after ureterolysis include the development of ureteral stricture, which has required subsequent management by autotransplantation, ileal substitution, or ureteral reimplantation with bladder flap.

SUGGESTED READING

Baker LRI, Mallinson WJW, Gregory MC, et al. Idiopathic retroperitoneal fibrosis. A retrospective analysis of 60 cases. Br J Urol 1988; 60:497–503.

Higgins PM, Bennett-Jones DN, Naish PF, Aber GM. Non-operative management of retroperitoneal fibrosis. Br J Urol 1988; 75:573–577.

Koep L, Zuidema GD. The clinical significance of retroperitoneal fibrosis. Surgery 1977; 81:250–257.

Lepor H, Walsh PC. Idiopathic retroperitoneal fibrosis (review article). J Urol 1979; 122:1–6.

Smith SJ, Bosniak MA, Megibow AJ, et al. CT demonstration of rapid improvement of retroperitoneal fibrosis in response to steroid therapy. Urol Radiol 1986; 8:104–107.

Tiptaft RC, Costello AJ, Paris AMI, Blandy JP. The long-term follow-up of idiopathic retroperitoneal fibrosis. Br J Urol 1982; 54:620–624.

I BLADDER

INTERSTITIAL CYSTITIS

ALAN J. WEIN, M.D.
PHILIP M. HANNO, M.D.

Interstitial cystitis (IC) is a chronic inflammation of the bladder wall of unknown cause. Most current theories of pathogenesis involve access of a component of urine to the interstices of the bladder wall, resulting in an inflammatory response induced by toxic, allergic, or immunologic means. The urinary substance either can be a naturally occurring one, but one that acts as an initiator only in particularly susceptible individuals, or may act like a true toxin, gaining access to the urine by a variety of mechanisms or metabolic pathways. Access to the bladder interstitium is gained through a quantitative or a qualitative defect in the cytoprotective urothelium. To achieve the best therapeutic results for an individual patient, both patient and physician must understand that there is no cure for IC, nor is there a single treatment that is effective in reducing symptoms for every patient. Most patients, however, can be benefited by one treatment or another, or a combination of treatments, and most can be maintained in a satisfactory, although definitely not asymptomatic, state, punctuated by exacerbations and remissions.

INITIAL EVALUATION AND DIAGNOSIS

The first rule in obtaining the most success possible with this difficult group of patients is that if one as a physician does not believe that this disease exists, or if one believes the symptoms to be entirely a psychosomatic manifestation, one is doing no one any service by trying to treat it. It is necessary not only to be knowledgeable, but also to be sympathetic, empathetic, tolerant of long descriptions of symptoms and previous failed courses of therapy, and willing to return calls promptly.

How is the diagnosis of IC made? Not surprisingly, there is a considerable lack of agreement. Because recognition that the disease exists in a given patient is the first step in successful management, it is important to have at least some criteria on which to base the diagnosis. The current NIDDK criteria are helpful in defining a group of patients that most would agree have IC, and thus these criteria comprise a de facto definition of the disease. Patients have pain associated with the bladder or urinary urgency, and they must have either glomerulations on cystoscopic examination or a classic Hunner's ulcer. The cystoscopic examination for glomerulations is undertaken after distention of the bladder under anesthesia to 80 to 100 cm water pressure for 1 to 2 minutes. The bladder may be distended up to two times before evaluation. The glomerulations must be diffuse: at least ten per quadrant and present in at least three quadrants of the bladder. Any of the following generally excludes the diagnosis of IC: a bladder capacity of over 350 ml on awake cystometry using either gas or liquid; absence of urgency on filling cystometry at 100 ml of gas or 150 ml of water using a fill rate of 30 to 100 ml per minute; involuntary bladder contractions demonstrated on cystometry; absence of nocturia; awake urinary frequency of less than eight times per day; symptoms relieved by antimicrobial, urinary antiseptic, anticholinergic, or antispasmodic agents; or a concomitant diagnosis of bacterial cystitis/prostatitis, vaginitis, bladder or lower ureteral calculi, genital herpes, lower urinary tract cancer, gynecologic cancer, urethral diverticulum, and chemical, tuberculous, or radiation cystitis. IC is rarely diagnosed in individuals younger than 18 years of age or older than 65 years of age.

With this history in mind, the possibility of IC can be considered and its further evaluation discussed with the patient. We consider a urodynamic evaluation important to rule out relative urinary retention, and particularly phasic involuntary bladder contractions during filling. Patients with either detrusor hyperreflexia or instability are not diagnosed as having IC and are generally treated with anticholinergic or antispasmodic medication with a reasonable degree of success. In the IC population, the urodynamics generally demonstrate hypersensitivity, normal compliance, and adequate emptying with low flow rates because of the low volumes voided.

The next step is both diagnostic and therapeutic, and involves cystoscopy with hydraulic distention of the bladder under general or spinal anesthesia. After initial inspection, bladder washings for cytology are obtained, and hydraulic distention is carried out for 1 to 2 minutes at a water pressure of 80 to 100 cm. The bladder is emptied and then refilled to establish the diagnosis as described previously, and then a more therapeutic hydraulic distention can be performed for another 6 to 8 minutes. If the bladder is to be biopsied, it is done after the second hydraulic distention.

We recently evaluated our results with a number of therapies that we routinely use, and found a 28 percent success rate with hydraulic distention alone in patients whose bladder capacity under anesthesia was less than 600 ml, and a 56 percent success rate in those with a bladder capacity under anesthesia of more than 600 ml. Most favorable responses were extremely brief, with the exceptional patient noting improvement for 6 months. In such patients, however, intermittent hydraulic distention may be requested as the mainstay of treatment, and under these circumstances is successful. There are other methods, generally involving prolonged distention under anesthesia for up to 3 hours at a pressure that approximates systolic blood pressure. We have little experience with this, and would caution that the incidence of bladder rupture with such treatment approaches 10 percent.

In the unusual patient with a discrete Hunner's ulcer, a complete transurethral resection may be carried out; though reported series are understandably small, but success rates of up to 50 percent have been reported. Patients with localized lesions have also been reported to show good responses to neodymium-YAG laser irradiation, although the risk of forward laser scatter with small bowel damage should always be kept in mind, especially in the "typical" patient with a very thin walled bladder.

INITIAL APPROACH TO TREATMENT

When the diagnosis of interstitial cystitis is made, either after endoscopic examination or before referral, or if such a diagnosis appears likely, it is helpful to discuss the condition with the patient and family members. Such a discussion should be frank, but sympathetic and supportive. It should be emphasized that IC is not "in your head," not a life-threatening disorder, and not related to cancer, but can be one of the most difficult diseases to treat. Certain self-help possibilities exist and should be employed.

Self-Help

It is useful to have patients keep a voiding diary, recording their frequency for two weekdays and one weekend day every week. Any improvements will become apparent in the diary. Although some tend to discount the effect of certain foods and beverages on the symptoms of patients with IC, there is no doubt that some of these consistently aggravate the condition in some patients. It is helpful to provide a list of potential foods and drinks to avoid, and to encourage patients to try to find a diet that seems best for them. Alcohol, caffeine-containing beverages, chocolate, citrus fruits, tomatoes, and spicy foods seem to be the prime offenders.

Other self-help strategies include bladder training (trying to increase the interval between urinations by a fixed amount every week) and stress reduction. It is often useful to give the patient a package containing general information about the disease, all the self-help possibilities, and the address of the Interstitial Cystitis Association (P.O. Box 1553 Madison Square Station, New York, NY 10159) and of any local chapter.

Intravesical Therapy

Our next line of treatment is generally the intravesical instillation of dimethylsulfoxide (DMSO), a product of the wood pulp industry and a derivative of lignum. Its pharmacologic properties include membrane penetration, enhanced drug absorption, anti-inflammatory and analgesic effects, collagen dissolution, muscle relaxation, and mast cell histamine release. Our DMSO "cocktail" consists of 50 ml of 50 percent drug to which is added, for theoretical reasons, 5,000 to 10,000 U of heparin, 10 mg of triamcinolone acetonide or its equivalent, and 44 mEq of bicarbonate. Six to eight weekly instillations constitute our treatment course. Of the patients we have treated, 53 percent have had an excellent or fair response. The average length of response was 10 months. If there is a good initial response, we consider placing patients on monthly maintenance for 8 to 12 additional months; this is done in about one in four patients. The details of the treatment are simple. After the mixture is placed in the bladder, the catheter is removed, and the patient is asked to hold the medication for 15 to 40 minutes and then void. Almost everyone is familiar with the garlic-like breath odor that DMSO imparts, and many patients experience increased vesical irritability after instillation, especially after the first few. The manufacturer recommends slit lamp eye examinations before and during treatment, presumably because of results with animal experimentation, although extensive human studies have demonstrated no changes in the ocular refractive index and no development of lens opacities to our knowledge. DMSO should not be used in pregnancy. DMSO or a DMSO cocktail is safe, effective, and generally free of local or systemic true toxicity. It is relatively inexpensive and does not require anesthesia to administer.

Other groups have promoted the initial intravesical instillation of different agents. Results equivalent to those from DMSO have been reported with oxychlorosene sodium (Chlorpactin WSC-90), generally in a 0.4 percent concentration. The instillation requires anesthesia because of intense discomfort, and a preliminary voiding cystourethrogram to rule out ureteral reflux, which we believe contraindicates this therapy because of reported ureteral complications. If oxychlorosene sodium is used, most authors recommend overnight catheter drainage for maximal patient comfort. Intravesical silver nitrate administration in varying concentrations (1:5,000 to 1:1,000) has been reported to yield similarly good results, but we have no experience with this.

Oral Drug Therapy

In patients who have failed to respond to hydraulic distention, resection or laser irradiation, or intravesical therapy, we have found amitriptyline to be useful. Patients are begun on a dosage of 25 mg at bedtime, gradually increasing by weekly increments to a maximal dose of 75 mg. Overall, in patients with an anesthetized bladder capacity of more than 600 ml, excellent and fair results were achieved in 26 and 28 percent, respectively; in those with capacities of under 600 ml, the corresponding figures were 22 and 17 percent. Amitriptyline is the most potent tricyclic antidepressant in terms of blocking H_1 histamine receptors. It has also been reported to be a mast cell stabilizer in vitro. It has analgesic actions that are not clearly understood, and theoretically could decrease the excitability of smooth muscle in the bladder body. It has a sedative effect that is adverse in some patients, but is therapeutic in others.

Sodium pentosan polysulfate (Elmiron) is a synthetic sulfated polysaccharide that has been extensively studied as another oral therapeutic agent for IC. Although there is some disagreement as to the magnitude of its therapeutic effects, and whether these are different from placebo, the latest data seem to show a modest response rate in excess of placebo. In our studies, 100 mg of the substance was administered orally three times daily for a minimum of 3 months. In patients with capacities of more than 600 ml we obtained excellent and fair results in 25 and 18 percent, of patients respectively; in those with capacities of less than 600 ml under anesthesia, the corresponding numbers were 20 and 0 percent. By the time this is published the drug will probably have FDA approval, it appears to be a potentially safe, easily administered drug that could be given to patients as initial therapy or to those who have failed other simpler types of standard therapy. Side effects are few, predominantly peripheral edema and diarrhea. Only a small amount of the drug is excreted in the urine, which supposedly is why there is a relatively long time lag before clinical improvement is noted. The rationale for such therapy rests on the hypothesis of a deficient glycosaminoglycan (GAG) layer in the bladder urothelium that the synthetic GAG is hypothesized to replenish. Using a similar rationale, Lowell Parsons has described intravesical heparin as another conservative method of treatment. Direct intravesical instillation of this synthetic GAG seems at least as reasonable as oral administration of such an agent with a poor urinary excretion. Ten thousand units of heparin are placed into 10 ml of sterile water, instilled by the patient three times a week, and held for as long as possible. It is recommended that 12 weeks elapse before treatment is considered a failure.

Other Therapies

Other conservative therapies are available, but there is less consensus as to their benefits. Transcutaneous electrical nerve stimulation (TENS) is used more frequently overseas than in the United States. The stimulation is delivered by suprapubic electrodes, and the rationale is to block afferent noxious impulses from the bladder. The generally recommended regimen is stimulation for 2 hours twice daily, although it would seem logical that longer periods of use would produce better results. The best results have been reported after treatment periods ranging up to 6 months. TENS has a negligible risk and is extremely noninvasive, and therefore can be considered as isolated or concomitant treatment, especially in patients whose main complaint is discomfort.

Other noninvasive therapies that have been recommended, in a serious or anecdotal fashion, include nonsteroidal anti-inflammatory agents, steroids, antihistamines (H_1 and H_2 blockers), alpha-adrenergic antagonists, anticholinergics, antispasmodics, and urinary analgesics. Acupressure and acupuncture have also been mentioned as potential treatments, and the administration of caudal steroids by an experienced anesthesiologist may be considered. The use of intravesical capsaicin is undergoing trials overseas, and the results will certainly be watched closely. Capsaicin is a compound that depletes candidate sensory neurotransmitter substances from certain populations of afferent neurons. Finally, nalmefene is an orally administered opioid antagonist currently undergoing clinical trials for the treatment of IC. Opioids have been shown to cause mast cell degranulation in certain in vitro circumstances, and if mast cell degranulation has a role in the pathophysiology of IC symptomatology, inhibition of this process theoretically should prove beneficial.

SURGICAL THERAPY

It is worthwhile to exhaust all reasonable conservative measures before proceeding to surgical treatment in a disease such as IC, which is chronic, not life-threatening, and subject to spontaneous changes in symptoms. Of the available surgical therapies, we have found augmentation cystoplasty with supratrigonal cystectomy to be the procedure of choice in patients who have a small-capacity bladder under anesthesia. The bowel segment used is best detubularized to create a low-pressure capacious reservoir and to prevent mass contraction with resultant incontinence. Webster has collected 19 such patients and reported that 12 were cured of pain and frequency while four experienced improvement. This coincides with our impression of the results in our own patients. If this avenue of therapy is chosen, a thorough discussion of the procedure and its risks must be carried out with patient and family. It should be emphasized that there are no guarantees with respect to either pain or frequency, and that intermittent self-catheterization may be required afterward on a permanent basis. We generally quote the patients a figure of a 20 percent possibility of this eventuality, and it is a sound idea to have these patients taught CIC beforehand as part of the "informed consent" process.

Urinary diversion with or without cystectomy is definitely a treatment of last resort. Although recent configurations of continent reservoirs may make diversion and cystectomy a more attractive alternative, we view this as a desperate measure for a desperate patient and would still be unwilling, in a patient who has failed other forms of therapy, to try to predict relief of pelvic pain.

In summary, IC is a difficult condition to manage. The results of treatment can range from spectacular to awful and may change over a short period. Nevertheless, most patients with IC can be helped to live relatively normal lives and, with the aid of various forms of treatment modalities, including self-help, to tolerate their disability.

SUGGESTED READING

Hanno PM. Interstitial Cystitis. In: Lytton B, McGuire E., eds. Advances in urology. Chicago: Year Book Medical Publishers, 1990:91.

Hanno PM, Staskin DR, Krane RJ, Wein AJ. Interstitial cystitis. New York: Springer Verlag, 1990.

Hanno PM, Wein AJ. Interstitial cystitis (Parts 1 and 2). American Urological Association Update Series, Lessons 9 and 10, Volume 6, Houston, TX 1987.

Parsons LC. Interstitial cystitis: clinical manifestation and diagnostic criteria in over 200 cases. Neurourol Urodyn 1990; 9:241.

Sant G. Interstitial cystitis: pathophysiology, clinical evaluation and treatment. In: Rous SN, ed. Urology annual. Norwalk, CT: Appleton & Lange, 1989:171.

HEMORRHAGIC CYSTITIS INDUCED BY CYCLOPHOSPHAMIDE AND RADIATION THERAPY

TIMOTHY G. WILSON, M.D.
JEFFRY L. HUFFMAN, M.D.

A few medical conditions are routinely problematic and frustrating for both patient and clinician. Hemorrhagic cystitis caused by cyclophosphamide or radiation therapy is one of these conditions. A routine systemic approach to this condition is necessary to optimize resources and achieve the best possible results.

Cyclophosphamide, an oxaphosphorine alkylating agent, was introduced in 1958 and is currently used in the systemic treatment of several solid tumors, B-cell malignancies, and other non-neoplastic disease such as thrombocytopenic purpura, rheumatoid arthritis, lupus, nephrotic syndrome, and Wegener's granulomatosis. Another common use is as a conditioner for bone marrow transplantation. Hemorrhagic cystitis may occur in up to 70 percent of patients who have received cyclophosphamide, and commonly has a high morbidity rate and an estimated associated mortality rate as high as 4 percent.

The urotoxicity of cyclophosphamide is a result of its aldehyde hepatic metabolite, acrolein, which is excreted by the kidneys and is directly toxic to the urothelium. Hemorrhagic cystitis may occur at any time during cyclophosphamide therapy and up to several months afterward. Hematuria may range from mild and benign to severe and life threatening.

With the elucidation of acrolein as the toxic agent in 1979, it became clear that prevention was a possibility. During cyclophosphamide therapy, it is important that patients receive continuous bladder irrigation and vigorous diuresis to reduce toxicity. Also, MESNA (2-mercaptoethene sulfate) should be given prophylactically. This agent is oxidized to a stable inactive disulfide and excreted in the urine, and binds with acrolein, reducing its toxicity. MESNA is given just before the cyclophosphamide at a dosage of 20 mg per kilogram every 4 hours for three or four doses. Despite these measures, however, patients still occasionally acquire cyclophosphamide-induced hemorrhagic cystitis.

External beam radiation therapy may also induce hemorrhagic cystitis. Pelvic malignancies such as prostate cancer in males or cervical cancer in females may be amenable to external beam radiation therapy. The proximity of the bladder in these conditions may have significant effects on the bladder, one of which is hemorrhagic cystitis. Careful treatment designs minimize bladder dosage, but most patients experience bladder symptoms ranging in severity from mild dysuria and frequency to hemorrhagic cystitis.

EVALUATION

The initial evaluation of a patient for hemorrhagic cystitis is similar in many respects to that for gross hematuria. A complete history taking and physical examination, urinalysis for culture (including viral), serum chemistries, BUN, creatinine, prothrombin time, partial thromboplastin time, hematocrit, and platelet count should be checked. Normal renal anatomy is verified by a baseline renal ultrasonography (Table 1).

TREATMENT

A multieyed Robinson catheter is initially placed into the bladder and irrigated by hand until the bladder is free of clots. A three-way Foley catheter is inserted for continuous bladder irrigation, and the hematocrit and vital signs are followed closely. Transfusions are given as needed, coagulopathies corrected, and positive urine cultures treated with appropriate antibiotics. Depending on the patient's condition and the stability of the hematocrit, the patient is taken to the operating room either emergently or electively to undergo cystoscopy. The bladder is irrigated free of clots and examined carefully, and any bleeding points are fulgurated with the resectoscope. Since a significant number of patients resolve with fulguration only, we stop at this point and continue with continuous bladder irrigation. We have not had success using other forms of treatment such as AMICAR or irrigation with silver nitrate or prostaglandin.

Patients with unresolved mild hematuria after fulguration receive continuous irrigation with alum, which is available as either the potassium or the ammonium salt of aluminum sulfate; each has equal efficacy. Its action is through protein precipitation, and it may be used safely without anesthesia and in the face of vesicoureteral reflux. Few, if any, side effects occur. However, patients with renal insufficiency should have serum aluminum levels monitored, since encephalopathy and acidosis have been reported. A 1 percent alum solution in sterile water is instilled through a large-bore catheter as continuous bladder irrigation, alternating each hour with normal saline to keep the catheter patent. This is continued for 48 to 72 hours.

Patients who fail alum irrigation or have persistent moderate to severe hematuria after fulguration go on to receive bladder instillation of formalin. Formalin acts by hydrolyzing protein and coagulating tissue on a superficial level, controlling bleeding from the mucosa and submucosa; 100 percent formalin is a 30 percent formaldehyde solution. It must be used under anesthesia.

The patient is taken to the cystoscopy suite and placed under adequate general or spinal anesthesia. A gravity cystogram is taken to rule out vesicoureteral reflux. The patient is cystoscoped and the bladder irrigated free of clots or clumps of alum. If reflux is observed on the cystogram, a No. 6 French whistle-tip catheter or a 5-mm ureteral balloon catheter is passed up

Table 1 Treatment of Cyclophosphamide- or Radiation-induced Hemorrhagic Cystitis

1. Transfuse as needed and correct coagulopathies

2. Insert multieyed Robinson catheter, hand irrigate clots, and begin continuous irrigation with saline through three-way Foley catheter

3. If bleeding persists, perform cystoscopy and fulgurate bleeding points

4. For persistent bleeding, irrigate bladder with 1% alum

5. If bleeding still persists, perform cystoscopy under anesthesia and instill 2.5% formalin

6. Urinary diversion may be required if hemorrhage continues after repeat formalin instillation

each refluxing ureter and left exiting from the urethral meatus. If catheters cannot be passed, the patient is placed in the reverse Trendelenburg position during the actual instillation of formalin. If under general anesthesia, the patient is paralyzed to prevent bladder spasms, and 2.5 percent formalin is introduced under gravity and left to dwell for 15 minutes. The bladder is then drained and continuous bladder irrigation restarted. The perineum is washed with copious amounts of irrigation to prevent skin irritation, and the patient is returned to the ward. Continuous bladder irrigation typically is continued for 24 to 48 hours and slowly stopped, and the catheter is removed if the urine remains clear. Some patients may require two or three instillations. If gross hematuria continues, the formalin is increased to 5 percent and left to dwell for 10 minutes. Side effects of formalin include bladder fibrosis and contracture, intramural ureteral fibrosis and obstruction, and vesicoureteral reflux with papillary necrosis. These side effects can be minimized by using the lower concentrations of formalin, which are usually effective.

Rarely, despite the above measures, hemorrhage continues. The decision to proceed with more aggressive therapy is made only after other causes of bleeding have been eliminated and the patient's overall prognosis permits. Usually, urinary diversion without cystectomy relieves the bleeding and leaves open the option of undiversion in the future. Nephrostomy diversion alone is usually inadequate because urine generally is not completely diverted from the bladder. On rare occasions, we ligate the ureters via a lumbodorsal approach and place a nephrostomy tube for palliation in patients who have had multiple abdominal surgeries or who have documented carcinomatosis.

PROSTATIC ABSCESS

MARC S. COHEN, M.D.

Prostatic abscess is encountered infrequently. A discussion of current therapy is affected, therefore, by the fact that despite significant change in the ability to diagnose and treat prostatic abscess, little information other than anecdotal experience is available regarding the most appropriate treatment options.

The clinical findings in the patient with a prostatic abscess are often nonspecific. The patient may note frequency, urgency, difficulty in voiding, or urinary retention. There may be perineal, rectal, or suprapubic discomfort. The patient may be without genitourinary complaint but may present with constitutional findings (fever, weakness, fatigue, malaise) or evidence of sepsis. A relationship with immunocompromise, diabetes mellitus, adenocarcinoma of the prostate, maintenance hemodialysis, urethral instrumentation, and urethral catheterization has been described. Rectal examination may classically reveal fluctuance in the prostate gland, but this is noted in only about 25 percent of cases. Nonspecific findings on rectal examination are more common, such as tenderness, edema, and asymmetry. These are often seen with acute and chronic prostatitis, and prostatic abscesses are probably a sequela of such infection, although metastatic infections from other sites have also been described. Urine cultures may be positive in association with a prostatic abscess, but a negative culture may occur in approximately 25 percent of patients; a negative culture therefore does not exclude the possibility of abscess. Nonspecific findings and risk factors such as those mentioned above in a patient who has unexplained bacteremia or who is responding poorly to antimicrobial therapy should warrant further diagnostic evaluation for a possible prostatic abscess.

Diagnostic evaluation may be accomplished by either computed tomography (CT), magnetic resonance imaging (MRI), or transrectal ultrasonography (TRUS). It is also possible that a radiolabeled white blood cell test or gallium scan may suggest a prostatic abscess. CT, MRI, or radionuclide studies are most frequently employed in the evaluation of infection without a clinically suspect source. Thus, prostatic abscess in such a scenario is often an unsuspected finding. When there is a high index of clinical suspicion, TRUS is the diagnostic test of choice. Prostatic abscesses tend to present as focal inhomogeneous areas of decreased or mixed echogenicity. Hypoechoic, multiseptate, or purely cystic appearances have also been described. Findings that may help differentiate a prostatic abscess from other hypoechoic lesions of the prostate (e.g., prostatic carcinoma) include its size, a central location within the prostate gland, and lack of a hyperechoic rim.

THERAPEUTIC ALTERNATIVES

Conservative Treatment

A wide variety of treatments have been suggested, practiced, and condemned (Table 1). Conservative alternatives (with the exception of the preoperative use of antibiotics as discussed below) in anticipation of spontaneous rupture into the urethra are not recommended, because disastrous consequences such as rectal, perineal, vesical, and peritoneal fistulas and death have been described. Also, incomplete spontaneous drainage may result in recurrent abscess formation.

Table 1 Prostatic Abscess: Alternative Therapies

Conservative Treatment

  Heat*
  Rest*
  Urinary antiseptics*
  Antibiotic therapy

Surgical Treatment

  Rupture with urethral sound or catheter*
  Perineal urethrotomy with digital rupture*
  Perineal incision and drainage*
  Prostatectomy (suprapubic, retropubic, perineal)
  Transurethral resection ("radical" TURP)[†]
  Transurethral incision
  Percutaneous drainage

  *Historical interest.
  [†]Transurethral resection.

Surgical Treatment

Surgical intervention is usually necessary once the diagnosis of prostatic abscess is established and antibiotic coverage initiated. Several surgical approaches have been entertained in the past and, in view of recent technologic advances, are of historical significance only (see Table 1). Among these are blind rupture with a urethral sound, perineal urethrotomy with rupture by digitalization of the prostatic urethra, perineal incision with direct or indirect incision, and perhaps suprapubic, retropubic, or perineal prostatectomy. Although all these methods have been employed with varied success in the past, they are associated with significant compromising risks. In the case of blind rupture, incomplete drainage may result. With urethrotomy, fistulization and sphincter injury may accompany incomplete drainage. Perineal incision may compromise normal adjacent tissues, and without proper localization of the abscess cavity, incomplete drainage may result. Open prostatectomy remains a viable treatment alternative, but there is a risk of spread of infection to normal tissues. Open prostatectomy may also be technically difficult in the presence of infection and may be associated with an increased risk of morbidity related to sepsis and tissue compromise. Therefore, open prostatectomy is best used for prostatic abscess when other associated pathologic conditions warrant an open procedure (e.g., prostatic size, large bladder calculi, bladder diverticula) rather than the singular finding of a prostatic abscess.

PREFERRED APPROACH

Antibiotic Treatment

All patients with prostatic abscess should be started on broad-spectrum antibiotics as soon as the diagnosis is known or suspected.

It is likely that many patients, by the nature of their presentation, will have already been started on an oral or intravenous antimicrobial agent. Previous studies have demonstrated that in the era before antibiotic use, the most often recognized organism in prostatic abscesses was *Neisseria gonorrhoeae*. More recent studies show that *Escherichia coli* is currently the predominant organism identified in prostatic abscess, although others (*Proteus* spp., *Pseudomonas, Salmonella, Staphlococcus* spp., *Bacteroides,* and *Peptostreptococcus*) have been encountered, with mixed cultures frequently identified. These different organisms necessitate broad-spectrum antibiotic coverage with an aminoglycoside (gentamicin, tobramycin) (3 to 5 mg per kilogram per day every 8 hours) and penicillin agent (penicillin G, 2.5 to 3 million units every 4 hours) until culture results can be obtained. If there is evidence to suggest the presence of anaerobic organisms (gas formation in tissues, foul-smelling aspirate or discharge), the inclusion of clindamycin hydrochloride (600 to 1,200 mg per day every 6 to 12 hours) or chloramphenicol hydrochloride (50 to 100 mg per kilogram per day every 6 hours) is recommended. These

latter agents provide excellent coverage of anaerobic organisms, including *Bacteroides fragilis,* which is the most common anaerobic organism isolated from prostatic abscesses. Antibiotic coverage should be altered when culture information demonstrates inadequate coverage or a more efficacious antimicrobial agent. Antibiotics are continued until the abscess has been resolved.

Surgical Treatment

Current therapy revolves around endoscopic (transurethral resection [TURP], transurethral incision [TUIP]) and percutaneous (ultrasonographic) approaches (Fig. 1). A thorough understanding of the best application of these techniques is compromised by the relatively small number of cases reported in the literature. It also has yet to be determined what impact the use of postprocedure CT, MRI, and especially ultrasonographic technology may have on determining how successful a particular treatment protocol might be in long-term follow-up.

Transurethral Resection

Prostatic resection has been considered the treatment of choice by many authors. This belief is founded in data suggesting that less radical therapy such as transurethral incision can result in the possibility of missing an abscess cavity and leaving it undiagnosed and undrained. With more conservative treatment (percutaneous drainage or transurethral incision), there is also a possibility of abscess reformation. Preoperative use of CT, MRI, and particularly ultrasonography to localize and identify the prostatic abscess cavity, and their usefulness in determining the size, number, and extent of prostatic involvement (one or both lobes), allows a better application of transurethral and percutaneous techniques. The further use of these diagnostic techniques postoperatively enables better assessment of the results, and the above difficulties may be minimized. It is now my custom to limit the use of transurethral resection to (1) patients with evidence of associated benign prostatic hyperplasia and/or obstructive symptoms that predate abscess formation; (2) patients with multiple or small abscess cavities seen on ultrasonography, which would be poorly drained by incision or percutaneous drainage alone; and (3) patients medically stable enough to undergo anesthesia. The technique employed is no different from that employed in standard TURP, with the exception that a concentrated effort is made to remove all prostatic tissue down to the level of the surgical capsule (i.e., "radical" TURP). This lessens the risk of leaving residual infected tissue or an undrained abscess cavity.

Transurethral Incision

Incision and drainage with a knife electrode, resectoscope loop, or urethrotomy knife have all been described as poor means for drainage of the prostatic

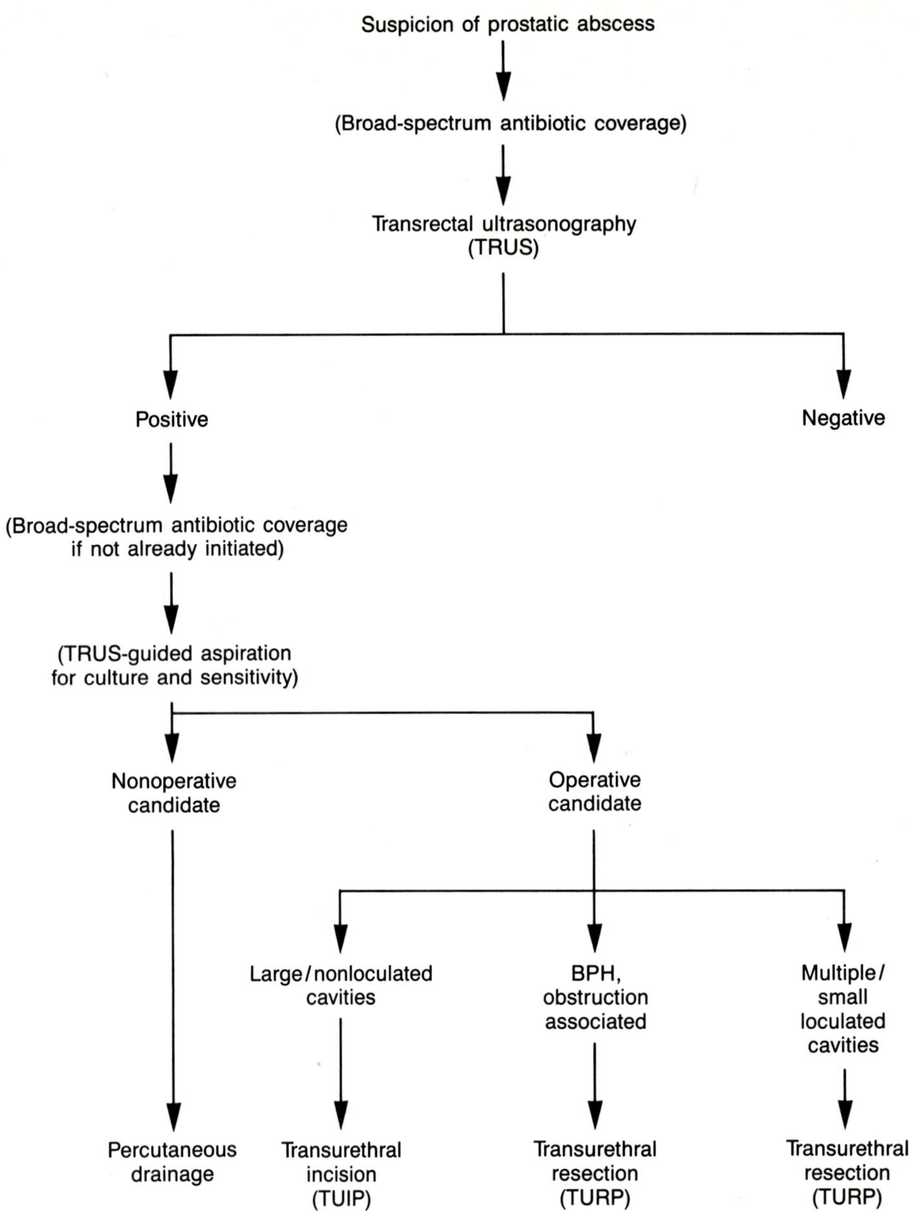

Figure 1 Management of prostatic abscess.

abscess. The potential for undrained abscess exists, as described above. Again, the impact of current diagnostic technology in determining the extent of abscess formation and the subsequent application of therapy remains to be defined. Transurethral incision is most applicable in patients with (1) large solitary abscess formation without septation, (2) minimal periurethral tissue intervening between the abscess and urethral lumen, (3) no evidence of prostatic hyperplasia or obstruction, (4) a desire to maintain fertility, or (5) no contraindication to anesthesia. The incision is accomplished endoscopically by first visualizing the affected lobe, which may present as an asymmetric, bulging lobe. The surface may be tense but compressible, depending on the depth of the abscess and the amount of surrounding prostatic tissue. An incision is made from the bladder neck distally with the resectoscope loop or knife electrode, and is deepened as necessary until the abscess cavity is entered. Alternatively, a urethrotomy knife can be plunged into the distal aspect of the abscess and the cavity opened proximally with the blade. After evacuation of the abscess the cavity may often be inspected for loculations or septations, which may be destroyed with the resectoscope beak or loop.

Percutaneous Transperineal Aspiration With Ultrasonographic Guidance

Transperineal percutaneous drainage using transrectal ultrasonography can be used to obtain an aspirate for culture identification and to effect drainage in certain instances. Although it is possible to drain the prostate percutaneously by digital guidance in a fashion similar to transperineal prostatic biopsy, transrectal ultrasonography improves the accuracy of the technique. The procedure may be undertaken in (1) patients under local anesthesia deemed to be poor surgical risks, (2) patients with solitary or few abscesses without septation or loculation, and (3) patients with peripheral abscesses not easily incised by a transurethral route.

The technique of percutaneous aspiration and drainage is best performed using a transrectal ultrasonographic probe with perineal needle guide. The patient is placed in a dorsal lithotomy position and the perineum prepared, scrubbed, and draped in a sterile fashion. One percent lidocaine (Xylocaine) is used to anesthetize the perineal skin. With the transrectal probe in position and the abscess cavity visualized, the prostatic abscess may be evaluated with regard to size, appearance, position, and the presence of loculation. Using the perineal needle guide, an 18-gauge needle (e.g., a spinal needle) is directed through the guide into the abscess cavity (the needletip being visible on ultrasonography). Once positioned, the needle obturator is removed and aspirate may be obtained for culture. With continued ultrasonographic or fluoroscopic guidance (the latter accom-

plished by injecting 2 to 5 ml of contrast material), a floppy tip guidewire (0.032 inch) may be directed through the needle into the abscess cavity. The tract may be dilated with a No. 4 to No. 10 French fascial or Van Andel catheter and a No. 4 to No. 8 French pigtail, accordion, or Cope loop catheter placed in the abscess cavity. The subsequent resolution of the abscess cavity can be monitored by follow-up fluoroscopic or ultrasonographic study. Catheters may be removed when the cavity is no longer present and purulent drainage has ceased. Anecdotal reports of this approach suggest that abscess recurrence after percutaneous drainage is rare.

SUGGESTED READING

Chitty K. Prostatic Abscess. Br J Surg 1957; 44:599–601.

Cytron S, Weinberger M, Pitlik SD, Servadio C. Value of transrectal ultrasonography for diagnosis and treatment of prostatic abscess. Urology 1988; 32:454–458.

Kadmon D, Ling D, Lee JKT. Percutaneous drainage of prostatic abscess. J Urol 1986; 135:1259–1260.

Thornhill BA, Morehouse UT, Coleman P, Hoffman-Tretin JC. Prostatic abscess: CT and sonographic findings. AJR 1987; 148: 899–900.

Trapnell J, Roberts M. Prostatic abscess. Br J Surg 1970; 57:565–569.

PERIURETHRAL ABSCESS IN MALES

PETER T. NIEH, M.D.

Periurethral abscess usually originates in periurethral glands as a localized infection within Buck's fascia. Because urethral stricture is often an associated finding, the increased intraurethral pressure rapidly promotes the abscess to extend beyond this fascial layer to involve the subcutaneous tissues of the penis, scrotum, and perineum. This necrotizing synergistic infection may extend beneath Scarpa's fascia onto the abdominal and chest walls, presenting as fulminant Fournier's gangrene.

Although most periurethral abscesses are associated with urethral strictures and infection of the urinary tract, any urethral injury (e.g., false passage created by traumatic instrumentation or catheterization, foreign bodies, a chronic indwelling urethral catheter, self-manipulation, or external blunt trauma) may result in disruption of the mucosa, urinary extravasation, and local sepsis. Urethral carcinoma should be suspected in a patient presenting with urethral "stricture" and bloody urine or urethral discharge. Malnutrition, alcoholism, diabetes, or any immunocompromised state increases the possibility of progression.

The diagnosis is made on the basis of localized tenderness, swelling, and sometimes crepitus of the base of the penis and perineum (Fig. 1); infected urine; a history or symptoms of urethral stricture disease; and extravasation as seen on retrograde urethrography.

The therapeutic alternatives to surgical intervention are limited. Although patients with early well-localized periurethral abscess confined within Buck's fascia can be treated with antibiotics alone, most present with more advanced soft tissue infection. Delay in treatment endangers the viability of the entire genitalia as well as the patient. Thus, prompt diagnosis, urinary diversion, and aggressive surgical management are mandatory.

PREFERRED APPROACH

Broad-Spectrum Antibiotic Coverage

Multiple organisms are often cultured from these wounds at operation. Thus, intravenous broad-spectrum antibiotics with effective gram-positive, gram-negative, and anaerobic coverage are required. A good initial choice would be an aminoglycoside, such as gentamicin, 1 mg per kilogram every 8 hours, or tobramycin, 1 mg per kilogram every 8 hours, provided that the patient has normal renal function; this should be combined with mezlocillin (Mezlin), 200 to 300 mg per kilogram per day in four to six divided doses, or a second-generation cephalosporin. For additional anaerobic coverage, metronidazole, 15 mg per kilogram over 1 hour then 7.5 mg per kilogram over 1 hour every 6 hours, is added. Administration of these antibiotics is continued until results of culture and sensitivity studies have identified more selective agents to replace these drugs.

Stabilization of Patient

Metabolic abnormalities, such as hyperglycemia or metabolic acidosis, must be corrected. Patients with anemia of chronic disease or poor nutrition should receive transfusions preoperatively. Hypotensive patients with a septic abscess must be resuscitated aggressively with fluids, central venous pressure monitoring, and judicious use of appropriate pressor agents, colloids or other volume expanders, and blood products. In these ill patients, the use of corticosteroids is controversial but may be beneficial.

Anesthesia

Spinal or epidural anesthesia is preferred because the postoperative analgesia is superior to that achieved with general anesthesia. Morphine given epidurally can provide excellent control of pain during the first postoperative day. Control of pain is especially important during dressing changes and care of the wound on the first day when it is critical to monitor progression of soft tissue infection.

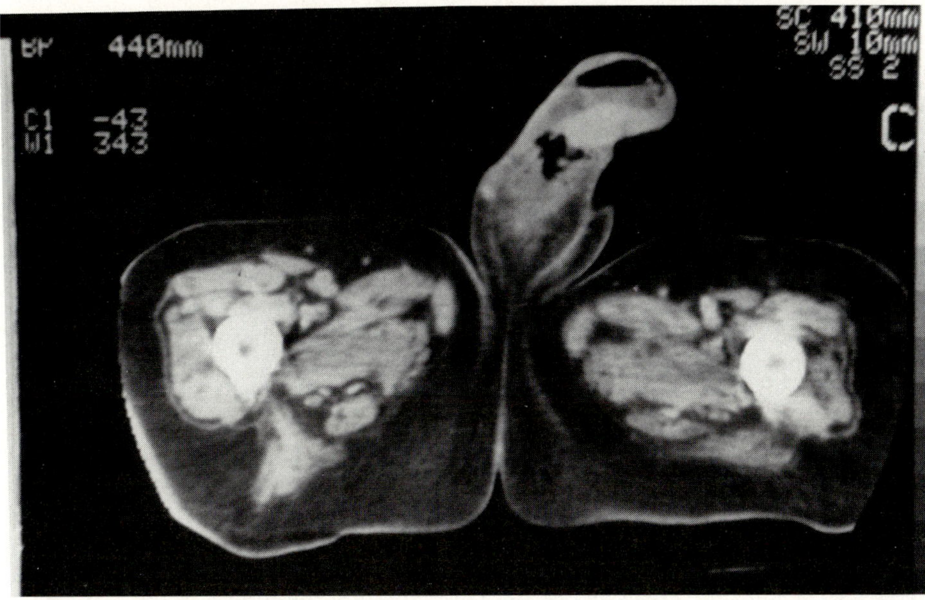

Figure 1 Computed tomographic scan of a 55-year-old man with insulin-dependent diabetes who presented with dysuria, fever, and a painful, edematous, inflamed penis and scrotum. Air-fluid levels in penile tissue demonstrated the gas-forming infection. A phlegmon was found near the deep bulbar urethra. Staged urethroplasty and scrotal flap grafts were eventually required.

Positioning for Operation

A modified dorsal lithotomy position in which the thighs are spread with the legs extended using heel supports or stirrups, permits access to the perineum, scrotum, and suprapubic region. This position also allows exposure of the abdominal wall or chest when the infection has extended that far. A careful digital rectal examination should be performed to exclude perirectal sources of infection.

Surgical Precautions

As in other surgical situations, and in this era of awareness of acquired immunodeficiency syndrome (AIDS) when the physician is possibly dealing with immunocompromised individuals, the usual precautions regarding potential human immunodeficiency virus (HIV) infection should be taken by the surgeon and the entire operating team.

Urethral Anatomy Defined Cautiously

Retrograde urethrography is performed very gently to demonstrate the site of extravasation and the extent of often coexisting urethral strictures. Cystoscopes, urethral sounds, urethral catheters, or filiforms and followers are not passed at this time because such urethral manipulation may result in full-blown septic shock.

Diversion of Urine

Urinary diversion is one aspect of management that differs from that of Fournier's gangrene, which can be managed safely with a urethral catheter. Urethral pathologic findings are invariably associated with periurethral abscess and are best dealt with by a bypass procedure using suprapubic drainage. I have used a No. 12 French suprapubic cystocatheter* in this situation. Although these catheters are satisfactory for short-term drainage, the tip tends to migrate beyond the neck of the bladder, and the relatively soft silicone tubing can kink or dislodge easily when the adhesive or sutures loosen.

A more reliable suprapubic catheter can be introduced by trocar cystostomy using a No. 12 or 16 French catheter held securely by a balloon or coiled loop. Examples of these newer devices are the Stamey percutaneous loop suprapubic catheter No. 12 or 14 French or Rutner percutaneous suprapubic balloon catheter No. 10 or 16 French.† These catheters may be exchanged over a guide wire or replaced with Foley catheters after 2 weeks when the tract will have matured.

When the patient has a greatly enlarged prostate (open prostatectomy size), especially with a large middle lobe, a small incision is made to expose the anterior

---

*Cystocath Suprapubic Drainage System, Dow Corning Corp., Medical Products, Midland, Mich.

†Cook Urological, Spencer, Ind.

bladder wall to place the tube safely (Nos. 20 to 24 French Foley catheter with 5-ml balloon) under direct vision.

Drainage of Sepsis

Loculated collections are incised and drained. Although healing of the scrotal wall occurs regardless of the placement of the incision, longitudinal incisions on the penile shaft may be less injurious to lymphatic drainage than transverse or circumferential incisions. Material should be obtained for Gram stain smears and cultures (aerobic and anaerobic and gonorrhea).

Debridement of Frankly Nonviable Tissue

The debrided tissue is sent for histologic analysis because underlying carcinoma may be detected. Scrotal and shaft skin and urethral tissue are preserved when possible. An eye should be kept toward eventual reconstruction. Even with significant subcutaneous purulence in which the picture may resemble Fournier's gangrene, the cord structures and testes can usually be preserved. Penrose drains are placed through and through and secured with sutures of chromic catgut.

The wound is packed loosely using wide mesh gauze sponges soaked with iodine solution, half-strength hydrogen peroxide, or Dakin's solution.

Identification of Site of Urethral Defect

The site of the urethral defect is identified if possible. The urethral edges are freshened carefully, and the first stage of urethroplasty is performed by marsupialization of the urethra to surrounding penile shaft or scrotal skin. This may not be possible until the wounds are cleanly granulating.

POSTOPERATIVE CARE

The dressings are changed every 8 hours, care being taken to apply the moistened wide mesh gauze to the wound surface to debride effectively. The packing material should be kept loose enough to prevent loculation of purulent debris. The Penrose drains are advanced slowly when purulent drainage ceases. Should areas of necrosis appear, further surgical debridement is performed with the patient in the operating room under anesthesia if necessary.

Hydrotherapy and debridement in a whirlpool bath are performed to obtain fresh granulation tissue. When management of the wound is aggressive, a healthy bed is obtained for future grafts. Patients find these sessions relaxing and soothing, permitting the surgeon to debride necrotic tissue with minimal analgesia.

Although I have had no experience with hyperbaric oxygen, application of this adjunctive modality would hasten recovery in patients with extensive anaerobic infections and subcutaneous crepitus.

Nutrition with multivitamins, especially in debilitated individuals, alcoholics, or other high-risk patients, must be adequate. When gangrene resembling Fournier's gangrene results in an extensive perineal wound, a low-residue, high-protein, high-calorie diet may be necessary to achieve an anabolic state with minimal fecal soilage of the wound.

Delayed Wound Coverage and Reconstruction

Implantation of the exposed testes into subcutaneous thigh pouches will safely protect them until the final stages of genital reconstruction. Patience with wound management will provide pliable well-vascularized tissue for eventual reconstruction. The various options for coverage include split-thickness skin grafts for the superficial areas, vascularized pedicle scrotal skin flaps for more extensive exposed areas, and myocutaneous gracilis muscle flaps for the most severe defects in the highest risk patients, such as those with wounds after radiation therapy.

Underlying Conditions

Underlying conditions that may have contributed to the abscess, such as distal urethral stricture, urethral diverticulum, and urethral carcinoma, must be treated. Perineal urethrostomy is a satisfactory alternative to permanent suprapubic catheterization when the patient is not a candidate for total reconstruction.

Complications

The complications and sequelae of periurethral infections are recurrent abscesses, progression to Fournier's gangrene, fistulization, and erectile dysfunction. Recurrent abscess may occur, especially when underlying conditions such as distal stricture, urethral diverticula, or neurogenic bladder, are unrecognized. Recurrent periurethral infection may occur in conjunction with an obstructed suprapubic catheter. An inadequately treated abscess may progress to Fournier's necrotizing gangrene. Chronic periurethral abscess may progress to multiple cutaneous fistulas, especially fistulas associated with gonococcal urethritis, resulting in the "watering pot perineum." Infection rarely may penetrate the tunica albuginea of the corpus cavernosum, producing cavernositis and subsequent erectile impotence.

SUGGESTED READING

Gray JA. Gangrene of the genitalia as seen in advanced periurethral extravasation with phlegmon. J Urol 1960; 84: 740–745.

Walther MM, Mann BB, Finnerty DP. Periurethral abscess. J Urol 1987; 138:1167–1170.

Wilkey JL, Barson LJ, Portney FR. Urinary extravasation and periurethral phlegmon: clinical analysis of 100 cases. J Urol 1959; 82:657–658.

FOURNIER'S GANGRENE

J. PATRICK SPIRNAK, M.D.

In 1882, Jean Alfred Fournier, a French venereologist, reported five patients with unexplained gangrene of the penis and scrotum. All five demonstrated three common characteristics: (1) an abrupt onset in a previously healthy individual, (2) rapid progression of the infectious process to gangrene, and (3) absence of a specific causative agent or factor. Today, the eponym Fournier's gangrene is applied to any gangrenous infectious process involving the external genitalia and perineum. It is rarely idiopathic and typically arises from either an infection involving the urinary tract or a direct involvement from a perirectal source. Fournier's gangrene represents a true urologic emergency requiring prompt administration of broad-spectrum antibiotics and immediate surgical drainage and debridement of all devitalized tissues.

Patients usually present with pain and swelling of the external genitalia in addition to signs and symptoms of a systemic illness, including fever, chills, and generalized malaise. The onset of symptoms may be insidious, requiring several days before the individual seeks medical help, or abrupt and of such a fulminant nature that the patient presents in shock. A complete urologic history is obtained, with particular emphasis placed on the presence of obstructive or irritative voiding symptoms. Complaints of dysuria, hesitancy, and slow stream coupled with a history of urethral stricture disease, urologic trauma, previous catheterizations, or urologic surgery should alert the physician to the possibility of coexisting urethral pathology and warrants additional urologic evaluation consisting of urethrography. Similarly, a history of colorectal complaints or previous colorectal surgery may implicate a perirectal source as the cause. In my experience, most patients present with other coexisting systemic conditions such as diabetes or chronic ethanol abuse that may affect the immune system, making them particularly vulnerable to this type of overwhelming infectious process.

Physical examination is diagnostic. If the patient presents early during the initial phase of the disease, physical findings may be limited to swelling and erythema of the penis or scrotum. As the process progresses, there may be crepitus in addition to obvious necrosis of the involved skin. A foul feculent odor is common, usually indicating an anerobic infection.

Bacterial cultures of the necrotic tissue or pus usually yield multiple organisms, including anaerobic and aerobic bacteria. Clostridia should be suspected in the presence of concomitant colorectal disease or when subcutaneous emphysema is palpated or identified on radiographic examination. Aggressive broad-spectrum intravenous antibiotics are indicated. Tobramycin, 3 to 5 mg per kilogram for 1 day, is administered in divided doses (every 8 hours) and will cover most gram-negative rods. Daily peak and trough levels are obtained routinely and the tobramycin dosage is adjusted as necessary. Clindamycin, 600 mg, is administered intravenously every 8 hours to provide anaerobic coverage. If clostridia are suspected, 3 million U of penicillin G is also given every 6 hours.

After the patient has been stabilized with fluids and antibiotics have been given, surgical management is undertaken. When a urethral source is suspected, retrograde urethrography is performed. If there is urinary extravasation or a tight urethral stricture, urinary diversion in the form of a suprapubic cystostomy is performed. A proctoscopic examination will help rule out an anorectal source. If significant rectal pathology is identified, consideration is given to a temporary diverting colostomy.

Surgical debridement of all necrotic and devitalized tissue is carried out with the patient in the dorsal lithotomy position. Questionable areas of viability are best left to be re-evaluated after 24 hours. The blood supply of the testes is different from that of the penis and scrotum, and therefore they are rarely involved in the gangrenous process. If significant loss of scrotal skin has occurred, the testes are preserved by placing them into subcutaneous thigh pouches. The wound is irrigated with a 25 percent sodium hypochlorite Dakin's solution and packed with fine-mesh gauge soaked in Dakin's. Frequent dressing changes are performed, and if needed, further debridement is carried out in the operating room. Daily whirlpool therapy is instituted once the patient's condition has stabilized and provides an excellent means of mechanical debridement. The use of hyperbaric oxygen has been reported to reduce morbidity in patients with extensive myonecrosis or subcutaneous emphysema, or in those who fail to respond to standard therapy.

The wounds are closed after a clean bed of granulation tissue has been achieved. Areas of extensive skin loss are covered with split-thickness skin grafts.

In spite of aggressive surgical and medical management, Fournier's gangrene is associated with a significant mortality rate, ranging from 7 to 50 percent. In a retrospective review conducted at my institution, nine of 20 patients (45 percent) died of complications associated with this infectious process.

SUGGESTED READING

Flanigan RC, Kursh ED, McDougal WS, et al. Synergistic gangrene of the scrotum and penis secondary to colorectal disease. J Urol 1978; 119:369–371.

Kearney GP, Carling PC. Fournier's gangrene: an approach to its management. J Urol 1983; 130:695–698.

Spirnak JP, Resnick MI, Hampel N, et al. Fournier's gangrene: report of 20 patients. J Urol 1984; 131:289–291.

SCROTAL ABSCESS

EUGENE F. FUCHS, M.D.

The scrotum is a cutaneous pouch that normally contains the testis, the epididymis, and the spermatic cord structures. It is divided into two compartments by a septum that is manifested on the surface as the median raphe. The skin has a characteristic rugated appearance and typically is sparsely haired. The hair follicles usually are clearly visible.

The multiple layers of the scrotum and spermatic cord are continuations of homologous layers of the abdominal wall. Just below the scrotal skin, and virtually inseparable from it, is the dartos layer, or Colles' fascia, which fuses to Scarpa's fascia on the anterior abdomen, the fascia lata of the thigh, and the fascia of the perineum. The anatomic barrier created by Colles' fascia forms a closed space that tends to contain any blood, edema fluid, or pus that forms within it. It will also contain any urine that may leak from the bulbous urethra in the event of a urethral perforation posteriorly. Colles' fascia also prevents superficial scrotal abscesses from easily penetrating the scrotal compartment.

The layers of the spermatic cord are also continuations of the anterior abdominal layers, but are only loosely attached to the interior surface of the scrotum. The external spermatic fascia is a continuation of the aponeurosis of the external oblique at the external inguinal ring. The cremasteric muscle and fascia correspond to the internal oblique muscle. The internal spermatic fascia is an extension of the transversalis fascia at the level of the internal inguinal ring. Finally, the processus vaginalis is ordinarily an obliterated tongue of peritoneum that extends with the spermatic cord to drape over the testicle superiorly. The portion covering the testis is the tunica vaginalis and normally contains a small amount of fluid, allowing for relatively free movement of the testicle.

The route of the spermatic cord is important because intra-abdominal abscesses can track along a patent processus vaginalis and present as a scrotal mass. Traumatic disruption of the inguinal canal or the attachments of Colles' fascia can contribute to accumulation of intrascrotal blood from retroperitoneal, pelvic, or even lower extremity bleeding. The intrascrotal blood can become secondarily infected and present as a scrotal abscess.

The anatomic barrier of the scrotum and spermatic cord generally prevent superficial infection from invading the scrotal compartment. Conversely, infections arising from within the testis or epididymis remain confined for prolonged periods before finally penetrating the scrotal wall and "pointing" at the surface.

SKIN ABSCESSES

The scrotal skin is colonized with skin flora and is subject to repeated exposure to coliform bacteria from the perianal area. The warm, moist environment of the scrotum is ideal for bacterial growth, but scrotal skin infections are rare, even in debilitated or immunosuppressed men.

When superficial scrotal abscesses do arise, they usually present as infected hair follicles, infection of superficial scrotal lacerations, or similar minor injuries. The involved area is typically surrounded by an area of erythema. The patient rarely has a fever, and pain is minimal. There may be swelling and tenderness of the superficial inguinal lymph nodes. If antibiotics are used, acute selection must be made without benefit of a culture, so it is important to use a broad-spectrum drug to attack the gram-positive cocci and the gram-negative coliform bacteria. The abscess may spontaneously drain with hot compresses or hot baths. It rarely is necessary to place drains or pack the abscess cavity, but local cleaning is important; thus, proper patient education needs attention. Antibiotics may not be needed after drainage occurs. Superficial wound infection following minor scrotal surgery, such as a vasectomy, is unusual.

Such abscesses are best treated by removing the skin sutures to allow wound drainage.

PRIMARY INTRASCROTAL ABSCESSES

Intrascrotal abscesses usually arise from a primary bacterial epididymal orchitis. My experience with this rare problem has been confined to younger men with neglected primary *Escherichia coli* epididymitis, or elderly men who develop acute epididymal orchitis after transurethral resection of the prostate, prolonged urethral catheterization, or even such a minor procedure as a cystoscopy. The presumed mechanism in all cases is retrograde passage of bacteria through the vas and into the epididymis, or possibly via lymphatic or hematogenous spread to the epididymis. If the condition is diagnosed early and appropriate treatment with antibiotics started, abscess formation may be averted. These men usually have a urinary tract infection with the same organism, affording guidance for proper antibiotic selection.

Scrotal ultrasonography is an excellent diagnostic tool to evaluate a possible abscess in men who have an inflammatory mass, or to monitor for abscess formation in patients who may not be responding to appropriate antibiotics. In addition to demonstrating the typical echo pattern of an abscess, the ultrasound examination can determine whether the testis is involved or whether the abscess is confined to the epididymis.

An intrascrotal abscess, regardless of its cause, requires surgical treatment. If preservation of testicular function is essential, an incision and drainage procedure is required. If the contralateral testicle is normal, an orchiectomy may be the most expeditious treatment. In the old or debilitated, an orchiectomy may be the best treatment even in patients with a solitary testicle.

If preservation of testicular function is important, it should be remembered that epididymal function will be destroyed by the abscess. After recovery the testicle may continue spermatogenesis, but the ductal system will be ablated and unable to transport sperm during ejaculation. In cases of *severe* epididymo-orchitis it is unlikely that the germ cell population will survive or that the interstitial cells will escape damage. Continued production of sperm and testosterone after recovery is unlikely.

Incision and Drainage of Scrotal Abscess

An incision and drainage procedure should be performed in the operating room with the patient under general or regional anesthesia. An ample scrotal incision is required. All abscess cavities must be opened and thoroughly drained. If the abscess involves the testicle, it too must be opened. The cavity must be drained with small Penrose drains or packed open with gauze. Drains are difficult to keep indwelling, but they avoid the painful packing changes required if wound packing is chosen. If drains are used, they should remain in place until all drainage has stopped and the inflammatory process has been substantially reduced.

Primary Wide Excision of the Inflammatory Mass and Orchiectomy

When preservation of testicular function is not a concern, it has been my practice to perform an orchiectomy with wide excision of the inflammatory mass and the involved overlying scrotal skin. In some cases, the scrotal skin may be so extensively involved that a hemiscrotectomy is required.

The procedure requires regional or general anesthesia. In a patient who is an extreme anesthetic risk, it is possible to perform the procedure with a high cord block and supplemental local anesthesia. After the usual skin preparation and draping, the limits of the skin incision should be determined (Fig. 1). A circumferential skin incision is made with care to avoid entering the abscess cavity. By blunt and sharp dissection the inflammatory mass can be easily freed from the surrounding scrotal wall and delivered through the scrotal incision. The spermatic cord is dissected free for several centimeters beyond the involved area, but at least to the external inguinal ring, where it is ligated and transected in the usual manner (Fig. 2). To avoid the problem of secondarily infecting the suture, which could be a source of continuing infection postoperatively, I would caution against using braided nonabsorbable ligatures. After the mass is removed the skin should be loosely approximated over a Penrose drain, which can be removed after 36 to 48 hours.

This approach proved efficient and cost effective. Patients recover rapidly and are usually discharged

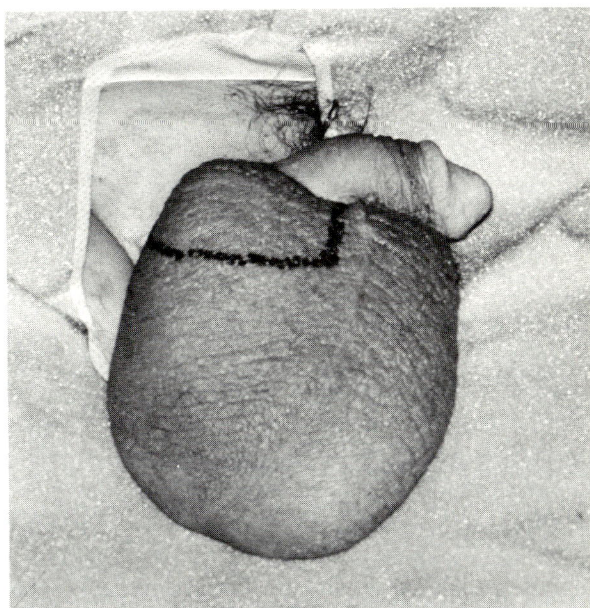

Figure 1   The involved skin has been outlined in preparation for removing a large abscess of the testis and epididymis and the surrounding inflammatory mass.

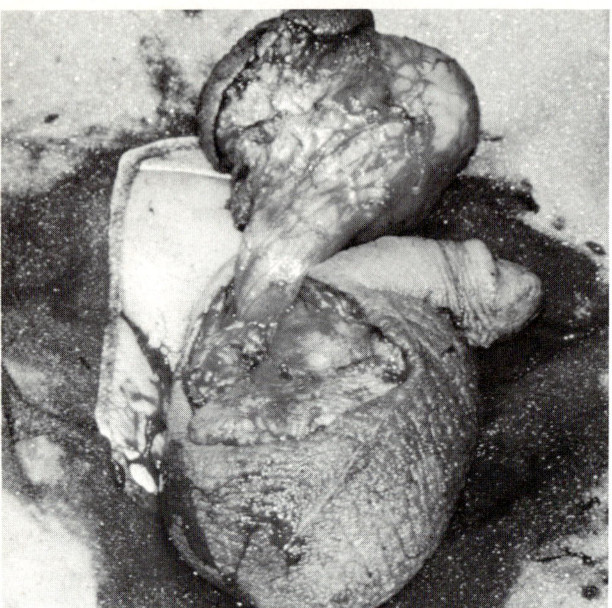

Figure 2 The epididymal testicular abscess, its surrounding inflammatory mass, and the overlying involved skin has been removed en bloc. The spermatic cord has been dissected to the level of the external ring and is about to be ligated and transected.

within a day or so. In no cases, in my experience, has the abscess reaccumulated, nor has there been delayed wound healing. All patients received oral antibiotics for 7 to 10 days postoperatively.

SECONDARY ABSCESSES

Secondary scrotal abscesses occur when an extrascrotal source of infection spreads into the scrotum to present as an infected scrotal mass. Appendiceal abscesses have been reported to present as a scrotal abscess after tracking along a patent processus vaginalis. My personal experience with this problem has been confined to trauma patients who have major posterior disruption of the inguinal canal, so that they accumulate an intrascrotal hematoma that becomes secondarily infected, or a retroperitoneal abscess that spreads along the disrupted inguinal canal to enter the scrotum. When confronted with what appears to be a primary intrascrotal abscess in a patient who has had major abdominal trauma or who has no history suggesting a primary intrascrotal abscess, one must always consider the possibility of a secondary scrotal abscess.

Typically, these patients have a palpable mass that extends along the cord and into the inguinal canal. Ultrasonography and computed tomography (CT) are valuable in correctly diagnosing a secondary abscess. The epididymis and testis are rarely involved, although the abscess cavity may extend to that level and even superficially involve those structures.

Treatment is directed to the primary source, with complete drainage of the infected material. An incision may be required in the inguinal canal or scrotum to drain all the involved tissue layers adequately. Postoperatively, the drains may be removed when the drainage has stopped and the inflammatory reaction has been resolved.

TESTICULAR ABSCESS

LAURENCE B. KANDEL, M.D.
LLOYD H. HARRISON, M.D.

Although suppurative orchitis, or testicular abscess, has probably been known since the time of Hippocrates, it has not been a common medical problem in the 20th century. Urologists occasionally see it in clinical practice, and this chapter describes the presentation, diagnosis, and treatment of this disease.

PATHOGENESIS

Before the advent of antibiotics and immunizations, testicular abscess was seen primarily in patients with gonococcal epididymitis, syphilis, typhoid fever, pneumonia, tuberculosis, leprosy, scarlet fever, mumps, smallpox, chickenpox, influenza, and dengue fever. Now, testicular abscess related to associated bacterial and viral illnesses is nearly extinct. However, invasive support devices (endotracheal tubes, arterial lines, Foley catheters), immunosuppressive chemotherapy, and the liberal use of antibiotics have increased the frequency of fungal testicular abscesses as well as those caused by more resistant bacteria. The wide variety of infectious organisms that have been associated with suppurative orchitis is apparent in Table 1.

Because of the rarity of testicular abscess today, the most common mechanism for infection is difficult to assess. Before the advent of antibiotics, most cases were related to direct extension of suppurative epididymitis. Other known mechanisms range from retrograde seeding of the testicle through the urinary tract to systemic seeding of the testicle from both primary and secondary infections of the bloodstream (Table 2). Although current concepts of pathogenesis do not differ widely from those of 50 years ago, the one-time controversy over whether the testicle infected the urinary tract or became infected from the urinary tract is no longer a focus of discussion, since it is no longer generally accepted that the testicle, like the kidney, serves an excretory function, filtering organisms from the bloodstream and then excreting them into the urinary tract through the ejaculatory ducts.

DIAGNOSIS

Clinical History

Because testicular abscess occurs so infrequently, it is difficult to diagnose early in its course. Clinical suspicion is therefore important for diagnosis. The history may be helpful, and the histories of patients presenting with testicular abscess can be as varied as their ages. What follows is a representative summary of different cases occurring in different age groups.

Neonates and Infants

Interestingly, reports of suppurative orchitis in the newborn continue to appear in the literature. In 1975, a 5-lb 7-oz boy developed *Escherichia coli* septicemia on the second day of life and, even after treatment with antibiotics, underwent orchiectomy 2 weeks later for an *E. coli* testicular abscess. In 1983, testicular suppuration

in an infant aged 1 month was diagnosed and treated with surgical debridement, drainage, and antibiotics. Although the infant had no clinical evidence of disease other than a scrotal mass, *Salmonella enteritidis* was cultured from the abscess.

In the 1920s congenital syphilitic orchitis and testicular tuberculosis in neonates were not all that uncommon; today, these organisms rarely infect newborns in industrialized countries, but they remain potential medical problems for newborns in Third World nations.

Preadolescents and Adolescents

Like the infant, the preadolescent and the adolescent are susceptible to suppurative orchitis. On occasion, a missed testicular torsion may become secondarily infected and present as a testicular abscess; primary infections, although uncommon, also occur. Overall, however, bacterial abscesses are rare in this age group. Most cases of preadolescent testicular abscess appear to be caused by parasitic infections. Naturally, only children in endemic areas are so affected, but this age group in those areas seems highly susceptible because of its inquisitive and exploratory nature.

Adults

The third, fourth, and fifth decades of life are those of greatest sexual activity. Venereal disease with associated epididymo-orchitis is therefore the leading cause of testicular suppuration in this age group.

In the elderly, other disease entities come into play. Generalized illness, cancer, immunosuppression, and bodily invasive diagnostic and therapeutic modalities compromise these patients to resistant bacterial and fungal infections. Three cases of nocardial testicular abscess have been cited in the literature, the two most recent within the last 15 years. One patient, a man of 70 years, had a lymphoproliferative disorder, and the other, a man aged 61 years, had a myeloproliferative disorder; both were being treated with corticosteroids.

Thus, no "classic history" exists for the diagnosis of testicular abscess like those for the diagnosis of diseases

Table 1 Causative Agents of Testicular Abscess

Bacterial
  Gonorrhea (*Neisseria gonorrhoeae*)
  Syphilis (*Treponema pallidum*)
  Tuberculosis (*Mycobacterium tuberculosis*)
  Leprosy (*Mycobacterium leprae*)
  Typhoid (*Salmonella typhi*)
  Gastroenteritis (*Salmonella enteritidis*)
  Undulant fever (*Brucella abortus*)
Viral
  Mumps (*Paramyxovirus mumps*)
  Smallpox (*Orthopoxvirus variola*)
  Dengue fever (*Flavivirus dengue*)
Fungal
  Nocardiosis (*Nocardia asteroides*)
  Actinomycosis (*Actinomyces bovis*)
Parasitic
  Dracunculosis (*Dracunculus medinensis*)
  Bilharziasis (*Schistosoma haematobium*)

Table 2 Etiology of Testicular Abscess

Direct extension of infection
  Suppurative epididymitis
Retrograde seeding from urinary tract
  Cystitis
  Prostatitis
  Epididymitis
Vascular compromise
  Torsion
  Orchitis
  Trauma
  Iatrogenic (inguinal hernia repair)
Systemic infection (bacterial, viral, fungal, parasitic)
  Primary
  Secondary

such as angina pectoris and cholelithiasis. Important considerations focus on a patient's age and on related factors such as sexual activity, geographic location, underlying illness, and the patient's current medical therapy (e.g., steroids, antibiotics).

Signs and Symptoms

Depending on the pathogenesis of the abscess, early associated signs and symptoms are the same as would normally be manifested by the primary disease, e.g., epididymitis, torsion, and mumps. Once the abscess becomes established, high fever, chills, testicular pain (often with radiation to the inguinal canal), and a testicle exquisitely tender to palpation are the usual presentation. Nausea and vomiting may also be present. Rapid cessation of the pain usually indicates that the abscess has ruptured. The exception to this presentation is an abscess secondary to syphilis, when painless enlargement of the testicle is the rule.

Physical Examination

The involved hemiscrotum is erythematous and edematous. If the abscess is long-standing, a draining sinus tract may be present. Palpation of the scrotum and its contents may be difficult because of the extreme sensitivity of the inflamed scrotal wall. The testicle itself is usually swollen, tense, and very tender. If the abscess is large, the testicle may be fluctuant; however, reactive hydroceles are not uncommon and can easily be confused with fluctuance.

Ancillary Tests

If the degree of pain is high, physical examination may not be possible, and although surgical exploration is 100 percent diagnostic, less invasive approaches are available. Testicular ultrasonography has been used, but in most cases it cannot distinguish between an abscess, a neoplasm, orchitis, and a hematoma of the testicle. In contrast, the radionuclide appearance of a testicular abscess is dramatic. There is a marked increase in perfusion of the spermatic cord vessels and throughout the involved hemiscrotum, with the "cooler" area representing the abscessed testicle.

Differential Diagnosis

The diseases to be considered in differential diagnosis are primarily epididymitis, torsion of the spermatic cord, and neoplasm. Epididymitis, as opposed to epididymo-orchitis, does not involve the testicle, and the differential diagnosis can often be made by physical examination alone. Urinalysis, sexual history, and if necessary, a nuclear scan all help to distinguish between the two. By contrast, torsion of the spermatic cord involves both the testicle and the epididymis. By history, the onset of torsion is acute, and more often than not the pain is more severe than that associated with abscess.

Radionuclide scanning usually allows differentiation between abscess and torsion.

Testicular neoplasms classically are not painful and therefore are confused only with granulomatous testicular abscess (i.e., tuberculosis, syphilis, leprosy). Systemic manifestations, skin testing, or serology should resolve any diagnostic dilemmas.

TREATMENT

Once frank abscess has occurred, chemotherapy (antibiotics, antifungal agents) rarely salvages the testicle, and in almost all cases the treatment is surgical. Whether to incise and drain the abscess or to perform an orchiectomy can be decided only at the time of scrotal exploration. Controversy still exists concerning the testicular salvage rate from incision and drainage. Many believe that incision of the tunica albuginea leads to testicular destruction because of complete herniation of the tubules. If, at exploration, the abscess is found to be localized and there is good reason to attempt to salvage testicular tissue, consider incision and drainage as a primary mode of treatment. In support of this, note that spontaneous rupture of an abscess with drainage through a cutaneous sinus and resulting testicular salvage has been reported.

Although chemotherapy remains only an adjuvant to treatment of most abscesses, patients with syphilitic and tubercular abscesses have been reported to be cured without surgical intervention. Nevertheless, regardless of the etiology of the suppuration, most patients require orchiectomy, and it remains the standard treatment.

Once the decision to explore the scrotum has been made, start broad-spectrum intravenous antibiotic coverage if it is not already in progress. Naturally, after culture and sensitivity results become available, employ specific chemotherapy.

Before exploration, obtain answers to the following questions: Has the patient fathered children? If so, does he desire to conceive more children? Has the patient a history of mumps, orchitis, or undescended testicle? What is the status of the contralateral testicle?

If testicular salvage bears weighted consideration, keep this in mind at the time of exploration. If the abscess is small and localized to a well-demarcated area of the testicle, consider incision and drainage as opposed to orchiectomy. If the testicle cannot be salvaged, perform orchiectomy without reservation.

Surgical Technique

Incision and Drainage

With the scrotum shaved of all hair, the surgical field should be thoroughly cleansed with antimicrobial scrub solution. Place the patient either in the supine or in the dorsal lithotomy position according to preference. Make a longitudinal incision over a non–vein-bearing area of the involved hemiscrotum so that the median scrotal raphe is not violated. Make a generous incision so that the entire hemiscrotum along with its contents can be inspected thoroughly. Cultures of the abscess should include routine bacterial (aerobic and anaerobic), fungal, acid-fast, and, if indicated, *Treponema* cultures. Once the testicle has been delivered through the incision, estimate the extent of its damage. Assess the epididymis, vas deferens, and spermatic cord vessels for potential viability. If incision and drainage is elected, remove all necrotic tissue. Irrigate the testicle and the involved hemiscrotum with copious amounts of sterile saline. Remaining tunica albuginea can be *very loosely* reapproximated with a 3-0 or 4-0 chromic suture. Then, place the testicle and cord structures back into the scrotum, inserting a 1-inch Penrose drain into a dependent position in the involved hemiscrotum. Close the most superior aspect of the wound and exteriorize the Penrose drain through the most inferior portion of the wound to allow for adequate dependent drainage. Close the dartos with a running 3-0 chromic suture. The scrotal skin is not sutured, but is dressed with wet-to-dry saline soaks and allowed to heal by secondary intention. Give the patient broad-spectrum antibiotics until the suitability of a specific drug is determined from the results of the intraoperative cultures. This antibiotic is administered until the Penrose drain is removed, on about the seventh postoperative day. By this time the drainage tract should be well established.

Further drug therapy is based on the patient's clinical condition. If at any time the abscess appears to be recurring, do not hesitate to re-explore the scrotum and perform an orchiectomy.

Orchiectomy

For the vast majority of patients, guillotine orchiectomy will be indicated. Preoperative preparation is the same as previously described, and details of the surgical procedure can be found in any of the major urologic surgical textbooks.

If the hemiscrotal wall is abscessed, perform wide excision of the involved tissue. Closure of the debrided hemiscrotum should not be difficult because of the dilatation from the abscess as well as the loss of intrascrotal contents following orchiectomy. Closure of the hemiscrotum may allow placement of a testicular prosthesis at a later date if the patient so desires. If, however, reapproximation of the hemiscrotum is not possible, perform a hemiscrotectomy at the time of orchiectomy.

BLUNT RENAL TRAUMA

CHRISTOPHER M. DIXON, M.D.
JACK W. McANINCH, M.D.

Blunt trauma to the kidney is the most common genitourinary injury. It has many causes, including motor vehicle accidents, assaults, falls, and contact sports. Although the great majority of these injuries are minor (>90 percent), life-threatening renal injuries do occur. The urologist must decide which patient needs radiographic evaluation, which imaging study should be performed, and whether surgical intervention is required. Our management is based on individual case evaluation, accurate injury staging, and selective renal surgery.

PATIENT EVALUATION AND INJURY STAGING

In the traumatized patient, a renal injury is diagnosed by the presence of hematuria (>5 RBC/HPF), assuming that a lower tract injury has been excluded. It is well established that the degree of hematuria does not correlate with the severity of renal injury.

The process of defining the extent of injury is termed "staging" and begins with radiographic imaging, but selected patients may require renal exploration. The purpose of accurate staging is to determine appropriate management (Fig. 1). A renal injury scale has recently been established by the Organ Injury Scaling Committee of the American Association for the Surgery of Trauma (Fig. 2). Minor renal injuries include contusions and parenchymal lacerations confined to the cortex; major renal injuries include vascular, parenchymal, and collecting system injuries. A major laceration is defined as a parenchymal disruption through the corticomedullary junction, with or without violation of the collecting system. Vascular injuries include thrombosis or avulsion of the renal pedicle (main artery or vein) or segmental vessels. Collecting system injuries are usually associated with major lacerations; rarely, the ureter is avulsed at the ureteropelvic junction.

Not every patient with hematuria from blunt trauma requires radiographic investigation. The criteria have been defined. Imaging should be performed if there is gross hematuria, shock, or a clinical indicator of flank trauma. Shock is defined as an initial systolic blood pressure of less than 90 mm Hg and is often determined in the field. Clinical indicators of renal trauma include major intra-abdominal organ injury, physical signs of flank trauma, and deceleration accidents. In such patients, imaging should be considered even in the absence of gross hematuria or shock. Adult patients with microscopic hematuria but no shock generally do not require radiographic imaging; however, clinical assessment is important. These imaging criteria do not apply to children (younger than 16 years of age) or to patients with penetrating injuries.

The choice of radiographic study depends on the clinical situation. In a stable patient, high-dose infusion pyelography (2 ml per kilogram, maximum 150 ml) is performed. If the intravenous pyelogram (IVP) is indeterminate, computed tomography (CT) should be performed. If the trauma surgeon prefers CT or abdominal aortography as an initial study to evaluate possible associated injuries, the kidneys can be imaged simultaneously and the IVP is not needed. CT is being used more frequently as a first study because it accurately stages renal injuries and provides additional information about associated intra-abdominal injuries. Arteriography is most useful for a suspected pedicle injury, but this can also be accurately diagnosed by CT. Ultrasonography has limited usefulness.

Frequently, the urologist is consulted intraoperatively to evaluate a retroperitoneal hematoma found during emergency laparotomy. Under these conditions the IVP is the only imaging study possible and should be done to evaluate the injured kidney and establish a functioning contralateral kidney. Often the IVP will be of poor quality and the kidney must be explored to stage the injury accurately and permit repair. The initial laparotomy is the best time for exploration, because delays carry a reported nephrectomy rate of up to 50 percent.

TREATMENT

Successful management of renal injuries depends on accurate staging. The goals of treatment are to preserve renal function and limit complications. Contusions and

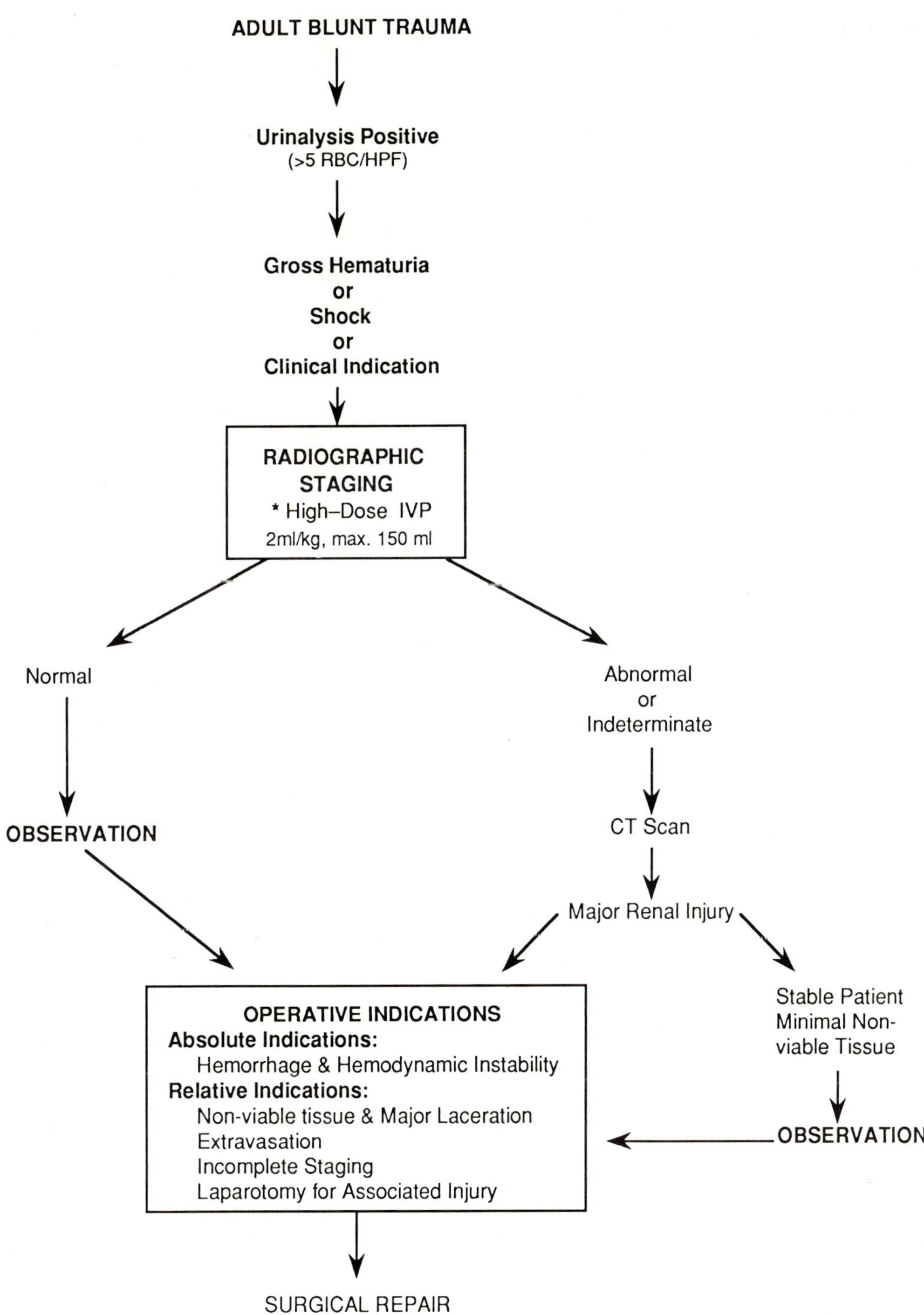

Figure 1 Management protocol for adults in whom a renal injury from blunt trauma is suspected.

minor lacerations should be managed expectantly; major renal injuries require observation or surgery. Our indications for operation are based primarily on clinical findings complemented by results of imaging studies. Absolute indications include continued bleeding with hemodynamic instability, or an expanding or pulsatile hematoma discovered at laparotomy for associated injuries. Relative indications include urinary extravasation, nonviable tissue, laparotomy for associated injury, or incomplete staging of the renal injury.

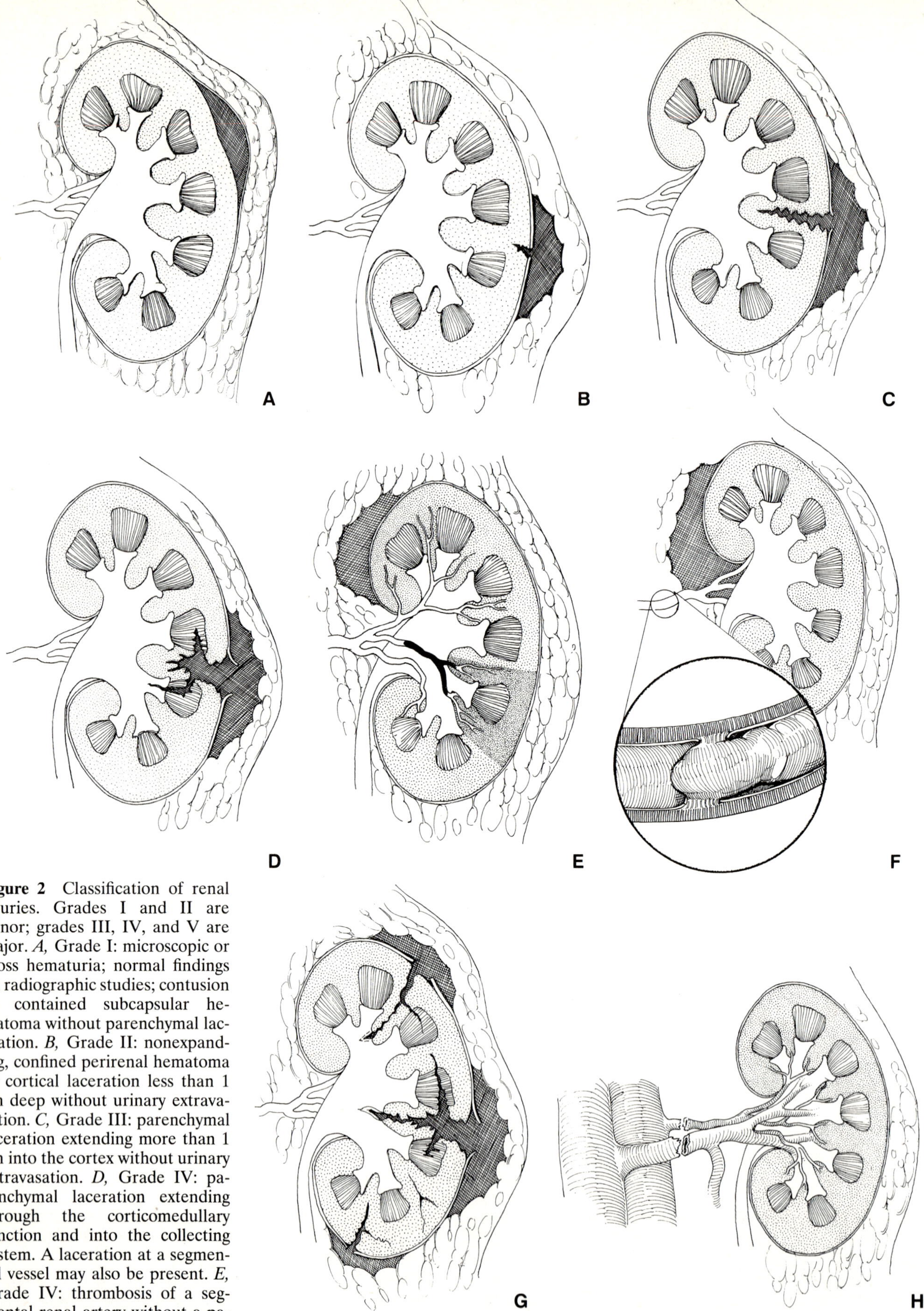

Figure 2 Classification of renal injuries. Grades I and II are minor; grades III, IV, and V are major. *A,* Grade I: microscopic or gross hematuria; normal findings on radiographic studies; contusion or contained subcapsular hematoma without parenchymal laceration. *B,* Grade II: nonexpanding, confined perirenal hematoma or cortical laceration less than 1 cm deep without urinary extravasation. *C,* Grade III: parenchymal laceration extending more than 1 cm into the cortex without urinary extravasation. *D,* Grade IV: parenchymal laceration extending through the corticomedullary junction and into the collecting system. A laceration at a segmental vessel may also be present. *E,* Grade IV: thrombosis of a segmental renal artery without a parenchymal laceration. Note the corresponding parenchymal ischemia. *F,* Grade V: thrombosis of main renal artery. Inset shows intimal tear and distal thrombosis. *G,* Grade V: multiple major lacerations, resulting in a "shattered" kidney. *H,* Grade V: avulsion of main renal artery and/or vein.

Management of major parenchymal lacerations is controversial. After diagnosis, our choice between expectant management or surgery is determined by clinical and radiographic factors. If a major laceration is identified in a hemodynamically stable patient who does not require laparotomy for associated injuries, close observation by serial hematocrits and blood pressure monitoring is recommended. A notable exception is the patient with both a major parenchymal laceration and large devascularized segments of renal tissue, as in a completely transected or shattered kidney. The IVP will be indeterminate because the parenchyma is functioning poorly and the hematoma obscures the renal margins. Because the patient is stable with an indeterminate IVP, we would obtain a CT scan to define the injury accurately and complete the staging process. With a large amount of nonviable tissue and associated major laceration, surgical repair is recommended because of the high risk of delayed bleeding, urinary extravasation, and abscess formation.

Occasionally, a hemodynamically stable patient with a well-staged major renal laceration that would be managed expectantly will undergo a laparotomy for associated intra-abdominal injury. Because delayed bleeding from a major laceration is unpredictable, but renal repair is safe and reliable, we would repair the kidney in such a patient.

Renal pedicle injuries are problematic. Early diagnosis and repair are necessary to preserve renal function. Despite prompt treatment, nephrectomy is common and salvage rare.

Technique of Renal Exploration and Repair

After the decision is made to explore an injured kidney, constant awareness of the patient's clinical condition will determine whether the kidney should be reconstructed or an expeditious nephrectomy performed. (Before nephrectomy, a functioning contralateral kidney must be confirmed by IVP.) In most situations, renal salvage is possible.

The preferred surgical approach is a midline, transabdominal incision. This allows intra-abdominal exploration and access to the aorta and vena cava. After radiographic imaging, renal exploration begins with control of the main renal vessels. Only about 12 percent of renal explorations require clamping of the artery, but because it is impossible to predict which injuries will require pedicle occlusion, early vascular control should be the first step in renal exploration. The transverse colon is lifted superiorly and the small intestines are placed in a transparent "bowel bag" on the right chest. This allows periodic inspection of the intestines and provides excellent exposure of the retroperitoneum. The posterior peritoneum is incised in the midline over the aorta; if the aorta is not palpable because of a large hematoma, the incision is made medial to the inferior mesenteric vein (Fig. 3). The incision should extend to the ligament of Treitz, and dissection proceeds cephalad along the aorta, exposing

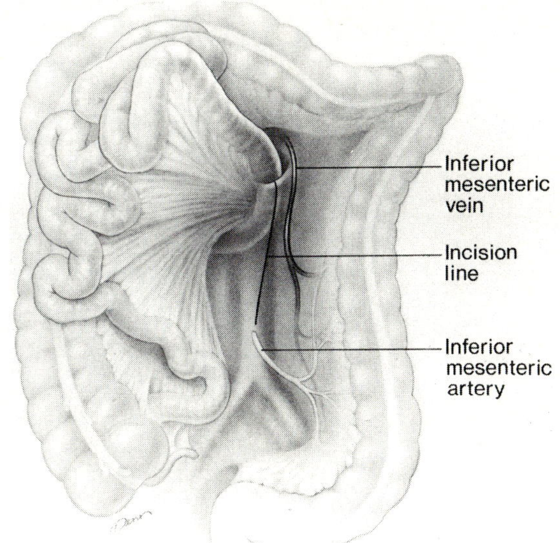

Figure 3 Incision into the posterior peritoneum. Note the location of the inferior mesenteric vein.

an important landmark, the left renal vein, which crosses anteriorly. The left renal artery is identified superior and posterior and the right renal artery superior and medial to the left renal vein. The right renal artery can be controlled between the aorta and the vena cava. Figure 4 depicts the usual anatomic relationships of the renal vasculature. By following the anterolateral borders of the aorta, accessory renal arteries may also be identified and controlled. The arteries can be circled with a vessel loop near their origin from the aorta. Control of the veins is not as essential and is more difficult on the right because the renal vein is shorter on that side.

Complete mobilization of the kidney and exposure of the injury are essential to successful repair. After the colon is reflected, Gerota's fascia is sharply incised and the anterolateral surface of the kidney exposed through the hematoma. Occasionally, there are small vessels in the perirenal space that must be ligated or coagulated. If hemorrhage is going to be significant, it often begins shortly after Gerota's fascia is opened; therefore, the injured kidney should be mobilized quickly by a combination of blunt and sharp dissection. If the renal capsule has been disrupted, care must be taken to avoid inadvertent subcapsular dissection, particularly if the laceration is located posteriorly and is not directly visible. The adrenal gland is dissected superiorly by staying close to the renal capsule; on the left, the tail of the pancreas must also be avoided. If bleeding is excessive, the main artery should be occluded. This can be done by applying Rumel tourniquets to the vessel loops or using bulldog vascular clamps. If the repair is anticipated to take longer than 30 minutes, the kidney should be cooled with slush. After complete mobilization, the assistant can hold the kidney so that gentle compression along the laceration margin will control bleeding and allow inspection but permit circulation to

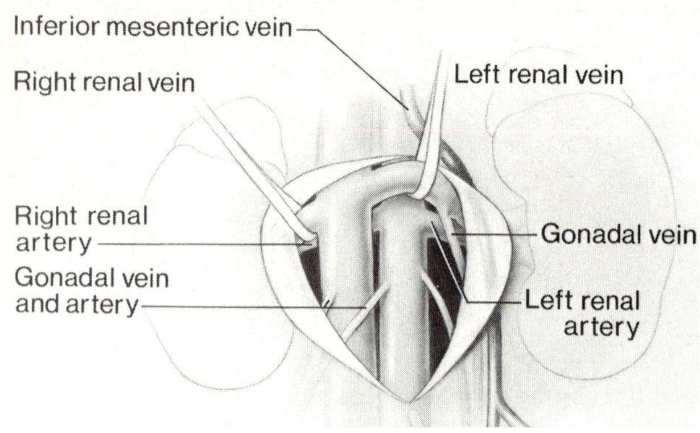

Figure 4 Anatomic relationships of the renal vasculature.

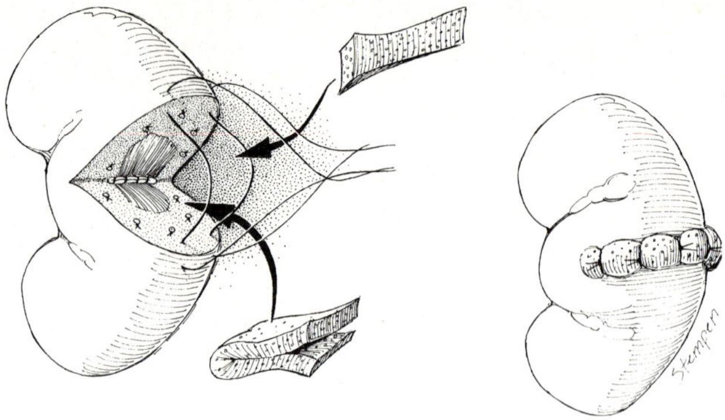

Figure 5 Reconstruction of a midparenchymal laceration.

the parenchyma. Actively bleeding vessels should be suture ligated with absorbable material. Nonviable tissue should be debrided and the collecting system closed with running 4-0 chromic sutures.

Major polar lacerations are best treated by partial nephrectomy. Midportion injuries can be reconstructed with an absorbable bolster. After all nonviable tissue has been debrided and the collecting system closed and bleeding points have been controlled, a first layer of an absorbable bolster (Gelfoam) is packed into the defect. The defect is closed by reapproximating the renal capsule with 2-0 chromic sutures. These are tied over a second layer of the bolster, which prevents them from tearing through the capsule. The bolster also effectively seals the defect (Fig. 5). A mobilized flap of omentum is useful after partial nephrectomy and to cover large parenchymal defects. Usually, this can be done by dividing the omentum without taking down the short gastric vessels and bringing it through a small window in the mesentery of the colon.

Injuries of the main renal artery or vein are the most difficult to repair successfully. Vascular control is essential. Partial lacerations of the main vessels can be repaired with 5-0 vascular suture. Avulsion or thrombosis of the artery from intimal tearing requires arterial repair, autotransplantation, or nephrectomy. Segmental renal vessels are usually too small for reconstruction and should be ligated. If there is an associated major laceration involving a thrombosed segmental artery, a partial nephrectomy should be performed.

After the repair has been completed, the kidney is returned to its normal position inside Gerota's fascia, but the fascia is not closed. Drainage should be considered if the collecting system has been violated or if there is an associated bowel injury.

Postoperative Management

Gross hematuria usually clears within 24 hours, but microscopic hematuria may take weeks to resolve. Ambulation is encouraged as soon as gross hematuria resolves. If a retroperitoneal drain has been used, the drainage can be checked for creatinine to determine whether urine is leaking. Usually the drain should be removed in 24 to 72 hours to prevent infection of the retroperitoneum. Frequent blood pressure and daily hematocrit determinations should be obtained until they stabilize.

Functional studies of the injured kidney are routinely performed 10 days and 3 months after injury. These include a dimercaptosuccinic acid (DMSA) or glucoheptanate renal scan and IVP. Blood pressure should be measured every 2 months for the first year and annually thereafter.

Complications

Postoperative complications include renal bleeding, urinoma with abscess formation, and hypertension. Renal failure is uncommon unless a solitary kidney has been injured.

Because of limited long-term follow-up data, the incidence of hypertension after renal injury is unknown. Available literature suggests an incidence of about 5 percent, but, depending on the type of renal injury, a range of 1 to 57 percent has been reported. Presumably, hypertension after renal injury is caused by elevations of renin and angiotensin II from parenchymal ischemia. This can have several causes: thrombosis or occlusion of the main renal artery (Goldblatt model), segmental arterial thrombosis, renal compression from a perinephric hematoma (Page kidney), an arteriovenous fistula, or parenchymal injuries. Hypertension usually develops within the first year of injury, but cases have been reported as long as 14 years later. The clinical presentation varies from mild blood pressure elevation to hypertensive encephalopathy. When hypertension develops several days after injury, it usually resolves spontaneously; when it persists or occurs beyond the hospitalization period, it should be aggressively investigated and treated, particularly in young patients. Persistent hypertension seems to respond better to conservative surgery in the first year than at a later time. Frequent blood pressure determinations are therefore most important during the first year, but lifelong follow-up is advisable.

Clinically significant extravasation often becomes manifest as prolonged ileus or fever. Usually, percutaneous drainage is attempted, but surgical drainage and renal repair may be required. Small amounts of extravasation seen on early postoperative radiographic studies, particularly CT scans, often resolve without intervention. Ureteral stents generally are not needed.

SUGGESTED READING

Carroll PR, Klosterman P, McAninch JW. Early vascular control for renal trauma: a critical view. J Urol 1989; 141:826–829.

Carroll PR, McAninch JW. Staging of renal trauma. Urol Clin North Am 1989; 16:193–202.

Cass AS. Renovascular injuries from external trauma: diagnosis, treatment, and outcome. Urol Clin North Am 1989; 16:213–220.

McAninch JW, Carroll PR. Renal exploration after trauma: indications and reconstructive techniques. Urol Clin North Am 1989; 16:203–212.

Mee SL, McAninch JW, Robinson AL, et al. Radiographic assessment of renal trauma: 10-year prospective study of patient selection. J Urol 1989; 141:1095–1098.

Peterson NE. Complications of renal trauma. Urol Clin North Am 1989; 16:221–236.

Watts RA, Hoffbrand BI. Hypertension following renal trauma. J Hum Hypertens 1987; 1:65–71.

PENETRATING RENAL TRAUMA

J. PATRICK SPIRNAK, M.D.

Renal trauma is classified according to the mechanism of injury as either penetrating or blunt. Penetrating renal injuries are further divided into those caused by gunshot and those caused by knife wounds. The incidence of penetrating renal injuries varies, depending on the urban location and the number of violent crimes committed in that area. Blunt renal injuries are usually more common in a civilian population and account for up to 80 percent of all cases of renal trauma. Although penetrating renal injuries account for only approximately 20 percent of all renal trauma cases, they represent 80 to 90 percent of all renal injuries that require surgical exploration. All patients with penetrating gunshot injuries to the chest or abdomen and a concomitant renal injury have at least one other significant organ injury; therefore, surgical exploration is required in all cases. At the time of surgery the kidney is explored and repaired. Because renal stab wounds are more likely to occur without concomitant organ injury, a course of careful clinical observation may be warranted in selected patients.

EVALUATION

All clinically stable patients presenting to the emergency room with abdominal or lower thoracic gunshot wounds undergo an emergency intravenous pyelogram (IVP) as part of the initial clinical evaluation. The study is performed in the emergency room while resuscitation is being performed. To maximize the amount of clinical information obtained by the study, sufficient contrast material must be administered: 1 ml per pound body weight is rapidly injected intravenously (150 ml of contrast for the average 70-kg person). Abdominal x-ray films are obtained at 1, 5, and 10 minutes; the quality of these is often suboptimal, but usually is adequate to document the presence of either one or two functioning kidneys. Since I believe that all renal gunshot wounds with concomitant abdominal penetration must be surgically explored, additional radiographic studies to better delineate the severity of the injury are seldom if ever required. The emergency IVP is best thought of as providing information regarding the presence and function of the noninjured kidney rather than as a means to stage the extent of the renal injury because visual inspection of the injured kidney will be performed at the time of surgery. When renal injury is suspected, the bullet's path is retroperitoneal, and a peritoneal lavage is negative, computed tomography (CT) is useful to stage the extent of the renal injury further. CT is also extremely helpful in staging the extent of parenchymal laceration associated with stab wounds.

A urinalysis is performed in all trauma victims. The presence of hematuria suggests a urologic injury, but its absence does not exclude renal involvement. Renal pedicle injuries may occur with minimal or no hematuria.

GUNSHOT WOUNDS

Patients with gunshot wounds are examined and the entrance wound is noted. The presence of an exit wound suggests a high-velocity injury and should alert the physician to more extensive tissue injury than is readily apparent because of the blast effect of the missile. In such patients extensive tissue debridement may be required to avoid tissue necrosis and delayed hemorrhage.

All patients with penetrating abdominal gunshot wounds are explored through a xiphoid-to-pubis midline incision. This approach allows for adequate exposure regardless of the organ injured. Mortality in renal trauma patients, with rare exceptions, is determined by the severity of associated nonrenal injuries. In the absence of a pulsatile hematoma or transection of the renal pedicle, all nonurologic injuries are managed prior to renal exploration. Proximal control of the renal pedicle is obtained before the kidney is explored. The posterior peritoneum directly over the aorta is incised vertically, and the dissection is carried cephalad until the left renal vein is identified. The right renal artery is identified between the vena cava and aorta; the left is usually identified just cephalad to the left renal vein as it crosses the aorta. A vessel loop is placed around the renal artery. The colon is reflected medially and Gerota's fascia opened. If excessive bleeding occurs, temporary occlusion of the renal artery will allow for the exploration and repair to proceed in a bloodless field.

It is important to mobilize and inspect the entire kidney. All devitalized tissue is debrided, bleeding vessels are ligated, the collecting system is closed, and parenchymal edges are reapproximated with absorbable suture. Significant tissue defects are filled with a pedicle graft of omentum or perinephric fat. Extensive polar injuries are managed by partial nephrectomy. The retroperitoneum is then drained.

STAB WOUNDS

The management of renal stab wounds continues to evolve. In general, renal stab wounds anterior to the anterior axillary line are associated with a high incidence of other intra-abdominal organ injuries and require prompt surgical exploration and repair. The management of renal stab wounds confined to the flank is controversial. Since there is a low incidence of associated retroperitoneal or intra-abdominal injuries when the renal stab wound occurs posterior to the anterior axillary line, a nonoperative approach may be indicated in selected patients. Such an approach is considered when the peritoneal lavage is negative, there is no evidence of severe blood loss, the vital signs are stable, and CT findings are suggestive of a superficial renal laceration. The patient is placed at bed rest until the urine is grossly clear. Frequent physical examinations and serial hematocrit readings are obtained. Broad-spectrum intravenous antibiotics are administered. If hemodynamic instability (shock) occurs or signs of peritoneal irritation develop, surgery is performed.

POSTOPERATIVE CARE

Postoperative management is similar to that of other urologic patients who undergo major renal surgery. The drain is usually removed in 2 to 3 days or when drainage has ceased. A follow-up IVP is obtained 2 to 3 months after discharge. The patient's blood pressure is followed closely for the first year. The onset of gross hematuria suggests the possibility of an arteriovenous fistula, which is investigated by arteriography, and if present is managed by embolizing the involved renal vessel.

TRAUMATIC URETERAL INJURY

WINSTON K. MEBUST, M.D.

Blunt trauma that causes ureteral injury is rare. It usually occurs in a young child from a hyperextension injury to the back (e.g., being hit from behind by a car). Classically, there is an evulsion of the ureter from the ureteropelvic junction. Penetrating injuries are significantly more common. Approximately 2.2 to 5 percent of abdominal gunshot wounds have associated ureteral injuries. The ureter is somewhat difficult to injure because it is small and deep in the retroperitoneum. Stab wounds account for only about 4 to 5 percent of ureteral injuries from penetrating trauma, compared with 95 percent from gunshot wounds.

The site of the penetration should raise suspicions of a possible ureteral injury when it is near the area of the ureter. Microscopic hematuria is a common finding in ureteral injuries from penetrating abdominal trauma, but occasionally, there is gross hematuria. However, in 10 to 35 percent of patients the urinalysis is normal.

At my institution, intravenous pyelography (IVP) is performed for all penetrating injuries associated with hematuria, either gross or microscopic. Many authors have suggested that visualization of the urinary tract is necessary only in patients who have either gross or microscopic hematuria associated with shock. However, we believe that the urologist, who has only modest exposure to trauma patients, should still obtain an IVP if possible in such situations. The most common finding on IVP is extravasation of the contrast material. Other signs of possible ureteral injury are ureteral dilatation and deviation of the ureter by a massive hematoma. Although 20 to 40 percent of IVPs may be read as normal, I believe that IVP is necessary, not only to ascertain the extent of possible renal injury but also to be sure of the functional status of both kidneys.

If there is a suspicion of ureteral injury and the patient is stable, a retrograde pyelogram can confirm the diagnosis. However, this is rarely the case, because many patients need exploration for injury to other intra-abdominal organs. Often, an IVP is not obtained when the patient is admitted to a smaller hospital. The injury is then found at the time of surgical exploration; this has been reported in as many as 50 percent of ureteral injuries. The surgeon's attention is called to the possibility of a ureteral injury because of the site of the penetration. The site of injury is usually the upper or middle ureter.

The type of gunshot wound is also of importance. High-velocity missiles can cause a cavitation defect of 30 to 40 times the volume of the missile. Such missiles classically are hunting rifles (i.e., as a 30-06) and military weapons (M-16 or AK-47). Handguns are not necessarily low-velocity missiles. A 22-caliber missile has a muzzle velocity of 1,120 feet per second compared with a 38-caliber bullet, which has a muzzle velocity of 855 feet per second. Therefore, the extent of injury to a ureter from a high-velocity missile may not be apparent when evaluated at surgery. With the cavitation effect of the missile, the small vessels to the ureter can be injured. The surgeon can be suspicious of a high-velocity missile injury if the type of weapon is known or suspected or if there is extensive retroperitoneal hemorrhage from the penetrating bullet. With a high-velocity missile injury to the ureter, more extensive debridement is indicated. Occasionally, the ureter will appear only contused. Depending on the surgeon's judgment, this contusion should probably be excised and a ureteroureterostomy performed. A stent is always used. If there is minimal contusion, it is safest to perform a proximal ureterotomy and insert a double-J stent. The area should also be carefully drained.

For a frank injury from a high-velocity missile, even with extensive debridement and use of an internal stent, I also recommend proximal diversions with a nephrostomy, or use the universal stent, which can act as an indwelling stent as well as a nephrostomy tube. This can be a percutaneous nephrostomy, done in the immediate postoperative period, if the patient's condition makes it inadvisable to take the additional time to mobilize the kidney.

REPAIR OF MIDDLE AND UPPER URETERS

At our institution, all penetrating gunshot wounds are explored through a midline abdominal incision.

Ureteral injuries are almost always associated with other intra-abdominal organ injuries that usually take priority over the repair of the ureter. Once these organs are repaired, however, the site of ureteral injury should be ascertained. If there is a large retroperitoneal hematoma, it may be necessary to dissect from the renal pelvis down through the hematoma. The ureter should be carefully mobilized, preserving its blood supply as much as possible. If the injury was not documented with IVP before surgery, it may be necessary to induce a brief diuresis with Lasix and saline and give the patient intravenous methylene blue to identify the site of injury.

Penetrating injuries to the upper and middle ureter are then repaired by a ureteroureterostomy. The damaged tissue is resected back to freely bleeding viable tissue. By mobilizing the ureter, and if necessary, the kidney, as much as 3 to 5 cm of additional length may be obtained. The ureteral ends are spatulate for a distance of 1 cm (Fig. 1) and then reapproximated. The closure is a watertight and mucosa-to-mucosa anastomosis with running 5-0 chromic sutures (more recently, PDS). This is done over a No. 7 French pigtail catheter or double-J stent. Magnifying loops are useful. Some surgeons prefer an interrupted suture line to a running suture.

The use of proximal diversion also is somewhat controversial. If there has been pancreatic or duodenal injury, a proximal diversion is performed. Again, a universal stent, which can function as a nephrostomy tube, and a ureteral stent are useful. If possible, the ureteral repair should be wrapped with omentum, especially if there is a suture line repairing another organ in the immediate vicinity and when there are vascular injuries. The vascular suture line and ureteral suture line should not be in proximity. I then prefer to drain the area with a suction type of drain (Jackson-Pratt).

The principles of ureterostomy are (1) adequate debridement; (2) watertight anastomosis without tension; (3) isolation of the anastomosis from associated injuries whenever possible; (4) a ureteral stent; and (5) proximal diversion when circumstances warrant it.

LOWER URETERAL INJURIES

Lower ureteral injuries are rarely, if ever, managed by a ureteroureterostomy. I prefer to perform a ureteroneocystostomy and, if possible, to tunnel the ureter into the bladder to prevent vesicoureteral reflux. A stent (No. 8 infant feeding tube) is placed up to the kidney and brought out through a separate stab wound in the bladder. If there has been loss of ureteral substance, it may be necessary to perform a simple end-on anastomosis into the dome of the bladder. This is acceptable if the patient is male, because males are less prone to infections than females.

I prefer, however, to mobilize the bladder, as for a psoas hitch, taking down the vascular pedicles on the contralateral side to provide additional mobility to bring the bladder up to the psoas. This permits a tunnel, antirefluxing anastomosis. A Boari flap may be necessary, or a combination of the psoas hitch and Boari flap. A transureteroureterostomy is also a possibility in a lower ureteral injury, but this places at jeopardy the contralateral kidney and ureter.

PROBLEM SITUATIONS

Extensive loss of ureteral substance in the middle and upper ureter may rule out a primary ureteroureterostomy. A transureteroureterostomy also is usually not possible. Substituting bowel for ureter or an autotransplant procedure may be considered, but usually the patient's condition makes this inadvisable. At this point, a staged repair is preferable. One can simply tie off the ureter and perform a percutaneous nephrostomy during the immediate postoperative period. If the kidney has already been mobilized, a simple intraoperative nephrostomy can be done. If it is apparent that a percutaneous nephrostomy probably cannot be performed in the immediate future because of patient status, a No. 8 infant feeding tube can be placed up to the kidney and the ureter tied around the tube. The tube is brought out laterally through a separate stab wound, bringing the ureter toward the skin. If a primary cutaneous ureterostomy is possible, this is advisable. However, leaving the stent in place, with the ureter being drained by the infant feeding tube, offers a temporary solution. Every attempt should be made to repair to retroperitonealize the ureter in such a situation.

A nephrectomy is rarely indicated. Sometimes, however, a vascular graft has been put in place and it is apparent that a primary ureterostomy cannot be accomplished. If there is concern over possible leakage of urine, even with a nephrostomy tube in place, a nephrectomy should be considered.

The use of proximal diversion with a nephrostomy

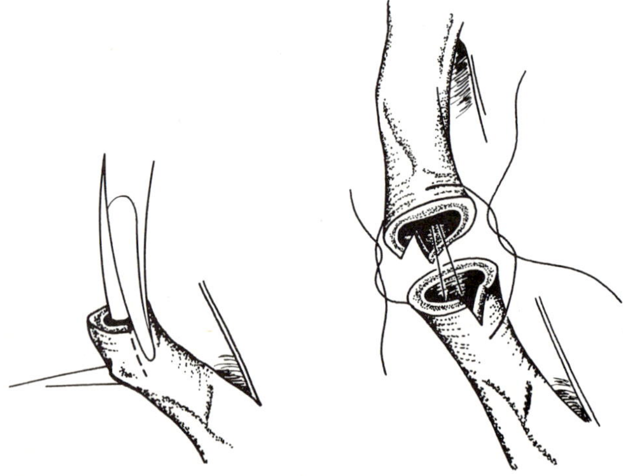

Figure 1 A ureteroureterostomy is done by first excising the devitalized ureteral tissue. The ureters are then spatulated and reapproximated with a mucosa-to-mucosa anastomosis, using a fine absorbable suture.

tube is controversial. This has usually been reserved for situations in which there is an associated pancreatic or duodenal injury or a high-velocity missile injury to the ureter. Certainly, the reported complications are less when it is done routinely compared with a simple indwelling ureteral stent or when neither a stent nor a nephrostomy tube is used.

LATE COMPLICATIONS

Late complications can occur at a rate as high as 18 percent, depending on the type of injury, the type of repair, and whether stenting and proximal diversion have been performed. The more common problems are ureterocutaneous urinary fistula, stricture, and hydronephrosis.

I use ureteral stents routinely and leave them in place for approximately 4 weeks. At that time, an IVP is performed, or if a nephrostomy has also been done, a nephrostomy tube injection is performed to determine the status of the ureteral repair. If there appears to be no leakage, the stent is removed. A repeat IVP is carried out after approximately 4 months.

IVP or ultrasonography of the kidneys is performed at 4 months to ensure that hydronephrosis is not developing. This is repeated 1 year after the injury. If a ureteral stricture develops, it may be treated with balloon dilatation, either antegrade or retrograde, as the situation may warrant, or a formal repair may be necessary.

BLUNT URETERAL TRAUMA

As previously noted, this classically occurs in the young child from a hyperextension injury as in being struck from the rear by an automobile. The ureter is avulsed at the ureteropelvic junction. The diagnosis usually becomes apparent because of persistent fever and a palpable mass and is confirmed by an IVP. The urinoma is drained percutaneously and the patient is placed on appropriate antibiotics. A percutaneous nephrostomy is performed. The decision whether to repair the injury at this time or later is dependent on the status of the child and the surgeon's experience with this type of injury. There are no extensive series comparing delayed or immediate repair in this situation. Usually the status of the child dictates a delay in the repair, after which delay it may be impossible to do a primary ureteropelvic anastomosis. At this time a lower caliceal ureteral anastomosis should be considered. At the time of repair, I usually stent the anastomotic repair with an infant feeding tube or a double-J stent and also use a nephrostomy tube. A universal stent again may be useful, functioning both as a ureteral stent and a nephrostomy tube.

SUGGESTED READING

Franco I, Eshghi M, Schutte H, et al. Value of proximal diversion and ureteral stenting in management of penetrating ureteral trauma. Urology 1988; 32:99–102.
Guerriero WC. Ureteral injury. Urol Clin North Am 1989; 16:237–248.
Pitts JC III, Peterson NE. Penetrating injuries of the ureter. J Trauma 1981; 21:978–982.
Rober PE, Smith JB, Pierce JM Jr. Gunshot injuries of the ureter. J Trauma 1990; 30:83–86.

IATROGENIC URETERAL INJURY

GILBERT ROSS, Jr., M.D.

Iatrogenic ureteral injuries most frequently involve the pelvic ureter, generally when a hysterectomy or some other pelvic procedure is complicated by an inflammatory process. If possible the ureter must be visualized, or at least its relationship clarified, before clamping, cutting, or ligation in areas where it is particularly vulnerable to injury: behind the ovary in the ovarian fossa, within the ureterosacral ligaments, or (most often) in the juxtavesical portion of the ureter where it is crossed anteriorly by the uterine artery lateral to the cervix.

A relatively large number of minor injuries to the lower third of the ureter are related to various endoscopic procedures. Most of these are recognized and dealt with appropriately, and generally heal uneventfully. By the same token, endourologic procedures and techniques have been valuable in dealing with a ureteral injury either definitively or as a temporizing measure when definitive correction cannot be undertaken at the time of diagnosis. Along with the great expansion of endourologic techniques in patient management has come the realization that earlier caveats regarding the necessity for waiting as long as 6 months before undertaking definitive repair of an injury not recognized within the first day or two are quite unnecessary. Such injuries can often be dealt with expeditiously, producing enhanced patient comfort and sometimes a superior clinical outcome.

Many absorbable suture materials are available for ureteral repair. Chromic catgut is often selected because of its reported resistance to premature dissolution in infected urine. Recent in vitro studies have failed to confirm the superiority of chromic catgut in this context, and the synthetic materials polyglycolic acid (PGA) and polyddioxanone (PDS) may be equally acceptable. In fact, the resistance of such sutures to urinary pathogens may be organism specific. The size of the suture should be the smallest compatible with the requisite tissue strength and resistance to tension required (4-0 chromic has long been standard). Some of the smaller synthetics may do equally well, but PDS remains in tissue long after losing tensile strength and may therefore be a consideration with regard to foreign body stone formation.

When there are no known urinary pathogens, the use of antibacterial agents may be irrational; however, we typically use an aminoglycoside and first-generation cephalosporin preoperatively and for a day or two after surgery. When bowel is used, both mechanical (GoLytely) and antibacterial (erythromycin base and neomycin) bowel preparation is advisable.

ENDOUROLOGIC INJURIES

Several injuries, generally minor perforations, of the lower ureter attend various forms of stone manipulation, particularly ureteroscopy. Such injuries may be avoided, or their impact ameliorated, by certain procedures: a good quality x-ray examination that defines the anatomy prior to the procedure; use of a safety guidewire that will virtually assure the passage of a ureteral stent in the event of a perforation; use of the smallest ureteroscope that will accomplish the job at hand; use of the C-arm, or over-the-table fluoroscopy, during ureteroscopy if it is available; minimization of ureteral trauma during dilatation; and finally (and most important), immediate discontinuation of the procedure if a perforation is recognized, leaving a ureteral stent in place for 3 or 4 days. A sizeable perforation and the inability to place a stent generally necessitate a percutaneous nephrostomy.

Less commonly encountered is a ureteral avulsion. This may be a simple sleevelike mucosal avulsion that will respond to stent placement and internal diversion, notwithstanding the possibility of a late ureteral stricture. Alternatively, full-thickness avulsion of the ureter generally involves the lower ureter, and if feasible, should be corrected on the spot with reimplantation into the bladder. Avulsion of most of the ureter presents a formidable problem in repair that initially, at least, requires the placement of a nephrostomy and possibly percutaneous drainage of any areas of urine collection. Balloon occlusion of the proximal ureter may be attempted in the event of continued extravasation.

Nephrectomy may have to be considered as an early alternative to an extensive reconstructive procedure such as autotransplantation of the kidney or the construction of an ileal ureter.

With the expansion of laparoscopic abdominal surgery to include cholecystectomy, and pelvic lymph node biopsy, it is inevitable that occasional ureteral injuries will occur. Most will be unrecognized initially, and their management is discussed later in the chapter.

INJURIES TO THE PELVIC URETER

Injuries to the pelvic ureter are particularly prone to occur when it is involved with significant distortion or inflammatory disease. Occasionally the ureter may be injured during the performance of a radical prostatectomy or diverticulectomy, but reports indicate that injuries to the pelvic ureter in the male are distinctly uncommon during open surgery.

The injury may result from a laceration, delayed ischemic necrosis from skeletonization of the ureter, clamping in the vicinity of the ureter (usually during an attempt to control bleeding), partial or complete ligation, or kinking.

Intraoperative Treatment

The results of immediate treatment are excellent, so if there is even a faint possibility that the ureter has been lacerated, indigo carmine and furosemide should be given intravenously to identify a possible leak. If there is a question of ureteral ligation, it should be investigated by either cystoscopy and retrograde passage of a ureteral catheter, or by a ureterotomy somewhat above the point of suspected ligation with the antegrade passage of a ureteral catheter. Ureteral catheters may also be passed through the flexible cystoscope without repositioning the patient, but this is time consuming. It is often most expeditious simply to open the bladder and pass a catheter retrograde; this will permit the subsequent passage of a double-J stent if necessary.

If the ureter has been ligated with a substantial amount of periureteral tissue for a few minutes, a simple deligation may be all that is required, although prudence would advocate stenting the area for several weeks. When little periureteral tissue is involved in the ligation or particularly when the ureter has been directly crushed, 1 ampule of fluorescein dye injected intravenously and inspection of the area using a Woods light to assess the blood supply may be helpful but is often indeterminate. In this instance, it is best to proceed on the assumption that the ureter will become ischemic and to take steps to avoid a ureteral fistula by performing a definitive repair.

Small ureteral leaks should be stented with a double-J stent and closed with fine interrupted sutures of 4-0 chromic catgut. If the ureter is largely or completely divided, the safest course of action is to reimplant it into the bladder via an intravesical approach and submucosal tunnel. If there is some reduction in ureteral length or, as a matter of surgical preference, an extravesical reimplantation on the anterolateral surface of the bladder may be performed as an alternative. This requires less ureteral length and has provided good results in renal transplantation surgery. Two parallel incisions about 2 to 3 cm apart are made perpendicular to the anticipated course of the ureter and are deepened to expose the mucosa, which is then dissected free from the overlying flap of muscle and adventitia. The ureter is drawn below the spermatic cord in the male, distally beneath this flap. The distal mucosa is opened, and a direct anastomosis is made between the full thickness of the ureter and the mucosa of the bladder with interrupted 4-0 chromic catgut sutures. During the anastomosis, a feeding tube should bridge the anastomosis until the last stitch or two is taken, to eliminate any possibility of ureterovesical junction occlusion. The distal portion of the isolated myoadventitial flap is then approximated to the adjacent distal bladder wall over the ureteral anastomosis, using the same suture material. This procedure is satisfactory because it does not require opening the bladder, requires relatively brief periods of Foley catheter drainage, and seems to be trouble-free for the most part. Regrettably, it may be hard to catheterize if late ureterovesical junction obstruction develops.

If the ureteral injury is some distance above the bladder, precluding a tension-free anastomosis, either form of reimplantation may be augmented with a psoas hitch using heavy, long-lasting absorbable suture. Alternatively, if the injury occurs high in the pelvic ureter, the choices are a Boari flap repair or ureteroureterostomy. If there has been much loss of the ureter below the level of injury, ureteroureterostomy may not be feasible, although it is by far the fastest of the two methods. Transureteroureterostomy, discussed later in this chapter, also has broad applications to many reconstructive problems in the pelvis.

A bladder flap repair can be used to replace large losses of the ureter up to the pelvic brim and sometimes virtually the entire ureter if the kidney is mobilized and deflected downward. There is inevitably some reduction in the size of the bladder, and therefore the potential length of the flap must take into consideration residual bladder volume. Typically, the base of the flap should be about 4 cm in width and located somewhat above the trigone, with the flap directed toward the anterior contralateral side of the bladder where it narrows somewhat toward its tip. If greater length is required, it may be made in a spiral, circumferential fashion to provide a long flap. The flap is closed on itself in several layers using 3-0 chromic catgut. I prefer to close the mucosa with a running stitch, with a second running stitch to close the muscular coat of the bladder, reinforced with interrupted seromuscular sutures. If this narrows the flap too much, the second layer should be interrupted, excluding the mucosa. This closure will be contiguous with the bladder closure, which may be made in two or three layers. The ureter can be implanted into the tip of the flap, end to end or end to side, advancing

the ureter beneath a submucosal tunnel before finishing the closure of the flap. The ureteral anastomosis is done with 4-0 chromic catgut. I prefer this latter method, but even with an end-to-end anastomosis, reflux is not inevitable. The flap is usually edematous and the anastomosis should be stented for several weeks, using a double-J stent. It is well to protect the closure with a urethral catheter on an interim basis and a suprapubic catheter and wound drains. I advocate anchoring the flap to the psoas muscle. Even if reflux occurs, any long-term deleterious effect is unlikely if the upper tracts are normal.

Ureteroureterostomy is a much faster procedure if there is little loss of ureteral length. The ends of the ureter should be trimmed back until there is good bleeding, and the ureteral ends are spatulated on opposite sides of each other; a double-J stent is passed into the bladder and up into the renal pelvis with approximation of the ureter using closely spaced, interrupted 4-0 or 5-0 chromic catgut. This anastomosis should be stented for 2 or 3 weeks. Again, some leakage of urine is not uncommon and the wound should be drained.

Delayed Recognition and Management

In the event of a ureteral ligation, there may be flank pain, an abdominal mass, or no symptoms whatever, unless both ureters have been ligated. The diagnosis can generally be made by intravenous urography, but occasionally ultrasonography and radionuclide studies are required to assess the amount of residual renal tissue and the functional capacity of the involved kidney. If ureteral ligation appears likely, either cystoscopy with bulb ureterograms and attempted ureteral catheterization, or preferably percutaneous nephrostomy, is required. Nephrostography will show the failure of passage of contrast material into the bladder if the obstruction is complete; it should be repeated after an interval of several weeks to look for evidence of transport into the bladder. Because I have seen instances of spontaneous resolution of what appeared to be a complete obstruction after simple nephrostomy drainage for a month or so, I suggest waiting for at least that length of time before making the assumption that a delayed repair will be required.

If there is loss of ureteral continuity, there may be leakage through the vaginal cuff, an abdominal mass due to a urinoma, or a more vaguely defined symptom complex with prolonged ileus, which may attend the slow leakage of urine into the retroperitoneal space and peritoneal cavity. An intravenous urogram may show either more or less dilatation than in the presumed normal contralateral side.

When these injuries are identified within the first several days, definitive early correction may be in order if there appears to be a total loss in ureteral continuity. If, however, the patient is in relatively tenuous condition, a period of nutritional support may be necessary. In this instance, or if there is any uncertainty regarding the extent of the injury, percutaneous nephrostomy will relieve any urgency about dealing with the matter more definitively. In fact there is a natural tendency toward procrastination because one or more of these factors often impact on clinical decision making. These injuries are often partial, sometimes permitting a retrograde ureteral stent to be passed, or percutaneous nephrostomy with antegrade stenting. If the patient is completely dry with a stent, a nephrostomy, or both, I generally advocate waiting 6 weeks before removing the stent and proceeding with surgical repair if leakage persists. If the patient with a nephrostomy or stent, singly or in combination, is not dry after 3 weeks or so, open surgical correction may be performed, generally without undue difficulty. During the operation, the ureter should be identified above the level of the injury and traced distally until it disappears into a necrotic mass or is inexorably trapped in a sheet of fibrous reaction. The procedure will be dictated by the length of available ureter and the amount of inflammation in the pelvis due to urinary extravasation and fibrosis. There may be less ureteral length than would be available in an immediate repair, and therefore more reliance on a bridging procedure such as a Boari flap or transureteroureterostomy than on simple reimplantation.

There are no hard and fast rules with regard to the exact timing of the definitive repair of a ureteral injury. If percutaneous methods appear to be working, however, it is reasonable to persist with them if there is a reasonable chance of spontaneous closure. Moreover, there are no guidelines regarding which partial ureteral disruptions will heal without the formation of a ureteral stricture, and which strictures will subsequently lend themselves to endoscopic dilatation.

INJURIES TO THE ABDOMINAL URETER

Treatment

Iatrogenic injuries to the abdominal ureter are much less common than those to the pelvic ureter, but are more often unforgiving and may more frequently lead to the performance of a nephrectomy. When an injury occurs in the upper two thirds of the ureter and is immediately recognized, and no more than a few centimeters of ureter have been lost, the simplest way to deal with the situation is ureteroureterostomy. If the kidney is readily accessible and the defect is of more than several centimeters, some additional length for bridging can be obtained by mobilizing the kidney. Such mobilization and downward deflection of the kidney may provide the extra length required for a tension-free anastomosis. When the injury is not too high and is too long for direct ureteroureterostomy, a Boari flap may be considered if the bladder is capacious.

Another alternative is transureteroureterostomy. This usually requires enough ureteral length for the ureter to be swung behind the posterior peritoneum to the contralateral side without any tension or angulation, avoiding trapping by the inferior mesenteric artery. Good exposure to both ureters is required, and if this is a delayed repair, some form of transabdominal approach is required. The anastomosis is done tangentially by trimming the end of the donor ureter at about 45 degrees. The recipient ureter is exposed through an incision in the posterior peritoneum and mobilized just enough to permit an easy ureteral juxtaposition for the end-to-side anastomosis. The recipient ureter is opened along its medial side for a distance of about 2 cm, and the donor ureter is brought into position. Interrupted or running suture technique is used to complete the anastomosis with 4-0 chromic catgut with knots on the outside. Traditionally, I have left a double-J stent in the recipient ureter, and a No. 5 French feeding tube may be threaded into the donor kidney and brought out through a tiny stab wound just opposite the point of the anastomosis, and then extraperitoneally out to the skin. Two very small double-J stents could also be used for drainage, but at least the recipient ureter should be stented. In most instances, there is a nephrostomy on the side of the donor ureter, which is invaluable for temporary drainage and periodic assessment of anastomotic healing. The feeding tube can be removed at this point, and the double-J stent several days later. A final nephrostogram should be performed before removal of the nephrostomy tube.

Transureteroureterostomy is a very useful operation when it is not possible to get back into the pelvis for direct reimplantation, when there has been substantial loss of lower ureteral length, or as a secondary operation after failure of a previous repair.

Delayed Treatment of Extensive Injuries

Autotransplantation of the kidney or substitution of ileum for the ureter may be used in those rare instances of extensive ureteral loss in which less drastic measures will not suffice. If the kidney is not densely bound down and if virtually the entire ureter is destroyed, autotransplantation is preferable, assuming reasonable pelvic vessels, normal renal parenchyma, and no undue difficulty in exposing the pelvic side wall. Nephrectomy must be just as meticulous as for a living related donor transplant, obtaining the maximal length of vessels and using vascular clamps for the renal artery and vein. The kidney should be immersed in saline slush and flushed with chilled Collins solution. When it is prepared in this manner, there is ample time to make repairs at the back table and to replace the kidney through a standard extraperitoneal incision.

In the patient with vascular disease or long-standing type I diabetes, it is necessary to obtain a pelvic arteriogram before autotransplantation is considered. However, if there are no risk factors in the history and if femoral and peripheral pulses are good, the condition of the pelvic vessels is generally suitable for transplantation. The venous anastomosis is between the donor renal vein and the recipient external iliac vein. I prefer to use running 5-0 Prolene or an equivalent suture. The renal artery is spatulated and implanted into the end of the hypogastric artery or, if there is plaque at the bifurcation, into the side of the external iliac artery with running Prolene. I advocate systemic heparinization before cross clamping of the external iliac artery. An extravesical ureteral reimplantation is generally used.

Assuming appropriate cooling and preparation and in the absence of any kind of vascular calamity such as arterial thrombosis, the autotransplant should function well and should avoid some of the inherent problems of ileal substitution—e.g., fluid and electrolyte disturbances related to the absorption of urinary solutes, particularly in patients with impaired renal function.

If there is substantial fibrous reaction around the kidney, particularly in the area of the hilum, it may be difficult to perform a good nephrectomy that will permit autotransplantation. In this event, it may be best to use the ileum for total or partial replacement of the ureter. It is often unnecessary to replace the entire ureter, and segmental ureteral replacement has worked well. Ureteral substitution with ileum may be used in conjunction with a Boari flap to further reduce the total amount of ureter requiring substitution with ileum. All of these possibilities inevitably reduce the likelihood of acidosis and electrolyte disturbances, although such complications do not generally occur if the serum creatinine level is below 2.0 mg per deciliter.

The appendix may also be a useful organ for replacement of partial ureteral loss, if it is long enough to bridge the defect. The mesoappendix, including the appendicular artery, needs to be preserved and separated from the mesoileum. The appendix can then be interposed between the proximal and distal ends of the ureter with an end-to-end anastomotic technique after first trimming off the closed end of the appendix.

URETERAL INJURY IN THE PRESENCE OF A PROSTHETIC VASCULAR GRAFT

When a ureteral injury occurs in conjunction with creation of an aortic or iliac graft, the circumstances are unique, because of the possibility of a late mycotic rupture if a fistula develops. Any anastomoses should be stented and consideration given to the simultaneous establishment of a nephrostomy. This carries the possibility of eventual urinary tract infection, potentially deleterious in the event of leakage, but also provides an effective form of diversion during the healing phase and easy access for x-ray studies to confirm healing. If there is delayed urinary leakage, the injury must be rapidly assessed and, by whatever means (including nephrostomy and stenting), the drainage must be brought to a halt. If it is not readily apparent that this is the case, early nephrectomy is in order. If urinary leakage stops, consideration can be given to secondary reconstruction at a later date. However, on balance, many of these patients are eventually treated with nephrectomy because of the well-founded concern about urine around a vascular graft. The adverse effect of sterile urine on a prosthetic graft is not clear, but infected urine poses a definite hazard, and there is an understandable reluctance on the part of vascular surgeons to advocate procedures that may involve persistent urinary contact with the graft.

SUGGESTED READING

Hefty T. Experience with parallel incision extravesical ureteroneocystostomy in renal transplantation. J Urol 1985; 134:455.

Hodges CV, Barry JM, Fuchs EF, et al. Transureteroureterostomy: 25-year experience with 100 patients. J Urol 1980; 123:834.

Juma S, Nickel JC. Appendix interposition of the ureter. J Urol 1990; 144:130.

Thompson IM, Ross G Jr. Long-term results of bladder flap repair of ureteral injuries. J Urol 1974; 111:483.

Weinberg JJ, Synder JA, Smith AD. Mechanical extraction of stones with rigid ureteroscopes. Urol Clin North Am 1988; 15.

BLUNT BLADDER TRAUMA

BARRY S. STEIN, M.D., F.A.C.S.

ETIOLOGY AND CLASSIFICATION

Most cases of blunt trauma to the bladder are the result of injuries sustained in vehicular accidents: a lesser number are caused by falls or a direct blow to the abdomen. Three classifications of bladder injury are recognized: (1) contusion, (2) extraperitoneal rupture, and (3) intraperitoneal rupture. The type of bladder injury sustained varies according to the degree and mechanism of injury, as well as the amount of urine in the bladder at the time of trauma. The bladder contusion is associated with hematoma formation in the perivesical space and with gross hematuria with no sign of extravasation (Fig. 1). The extraperitoneal rupture is associated with a pelvic fracture in 95 to 97 percent of cases. Most of these injuries occur when a bone fragment punctures the bladder wall (Fig. 2). The lateral wall is the area most often injured. Five to 10 percent of patients with pelvic fractures sustain extraperitoneal bladder ruptures, which constitute 45 to 60 percent of bladder ruptures. Intraperitoneal rupture is most often due to indirect injury to a full bladder, not to direct puncture by a bone fragment (Fig. 3). In this case, the increased pressure to the bladder leads to a rupture at its weakest point, the dome. This represents 25 to 45 percent of bladder ruptures. Combined injuries occur in 2 to 8 percent of cases. This is thought to occur with rupture of the dome due to the pressure increase, followed by a puncture wound of the bladder by a bony spicule.

DIAGNOSIS

Some of these patients experience suprapubic pain, while others may be unable to void. However, these

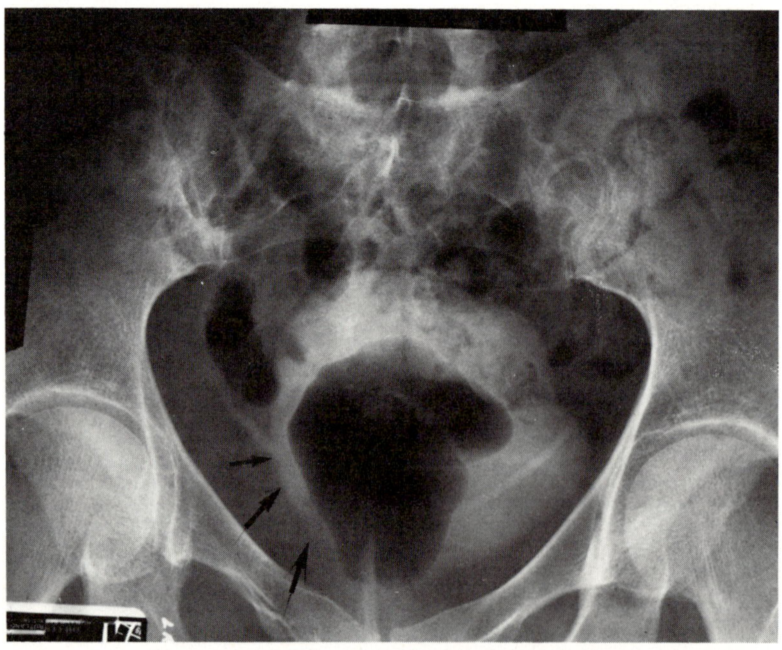

Figure 1 Contusion of the bladder. Arrows indicate deviation of the bladder wall due to pelvic hematoma.

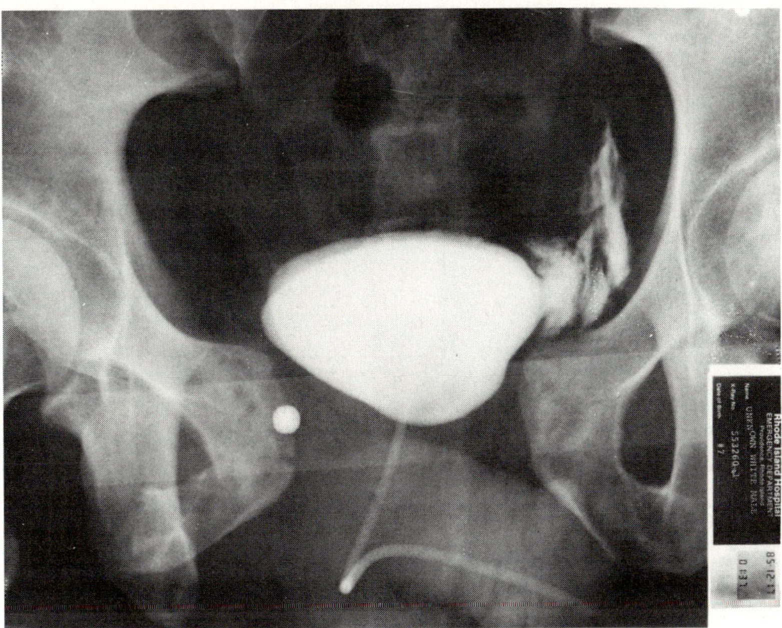

Figure 2 Cystogram of extraperitoneal bladder rupture.

classic textbook features are often not helpful in the emergency department setting. Most patients have pelvic fractures and other injuries, which are potential causes of nonspecific pain. Others will be in shock and unable to provide any responses to the examiner. Often these patients have catheters inserted in the emergency department before the urologist is even called. In such cases, other guidelines are needed.

HEMATURIA

The degree of hematuria appears to be a reliable index of the degree of bladder injury, unlike the situation in other areas of genitourinary trauma. Fifty to 60 percent of patients with gross hematuria and pelvic fracture have a major lower genitourinary tract injury. Thus, this group of patients requires radiographic evaluation. In patients with microscopic hematuria, only 1 of 77 patients in one study and none of 120 patients in another study were found to have had significant lower tract genitourinary pathology. This suggests a conservative approach to further evaluation of the clinically stable patient with microscopic hematuria.

Cystography

Before a cystogram is performed, it is imperative to consider the possibility of urethral injury. In patients with bladder rupture due to pelvic fractures, urethral injury may coexist in 15 to 20 percent of cases. If any question exists then, a retrograde urethrogram must be performed prior to the cystogram. Only if no urethral injury is present should the catheter be placed for cystography.

Great attention must be paid to the proper performance of cystography in this setting. A properly performed cystogram is 90 to 100 percent diagnostic; however, failure to fill the bladder fully and obtain an emptying film may increase the false-negative rates to 20 percent. A plain film of the pelvis is first obtained. Iodinated contrast medium is then instilled to bladder capacity (approximately 400 ml). In some situations, extravasation may be missed by underfilling of the bladder. Drainage films are then needed, since extravasated contrast may "hide" behind the full bladder. In selected cases, oblique films may also be of help to examine areas of possible extravasation behind bone fragments. If extravasation is present, sufficient contrast material should be used to allow for classification as extraperitoneal, intraperitoneal, or combined rupture. Intravenous urography should be performed only after the cystogram, and as indicated by the nature of the injury.

TREATMENT

The treatment is dependent on the type of rupture present (Fig. 4). In my opinion, all cases of intraperitoneal rupture warrant exploration. Although less often than seen in cases of extraperitoneal rupture, most of these patients have associated pelvic fractures, and often other visceral organ injuries as well. In these cases, it is imperative to close the bladder wall and peritoneum, drain the perivesical space, and institute good catheter drainage. In males, good catheter drainage means a suprapubic tube, while in females, a large catheter may be used per urethra. Cases of combined injury with both intra- and extraperitoneal rupture should be treated as intraperitoneal rupture with exploratory laparotomy, debridement and closure, and drainage.

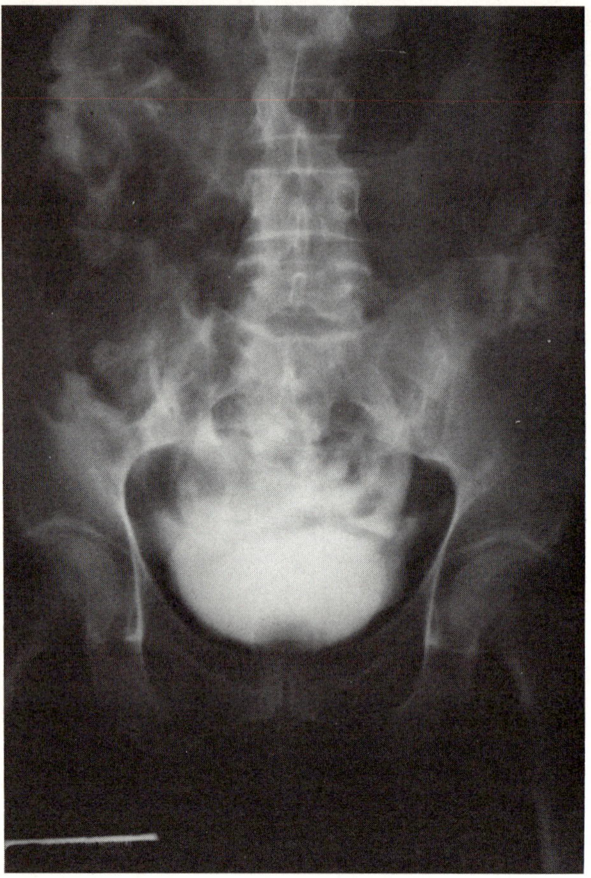

Figure 3 Cystogram of intraperitoneal bladder rupture with loops of bowel outlined by contrast medium.

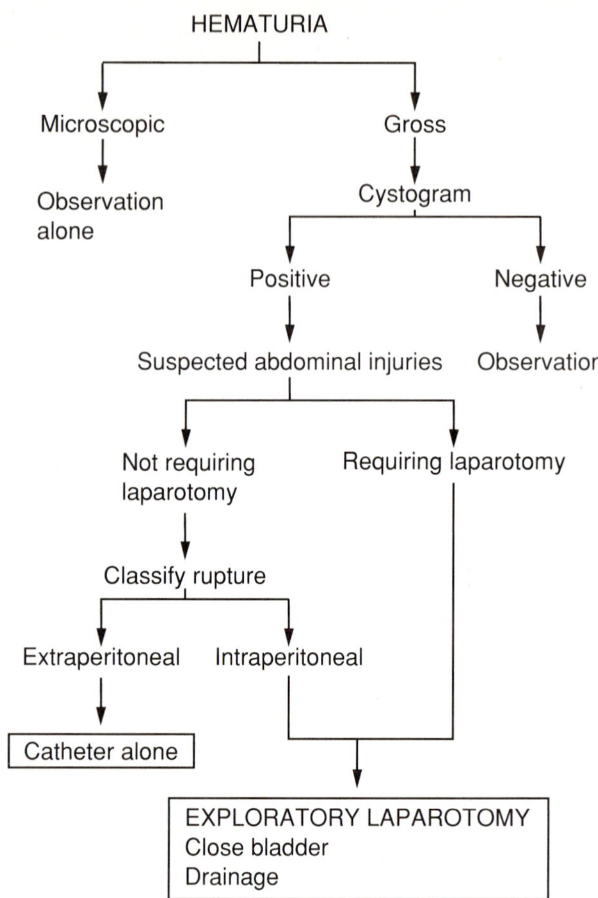

Figure 4 Algorithm for suspected bladder rupture.

The treatment of extraperitoneal rupture is controversial. There are proponents of both the nonoperative approach advocating catheter drainage alone, and the operative approach, which treats extraperitoneal rupture the same as intraperitoneal rupture. Unfortunately, the degree of extravasation seen on cystography does not correlate with the size of the bladder rent, and thus cannot be used to decide the treatment approach. I believe that in many cases the decision is made for us by general surgeons who perform exploratory laparotomy to rule out concomitant visceral organ injury, since a large number of these patients have severe multisystemic injuries, and the genitourinary trauma constitutes only a small portion of their care. Many have associated injuries. to the chest, central nervous system, abdominal visceral organs, or other genitourinary organs, (e.g., kidney or urethra). Bladder perforation alone is unlikely to cause shock in these patients, and vigorous evaluation of other sources must be sought in the hypotensive patient. The mortality rates today vary from 12 to 22 percent.

However, the bladder perforation is rarely if ever the cause of death, and the likelihood of coexisting injury must be kept in mind.

If the patient is to undergo an abdominal exploration, I prefer in that setting to close the bladder and insert a drain as described above. However, in patients not undergoing abdominal laparotomy, I believe that Foley catheter drainage and observation is sufficient. Repeat cystograms can be performed 7 to 10 days later, or sooner if the clinical course dictates. The catheter is removed when the bladder no longer demonstrates extravasation. Clinical parameters such as temperature, suprapubic tenderness, or abdominal distention may indicate the need for earlier re-evaluation.

In summary, most patients with blunt trauma of the bladder still undergo operative repair whether because of intraperitoneal rupture or because of concomitant general surgical injuries. In the selected cases of extraperitoneal rupture, however, catheter drainage alone may be sufficient.

PENETRATING BLADDER TRAUMA

STANLEY A. BROSMAN, M.D.

Bullet wounds, gunshot injuries, and stabbings are the cause of most instances of penetrating bladder trauma. High-velocity guns and semiautomatic weapons have become a part of the arsenal of the street gangs and narcotics dealers. Emergency rooms and trauma centers are the recipients of these patients, many of whom are children and adolescents.

Although bladder injuries per se are not lethal, failure to recognize and manage them properly may lead to serious and potentially fatal complications. During the early assessment and stabilization of patients with penetrating trauma, an indwelling urethral catheter is usually placed. The appearance of dried blood at the meatus or fresh bleeding from the urethra suggests urethral trauma, and urethrography should be considered before placement of an indwelling catheter. When the catheter has been placed, the presence of hematuria indicates the possibility of an injury somewhere in the urinary system. Even microscopic hematuria may presage a serious injury. Because bullets are notorious for their unpredictable course through the body, there is a need to assess the entire urinary tract with some type of radiologic study. Bullet fragments may be found in the bladder even though the entrance wound is in the upper abdomen.

The excretory urogram and computed tomographic (CT) scan with contrast material may be used to evaluate the integrity of the bladder, but the best study is still cystography. This can be done at the same time that an abdominal series or intravenous pyelography (IVP) is in progress. The study can be done with routine x-rays or combined with fluoroscopy. A commercially prepared bottle of contrast can be attached to the catheter with intravenous tubing, or a solution can be prepared by mixing an injectable contrast agent with saline and instilling this by gravity through an open catheter syringe. There should be 300 to 500 ml of solution available for instillation. Three vials of contrast material are mixed with 400 ml of saline when a prepackaged solution is not available.

The trick to diagnosing a bladder perforation is to fill the bladder with enough contrast. It is convenient to observe the bladder with fluoroscopy during filling and obtain 14 × 17 films centered over the pelvis when there is about 200 ml in the bladder, and again at 100-ml increments. Filling is stopped when extravasation is apparent, when the bladder will accept no more fluid, or when the bladder has been filled with 500 ml of contrast solution. If possible, films are obtained in the oblique positions. The contrast is drained from the bladder and additional films are obtained to identify contrast outside the bladder.

If the patient is already in the operating room and the abdomen is open, the bladder can be filled through the catheter, using saline mixed with methylene blue or indigo carmine. Standard cystography can also be performed if x-ray studies can be obtained.

Penetrating bladder injuries are unlikely to represent solitary organ trauma, with the exception of some patients with stab wounds that occurred when the bladder was full. Ice picks, knitting needles, and a variety of knives and bayonets have been associated with bladder trauma. Repair involves opening the bladder and identifying and debriding the sites of injury before closing them with two layers of suture material. The repair is usually done from within the bladder, using 2-0 or 3-0 PGA or chromic interrupted sutures on the muscle layer and 3-0 or 4-0 continuous sutures on the epithelium. In some instances, a partial cystectomy is necessary to remove devitalized tissue. The lower ureters require careful examination to be certain they have not been traumatized. If radiography is available, bulb ureterography using dilute methylene blue or contrast material helps ascertain the integrity of the ureters. Merely passing a catheter up the ureter does not rule out the presence of an injury. When trauma to the lower ureter is associated with a bladder injury, reimplantation and stenting of the ureter has worked better for me than trying to repair and anastomose the ureter.

The other structures requiring careful assessment are the lower colon and rectum. Unrecognized perforations of the bowel can be disastrous. If one cannot be certain that these structures are intact, a colostomy may be performed.

The bladder is drained with a large Malecot suprapubic tube and a urethral catheter. A drain is left in the suprapubic area for 5 days or until drainage has ceased. Cystography is performed at 10 to 14 days, and if the bladder has healed, the catheters are removed. I usually remove the suprapubic tube first and wait a day before taking out the urethral catheter. Although the patient may have been on antibiotics during the early postoperative period, I do not usually maintain this therapy when the catheters are in place. A urine culture is obtained at the time of cystography, and appropriate antibiotics are started as the catheters are being removed. Patients are followed until the urine is normal and bladder function has returned. In practice, most of these patients do not return for follow-up care.

IATROGENIC BLADDER TRAUMA

EARL F. WENDEL, M.D.

Iatrogenic bladder trauma is an injury to the bladder induced inadvertently by a physician or by the treatment. By definition this injury is unintentional, although one definition of the word "iatrogenic" implies that the injury may be the result of inattention. The recognition that bladder injury can occur during a variety of treatments or procedures can aid in prevention. Most iatrogenic bladder injuries occur during gynecologic surgery or obstetric, urologic, or general surgical procedures.

While the urinary bladder in the infant is primarily an abdominal organ, the adult bladder lies deep in the pelvis, and is protected by the anterior abdominal muscles and the bony pubis and posteriorly by the rectum and the sacrum. In males the inferior aspect is attached to the prostate, whereas in females the pelvic muscles are inferior and the uterus and vagina posterior. The superior aspect of the bladder is covered in part by the pelvic peritoneum. The extensive blood supply to the bladder may contribute to bleeding at the time of any injury, but also contributes to good healing. A distended bladder is much more susceptible to injury than is a decompressed bladder, and in most surgical procedures the bladder is decompressed with a catheter. Therefore, iatrogenic injuries are not common, although in one series of penetrating trauma to the bladder, five of 19 injuries were classified as iatrogenic and one additional injury was secondary to catheterization.

The approach to this problem consists of awareness of the risk of bladder injury during each specific surgical procedure, recognition that an injury may have occurred, careful documentation of the injury and its extent, and institution of appropriate treatment. The principles of treatment of these bladder injuries may involve urinary bladder diversion, drainage of extravasated urine and irrigating fluid, and possible closure of the bladder defect.

BLADDER INJURY DURING INSTRUMENTATION

The ability of bladder muscle to stretch and distend, which leads to its storage capacity, also lends some protection against penetrating injury due to instrumentation via the urethra. On the other hand, instrumentation of the bladder is a common procedure in medical office settings, hospitals, and nursing home facilities. In addition, a large number of patients are using the technique of intermittent self-catheterization to empty their bladders. Factors that may increase the likelihood of bladder injury secondary to instrumentation include conditions that may restrict the elasticity of the bladder or decrease the sensation of the bladder wall, or forceful instrumentation. Radiation to the pelvic area for a variety of reasons may limit the distensibility of the bladder wall. In addition, surgical procedures such as cesarean sections may cause scarring in the area of the bladder. Patients who have undergone augmentation cystoplasties do not have a normal bladder reservoir and have reportedly perforated their bladders with self-catheterization.

As most urologists are aware, the risk of bladder injury is decreased by instrumenting the bladder when it is distended to allow for passage of the instrument above the bladder neck before striking the bladder wall. When changing suprapubic or urethral catheters, it is often helpful to distend the bladder before removing the indwelling catheter and inserting a new catheter. It is not unusual, however, for instrumentation of the bladder to be required in the office after the patient has voided for a urine specimen. The passage of catheters or, more particularly, rigid instruments such as the van Buren urethral sounds in males or Walther catheter dilators in females should be carried out with as much gentleness and care as possible. If the urologist is attuned to this, it is not unusual, particularly in females, to actually feel the instrument encountering the superior wall of the bladder after passing through the bladder neck. The rapid passage of a rigid instrument such as a urethral sound or a cystoscope into the bladder in a cavalier fashion has been known to cause perforation. As is well-known, most lower urinary tract injuries secondary to instrumentation in males are in the urethra rather than the bladder. Several cases of spontaneous perforation of the bladder during long-term catheterization have been reported.

DIAGNOSIS OF BLADDER INJURY

The signs and symptoms of bladder injury vary according to the manner in which the bladder is injured and the state of distention or decompression of the bladder. In addition, if the patient is awake, symptoms may be elicited that are not available in an anesthetized patient. If the bladder is perforated during a cystoscopic examination, the urologist may notice hematuria, a lack of return of the irrigating fluid, and difficulty in visualization due to bleeding plus the collapse of the bladder wall. Under local anesthesia, severe and increasing pain may be present, and distention of the abdomen due to irrigating fluid also occurs. If the bladder is penetrated during an open pelvic operative procedure and the bladder is not decompressed, a rapid gush of urine may ensue, alerting the surgeon to this problem. If a urethral catheter is indwelling, only a small amount of urine may leak into the operative site, although it probably will continue to do so, or the urine in the drainage system may become bloody. If the bladder is opened during a vaginal operative procedure, a similar leaking of urine into the vagina may occur. A prompt cystogram with methylene blue should establish the diagnosis. If no methylene blue leaks into the operative field, but there is continuing extravasation of urine, one should suspect ureteral injury. Intravenous indigo carmine can then be administered to establish this diagnosis.

Retrograde cystography is the definitive means of establishing the diagnosis of bladder injury with extravasation. This is the most appropriate means in the setting of cystoscopy or transurethral resection. A preliminary film in the anteroposterior projection is taken. The bladder is then filled under gravity pressure. Fluoroscopy adds immeasurably to the diagnosis of injury. If fluoroscopic examination reveals extravasation of 50 or 100 ml of contrast medium, no further filling is required. If there is no evidence of extravasation, the bladder should gradually be filled up to approximately 400 ml under gravity. Anteroposterior films are not always sufficient; if injury is suspected and none seen on the film, oblique films may add to the diagnosis. One of the most crucial aspects of cystography is the drainage film, which may reveal contrast media in tissues outside of the bladder after the bladder is emptied of contrast media. The filled bladder and the anteroposterior projection may well obscure some smaller or posterior extravasations. Although bladder injury with urine extravasation may be seen on computed tomographic (CT) scans of the pelvis, or occasionally even documented by ultrasonography of the bladder, neither of these studies is the procedure of choice, but rather retrograde cystography.

BLADDER INJURIES IN OBSTETRICS

The urinary tract is commonly distended during pregnancy, and the bladder also may have a large capacity and may empty poorly at the time of delivery. The incidence of bladder injury during delivery may be diminished by catheterization of the bladder to avoid overdistention. This is particularly important with prolonged delivery, the use of intravenous fluids, and concomitant use of epidural anesthesia. The incidence of obstetric bladder injury has decreased owing to the increased use of cesarean section in prolonged labor as well as the decrease in high- or mid-forceps deliveries. Injury to the bladder due to pressure of the fetal head compressing the bladder against the symphysis in prolonged labor can result in pressure necrosis, but generally presents on a delayed basis as a vesicovaginal fistula. This subject is discussed in another chapter.

Injuries to the bladder as a result of forceps deliveries are usually the result of errors of judgment or inexperience. The incidence of these bladder lacerations varies from minimal for simple outlet forceps delivery to a significantly increased risk for midforceps deliveries, particularly with rotation and delivery performed by an inexperienced obstetrician.

In general, mid- or high-forceps deliveries have given way to the increased use of cesarean section. Although many cesarean sections may be done on a scheduled basis, a significant number are of an emergent nature. Since the bladder is commonly distended and is in an abdominal position, bladder injury is increased if the bladder is not decompressed. The bladder may be injured during lower segment or classic fundal cesarean section, particularly if a previous cesarean section has resulted in fibrosis and adherence of the bladder to the uterus. Extension of the uterine incision into the bladder should generally result in a sudden leak of urine, which should be easily identifiable and can be confirmed by instillation of methylene blue via a urethral catheter or by the use of intravenous indigo carmine dye. With an injury such as this, which may be recognized immediately, the bladder can be repaired before closure of the uterine incision. Identifying the ureteral orifices and their proximity to the injury may be aided with ureteral catheter passage or with intravenous indigo carmine. The edges of the bladder injury are then debrided and closed in two or three layers with running sutures of absorbable material. In these women, an indwelling ureteral catheter is generally satisfactory for drainage and should be left in place for 7 to 10 days. Cystography is carried out before removal of the catheter to document the absence of extravasation.

The bladder may also be injured during delivery at the time of rupture of the gravid uterus. This complication of obstetrics also has decreased significantly with the increased use of cesarean section. Associated rupture of the bladder with rupture of the gravid uterus apparently occurs in less than 10 percent of these cases, but should be sought at the time of repair of the uterus and repaired appropriately at that time.

Other injuries to the bladder may also occur during abortions, either with dilatation and curettage procedure or with suction curettage. Although the frequency of uterine perforation and bladder injury is low with these procedures, the increase in the number of abortions may result in a numerical increase in this complication.

Although bladder laceration during cesarean section may be promptly recognized, the injuries to the bladder from obstetric procedures with an essentially closed pelvis may go unrecognized at the time of injury, with resultant extravasation, the formation of an abscess, and/or a fistula on a delayed basis. It may be anticipated that most, but not all, patients with bladder injuries will have gross hematuria. Minor levels of hematuria after obstetric maneuvers are generally observed with or without Foley urethral catheter drainage until they clear. More severe levels of gross hematuria should be investigated primarily with cystography.

BLADDER INJURIES IN GYNECOLOGY

The incidence of bladder injury in gynecology is low. However, gynecologic surgery is the most common cause of vesicovaginal fistula in up to 70 percent of cases. The bladder is injured twice as often as are the ureters. Most of these bladder injuries occur during anterior vaginal repairs or during hysterectomy by either the abdominal or vaginal approach. The base of the bladder lies immediately in front of the anterior vaginal wall and the cervix. Scarring in this area as a result of previous cesarean section or pelvic surgery or secondary to infection, endometriosis, or radiation therapy may increase the likelihood of bladder injury during dissection in this area. Obliteration of the anatomic plane between the bladder and the uterus may result in tearing of the bladder during downward displacement, with isolation of the uterine vessels or with clamping of the lateral cervical attachments. This may result in immediate leakage of urine into the incision. This also should be recognized at once if the bladder is injured during electrocautery dissection in this area. Devascularization of the bladder during dissection, or inadvertent perforation with sutures or clamping of the bladder wall, result in a delayed injury, an abscess, or a vesicovaginal or vesical cutaneous fistula.

Since the immediate repair of the bladder is relatively uncomplicated, whereas delayed injuries with fistula formation represent a more major surgical undertaking, it is important to be aware of the possibility of injury. If there is any question that injury to the bladder may have occurred, instillation of methylene blue with distention of the bladder should be carried out. The bladder should be adequately distended to document even small leaks. If no leak is noted, it is advisable to document that this test was done. If a bladder tear is recognized, a two- or three-layer running absorbable suture closure can be made. The area is drained to prevent accumulation of any urine, the bladder is decompressed for the next 7 to 10 days, and a cystogram is done before removal of the catheter.

Pelvic surgery is a difficult undertaking at best and may be even more difficult when there are adhesions or previous infection or radiation. Even the most meticulous gynecologic surgeon can anticipate that this injury will occur during his or her practice. The most important principles in this regard are to be aware of the possible occurrence of bladder injury and to perform cystography with contrast media or methylene blue if the question of injury exists. The presence or absence of urine extravasation should be documented and treated appropriately. The excellent blood supply to the bladder generally results in rapid healing of these injuries, so that the catheter can be removed in 7 to 10 days if the cystogram reveals no leakage. A small drain brought out to the skin away from the incision virtually eliminates urinoma formation or abscess. Prolonged leakage after primary closure of the bladder and drainage of the perivesical area is uncommon, but can be treated with continued bladder decompression. If urinary extravasation is prolonged, radiographic studies should be carried out to ascertain that the perivesical drain is not too near the closure, and the drains moved if necessary. Prolonged drainage and even persistence to fistula may be increased in patients who have had radiation therapy to the pelvis, particularly therapy for cervical carcinoma. In addition, primary radiation therapy alone for carcinoma of the cervix has resulted in vesicovaginal fistula in up to 2 percent of these patients.

BLADDER INJURIES IN GENERAL SURGERY

Injuries to the bladder during general surgical procedures are relatively uncommon. This may be due less to the skill of the general surgeon as opposed to other surgeons than to the lower frequency of dissection in the pelvis near the bladder. Injuries to the bladder can occur during repair of an inguinal hernia, particularly if the bladder is one component of a sliding hernia. More commonly, the bladder may be injured in dissection from the sigmoid colon or rectum, which is involved with carcinoma, with inflammatory disorders such as Crohn's disease or diverticulitis. These inflammatory processes cause marked adherence of the bowel to the bladder, and the risk of injury is increased.

Once again, awareness of the risk of injury and prompt use of a methylene blue cystogram are the general surgeon's best approaches. If a bladder laceration is recognized, it may be repaired as previously discussed. A two- or three-layer running absorbable suture closure is appropriate. Most of these patients have an indwelling urethral catheter, and therefore both identification of the injury by cystogram and decompression of the bladder subsequently are relatively easy to obtain. Drainage of the perivesical space, however, must be adhered to in order to prevent urinoma formation or abscess. A three-layer closure is usually easier to obtain in men than in women, and the surgeon may also opt for suprapubic cystotomy drainage in these men to avoid urethral catheterization.

BLADDER INJURIES IN UROLOGIC SURGERY

The bladder is probably injured by urologists more frequently than by any other physician or surgeon. This generally is due not to lack of skill or lack of care on the part of urologists, but to the frequency with which they approach the bladder. These injuries may occur with a variety of instruments and procedures. In an awake patient in an office setting, several factors may influence the risk of bladder perforation. The introduction and use of instruments by the urologist is a skill learned over time. The gentleness with which the instruments are used, respect for the delicate tissues involved, and the sensitivity and comfort of the patient also contribute to lessening the risk of injury. Communication with patients regarding the procedures being employed, both to inform them and to help them relax during these procedures, is extremely important. The combination of an anxious patient who tenses muscles and resists the passage of an instrument with insensitive and forceful passage of an instrument markedly increases the risk. No instrument, either flexible or rigid, should be passed against the marked resistance of a tense muscle, against scar, or through a tortuous channel. The passage of an instrument into a somewhat distended bladder may lessen the risk of perforation through the wall. In addition, a cystoscope or other instrument should never be moved in the bladder if vision is impaired.

The practice of blind litholapaxy has fortunately disappeared. The instruments used, which had no endoscopic component, were passed in a blind fashion into the bladder with the jaws closed. The jaws, which were quite strong, were then opened, and the stone, which was generally very hard, was engaged and "cracked" after an attempt was made to remove the instrument from the area of the bladder wall. Fortunately, this type of instrumentation for bladder stones has been replaced by the crushing of soft bladder stones with a Lowsley grasping forceps with an endoscopic component, and by the use of ultrasonic or electrohydraulic cystolitholapaxy. Smaller stones, of course, can often be evacuated through a resectoscope sheath. Although the risks of bladder injury have diminished with these instruments, bladder perforation can still occur. Perforation of the bladder is probably most common during treatment of bladder tumors. It can also occur during transurethral resection of the prostate. This may happen when the resectoscope loop is inadvertently left extended and the resectoscope is within the bladder. At this time, if either the surgeon or a bystander inadvertently activates the cutting current of the electrode, bladder perforation may occur.

An unusual cause of bladder rupture is that of intravesical explosion of hydrogen formed from electrolysis or the cauterization of tissue. Although this is unusual, it has been reported, and lesser explosions without bladder damage, but with a characteristic popping sound during resection, have probably been noticed by most urologists. Since this gas collects in the anterior aspect of the bladder over time before apparently reaching a critical volume, the occasional emptying of the anterior wall or dome of the bladder, by occasionally positioning the resectoscope in this area during emptying of the bladder, may help prevent this complication.

An inexperienced resectionist who encounters heavy bleeding from the prostate, loses the normal landmarks, and proceeds with panic rather than caution may not only perforate the prostatic capsule, but also wander into the bladder and resect the bladder wall as well. Most bladder injuries, however, occur during the treatment of transitional cell carcinoma of the bladder. This risk appears to be lower in the superficial bladder tumors treated with cup biopsy and simple fulguration. However, full-thickness perforations of the bladder with simple cup biopsies of small bladder tumors do occur. In addition, prolonged coagulation of the bladder tumors, particularly in their depths, may result in an evolving injury with subsequent bladder leak. The use of newer modalities, such as laser treatment of these tumors, has also been shown to cause full-thickness injury and necrosis of the bladder wall, although not on an immediate basis.

At times, a bulky but superficial-appearing bladder tumor must be resected. Patience is required in carefully paring down or resecting this tumor to its base. At this point, bleeding should be scrupulously managed to maximize visualization of the base of the tumor. Resec-

tion of the base of the tumor into bladder muscle is generally done at this point to stage the level of invasion. Most bladder injuries occur at this time. The depth of the bladder wall is notoriously variable. If bleeding is well controlled and visualization is good, the surgeon can minimize the changes in the depth of the bladder wall by keeping irrigation at a minimum, or even having irrigation turned off during part of this resection. This decreases movement of the bladder wall and maintains a consistent bladder wall thickness.

In spite of the most meticulous technique, however, the instrument may go deeper than intended and cause a full-thickness perforation of the bladder. Most of these injuries are extraperitoneal rather than intraperitoneal, which may simplify their management. The continued use of high volumes of irrigating fluid at this point can worsen the problems. If the irrigating fluid used is sterile water, the problems of hemodilution and hemolysis and water intoxication may arise. If the irrigating fluid used is glycine, hypervolemia syndromes may occur, and in addition glycine itself may be toxic in high amounts. The absorption of these fluids may be more rapid if the injury is intraperitoneal rather than extraperitoneal.

In addition to the difficulty of maintaining constant depth of resection into the bladder wall during tumor staging, the urologist is perplexed by two other technical problems. One is that the resectoscope loop arrangement makes it difficult to resect with safety certain areas of the bladder, particularly the superior aspects or dome of the bladder. Although resections can at times be carried out by simply sweeping or moving the instrument with the loop extended and activated, this is a hazardous maneuver. The areas immediately adjacent to the bladder neck are also at time difficult to reach.

Another dangerous occurrence that can lead to inadvertent bladder penetration with the resectoscope is obturator nerve spasm. This generally occurs during resection laterally either in the bladder wall or even in the prostate, although it can happen at almost any time. Stimulation of the obturator nerve by high-frequency current causes adductor muscle spasm, sudden violent movement of the leg on the affected side, and passage of the activated resectoscope loop completely through the bladder wall. When this has occurred during resection, but without significant injury to the bladder wall, several maneuvers may decrease the problem. The resection may continue at a lower volume of bladder filling to avoid high-volume expansion and placement of the loop closer to the obturator space. In addition, the current settings can be reduced to the lowest level that allows adequate cutting and cautery. A further sometimes helpful maneuver has been to move the electrocautery grounding pad from the leg on the side involved to either the other leg or a different portion of the body in an attempt to change the current pathway.

Once the suspicion of bladder perforation arises, the procedure should be terminated as quickly as possible. The irrigation fluid should be kept to a minimum, the level of gravity filling of the bladder through the instrument lowered, bleeding managed expeditiously, and the procedure terminated as quickly as possible. Cystography with contrast medium may then be carried out. In addition, endoscopic visualization should give some idea of the size of the opening. If the amount of extravasated fluid is not too large and if the penetration of the bladder is relatively small, many of these injuries may be managed with simple urethral catheter drainage, particularly if the injury is in an extraperitoneal position. If the opening in the bladder is large or if a large amount of fluid has been extravasated before recognition of the injury, a suprapubic Penrose drain may be inserted at this time in addition to catheter drainage. This is usually easy to carry out by preparing the suprapubic area with antiseptic and making a small midline incision. Once the rectus sheet is penetrated, the opening in the fascia can simply be enlarged with curved 6-inch clamps or with the finger, and a Penrose drain passed bluntly down with the clamp to the site of the injury. Formal incision and drainage is not required in this case. If a truly severe bladder resection has occurred and the opening is large and irregular, it is possible that in these unusual circumstances a formal open incision with identification, debridement, and repair of the bladder wall, plus drainage of the perivesical space and either suprapubic cystostomy or urethral catheter drainage, may be necessary.

One other urologic procedure that may result in inadvertent bladder rupture is hydrodistention of the bladder. This is generally carried out in an attempt to mechanically enlarge bladder capacity in patients with interstitial cystitis. These procedures carry a definite risk of bladder rupture, whether performed with hydrodistention or the Helmstein balloon. Fortunately, this risk is well known and the rupture is often recognized as soon as it has occurred, generally by the sudden influx of the irrigating fluid. In addition, the influx of a large amount of irrigating fluid during this procedure, as well as during transurethral resection of bladder tumors or prostate, may result in a definite feeling of coolness and prominent suprapubic swelling. With the rupture of the bladder associated with hydrodistention, the procedure is generally terminated at this time. Cystography may then be performed. It is unusual to require any treatment other than simple catheter drainage for several days to allow healing, and in general no perivesical drain need be inserted.

SUGGESTED READING

Carroll PR, McAninch JW. Major bladder trauma: the accuracy of cystography. J Urol 1983; 130:887–888.

Mulkey AP Jr, Witherington R. Conservative management of vesicle rupture. Urology 1974; 4:426–430.

Spees EK, O'Mara C, Murphy JB, Newton CG. Unsuspected intraperitoneal perforation of the urinary bladder as an iatrogenic disorder. Surgery 1981; 89:224–231.

URETHRAL STRADDLE INJURIES

ALEXANDER S. CASS, M.B.B.S., F.R.C.S.

Blunt trauma causes urethral straddle injuries and can result from a fall astride injury, such as from the crossbar of a bicycle, or from a kick in the perineum. The injury is usually the sole one, and no associated injuries are seen in these patients. The injury to the urethra can be a contusion or a partial or complete rupture of the bulbous part of the anterior urethra. The patient complains of perineal pain and bruising and has difficulty voiding. Examination reveals blood at the external urinary meatus, or hematuria in the voided specimen. There is a butterfly hematoma in the perineum (Fig. 1). If the diagnosis is delayed, there is swelling, redness, and induration from extravasation of urine. The diagnosis of a urethral lesion is made by retrograde urethrography, which will reveal some extravasation at the site of the partial (Fig. 2) or complete rupture, but is normal in the case of a contusion. The urethral catheter should not be passed, because it may extend the laceration in the urethra or even convert a partial rupture into a complete one.

When diagnosis is delayed, there is extravasation of urine through the ruptured Buck's fascia, extending into the scrotum and posteriorly in the perineum, where it is limited by the fusion of Colles' fascia to the triangular ligament (Fig. 3). Extravasation extends down into the upper thighs, where it is limited by the fusion of Scarpa's fascia to the deep fascia (fascia lata) of the thigh. It can extend up the abdominal wall, where it is limited by Scarpa's fascia.

TREATMENT

Early intervention is needed to prevent extravasation of the urine and minimize formation of the urethral stricture with partial and complete rupture of the urethra. The early surgical intervention should consist of suprapubic cystostomy with urinary drainage. This will allow the urethral rupture to heal without a significant

stricture, especially in a partial rupture, which is the most common lesion. At 2 weeks, voiding cystourethrography via the suprapubic tube is performed. If the rupture has healed, the suprapubic tube is removed. If some extravasation occurs at the site of rupture, the suprapubic drainage is continued for another 2 weeks and a voiding cystourethrogram repeated. This is repeated each 2 weeks until the rupture has healed, after which the suprapubic tube is removed. The patient is then followed at 3-month intervals for possible stricture formation. The evaluation requires a voiding history and a uroflow voiding rate. Retrograde urethrography is performed at 12 months or earlier if a urethral stricture

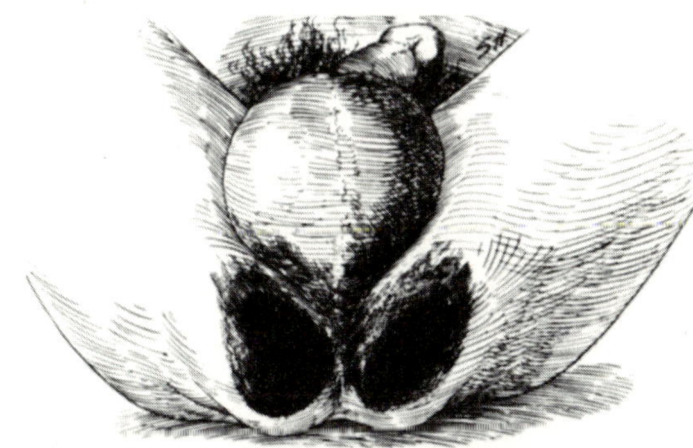

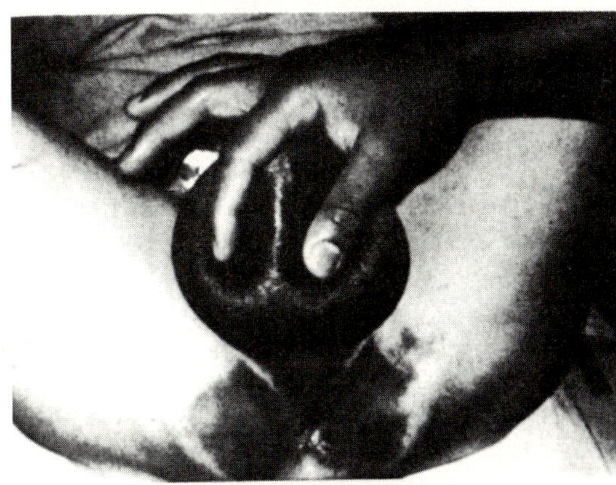

Figure 1 Butterfly hematoma in the perineum. (Republished with permission by Blackwell Scientific Publications, Inc. Morehouse DD. Delayed management of enteral urethral injury. In: Cass AS, ed. Genitourinary trauma. Boston: Blackwell Scientific Publications, 1988:211.)

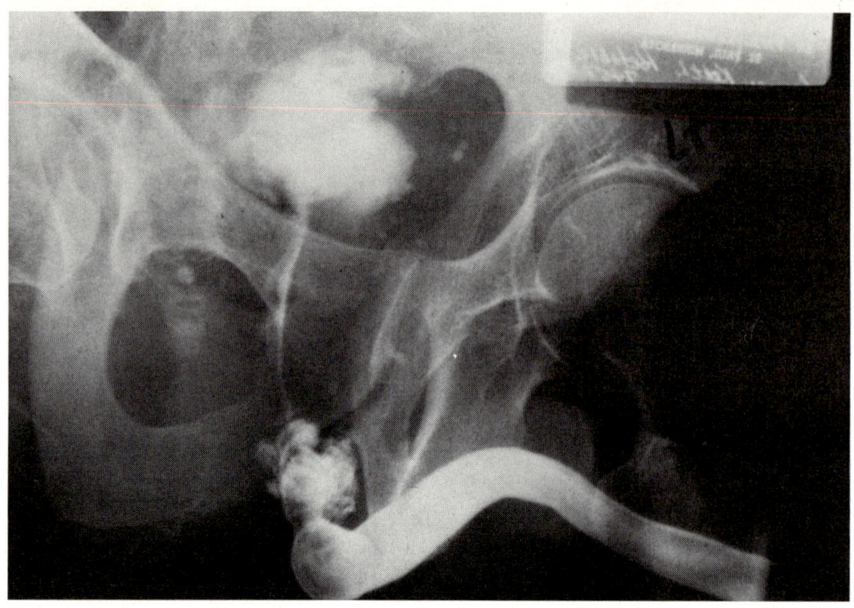

Figure 2 Retrograde urethrogram showing limited extravasation of dye at the site of partial rupture of the urethra, and dye extending into the bladder.

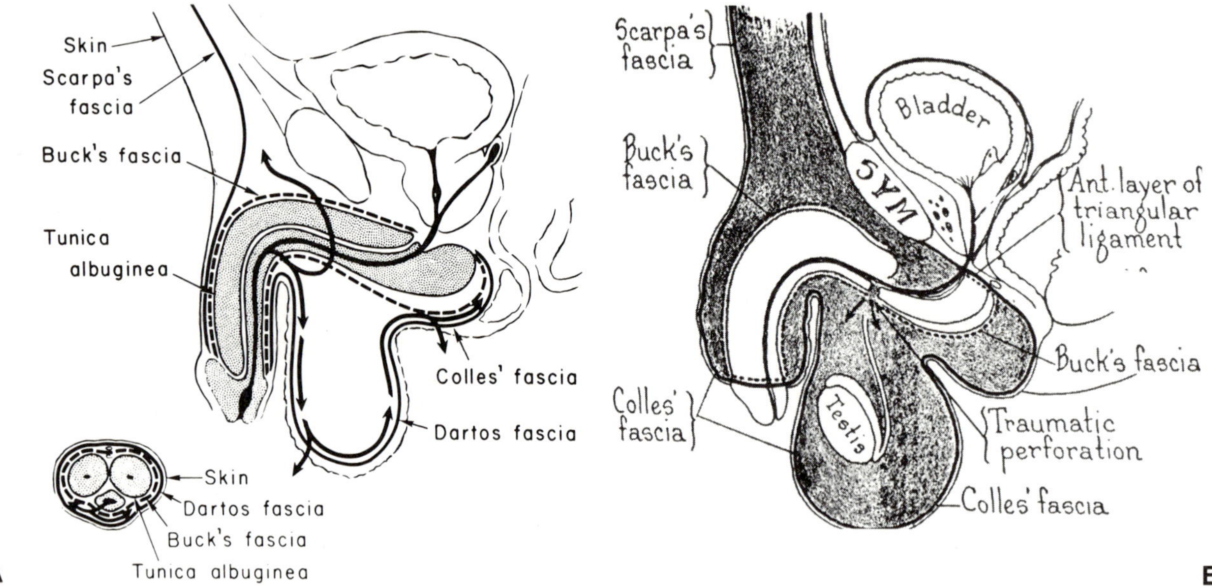

Figure 3 *A,* Route of extravasated urine from urethral injury. *B,* Extent of full extravasation.

is suspected. When such a stricture is seen on a retrograde urethrogram, it is confirmed at endoscopy and an internal visual urethrotomy performed. If the stricture recurs after one or two urethrotomies, urethroplasty is indicated. Since urethral rupture injuries produce a short stricture, excision of the stricture with spatulated end-to-end anastomosis is performed, using 4.0 or 5.0 suture material.

An alternative treatment is the passage of a urethral catheter to divert the urinary flow. Although this can be successful, it usually results in a high complication rate, with increased incidence of severe urethral stricture and

an increased risk of urethral bleeding from secondary infection at the site of the laceration. If a urethral catheter is used, retrograde urethrography is performed at 2 weeks by placing a feeding tube into the fossa navicularis beside the catheter, clamping the glans penis, and then injecting dye to visualize the urethra. When no extravasation is seen at the site of injury, the urethral catheter is removed.

When a large hematoma and swelling are present from bleeding or extravasation, exploration of the bulbous urethra may be indicated, with evacuation of the clot, debridement of the ruptured ends of the urethra, and spatulated end-to-end anastomosis using 4 or 5.0 suture material over a No. 24 French catheter. The catheter is then removed, a small urethral stent placed, and a suprapubic cystostomy performed. The stent is removed after 2 weeks, and voiding cystourethrography is performed to determine whether the anastomosis has healed. If extravasation is present, the suprapubic drain is continued, and a voiding cystourethrogram is repeated every 2 weeks until healing has occurred. Possible stricture formation is evaluated at 3-month intervals with a voiding history and uroflow voiding rate, and retrograde urethrography if stricture is suspected.

SUGGESTED READING

Dixon CM, McAninch JW. Minimizing consequences of urethral trauma. Contemp Urol May 1990; 25.

McAninch JW. Traumatic injuries to the urethra. J Trauma 1981; 21:291–297.

Morehouse DD. Delayed management of external urethral injury. In: Cass AS, ed. Genitourinary Trauma. Boston: Blackwell Scientific Publications, 1988:209.

Pontes JE, Pierce JM Jr. Anterior urethral injuries: four years of experience at the Detroit General Hospital. J Urol 1978; 120: 563–564.

REPAIR OF PENIS AMPUTATION

CHARLES J. DEVINE, Jr., M.D.
GERALD H. JORDAN, M.D.

In our culture, penile amputation, if not accidental, is usually the result of self-emasculation by a psychotic individual with long-standing mental illness, the act of self-mutilation occurring during acute psychotic decompensation. If not psychotic, the individual usually has a severe character disorder or pre-existing conflict about his role as a male. He will obey a hallucination that commands amputation of all or a portion of the genitalia during his first acute psychotic break, often while under the influence of drugs or alcohol. In other situations the penis is amputated by a jealous rival or a heterosexual or homosexual lover. Blacker and Wong described a characteristic background for patients with poor gender identity. Often with a domineering older mother and no male influence in the home during their childhood, they have been or are made to feel guilty and inadequate as males. In many cases these patients have been born into impoverished families, severely limiting the influence of other adults.

Stewart and Lowrey indicated that self-inflicted injury is not an absolute contraindication to replantation, and the literature supports this concept. Mental rehabilitation of these patients is usually successful, and if feasible, replantation should be accomplished without delay. In a review of more than 40 patients with penile amputation, Greilheimer and Groves found only one postoperative suicide and one repeated attempt at emasculation.

PENILE ANATOMY

The vasculature of the deep structures of the penis is derived from branches of the internal pudendal arteries. These distal branches of the hypogastric artery arrive in the perineum through the lesser sciatic foramen, passing into Alcock's canal. In the perineum the terminal branches of the artery form the artery to the corpus spongiosum, the circumflex arteries of the crus of the corpus cavernosum, the cavernosal artery, and the dorsal artery of the penis. Small vascular connections exist in the "urethral groove" linking the corpora cavernosa with the corpus spongiosum. The genital skin has a dual blood supply, also based in part on branches of the pudendal artery. Quartey nicely documented the fasciocutaneous vascular supply of the genital skin.

The venous drainage of the penis has been well described. First, the superficial dorsal venous system is located in the dartos fascia layer and communicates with the femoral, and eventually the iliac, arteries. Second, there is the intermediate system consisting of the emissary and circumflex veins that join the deep dorsal vein coursing in the midline on the dorsum of the penis beneath Buck's fascia, and eventually joining the periprostatic plexus. Third, the deep system contains (1) the crural vessels departing the corpora cavernosa at the crus and draining into the periprostatic plexus and (2) the cavernosal veins draining the corpora proximal to the crus into the pudendal veins.

With microvascular re-establishment of the continuity of the dorsal arteries and/or the cavernosal arteries and the deep dorsal vein and some of the superficial veins of the penis, the amputated portions of the penis survive reliably. However, even without the use of microvascular techniques, simple reattachment of the corporeal structures safely preserves the corpora cavernosa, the corpus spongiosum, and the spongy erectile tissue of the glans penis. It may be surprising that after replantation of the penis by microvascular or nonmicrovascular techniques, erectile function is often unchanged. In the past corporeal reapproximation (referred to as a composite graft) was fraught with complications. In the long run, most of these patients ended up with salvage of a portion of the penis, but the pattern of survival does not fit with what we know about graft take.

The take of a graft occurs in two phases. The first phase, lasting for about 48 hours, is termed imbibition. There is no active blood flow in the graft, and the grafted tissues live by imbibing nutrients from the plasma of the underlying host graft bed. The graft is pale and exists at a temperature below core body temperature. Some authors consider that the graft is only in suspended animation, protected from desiccation by imbibing the tissue fluids, but during this period of anaerobic metabolism the vessels in the graft produce a growth factor inducing angiogenesis, leading to the second stage of graft take, termed inosculation. During this phase, budding vessels from the host graft bed penetrate the graft and, "kissing" the vessels of the grafted tissue, re-establish its microcirculation. As the microcirculation is restored, the graft becomes pink and assumes normal body temperatures. It has taken.

Virtually all the case reports of penile "composite graft" describe the amputated tip of the penis as becoming pink and warm immediately, or at least within several hours. Thus, it appears that an amputated penis repaired by corporeal reapproximation survives because of the truly different vascular properties of the penis, not by the process of imbibition and inosculation.

We know of no studies examining the P_{O_2} or the P_{CO_2} of the blood in the sinuses of the corpora cavernosa or corpus spongiosum. However, we believe that these parameters in penile blood probably approximate those of arterial blood. Procedures that approximate only the corporeal structures probably owe their success to the fact that the corpora are largely lakes of nearly arterialized blood. While processes of angiogenesis may form new collaterals within the amputated portions of the penis, survival of the amputated part probably depends on the dynamics of flap transfer. The portions with access to the blood in the erectile space survive. The skin loss and glanular slough seen in these nonvascularized penile reanastomosis techniques occur because tissues are not vascularized by this process. With re-establishment of the circulation by microvascular anastomosis of the identified arteries and veins, one can expect extremely reliable survival of the amputated penis.

EFFECTS OF ISCHEMIA ON TISSUES

It is well established that hypothermia prolongs the ischemic survival time of all tissues, but the precise response of penile tissues has not yet been studied. Hayhurst and colleagues showed that hyperthermia prolongs the ischemic time compatible with eventual survival after replantation from 6 hours to 24 hours. May and colleagues, evaluating survival of rabbit flaps, determined that 12 hours of normothermic ischemia led to flap loss. Their experiments looked at the "no-reflow phenomenon," which is clearly related to ischemia time in a number of flap models.

Successful penile replantation after 16 hours, much of which was normothermic ischemic time, has been documented. Again, it seems that penile tissues are unique and survive ischemia well. Replantation should always be considered if hypothermic ischemia has existed for less than 24 hours or perhaps a little longer.

Although the first successful penile replantation patients were treated perioperatively with anticoagulant therapy, there is no real indication for the routine use of such therapy in elective microsurgery. It has been suggested that the many vascular planes in the penis may predispose to hematomas that may compromise the surgical repair. The use of anticoagulants in penile replantation must be addressed as individual cases arise.

REPAIR OF PENILE AMPUTATION BEFORE THE USE OF MICROSURGERY

In 1929 Ehrich reported the first case of "replantation" of an amputated penis. The patient, a factory worker, had moved too close to a radial saw. The corpora were reapproximated with chromic suture, the urine being diverted by a urethral catheter. The skin of the penis had been avulsed by the accident, and the penis was buried beneath the scrotal skin for coverage. After 2 years, the man reported some shortening of his penis, although it had an almost normal appearance, and he was having erections and was sexually active. Since that time, about 40 cases of penile reattachment by nonmicrovascular techniques have been reported. Many variations in management have been devised in an effort to avoid the frequent complications of skin and distal glans slough.

In 1944 Dodson reported reattachment of a partially amputated penis, but the details of management are not clear. Price in 1952 described reattachment of a near-total penile amputation. The corpora were meticulously reapproximated as Ehrich had done, and postoperatively the penis was packed in ice to "retard metabolism." One and one-half years later the patient had a small urethrocutaneous fistula, but otherwise was doing well and was sexually active. Subsequently, three cases of partial amputation were documented in which the corpora cavernosa were damaged but the corpus spongiosum spared. The corpora were meticulously reapproximated after ligation of the dorsal vessels. In all cases the cosmetic results were good, but two patients were potent and one was impotent after repair.

In 1962, Best and colleagues reported a case of complete amputation of the penis in which reattachment was accomplished by meticulous reapproximation of the corporeal structures and diversion via a urethral catheter. In an effort to "preserve all the blood supply of the base of the corpora and adjacent structures," they did not ligate the vessels. Postoperatively, the distal penile, preputial, and glanular skin and a major portion of the urethra sloughed, although the other deep structures were preserved. The patient eventually did well; the urethra was reconstructed with a full-thickness skin graft, and penile coverage was accomplished by burying the shaft beneath the scrotal skin. At a subsequent procedure, the penile shaft was liberated from the scrotum and grafted. At follow-up, the patient claimed to be sexually active.

In 1968 McRoberts and associates reported a case of complete penile amputation with skin avulsion, managed by corporeal reapproximation. The avulsed skin was debrided and the shaft buried in the scrotal skin. In this and in Ehrlich's patient an avulsion injury had accompanied the trauma, but McRoberts and associates mentioned another patient managed by Osborne in whom after corporeal reapproximation the distal penile shaft was intentionally denuded and buried in the scrotum. In these cases, there was some loss of the glanular epithelium, but overall the outcomes were excellent. A review of the cases led McRoberts and associates to propose the following management principles: (1) the distal penile skin should be removed; (2) the anastomosed penile shaft should be buried in the scrotum, with the glans protruding from its dependent portion and the glanular epithelium anastomosed to the scrotal skin; and (3) the urine should be diverted suprapubically, with the urethral catheter removed at the end of the operation.

Tuerk and Weir in 1971 and Mendez and colleagues in 1972 added several more cases of partial and complete penile amputation managed by corporeal reapproximation. They did not bury the penis in the scrotum; Mendez and colleagues said they feared that burying the penis might place tension on the corporeal sutures. They felt that survival of the penis was based on corporeal blood flow, and were the first to attempt reapproximation of the dorsal vein in an effort to avoid distal vascular congestion. A number of other cases were described in which the penis was not buried; in these, there were adequate results despite variable amounts of skin loss.

In 1974, Engleman and associates described cases of penile amputation and reviewed previous reports. They concluded that the viability of the distal penile skin was a function of the extent of laceration, the delay until reattachment, and the type of repair. With incomplete laceration, even when only a narrow skin bridge persisted, there was a much lower incidence of skin necrosis. This phenomenon was thought to be a function of the extensive collateralization seen between the deep vessels and the fasciocutaneous vessels of the dartos layer. These authors debated the option of microvascular anastomosis of the dorsal vessels, theorizing that microvascular repair would avoid skin necrosis because of the immediate re-establishment of the subcutaneous blood flow, instead of depending on the perforators to the dartos fascial vessels and subdermal plexus of the penile skin. They also suggested that hypothermic storage of the amputated penis might improve results by prolonging vitality from the time of injury to reattachment, and proposed the reapproximation of the sensory nerves of the penis via microneurosurgical techniques.

In 1978, Bux and associates reported cases of penile reattachment managed by corporeal reapproximation. Their report appeared after the first reports of microvascular replantation of the amputated penis, but these cases were not cited and presumably must have become available after their manuscript was submitted. They stated, however, that neither microanastomosis of the dorsal vessels and nerves nor burying the penis is necessary or desirable, if a meticulous corporeal reapproximation has been accomplished.

Since 1977, papers describing corporeal reapproximation in the treatment of penile amputation have continued to be published, although these reports indicate that microreplantation is probably superior to simple corporeal reapproximation. These patients have been managed by corporeal reapproximation because of the inability to get them to centers performing microvascular and microneurosurgery.

HISTORY OF MICROREPLANTATION TECHNIQUES

In 1976, Tamai and associates and Cohen and associates reported successful replantation of an amputated penis. Tamai and associates reanastomosed the dorsal vein of the penis, both dorsal arteries, and several of the dorsal nerves. The patient was given low-molecular dextran perioperatively. Cohen and associates reanastomosed one cavernosal artery, the dorsal vein, both dorsal arteries, and a number of the dorsal nerves. The patient was treated with urokinase perioperatively. Both groups of surgeons used microvascular and microneurosurgical techniques with excellent results; neither group had knowledge of the other's accomplishment until the reports of their success were published.

Since these landmark cases, a number of repairs using microvascular and microneurosurgical techniques with uniformly good results have been reported. Carroll and colleagues reviewed a number of these cases in 1985. Sensation was present uniformly. Most authors reported that erections occurred beyond the area of repair, but the ability to achieve intromission was not specifically addressed. Skin was lost in some patients despite microreplantation, but in only one man in whom a urethrocutaneous fistula occurred did the amount of skin loss essentially alter the postoperative course. On the basis of this review, these authors proposed a logical sequence of care for a patient who presents with a penile amputation injury. The uniform success of microreplantation in treatment of penile amputation has changed the status of this unusual injury from reportable to essentially nonreportable.

HISTORY OF REPLANTATION OF THE TESTIS

Evins and associates in 1977 reported a paranoid schizophrenic who presented with bilateral amputation of the testicles and an abortive attempt at penile amputation. After stabilization of the patient, the testicles were debrided, filleted, and placed into subcutaneous thigh pouches. Postoperatively, the patient appeared to be anorchidic, and biopsy of the testicles showed total coagulation necrosis. Although unsuccessful, this was the first attempt at testicular salvage after amputation. In 1976, Silber and Kelly reported the successful autotransplantation of an intra-abdominal undescended testicle. Since that report, many others have further documented the feasibility of microvascular anastomosis of the vessels of the spermatic cord. By this time the use of the microscope for vasovasostomy was also well established.

In 1979 Abbou and colleagues replanted the testicles and the penis by microvascular-microneurosurgical techniques. Subsequent reports have documented the successful application of microreplantation techniques to traumatically amputated testicles.

CURRENT CONCEPTS OF MICROREPLANTATION

It is clear from the literature that the length of time that amputated organs can remain ischemic can be extended by means of hypothermia. The amputated penis and/or testicle should be preserved by the bag-within-a-bag technique in which the amputated part is placed on saline-soaked gauze inside a clean ziplock plastic bag. The bag is sealed and placed into a second bag containing an ice slush. The amputated organ can then be transported with the patient to a center for replantation; this should be done within 18 hours. However, experience has shown the remarkable resilience of the penis to ischemia, and thus cold ischemia times of more than 24 hours do not make replantation out of the question.

Penile replantation should proceed in a systematic fashion. Exploration of both of the severed ends should identify the structures that need to be reanastomosed (Fig. 1). Debridement, if necessary, should be accomplished judiciously (Fig. 2). Mechanical stabilization of the penis is achieved by stenting the urethra and proceeding with a two-layer spatulated urethral anastomosis. The mucosa is approximated edge to edge with interrupted 6-0 chromic sutures. The adventitia and spongy erectile tissue are then approximated with running sutures of 4-0 or 5-0 PDS. When the penis has been stabilized, the corpora cavernosa are approximated. In proximal injuries, reanastomosis of the cavernosal artery may be possible and if so should be accomplished. This requires some dissection of the artery within the spongy erectile tissue with reanastomosis, using 11-0 nylon suture. Careful reapproximation of the tunica albuginea of the corpora cavernosa is then performed, also reapproximating the septal fibers of the corpora cavernosa with 4-0 or 5-0 PDS suture.

The dorsal neurovascular structures can then be addressed. Both arteries should be repaired, reanastomosing them with 11-0 nylon sutures (Fig. 3). The dorsal vein can then be reanastomosed with 9-0 or 10-0 nylon suture. After vascular anastomosis, the arborized nerve should be dissected and reanastomosed with 9-0 or 10-0 nylon suture. Fascicular reapproximation is not necessary; the stitches can be placed in the epineurium, thereby reapproximating the ends of the severed fascicles. Dartos fascia is then closed, and 5-0 or 6-0 Vicryl serves well in this layer. Any large superficial veins present in this layer should also be reanastomosed. The skin is approximated with 4-0 or 5-0 chromic suture. A suprapubic cystostomy catheter should be placed while the urethral anastomosis is stented with a small silicone catheter (Fig. 4). To simplify postoperative monitoring, sites where the pulse in the dorsal arteries can best be identified with a Doppler probe are marked on the skin of the replanted end of the penis.

The patient must be kept well hydrated with a normal body temperature throughout the procedure and in the postoperative course. Heat lamps should be used to keep him warm and thus peripherally vasodilated. The

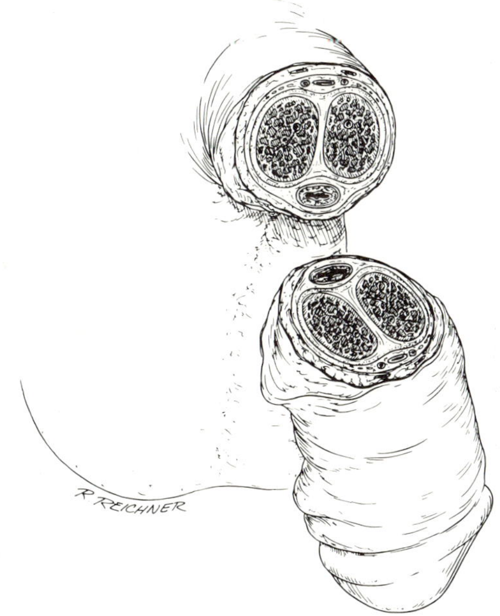

Figure 1 The amputated portion of the penis should be cooled as quickly as possible. The structures are readily identifiable as they are cut in cross section. (Republished with permission by Jordan GH, Gilbert GA. Management of amputation injuries of the male genitalia. Urol Clin North Am 1989; 16:359–367.)

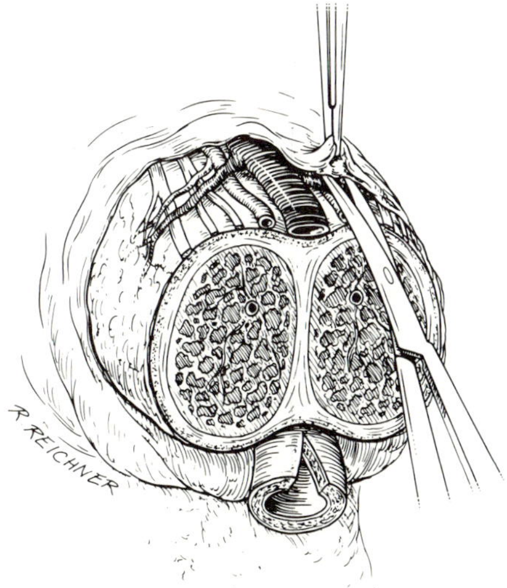

Figure 2 Minimal debridement exposes the arborized nerves, the arteries, and the deep dorsal vein. The urethra has been spatulated. (Republished with permission by Jordan GH, Gilbert GA. Management of amputation injuries of the male genitalia. Urol Clin North Am 1989; 16:359–367.)

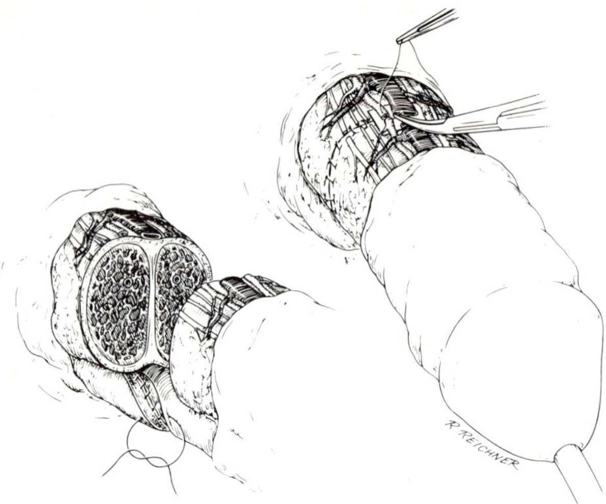

Figure 3 The repair is stabilized by placing a catheter through the urethra, which has been anastomosed in a two-layer spatulated fashion. The tunica albuginea and septal fibers of the corpora cavernosa are reapproximated, and microanastomosis of the dorsal arteries, dorsal vein, and arborized nerves is begun. In some cases of very proximal amputation, the cavernosal artery or arteries can also be reanastomosed. (Republished with permission by Jordan GH, Gilbert GA. Management of amputation injuries of the male genitalia. Urol Clin North Am 1989; 16:359–367.)

patient should be kept at bed rest for at least 1 week and, as noted, close monitoring of the penile circulation with the Doppler is necessary.

Urinary diversion should be continued for 2 to 3 weeks, depending on wound healing and the presence or absence of skin loss. The stenting catheter can then be removed and voiding urethrography performed to document the integrity of the repair site. Anticoagulation is controversial, but the use of one baby aspirin per day is probably warranted.

The advantages of microreplantation are obvious, and if this is not available locally, we recommend transfer to a facility with such capabilities. However, if transfer is impossible, the penis should be reattached by corporeal reapproximation. The literature shows that in most cases, penile salvage is possible despite the lack of microsurgical technology, although the incidence of postoperative complications may be greater. Denuding the penis and burying the penile shaft in the scrotum, as recommended by McRoberts and colleagues, has yielded acceptably good results.

It appears that a sharply amputated testicle is also reliably salvageable. Identification of the proximal artery may be tricky, but the vessel can be reanastomosed by microsurgery using 11-0 nylon suture. The literature suggests that the distal venous stumps can be identified by observing back-bleeding. When the bleeding veins have been identified, two to three venous anastomoses can be accomplished using 9-0, 10-0, or 11-0 suture, depending on the vessel diameter. The vas deferens is then anastomosed in an end-to-end fashion. We favor an

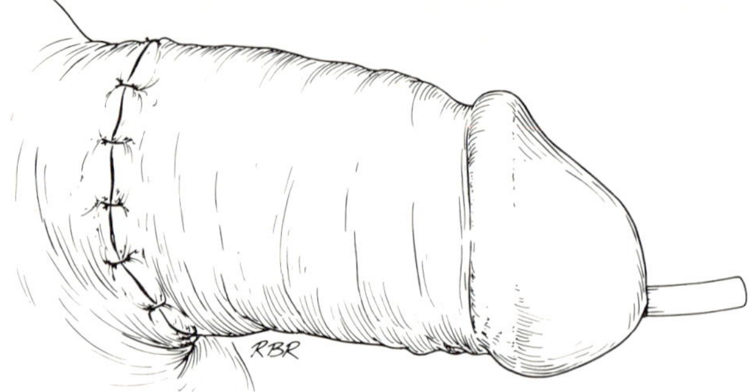

Figure 4 Meticulous anatomic closure of the layers superficial to the neurovascular bundle and urethra has been accomplished, and the skin closed with interrupted chromic sutures. A suprapubic tube has been installed and the urethral repair stented with a soft silicone catheter. (Republished with permission by Jordan GH, Gilbert GA. Management of amputation injuries of the male genitalia. Urol Clin North Am 1989; 16:359–367.)

unstented two-layer microtechnique, approximating the mucosa with 10-0 or 11-0 nylon suture and the muscularis with 9-0 suture.

An avulsed testicle is rarely, if ever, suitable for microreplantation owing to the damage and vascular spasm caused by the stretch before the snap phenomenon that occurs. The scrotal skin, unlike that of the penis, is not vascularized by the underlying deep structures. If scrotal skin is lost, the replanted testicles should be placed in superficial thigh pouches. They can be liberated at a second procedure and covered with a split-thickness skin graft.

If a patient presents without the amputated part, hemorrhage should be controlled. In the case of the penis, often more skin than penile shaft is amputated, and coverage of the shaft with a split-thickness skin graft may yield better results than burying the shaft and closing the remaining skin. The neomeatus must be widely spatulated in the fashion of a partial penectomy to avoid subsequent meatal stenosis.

DISCUSSION

Development of modern tissue transfer techniques has markedly modified the approach to reconstructive surgery in general, and the management of traumatic genital amputation is no exception. The unique nature of the vascularity of the penis has allowed for exceptionally good results in a number of cases in which simple replantation followed genital amputation. Microvascular and microneuroreplantation can provide uniformly better results while minimizing postoperative complications. After penile amputation and microreplantation a patient can be left with a penis cosmetically normal and functionally nearly normal or undetectably abnormal. Microreplantation offers the best results after penile amputation, but if such technology is not available and the patient cannot be moved within 18 hours to a facility offering this procedure, the older corporeal reattachment techniques should be carried out as soon as possible.

SUGGESTED READING

Abbou CC, Servant VM, Bonnet F, et al. Replantation du penis et des deux testicules apres autoemasculation complete. Chirurgie 1979; 105:354–357.

Best JW, Angelo JJ, Milligan B. Complete traumatic amputation of the penis. J Urol 1962; 87:134–138.

Blacker KH, Wong N. Four cases of autocastration. Arch Gen Psychiatry 1963; 8:169–176.

Bux R, Carroll P, Berger M, Yarbrough W. Primary penile reanastomosis. Urology 1978; 11:500–503.

Carroll PR, Lue TF, Schmidt RA, et al. Penile replantation: current concepts. J Urol 1985; 133:281–285.

Cohen BE, May JW, Daly JS, Young HH. Successful clinical replantation of an amputated penis by microneurovascular repair. Plast Reconstr Surg 1977; 59:276–288.

Dodson AI. Urologic surgery. St. Louis: CV Mosby, 1944.

Ehrich WS. Two unusual penile injuries. J Urol 1929; 21:239–241.

Einarsson G, Goldstein M, Laungani G. Penile replantation. Urology 1983; 22:404–405.

Engelman ER, Polito G, Perley J, et al. Traumatic amputation of the penis. J Urol 1974; 112:774–778.

Evins SC, Whittle T, Rous SN. Self-emasculation: review of the literature, report of a case and outline of the objectives of management. J Urol 1977; 118:775–776.

Greilsheimer H, Groves JE. Male genital self-mutilation. Arch Gen Psychiatry 1979; 36:441–446.

Izzidien AY. Successful replantation of a traumatically amputated penis in a neonate. J Pediatr Surg 1981; 16:202–203.

McRoberts JW, Chapman WH, Ansell JS. Primary anastomosis of the traumatically amputated penis: case report and summary of literature. J Urol 1968; 100:751–754.

Mendez R, Kiely WF, Morrow JW. Self-emasculation. J Urol 1972; 107:981–985.

Price KA. Accidental transection of all corpora of the penis: repair with good results. J Urol 1952; 68:620–622.

Schulman ML. Reanastomosis of the amputated penis. J Urol 1973; 109:432–433.

Silber SJ, Kelly J. Successful autotransplantation of an intra-abdominal testis to the scrotum by microvascular techniques. J Urol 1976; 115:452–454.

Stewart DE, Lowrey MR. Replantation surgery following self-inflicted amputation. Can J Psychiatry 1980; 25:143–150.

Tamai S, Nakamura Y, Motomiya Y. Microsurgical replantation of a completely amputated penis and scrotum. Plast Reconstr Surg 1977; 60:287–291.

Tuerk M, Weir WH Jr. Successful replantation of a traumatically amputated glans penis. Plast Reconstr Surg 1971; 48:499–500.

PRIAPISM

DONALD R. BODNER, M.D.

Priapism is a persistent, painful penile erection that occurs without sexual stimulation or desire. The etiology may be idiopathic or secondary to medication or underlying illness. There may be one or more previous episodes of sustained, painful erections of shorter duration that resolved spontaneously or responded to intervention. Priapism can occur at any age from early childhood on; most occur after puberty. In adults, most cases are idiopathic. However, there is growing evidence that a number of drugs such as the psychotropics, antihypertensives, and heparin may be responsible.

In children, sickle cell disease and leukemia are the two leading causes of priapism. In sicklers, the red blood cells sickle as oxygen is consumed during the erection. The increased viscosity of the blood then leads to mechanical obstruction of the vessels, preventing venous drainage. Two thirds of children with priapism have sickle disease. In the remaining third, the etiology is equally divided among leukemia, trauma, and idiopathic causes. In leukemia, leukemic infiltrates may involve the dorsal vein and corpora cavernosa, leading to mechanical obstruction to venous drainage from the penis.

In contrast, in the vast majority of adults with priapism there is an idiopathic etiology. Sickle trait may be associated in adult black males, while leukemia, trauma, and tumor each play a minor role in adults. Priapism is also seen in adults as a complication of intracorporeal injection of vasoactive medications used to restore erections. Patients with neurogenic impotence are particularly prone to this complication. When rigid erections persist for more than 4 hours after intracorporeal injection therapy, they must be reversed to prevent long-term complications of priapism.

THERAPEUTIC ALTERNATIVES

A careful history taking and physical examination may help to uncover the cause of the priapism. Sickle status should be determined. Except when a sickle cell disorder is the etiology, intervention generally is surgical. With sicklers, medical intervention should be begun immediately with hydration, oxygenation, alkalinization, blood transfusion, and exchange transfusion when necessary. Only when these conservative measures have failed in the sickle cell patient should more invasive measures be considered.

For individuals without sickle cell disease, early surgical intervention should be instituted. Patients should be advised of an approximately 50 percent incidence of permanent impotence after priapism whatever the type of intervention. A multitude of conservative methods have been attempted to avoid surgical intervention, including ice and warm enemas; general, spinal, and epidural anesthesia; fibrinolysins; and sequential tourniquets. Because these techniques are generally ineffective, limited time should be expended with them before more invasive and effective procedures are begun. The patient's subsequent ability to have erections may be influenced by the expediency with which the priapism is corrected, and therefore early intervention is necessary. Intervention within 72 hours of onset of priapism is advisable.

Aspiration and Irrigation

Approximately half of the patients with priapism can be effectively treated with aspiration and irrigation of the corpora cavernosa. An 18-gauge needle attached to a 10-ml syringe is placed from the dorsal tip of the glans directly into the ipsilateral corporeal body. Blood is aspirated from the corporeal body, which is then gently irrigated with normal saline. The corporeal body can be massaged to evacuate the old blood. The aspirated blood may appear old and dark, and aspiration and irrigation should be continued until the blood appears red and no old blood remains. Generally about ten irrigations are performed, under local anesthesia at the bedside or under local, general, or spinal anesthesia in the operating room. If the penis remains flaccid, no further treatment is required. However, if priapism reoccurs or if the penis is not flaccid after aspiration and irrigation, one should proceed to a shunt.

Priapism Secondary to Intracorporeal Injection of Vasoactive Medications

When erections persist for more than 4 hours after injection of vasoactive medications, they must be reversed. Pharmacologic reversal of drug-induced erections has nearly always been successful when the erection has lasted less than 14 to 16 hours. This can often be accomplished simply by aspirating the corpora cavernosa and irrigating them with saline. If detumescence is not achieved by this technique, irrigation with a variety of alpha-stimulants can be tried. During this irrigation, blood pressure must be carefully monitored. Phenylephrine hydrochloride is effective and can minimize the cardiac side effects of agents such as epinephrine. The phenylephrine (10 mg) is diluted in 500 ml of normal saline. The corpora are then irrigated with 10 to 15 ml of the irrigant and the process is repeated several times until detumescence is accomplished. Surgical shunting is rarely required if corporeal irrigation is unsuccessful. The same technique can be performed using epinephrine (1 mg epinephrine mixed in 1,000 ml of normal saline) or metaraminol, using from 0.1 to 0.3 ml (1 to 3 mg).

Glans Penis to Corpora Cavernosa Shunt (Winter's Shunt)

After aspiration and irrigation of the penis, shunts can be created between the spongiosum of the glans penis and the corpora cavernosa. One of the most popular methods is the percutaneous technique described by Winter. The irrigation needle is removed from the glans and a TruCut needle is inserted from the glans into the corpora cavernosa. Several cores are obtained, taking tissue from the septum between the glans and the corpora. The procedure can be performed with the patient under local anesthesia (1 percent lidocaine) infiltration or under general or spinal anesthesia. The needle should be rotated 360 degrees, and excess tissue can be removed with a rongeur. A small incision can be made in the glans penis, and the septum between the glans and the corpora cavernosa excised with a rongeur. At the end of the procedure, a 3-0 chromic figure-of-eight suture is placed in the glans at the incision site for hemostasis. The penis should remain flaccid. This can be accomplished by having the patient squeeze it every few minutes, or a pediatric blood pressure cuff can be applied and inflated every few minutes for the first 12 hours. A compression dressing should not be applied directly to the penis, as this can lead to necrosis. If the penis remains more than 50 percent rigid after 12 to 24 hours, the above procedure can be repeated or an alternative shunt can be performed.

Corpus Cavernosum to Corpus Spongiosum

An alternative procedure for the treatment of priapism is the creation of a shunt between the corpus cavernosum and the corpus spongiosum. The incision is best made in the perineum or at the base of the penis, where inadvertent injury to the urethra can be avoided. The bulbocavernous muscle is incised in the midline in a longitudinal direction and then retracted laterally. The corpus cavernosum and corpus spongiosum are identified. A running suture is placed between the fascia of these two corpora. A catheter should be in place to identify the depth of the urethra. A 1-cm round window of tunica albuginea is removed from the corpus spongiosum and from the adjacent corpus cavernosum at the level of the bulbous urethra. Old blood is evacuated from the corpus cavernosum, which is then irrigated with saline. The two corporeal windows are anastomosed together, using a running 2-0 chromic suture to create the fistula. Unilateral anastomosis may be sufficient, but the creation of a fistula with the other corpus cavernosum may provide optimal shunting.

Corpus Cavernosum to Saphenous Vein

Anastomosis of the corpus cavernosum to the ipsilateral saphenous vein allows blood to drain directly from the penis and avoids the venous obstruction. Intervention should be instituted within 72 hours of the onset of priapism, although some successes have been reported when intervention has been delayed. An incision is made over the saphenous vein, which is isolated and dissected from its insertion in the femoral vein to the midthigh. The saphenous vein is divided in the midthigh and the proximal end is tied. A separate incision is made at the base of the penis. The saphenous vein is tunneled to the incision at the base of the penis, and then anastomosed to one of the corpora cavernosa with a running vascular suture.

Complications

With time, most of the shunts created to treat priapism spontaneously close off, permitting the patient to obtain an adequate erection. Virtually all of the corpora cavernosa to saphenous vein shunts also close. However, as many as 40 percent of patients may have problems with erection after appropriate treatment for priapism. Complications of open shunt operations occur in approximately 15 percent of cases, including urethrocutaneous fistula, urethrocavernous fistula, hematoma, abscess, gangrene of the distal penis, and occasional pulmonary emboli. The risk of these complications arising must be taken, because long-standing untreated priapism almost always leads to impotence.

SUGGESTED READING

Grayhack JT, McCullough W, O'Conor VJ Jr, et al. Venous bypass to control priapism. Invest Urol 1964; 1:509.

Kursh ED, Bodner DR, Resnick MI, et al. Injection therapy for impotence. Urol Clin North Am 1988; 15:625–629.

Sidi AA. Vasoactive intracavernous pharmacotherapy. Urol Clin North Am 1988; 15:95–101.

Winter CC. Priapism. In: Glenn JF, ed. Urologic surgery. 3rd ed. Philadelphia: JB Lippincott, 1983:803.

I SCROTUM AND ITS CONTENTS

SCROTAL LACERATION AND AVULSION

EDWARD W. CAMPBELL, Jr., M.D.

Scrotal lacerations and avulsion injuries vary greatly in severity and may involve underlying structures such as the urethra and rectum. Staged repair is necessary in more extensive injuries or grossly contaminated wounds. Guidelines are offered to aid in the selection of appropriate surgical techniques for reconstruction of the denuded penis and avulsed scrotum.

SCROTAL LACERATION

Simple lacerations of the scrotum and penis are seen frequently and may result from industrial, vehicular, and sporting accidents. Superficial lacerations are appropriately managed in the emergency room setting, but more extensive injuries are better dealt with in the operating room. Injury to the underlying structures, including the spermatic cord, testis, urethra, and corporal bodies, is common in the latter instance. Preliminary urethrography is indicated if blood is apparent at the meatus or if urethral injury is otherwise suspected. If corporal injury is of concern, the penis may be circumcised just proximal to the coronal margin and the penile skin and superficial fascia reduced in glovelike fashion to its base, affording good exposure of the erectile bodies and the urethra. Injuries to these structures are closed with absorbable suture material after appropriate debridement. The skin laceration should be thoroughly irrigated, cleansed with povidone-iodine, and closed with absorbable suture material, care being taken to evert the skin edges with mattress sutures. Grossly contaminated wounds are drained or left open and packed, awaiting secondary closure in 5 to 7 days. Patients with significant scrotal lacerations routinely receive a cephalosporin antibiotic. A loose sterile scrotal dressing is held in place with an athletic supporter or elastic hose. Sitz baths are begun 4 days after the repair.

SCROTAL AVULSION

Currently, most scrotal injuries associated with skin loss seen in my trauma center result from motorcycle deacceleration injuries. Industrial, farming, and even sporting accidents may predominate in other areas of the United States. The extent of genital skin loss varies greatly and may, in its more severe forms, be associated with testicular loss or laceration as well as urethral and rectal injuries. I have assisted in the management of several patients with massive perineal injuries involving loss of portions of the urethra, scrotal contents, and lower rectum. These patients have required urinary and fecal diversion and extended wound cleansing before coverage with gracilis muscle flaps and skin grafts. Fortunately, most skin loss is more limited and the surgeon can institute definitive or staged repair immediately.

One must always rule out injury to the underlying tissues, including the urethra, corpora, testes, and rectum. Urinary and fecal diversion with suprapubic tube and colostomy may be required in the course of urethral reconstruction and rectal injury.

Having assured the integrity of these structures, the surgeon must carefully assess the degree of penile, scrotal, and perineal skin loss and soft tissue loss. Degloving injuries of the penis commonly result in loss of the skin and dartos fascia, the underlying Buck's fascia affording an excellent base for primary grafting. Remaining skin flaps arising from the base of the penis may be extended distally on the shaft to provide partial coverage. However, distal flaps, when circumferentially separated from the suprapubic skin and penile base, often become edematous. It is therefore advisable to trim this skin to within 1 cm of the glans and cover the shaft with grafted skin. In one instance it was possible to cover the entire dorsum of the penis with a distally based penile flap and achieve a favorable cosmetic result without edema. Partial or total replacement of penile skin with split-thickness skin grafts provides excellent results in most instances. Buck's fascia affords a good base for the acute application of a skin graft; granulation tissue, if unhealthy, should be removed by sharp scraping in delayed grafting. The anterior lateral aspect of the thigh is most commonly chosen as a donor site and is shaved, prepared with povidone-iodine, and draped into

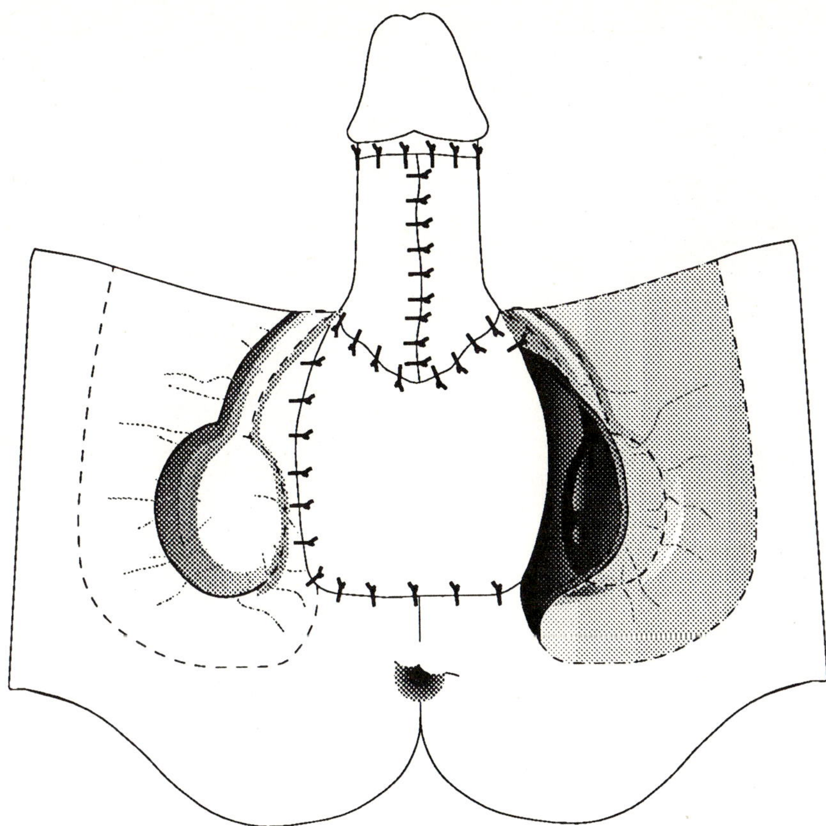

Figure 1 The testes are buried in superficial thigh pouches and the penis and perineum covered with skin grafts. Note that the encircling penile graft is approximated ventrally and that the perineal wound forms the medial aspect of the potential thigh flaps.

the operative field. Most air dermatomes produce a 10- to 12-cm wide graft. This comfortably encompasses the erect penis and is sutured longitudinally on the ventral surface (Fig. 1). Narrower grafts may be used to wrap the penis in a "barber pole" fashion and achieve good coverage. While this is thought to prevent chordee formation, a graft wrapped vertically and sutured ventrally has not been associated with significant postoperative curvature. A thin meshed graft is preferred as this is suitable for a high percentage of patients and leaves a rapidly healing donor site. Thicker nonmeshed split-thickness grafts, however, provide more elasticity and a better cosmetic appearance, obvious advantages in a potent patient. The penis is dressed erect with a bolster, and urinary drainage is achieved with a urethral catheter. Skin flaps based on the thigh or abdomen may also be used to cover the denuded penis, but generally with less pleasing cosmetic results. Skin grafting in my opinion provides the most satisfactory form of coverage. If the scrotum remains intact, one may elect to use an anterior scrotal tunnel to bury the denuded penis while exteriorizing the glans through a small transverse midline incision, enabling the patient to direct his urinary stream and affording a rapid and acceptable means of skin coverage (Fig. 2). The penis may be mobilized at a later date with its overlying scrotal skin for circumfer-

ential integument replacement. The elastic scrotal skin is then easily mobilized to close the resulting defect.

Avulsion of the scrotal skin will vary considerably in degree, and when complete, may also include perineal skin loss. The avulsed tissue most often includes skin, the loose dartos fascia of the scrotum, and Colles' fascia of the perineum, while sparing the testicular tunics. The unusual elasticity of the scrotal skin provides an opportunity to cover extensive skin loss with seemingly small residual integument. Thus, partial and even moderately severe injuries may be managed primarily with debridement and closure, developing scrotal flaps as necessary.

Complete loss of scrotal and penile skin is more likely to involve deeper structures such as the urethra, testes, and scrotum. Initial efforts are directed at identification and repair of these injuries, and may necessitate suprapubic cystostomy and colostomy. Multiple factors must be considered in planning the approach to the skin loss: the nature of the wound and contamination, the degree of integument loss, the age of the patient, and his erectile and reproductive potential.

Traditionally, the testes are either immediately, or after a period of cleansing, placed in medial thigh pockets and the penile and perineal defects covered with meshed split-thickness grafts. This position provides an optimal environment for the injured testes and a

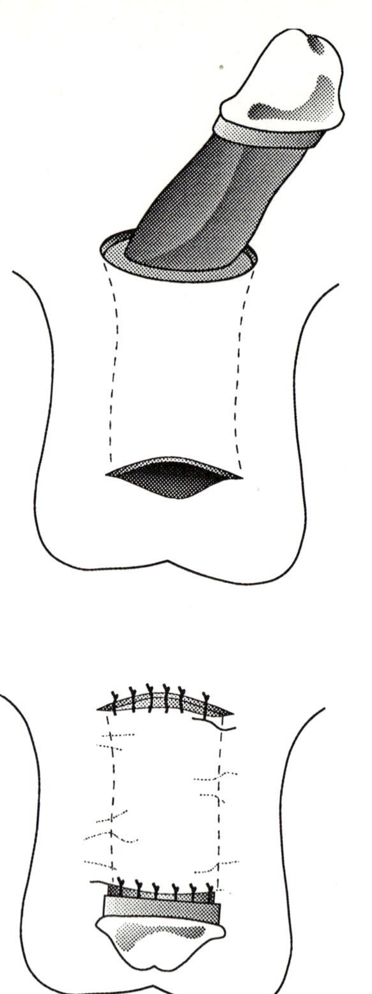

Figure 2 The denuded penile shaft is buried in an anterior scrotal compartment and the normal glans exteriorized.

temperature conducive to the preservation of spermatogenesis and fertility when this is of concern. The testes should be placed just beneath the skin, in the center of the proposed thigh flaps and at different levels in each thigh (see Fig. 1). Attention to these details will provide optimal temperature, aid in the subsequent development of flaps encompassing the testes, and prevent "bumping" once the testes are brought to the midline for reconstruction with their respective flaps.

Thigh flaps may be developed and transferred to the midline to cover the testes as a primary procedure. However, if the testes have been initially placed in thigh pockets, thigh flaps may be mobilized 4 or more weeks later with their underlying testes and brought to the perineum to form a new scrotum (Fig. 3). In either instance the flaps are based superiorly, ensuring adequate blood and neural supply. The perineal wound will define the medial aspect of the flap. The flap is raised by incising through to the superficial fascia of the thigh. There should be no subcutaneous tissue overlying the back of the testes, if these are being mobilized with the flaps. The flaps are rotated medially and sutured around

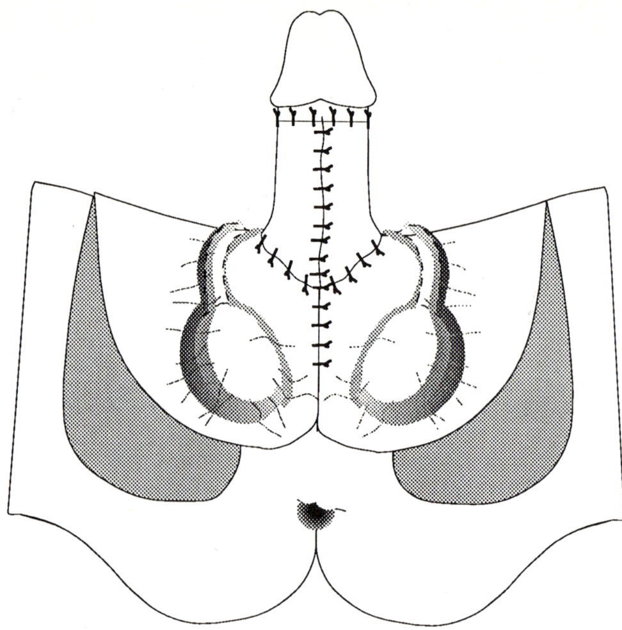

Figure 3 The testes are mobilized with their covering skin flaps and approximated in the midline to form a new scrotum. The thigh defects are closed primarily or covered with split-thickness skin grafts.

the base of the penis and subsequently to each other in the midline, with absorbable suture material (Fig. 3). The thigh defects are closed primarily if possible. Both the thigh and scrotal wounds are drained.

Thigh flaps offer a cosmetically acceptable reconstruction of the scrotum. However, the procedure does require loose, pliable thigh skin with limited subcutaneous fat to ensure free mobilization of the flaps and primary closure of the thigh defects. Undesirable thigh scars may result from this procedure. Further, the dislocated testes are often a source of discomfort for the patient, even though temporary in nature. As an alternative to the transfer of the testes with encompassing flaps, one may mobilize the testes from their pockets through medial incisions, suture them in the midline, and apply a meshed split-thickness graft.

The most expeditious approach involves immediate application of meshed split-thickness grafts to the scrotum and perineum and a moderately thick graft to the penis, assuring that all nonviable tissue is recognized and removed. Gross wound contamination and extensive soft tissue damage require 2 to 4 weeks of debridement, and intensive wound care before split-thickness skin coverage. Such delay may actually improve scrotal graft take as granulation tissue fills in acute angles presented by the approximated testes, which may otherwise make coverage difficult. In either instance, the meshed graft is applied so as to cover the entire surface of the spermatic cords and the approximated testes. A fine-mesh petrolatum gauze covers the graft to help immobilize it during the initial healing period. This in turn is reinforced with a large fluff dressing held in position with a tight-fitting

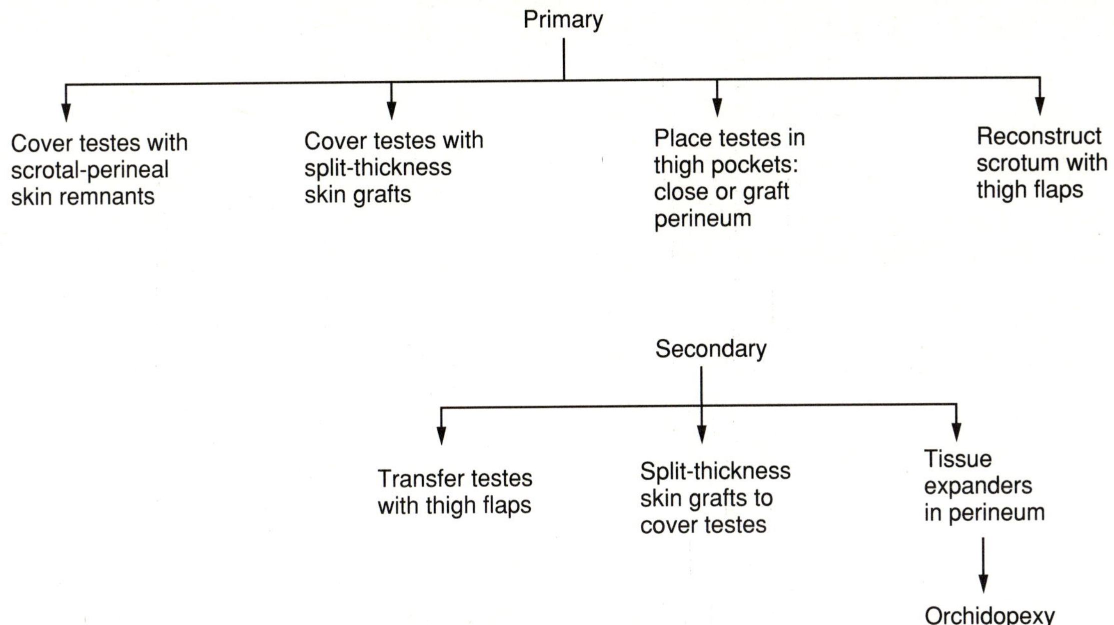

Figure 4 Options in the surgical management of the avulsed scrotum.

elastic undergarment. Immobilization for 5 to 7 days is desirable, because displacement of the graft would jeopardize a successful take. Early grafting provides a relatively simple, single-stage procedure that offers satisfactory cosmetic and functional results in most surgeons' hands. Complications include hematoma formation and infection with graft loss. Scar contraction and lymphedema have posed manageable problems.

A delayed approach can be rewarded with the development of residual scrotal and perineal skin adequate for coverage of the denuded testes. In injuries associated with extensive scrotal skin loss and contamination, the wounds are initially debrided and all viable tissue is preserved. No attempt is made to bury the testes in thigh pockets or to immediately cover them with split-thickness grafts. After 3 to 4 weeks of intensive wound care and careful debriding, adequate, healthy scrotal and perineal skin may be available for coverage of the testes. This is further evidence of the remarkable pliability of these tissues, which can, with careful selection, provide adequate tissue for coverage.

Tissue expanders can be used, taking advantage of the recuperative capability of the perineal skin. The testes are initially transplanted to medial thigh pockets and the penis is covered with split-thickness skin grafts. Perineal closure is performed initially by advancement flaps, or delayed until the residual skin has better defined itself. Five months later, tissue expanders are inserted on either side of the midline, achieving volumes of 300 ml within several additional months. Orchidopexy completes the procedure. A time-consuming and multistage reconstruction, this appears capable of achieving a satisfying two-compartment scrotum and should find

application in reconstruction after certain cases of scrotal skin avulsion.

SURGICAL OPTIONS

Surgical procedures appropriate for reconstruction of the denuded genitalia have been discussed, and management is outlined in an algorithm (Fig. 4). Residual scrotal and perineal skin can often be salvaged in a primary or delayed approach to provide adequate reconstruction of the scrotum. Primary skin grafting of the penis and testes affords a one-stage procedure that is applicable in the face of more extensive skin loss. The testes may be transferred to thigh pouches under the same circumstance, awaiting perineal healing and the secondary application of split-thickness skin grafts or the formation of a new scrotum with thigh flaps. Tissue expanders offer a new and effective technique for constructing a cosmetically appealing scrotum, but require a multistage procedure.

SUGGESTED READING

Bertini JE Jr, Corriere NJ Jr. The etiology and management of genital injuries. J Trauma 1988; 28:1278–1281.

Furnas DW, McCraw JB. Resurfacing the genital area. Clin Plast Surg 1980; 7:235–238.

McAninch JW. Management of genital skin loss. Urol Clin North Am 1989; 16:387–397.

McDougal WS. Scrotal reconstruction using thigh pedicle flaps. J Urol 1983; 129:757–759.

Still EF 2nd, Goodman RC. Total reconstruction of two-compartment scrotum by tissue expansion. Plast Reconstr Surg 1990; 85:805–807.

Tripathi FM, Sinha JK, Bhattacharya U, Bariar LM. Traumatic avulsion of penile and scrotal skin. Br J Plast Surg 1982; 35:302–303.

TESTICULAR TORSION

GEORG BARTSCH, M.D.
GREGOR MIKUZ, M.D.
OTMAR ENNEMOSER, M.D.
GÜNTER JANETSCHEK, M.D.

Torsion of the testicle or the spermatic cord is an acute urologic emergency; the twisted testis suffers severe tissue damage within a few hours owing to anoxia. Only its proper and timely diagnosis can prevent necrosis and, hence, irreversible testicular damage. Fortunately, the anamnesis and clinical findings are usually typical in the therapeutically important early phase so that early diagnosis is possible. Nevertheless, the clinical picture is not always recognized early.

TYPES OF TORSION

Extravaginal (Neonatal) Torsion

This type represents approximately 6 percent of the entire group of torsions. The normal testis is not free to twist on its own spermatic cord except in the newborn, when the testis and its large gubernaculum have only recently entered the scrotum and are still free to rotate (Fig. 1). In neonatal torsion, epididymis and tunica vaginalis twist together in a vertical axis on the cord at the external inguinal ring. The clinical picture shows a firm, or stony hard, enlarged scrotal mass. It does not transilluminate, it is not apparently tender, and the child is surprisingly little disturbed; systemic signs are rare.

Intravaginal (Adolescent) Torsion

In adolescence, torsion of the testis almost invariably takes place within the tunica vaginalis and can occur only if there is a deficiency of the suspension of the testicle (capacious tunica, small bare area) (Fig. 2). The classic presentation following violent exercise, with severe testicular pain and swelling, is relatively uncommon. The initial pain is commonly felt in the groin or lower abdomen and may not be particularly severe. The onset may be at night, the boy being awakened with groin pain, only to discover later that the testis is swollen and tender. Within a few hours the scrotum becomes edematous and red, an appearance that often suggests bacterial infection. Even in the case of hemorrhagic infarction, the temperature is usually normal or subnormal. There are no urinary symptoms, and the urine contains neither cells nor bacteria.

Torsion of the Testicular Appendages

Attached to the testis, epididymis, and cord are a group of polypoid structures of mesonephric and müllerian origin. There are five testicular appendages: the paradidymis or "organ of Giraldés," the appendix

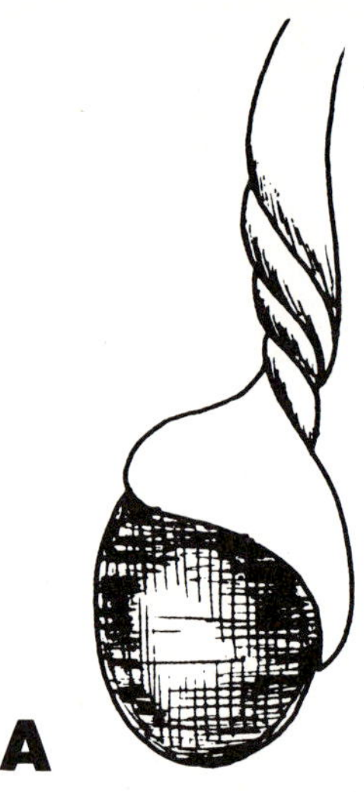

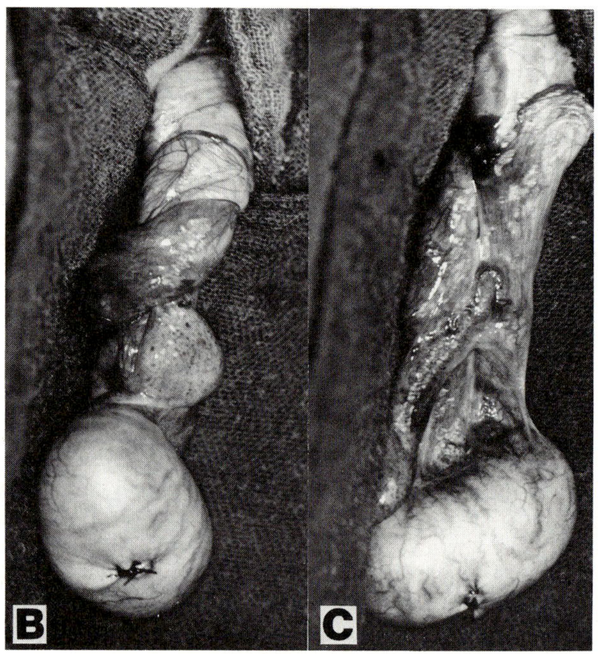

Figure 1 *A* and *B,* Extravaginal torsion. *C,* After detorsion.

epididymidis, and the superior and the inferior vas aberrans of Haller, all of which are vestiges of the mesonephric tubules (Fig. 3); the appendix testis or "hydatid of Morgagni" is derived from müllerian ducts and is by far the most common of these appendages, being present in one or both testes in over 90 percent of the patients. The appendix epididymidis is encountered in about 30 percent of the patients; the collective incidence of the other appendages totals no more than 1 to 3 percent (Fig. 3).

If these remnants have only a slender attachment, they are liable to undergo spontaneous torsion (Fig. 4). The clinical picture is frequently indistinguishable from that of true testicular torsion. First, the scrotal swelling may not be evident, although careful examination may

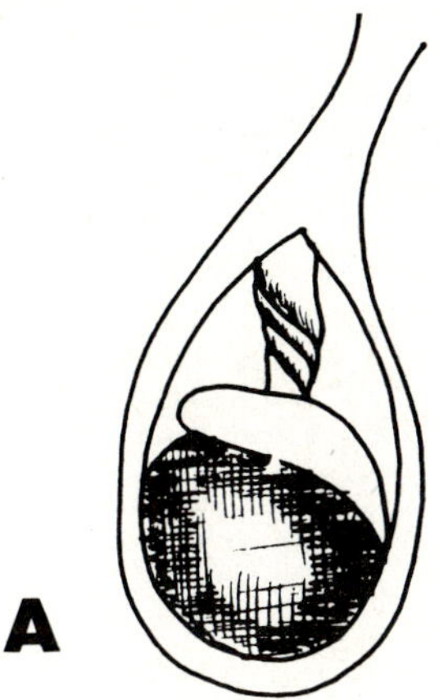

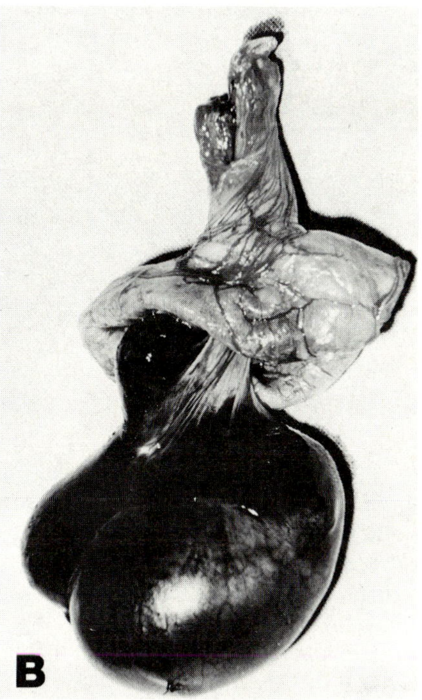

Figure 2 *A* and *B,* Intravaginal torsion.

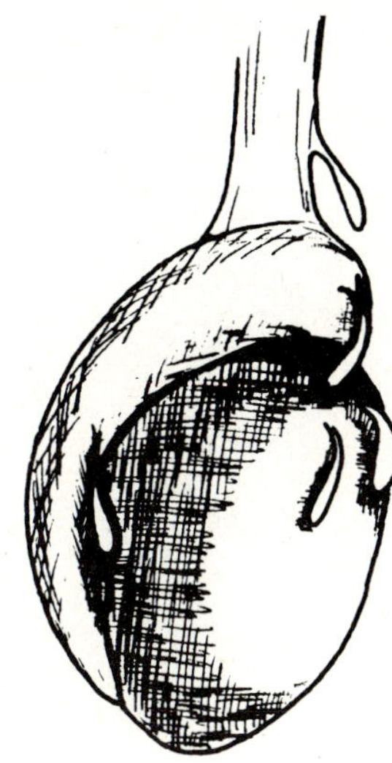

Figure 3 Testicular appendages.

disclose the twisted appendage as a tender mass, 3 to 5 mm in diameter, near the upper pole of the testis. As time passes, scrotal edema and redness appear. A small sympathetic hydrocele may then mask the presence of the localized lesion.

DIAGNOSIS

Torsion of the testis can be diagnosed within the first hours after onset of symptoms by thorough questioning and a detailed clinical examination without the need for further laboratory investigation. Generally, the patient initially perceives a sudden, violent, colicky pain in the groin or in a testis after exercise or minor trauma. More often, the onset is at night, the patient being awakened with sharp pain. The classic presentation of testicular torsion is an increasingly painful swelling of the testis in conjunction with an extreme sensitivity to touch and pressure. In such cases, owing to the reflex contraction of the cremaster muscle, a high position of the testis (Brunzel's sign) is observed. Sometimes, especially in the early phase, the epididymis still can be distinguished from the testis and be palpated regardless of the degree of torsion. In contrast to epididymitis, the lifting of the twisted testis produces increased pain (positive Prehn's sign). Occasionally, the point of torsion can be localized owing to a thickening of the spermatic cord.

Doppler stethoscope examination and sodium pertechnetate blood flow scintiscans of the testicle have been suggested as methods for determining the diagnosis, but if uncertainty exists, scrotal exploration should be done.

Frequently, general symptoms, such as peritonism, pain in the lower abdomen, collapse, profuse sweating, and tachycardia prevail; however, leukocytosis and fever are considered late symptoms, and together with the local findings may give rise to the wrong diagnosis of epididymitis.

Differential Diagnosis

The longer the torsion lasts and the more violent its course, the more difficult becomes the differential diagnosis. The most frequent false diagnosis is certainly epididymitis. Its characteristic symptoms are the sole enlargement of the epididymis without pathologic findings in the testis, the extreme sensitiveness of the epididymis to touch, as well as the early rise in temperature, the high leukocytosis, and the almost always accompanying dysuric complaints. The age distribution of the two diseases (epididymitis and torsion) is different (Fig. 5). The torsion of the testicle is mainly a disease of the first and second decade of life, whereas

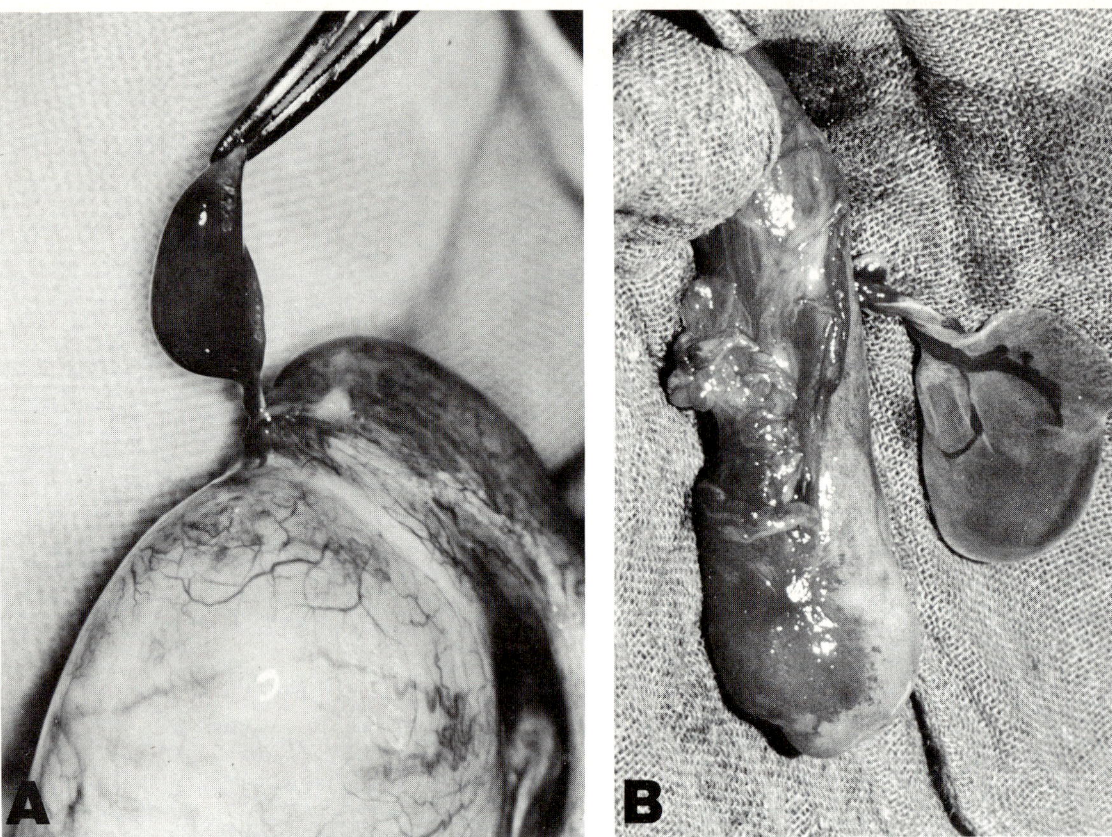

Figure 4 *A* and *B,* Torsion and testicular appendages.

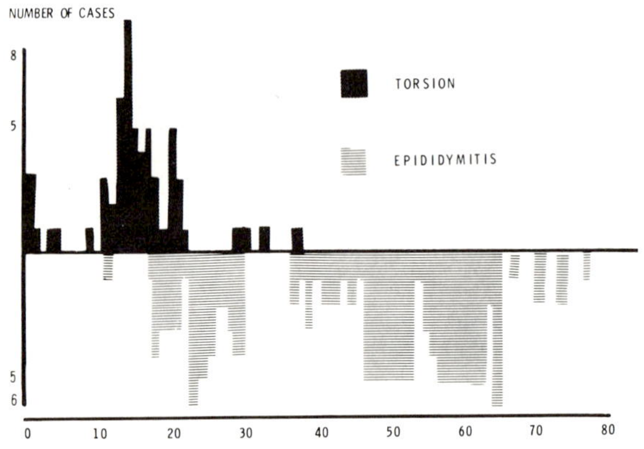

Figure 5 Patient age distribution.

epididymitis seldom occurs in infancy. Acute orchitis occurs predominantly in the wake of epidemic parotitis. The local findings are similar to those observed in testicular torsion. However, the history and the lower position of the testis permit a correct diagnosis. The differential diagnosis between incarcerated inguinal hernia and twisted testis is difficult. However, the empty scrotal space and the local finding of an extremely painful swelling in the inguinal canal indicate torsion of an inguinal testis.

Greater and smaller parenchymatous hermorrhages after contusion also cause painful swellings of the testis and the epididymis. Generally, however, they can be diagnosed if a proper anamnesis is obtained. It is also difficult to differentiate between testicular torsion and the somewhat rare infarct of the testis. The latter is caused by thrombosis or embolism of an afferent artery in the wake of different primary diseases. Whereas complete torsion of the testicle evokes an acute process and requires prompt medical help, the course of testicular infarction is far more insidious.

TREATMENT

Every torsion of the testicle or even the sole suspicion of testicular torsion demands immediate surgery. In order to ensure a successful operation, it should be performed within the first hours after the occurrence of testicular torsion. Only then can a restitutio integrum of the testicular parenchyma be expected.

In a review of 500 cases from the literature, loss of the testis was noted in 90 percent. More recent investigations have shown that early diagnosis and treatment improve the testicular salvage rate from 42 to 68 percent. A significant correlation of the duration of the torsion with the degree of histologic changes and the salvage rate has been reported (Fig. 6). Patients in whom surgery was performed 8 hours after the onset of symptoms had normal-sized testicles and only slight changes in testicular morphology.

Detorsion of the testis as well as its lasting fixation in the scrotal space are the objectives of surgery. Since the contralateral testis generally also tends to twist, both testes should be fixed in a bilateral surgical approach. In the early and obvious case, the testicle should be explored through the scrotal approach. In the late, neglected case, when the differential diagnosis consists of chronic granuloma, neglected torsion, or an inflammatory variety of testicular tumor, the exploration should be performed through the inguinal canal as for testicular cancer.

Efforts to reduce the torsion manually before surgery are fine in theory, but of doubtful value in practice. The testis may twist in either direction internally or externally, any number of times, so that the examiner has no real idea of which way to twist it or how many rotations to give it.

After an anterior transverse scrotal incision, the incision is carried out to the tunica vaginalis, and the testis is delivered from the scrotum (Fig. 7); the

hydrocele fluid, which is often serosanguineous, is removed, and then the twist is undone, possibly by means of more than one complete turn; afterward the testis is inspected (Fig. 7). Some authors emphasize the necessity of testicular fixation, opening the parietal tunica vaginalis, everting it, and suturing the cut edges around the epididymis as in hydrocelectomy. Another technique involves fixation of the abnormally suspended testicle by a longitudinal row of sutures attaching the anterior margin of the testis to the overlying dartos fascia. In contrast to these techniques, we rely on two sutures; at the caudal pole as well as the medial aspect of the testis, the tunica albuginea is sutured and fixed to the dartos fascia (Fig. 7). Scrotal drainage is not necessary. If the testis has to be removed, a Silastic prosthesis can be placed during the same procedure. If torsion occurs in an undescended testis after puberty, the organ should be removed and a Silastic prosthesis sutured into the scrotum. Before puberty, however, torsion of an undescended testis is treated by orchidopexy and hernia repair.

Even when torsion of a testicular appendix is not determined beyond doubt, surgical intervention is recommended, because conservative management produces prolonged disablement and continued discomfort, particularly when the patient is walking. Surgical removal of the twisted structure through a small incision accelerates recovery. Exploration of the contralateral testis has been recommended but seems unnecessary.

Numerous reports of recurrent torsion of the spermatic cord have appeared. From the prognostic viewpoint, these are probably the more important cases, because their early surgical correction produces a higher percentage of patients with preserved spermatogenesis. Thus, surgery is imperative.

THE TESTES AFTER TORSION

Fertility

Testicular torsion may reduce fertility. In one study, the semen quality, as judged by two semen analyses, was normal in 15 patients, doubtful in three, and pathologic in 12. Correlation of the duration of torsion with the percentage of pathologic semen analyses was noted.

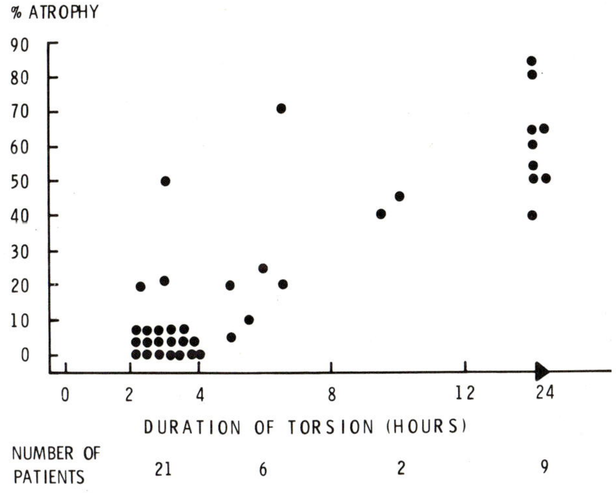

Figure 6 Degree of atrophy of twisted testis in relation to duration of torsion (adapted to data of Krarup).

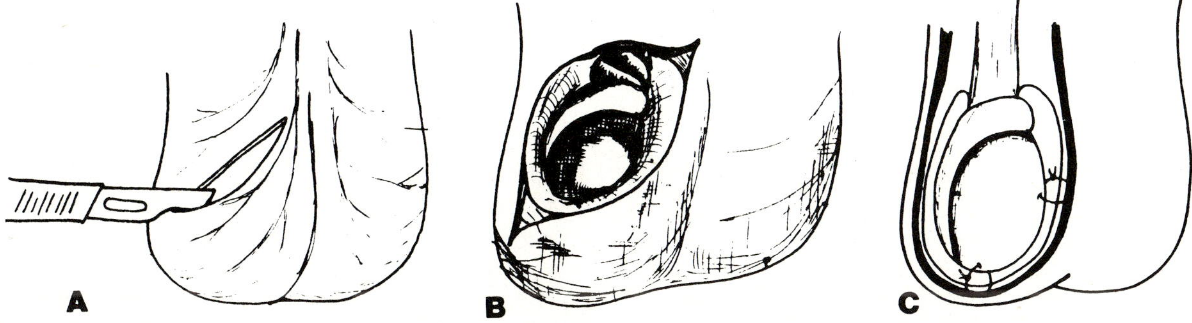

Figure 7 Surgery in testicular torsion.

With the exception of four patients, sperm characteristics were pathologic in all patients in whom detorsion had been performed later than 4 hours after the onset of symptoms. However, a strikingly high percentage (9 percent) of doubtful and pathologic semen analyses could be found even in the group of patients in whom detorsion had been done within 4 hours after the onset of symptoms and whose testicular size had been normal. This is corroborated elsewhere in the literature, which suggests that patients treated for unilateral testicular torsion seem to have bilateral testicular abnormalities. In this connection, it is of interest that in our study, although performed in a small population, semen analyses were normal in three patients in whom orchiectomy had been done, and pathologic in four patients in whom detorsion and contralateral fixation had been performed because the torsion had persisted for more than 24 hours.

In five patients, testicular biopsies were done at follow-up; in three patients in whom torsion had persisted for more than 24 hours, atrophic changes were noted in the twisted testis and hypospermatogenesis in the contralateral (untwisted) testis. The semen analyses obtained from these patients were pathologic. In one patient in whom torsion had persisted for 2 hours, the twisted testis showed slight hypospermatogenesis, whereas spermatogenesis was normal in the untwisted testis in spite of a pathologic semen analysis. In one case, the twisted testis was removed because of hemorrhagic infarction. Biopsy of the contralateral untwisted testis

showed a normal spermatogenesis. Consecutive semen analyses were normal.

Effect of Testicular Torsion on the Contralateral Testis

The cause of pathologic sperm characteristics in unilateral testicular torsion is not yet clear. In a similar condition, unilateral cryptorchidism, three possible causes have been put forth: (1) one normal testis cannot inhibit follicle-stimulating hormone secretion to the same degree as two normal tests, (2) the abnormal testis produces a substance that impairs the function of the so-called normal testis, and (3) both testes are abnormal. In connection with testicular torsion, a bilateral testicular abnormality has been suggested. However, histologic investigations in our follow-up study showed a pathologic spermatogenesis in the contralateral testis when detorsion and fixation of the twisted testis were done later than 24 hours after torsion. On the other hand, although castration of the twisted testis was performed in only one patient, normal spermatogenesis was found in the contralateral testis. Further correlative studies with regard to duration of the torsion and follow-up testicular biopsies in patients with unilateral testicular torsion should elucidate whether testicular torsion is a bilateral disease with a chronic torsion of both testes, or whether there are similar conditions, such as unilateral cryptorchidism or unilateral testicular tumor, in which spermatogenesis often is impaired.

TESTICULAR RUPTURE

ELI K. MICHAELS, M.D.

Testicular rupture is an infrequent complication of blunt or penetrating trauma to the external genitalia and has been reported to occur spontaneously, albeit rarely, in the presence of testicular neoplasm. The true incidence of testicular rupture is not known because nonoperative management of blunt genital trauma was previously common. The strength of the tunica albuginea and the mobility of the gonad make injury infrequent unless there is compression against the pubic bone, most commonly during athletic or social confrontations or from motor vehicle accidents. Testicular rupture implies disruption of the tunica albuginea and extrusion of seminiferous tubules; accumulation of blood within the tunica vaginalis (hematocele) results in a painful scrotal mass that usually precludes accurate physical examination of the testis.

Testicular rupture must be differentiated from other

causes of a painful, swollen scrotum (Table 1). An accurate history of trauma, and the presence of a hematocele characterized by ecchymosis and scrotal swelling without transillumination, suggest testicular rupture; spontaneously occurring pain and scrotal swelling with erythema are more typical of epididymo-orchitis with reactive hydrocele or abscess, while spontaneous torsion usually presents without a scrotal mass. An underlying testicular neoplasm should be suspected when there are findings of testicular rupture and a history of relatively trivial trauma.

PATIENT SELECTION

The goal of treatment for testicular rupture is preservation of seminiferous tissue and endocrine function. Historically, nonoperative treatment of traumatic hematocele (probably from testicular rupture) by aspiration, bed rest, ice packs, antimicrobial agents, and proteolytic enzymes was accompanied by significant testicular loss. Nonoperative management cannot ensure that the testis is intact, and continued hemorrhage and extrusion of parenchyma may result in subsequent

Table 1 Patient Selection

History	Diagnosis	Physical Findings	Sonogram	Nuclear Scan
Genital trauma	1. Testicular hemorrhage	Tenderness	Testis nonhomogeneous 1 ± 3	Decreased uptake testis 1 ± 3
	2. Testicular rupture ± hematocele	Tenderness ± scrotal mass		
	3. Simple hematocele	Scrotal mass	Low-level echoes around testis	Decreased uptake around testis
	4. Testicular dislocation ± 1, 2, 3	Ectopic testis ± 1, 3	Ectopic testis ± 1, 3	Ectopic testis ± 1, 3
Spontaneous pain	5. Testicular torsion	Tenderness ± mass	Testis enlarged and hypoechoic	Decreased uptake testis
	6. Epididymitis	Tenderness ± mass	Epididymis enlarged and hypoechoic	Decreased uptake testis and epididymis

atrophy. Aspiration of the hematocele may introduce secondary infection, and pain and disability from continuing hemorrhage may be prolonged. All patients with penetrating trauma and most of those with significant hematocele from blunt trauma therefore require surgical exploration. When trauma is less severe and only a small hematocele is present, the possibility that there is no testicular injury warrants a period of observation during which imaging studies may be obtained and expansion of the hematocele monitored. If imaging studies suggest more severe injury or if the patient's condition worsens, surgery within 48 to 72 hours of injury gives the best results.

There may be testicular rupture without hematocele or testicular hematoma contained within the tunica albuginea; delay in surgical repair or decompression in this event will result in testicular infection or atrophy. An abnormal sonogram or nuclear scan in these circumstances indicates the need for surgical exploration. Ultrasound evaluation of the scrotum will reveal focal areas of increased or diminished echogenicity within the testis corresponding to infarction or hemorrhage, with or without rupture; actual fracture lines are not visualized unless there is major disruption. If hematocele is present, it will appear as an area with low-level echoes surrounding the testis, in contrast to a reactive hydrocele, which would be echo free. Radionuclide scanning with ^{99m}technetium pertechnetate will demonstrate decreased testicular uptake because of necrotic parenchyma or hemorrhage; a photon-deficient area around the testis will correspond to the hematocele, if present. These findings are not dissimilar to those of untreated torsion or testicular abscess, which also require exploration but are usually differentiated by an accurate history.

Blunt genital trauma may also cause dislocation of one or both gonads into superficial inguinal, prepubic, perineal, or crural locations and cause rupture of the testis or compromise of its blood supply. The extent of injury may not be apparent; patient discomfort will preclude adequate physical examination, hematocele may not be present, and testicular imaging studies may not be reliable with the gonad in an ectopic location. Inguinal exploration of dislocation is required except in the rare patient in whom closed manipulation of the gonad into the scrotum is successful and results in relief of pain. Documentation of an intact testis with normal blood flow by radionuclide studies is then required.

TIMING OF SURGERY

The mechanism of blunt injury causes compression of the gonad against the bony pelvis, followed by explosion and extrusion of parenchyma. Damage to the microvascular and ductal systems of the seminiferous tubules occurs at the time of impact, and necrosis is seen histologically even in tissue that may appear viable at surgery. The goals of immediate exploration are to repair the testicular defect, preventing continued extrusion of parenchyma, and to control bleeding. Early evacuation of the hematocele will reduce patient discomfort and prevent further testicular damage from pressure by the tense hematocele within a closed space, and is required even when testicular rupture is not the source of the hematocele.

Patients with testicular rupture and hematocele who delay for some days or weeks before urologic consultation should also be explored. Whereas there is no evidence that delayed exploration improves testicular salvage compared with no exploration, surgical drainage of the hematocele and proper debridement of devitalized tissue may lessen the risk of secondary infection and reduce patient morbidity. When presentation is delayed, differentiation must be made between testicular rupture with hematocele and simple post-traumatic hydrocele without testicular rupture, which may not require exploration. Sonography will demonstrate a hydrocele to be devoid of internal echoes; simple needle aspiration is then performed, and if the fluid is clear, hydrocele is proved. If blood-stained fluid is retrieved, testicular injury with hematocele is presumed and exploration required to prevent further complications.

SURGICAL TECHNIQUE

The patient is prepared for general or regional anesthesia and consent to include possible orchiectomy

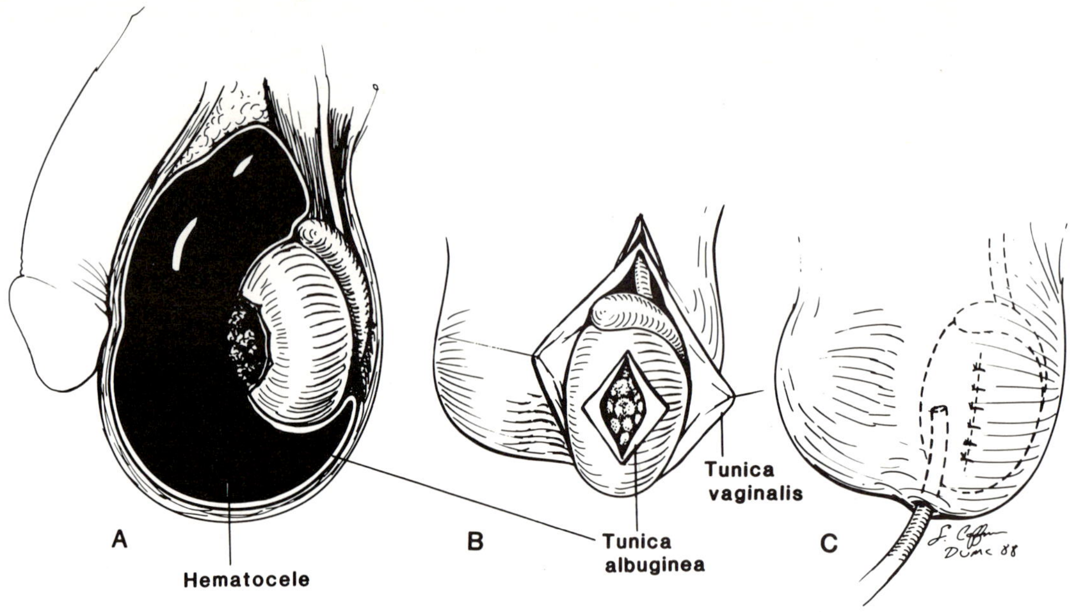

Figure 1 Treatment of testicular rupture. *A,* Testicular rupture with hematocele. *B,* Exposure through transscrotal incision. *C,* Repair with drainage. (Republished with permission by Fowler JE Jr. Mastery of surgery: urology. Boston: Little, Brown & Co. In press.)

obtained. Associated injuries of the penis, urethra, and bladder having been ruled out, the patient is explored through the scrotum on the affected side. After incision of the tunica vaginalis and evacuation of the hematocele, the testis, adnexa, and cord structures are inspected for injury. An intact testis under tension from a subcapsular or parenchymal hematoma is decompressed by incision over the hematoma; debridement of necrotic tissue and hemostasis are then required before closure of the tunica albuginea. When the testis is ruptured, nonviable extruded parenchyma is sharply debrided and the tunica albuginea closed with a continuous absorbable suture. A large or irregular defect of the tunica albuginea is managed by suturing edges of the defect to adjacent tunica vaginalis. Orchiectomy is indicated when viable parenchymal tissue cannot be found. Maintenance of endocrine function is possible if viable tissue adjacent to the tunica albuginea is preserved, making subcapsular orchiectomy preferable in younger patients or those with bilateral injury. After appropriate management of the testicular injury, dartos and skin layers are closed with absorbable interrupted sutures, and a Penrose drain is left in place for 2 to 3 days (Fig. 1). Antimicrobial agents and scrotal support may prevent further complications.

Bilateral testicular injury occurs in 1 to 5 percent of patients, but may not be apparent preoperatively because of scrotal distortion from a tense hematocele. For this reason, a preoperative sonogram or nuclear scan must also investigate the contralateral testis. Regardless of radiographic findings, the contralateral testis is always palpated after scrotal decompression and explored if abnormal. Separate scrotal incisions are used for bilateral injuries in anticipation of possible complications of infection.

An inguinal approach is indicated for patients with rupture due to testicular dislocation. This allows control of the spermatic vessels and detorsion if necessary and provides access to the ectopic position of the gonad. Inguinal exploration is also mandatory for patients with testicular rupture due to suspected underlying carcinoma. The vessels are controlled at the inguinal ring and the testis is delivered within the intact tunica vaginalis, if possible, to contain tumor spillage.

COMPLICATIONS

Surgical treatment of testicular rupture is straightforward and the postoperative course generally uneventful. Attention to hemostasis and drainage of the scrotum eliminate secondary bleeding or infection. Testicular atrophy is significantly more common when exploration is delayed, owing to continued extrusion of seminiferous tubules and the pressure effect of the hematocele under tension. When exploration is delayed beyond 3 days, testicular abscess is more frequently encountered and orchiectomy often required.

The reproductive function of the injured gonad is most likely impaired even if treatment is prompt and atrophy does not ensue, because of microvascular damage and ductal disruption from the impact of the original injury. Endocrine (and therefore sexual) function is not compromised as long as viable tissue remains. No data are available to address the question of fertility after unilateral injury, with or without orchiectomy. Bilateral testicular rupture is more commonly a result of penetrating injury or more severe blunt injury, including pelvic fracture, and the few reported patients with gonadal salvage usually have impaired sexual function and an abnormal semen analysis.

In conclusion, urgent surgical exploration is recommended for patients with suspected testicular rupture or contusion and/or hematocele resulting from blunt or penetrating trauma. Greatly reduced morbidity and testicular salvage of 90 percent may be expected when patients are treated within 3 days, in contrast to testicular salvage of only 55 percent when exploration is delayed.

SUGGESTED READING

Atwell JD, Ellis H. Rupture of the testis. Br J Surg 1961; 49:345–346.

Cass AS. Testicular trauma. J Urol 1983; 129:299–300.

Cass AS, Ferrara L, Wolpert J, Lee J. Bilateral testicular injury from external trauma. J Urol 1988; 140:1435–1436.

Jeffrey RB, Laing FC, Hricak H, McAninch JW. Sonography of testicular trauma. AJR 1983; 141:993–995.

McConnell JD, Peters PC, Lewis SE. Testicular rupture in blunt scrotal trauma: review of 15 cases with recent application of testicular scanning. J Urol 1982; 128:309–311.

RENAL CALICEAL CALCULI

MICHAEL MARBERGER, M.D.

Traditionally, urologists have approached caliceal calculi with reluctance, since the magnitude of the open surgical procedure required for removing them usually correlates poorly with the symptoms they cause respective to the obstructive potential they have for the kidney. In contrast to surgery for stones within the renal pelvis, mobilization of the kidney and nephrotomies are often needed, with all the inherent risks of parenchymal damage and perirenal scarring. With the advent of extracorporeal shock wave lithotripsy (ESWL) and percutaneous stone manipulation, the situation has completely changed in the past 10 years. Ninety-eight percent of all caliceal calculi can now be treated with these techniques with minimal morbidity, complication rates of less than 5 percent, and virtually no alteration of renal function and morphology. As another important step in this development, we acquired a second-generation lithotriptor in August 1986, which now routinely permits extracorporeal lithotripsy without the need for any anesthesia.

Although stones in the renal calices rarely cause symptoms as acute as those caused by pelveceal and ureteral calculi, they may be the reason for dull, chronic flank pain, recurrent hematuria, and persistent urinary tract infection. However, even when primarily asymptomatic, they are a latent source for urologic problems. Hübner, in Vienna, reviewed the fate of 63 patients with primarily asymptomatic caliceal stones over a mean follow-up period of 7.4 years. The calculi migrated to the pelvis and ureter in 52.5 percent of the patients, and there they almost always became symptomatic. Only 16.3 percent of the stones were passed spontaneously, usually with renal colics; 45 percent grew in size; and 40 percent of the patients eventually required surgical intervention to remove the stones (usually from the ureter). In six patients, obstruction and infection had damaged the kidney so severely by this time that it had to be removed.

In terms of patient discomfort and renal damage, the overall impact of this delayed treatment appears considerably higher than that of early therapy with less invasive methods. With the availability of pain-free extracorporeal lithotripsy, I have therefore adopted an aggressive approach to management of caliceal calculi. Provided the patient's general state of health justifies the effort, I treat all caliceal stones if they are radiopaque and large enough to be well visualized by ultrasonography or fluoroscopy (i.e., in general, larger than approximately 4 mm in diameter). Smaller stones are difficult to focus during treatment and are often passed spontaneously without symptoms. In special situations, such as in pilots who are grounded for even the smallest renal stone, this limit may of course be lowered at the price of a more difficult procedure. Expectant therapy is reserved for patients with small peripheral calculi in multiple calices and for patients with nephrocalcinosis. These patients frequently have gross metabolic disorders, the correction of which often promotes spontaneous stone passage without any further symptomatic treatment.

DIAGNOSTIC WORK-UP

The topography of all calculi within the kidney should be delineated preoperatively as precisely as possible. In general, this is accomplished with a good-quality plain film of the kidneys, ureters, and bladder and with an intravenous pyelogram. If the position of the affected calix remains unclear, oblique views are helpful, but renal ultrasonography is usually simpler and more efficient in confirming the diagnosis. Since it also depicts calculi down to a diameter of approximately 2 mm regardless of their density, it should routinely be used in patients with poorly radiopaque stones or kidneys with impaired function. Extracorporeal lithotripsy requires unobstructed urinary drainage for the spontaneous passage of the disintegrated calculous material. Obstructed calices and caliceal diverticula can usually be identified on the intravenous pyelogram. They are approached by percutaneous lithotripsy, and if any further information is required this is obtained by retrograde pyelography at the time of the definite procedure, prior to the percutaneous puncture, and by using the ureteral catheter routinely placed with this technique.

Urinary tract infection should be treated for at least 48 hours before the intervention, using antimicrobial agents chosen according to culture identification of the organism and sensitivity testing. A clotting screen, including at least a platelet count, the bleeding time, the prothrombin time, and the partial thromboplastin time, is routinely obtained. Hypertension should be controlled prior to the intervention.

Otherwise, the preoperative preparation is identical to that for other kidney stone procedures. Of course this also includes a metabolic work-up.

EXTRACORPOREAL SHOCK WAVE LITHOTRIPSY

Since most caliceal stones are small and in calices with unobstructed infundibula, ESWL is the treatment of choice for most patients. Clotting disorders are contraindications to this approach, but the indication for a therapeutic intervention for caliceal stones is naturally then very limited. With caliceal clubbing, strictured infundibula, or calculi larger than 20 mm in diameter, the stone fragments tend to be poorly cleared from calices, particularly in the basilar pole, so that percutaneous removal is preferable. For the same reason I always treat calculi in caliceal diverticula or horseshoe kidneys percutaneously. Branched staghorn calculi with extensions into multiple calices are best managed by percutaneous removal of the major stone mass in the lower-pole calices and pelvis, and subsequent ESWL of the residuals in the poorly accessible superior-pole and middle calices.

Whenever possible, we use our second-generation lithotriptor (Piezolith 2200, R. Wolf Co., Knittlingen, Germany), since its use is pain free and requires no anesthesia or analgesia (Fig. 1). With this unit, piezoceramic elements mounted on a concave-spherical plate produce high-energy sound pulses at a repetition frequency of 2 to 20 Hz, which are self-focused to provide pressures of 20 to 100 MPa in the focus of the system (Fig. 2). By use of a diagnostic ultrasonographic sector scanner integrated into the plate, which is freely movable along all three coordinates, the calculus is brought into the focus of the lithotripter. To prevent energy losses at acoustic interphases, the patient's flank is immersed into a confined bath of degassed water, which is sealed against the patient's body with a rubber dam. Caliceal calculi 7 to 15 mm in diameter are usually disintegrated with 700 to 1,000 shots in approximately 30 minutes. During disintegration, the stone is continuously monitored with the sector scanner and refocused as needed. Disintegration is readily visible by the changing contour of the stone shadow, but can also be controlled fluoroscopically by sliding a C-arm over the table, or by simply asking the patient to step down from the unit for a standard plain film. If stone disintegration is incomplete, the procedure is simply continued. For smaller stones, we do not routinely place a ureteral stent.

The results of Ziegler and colleagues at the University of Homburg/Saar Medical School, where the unit

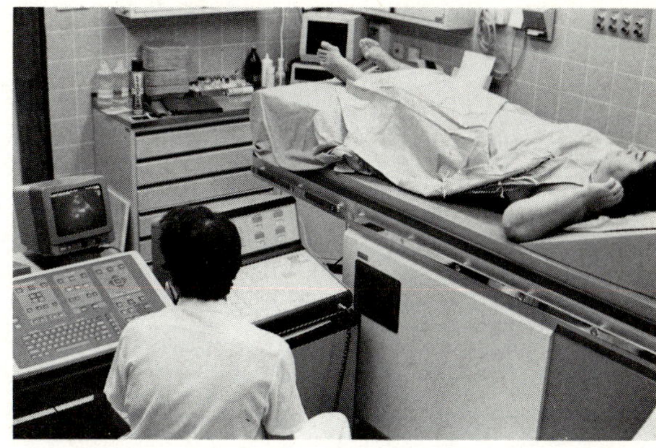

Figure 1 Mobile second-generation lithotriptor (Piezolith). The patient lies on the table with the flank over the shock wave generator, which is focused on the stone with an integrated ultrasound sector scanner.

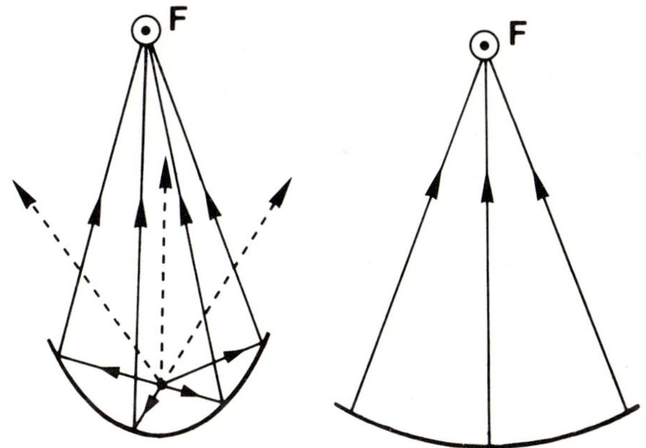

Figure 2 With conventional lithotriptors *(left),* the shock wave is produced in the first focus of an ellipsoidal reflector system and focused on the stone in the second focus. With the piezoceramic lithotriptor *(right),* the entire shock wave is focused on the stone; because of the low pressure intensity at the skin level ESWL is pain free.

was developed, and our preliminary experience suggest that at least 80 percent of all caliceal stones can be treated successfully with this instrument. Complete stone clearance may take several months, especially from basilar calices, but symptoms originally caused by the caliceal stone usually disappear within 2 to 3 days. The main limitations arise from difficulties in localizing small peripheral calculi in very obese patients or in upper-pole calices of a very high kidney, where the stones may be masked by the ribs. In these situations the patient is treated with ESWL using biplane fluoroscopy; the procedure is then performed with epidural anesthesia as described extensively elsewhere.

Because of the smaller volume of caliceal calculi, the complication rate of ESWL is significantly lower than that for larger pelveceal stones, but similar in type. Renal pain and fever are usually transient and rarely require auxiliary interventions, such as percutaneous nephrostomy or ureteral instrumentation. The main

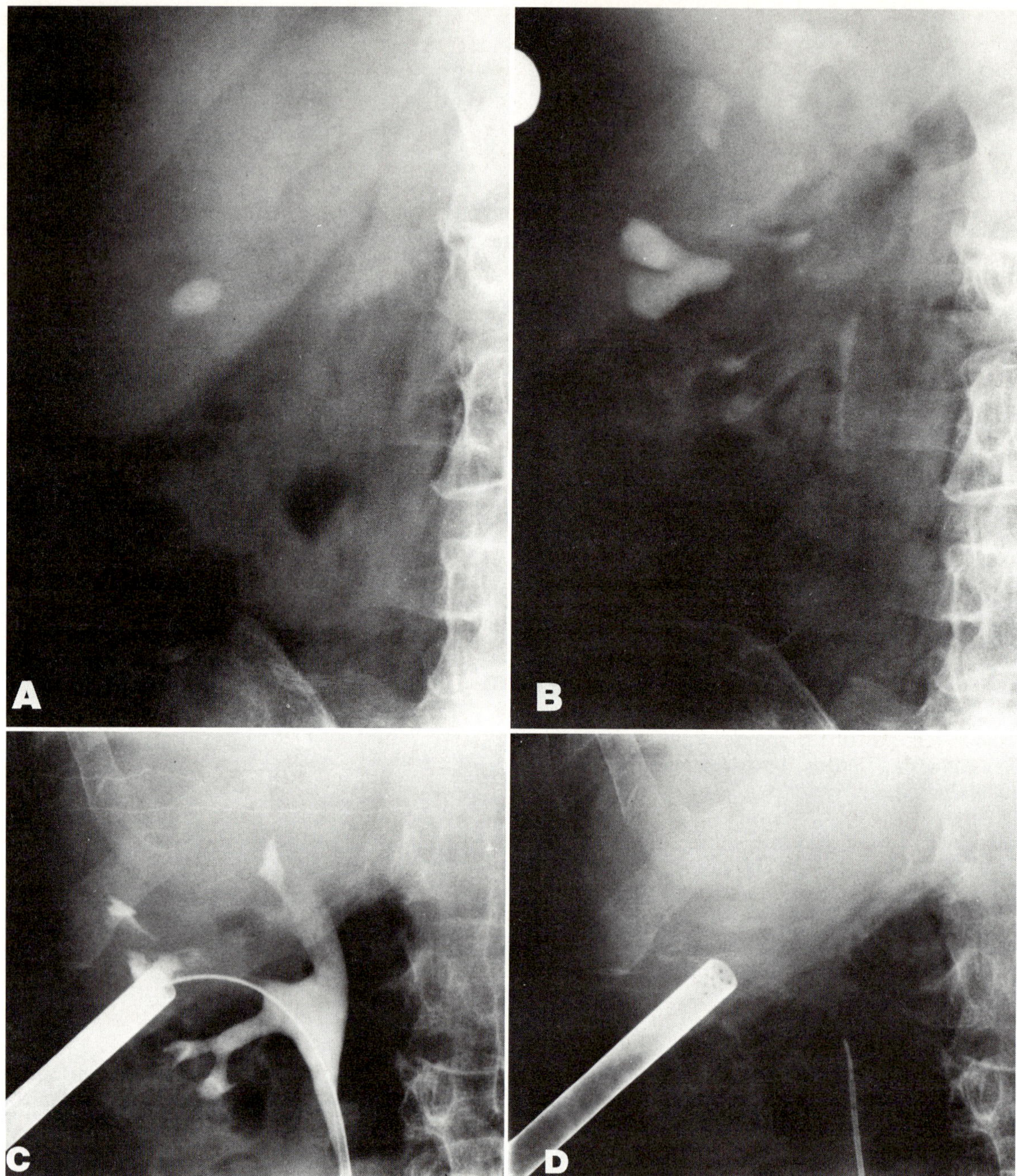

Figure 3 Caliceal calculus severely obstructing the middle calices. *A,* Preoperative plain film. *B,* Preoperative intravenous pyelogram. The calix was punctured directly and the stone removed by ultrasonic lithotripsy. *C,* The infundibula are cleared; note the safety guidewire in the ureter. *D,* Plain film showing complete stone removal.

cause of concern arises from the incomplete passage of stone fragments, which is observed in over 25 percent of caliceal stones in most large series, particularly for stones in basilar calices. The pattern seems to be identical for first- and second-generation lithotripters. Although conclusive evidence that this debris acts as a nidus for rapid stone regrowth is not available, I prefer percutaneous removal of caliceal stones that are larger than 20 mm in diameter, or stones that are in borderline obstructed calices.

PERCUTANEOUS NEPHROLITHOTRIPSY

Caliceal calculi unsuited for ESWL are treated percutaneously. In the past I tended to prefer percutaneous techniques to ESWL in ambiguous cases, but with the advent of pain-free lithotriptors, my attitude has changed. I now prefer ESWL for larger caliceal stones in the apical and middle calices. If the calculus cannot be visualized or disintegration appears incomplete, percutaneous lithotripsy may even be performed on the same table after anesthetizing the patient. With evidence for obstruction at the level of the infundibula, in particular in basilar calices, percutaneous lithotripsy is always preferred because of the high rate of incomplete stone clearance from these calices after ESWL.

I routinely perform percutaneous nephrolithotripsy as a one-stage procedure with the patient under general anesthesia. A ureteral catheter is always placed. The stone-bearing calix is punctured directly using the three-part coaxial Günther needle. After scanning the kidney with a sector scanner to determine the depth of the kidney and the optimal angle of puncture, I usually advance the needle directly onto the stone under anteroposterior beam fluoroscopy without injecting contrast dye. As soon as the stone is contacted, the inner needle is exchanged against a floppy-J guide wire, which is preferably threaded through the infundibulum and advanced into an apical pole calix or down the ureter (Fig. 3). If the calix cannot be punctured with this technique, it is delineated and even dilated by injecting contrast dye via the ureteral catheter, and the procedure is repeated. Once a correct tract is established, a Lunderquist guide wire is inserted and the tract is dilated with metal telescope dilators. If any doubt exists as to the correct position of the tract, this is confirmed by inspecting the punctured calix with a 12 Fr miniature nephroscope, which was specially developed for this purpose (Fig. 4). If the nephrostomy reaches the stone-bearing calix, the tract is dilated to 24 Fr to admit the standard No. 24 Fr continuous-flow nephroscope; to reduce renal trauma I never use a thicker instrument for caliceal stones, and with very delicate structures I may even use the No. 18 Fr pediatric nephroscope (Fig. 5).

Most caliceal stones can be extracted with forceps through the sheath of the No. 24 Fr nephroscope. Otherwise, they are disintegrated with ultrasonography, and the fragments are aspirated through the sonotrode; if the No. 18 Fr nephroscope is used, ultrasonic lithotresis is performed with the 2.4-mm sonotrode designed for the No. 12.5 F ureterorenoscope. The tract is usually dilated only to the calix. If the caliceal neck appears strictured, or if the stones are in a diverticulum, the narrow segment is also dilated to about 16 Fr. This usually relieves obstruction. I avoid direct incision of interposing parenchyma or scar tissue, since this may provoke brisk hemorrhage and in my experience does not give better results than plain dilatation. However, the key to safe dilatation is a guidewire threaded through the caliceal neck and into the adjacent collecting system. With a caliceal diverticulum it may be necessary to identify the draining channel under vision, because it may be impossible to advance the guidewire through it other than under endoscopic control. After complete stone removal a No. 14 Fr nephrostomy tube is left in the collecting system for 24 hours. Multiple stones in different calices can be approached via multiple nephrostomy tracts. Although we have not observed significant damage from the multinephrostomy technique, the need for this has virtually been eliminated by pain-free piezo-ESWL.

I have found percutaneous lithotripsy for caliceal stones to be highly successful. Some time ago I analyzed my first 1,000 patients subjected to percutaneous stone manipulations. There were 178 patients treated for isolated caliceal calculi. The procedure failed because the stone-bearing calix could not be punctured in 2 percent. In 8 percent, residual calculous material was noted on follow-up films, but this consisted of minute fragments termed *dust* in 6 percent. My experience with ultrasonic stone disintegration has shown that residuals of this type are usually passed spontaneously and do not justify additional interventions to remove them. One patient experienced hemorrhage that required superselective angioinfarction, but there was no nephrectomy or mortality among the patients. Data on postoperative hospitalization, which averaged 2.4 days, could be compiled only in the last 100 patients because of a changed technique. Follow-up studies revealed no significant late sequelae. Nevertheless, percutaneous nephrolithotripsy is more invasive than ESWL, and most

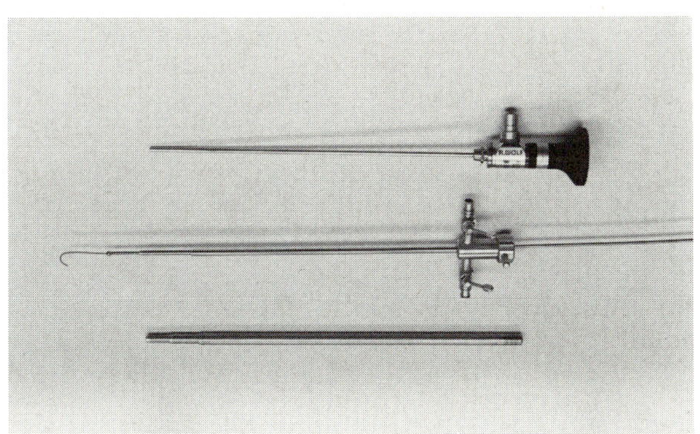

Figure 4 Miniature No. 12 Fr nephroscope (Wolf). *Top,* Telescope. *Middle,* Sheath of the instrument advanced over a Lunderquist guidewire and rigid rod and No. 8 Fr dilator of all metal telescope dilator. *Bottom,* Nos. 15, 18, and 21 Fr dilators for further dilatation.

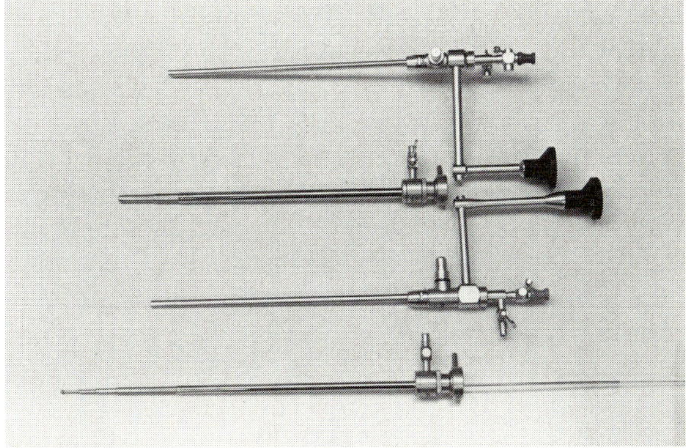

Figure 5 Nos. 18 and 24 Fr nephroscope (Wolf). *From bottom to top:* Telescope dilator Nos. 8 to 15 Fr, with No. 18 Fr sheath advanced over them; pediatric nephroscope; Nos. 18 and 21 Fr dilators with No. 24 Fr sheath advanced over them; and standard nephroscope.

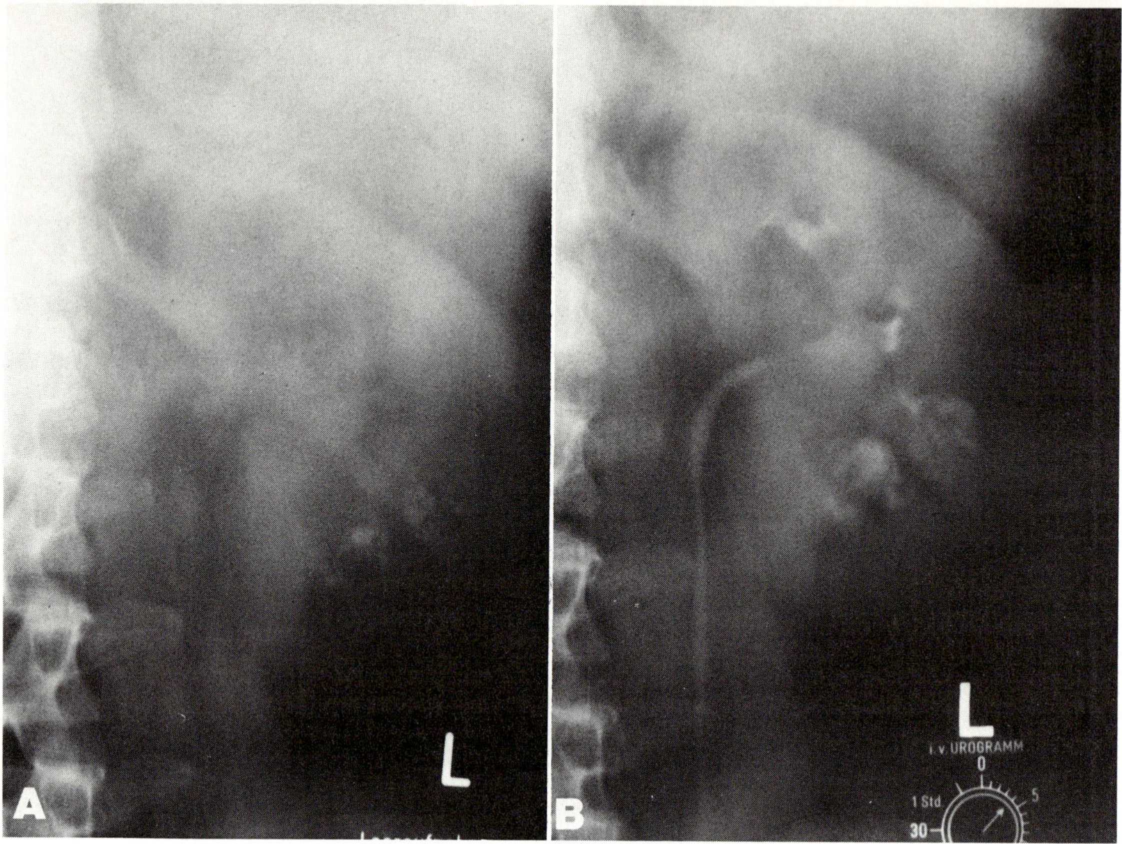

Figure 6 Renal tuberculosis with calcified caseous masses and strictured infundibula in the basilar pole requiring partial nephrectomy. *A,* Plain film. *B,* Intravenous pyelogram.

caliceal stones today should be managed with the latter technique.

OPEN SURGERY

Prospective studies have clearly shown that the concept of resecting the basilar pole of kidneys with caliceal calculi in this region does not reduce the recurrence rate, yet results in a significant loss of renal parenchyma and function. Partial nephrectomy is therefore indicated only when severe obstruction of a complete group of calices has resulted in segmental hydronephrosis with complete destruction of the related parenchyma. In my experience, this is extremely rare and mainly found in conjunction with urogenital tuberculosis (Fig. 6). Since the calculous material in the dilated calices usually represents caseous masses, partial nephrectomy is warranted.

DISCUSSION

The low morbidity of the new techniques for treating renal stones, in particular pain-free ESWL with second-generation lithotriptors, has changed the urologist's approach to management of caliceal calculi. Even primarily asymptomatic stones have a tendency to grow, to migrate to the pelvis and ureter, and ultimately to cause pain and obstruction. Early elective therapy therefore appears justified, provided the stones are of a size that makes them amenable to the new therapeutic modalities. This concept receives additional importance from the observation that with the world-wide improvement in diagnosis and therapy of urolithiasis, the number of large stones requiring intervention is rapidly dwindling. A growing number of patients today first see the urologist with small and frequently asymptomatic caliceal stones.

SUGGESTED READING

Coury TA, Sonda LP, Lingeman JE, Kahnoski RJ. Treatment of painful caliceal stones. Urology 1988; 32:119.

Hübner W, Porpaczy P. Treatment of caliceal calculi. Br J Urol 1990; 66:9.

Marberger M, Fitzpatrick FM, Jenkins AD, Pak Ch.D. Stone surgery. Edinburgh-London-Melbourne-New York-Tokyo, Churchill Livingstone, 1991.

Mee SL, Thüroff JW. Small caliceal stones: is extracorporeal shock wave lithotripsy justified? J Urol 1988; 139:908.

RENAL PELVIC CALCULI

JEFFREY N. WEISS, M.D.
ARTHUR D. SMITH, M.D.

The treatment of renal pelvic calculi has evolved over the past 10 years from open surgery to either extracorporeal shock wave lithotripsy (ESWL) or percutaneous stone extraction. Today, no one single method is suitable for removal of all renal pelvic calculi. Rather, the broad spectrum of stone disease demands that urologists use a variety of modalities. The indications for treating renal pelvic calculi have remained relatively constant, however, despite the use of numerous new techniques. A renal pelvic calculus that warrants removal should be either symptomatic, obstructive, in danger of becoming so, or the source of infection. Stones that do not fit these criteria should not be removed routinely simply because of the availability of less invasive methods.

Our role as urologists is to provide the most effective therapy to render the patient stone free. We must educate the patients about the risks and benefits of each form of treatment for their particular situation; they can then make an informed choice. For example, patients who are interested in avoiding manipulation may request ESWL monotherapy for a large stone, even though the results may not be as good as those obtained from concomitant manipulation or from percutaneous techniques alone.

MERITS AND DRAWBACKS OF AVAILABLE METHODS

Both ESWL and percutaneous nephrolithotomy have advantages and disadvantages. ESWL is attractive in that it can be performed on an outpatient basis and is noninvasive. In certain lithotripsy units, the procedure can be performed under intravenous sedation alone. The disadvantage of ESWL is that the failure rate is higher than with percutaneous lithotomy (PL) for similar-size calculi. This may be particularly true when intravenous sedation rather than anesthesia is used, because to provide patient comfort the kilovoltage may be lowered. This will result in lower stone-free rates at 3 months. Moreover, selection of ESWL does not guarantee the absence of manipulation, because 15 to 20 percent of patients treated with ESWL monotherapy require ancillary procedures such as stent insertion or ureteroscopy. Also, an estimated 20 percent of patients have substantial discomfort or even urinary obstruction from the passage of calculi fragmented by ESWL. Stenting may be used in an attempt to prevent these problems, but the possible complications of stents must then be taken into consideration: reflux, cystitis, bladder spasms, incontinence, and iatrogenic bladder and ureteral injury.

The advantages of percutaneous stone extraction are that there is a 98 to 100 percent success rate with renal pelvic stones irrespective of the type. Patients may be discharged from the hospital stone free; unlike the situation with ESWL therapy, they do not have to wait for stone fragments to pass (or, on occasion, not pass). Less than 2 percent of patients need to undergo ancillary procedures after percutaneous nephrolithotomy for renal pelvic stones. The obvious disadvantage is that percutaneous procedures are invasive, and patients experience substantially more pain than with ESWL and are hospitalized for several days. Also, percutaneous stone extraction has a greater morbidity than ESWL. However, patients usually can resume their usual activities soon after hospital discharge.

COMPLICATIONS

Significant post-ESWL bleeding occurs in no more than 1 percent of patients. These intrarenal, subcapsular, or perinephric hematomas usually can be managed with bed rest, transfusion, and correction of any unrecognized coagulopathy. We have had no significant complications to date after treating renal pelvic calculi by ESWL.

Many percutaneous nephrolithotomy–related complications are caused by faulty technique or inexperience. However, hemorrhagic complications certainly occur more frequently than after ESWL. In 1987 we reported a 1.2 percent incidence of significant bleeding in 582 patients. Intra- or postoperative bleeding usually can be controlled by nephrostomy tube clamping and a pressure dressing. If these methods fail, arteriography with embolization or even renal exploration may be necessary. Other complications include hemothorax, sepsis, and renal pelvic perforation with extravasation. In treating renal pelvic calculi 2 to 3 cm in size, we have had an overall complication rate of less than 1 percent and almost 99 percent success in rendering the patient stone free. Not unexpectedly, the success rate decreases and the complication rate increases with larger calculi. These are usually staghorn calculi, which also are problematic to remove with ESWL.

CONTRAINDICATIONS

The only absolute contraindication to either ESWL or PL is an uncontrolled bleeding diathesis. Patients receiving aspirin or dipyridamole (Persantine) should stop taking these medications before the procedure, which is then performed only if the bleeding time is normal. Also, neither ESWL nor PL should be performed in the face of acute infection, because stone removal by either method may lead to bacteremia, which can result in sepsis and septic shock, especially if the urinary tract is obstructed. Percutaneous nephrostomy tube placement or retrograde placement of a ureteral catheter may be therapeutic in obstructed patients who are infected.

Certain patients have anatomic abnormalities that can contraindicate percutaneous stone extraction. These include marked scoliosis, splenomegaly, and hepatomegaly. Morbid obesity is a relative contraindication to ESWL because the kidney may be a considerable distance from the skin, placing the stone beyond the focal point of the ESWL machine. These patients are best treated with PL.

TREATMENT SELECTION ACCORDING TO STONE TYPE AND PATIENT ANATOMY

Stone Size

Renal pelvic stones that are 2 cm or smaller generally are removed with ESWL. Most centers report a 3-month stone-free rate ranging from 78 to 91 percent. The residual fragments typically are small (less than 2 mm) and further treatment for these patients is not often necessary. However, in about 10 percent secondary procedures are required for renal pelvic stones of this size, including repeat ESWL, ureteroscopy with stone extraction, ureteral stent insertion, and percutaneous stone extraction.

Renal pelvic calculi of less than 2 cm have a residual stone rate of only 1 to 2 percent when treated percutaneously. Generally, PL is an excellent choice when it is essential to render the patient stone free, such as in cases of infected calculi and when there are occupational considerations (i.e., an airline pilot).

The area of controversy in the treatment of renal pelvic calculi is when the stone burden is greater than 2.5 to 3.0 cm. The debate continues over whether monotherapy with ESWL, PL, or combination therapy should be used. In the face of a large (> 2 cm) stone burden, ESWL monotherapy has shown only a 63 to 67 percent stone-free rate at 3 months. Moreover, the need for additional ESWL sessions increases with enlarging stone burden, and 32 percent of these patients require more than one session. There is a concomitant increase in the number of shock waves administered: patients receive an average of 1,574 shocks for stones larger than 2.0 cm versus 1,249 shocks for stones no bigger than 2.0 cm. Furthermore, the postoperative morbidity related to clearance of stone debris is greater. Despite additional sessions of ESWL, there is a strong possibility that a percutaneous procedure will be required to remove residual fragments if the original stone is 2.5 to 4.0 cm in size.

If the stone burden is greater than 2.5 cm, the pre-ESWL placement of an indwelling silicone double-J stent significantly reduces the complication rate from ureteral obstruction and urosepsis from 26 to 7 percent. The ability to perform retrograde studies to help delineate ureteral anatomy is another advantage of ureteral stenting. The stent may also help to localize radiolucent stones for ESWL, especially in fluoroscopically guided units. At Long Island Jewish Medical Center we routinely stent all patients with stone burdens greater than 1.5 cm before performing ESWL. We have noted a 3-month stone-free rate of 85 to 90 percent.

In our view, PL is the preferred method of treatment of renal pelvic calculi larger than 2.5 cm. The success rate for complete stone removal is high, and freedom from stones can usually be accomplished in one sitting. The morbidity of PL is higher with increasing stone burdens (i.e., staghorn calculi), but for renal pelvic calculi of 2.5 to 4.0 cm successful stone removal can be accomplished with little morbidity.

Stones of intermediate size (2.0 to 2.5 cm) may be treated with either modality. In these cases, treatment should be selected on an individual basis, taking into account the complications and stone-free rates and the type of stone.

Obstructive Uropathy

The success of ESWL for renal pelvic calculi depends on the ability of stone fragments to pass easily from the kidney to the bladder. Therefore, patients with renal pelvic stones and a narrow ureteropelvic junction (UPJ) need to be managed differently from those with normal anatomy. Often, secondary UPJ obstruction occurs because of the edema and spasm attributable to the presence of the stone. In these cases, placement of an internal stent followed by ESWL therapy should be adequate, especially if the stone is smaller than 2.0 cm.

If there is a primary obstruction of the UPJ, the patient is best managed by percutaneous nephrostomy and ultrasonic lithotripsy followed by an endoscopic pyeloplasty (endopyelotomy). Our success rates with endopyelotomy have been 84 and 90 percent for 45 primary and 70 secondary obstructions, respectively. Relief of the obstruction should reduce the risk of stone recurrence.

The possibility that previous ureteral surgery will influence the ureter's capacity to handle fragments should be considered. If there is a ureterocele or a megaureter or if there has been previous surgery at the ureterovesical junction, the renal pelvic calculi probably should be managed percutaneously, otherwise fragment passage after ESWL may be impeded.

Stones often become fixed in the UPJ. If they are treated in situ by ESWL, removal is successful in 80 to 90 percent of cases. However, even better stone-free rates (85 to 92 percent) can be achieved if these stones are manipulated into the renal pelvis or bypassed with a ureteral stent before ESWL.

Stone Composition

Stone composition affects the likelihood of success with certain stone removal procedures and the adjunctive measures needed. Generally, struvite-apatite and calcium oxalate dihydrate stones respond well to either ESWL or PL. The choice of treatment in these cases is dictated by other considerations, such as stone volume and the presence of obstructive uropathy.

Only 1 to 2 percent of stones (excluding cystine) fail to fragment with ESWL therapy, and these are usually calcium oxalate monohydrate. Percutaneous nephrolithotomy usually is highly effective in the treatment of these calculi. It is virtually impossible to predict which stones will be unresponsive to ESWL therapy, although by using factors such as clinical features (urinary crystals, urine pH, presence of infection), patient history (recurrent stone formation), as well as the radiographic appearance, the chances of successful ESWL therapy can be increased.

Uric acid calculi account for 5 to 13 percent of urinary calculi. The first-line treatment in these cases should be medical therapy: urinary alkalinization, increasing urinary volume, and reducing uric acid excretion. After medical therapy has been given for a time, the stone burden should be reassessed. As a renal pelvic calculus dissolves, pieces large enough to cause obstruction may pass into the ureter.

Patients who are unable to tolerate or who fail medical therapy usually can undergo successful ESWL for stones smaller than 2 cm. Ureteral catheters placed preoperatively are necessary for larger stones, as well as for patients who are to undergo treatment on a fluoroscopically guided lithotripter, because in the latter case, a retrograde pyelogram may be necessary to localize the stone. Ultrasonography-guided lithotripsy units can localize radiolucent stones without the aid of a ureteral catheter. Stones larger than 2.5 cm should be treated percutaneously, stone-free rates being similar to those obtained with stones made of calcium oxalate or struvite.

Patients with cystine calculi should undergo a trial of medical therapy. However, only 30 to 40 percent can be rendered stone free by long-term medical therapy. Further intervention is required in most patients, especially if there is a large stone burden. Cystine calculi generally do not respond well to ESWL because of their unique crystalline structure, although small renal calculi (less than 1 cm) can be destroyed with ESWL. An internal stent may be necessary. Any residual fragments can be managed by oral dissolution therapy or by placement of a nephrostomy tube for chemolytic irrigations.

In contrast, cystine stones readily fragment during ultrasonic lithotripsy performed percutaneously. Therefore, cystine stones larger than 1 cm are best managed initially by a percutaneous procedure. Even if such stones are fragmented by ESWL, the fragments will be large and will produce a difficult-to-manage Steinstrasse. An alternative to percutaneous stone extraction for large cystine stones is dissolution, but this necessitates lengthy hospitalization until the stone dissolves completely.

Ectopic Kidneys. Horseshoe kidneys often contain calculi, as many as 21 percent in certain series. ESWL therapy may be worthwhile for small pelvic stones in a nondependent portion of the kidney. If the initial session is unsuccessful, a percutaneous approach should be tried. Also, PL should be applied *initially* to patients with a large stone burden, obstruction, or stones in a dependent position. Good results have been obtained.

Calculi in ectopically located kidneys can be treated successfully with both ESWL and percutaneous techniques. Our success rate in removing calculi from pelvic kidneys percutaneously has exceeded 90 percent. Laparoscopic visual monitoring of the bowel has enabled a safe retrograde nephrostomy puncture and subsequent ultrasonic lithotripsy in these cases. ESWL therapy can also be successful in pelvic kidneys, although it requires the aid of special techniques.

Stones in a Renal Allograft. Calculi in a renal allograft pose a unique problem. Fortunately, they do not occur frequently, as they can be a cause of renal deterioration, and their effects can mimic a rejection episode. Both ESWL and percutaneous methods have been successful in treating such renal pelvic calculi.

Children

Childhood renal calculi are uncommon in the United States. The indications for surgical intervention are the same as for adults.

Endourologic procedures cannot always be applied to pediatric patients because of size limitations. However, the development of small-diameter pediatric scopes and equipment permit safer instrumentation for percutaneous nephrolithotomy.

ESWL has proved safe and effective in children. If the Dornier HM3 lithotripter is used, the gantry may need to be modified. Special consideration should be given to patients with a large stone burden, as Steinstrasse can be particularly difficult to manage in children.

TECHNIQUES

Extracorporeal Shock Wave Lithotripsy

We currently use a Technomed 3000 lithotripter at Long Island Jewish Medical Center. This unit is a ultrasonographically directed machine allowing prompt imaging of both radiopaque and radiolucent calculi. Renal pelvic stones up to 2 cm in size are generally treated by ESWL. We routinely use a ureteral stent for all patients with stones larger than 1.5 cm. Our philosophy is to overtreat rather than undertreat renal pelvic calculi. The mean number of shocks is approximately 3,000 per patient at 16 kV.

All ESWL procedures are performed under intravenous sedation with alfentanil and on an outpatient basis. Patients are discharged with oral pain medication, oral antibiotics, and a urine strainer. Initial follow-up is 2 weeks after ESWL to assess the amount of residual stone burden.

Percutaneous Lithotripsy

In percutaneous stone extraction, all patients are treated under general anesthesia. Preoperatively, urine cultures are obtained and intravenous antibiotics given. In the operating suite, cystoscopy with insertion of a No. 6 French ureteral catheter is performed. The catheter is connected to a syringe filled with 50 percent diatrizoate (Hypaque), which will be used to opacify the collecting system. After the patient is placed in the prone position, we gain access to the collecting system with a standard percutaneous technique and then dilate the tract to 34 Fr with the Amplatz renal dilators. The precise way in which a renal pelvic calculus is removed differs from patient to patient, although we generally use ultrasonic lithotripsy, which is highly effective for most stones. Once the stone is fragmented into small pieces, we routinely use grasping forceps to remove the fragments.

A No. 24 Fr nephrostomy re-entry tube is always left in place for both drainage and hemostatic purposes. On postoperative day 2, a nephrostogram with plain tomograms is obtained. If there are no residual stone fragments, no distal obstruction, and no extravasation, the nephrostomy tube is removed and the patient is discharged the following day. Residual fragments can be treated with ESWL, percutaneous extraction, or chemolysis.

SUGGESTED READING

Drach GW, Dretler S, Fair W, et al. Report of the United States Cooperative Study of Extracorporeal Shock Wave Lithotripsy. J Urol 1986; 135:1127.

Segura JW, Patterson DE, Leroy AJ, et al. Percutaneous removal of kidney stones: review of 1,000 cases. J Urol 1985; 134:1077.

Motola JA, Smith AD. Therapeutic options for the management of upper tract calculi. Urol Clin North Am 1990; 17:191.

Segura JW. Role of percutaneous procedures in the management of renal calculi. Urol Clin North Am 1990; 17:207.

STAGHORN CALCULI

MARTIN I. RESNICK, M.D.

Staghorn calculi can be defined as urinary stones occupying the renal pelvis and one or more infundibula with or without extension to the calices. Partial staghorn calculi have generally been defined as those occupying one or two infundibula, and complete staghorn calculi are those that totally fill the intrarenal collecting system. Although most of these stones are in part or completely composed of magnesium ammonium phosphate and carbonate apatite, and their formation is secondary to infections with urease-producing bacteria, staghorn calculi can also be composed of calcium oxalate, calcium phosphate, cystine, and uric acid and can be completely unrelated to urinary tract infections. More commonly, infection is an overriding causative factor in staghorn stone formation, but patients must be evaluated to identify the presence of any other predisposing factors. In approximately 50 percent of patients with infection due to staghorn stones, there is a readily identifiable metabolic cause that can be adequately treated so that the chance of recurrent disease is diminished. These concepts are addressed in more detail elsewhere in this volume.

The treatment of staghorn calculi has undergone many changes over the past two to three decades. In the late 1960s and early 1970s, surgical procedures, particularly anatrophic nephrolithotomy, were perfected, and improved results after removal of these large stones were realized. Percutaneous techniques were developed in the late 1970s, and extracorporeal shock wave lithotripsy (ESWL) became a reality in the early 1980s. These two techniques, used either alone or in combination, have been successfully employed for removal of these large stones.

Although the procedures have changed over the years, the objectives of surgery for removal of large staghorn calculi remain the same: primarily, removal of all stones; improvement of intrarenal drainage with reconstruction of the collecting system, when necessary; preservation of the maximal number of functioning nephrons; and, when present, eradication of upper urinary tract infection so as to reduce the rate of recurrence. Today, most stones that require removal can be managed by ESWL or percutaneous nephrostolithotomy. The role of open surgery is reduced and in some respects remains controversial.

Most would agree that the traditional pyelolithotomy and extended pyelolithotomy for treatment of partial staghorn calculi will now be infrequently employed. The anatrophic nephrolithotomy described by Boyce is likely to continue to have a role in the treatment of this problem because of the ability of the procedure to allow for both complete stone removal and reconstruction of the intrarenal collecting system. As mentioned, most smaller or partial calculi can be treated with ESWL, percutaneous nephrostolithotomy, or a combination thereof. Indications for open surgery remain controversial and include the following: (1) partial nephrectomy is required, (2) intrarenal reconstruction is necessary to improve intrarenal drainage, (3) coexisting problems are present in the kidney (e.g., ureteropelvic junction obstruction, caliceal diverticulum), (4) extensive stone disease is present that necessitate multiple percutaneous or ESWL procedures, (5) very hard stones are present that are not amenable to ESWL or percutaneous procedures, (6) there is an infected nonfunctioning kidney that necessitates nephrectomy, and (7) the surgeon must be experienced in the technique. This aspect of stone management is continually changing, and only with prolonged follow-up can one make reasonable comparisons among these multiple techniques.

When trying to compare the efficacy of open stone surgery with percutaneous nephrostolithotomy and/or ESWL, it becomes evident that the advantages of these newer techniques are fewer when treating patients with a large stone burden. Because in many instances multiple procedures are required (ESWL, percutaneous nephrostolithotomy, or both), the reduced hospitalization cost and recuperative time that was a distinct advantage in patients with smaller stones do not necessarily remain. Because of the need for multiple procedures, the average length of hospitalization of patients with full staghorn calculi has averaged 11 days, which is similar to the duration for patients having open surgical procedures. The cost factor between these newer techniques and traditional surgical approaches also becomes similar when multiple operative sessions are required. Data on recuperative time vary, and comparisons are at times difficult to establish.

It also becomes evident that, with the application of these newer techniques in the management of larger stones, the complication rate rises with the stone burden. With percutaneous nephrostolithotomy, the transfusion rate approaches 50 percent in the management of patients with staghorn calculi, and the stone remnant rate also averages 15 to 20 percent. The problem associated with ESWL when used alone in these patients is the high degree of obstruction secondary to the passage of a large number of fragments. In addition, the remnant rate has been reported to be as high as 40 percent. It must be remembered that comparisons of remnant rate are difficult. The percentage of retained stones in patients undergoing open surgical procedures averages 10 percent. The remnant rate in patients with large stones undergoing percutaneous procedures averages 15 to 20 percent and is probably double that when ESWL is used alone. The remnant rate for patients undergoing open surgical procedures has been based on intraoperative radiographic data, which are more accurate than the kidney-ureter-bladder views or tomograms that are obtained when monitoring patients undergoing the other two procedures. Because of the inability of tomography to identify very small stones, it is likely that the retained stone rate is much higher with these newer techniques.

Another area of controversy relates to the stone recurrence rate, about which there are few data in patients treated with these newer techniques. In patients with infectious stone disease undergoing open surgical procedures, the recurrence rate approximates 20 percent in 10 years. Because of the development of new antibiotics for treating *Pseudomonas* and *Proteus* infections that were not available a decade ago, it is believed that this number will decline. The recurrence rate with percutaneous nephrostolithotomy and/or ESWL is unknown, but one report places it at 7 percent in 1 to 2 years. Whether these rates will be comparable with those of open surgical procedures is unknown.

For the reasons discussed, there is no consensus as to the most appropriate management of patients with a staghorn stone. Many agree that patients with small staghorn stones occupying one or possibly two infundibula that are free of intrarenal scarring can be best managed by ESWL, either alone or in combination with percutaneous techniques. The placement of a percutaneous nephrostomy prior to treatment has been beneficial in controlling infection and maintaining drainage of the kidney that could be obstructed from the passage of many fragments. If reconstruction of the kidney is required, most agree that anatrophic nephrolithotomy with an intrarenal reconstructive procedure is probably the most appropriate approach.

More controversy exists over patients with full staghorn calculi. It is evident that patients can be rendered stone free with both percutaneous nephrostolithotomy and ESWL. Current experience indicates that the best approach is to debulk the stone with percutaneous nephrostolithotomy, and in most instances 80 to 90 percent of the stone can be removed with this approach. Many clinicians are initially performing a nephrostomy through an upper-pole infundibulum so as to gain greatest access to the collecting system. ESWL is then used to fragment any remaining stones. It has been reported that with this approach 78 to 92 percent of patients will be rendered stone free at 3 months. Although this rate of retained stones is greater than in the experience with anatrophic nephrolithotomy, a more important factor that is yet unknown is whether the recurrence rates between these two approaches are comparable. As in patients with partial staghorn calculi, the open surgical approach is generally preferred if intrarenal reconstruction is required.

In conclusion, many new approaches are available for the management of patients with staghorn calculi. It appears evident that patients with small or partial staghorn calculi can be treated with the newer, less invasive techniques, and open surgical techniques can be avoided. These patients do well, but it is unknown whether the recurrence rate associated with these techniques will be comparable with those experienced with open surgical procedures. More controversy exists over the treatment of the full staghorn stone, and it is only with increased experience that the best approaches will become evident. It does appear, however, that if ancillary procedures are required or intrarenal reconstruction is necessary, an open surgical approach is the more prudent course to follow. It must be remembered that no one approach is correct. Surgeons must decide on the best technique on the basis of the clinical situation and their own expertise.

SUGGESTED READING

Boyce WH, Elkins IB. Reconstructive renal surgery following anatrophic nephrolithotomy: follow-up of 100 consecutive patients. J Urol 1974; 111:307.

Griffith DP, Khonsari F, Skurnick JH, James KE. VA cooperative study Group A: a randomized trial of acetohydroxamic acid for the treatment and prevention of infection induced urinary stones in spinal cord injured patients. J Urol 1988; 140:318.

Patterson DE, Segura JW, LeRoy AJ. Long-term follow-up of patients treated by percutaneous ultrasonic lithotripsy for struvite calculi. J Endourol 1987; 1:71.

Winfield HN, Clayman RV, Chaussy CG, et al. Model therapy of staghorn renal calculi: a comparative study between percutaneous nephrolithotomy and extracorporeal shock wave lithotripsy. J Urol 1988; 139:895.

URETERAL CALCULI

SANJAYA KUMAR, M.D.
MANI MENON, M.D.

Ureteral calculi are predominantly seen in the third and fourth decades of life and are more often encountered in men than in women. Almost exclusively, the calculus originates in the kidney. A primary ureteric calculus is rare and occurs only when a foreign body, such as a suture, is present in the ureter.

DIAGNOSIS

It is not difficult to diagnose ureteral calculi. The patient presents with excruciating pain radiating from the loin to the groin, the genitalia, and the medial aspect of the thigh. The pain occurs in waves, corresponding to the waves or ureteral peristalsis, but the sufferer is seldom pain free between the spasms. There is an element of fixed loin pain that is due to renal capsular distention. Occasionally, however, the patient presents with nonspecific symptoms mimicking those of peritonitis or acute appendicitis. The wary clinician should consider ureteral calculus in any patient with microscopic hematuria and abdominal pain.

In a patient with suspected ureteral calculus, the diagnosis is traditionally established with a plain roentgenogram of the abdomen. Most urinary calculi (90 percent) are radiopaque. However, they must be about 2 mm in their longest diameter to be visualized on an optimal-quality abdominal roentgenogram. Calculi can be obscured by overlying bony structures and bowel gas. Since other conditions such as radiculitis can mimic ureteral colic, nonvisualization of the stone on a plain film despite a strong clinical history necessitates the performance of excretory urography. Most calculi too small to be seen on a plain abdominal film are situated at the ureterovesical junction, so a postvoiding oblique film to look for hang-up of contrast material at the ureterovesical junction is often critical. If the kidney is not visualized 15 minutes after injection of the contrast medium, delayed films need to be obtained at 1, 4, and 24 hours. Oblique films are useful in distinguishing ureteral calculi from phleboliths.

Other imaging techniques are rarely necessary for the diagnosis of ureteral calculi, the exception being computed tomography (CT). In situations in which a radiolucent filling defect is present in the ureter, a ureteral calculus will be densely opaque on a nonenhanced CT scan. In expert hands, real-time ultrasonography is as useful as excretory urography for the detection of ureteral calculi, but most hands are not so expert. Ultrasonography or radioisotope scanning may be needed in patients allergic to contrast media.

INITIAL MANAGEMENT

Analgesics are administered and the patient is hydrated. We have not found smooth muscle relaxants or prostaglandin synthetase inhibitors of much use either in decreasing pain or in promoting stone passage. If the calculus is less than 5 mm in diameter, under ordinary circumstances the patient can be managed on an ambulatory basis. If, however, the patient is febrile and has leukocytosis or bacteriuria, an intravenous antibiotic is given and the patient is admitted. An obstructed, infected kidney is a powerful focus for disseminated sepsis.

More than 90 percent of patients with ureteral calculi can be managed on an ambulatory basis. The indications for hospitalization are as follows: (1) stone in a solitary kidney; (2) stone in a patient with fever, leukocytosis, or bacteriuria; (3) stone greater than 6 mm in diameter (unlikely to pass spontaneously); (4) stones and azotemia; and (5) symptoms too severe for ambulatory management.

Most calculi less than 5 mm in width pass spontaneously within 4 weeks of the onset of symptoms. Nonetheless, 65 percent of calculi greater than 6 mm in diameter and almost all calculi greater than 8 mm will be in the ureter after 1 year. Under ordinary circumstances, therefore, we observe patients with stones less than 5 mm and intervene in patients with stones greater than 6 mm. Since obstruction untreated for more than 4 to 6 weeks can cause irreversible renal damage, we recommend intervention in all stones if obstruction is present after 4 weeks and the stone is not moving down the ureter (Table 1).

Table 1 Treatment of Ureteral Calculi

Stones <6mm		Wait 4 weeks
Stones >6mm	Upper or mid ureter	Proximal dislodgement and ESWL OR
		In situ ESWL with indwelling stents THEN
		Ureteroscopic maneuvers
	Distal Ureter	Ureteroscopic stone extraction
Stones associated with ureteral pathology		Ureteroscopy if possible THEN
		Open ureterolithotomy

Complete urinary tract obstruction with infection is a true surgical emergency. If the patient does not rapidly become afebrile, the urinary tract should be decompressed immediately. This is best done by means of a percutaneous nephrostomy, although cystoscopic placement of a ureteral stent is a reasonable alternative.

SURGICAL MANAGEMENT

Options for the treatment of ureteral calculi include stone dissolution, endourologic stone extraction, extracorporeal shock wave lithotripsy (ESWL), and open surgery.

The treatment of calculi by stone dissolution is discussed elsewhere in this book and will not be elaborated on here, except to mention that dissolution techniques are less successful in the treatment of ureteral calculi than in renal calculi.

Ureteral calculi can be removed endoscopically from above through a percutaneous nephrostomy or from below via the transurethral and transureteral route. In principle, stones in the upper third of the ureter are best managed through a percutaneous nephrostomy, and stones in the lower third of the ureter are best managed transurethrally. Stones in the midureter may be managed by either route. Despite these generalizations, ureteropyeloscopic techniques can be used to extract stones anywhere in the ureter. Because percutaneous techniques were developed primarily for the treatment of renal rather than ureteral calculi, they will not be discussed here. We will however, discuss techniques of ureteropyeloscopy and stone removal.

Ureteropyeloscopic Stone Extraction

A plain abdominal roentgenogram is obtained just before the procedure. Ureteroscopic stone extraction is painful and must be done with the patient under general anesthesia. It is important that the anesthesiologist be made aware that the procedure is significantly more involved than a cystoscopy. The operation is done with the patient in the lithotomy position and under fluoroscopic monitoring. It is strongly recommended that prophylactic antibiotics be used.

Cystoscopy is performed with a No. 23 to 25 Fr cystoscope. The ureteral meatus is visualized and the intramural ureter dilated. Dilatation can be done with metallic ureteral dilators that come in sizes 10 to 15 Fr. The dilator is passed through the cystoscopic sheath under direct vision and slowly advanced through the intramural ureter. It is not necessary to dilate the extravesical ureter, since this usually distends easily with irrigation and passage of the ureteropyeloscope. An alternative way to dilate the ureter is to use an angioplastic balloon catheter. We have found this technique to be better than ureteral dilatation with metal dilators. A 0.038-inch floppy-tipped guidewire is passed retrograde into the renal pelvis. The angioplasty balloon catheter is then passed, either over or by the side of the guidewire. It is often necessary to disconnect the telescope to thread the catheter over the guidewire. Under endoscopic vision, the balloon is inflated for 60 seconds, then deflated and removed. This method of dilatation is greatly preferred in patients with a history of lower ureteral surgery or injury.

The key to success in ureteroscopic stone removal is adequate dilatation of the intramural ureter. Once the ureter is dilated, the ureteropyeloscope can be introduced. These instruments are longer, thinner cystoscopes with external diameters ranging from No. 9 Fr to 13.5 Fr. They come with interchangeable bridges to accommodate 0-, 5-, and 70-degree lenses or with a fixed telescope. The larger-diameter ureteropyeloscopes have working channels for the passage of forceps, electrodes, or ultrasonic probes. In general, it is easier to pass a smaller ureteropyeloscope than a larger one.

The ureteropyeloscope is placed transurethrally into the bladder. The ureteral orifice is approached with the instrument directed inferiorly and laterally, in the direction of the intramural tunnel. Rotation of the instrument 180 degrees often allows the beveled tip to slip underneath the superior lip of the ureteral orifice. The instrument is then rotated again and the guidewire visualized. Once the intramural ureter has been traversed, the flow of irrigation is decreased to a bare minimum so that the stone is not pushed upward by the force of the irrigating fluid. The instrument is advanced proximally, always keeping the lumen in the center of the viewing field. The extramural portion of the pelvic ureter is easily distensible, and no difficulty should be encountered in passing the ureteropyeloscope once the intramural ureter has been traversed. However, the ureter at the level of the pelvic brim is more rigid and it may be difficult to pass the ureteroscope through it. In such an instance, the ureter should be dilated with a small balloon catheter.

Once the calculus is identified, the patient is placed in the reverse Trendelenburg position. A stone basket is passed and opened, and the stone is engaged under endoscopic monitoring. The basket is then closed, and if the stone is small enough, ureteroscope, basket, and stone are removed under direct vision. A double-J stent is then inserted so that the ureter is not occluded with edema.

Ultrasonic Lithotripsy

If the stone is too large to be removed intact, it should be disintegrated using an ultrasonic probe. This probe has a hollow lumen so that irrigation and suction may be applied to it. The ultrasonic probe is passed through the working channel of the ureteropyeloscope and brought into direct contact with the stone, held in position by the stone basket. Ultrasonic waves are not diffused by the wires of the stone basket, nor do they damage the ureteral wall; they are therefore very safe for intraureteral use. The stone is disintegrated under direct vision using short bursts of ultrasonic energy. Irrigation fluid is run through the probe, and suction is applied to it. This dissipates the heat generated by the ultrasonic waves and aspirates the stone fragments. Application of suction also serves to keep the stone in contact with the probe and prevent its proximal migration. Nonetheless, if the stone is initially fragmented into two pieces, one of the smaller pieces may break away and be pushed proximally. It is sometimes necessary to remove the stone basket and place a Fogarty balloon catheter to occlude the ureter proximal to the stone and prevent stone migration.

Electrohydraulic Lithotripsy

Ultrasonic destruction of ureteral calculi can sometimes be difficult and tedious. Instead, electrohydraulic lithotripsy can be used to fracture the stones. The rapid expansion of vapor generated by a high-voltage spark across two copper wires produces the shock wave that disintegrates the stone. The electrohydraulic lithotriptor probe is a No. 5 Fr diameter and flexible.

The advantages of electrohydraulic lithotripsy over ultrasonic lithotripsy are that the procedure is quicker and that harder stones can be fragmented. The electrohydraulic probe can be passed through a No. 9.5 Fr ureteroscope, whereas the ultrasonic probe requires a No. 13 Fr. The disadvantages include a much greater risk of ureteral injury—the electrohydraulic probe cannot be used with a wire basket. In addition, the fragments are not sucked away and tend to disperse in the ureter. Therefore, it is important to place a ureteral occlusion catheter proximal to the stone prior to the disintegration. Because of these difficulties, we prefer to use the ultrasonic lithotriptor and reserve the electrohydraulic lithotriptor for patients in whom ultrasonic lithotripsy has failed.

Flexible Ureteropyeloscopy and Laser Lithotripsy

Many varieties of flexible ureteropyeloscopes are now available. These instruments range in diameter from 5 Fr to 11 Fr. The smaller instruments are used primarily for diagnostic procedures, whereas the larger ones have deflectable tips and working channels. Graspers, baskets, and even flexible electrohydraulic and laser lithotriptor fibers can be passed through these working channels. A pulse dye laser has recently become commercially available. The conventional Candela MDL-1 Laser Triptor delivers a maximum of 60 milijules of energy at the tip of a 200 micron core fiber. The discharge from the laser fiber creates a plasma of rapidly expanding ions and electrons around the stone. Collapse of this plasma following the laser pulse generates a mechanical shock wave. Repetitive pulses fragment the stone in a fashion quite similar to that of the electrohydraulic probe. However, unlike the electrohydraulic lithotriptor, it is more controlled in action and causes less ureteral injury. It is good for fragile stones—especially impacted ureteral stones—and for disimpaction of steinstrasse following extracorporeal shock wave lithotripsy (ESWL). More recently even the hard calcium oxalate monohydrate calculi have been successfully disrupted using the upgraded MDL 2,000 laser triptor that can deliver a maximum of 140 milijules of power at the tip of the 320 micron core laser fiber. The laser fiber is usually passed through a 7.5 Fr semirigid ureteroscope; however, the flexible fiber can be passed through most flexible ureteroscopes that have the ability to reach stones located in virtually any part of the collecting system.

Extracorporeal Shock Wave Lithotripsy

In the procedure of ESWL, shock waves generated electrically in a medium of water are focused through the body of the patient onto the ureteral stone, resulting in its gradual disintegration. ESWL is 70 to 80 percent effective in the treatment of ureteral calculi, but is more than 90 percent effective in the treatment of renal calculi. Stones in the upper ureter are broken up more easily than those in the lower ureter, probably because they can be localized more easily. There is no significant deleterious effect on the kidney, bone, or adjacent organs.

ESWL is not useful when stones have been impacted in the ureter for 4 weeks or longer. Impacted calculi are often encased in a mucoid or fibrous sheath. The outer layer of such a stone may be fragmented, but the shell of organic material holds the pieces intact like a mosaic, preventing them from dispersing and creating new interphases that reflect the shock waves. This prevents effective stone disintegration. The routine use of a ureteral stent has greatly increased the stone fragmentation rate by providing better visualization of the ureteral calculus, and perhaps by creating an interphase between the stone and the wall of the ureter. In addition, the ureteral catheter provides drainage of the upper tracts. Success rates are greatly improved by dislodging ureteral calculi into the renal pelvis and then submitting them to ESWL.

Open Ureterolithotomy

The indications for open stone surgery have become rare with the advent of the techniques mentioned previously. Open stone surgery is used primarily when there is ureteral pathosis in association with a stone. Thus, open ureterolithotomy is necessary in patients with ureteral stone associated with massive reflux, obstruction, or tumor. It also becomes necessary in patients in whom endourologic stone removal or ESWL has failed. Stones in the upper ureter are approached by means of a dorsal lumbotomy or through a subcostal flank incision. We favor the dorsal lumbotomy, since it is associated with much less postoperative pain and morbidity.

The patient is placed on the flank, but the table is not flexed. The up shoulder and the bony pelvis are allowed to drop forward at an angle of 45 degrees away from the surgeon. A vertical incision is made over the belly of the erector spinae. The posterior layer of the dorsolumbar fascia is incised, and the erector spinae retracted medially. The fused middle and anterior layers of the dorsal lumbar fascia and Gerota's fascia are incised sequentially, exposing the ureter.

Calculi in the midureter are approached through a muscle-splitting high-Gibson incision. Access to the lower third of the ureter is gained through a modified Gibson approach, the incision being placed in the lower quadrant and extending medially. Alternatively, a low midline (our preference) or Pfannenstiel incision can be employed. If the calculus is in the juxtavesical ureter, an anterior cystotomy is performed. The posterior wall of the bladder is then opened above and lateral to the intramural ureter, and the juxtavesical portion of the ureter is identified posterior to the bladder. In women with juxtavesical calculi in whom the stone can be palpated transvaginally, the stone can be grasped with a Babcock forceps and a small transvaginal, transureteral incision can be used to remove the stone. This approach has particular merits in pregnant women who need ureterolithotomy.

Irrespective of the incision used for ureterolithotomy, an extraperitoneal approach is employed. In any of these approaches, occluding the proximal ureter with Silastic tape before dissecting out the calculus prevents proximal migration. The ureter is incised longitudinally over the stone. After stone extraction, the distal and proximal ureter is flushed with saline to free it of any stone concretions. A pediatric feeding tube is passed proximally and distally to ensure that no residual fragments are present. The ureterotomy is then closed with fine absorbable sutures without tension. The ureterotomy is invariably drained. A ureteral stent is used if the tissues appear suboptimal.

URETERAL CALCULI IN PREGNANCY

Ureteral calculi are rare in pregnancy. The physiologic hydronephrosis seen in pregnant women does not predispose to stone formation. However, the diagnosis should be suspected in a patient with flank pain and microscopic hematuria. A screening ultrasound examination, if normal, excludes the diagnosis. However, the presence of hydronephrosis does not confirm the diagnosis. A plain abdominal roentgenogram and a limited excretory urogram (20-minute and 1-hour delayed film, imaging only the involved site) are then taken. Although there is increased risk of congenital malformations in the fetus if the pregnant mother receives a radiation dose greater than 5 rad in the first trimester, the technique described here usually delivers less than 1 rad.

In general, the management of ureteral calculi in pregnancy should be conservative. High-grade obstruction and infection should be drained by means of a percutaneous nephrostomy. Occasionally, an obstructing calculus in the ureter can be pushed back into the pelvis and a ureteral stent left indwelling. Stone extraction or ureterolithotomy are necessary only in the rare circumstance when the calculus is implicated as the cause of premature labor. Except for this, definitive therapy is deferred until the postpartum period.

SUGGESTED READING

Morse RM, Resnick MI. Ureteral calculi: natural history and treatment in an era of advanced technology. J Urol 1991; 145(2): 263–265.

Rassweiler J, Schmidt A, Gumpinger R, Mayer R, Eisenberger F. ESWL for ureteral calculi. Using the Dornier HM 3, HM 3+ and Wolf Piezolith 2,200. Journal D Urologie. 1990; 96(3):149–153.

Dretler SP. Ureteral stone disease. Options for management. Urol Clin North Am 1990; 17(1):217–230.

Dretler S, Watson G, Parrish J, and Murray S. Pulsed dye laser fragmentation of ureteral calculi: initial clinical experience. J Urol 1987; 137:386–389.

Vandeursen M, Pittomvils G, Boving R, and Baert L. High energy pulsed dye laser lithotripsy: management of ureteral calcium oxalate monohydrate calculi. J Urol 1991; 145:1146–1150.

BLADDER AND URETHRAL CALCULI

JEFF FEGAN, M.D.
GLENN M. PREMINGER, M.D.

Mankind has been plagued with bladder stones since antiquity. The earliest known case of this disease was discovered in a 7,000-year-old mummified Egyptian teenager. Treatment of bladder calculi by perineal lithotomy was described by Celcus nearly 2,000 years ago. Medical records show that the pattern of urinary stone disease has changed over the years. In medieval Europe, bladder stones had become so common that lithotomy became a surgical subspecialty. After the Industrial Revolution, the incidence of bladder calculi decreased significantly, with a concomitant rise in the incidence of renal and ureteral stones. Today the disease is found most commonly in children in the developing nations of Asia and the Middle East.

Thai children have a high incidence of primary bladder calculi. Studies have shown that a relatively low fluid intake, a hot climate, and the specific Thai diet predispose to concentrated urine, as well as increased urinary excretion of calcium, oxalate, uric acid, and ammonia. Bladder stones in these children are usually composed of ammonium acid urate and either calcium oxalate or calcium phosphate.

In the modern Western world, bladder stones are usually found in older men and are secondary to urinary stasis due to bladder outlet obstruction or concentrated urine due to low fluid intake. The spectrum of stone composition is similar to that seen in upper tract urolithiasis, but urinary stasis more frequently leads to infection stones consisting of struvite or calcium apatite. Such stones may also form in patients with poor bladder emptying due to diverticula or neurogenic bladder dysfunction.

Foreign bodies in the bladder can become encrusted with calcium phosphate or struvite and thereby act as a nidus for stone formation. The most common offending object is an indwelling Foley catheter. Other potential causes are ureteral catheters, bullet and bone fragments, pieces of catheter balloons, nonabsorbable sutures, and a myriad of other objects that have been self-inserted into the bladder via the urethra.

Although most urethral calculi originate in the bladder, primary urethral stones can form when a stricture is present, or in association with a diverticulum. Prostatic calculi can migrate from the prostatic ducts into the posterior urethra and be passed spontaneously. Stone formation is also a possible complication of urethroplasty when hair-bearing skin has been used in the procedure.

DIAGNOSIS

Patients with urethral or bladder calculi usually present with symptoms of outlet obstruction or urinary tract infection. They may complain of sudden, intermittent pain referred to the perineum or tip of the penis. Often these symptoms are positional, resulting from a vesical stone rolling into the bladder neck or prostatic urethra. The pain generally occurs when patients are in the upright position or performing such activities as descending a flight of stairs, and may be relieved when they recline. Some patients complain of dribbling or sudden interruption of the urinary stream. Acute urinary retention may also be caused by the intermittent changes in position of a vesical calculus. One of many famous historical figures afflicted with bladder stones, Emperor Napoleon III was once described as being forced to lean against a tree in an attempt to void.

A stone in a urethral diverticulum may be asymptomatic for long periods, or may present with only a urethral discharge, due to infection in the diverticulum. Patients may notice a palpable lump, which can be exquisitely tender at times. In females, pain during colitis is a prominent symptom of stones in a urethral diverticulum. Urethral calculi can usually be found with palpation of the penis, perineum, vagina, or rectum. Urinalysis usually reveals microhematuria or pyuria.

The diagnosis of bladder and urethral calculi is often difficult to make radiographically. Most bladder calculi are poorly opacified, and other pelvic calcifications may add to the challenge of stone identification. The physician may dismiss calcifications seen on a plain film of the abdomen as prostatic calculi or phleboliths in an asymptomatic patient with coexisting bladder stones. Oblique projections usually differentiate the conditions. For radiolucent stones, cystography performed with dilute contrast medium or carbon dioxide usually shows a filling defect. Often, however, cystourethroscopy is required to make the definitive diagnosis.

TREATMENT

Bladder Calculi

The ancient technique of perineal vesicolithotomy has been abandoned in favor of suprapubic removal or transurethral pulverization and extraction of bladder stones. It is also possible to dissolve certain calculi with chemolytic solutions. Suprapubic removal is preferred in children, owing to their small-caliber urethras, or in adults with extremely large (greater than 5 cm) or hard stones. Open vesicolithotomy is also recommended in patients with heavily trabeculated bladders or bladder diverticula, since stone fragments may become lodged within the diverticula.

Small-capacity bladders are more vulnerable to mucosal injury during endoscopic manipulation. The subsequent bleeding obscures vision and increases the risk of bladder perforation. An open surgical procedure is therefore the preferred technique in such patients. In patients with an associated large, obstructing prostate, the surgeon also may prefer an open surgical procedure. Such an approach allows rapid removal of all stone material as well as the performance of an enucleation prostatectomy.

Spinal anesthesia with intravenous sedation is usually sufficient for open vesicolithotomy, although some patients may require general anesthesia. Since most patients with bladder stones have infected urine, a urine sample for culture and sensitivity should be obtained, and culture-specific intravenous antibiotics initiated 24 hours preoperatively. If the urine is sterile, a single preoperative dose of a broad-spectrum antibiotic such as a third-generation cephalosporin is given.

Any suspicious mucosal lesions discovered intraoperatively should be biopsied, because mechanical irritation from a bladder calculus can lead to squamous metaplasia or squamous cell carcinoma. Although some surgeons drain the bladder with a Foley catheter, we prefer to place a suprapubic tube at the end of the procedure. When patients can tolerate a diet, they are switched from intravenous to oral antibiotics, which are continued until removal of the suprapubic catheter 5 to 7 days after surgery.

Most bladder calculi are best treated transurethrally. Methods include mechanical crushing of the stone with a lithotrite, or stone fragmentation, using ultrasonic, electrohydraulic, or microexplosive techniques. Some basic principles apply to all techniques. Antibiotics are started preoperatively in the same manner as for an open procedure. Topical anesthesia, with or without intravenous sedation, may be satisfactory for a patient with small stones and a normal-sized prostate. With larger stones, or when additional endoscopic manipulation is anticipated, spinal or general anesthesia is required. Suspicious lesions are biopsied endoscopically. After the procedure, we drain the bladder for 24 hours with a Foley catheter. If bleeding is encountered during surgery, a three-way Foley should be placed for irrigation. Intravenous antibiotics are continued until the patients tolerate a diet, at which point they are switched to oral antibiotics for 7 days if the preoperative culture revealed infected urine. Otherwise, no further antibiotics are necessary.

Transurethral crushing or litholapaxy was originally performed blindly, with a tactile lithotrite. Although older, experienced urologists may still use this technique effectively, it has essentially been replaced by various methods using direct vision. Visual litholapaxy entails engaging a stone between the two jaws of the device and mechanically crushing it until the pieces can be washed out with an Ellik evacuator. The technique is limited to stones less than 2 cm in diameter. Complications include bladder laceration or perforation, and hemorrhage due to incidental bladder or prostatic trauma. The risk of

bladder injury is increased if the calculus is adherent to the wall, as when associated with a foreign body or tumor. Prostatic bleeding usually subsides with irrigation.

Electrohydraulic or ultrasonic lithotripsy have become the preferred techniques for bladder stone fragmentation in most patients. Ultrasonic lithotripsy uses high-frequency sound waves to create vibrations of sufficient intensity to disrupt most calculi. The hollow steel ultrasound probe is passed through a rigid endoscope with an offset lens, and is placed directly in contact with the stone. Ultrasonic energy at a frequency of 26.5 kHz is delivered from the generator to the stone, while irrigant flows continuously into the probe tip. The resulting suction holds the stone in place and simultaneously evacuates the stone particles. Ultrasonic energy causes mucosal erythema and possible significant bleeding if applied directly to the bladder wall. The probe itself can perforate the wall if undue pressure is applied, so direct visual control is imperative. Struvite and most calcareous stones can be managed conveniently with ultrasonic lithotripsy. Uric acid, cystine, and large calcium-containing stones may be treated more effectively with the more powerful electrohydraulic lithotripsy.

Electrohydraulic lithotripsy (EHL) is our preferred technique for the treatment of most bladder stones. EHL makes use of hydraulic shock waves, created when high-voltage sparks are generated under water, to fragment stones. This technique uses the same principle as the electrohydraulic extracorporeal shock wave lithotripsy (ESWL) devices. EHL equipment consists of a power generator, a coaxial probe, and a standard rigid or flexible cystoscope. The EHL probe itself is actually a coaxial electrode, consisting of a central metal core and outer metal sheath separated by a layer of insulation. The probes are flexible and are available in Nos. 3 to 9 Fr sizes; No. 5 or 9 is the preferred probe size for bladder stones.

The EHL probe is passed through either a rigid or flexible cystoscope and advanced until the tip is 1 to 2 mm from the stone. Depressing the foot pedal discharges the current in short bursts at the probe tip, where a spark is generated. The intense heat production in the immediate area surrounding the probe tip results in a cavitation bubble, which produces a shock wave that radiates spherically in all directions. Collapse of the bubble causes a second shock wave. Repeat administration of these shock waves results in stone fragmentation.

Several important factors should be kept in mind when using EHL. Care must be taken to avoid contact with the bladder wall while the probe is discharging, otherwise significant mucosal injury or perforation will occur. The probe tip must also be advanced at least 5 mm beyond the end of the cystoscope, to avoid shattering the lens. After the probe is fired about 10 to 15 times, the tip should be inspected for signs of wear, including destruction of the central core or peeling of the insulation. If the probe appears worn, it should be discarded and replaced by a new one. Continuing to use a worn probe may result in shedding of either metal or insulation fragments, which are often difficult to identify and extract.

For most efficient stone fragmentation, the use of 1/6 normal saline solution at room temperature has been suggested. However, we have found EHL to be successful in fragmenting bladder calculi using normal saline. Our current procedure is to begin with normal saline; if no fragmentation is noted, we switch to 1/6 normal saline. It is important to remember that perforation and absorption of 1/6 normal saline solution has a much higher risk of complications than if isotonic irrigants are being used. If a perforation occurs, the 1/6 normal saline irrigation should be discontinued immediately. Intravenous furosemide or mannitol may be given to induce a diuresis.

The primary disadvantage of EHL is its inability to remove the stone fragments efficiently. All particles have to be either manually extracted or small enough to pass spontaneously. It is therefore advantageous to fragment the stone into the largest sized particles that will allow extraction with grasping devices. There is no virtue in transforming a large stone into numerous small particles, because a significant amount of time will be required to remove the debris.

Microexplosion lithotripsy entails drilling a hole in the calculus and inserting a lead azide pellet, which creates a small explosion to fragment the stone. This technique does not seem to offer any advantage over standard EHL or ultrasonic lithotripsy, and provides significantly less control during stone fragmentation.

Chemodissolution is theoretically applicable for struvite, cystine, or uric acid bladder calculi. However, the long time required for this therapy make it less attractive than others in most situations. However, for patients with struvite calculi and chronic indwelling Foley catheters, stone dissolution with acidifying agents such as Suby's Solution G or hemiacidrin may well be the treatment of choice. Moreover, acetohydroxamic acid given orally has been used prophylactically in such patients to prevent catheter incrustation, with some success.

ESWL has been used successfully to treat small bladder calculi. Patients must be in the prone position and fluoroscopy or ultrasonography is used for stone visualization. Further experience with ESWL will determine the efficacy and practicality of using this modality to treat bladder stones.

Urethral Calculi

Treatment of urethral calculi depends on the position of stone impaction. Stones at the meatus or fossa navicularis can sometimes be grasped with forceps or removed through a meatotomy incision. Small stones in the penile urethra can usually be removed with a cystoscope by using either stone graspers or a basket. Sometimes an internal urethrotomy incision is required, if a stricture is present distal to the stone. When a large stone has been impacted for some time in the urethra, an external urethrotomy may be necessary. This should be avoided if possible, however, owing to the danger of fistula formation if a previous traumatic attempt at transurethral extraction has been made.

A stone recently impacted in the posterior urethra can often be pushed or irrigated back into the bladder and then crushed. If it is large and fixed, transurethral ultrasonic or electrohydraulic lithotripsy (EHL) under direct visual control should be attempted. Failure of this approach necessitates suprapubic or perineal extraction.

In all cases, the underlying cause of the urethral stone should be sought and eliminated, including any metabolic abnormalities. Since urethral calculi are usually found in a diverticulum or urethrocele in women, surgical excision of the sac containing the stone is necessary. In the past, urethral calculi were associated with high recurrence rates. Correction of the underlying pathology and treatment of associated infections now lead to extremely satisfying results.

SUGGESTED READING

Bulow H, Frohmuller HGW. Electrohydraulic lithotripsy with aspiration of the fragments under vision: 304 consecutive cases. J Urol 1981; 126:454–456.

Burns JR, Gauthier JF. Prevention of urinary catheter incrustations by acetohydroxamic acid. J Urol 1984; 132:455–456.

Durazi MH, Samiei MR. Ultrasonic fragmentation in the treatment of male urethral calculi. Br J Urol 1988; 62:443–444.

Streem SB. Bladder calculi. In: Rous S, ed. Stone disease: diagnosis and management. Philadelphia: Grune & Stratton, 1987:335–345.

Watanabe H, Watanabe K, Shiino K, Oinuma S. Microexplosion cystolithotripsy. J Urol 1983; 129:23–28.

CALCIUM OXALATE STONES

CHARLES Y.C. PAK, M.D.

Nephrolithiasis is a common disorder, affecting 220,000 to 660,000 Americans annually and 2.2 to 11.0 million Americans in their lifetime. In approximately 80 percent of patients, the disease is due to formation of stones composed of calcium oxalate.

There are two general approaches to the management of nephrolithiasis. One is to remove existing stones; the other is to prevent recurrent stone formation. Existing stones should be removed if they cause bleeding, infection, intractable pain, obstruction, or deterioration of renal function. New innovative methods for stone removal are described in other chapters.

Removal of stones, however, does not avert recurrence of stone formation. There is emerging evidence that recurrent formation of calcium oxalate stones may be prevented in most patients medically by conservative measures (of dietary modification and fluids), as well as a variety of specific drug treatments (Table 1).

CONSERVATIVE TREATMENT

Conservative therapy should be provided to all patients with stones, whether with a single stone or multiple stones, or an active or an indeterminant disease. Some measures should be applied to all patients; others should be confined to certain patients, depending on their particular physiologic derangement.

High Fluid Intake. A general measure recommended for all stone-forming patients is high fluid intake, sufficient to ensure urinary volume of at least 2 liters per day. An individual without excessive sweating and diarrhea should drink ten glasses (10 oz each) of fluids per day: e.g., two glasses with each meal, one between meals and at bedtime, and another glass upon awakening during the night to urinate. Fluid intake should be increased when there is an unusual extrarenal fluid loss.

Fluids are effective in controlling stone formation, because by increasing urinary volume it decreases urinary concentration of stone-forming constituents, and thereby lowers urinary saturation of stone-forming salts.

Sodium Restriction. A high sodium intake increases the risk of stone formation by increasing urinary calcium, lowering urinary citrate, and enhancing sodium urate–induced calcium oxalate crystallization. Moreover, it attenuates hypocalciuric response to thiazide. Thus, dietary sodium restriction should be less than 100 mEq per day. Patients should be discouraged from salting foods at the table, or eating salty foods or snacks.

Oxalate Restriction. Urinary oxalate may increase substantially after a high oxalate intake, especially in patients with intestinal hyperabsorption of calcium. A moderate oxalate restriction is recommended in order to avert dietary hyperoxaluria. However, oxalate bioavailability of foods varies widely among oxalate-rich food items and among individuals. It is my practice to limit first the ingestion of spinach and similar dark greens, rhubarb, tea, nuts, and chocolate. If hyperoxaluria persists, a more rigorous dietary oxalate restriction may be applied. Vitamin C supplementation (>500 mg per day) should be prohibited, because ascorbic acid serves as a substrate for oxalate synthesis.

Animal Protein Restriction and Increased Intake of Citrus Fruits. Animal protein excess increases the risk of stone formation by raising urinary calcium and uric acid, and lowering urinary citrate and pH. Some of these disturbances may be overcome by ingestion of alkali contained in fruit juices. In patients with hyperuricosuria or hypocitraturia, reduced intake of meat products and increased ingestion of citrus juices may be helpful.

Table 1 Specific Medical Treatments

Condition	First Choice	Second Choice
Absorptive hypercalciuria		
Type I, severe	Sodium cellulose phosphate	Thiazide + K$_3$Cit
Type I, mild-to-moderate	Thiazide + K$_3$Cit	Orthophosphate
Thiazide-resistance	Sodium cellulose phosphate Orthophosphate	
Type II	Dietary calcium restriction	Thiazide
Hypophosphatemic (type III)	Orthophosphate	Thiazide
Renal hypercalciuria	Thiazide + K$_3$Cit	
Hyperuricosuric calcium nephrolithiasis		
Severe	Allopurinol	K$_3$Cit
Mild-to-moderate	K$_3$Cit	Allopurinol
Distal renal tubular acidosis	K$_3$Cit	
Chronic diarrheal syndrome	K$_3$Cit	
Thiazide-induced hypocitraturia	K$_3$Cit	
Idiopathic Hypocitraturia	K$_3$Cit	
Gouty diathesis	K$_3$Cit	
With hyperuricemia	K$_3$Cit + allopurinol	

K$_3$Cit, potassium citrate.

Dietary Calcium Restriction. In patients with absorptive hypercalciuria maintained on oxalate restriction, a high calcium intake may exaggerate stone formation by significantly increasing urinary calcium without substantially lowering oxalate excretion. Moreover, it may reduce inhibitor activity against calcium oxalate crystallization, possibly by binding negatively charged inhibitors. A moderate restriction of dietary calcium is advisable for patients with intestinal hyperabsorption of calcium; this may be accomplished by limiting dairy products and dark roughages.

Calcium restriction should be undertaken with caution in growing children and in postmenopausal women because of potential adverse effects on bone.

SPECIFIC DRUG THERAPIES

Calcium oxalate stones may develop in patients suffering from a wide variety of metabolic-physiologic disturbances, including hypercalciuria, hyperoxaluria, hyperuricosuria, hypocitraturia, and hypomagnesiuria. Thus, there are several drug treatments available for prevention of calcium oxalate stone formation. These are generally applied in patients with recurrent active stone formation who are recalcitrant to conservative treatment. Specific drug therapies should also be considered if they are known to correct adverse extrarenal manifestations complicating the stone disease.

Thiazide. Thiazide is the ideal treatment for renal hypercalciuria, since it can correct the renal leak of calcium, secondary hyperparathyroidism, and compensatory intestinal hyperabsorption of calcium. The restoration of normal urinary calcium reduces urinary saturation of calcium oxalate. There is no apparent loss of hypocalciuric action during long-term treatment.

In my experience, trichlormethiazide, 4 mg per day, is preferred to hydrochlorothiazide or chlorthalidone, because it is well tolerated and less likely to cause severe hypokalemia. However, all three diuretics may cause hypocitraturia. Thus, it is my practice always to provide potassium citrate (10 to 20 mEq twice a day) with trichlormethiazide (4 mg per day).

Although the combined formulation of hydrochlorothiazide (50 mg) and amiloride (5 mg) may produce a greater hypocalciuric action than hydrochlorothiazide alone, the amount of amiloride it contains is not always sufficient to prevent hypokalemia and hypocitraturia. The use of potassium citrate with a drug containing potassium-sparing agent (amiloride) is potentially hazardous. I therefore find it more convenient to provide trichlormethiazide with potassium citrate.

Thiazide with potassium citrate is my first-line treatment for mild-to-moderate absorptive hypercalciuria type I, especially in women. Unfortunately, thiazide does not correct the intestinal hyperabsorption of calcium. Thus, some patients with this condition may show an attenuation of hypocalciuric action of thiazide after more than 2 years of treatment. In such patients, a temporary replacement of thiazide by sodium cellulose phosphate or orthophosphate for 6 months may restore responsiveness to thiazide.

Thiazide is contraindicated in resorptive hypercalciuria, since it may provoke hypercalcemia. Thiazide may cause hypokalemia, volume depletion, hyperuricemia, impotence, and rarely hepatocellular damage.

Sodium Cellulose Phosphate. This nonabsorbable ion exchange resin may correct hypercalciuria by binding calcium in the intestinal tract and inhibiting calcium absorption. Its sole indication is absorptive hypercalciuria type I. It is my first-line treatment for severe absorptive hypercalciuria. It is also used in patients who are resistant to or intolerant of thiazide.

Sodium cellulose phosphate is not ideally indicated for absorptive hypercalciuria, since it does not affect the basic intestinal transport process. Thus, this agent may cause complications of hypomagnesiuria (by binding magnesium) and hyperoxaluria (by increasing free oxalate pool). Moreover, this drug is contraindicated in other forms of hypercalciuria because it can overstimulate parathyroid function. It should be used with caution in postmenopausal women and growing children, because of its potential for exaggerating bone loss and impairing skeletal growth.

For the above reasons, sodium cellulose phosphate (2.5 to 5 g with a calcium-rich meal) should be restricted to patients with severe absorptive hypercalciuria type I or those intolerant of or resistant to thiazide. Magnesium supplementation (magnesium gluconate, 1 g twice per day) should be provided separately from sodium cellulose phosphate, and a moderate dietary oxalate restriction is advised.

Orthophosphate. Orthophosphate (a neutral or alkaline salt of sodium and/or potassium, 0.5 g phosphorus three or four times per day) reduces urinary calcium by altering renal tubular reabsorption of calcium or by inhibiting calcium absorption. The level of urinary phosphorus is markedly increased owing to the absorbability of phosphate. Physicochemically, orthophosphate reduces urinary saturation of calcium oxalate but increases that of brushite. Moreover, urinary inhibitor activity is increased, probably owing to stimulation of the renal excretion of pyrophosphate and citrate.

This drug is indicated for hypophosphatemic absorptive hypercalciuria as a first-line treatment. It is also used in patients recalcitrant to thiazide therapy. It should be used with caution in hypercalcemic patients or those with impaired renal function, because of the dangers of soft tissue calcification. Orthophosphate is contraindicated in urinary tract infections. The rise in urinary pyrophosphate or citrate may not occur because of bacterial enzymatic degradation. Thus, the inhibitor activity may not increase sufficiently to oppose the rise in saturation of brushite. Minor gastrointestinal disturbances (including abdominal bloating and diarrhea) may develop during treatment.

Allopurinol. Allopurinol (300 mg per day) is the physiologically meaningful drug of choice for hyperuricosuric calcium nephrolithiasis if hyperuricosuria is severe (> 800 mg per day) or if hyperuricemia coexists.

Physicochemical changes ensuing from the restoration of a normal level of urinary uric acid by allopurinol include a reduction in the urinary saturation of monosodium urate, and a commensurate increase in the urinary limit of metastability of calcium oxalate. Thus, the spontaneous nucleation of calcium oxalate is retarded by treatment with allopurinol, probably because the treatment inhibits the calcium oxalate crystallization induced by monosodium urate.

When patients with stones are treated with allopurinol, side effects are rare, although hepatotoxicity, bone marrow depression, and rash have been reported. The complication of xanthine stone formation is also rare.

Potassium Citrate. Potassium citrate is indicated for stone formation due to distal renal tubular acidosis, hypocitraturia associated with chronic diarrheal syndrome, thiazide-induced hypocitruria, idiopathic hypocitraturia, gouty diathesis, and hyperuricosuric calcium nephrolithiasis.

Potassium citrate increases urinary pH and citrate, and sometimes lowers urinary calcium (in distal renal tubular acidosis). Thus, this treatment reduces urinary saturation of calcium oxalate and uric acid, and inhibits crystallization of calcium oxalate. The dosage of the drug depends on the severity of the condition: generally 10 to 20 mEq twice per day for thiazide-induced and idiopathic hypocitraturia, and 30 to 60 mEq twice per day for chronic diarrheal syndrome and renal tubular acidosis. For gouty diathesis, a modest dose of potassium citrate (generally 10 to 20 mEq twice per day) sufficient to maintain urinary pH between 6 and 7 is usually effective in preventing both complications of calcium stones and underlying uric acid stone formation.

In mild-to-moderate hyperuricosuric calcium nephrolithiasis (<800 mg per day), a moderate dietary restriction of purine may be helpful, although usually impractical. If hyperuricosuria and stone formation persist, allopurinol (300 mg per day) or potassium citrate (10 to 20 mEq twice per day) may be used. The latter drug is preferred if hypocitraturia is also present.

Potassium citrate is contraindicated in renal failure (glomerular filtration rate <40 ml per minute), hyperkalemia, peptic ulcer disease, and active urinary tract infection.

SUGGESTED READING

Pak CYC, Britton F, Peterson R, et al. Ambulatory evaluation of nephrolithiasis: classification, clinical presentation, and diagnostic criteria. Am J Med 1980; 69:19–30.

Pak CYC. Kidney stones. In: Foster DW, Wilson JD, eds. Williams textbook of endocrinology. Philadelphia: WB Saunders, 1985: 1256–1273.

Pak CYC. Medical management of nephrolithiasis. J Urol 1982; 128:1157–1164.

Pak CYC. Citrate and renal calculi. Miner Electrolyte Metab 1987; 13:257–266.

Pak CYC. Medical management of nephrolithiasis: update 1987. J Urol 1988; 140:461–467.

URIC ACID STONES

MARTIN I. RESNICK, M.D.

Uric acid calculi are relatively uncommon and make up 5 to 10 percent of all urinary stones in the United States. Interestingly, in some Middle East countries such as Israel the incidence of uric acid calculi approaches 25 percent. The reasons for this are probably related to several factors, including the higher uric acid excretion in the population at risk and the relatively warm climate, which likely results in excretion of a more concentrated urine. Dietary factors related to a high purine intake probably are also a significant factor. It is also of note that uric acid stones are associated with a history of gout, and experience has indicated that approximately 20 to 25 percent of patients with uric acid stones have gout. In addition, a comparable percentage of patients with gout form uric acid stones. Latent gout, a condition associated with increased urine acidity without hyperuricemia or hyperuricosuria, is probably present in a significant percentage of patients who form uric acid stones. These patients may form uric acid stones alone but are predisposed to calcium oxalate or calcium phosphate stones, or a combination of the two.

ETIOLOGY

Uric acid is an end product of purine metabolism, and the development of uric acid crystals and subsequent stone formation is a function of the supersaturation of urine in relationship to undissociated uric acid. If supersaturation occurs, uric acid precipitation generally follows. The factors affecting supersaturation include urinary pH and uric acid concentration. The latter is influenced by both urinary volume and uric acid excretion, in that a low volume and a high rate of excretion can have comparable effects. High excretion may be related to increased endogenous production or may follow the ingestion of purine-containing foods (e.g., meats, fish, chicken). Patients with low urinary volumes (e.g., those with an ileostomy or inflammatory bowel disease) are at risk for low urinary volume and hence concentrated urine.

Probably the most important factor, and the most

commonly encountered entity related to uric acid formation, is a persistently acid urine. The pH of urine is important because it has a significant effect on the urinary saturation of undissociated uric acid. The first proton of uric acid has a pKa of approximately 5.5, and below this level most of the uric acid remains in the undissociated form. Solubility is low and crystallization results. Elevations of urinary pH result in increased levels of dissociated uric acid, and above a urinary pH of approximately 6.5 all uric acid is in this form. It is also important to recognize that urate salts have variable solubility. For example, monosodium urate has a lower solubility than monopotassium urate, and increasing sodium concentration will result in a decrease in soluble urate concentration.

Uric acid concentration is another important factor in uric acid stone formation. As previously noted, this is related to both excretory levels and urinary volume. The saturation of uric acid is thus related to the ratio of total uric acid concentration and the solubility of uric acid at the specified pH. Therefore, the interaction of these variables influences uric acid crystallization and subsequent stone formation.

The cause of low urinary pH typically present in uric acid stone formers is unknown. It is recognized that patients with primary gout excrete relatively less ammonium and relatively more titratable acid than normal subjects, but the metabolic basis for the acid urine is unclear. Patients with uric acid stones and low urinary pH may have latent gout, in the form of a highly acid urine without hyperuricema or hyperuricosuria. Some clinicians believe that this may represent an early phase of primary gout without the other manifestations of the disorder. It has been observed that stone symptoms and formation may precede the joint manifestations of primary gout in 40 percent of patients. Some believe that latent gout resembles the disorder that has been termed idiopathic uric acid lithiasis.

Other causes of uric acid stone formation include inborn errors of uric acid metabolism, the presence of concentrated acid urine, and hyperuricosuria without hyperuricemia (Table 1).

DIAGNOSIS

Typically, patients with uric acid lithiasis present with acute pain or colic associated with stone passage and urinary obstruction. Routine x-ray examination fails to reveal any calcification, and contrast studies demonstrate the presence of filling defects. The differential diagnosis typically includes a nonopaque calculus, urothelial tumor, blood clot, or sloughed renal tissue. Many techniques have been used to attempt further assessment and diagnosis; the usual methods include clinical history, physical examination, serum chemistry, urinalysis, and urine culture. Nonspecific studies include urinary cytology and a variety of invasive and noninvasive techniques directed at differentiating between these various processes.

Table 1 Classification of Uric Acid Lithiasis

1. Gouty diathesis (primary gout)
   a. Urate overproduction
   b. Diminished urate clearance
   c. Latent gout

2. Urate overproduction with normal urinary pH
   a. Inborn errors of metabolism
   b. Tissue metabolism (myeloproliferative disorders)

3. Passage of concentrated and unduly acid urine
   a. Chronic diarrheal states
   b. Physical exercise
   c. Ileostomy
   d. Inflammatory bowel disease

4. Hyperuricosuria without hyperurisemia
   a. Uricosuric drugs
   b. Overindulgence in animal protein

Adapted from Pak CYC. Uric acid nephrolithiasis. In: Resnick MI, Pak CYC, eds. Urolithiasis: medical and surgical reference. Philadelphia: WB Saunders, 1990:105.

Ultrasonography is a noninvasive study that may be able to detect a nonopaque calculus not evident on plain film radiography. Calculi measuring 0.5 to 1.0 cm can be detected with this technique, but other studies are of comparable value. Computed tomography (CT) is relatively simple and noninvasive and is also able to detect small stones. It provides greater density discrimination than conventional radiography, and therefore most stones are readily visualized with this technique. CT is also helpful in monitoring patients to determine whether stone dissolution has been accomplished and to detect new stone formation. Other more invasive studies include retrograde pyelography and retrograde brushing in association with urinary cytology. Ureteroscopy is also of value in visualizing the defect and obtaining biopsy material if necessary.

After the diagnosis of uric acid stones is established and treatment instituted, patients should be evaluated to determine the cause of stone formation so that treatment can be instituted and the risk of recurrence reduced. Twenty-four-hour urine collections with measurement of urinary volume and uric acid are essential. Measurement of urinary pH is also of significant importance in determining the cause of stone formation and directing treatment.

TREATMENT

Uric acid stones are unique in that, of all the calculi encountered in the urinary tract, they are most easily dissolved with appropriate therapy. Treatment is generally directed at raising urinary pH and lowering uric acid concentration by decreasing excretion and increasing urinary volume.

As noted, urinary pH in the range of 5.0 to 5.5 is typically identified in patients with uric acid stone formation. A variety of agents can be used to alkalinize the urine in uric acid stone formers, and in many instances, the choice of product depends on the clinical situation. If patients require hospitalization because of associated pain, nausea, and vomiting, intravenous infusion with 1/6 molar lactate is often of value. Infusion of 50 to 75 ml per hour raises urinary pH to 7.0 to 7.5 within several hours. The sustained elevation in urinary pH and the enhanced urinary volume both aid in dissolution of stones. Ureteral stones can be managed in this manner, and experience indicates that many pass spontaneously within several days after alkalinization as described. The use of 1/6 molar lactate is safe and probably as effective as direct irrigation of the renal pelvis with sodium bicarbonate solution. Since interventional techniques such as nephrostomy are avoided, the risks of infection or complications associated with this invasive procedure are minimized. A disadvantage of infusion with 1/6 molar lactate is the increased sodium load administered. This is less than infusions with sodium bicarbonate, but patients must be monitored for fluid overload and congestive heart failure. It must also be remembered that sodium infusion can result in sodium urate deposition, which occurs more readily at an elevated pH than uric acid alone.

Oral alkalinization agents are also of value, particularly in the outpatient setting when intravenous administration is not practical. Most clinicians give potassium citrate in a dosage of 15 mEq three to four times a day. Because of the delayed release form of the agent, sustained elevations in urinary pH are often achieved. It is not necessary to raise the urinary pH above 6.5, and if elevations greater than this level are maintained for a sustained period, the patient may be predisposed to calcium oxalate or calcium oxalate stone formation. Other forms of citrate (e.g., sodium citrate) have been effective in alkalinizing urine, but because of dissociation of phosphate, urinary saturation for calcium phosphate increases. As noted, the saturation of monosodium urate increases as well because of the increased dissociation of uric acid and the presence of a high sodium load. The presence of these two substances increase the likelihood of calcium stone formation.

If patients have malabsorption problems or chronic diarrheal states (e.g., inflammatory bowel disease), a liquid preparation of potassium citrate or sodium-potassium citrate is of particular value. Because of the rapid transit time in the intestine, delayed-release pills often are not absorbed, and a liquid preparation is more effective.

If urinary volumes are low and increased uric acid concentration is related to this factor, attempts should be made to increase fluid intake, with subsequent effect on urinary volume. This is sometimes difficult, particularly in patients with chronic diarrheal states, but optimal urinary output should be achieved. Ideally, minimal urinary excretion should be 2 to 3 L per 24 hours, and if this can be maintained, supersaturation levels can often be reduced.

Finally, in hyperuricosuric patients, efforts should be made to reduce uric acid excretion. If the condition is related to dietary factors, patients should be instructed to reduce their intake of red meat, beef, chicken, and other high-protein foods such as peanuts. In my experience, patients with uric acid stones and hyperuricosuria rarely respond to this regimen, and medications are required to reduce uric acid excretion. Allopurinol, 300 mg daily, is effective in achieving this and is well tolerated. A small percentage of patients have an allergic reaction to allopurinol, but most tolerate it quite well.

Follow-up should include monitoring of urinary pH, urinary volume, and uric acid excretion. Attempts should be made to adjust these parameters so that urine is undersaturated for uric acid. If this is achieved, not only will new stone formation be prevented but existing stones will probably dissolve. If dissolution cannot be obtained, calcium components typically are present within the stone, and other forms of fragmentation (e.g., extracorporeal shock wave lithotripsy or percutaneous lithotripsy) are required.

In most instances stone prevention can be obtained by increasing urinary pH to 6.5 to 6.8 and increasing urinary volume. If hyperuricosuria is present, this also requires correction, but allopurinol is often required because many patients do not respond to dietary therapy. Patients should be followed and attempts made to measure important parameters associated with uric acid stone formation.

SUGGESTED READING

Goldman IL, Resnick MI. The diagnosis and management of uric acid lithiasis: a retrospective epidemiologic study. J Lithotripsy Stone Dis 1989; 1:107.

Gutman AB, Yu TF. Uric acid nephrolithiasis. Am J Med 1968; 45:756.

Kursh ED, Resnick MI. Dissolution of uric acid calculi with systemic alkalinization. J Urol 1984; 172:286.

Pak CYC. Uric acid nephrolithiasis. In: Resnick MI, Pak CYC, eds. Urolithiasis: a medical and surgical reference. Philadelphia: WB Saunders, 1990:105.

Pak CYC, Sakhae EK, Fuller C. Successful management of uric acid nephrolithiasis with potassium citrate. Kidney Int 1986; 30:422.

Pak CYC, Waters O, Arnold L, et al. Mechanisms for calcium nephrolithiasis among patients with hyperuricosuria: supersaturation with urine with respect to monosodium urate. J Clin Invest 1977; 59:426.

STRUVITE STONES

JOHN R. BURNS, M.D.

The role of infection in the formation of renal calculi is usually limited to phosphate calculi. Struvite is a crystalline compound composed of magnesium ammonium phosphate. Pure struvite calculi are known to form in some animal species, but human struvite calculi usually consist of a combination of struvite and carbonate apatite. In humans, struvite calculi form only when the urinary pH is higher than 7.0, which is not the case in normal urine. Only after the introduction of a urease-producing bacterial infection are conditions favorable for precipitation of struvite and carbonate apatite. Struvite calculi often fill the collecting system and assume a branched configuration. In this chapter, these calculi are referred to as infection-induced calculi.

MICROBIOLOGY

The enzyme urease is most often associated with *Proteus* infections. More than 90 percent of all *Proteus* species produce urease. Urease production is less common with *Pseudomonas* (32 percent of strains) and *Klebsiella* (64 percent). *Escherichia coli* rarely, if ever, produces urease. Several *Mycoplasma* species have been shown to produce urease and cause formation of infection-induced calculi.

Urease catalyzes the hydrolysis of urea into ammonia and carbon dioxide. This results in an increased concentration of ammonia and an alkaline pH, both conditions conducive to struvite and carbonate apatite precipitation. Bacteria are believed to secrete a glycocalix, which promotes their adherence to the urothelial surface. The increased concentration of urinary ammonia injures the protective glycosaminoglycan layer of the urothelium, facilitating the adherence of bacteria and tissue damage. Urinary microproteins and struvite and carbonate apatite crystals bind to the glycocalix, and eventually form a matrix calculus. Further crystal deposition results in progressive mineralization and formation of a dense radiopaque calculus.

INCIDENCE AND MODE OF PRESENTATION

About 15 percent of all renal calculi in the United States are infection-induced calculi. They are more common in females and in patients prone to urinary infection. Patients with neurogenic bladders, especially those secondary to spinal cord injury, are at increased risk for calculus formation. The presence of a foreign body, such as a nephrostomy tube or a urethral catheter, is also a risk factor, in that bacteria can adhere to a foreign body for a long period and thus allow crystallization.

A urease-producing infection can be superimposed on a pre-existing metabolic disease, especially in post-menopausal, multiparous black women with urinary calculi. Although the calculi in this group of patients are often struvite, a substantial portion of these individuals have hyperparathyroidism.

Most infection-induced calculi do not cause the renal colic typical in the presence of calculi. A patient with an infection-induced calculus most commonly has a history of recurrent febrile urinary infections and persistent dull flank pain.

DIAGNOSIS

Infection-induced calculi are usually diagnosed on either a plain abdominal x-ray film or an excretory urogram. The latter is necessary to define the anatomy of the collecting system and the degree of caliceal dilatation. Plain renal tomography should be part of excretory urography, because many infection-induced calculi are poorly opacified and not visualized on routine radiographs. When there is a question of function of the involved kidney, radionuclide differential renal scanning is helpful in formulating strategy. For example, if the involved kidney contributes less than 10 percent of total renal function and the contralateral kidney is normal, nephrectomy may well be indicated; this is especially true of an anatomically abnormal kidney with a large stone burden. A urine culture and sensitivity is obtained to provide proper antibiotic coverage before intervention. Routine blood studies should be performed to eliminate the possibility of primary hyperparathyroidism. If fasting serum calcium is greater than 10.2 mg per deciliter, a C-terminal parathyroid hormone assay (PTH) should be drawn. If hyperparathyroidism is diagnosed, it should be corrected before treatment for calculi is begun.

TREATMENT

Infection-induced calculi can cause considerable morbidity. For example, patients with an untreated infected staghorn calculus have a 50 percent chance of losing the involved kidney, and in those with bilateral untreated staghorn calculi there is a 40 percent mortality rate within 10 years. Conservative treatment is therefore indicated only in elderly patient or one with an otherwise reduced life expectancy; it can be dangerous, however, because there is a constant risk of bacterial seeding of the uninvolved kidney.

In a patient with a staghorn calculus in a poorly functioning kidney, nephrectomy is often the best option. This approach presupposes the presence of one normal kidney. The decision to perform a nephrectomy is based on the differential renal function of the kidney as determined by radionuclide renal scanning.

Acidification of Urine

As mentioned, struvite and carbonate apatite form only when the urine is alkaline. If one could effectively acidify the urine, these crystals theoretically would dissolve and surgery would not be necessary. However, this is impossible in the presence of a urease-producing infection. Moreover, for reasons that are not entirely clear, acidification often is not effective, even with proper antibiotic control of infection. Acidifying agents previously used are cranberry juice, methenamine mandelate, and ammonium chloride. Cranberry juice is a poor choice, because its high oxalate content can cause encrustation of an existing stone with calcium oxalate. Methenamine mandelate is ineffective in the presence of a urease-producing infection because its conversion to formaldehyde in alkaline urine is negligible. Ammonium chloride (750 mg four times a day) may be effective in keeping urine acidic, but only if the infection is suppressed. If only one kidney is infected, the pH of bladder urine can be an unreliable indicator of urinary acidification in the infected kidney.

When feasible, the treatment of infection-induced renal calculi in the absence of hyperparathyroidism begins with vigorous and protracted antibiotic therapy followed by removal of all calculous material. Bacteria can grow in the interstices of infection-induced calculi and persist even after long-term antibiotic therapy. Failure to remove all calculous material results in recurrent or persistent infection in almost 50 percent of patients, and recurrent calculi in 22 to 75 percent.

Nephrolithotomy

Open surgical removal is the most effective method of eliminating an entire branched calculus in a single procedure. Most of these calculi are large, so anatrophic nephrolithotomy is required. After open lithotomy by experienced surgeons, 78 percent of patients remained stone free for at least 8 years. However, anatrophic nephrolithotomy has been almost forgotten in the current push for minimally invasive surgical procedures. Today, many patients are reluctant to undergo a major open procedure and choose less invasive measures. Anatrophic nephrolithotomy is now rare, even in major teaching hospitals, and most urology residents are therefore poorly equipped to perform it. Complication rates after anatrophic nephrolithotomy in large series were acceptable, but will undoubtedly be much higher when the procedure is used only occasionally.

Percutaneous Nephrolithotomy

Percutaneous nephrolithotomy (PCN) has become the preferred procedure in most patients with branched infection-induced calculi. When PCN is used alone, multiple percutaneous punctures are usually required to ensure complete calculus removal. The bulk of the calculus can be removed with ultrasonic lithotripsy. Calices that are inaccessible to the rigid nephroscope can be treated with an electrohydraulic probe passed through a flexible nephroscope or flexible cystoscope. Infection-induced calculi usually are easily broken with ultrasonic lithotripsy, even if they appear densely radiopaque.

Extracorporeal Shock Wave Lithotripsy

The treatment of branched infection-induced calculi with extracorporeal shock wave lithotripsy (ESWL) has evolved over the last few years. After the introduction of ESWL in the United States, a tendency developed to treat all renal calculi with this technique. It usually takes several ESWL treatments to fragment a large staghorn calculus totally. It was soon apparent, however, that few patients become stone free after ESWL alone. In addition, the complication rate after ESWL used alone is unacceptable; a substantial percentage of patients develop ureteral obstruction from stone fragments (steinstrasse). Because the obstruction is often asymptomatic, urosepsis and loss of renal function can occur. The endoscopic treatment of steinstrasse is often unsuccessful, and nephrostomy drainage can be necessary. For these reasons, the use of ESWL by itself is not the preferred treatment for large branched calculi.

ESWL is currently used in conjunction with PCN in most patients with branched renal calculi. Percutaneous debulking is performed first, usually through a single puncture site. In a patient with normal renal anatomy, about 80 percent of the total stone burden can usually be removed with PCN. The patient is then allowed to rest for a week, and the remaining stone material is treated in a single ESWL procedure.

For patients with partial staghorn calculi, the use of ESWL alone versus PCN is controversial. Treatment of upper pole partial staghorn calculi with ESWL alone often yields acceptable stone-free rates. Some authors argue that ESWL can be used alone for a complete staghorn calculus if there is normal renal anatomy and no caliceal dilatation. I have found that very few patients so treated become stone free. For lower pole partial staghorn calculi, the treatment of choice is PCN, because ESWL leaves only 32 percent of patients stone free if they have lower pole calculi greater than 2 cm in diameter.

The success of ESWL is expressed in different ways in the current literature. In the days of open nephrolithotomy, surgical success was equated with achieving a stone-free status; if a fragment was missed in surgery, the procedure was considered a failure. Today, ESWL is commonly considered successful if the patient is left with "insignificant fragments," usually less than 4 mm in diameter. It has been shown that more than 20 percent of these insignificant fragments will grow within a year, this figure is based on a series of several thousand patients, most having sterile calcium calculi. In patients with infection-induced calculi, the incidence of growth of residual fragments is unknown, but is probably higher than 20 percent. Such fragments can therefore hardly be considered insignificant. Our goal should remain the same as with open nephrolithotomy: rendering the patient stone free.

Combination Therapy

Combination or sandwich therapy is often used in an attempt to improve the results of ESWL. It consists of percutaneous debulking followed by ESWL. Several days after ESWL, flexible nephroscopy is repeated, often without anesthesia or sedation, and residual fragments are then either removed or flushed out through the nephrostomy tract. The efficacy of this approach is unknown, but it probably lowers the recurrence rate. An alternative to repeated nephroscopy is chemolysis.

Chemolysis

Chemolysis is an important adjunct in the treatment of infection-induced calculi. A radiograph made after successful PCN often shows no residual calculi. If the collecting system is examined with a flexible nephroscope, however, minute stone fragments adherent to the mucosa are likely to be visible. The fate of these fragments is unknown, but it is reasonable to assume that they can lead to clinical recurrence. Rates of stone recurrence after open nephrolithotomy have been lowest in series in which routine chemolysis was used.

The agents currently used for chemolysis of infection-induced calculi are urologic-G solution and hemiacidrin. Both are buffered to a pH of 4.0, at which the solubility of struvite and carbonate apatite is markedly increased, and dissolution therapy is practical. Because the rate of dissolution is a function of surface area, chemolysis after ESWL is extremely effective. Urologic-G solution is approved for renal irrigation; hemiacidrin is approved only for bladder irrigation. In vitro studies have shown that hemiacidrin is the more effective in promoting struvite dissolution, and if proper precautions are used, is safe even though not approved for renal irrigation.

If chemolysis is to be used, a preirrigation nephrostogram should show good drainage and no extravasation. The urine should be sterile and the patient afebrile. Irrigation is started with normal saline solution at 30 ml per hour, increased to 120 ml per hour over 4 to 6 hours, with a maximal pressure head of 30 cm H_2O. Hemiacidrin irrigation is then started at 120 ml per hour. Urine is cultured daily and irrigation stopped if the culture is positive. Because hemiacidrin has a high magnesium content, serum is tested for magnesium concentration daily. A urethral catheter is often helpful to ensure patient comfort. The major precaution is to have a hemostat at the bedside and to ensure that the patient uses it to stop the irrigation at the first sensation of pain, fever, or other sign of lack of well-being. Irrigation is continued for 48 hours after the disappearance of calculi, as demonstrated on a plain renal tomogram.

Matrix Calculi

Although most infection-induced calculi are heavily mineralized and readily apparent on radiographs, a small percentage are composed primarily of protein matrix with minimal mineralization. Such calculi are either radiolucent or faintly radiopaque, have the consistency of putty, and can be difficult to treat. The lack of adequate mineralization makes ESWL ineffective. Large-matrix calculi can often be removed through a ureteroscope because the soft material will conform to the ureter. Large collections of matrix calculi in the kidney are best treated with PCN. I have been generally unsuccessful with postoperative irrigation with hemiacidrin. Irrigation with a mucolytic agent, such as acetylcysteine, should be effective, but there are no supporting clinical data.

Medical Therapy

The medical treatment of infected phosphate calculi is summarized in Table 1. The most important element of medical therapy is prevention of recurrent urinary infection. In a patient with a neurogenic bladder requiring chronic catheter drainage, one should consider either clean intermittent catheterization or external sphincterotomy followed by condom catheter drainage. If a patient does develop recurrent urinary infection, long-term antibiotic therapy is indicated. Most of these infections are caused by *Proteus* species and can be treated with one of the penicillins. Either oral penicillin (500 mg every 6 hours) or ampicillin (250 mg every 6 hours) can keep the urine sterile, even in the presence of a residual infected stone fragment. In patients with persistent *Pseudomonas* infections, long-term tetracycline can be effective.

The recurrence of phosphate calculi is minimally affected by dietary modification. The Shorr regimen consists of a low-calcium, low-phosphorus diet, supplemented with aluminum hydroxide gels, such as Amphojel or Basaljel. Although the regimen can effectively lower urinary phosphate levels, it is poorly tolerated and side effects are common. It is worthwhile to eliminate any unnecessary magnesium-containing medications, especially antacids, and patients should be encouraged to maintain a urinary output of more than 2 L per day.

Patients who continue to form calculi despite use of antibiotics are candidates for a urease inhibitor. Acetohydroxamic acid (AHA) is a urease inhibitor that decreases urinary pH and urinary ammonia, even in the presence of a urease-producing infection. AHA can prevent stone growth in many patients and has been

Table 1 Medical Treatment for Infected Phosphate Calculi

1. If possible, remove all infected calculi; this probably means using preoperative antibiotics and some combination of PCN, ESWL, and chemolysis
2. If possible, remove sources of infection, such as a urethral catheter
3. Vigorously treat any persistent or recurrent infection
4. Attempt to reduce urinary inorganic phosphate content with diet
5. Discontinue magnesium-containing medications
6. Encourage oral intake of fluids to ensure urinary output of more than 2 liters/day
7. Treat any underlying metabolic disease
8. Consider using acetohydroxamic acid (AHA) if above measures are not effective

reported occasionally to promote stone dissolution. In some patients, however, it has little effect. I have several compliant patients who have formed large staghorn calculi while on therapeutic doses of AHA. Approximately 20 percent of patients are unable to tolerate AHA, because of its vascular, neurologic, or hematologic side effects. In addition, AHA is contraindicated in pregnancy and in patients with renal insufficiency. Although AHA is thus far from the ideal drug, it should be considered in some patients with recurrent infection-induced renal calculi. It can also be useful in preventing the development of encrustation on chronic indwelling urethral catheters. Many patients who are prone to form catheter encrustation require frequent catheter changes. Encrustation can often be prevented by AHA (250 mg twice daily).

SUGGESTED READING

Eisenberger F, Rassweiler J, Bub P, et al. Differentiated approach to staghorn calculi using extra-corporeal shock wave lithotripsy and percutaneous nephro-lithotomy: an analysis of 151 consecutive cases. World J Urol 1987; 5:248.

Griffith DP. Struvite stones. Kidney Int 1978; 13:372.

Kahnoski RJ, Lingeman JE, Coury TA, et al. Combined percutaneous and extracorporeal shock wave lithotripsy for staghorn calculi: an alternative to anatrophic nephrolithotomy. J Urol 1986; 135:679.

Lerner SP, Gleeson MJ, Griffith DP. Infection stones. J Urol 1989; 141:753.

Nemoy NJ, Stamey TA. Surgical, bacteriological, and biochemical management of "infection stones." JAMA 1971; 215:1470.

CYSTINE STONES

CHARLES Y. C. PAK, M.D.

Cystine stones typically occur in approximately 10,000 persons in the United States who are homozygous for cystinuria. These persons excrete abnormal amounts of cystine in urine of over 250 mg per g of creatinine as well as excessive amounts of other dibasic amino acids (lysine, arginine, ornithine). In addition, they show varying intestinal transport defects for these same amino acids. The stone formation is the result of poor aqueous solubility of cystine.

PHYSICAL CHEMISTRY OF CYSTINE STONE FORMATION

Since there are no known inhibitors of the crystallization of cystine, the stone formation is dictated primarily by the urinary supersaturation of cystine. Thus, cystine stones could theoretically form whenever urinary cystine concentration exceeds the solubility limit. Dent and Senior established the solubility of cystine at various pH as approximately 300 mg per liter at pH 5, increasing to 400 mg per liter at pH 7 and 500 mg per liter at pH 7.5. However, the solubility for cystine in individual urine samples varies considerably, dependent on the amount and type of electrolytes and macromolecules. As much as 70 mg of additional cystine could be dissolved as the ionic strength increased from 0.005 to 0.3 M. In general, the actual cystine solubility limits in urine are considerably lower than those described by Dent and Senior, ranging from 170 to 300 mg per liter at pH 5, 190 to 400 mg per liter at pH 7, and 220 to 500 mg per liter at pH 7.5. Thus, the minimal cystine concentration required to elicit stone formation is lower than previously believed.

DIAGNOSIS

Table 1 summarizes the steps in diagnosis. One should examine the urinary sediment (preferably in fresh first-morning void) for the presence of typical hexagonal cystine crystals. Also, screen the urine sample for "qualitative" cystine by the cyanide-nitroprusside test. A positive reaction suggests that cystine excretion exceeds 75 mg per day. A false-positive test may be encountered in patients with homocystinuria and acetonuria. A similar qualitative measure of cystine excess may be obtained by the "paper strip" test developed by Santen Pharmaceutical Co., Ltd. and marketed by Mission Pharmacal Co. On x-ray film, cystine calculi are radiopaque as calcareous calculi, but are more rounded and homogeneous. They may attain a staghorn size.

If the above studies suggest the presence of cystinuria, quantitate urinary cystine excretion (e.g., by amino acid analyzer or Dionex ion chromatograph). The test procedure should be able to identify cystine itself, separately from a mixed disulfide. Urinary cystine exceeding 250 mg per g of creatinine is usually diagnostic of homozygous cystinuria. Analyze stones passed or

Table 1 Diagnosis

Presumptive
 Cystine crystals in urinary sediment
 Positive qualitative test for cystine in urine

Definitive
 Quantitative cystine determination (>250 mg/g creatinine)
 Cystine on stone analysis

Table 2 Therapeutic Considerations

Conventional therapy: applicable to all patients
 Dietary: avoidance of excessive methionine intake
 Fluids: sufficient to produce minimal urine output of 2 L/day
 Alkali: potassium citrate sufficient to maintain urinary pH at
  6.5–7

Specific therapy: applicable after failure of conventional therapy
 or in patients with severe cystinuria
  D-Penicillamine
  Alpha-Mercaptopropionylglycine

removed. The presence of cystine provides a definitive diagnosis of cystinuria.

Cystinuria is sometimes associated with hypocitraturia, hypercalciuria, or hyperuricosuria. A search for other abnormal risk factors is therefore indicated.

TREATMENT

The goal of therapy (Table 2) is to reduce the urinary cystine concentration below its solubility limit. This may be accomplished by dietary means aimed at reducing cystine synthesis and excretion, conservative measures directed at decreasing cystine concentration or increasing cystine solubility, and treatment with chelating agents that convert cystine to a more soluble form.

Dietary Manipulation

A low-methionine diet has often been recommended for the control of cystine nephrolithiasis because of the well-known requirement of this essential amino acid for cystine production. Although this dietary maneuver may reduce cystine excretion, a rigid methionine restriction is impractical. Patient compliance is often poor with a diet devoid or severely restricted in red meat, poultry, fish, and dairy products. Moreover, there may be long-term adverse consequences of such a diet on other organ systems, such as the skeleton. Thus, I recommend avoidance of excessive intake of the above food items, but do not severely restrict them. Sodium restriction may slightly lower urinary cystine. This effect may be offset by reduced solubility of cystine mentioned previously.

Conservative Measures

In patients with moderate cystinuria (250 to 500 mg per day) with cystine calculi, first attempt conservative measures of high fluid and alkali intake. Fluid therapy aims to increase urine volume sufficiently to reduce cystine solubility below the solubility limit. At least 3 L of fluid (ten 10-oz glassfuls) should be provided, including two glasses with each meal and at bedtime. Patients should expect to awaken at night to urinate; they should drink two more glasses of fluids before returning to bed. Additional fluids should be consumed if there is excessive sweating or intestinal fluid loss. Seek a minimal urine output of 2 L per day on a consistent

basis, a goal attainable by most patients with proper and persistent instruction.

All types of fluid are generally permissible, with the possible exception of milk (with high methionine content) and brewed tea (with high oxalate content, increasing risk of calcium oxalate nephrolithiasis, which sometimes complicates cystine nephrolithiasis). Fruit juices (e.g., grapefruit, orange, cranberry, apple, grape) may be particularly advantageous, because they provide not only water but alkali. For example, 600 ml of orange juice (one glassful with breakfast and again with dinner) may provide enough citrate and potassium to increase urinary pH by 0.5 unit.

The object of alkali therapy is to increase urinary pH to enhance cystine solubility. However, excessive alkali therapy is not indicated. Substantial increase in cystine solubility does not occur until the urinary pH exceeds 7.5. The provision of alkali, no matter how much, rarely raises urinary pH above 7.5. When urinary pH increases above 7 (with alkali therapy), the complication of calcium phosphate nephrolithiasis may ensue because of the enhanced urinary supersaturation of hydroxyapatite in an alkaline environment.

I recommend that a modest amount of alkali be provided to maintain urinary pH at a high normal range (6.5 to 7). Potassium alkali are better than sodium alkali because they do not cause hypercalciuria and are less likely to cause calcium stones. Citrate is preferable to bicarbonate because it produces a more constant and persistent elevation in urinary pH. The slow-release tablet preparation of potassium citrate is probably superior to the readily available liquid preparation in this regard. I prescribe potassium citrate (wax matrix tablets) at a typical dosage of 30 mEq twice a day. Adjust the dosage depending on the results of urinary pH.

Chelating Agents

D-Penicillamine (beta-beta-dimethyl-cysteine) and α-mercaptopropionylglycine (Thiola) are chelating agents, containing a free sulfhydryl group. Thus, they readily undergo thiol-disulfide exchange with cysteine to form a mixed disulfide (D-penicillamine-cysteine or Thiola-cysteine), which has a much higher aqueous solubility than cystine. After oral administration, a sufficient amount of D-penicillamine or Thiola could appear in urine to complex cysteine and thereby lower cystine excretion.

Chelating agents may be added to the conservative treatment program when the latter is ineffective in controlling stone formation in patients with moderate cystinuria. In patients with severe cystinuria (> 500 mg per day) in whom a customary conservative program alone is not likely to be effective, D-penicillamine or Thiola (*with* conservative measures) may be begun to start with.

D-*Penicillamine*

Base the dose of D-penicillamine on that amount required to reduce urinary cystine concentration to below its solubility limit (generally < 250 mg per liter). The extent of the decline in cystine excretion is proportional to the D-penicillamine dose. Each increment in D-penicillamine of 250 mg per day might be expected to reduce urinary cystine by 75 to 100 mg per day. Accordingly, assuming that a minimal desired urine output of 2 L per day has been achieved, the minimal effective D-penicillamine dose might be 1250 mg per day when cystine excretion is 1,000 mg per day or 750 mg per day when urinary cystine is 800 mg per day. The medication is generally given in divided doses before meals, since its absorption may be impaired when mixed with certain foods.

There is substantial evidence that D-penicillamine can favorably modify the course of cystine nephrolithiasis. If adequate amounts of the drug could be given to lower urinary cystine to desired levels, one could expect a reduction in rates of stone passage and new stone formation. When a sufficient fall in cystine excretion occurs to produce urinary undersaturation, dissolution of existing cystine stones could occur.

Unfortunately, a substantial number of patients develop adverse reactions to D-penicillamine treatment. Side effects include gastrointestinal complications (e.g., nausea, emesis, diarrhea, loose stools, anorexia, abdominal pain, bloating, or flatus), impairment in taste and smell (probably due to chelation of zinc), dermatologic complications (e.g., pharyngitis, oral ulcers, rash, ecchymosis, pruritus, urticaria, pemphigus, elastosis perforans serpiginosa, skin wrinkling), hypersensitivity reactions (e.g., laryngeal edema, dyspnea, respiratory distress, fever, chills, arthralgia, weakness, fatigue, myalgia, adenopathy), hematologic abnormalities (e.g., leukopenia, agranulocytosis, thrombocytopenia, anemia, eosinophilia), abnormal liver function tests, and renal complications (e.g., proteinuria, nephrotic syndrome, glomerulonephritis). In up to 50 percent of patients, the cessation of D-penicillamine therapy may be required because of these side effects. In some of them, D-penicillamine therapy may be reinstituted by desensitization. This technique entails restarting treatment at a low dose of D-penicillamine (10 to 25 mg per day), with a gradual increase in dosage at 3-day intervals until the desired dosage is reached over about 1 month.

During long-term therapy, D-penicillamine may cause vitamin B_6 deficiency by binding pyridoxine. Before the appearance of significant symptoms (e.g., dizziness, seizures, glossitis, seborrheic dermatitis), it may be prudent to provide pyridoxine supplementation (50 mg per day) in patients receiving large doses of D-penicillamine (> 1 g per day) chronically.

Alpha-Mercaptopropionylglycine

Thiola, now approved by the Food and Drug Administration, may serve as a reasonable alternative to D-penicillamine, especially in the setting of toxicity to the latter drug. It shares similar chemical properties with D-penicillamine. Because of its higher oxidation-reduction potential, α-mercaptopropionylglycine may be more efficient than D-penicillamine in undergoing thiol-disulfide exchange with cystine. The reduction in urinary cystine this drug provides is equivalent to that obtained during D-penicillamine therapy. Thus, the same comments regarding dosage schedule previously given for D-penicillamine apply to α-mercaptopropionylglycine treatment. Available data from Japan and Europe suggest that this drug is as effective as D-penicillamine in inhibiting cystine stone formation.

The major advantage of α-mercaptopropionylglycine appears to be its apparent reduced toxicity. A review of the literature disclosed ten reports entailing 120 cystinuric patients undergoing clinical trial with this agent. Minor gastrointestinal problems occurred in 35 patients, rash in 14, urticaria in 3, pemphigus foliaceus in 1, fever in 7, and nephrotic syndrome in 2. These adverse reactions were generally less common and less serious than those reported with D-penicillamine. Although serious side effects such as pemphigus and nephrotic syndrome have also been encountered during α-mercaptopropionylglycine therapy, they occurred less frequently. Thus, among 120 patients taking the drug, only two apparently had to stop taking the medication because of adverse reactions.

My own experience is compatible with the above findings. I have conducted a multiclinic trial with α-mercaptopropionylglycine in the United States to assess its therapeutic role as an alternative to D-penicillamine in the management of patients with cystine nephrolithiasis. The primary objective was to determine the safety and efficacy of the agent in patients with known toxicity to D-penicillamine.

Among 49 patients who took D-penicillamine first and later received α-mercaptopropionylglycine, 41 patients (83.7 percent) developed side effects to D-penicillamine and 37 (75.5 percent) to α-mercaptopropionylglycine. Adverse reactions involved all organ systems. Frequent adverse reactions to D-penicillamine were nausea in 36.7 percent, emesis in 28.6 percent, anorexia in 18.4 percent, rash in 34.7 percent, proteinuria in 12.2 percent, and fatigue in 16.3 percent. These reactions were also observed during α-mercaptopropionylglycine therapy but less frequently. Nausea was encountered in 24.5 percent of patients, emesis in 10.2 percent, anorexia in 8.2 percent, rash in 14.3 percent, proteinuria in 10.2 percent, and fatigue in 14.3 percent.

Moreover, serious side effects were less common

during α-mercaptopropionylglycine therapy. Thus, 69.4 percent of patients required cessation of D-penicillamine treatment, whereas only 30.6 percent had to stop taking the newer drug. Among 34 patients who could not tolerate D-penicillamine, 22 could tolerate α-mercaptopropionylglycine.

Seventeen patients with no history of taking D-penicillamine were offered the newer agent for the first time. Eleven patients (64.7 percent) had adverse reactions. However, many of these reactions were minor or nonspecific. Only one patient (5.9 percent) was forced to discontinue α-mercaptopropionylglycine treatment because of side effects.

The drug was as effective as D-penicillamine in reducing cystine excretion. During long-term treatment (average dose of 1,193 mg per day), urinary cystine was maintained at 350 to 560 mg per day and urinary saturation of cystine was kept undersaturated. Commensurate with these changes, the agent produced remission of stone formation in 63 to 71 percent of patients and reduced individual stone formation rate in 81 to 94 percent.

Recently, hepatotoxicity was reported during Thiola use in Japan, though not in the United States. Unlike D-penicillamine, Thiola does not cause depletion of copper, zinc, or pyridoxine. Thus, Thiola appears to be safer to use and just as effective in controlling cystinuria as D-penicillamine. It may be the first-line chelating agent.

SUGGESTED READING

Pak CYC. Kidney stones. In: Foster DW, Wilson JD, eds. Williams textbook of endocrinology. Philadelphia: WB Saunders, 1985:1256.

Pak CYC. Cystine stones. In: Resnick MI, Kursh ED, eds. Current therapy in genitourinary surgery, 1st ed. Philadelphia: BC Decker, 1987:412.

Pak CYC, Fuller C, Sakhaee K, et al. Management of cystine nephrolithiasis with alpha-mercaptopropionylglycine (Thiola). J Urol 1986; 136:1003–1008.

Sakhaee K, Poindexter JR, Pak CYC. The spectrum of metabolic abnormalities in patients with cystine nephrolithiasis. J Urol 1989; 141:819–821.

CHEMOLYSIS OF URINARY CALCULI

DEAN G. ASSIMOS, M.D.

Chemolysis of urinary calculi is a process in which the urinary environment is altered to promote stone dissolution. This is achieved by various methods, including decreasing the concentration of stone constituents and increasing their solubility by manipulating urinary pH or chemical conversion. This process can be accomplished systemically through oral or parenteral therapy (systemic chemolysis) or by directly changing the urinary environment with irrigation techniques (direct contact chemolysis). It is important to know stone composition, preferably by standard analytic techniques, before proceeding with either type of chemolytic therapy.

SYSTEMIC CHEMOLYSIS

Systemic chemolysis may be considered for patients with nonobstructing calculi, particularly if they are asymptomatic and do not have active urinary tract infection. Patients are monitored with periodic imaging studies to ensure that renal obstruction does not develop during therapy. The disadvantages of this approach are the long intervals to a stone-free status, the need for patient compliance, and mediocre success rates.

Uric Acid Calculi

Approximately 10 percent of patients with renal calculous disease have uric acid stones. Excessive urinary uric acid excretion and acidic urine promote uric acid stone formation. Treatment is aimed at reversing these abnormalities. The pKa of uric acid in urine at 37° C is 5.35, which means that at pH 5.35 one half of urinary urate is made up of undissociated uric acid and the other half consists of monovalent urate anions, which are more soluble. As urinary pH increases to 6.5 to 7.0, most of the urate assumes this more soluble form. Uric acid stone formers typically have a low urinary pH, and increasing the pH to this range promotes uric acid stone dissolution. This is accomplished with oral potassium citrate, sodium citrate, or sodium bicarbonate therapy. Potassium citrate is preferred in patients with normal renal function and serum potassium levels, especially those who are hypertensive, since monopotassium urate is more soluble than monosodium urate. Sodium bicarbonate or 1/6 molar lactate can be administered intravenously in selected patients to achieve urinary alkalinization. Patients monitor their urinary pH with narrow range pH strips (6.0 to 8.0) to ensure adequate alkalinization. Overalkalinization (pH 7.5 or higher) is not recommended, because this does not increase the solubility of uric acid significantly and may promote formation of calcium phosphate stones. The urinary concentration of uric acid is decreased by increasing daily urinary output to 2.5 to 3 L through increased fluid consumption. Uric acid excretion is reduced by allopurinol therapy and limiting consumption of animal protein.

Cystine Stones

In 1 to 3 percent of individuals with nephrolithiasis there are cystine stones caused by cystinuria, a rare autosomal recessive inherited disorder characterized by abnormal intestinal and renal transport of cystine, lysine, ornithine, and arginine. Except for cystine, these other amino acids are highly soluble in urine. Heterozygote adults usually excrete less than 350 mg of cystine daily, occasionally have problems with cystine stone formation, and may be predisposed to calcium oxalate nephrolithiasis, whereas homozygotes excrete larger quantities of cystine and are frequently plagued by cystine stones. Treatment goals include increasing cystine solubility and decreasing its urinary concentration. Cystine solubility increases substantially as urinary pH rises from 7 to 8. Approximately 400 mg of cystine is soluble in 1 L of urine at pH 7, while 1 g is soluble at pH 8. Urinary alkalinization to a pH range of 7.5 to 8 is accomplished by the methods described in the previous section. Increasing daily urinary output to 3 L with diurnal and nocturnal hydration decreases urinary cystine concentration. Cystine excretion is decreased with sulfhydryl medications such as D-penicillamine and alpha-mercaptopropionylglycine. Their mechanism of action is based on a thiol-disulfide exchange reaction in which cystine reacts with the sulfhydryl groups of these substances, forming a disulfide compound and cysteine that are both highly soluble. Since the side effects of alpha-mercaptopropionylglycine are less severe than those associated with D-penicillamine, this medication is preferred.

Infectious Stones

Approximately 10 percent of patients with nephrolithiasis have infectious stones. Stones form when the urinary tract is infected with urease-producing bacteria. This enzyme hydrolyzes urea, which generates bicarbonate and ammonia. The resulting alkaline urine promotes magnesium ammonium phosphate and calcium phosphate supersaturation, leading to struvite and carbonate apatite stone formation. Antibiotic therapy, administration of urease inhibitors, urinary acidification, and the Shorr regimen can be used to attempt struvite stone dissolution. However, results with these methods are usually poor.

DIRECT CONTACT CHEMOLYSIS

Direct contact chemolysis is mainly used as an adjunct for treatment of any residual calculi present after more definitive stone-removing procedures such as extracorporeal shock wave lithotripsy, percutaneous nephrolithotomy, ureterorenoscopic surgery, and open surgery. Primary treatment is not usually undertaken because of the often long intervals required to achieve a stone-free status. In addition, chemolysis may be more effective after some of these procedures. For example, lithotripsy increases the stone surface area, which theoretically should decrease chemolytic dissolution time. However, direct contact chemolysis may be employed initially for high-medical-risk patients who are not candidates for the above-mentioned procedures or for patients who express a preference for this therapy.

Certain aspects of patient preparation are germane to all types of direct-contact chemolysis. Daily urine cultures are performed to ensure that the urine remains uninfected. Serum creatinine and BUN levels are assessed every 24 to 48 hours. Patients are treated with broad-spectrum antibiotics throughout chemolysis. Two nephrostomy tubes (8 to 12 Fr) are inserted. One is used for inflow and placed in the targeted stone-containing area; the other tube is positioned in a dependent area to allow unimpeded outflow of the irrigant. Nephrostography is performed to make sure there is no extravasation before proceeding with infusion. An intravenous infusion pump is used to instill fluid at a steady prescribed rate. A central venous pressure manometer is attached to the inflow tube for close monitoring of infusion pressure, which is kept below 20 cm of water to prevent systemic absorption of the infusate. Vital signs are monitored frequently during infusion. All solutions must be sterile and are warmed to 37° C for infusion. Before the chemolytic solution is instilled, saline is infused, starting at a flow rate of 30 ml per hour and gradually increased to a maximum of 120 ml per hour over 36 to 48 hours. If the patient tolerates this trial infusion, the chemolytic instillation is begun in a similar gradual fashion. If fever, chills, malaise, flank, or abdominal pain develop, the infusion is promptly terminated. The patency and position of the nephrostomy tubes are reassessed and necessary readjustments made. If fever and the symptoms have resolved and the urine is not infected, the infusion is restarted, but it may be necessary to reduce the maximal flow. If the urine is infected, the infusion is restarted only after antibiotic therapy is appropriately adjusted and the urine becomes sterile. Systemic chemolysis is usually administered concurrently and is continued after termination of direct chemolysis to prevent recurrent stone formation. Radiographic studies are obtained every 48 to 72 hours to assess the progress of stone dissolution. Ultrasonography or computed tomography (CT) are used to follow patients with uric acid calculi, because these stones are radiolucent. If the calculi are refractory to chemolysis or if dissolution plateaus, the stone type may not have been accurately predicted, the stones may have mixed compositions also containing apatite or calcium oxalate, or there may be inadequate solution contact with the stone. If the latter is true, the nephrostomy tubes are repositioned. Chemolytic irrigation is continued 48 to 72 hours after radiographic confirmation of stone absence, to help eradicate small undetectable fragments. Direct contact chemolysis requires close monitoring and is usually performed in a hospital. In an effort to lessen the high costs of this therapy, some centers are treating selected patients in a controlled outpatient setting. Several provisions must be met to enact outpatient chemolysis successfully. The patient and a family member or friend must be well versed in perfusion techniques and their complications. A nurse must visit the patient every 24 to 48 hours to monitor progress, ensure that proper techniques are used, and obtain specimens for urine culture and specific serum chemistry testing. The patient should be in close proximity to the medical center and the treating physician should be readily available.

Uric Acid Calculi

Alkaline solutions are used for chemolytic dissolution of these calculi. Tromethamine E, an organic amine buffer with a pH of 10.2, is preferred to 0.1 to 0.2 molar sodium bicarbonate solutions that have a pH ranging from 8.4 to 9. The higher pH of this agent causes a more rapid breakdown of the organic stone matrix in these calculi, which accelerates dissolution.

Cystine Calculi

The best solution for direct contact chemolysis of cystine calculi is an alkaline solution of 2 percent N-acetylcysteine, a thiol that has been shown to be more effective than D-penicillamine and alpha-mercaptoproprionylglycine in in vitro studies. This agent is not effective for systemic chemolysis because it is rapidly deacetylated after oral ingestion, a process that does not occur with direct infusion. Tromethamine E is the preferred buffer for alkalinization of the N-acetylcysteine.

Infectious Calculi

Two commercially available acidic solutions, 10 percent hemiacidrin and Suby's G Solution G, which contain magnesium, citrate, and other substances outlined in Table 1, can be used for chemolytic dissolution of struvite and carbonate apatite calculi. Their mechanisms of action include inhibition of struvite and carbonate apatite crystallization from the resultant acidic milieu, formation of soluble phosphoric acid and calcium citrate complexes due to the available hydrogen and citrate ions, and magnesium and calcium ionic exchange. During early experiences with hemiacidrin irrigation of the upper urinary tract, a number of deaths were reported, and the Food and Drug Administration withdrew approval for use of this agent in locations proximal to the bladder. Close review of these cases indicated that the fatalities resulted primarily from sepsis. By following strict guidelines, both of these

Table 1 Comparison of Suby's Solution G and Hemiacidrin (1,000 ml)

Constituent	Suby's Solution G	Hemiacidrin
Citric acid (g)	32.3	28.2
Magnesium oxide (g)	3.8	0
Sodium carbonate (g)	4.8	0
Calcium carbonate (g)	0	1.0
D-Gluconic acid (g)	0	5.0
Magnesium hydrocarbonate (g)	0	14.8
Magnesium acid–citrate (g)	0	2.5
Water (ml)	1,000	1,000
pH	4.2	3.9

agents can be used safely for upper tract irrigation. Compliance with the general recommendations for direct contact chemolysis reviewed in the previous section is mandatory. In addition to these guidelines, serum magnesium levels are monitored daily because of the risk of hypermagnesemia. Patients with severe renal insufficiency (glomerular filtration rate of less than 10 ml per minute) are not candidates for this type of chemolytic therapy because their kidneys are not capable of excreting excess magnesium. Although increased magnesium absorption may occur in patients with interposed bowel in the urinary tract, hypermagnesemia is not usually a problem if renal function is normal. In patients with continent diversions, the conduit is catheterized during chemolysis to limit magnesium absorption across the bowel mucosa. When magnesium toxicity occurs, irrigation is promptly terminated, and the patient is given calcium gluconate and furosemide (Lasix) intravenously and vigorously hydrated with intravenous saline. In patients who do not respond to these measures, dialysis may be required. Patients may develop a chemical cystitis during chemolysis, which resolves if the irrigation is stopped. When symptoms abate, the bladder is catheterized to limit contact time with these solutions, and irrigation is resumed. These solutions can also cause uroepithelial irritation in the renal collecting system and ureter. Radiographic features of this include small, irregular, nodular filling defects and spiculation in these areas. If severe, this process may be obstructive and chemolysis should be terminated. These changes are transient, and resolution usually occurs within 7 to 10 days.

Calcium Oxalate Calculi

Calcium oxalate calculi are dissolvable in vitro with chelating agents that form soluble nonionic compounds with polyvalent cations such as calcium. There were some early reported clinical successes with disodium ethylenediaminetetraacetic acid (EDTA) dissolution of calcium oxalate calculi. However, its use was abandoned because of systemic toxicity and uroepithelial damage. These effects are not related directly to EDTA but arise as a consequence of chelation. Until these problems are solved, dissolution of calcium oxalate stones will remain an in vitro art.

SUGGESTED READING

Dahlberg PJ, Van Den Berg CJ, Kurtz SB, et al. Clinical features and management of cystinuria. Mayo Clin Proc 1977; 52:533–542.
Jenny DB, Goris GB, Urwiller RD, Brian BA. Hypermagnesemia following irrigation of renal pelvis. JAMA 1978; 240:1378–1379.
Palmer JM, Bishai MB, Mallon DS. Outpatient irrigation of the renal collecting system with 10 percent hemiacidrin: cumulative experience of 365 days in 13 patients. J Urol 1987; 138:262–265.
Rodman JS, Williams JJ, Peterson CM. Dissolution of uric acid calculi. J Urol 1984; 131:1039–1044.
Sheldon CA, Smith AD. Chemolysis of calculi. Urol Clin North Am 1982; 9:121–130.

RENAL TRANSPLANTATION

FISTULA AND OBSTRUCTION FOLLOWING RENAL TRANSPLANTATION

KENNETH A. KROPP, M.D.

Urologic complications are common nonimmunologic causes of morbidity and mortality in renal transplant recipients. The overall incidence of urologic complications varies from 3 to 34 percent and leads to graft loss in one out of every four instances. Most urologic complications are due to ureteral ischemia or to the ureteral reimplantation, and present as urinary extravasation, with or without fistula formation, or as an obstruction. The purpose of this chapter is to review the incidence, etiology, clinical presentation, and diagnosis of these urologic problems and outline a strategy for management.

OBSTRUCTION

Approximately 25 percent of the urologic complications seen after renal transplantation are due to obstruction. Most series report an incidence of 1 to 3 percent. Ureteral obstruction is rarely an immediate post-transplant problem, but is more often seen 30 or more days after transplantation. Although the differential diagnosis of immediate post-transplant anuria includes ureteral obstruction, which therefore must be excluded, it accounts for less than 10 percent of cases. Intrinsic causes of obstruction can occur at the ureteral mucosa–bladder mucosa junction as a result of faulty surgical techniques, or secondary to distal ureteral ischemia. Rarely, calculi can form in a transplant kidney and pass into the ureter to cause obstruction. Extrinsic causes of obstruction occur outside the bladder and are usually related to kinking, angulation, or compression by a lymphocele, a wound hematoma, or another type of fluid collection.

DIAGNOSIS

The diagnosis of obstruction is usually made during the work-up of renal allograft dysfunction, because there is no pain associated with allograft ureteral obstruction. When the obstruction is secondary to a lymphocele, the patient may be aware of an enlarging mass on the side of the transplant, or unilateral scrotal or labial edema. Although stone formation in the late post-transplant period is uncommon, I have seen three patients with a sudden onset of painless anuria months after transplantation, secondary to an obstructing ureteral calculus.

The differential diagnosis of decreasing allograft function includes ureteral obstruction. This is readily demonstrated by intravenous pyelography (IVP), ultrasonography, or isotope renography. An isotope renogram with furosemide (Lasix) frequently confirms the diagnosis. Additional studies such as computed tomography (CT) or retrograde/antegrade pyelography can localize the site of obstruction.

TREATMENT

Treatment depends on the cause of the obstruction. A lymphocele causing extrinsic ureteral compression is usually best managed by internal marsupialization, although percutaneous aspiration may occasionally result in cure. Other fluid collections, including wound hematoma or seroma, are best managed by exploration, but can be managed expectantly by placement of a ureteral catheter or stent.

Most intrinsic obstructions of the transplant ureter appear at the ureterovesical junction (UVJ). Treatment depends on the location and cause. Several authors have documented the feasibility of either transvesical or percutaneous ureteral balloon dilatation of a transplant ureteral stricture, but no long-term follow-up of a series of patients so treated is available for analysis. The most common treatment employed is elective open surgical revision with ureteral re-reimplantation, or use of the recipient's native ureter for ureteropyelostomy or ureteroureterostomy.

PREVENTION

Ureteral obstruction at the UVJ is primarily a result of faulty surgical technique. When urinary tract reconstruction is done through an open cystotomy using a modified Leadbetter-Politano technique, care must be taken to create a sufficiently wide tunnel through the bladder musculature and submucosa to accommodate the transplant ureter with all its adventitia. There is a trend to use a smaller and better constructed suture material such as 5-0 and 6-0 Vicryl for the ureteral reimplantation, plus loupe magnification. It is essential to be sure that proved ureteral patency is present before the bladder is closed. This can be accomplished by performing the anastomosis over a No. 5 to 8 French feeding tube, and by filling the transplant renal pelvis with enough saline before removing the feeding tube to observe the saline entering the bladder.

When ureteral reconstruction is performed by an external or a closed-bladder technique, such as a modified Lich or the Barry extravesical ureteral reimplantation, the chances of adequate tunnel construction and accurate suture placement are greater. These techniques are usually carried out in the dome of the bladder where there is no problem with exposure, and always under direct vision.

URINARY EXTRAVASATION/FISTULA

Urinary extravasation with or without fistula formation is a much more serious cause of post-transplant morbidity, graft loss, and death. In most large series, the incidence of urinary extravasation varies from 1 to 10 percent. Extravasation can occur from the bladder, the ureterovesical anastomosis, or the extravesical ureter. Probably the most common cause of urinary extravasation is ureteral necrosis from ischemic injury. Ischemic injury to the ureter can occur in a variety of ways. During organ recovery the ureters are generally dissected down to below the iliac vessels. With this dissection, great care must be taken to preserve a generous amount of periureteral tissue. Probably a longer segment of ureter than is theoretically viable is preserved, which means that the excess ureter must be amputated at the time of transplantation. (One must remember that the transplant ureter is receiving its blood supply solely from branches from the renal artery.) A second reason for ureteral damage resulting in ureteral ischemia necrosis is excessive hilar dissection during the freshening up of the kidney ex vivo. Most transplant surgeons like to know exactly how many renal vessels are present in imported kidneys, so recovery surgeons frequently do more hilar dissection than is necessary. Sometimes polar vessels are inadvertently ligated at the time of organ recovery. Kidneys with multiple vessels are more prone to late urinary extravasation from a calix owing to a ligation of a polar vessel leading to a polar infarct. Ureteral ischemia can also occur when a lower pole vessel is inadvertently ligated. All lower polar vessels should be revascularized, because one must assume that a lower pole vessel carries blood supply to the ureter. Ureteral problems are common in kidneys removed from pediatric donors under 6 years of age. The problem results from attempting to use too long a ureteral segment. My rule of thumb in pediatric kidneys is to consider that the maximal usable ureteral length is only 5 cm. After revascularization of a graft, attention should be paid to the ureteral blood supply. Fresh bleeding should occur from the end of the amputated ureter at the time of the ureteral reimplantation.

Landreneau and McDonald reviewed the literature on transplant urinary extravasation seen in the various forms of urinary tract reconstruction. They pointed out that the incidence of extravasation after either intra- or extravesicoureteral reimplantation is about 6 to 10 percent and has remained fairly constant since the 1960s. They believe that the technique of ureteral reimplantation probably plays a minor role compared with the vascular injury during organ recovery in contributing to urinary extravasation.

DIAGNOSIS

Urinary extravasation is a relatively early post-transplant complication, usually seen within the first 10 to 14 days. The diagnosis is suspected when the patient has increasing incisional pain, an enlarging wound mass (with or without scrotal or labial edema), or drainage of copious amounts of fluid from the incision. A rise in the serum creatinine level may be noted, but urinary output invariably falls. If wound drainage is present and ureteral leak is suspected, it is sometimes helpful to determine the creatinine level in the drainage fluid. When there is good renal function, intravenous indigo carmine will color the wound dressing blue. Sometimes it is difficult to determine whether drainage from a wound is urine or simply spontaneous drainage of a lymphocele or wound seroma. If the above tests fail to clarify the nature of wound drainage, a delayed CT scan (30 to 45 minutes) with contrast or radioisotope administration, and analysis of the dressing for the isotope, is usually confirmatory.

TREATMENT

Once the diagnosis of a urinary fistula is made, a cystogram may be helpful in deciding on treatment. In my opinion, cystography can encourage the transplant surgeon to be unwisely conservative. A cystogram showing no extravasation necessitates immediate reoperation. If the cystogram shows extravasation, one might consider simple replacement of the Foley urethral catheter. However, when a cystogram shows extravasation, it is difficult to determine whether the extravasation is from the site of the ureteroneocystotomy or from the bladder closure. It is my prejudice that extravasation from the bladder closure rarely, and extravasation from the ureteroneocystotomy never, stops with Foley catheter drainage. Therefore, my preferred method of management is reoperation, opening the entire transplant wound, copiously irrigating the wound, and then identifying the site and cause of the urinary extravasation.

It is reported that caliceal fistulas cannot be successfully treated with debridement and closure because sepsis is usually present. A recent study by Prompt and colleagues refutes that generalization.

Occasionally, a fistula is secondary to a necrotic area in the renal pelvis or ureter. The most likely explanation for this is a cautery/coagulation injury during attempts at hemostasis, or at the time of organ retrieval. If leakage occurs from the renal pelvis, the area can be debrided, stented, and closed with fine sutures. When extravasation occurs from the midureter because of coagulation injury or ischemic necrosis, the ureter must be resected back to healthy tissue. Occasionally, this requires removal of the entire transplant ureter back to the renal pelvis. In these situations, the urinary tract must be reconstructed using the recipient's ipsilateral native ureter. When some proximal ureter is left but is not long enough to reach the bladder, a Boari flap can be constructed for ureteroneocystotomy. If the urinary extravasation is from a distal ureteral necrosis, it may be possible to reimplant the ureter directly back into the bladder, but this is seldom possible.

Extravasation secondary to the reimplantation technique is best managed by removing the ureter completely from the bladder and doing a second ureteral reimplantation in a new location. Attempts to resuture the ureter at its initial reimplantation site are rarely successful and should be discouraged.

Sometimes, extravasation of infected urine has been prolonged and the diagnosis delayed. In these instances, after the diagnostic and localizing studies outlined above, the transplant wound is explored. A decision has to be made whether it is in the best interest of the recipient to proceed with transplant nephrectomy or to perform a salvage reconstructive procedure in the presence of infection and tissue induration. This is at times a difficult decision, especially when the kidney is beautifully vascularized, renal function has been excellent, and there has been no evidence of rejection. In most instances of extravasation with infection and a delay in diagnosis, the treatment of choice is transplant nephrectomy. If it is decided that one should proceed with reconstruction, ureteral stents, nephrostomy tubes, sump drains, and catheters are placed and the wound is packed open with povidone-iodine (Betadine)-soaked sponges in preparation for secondary closure or healing. These wounds eventually heal, but this may take months, requiring frequent return trips to the operating room for dressings.

SUGGESTED READING

Landreneau MD, McDonald JC. Genitourinary complications in renal transplantation. Transplant Rev 1987; 1:59–84.

Prompt CA, Manfro R, Ilha D de, Koff WJ. Caliceal-cutaneous fistula in renal transplantation: successful conservative management. J Urol 1990; 143:580.

LYMPHOCELE FOLLOWING RENAL TRANSPLANTATION

RAJA B. KHAULI, M.D.
MANI MENON, M.D.

A lymphocele is a retroperitoneal collection of lymph in a closed space. Lymphoceles following renal transplantation are relatively uncommon and occur in 1 to 18 percent of recipients. Most lymphoceles are detected on routine ultrasonography and are subclinical. However, some lymphoceles can reach large sizes with progressive accumulation of lymph, impinging on adjacent structures and resulting in ureteral, venous, and lymphatic obstruction.

PATHOPHYSIOLOGY

Controversy exists over the origin and pathophysiology of lymphoceles. It is believed that these collections most commonly arise secondary to technical errors of inappropriate ligation of the perivascular lymphatic channels surrounding the external iliac vessels, at the time of renal transplantation surgery. The transplanted kidney can also be the source of lymph, from the pericapsular or hilar lymphatics, transected at the time of harvesting. Thus, both the renal allograft and recipient lymphatics are believed to be underlying causes of lymphoceles, but the latter seems to be more important. Since renal transplantation is a retroperitoneal procedure, the continuous lymphatic leakage is not reabsorbed by the peritoneum and collects in the nonepithelialized closed cavity lined with fibromembranous tissue, the pseudocapsule. Symptoms range from suprapubic distention or pain, palpable abdominal mass, ipsilateral leg edema, edema over the graft and scrotal or labial edema, ipsilateral iliofemoral thrombophlebitis, clear drainage from the incision, ureteral compression and hydronephrosis, bladder displacement, and irritability mimicking urinary tract infection. Progressive azotemia and diminished urinary output mimicking graft rejection are common and may be caused by ureteral compression or the pressure effect of a large lymphocele surrounding the kidney creating

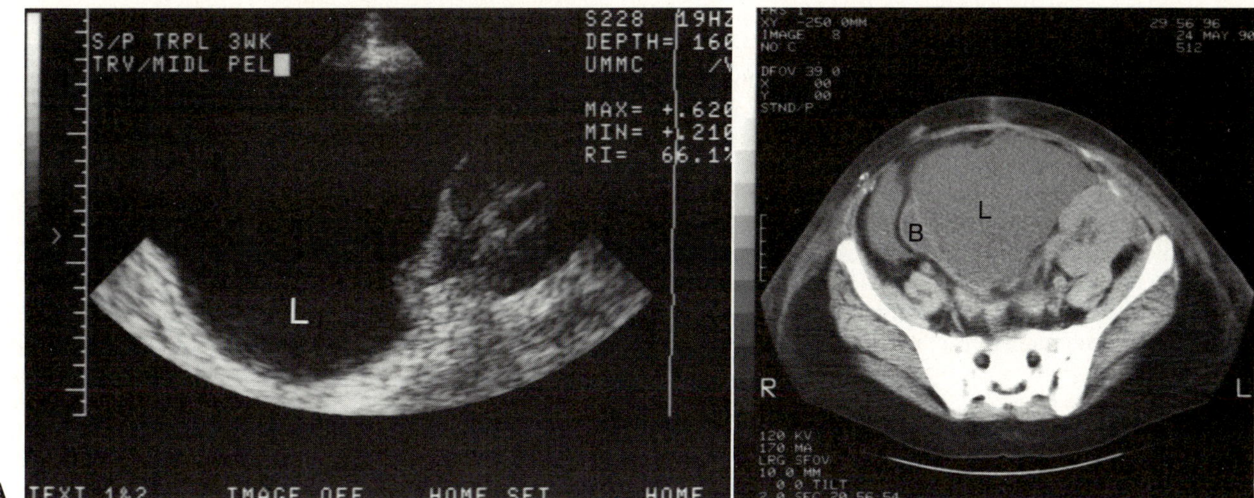

Figure 1 *A,* Ultrasonography shows a large, fluid-filled mass, a lymphocele (L), adjacent to the renal transplant in the left iliac fossa. *B,* Noncontrast CT image confirms a low-density fluid collection (L) contiguous with the transplanted kidney, and right lateral displacement of the urinary bladder (B).

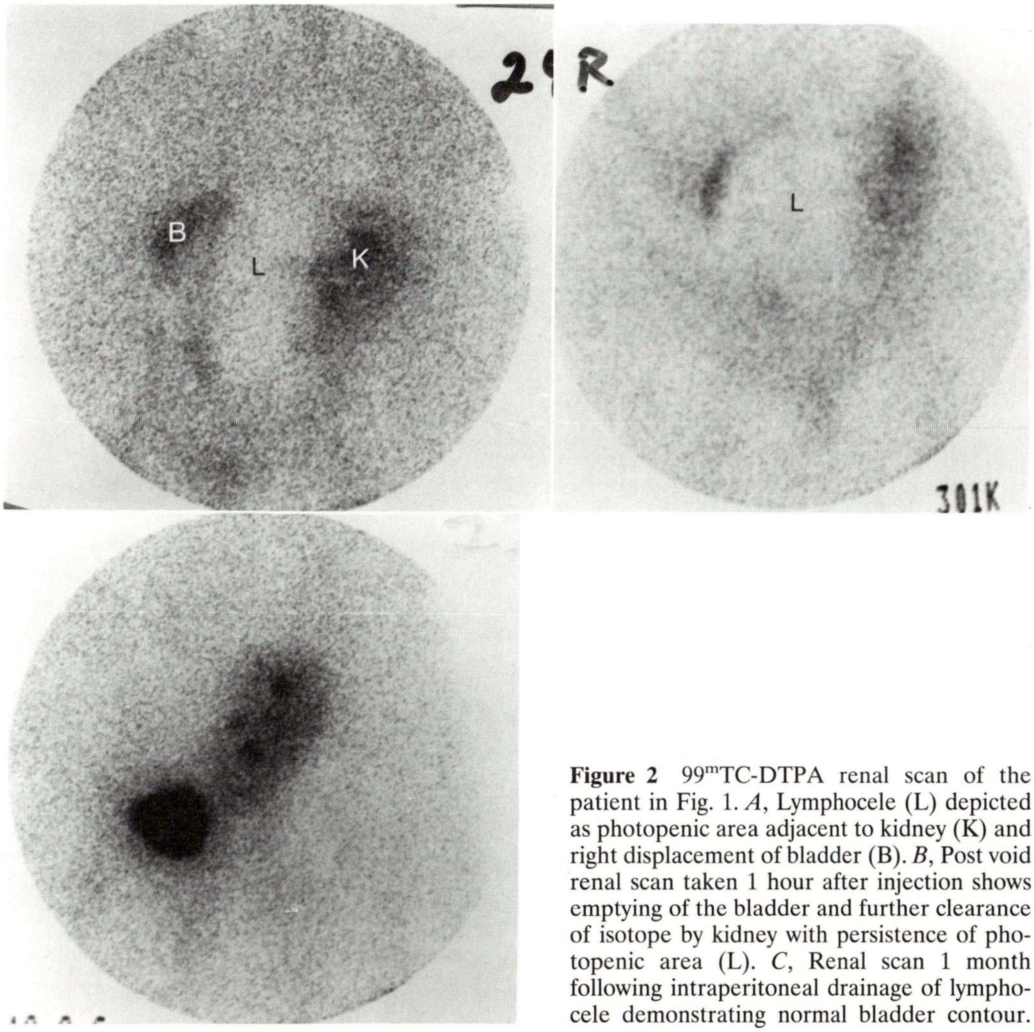

Figure 2 ^{99m}TC-DTPA renal scan of the patient in Fig. 1. *A,* Lymphocele (L) depicted as photopenic area adjacent to kidney (K) and right displacement of bladder (B). *B,* Post void renal scan taken 1 hour after injection shows emptying of the bladder and further clearance of isotope by kidney with persistence of photopenic area (L). *C,* Renal scan 1 month following intraperitoneal drainage of lymphocele demonstrating normal bladder contour.

a "Page kidney" phenomenon, with hypertension and renal dysfunction.

Lymphoceles usually present in the early months after transplantation, but may be detected as long as several years after surgery. The most important factors associated with lymphocele formation have included extensive perivascular dissection at the time of transplantation, capsular tear or decapsulation of the kidney, acute rejection episodes, performance of a graft biopsy, the presence of an ipsilateral lower extremity arteriovenous fistula, and the use of diuretics, high-dose corticosteroids, and anticoagulants.

PREVENTION

As there are two sources of lymphatic leakage, the recipient's lymphatics and the transplanted kidney, prevention is possible by directing attention to both these sources. Meticulous surgical technique at the time of vascular dissection for renal implantation, with careful ligation of all lymphatic channels, is probably most important in diminishing the rate of occurrence of lymphoceles. Extensive dissection of the iliac vessels should be avoided. When performing a hypogastric to renal artery anastomosis, the lymphatic channels along the external iliac and common iliac arteries should be left undisturbed, limiting the dissection to the iliac vein and hypogastric artery. Similarly, careful ligation of perihilar renal lymphatics and repair of capsular tears may further diminish the incidence of lymphoceles. Avoidance of systemic anticoagulation and high-dose steroids and the judicious use of diuretics will further reduce the rate of lymph exudation. Adherence to the above principles has been reported to limit the occurrence of lymphoceles to less than 1 percent.

DIAGNOSIS

Within a few months of transplantation, the diagnosis of lymphoceles relies on the presence of symptoms of abdominal pain, mass, edema of the extremity or genitalia, and deteriorating renal function. Confirmatory tests include ultrasonography and computed tomography (CT), which reveal a homogeneous hypoechoic fluid collection of low attenuation (Fig. 1). Ultrasonography is invaluable in detecting all collections, even very small ones, but is nonspecific for distinguishing lymphoceles from other fluid collections, e.g., hematoma, urinoma, or early abscess formation. Radionuclide scintigraphy using 99m-technetium diethylenetriaminepentaacetic acid (99^{m}Tc-DTPA), 99 m-technetium mercaptoacetyl-triglycine (99^m-Tc-MAG 3), or I-131 orthoiodohippurate (Hippuran) is noninvasive and can easily distinguish a lymphocele from a urinoma. A lymphocele is depicted on renal scan by a photopenic cold area of reduced activity adjacent to the graft, with

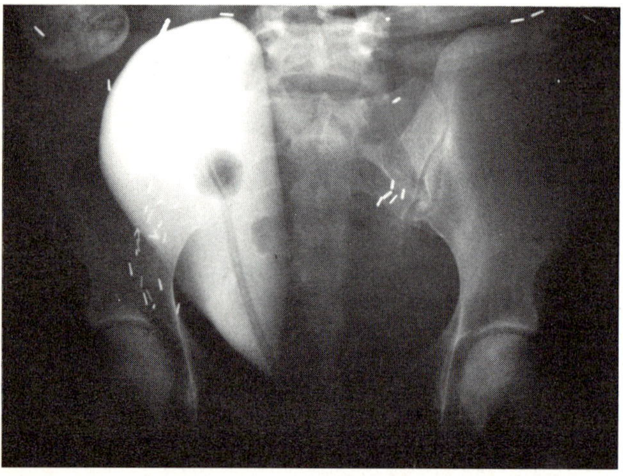

Figure 3 Cystogram of the patient in Figure 1 shows right lateral displacement of the bladder by a left-sided lymphocele.

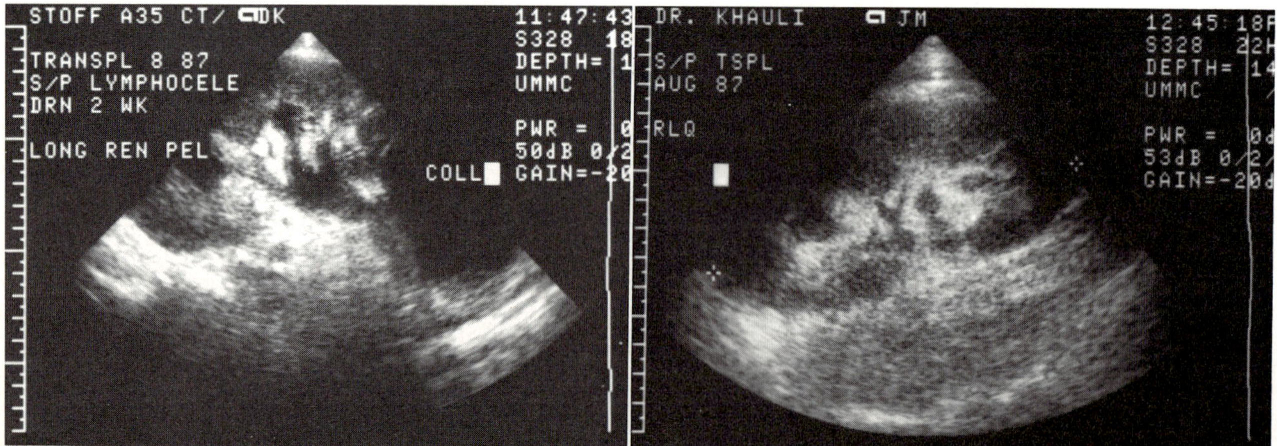

Figure 4 *A*, Ultrasonography shows a lymphocele inferior to a right renal transplant, with ureteral obstruction and hydronephrosis. *B*, Ultrasonography 3 months after peritoneal drainage demonstrates resolution of the lymphocele and hydronephrosis.

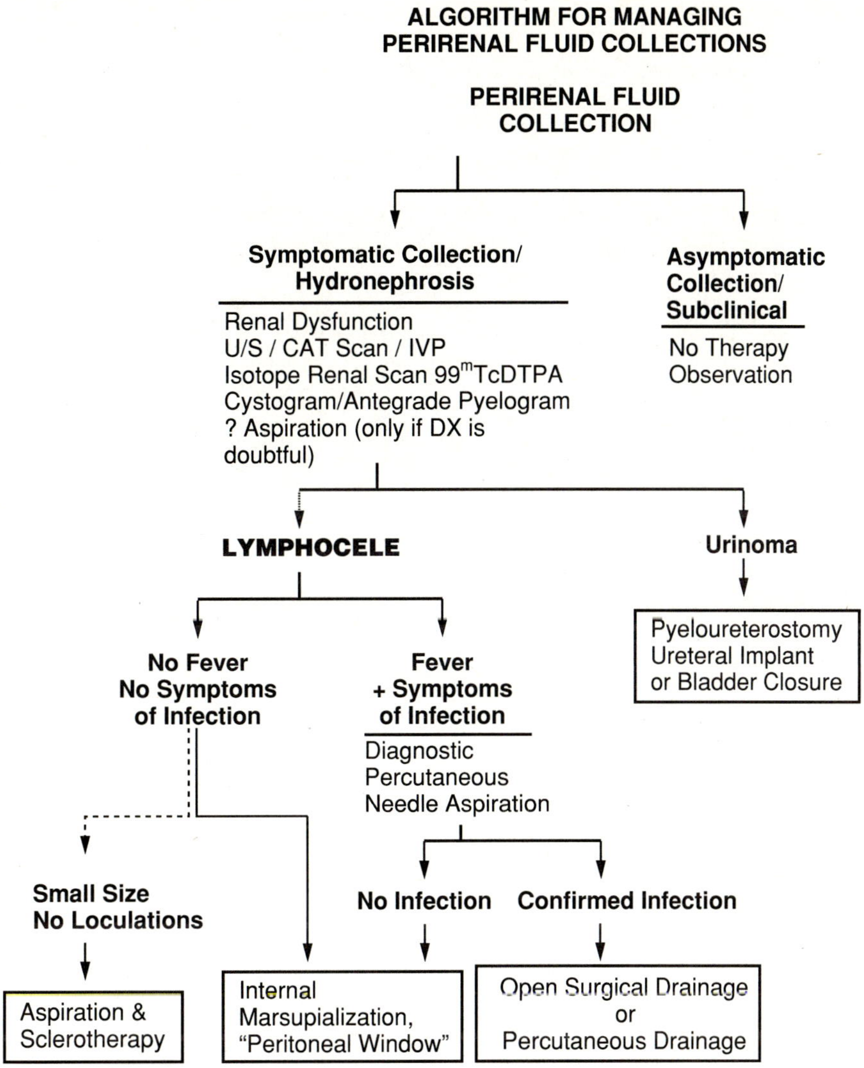

**ALGORITHM FOR MANAGING
PERIRENAL FLUID COLLECTIONS**

**PERIRENAL FLUID
COLLECTION**

**Symptomatic Collection/
Hydronephrosis**

Renal Dysfunction
U/S / CAT Scan / IVP
Isotope Renal Scan 99^{m}TcDTPA
Cystogram/Antegrade Pyelogram
? Aspiration (only if DX is
doubtful)

**Asymptomatic
Collection/
Subclinical**

No Therapy
Observation

LYMPHOCELE

Urinoma

Pyeloureterostomy
Ureteral Implant
or Bladder Closure

**No Fever
No Symptoms
of Infection**

**Fever
+ Symptoms
of Infection**

Diagnostic
Percutaneous
Needle Aspiration

No Infection   **Confirmed Infection**

**Small Size
No Loculations**

Aspiration &
Sclerotherapy

Internal
Marsupialization,
"Peritoneal Window"

Open Surgical Drainage
or
Percutaneous Drainage

Figure 5   Algorithm for the diagnosis and management of perirenal fluid collections.

displacement of the bladder and possible dilatation of the pelvicaliceal system and delayed excretion (Fig. 2). A urinoma, however, manifests as dispersion of the radionuclide activity adjacent to the kidney. Furthermore, this increased background activity is unchanged on the postvoid scan, indicating extravesical urine accumulation. Adjunctive tests to differentiate a lymphocele from a urinoma include high-dose intravenous pyelography and antigrade pyeloureterography to rule out ureteral leaks, or cystography to rule out bladder leaks (Fig. 3). Serial ultrasonography performed after drainage of a lymphocele are particularly helpful in documenting resolution of the collection and relief of ureteral obstruction (Fig. 4).

In our opinion, the use of lymphangiography is impractical and unwarranted. Needle aspiration is occasionally needed as a diagnostic tool but should rarely be used as a therapeutic procedure. The aspirate is analyzed for electrolytes, creatinine, urea nitrogen, cell count, Gram stain, and culture. Lymph constituents are similar to plasma, whereas urinary creatinine, potassium, and urea nitrogen are much higher than lymph. Aspiration is particularly important in cases of fever or suspected abscess formation. Figure 5 depicts an algorithm for diagnosing and managing symptomatic perirenal collections.

TREATMENT

The routine use of ultrasonography and meticulous follow-up protocols after renal transplantation have resulted in the identification of a significant subset of patients with small but asymptomatic lymphoceles. Intervention is not advised in these patients, because most of the lymphoceles either resolve spontaneously or remain subclinical. Patients with symptomatic lymphoceles, or evidence of impaired renal function as a result, should be treated to correct the renal dysfunction and ameliorate the associated symptoms.

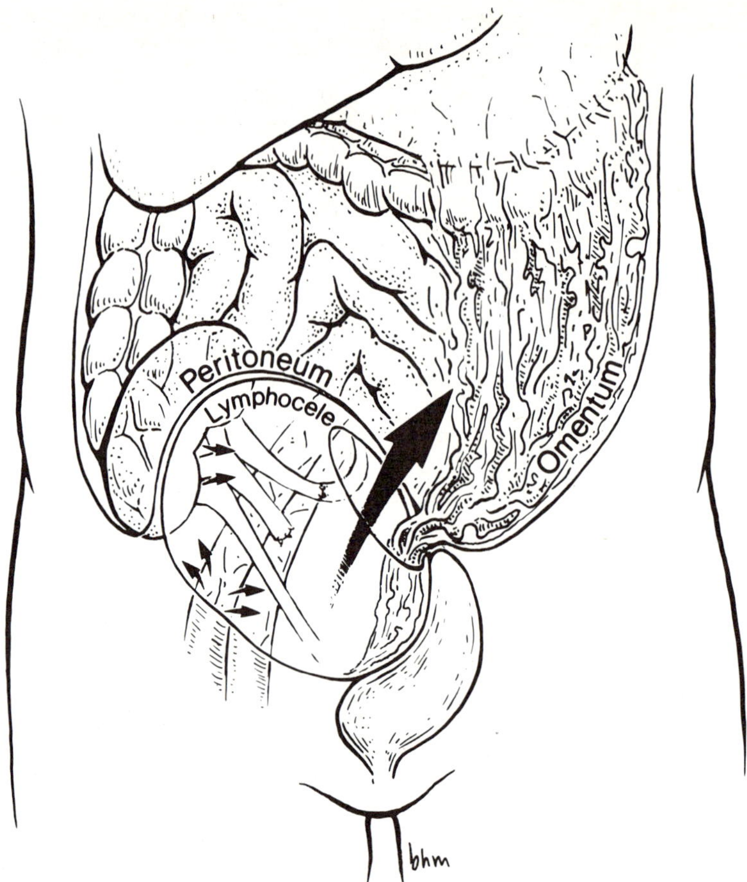

Figure 6 Internal marsupialization: "peritoneal window." The principle is to create an opening that allows escape of the continuously leaking lymph (*small arrows*) into the peritoneal cavity (*large arrow*) where it is reabsorbed.

Internal marsupialization ("peritoneal window") is the procedure of choice for large symptomatic lymphoceles that are not infected. The preferred surgical approach is through a median laparotomy. Exposure of the lymphocele is obtained transperitoneally, well away from the transplant incision, avoiding the risk of ureteral, vascular, or bowel injury. The procedure preserves the sterility of the lymphocele and peritoneal cavity, and is associated with low morbidity and insignificant recurrence rates. The basic principle is to create a window for lymph to pass freely and be reabsorbed by the peritoneum (Fig. 6).

While the most established approach for internal marsupialization is through a median laparotomy incision, we have recently applied the newer laparoscopic techniques for the internal drainage of a post transplant lymphocele. We believe that laparoscopic peritoneal drainage is the preferred method for many symptomatic lymphoceles that are amenable to this approach, and that it offers major advantages including faster recuperation and shorter hospital stay.

As mentioned above, needle aspiration should not be used as a therapeutic tool for the management of large lymphoceles, since this procedure is unreliable and is associated with an unacceptably high rate of infectious and hemorrhagic complications. Similarly, percutaneous insertion of drains or open surgical drainage is not recommended in the absence of infection and could result in prolonged drainage, chronic fistulous formation, and life-threatening infections.

Small symptomatic lymphoceles can be approached with careful needle aspiration and installation of sclerosing agents (sclerotherapy). Tetracycline, ampicillin, or povidine-iodine have been used. Despite some encouraging results from sclerotherapy, there may be rapid reaccumulation of fluid and bacterial contamination. Thus, this procedure should be reserved for patients with small symptomatic lymphoceles who understand and accept the limitations of this procedure and the need for serial follow-up ultrasound examinations.

Infected lymphoceles are treated by open surgical drainage and placement of sump drains in the retroperitoneal space. Preoperative needle aspiration is particularly important for confirming the diagnosis of infection and planning the surgery. Care is taken not to enter the

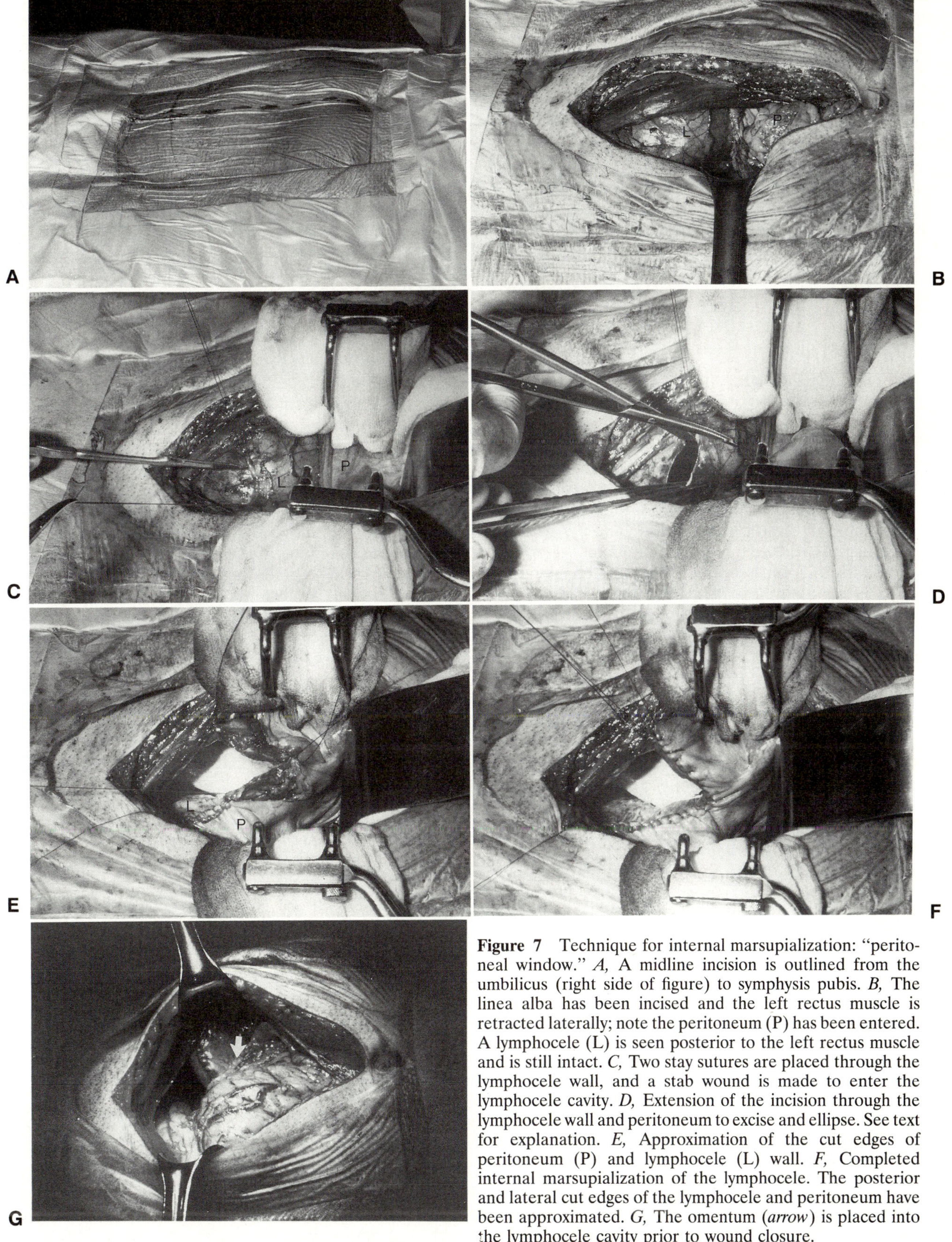

Figure 7 Technique for internal marsupialization: "peritoneal window." *A,* A midline incision is outlined from the umbilicus (right side of figure) to symphysis pubis. *B,* The linea alba has been incised and the left rectus muscle is retracted laterally; note the peritoneum (P) has been entered. A lymphocele (L) is seen posterior to the left rectus muscle and is still intact. *C,* Two stay sutures are placed through the lymphocele wall, and a stab wound is made to enter the lymphocele cavity. *D,* Extension of the incision through the lymphocele wall and peritoneum to excise and ellipse. See text for explanation. *E,* Approximation of the cut edges of peritoneum (P) and lymphocele (L) wall. *F,* Completed internal marsupialization of the lymphocele. The posterior and lateral cut edges of the lymphocele and peritoneum have been approximated. *G,* The omentum (*arrow*) is placed into the lymphocele cavity prior to wound closure.

peritoneum and risk its contamination, and to break all loculations to ensure complete drainage of the infected collection. Simple infected lymphoceles without any evidence of loculations are managed by needle aspiration and percutaneous placement of sump drains under ultrasonographic or CT guidance. These patients are maintained on appropriate parenteral antibiotics and followed with serial ultrasound examinations.

A lymph fistula is managed expectantly and the wound kept clean with frequent sterile dressing changes and topical antibiotics. These patients also may benefit from bed rest or limitation of activity, a high-protein diet, and discontinuation of any medications that could promote lymph exudation. Drainage usually ceases in 14 to 21 days.

Surgical Technique of Internal Marsupialization

The patient is placed in the supine position and a Foley catheter is inserted in the bladder. A ventral midline skin incision is made from just below the umbilicus down to the symphysis pubis (Fig. 7A). The linea alba is incised and the rectus muscles are separated and retracted laterally, exposing the supravesical space and lymphocele in the inferior aspect of the wound, and the peritoneum in the cephalad aspect. The peritoneal cavity is grasped with two forceps, elevated, and entered sharply and the incision is continued in a caudad fashion. Exposure is maintained with a self-retaining Balfour retractor, with a superior retractor blade holding the bowel loops cephalad (Fig. 7B). Inspection allows identification of the lymphocele as an encapsulated, blue-colored collection adjacent to the bladder (which may not be identified at this point). The transplanted kidney may be seen or palpated at a more cephalad and lateral position with respect to the lymphocele.

Two stay sutures are placed in a thin area of the lymphocele wall, and a stab incision is made to enter the lymphocele cavity and drain its contents (Fig. 7C). The incision is extended to remove a wide ellipse of lymphocele wall (with the attached peritoneum), care being taken not to injure the native or transplant ureter, which could be compressed along the medial wall of the lymphocele (Fig. 7D). We carefully palpate the internal wall of the lymphocele cavity at this point to identify the exact location of the bladder and the indwelling Foley balloon. After a wide peritoneal window is created to allow passage of the whole hand into the lymphocele cavity, the posterior aspect of the cut edges of the peritoneum and lymphocele wall are approximated using a running 3-0 chromic catgut suture (Fig. 7E). There is no need to complete the approximation anteriorly, as this may compromise the size of the peritoneal window upon closure of the wound. The completed marsupialization is shown in Figure 7F.

If the omentum is long enough and adjacent to the peritoneal window, we try to place it distally into the lymphocele cavity to ensure its patency (Fig. 7G). Surgical mobilization of an omental pedicle is not necessary except when dealing with a recurrent lymphocele after a marsupialization procedure. Similarly, we do not attempt to look for or ligate lymphatic channels overlying the iliac vessels.

The wound is copiously irrigated with antibiotic solution, and the closure is carried out with a continuous or interrupted 0 Prolene suture. The subcutaneous fat and skin are approximated and an antibiotic dressing is applied. No drains are left behind.

Internal marsupialization is a simple and effective procedure associated with little morbidity. Recurrences, although rare, may be noted and are related to inadequate size of the peritoneal window, or occlusion by bowel loops or the overlying renal allograft settling against the window after drainage. The redundant mesentery of the sigmoid colon may also contribute to herniation and occlusion of a left-sided "peritoneal window." Recurrent lymphoceles after surgical therapy are managed in a similar fashion, with a special effort to mobilize the omentum along a vascular pedicle and place it in the lymphocele cavity to enhance absorption and ensure continued patency.

SUGGESTED READING

Braun WE, Banowsky LH, Straffon RA, et al. Lymphoceles associated with renal transplantation: report of 15 cases and review of the literature. Am J Med 1974; 57:714.

Burleson RL, Marbarger PD. Prevention of lymphocele formation following allotransplantation. J Urol 1982; 127:18.

Greenberg RM, Perloff LJ, Grossman RA, et al. Treatment of lymphocele in renal allograft recipients. Arch Surg 1985; 120:501.

Pontes JE, McDonald FD, Migdal SD, et al. Lymphatic complications in renal allografts—a new look. Urology 1981; 17:26.

Schweizer RT, Cho SK, Kountz SL, Belzer FO. Lymphoceles following renal transplantation. Arch Surg 1972; 104:42.

CADAVERIC KIDNEY RECOVERY

RODNEY J. TAYLOR, M.D., F.A.C.S.

Urologists are frequently the designated local procurement surgeons for recovering cadaveric kidneys. With the increasing need for other organs for transplantation, such as heart and liver, it is not unusual for other procurement teams to be involved in the total donor operation. In this changing environment, the keys to a successful technique of cadaveric kidney procurement are flexibility and adaptability. It must be flexible to permit application to multiple organ procurement, including combinations of heart/liver, heart/lung, and pancreas, without compromising the viability of any organs procured. It must be adaptable to a change in donor status, allowing rapid access, stabilization, and in situ flushing and cooling to avoid unacceptable warm ischemia time. Over the past 5 years we have developed a technique for cadaveric organ procurement in general, and kidney procurement in particular, that we feel meets most needs of an ideal technique.

The criteria for brain death are well established and described and will not be repeated here, but it should be noted that at our institution all of our donors are brain-dead, heart-beating donors at the time of organ procurement. This allows for combined organ procurement with minimal warm ischemia time for all organs and maximal use of a rare resource.

The following criteria have been used for selection of donors for kidneys at the University of Pittsburgh Medical Center:

1. Donors selected are between the age of 1 and 60, without any known generalized atherosclerosis.
2. Donors are rejected if they have a history of moderate to severe hypertension or hypertension requiring medication, history of renal disease, history of malignancy other than a primary central nervous system tumor, history of sepsis, or history of hepatitis or drug use.
3. It is desirable for the serum creatinine level to be 2 mg/dl or less at the time of harvesting; however, it is more important to determine the direction in which it is going. If the patient has an elevated creatinine, but with hydration and stabilization the creatinine is coming down, we feel these kidneys will recover and these donors are not turned down. If with increasing hypotension and oliguria the creatinine continues to rise, these donors may be rejected.
4. All donors are prescreened for HTLV-3. If there is a positive screening elisa assay, the donor is rejected.

Once a donor has been identified and declared brain-dead, and permission obtained from the next of kin for organ procurement, the medical support of the donor is usually directed by an organ procurement coordinator. The goals at this point are to avoid hypoxia and to maintain a good cardiac output with minimal dependence on vasopressors through the liberal use of colloid and crystalloid resuscitation and diuretics such as furosemide and mannitol. The objective is to maintain a normal blood pressure and an adequate urinary output in the range of 100 ml or greater per hour. It is desirable to get the patient off all vasopressors if possible; if required, the vasopressor of choice is dopamine, and the dosage is decreased as rapidly as possible. Although it is not absolutely necessary, we have found that the presence of an arterial line, a central venous pressure (CVP) line, and several peripheral intravenous lines is helpful in the management of some unstable donors. This has become increasingly important in coordinating the arrival times of procurement teams from other institutions and other states in order to ensure organ viability.

The actual harvesting techniques for cadaveric kidney procurement depend on whether the donor is a kidney donor only or a multiple organ donor. The latter often involves careful orchestration of several surgical teams in order to ensure satisfactory organs for transplant. This is usually best handled by discussing the needs and concerns of all parties involved before beginning the procurement, in order to achieve the best possible results. Regardless of whether the patient is a multiple organ donor or only a kidney donor, a midline incision is made from the sternal notch to the symphysis pubis. The sternum is split to provide excellent exposure for removal of the heart, liver, kidneys, and other viscera as indicated. This approach permits access to, and control of, the supra- and infradiaphragmatic aorta and thus facilitates dissection and removal of the heart and liver before removal of the kidneys. Once the incision is completed, specially designed Hakala sternal and abdominal retractors are placed into the wound to increase exposure. If the kidneys alone are being removed, the right colon is mobilized and the duodenum kocherized, exposing the great vessels up to the level of the renal veins. On rare occasion, the left renal vein rises at the level of the bifurcation of the vena cava, and care must be taken to avoid injuring it. The dissection is continued on the anterior surface of the aorta above the renal veins cephalad to expose the superior mesenteric artery. Once identified, it is tied with 1-0 silk ties and divided. The dissection can be continued cephalad along the anterior surface of the aorta to expose the celiac axis, or by using a modification described by Rosenthal, the portal triad can be clamped and divided, allowing increased exposure to the celiac axis and aorta below the diaphragm. Once the celiac axis is identified and divided, an umbilical tape is placed around the aorta cephalad, providing for a wide, en bloc removal of the kidneys and decreasing the risk of inadvertent vascular damage. The aortic bifurcation is now exposed and clean enough to allow the aorta to be cannulated. If there are lumbar arteries arising in this area, they are divided between silk ties. The vena cava is cleaned and prepared in a similar fashion. It should be noted that when kidneys alone are being harvested, the infrahepatic vena cava is dissected around and umbilical tape is placed at this point. When all this is completed, if the donor continues to be stable, the ureters are identified and divided deep in the pelvis. Individual cultures are taken of both ureters and the ureters are mobilized, including all periureteral tissue to avoid any stripping of the vascular supply of the ureters. If a donor is unstable, this dissection can be done after flushing and cooling. Before the aorta is cross-clamped, the donor is given 20 to 30 thousand units of heparin and the vessels are cannulated. If desired, a vasodilator can be given at this point. The proximal aorta is clamped, and the flush with cold euro-collins started. The proximal vena cava is tied off and the distal vena cava is drained via the cannula. Approximately 2 liters of euro-collins is flushed through the cannula to allow complete central cooling of the kidneys. At no point is any dissection done in or around the renal hilum during procurement. This significantly decreases the possibility of damage to a vascular structure. After complete cooling and flushing, the kidneys are freed laterally and posteriorly. At this point the inferior mesenteric artery, if not divided already, can be divided well from the anterior surface of the aorta, thereby decreasing any risk of injury to a lower-pole vessel to a kidney. With an assistant gently holding the kidneys and ureters in his hands, the en bloc removal of the kidneys is completed by dissecting the aorta and vena cava off the spinal column and psoas muscles up to the level of the supraceliac aorta. The kidneys are placed in a cold Ringer's lactate solution at a back table. They are examined for any abnormalities; Gerota's fascia is opened and the surface of the kidney is inspected for any areas of incomplete flushing, pectechiae, or other abnormality that may preclude their transplantation. The kidneys are then turned over, and the separation of the organs is started by dividing the aorta posteriorly between the lumbar arteries. By dividing along this line, injury to the vascular structures to the kidneys is minimized. From the inside of the aorta, the number and location of the renal arteries is determined. The kidneys are then turned over, and along the anterior surface of the vena cava the veins are identified and separated, the left vein being taken with a cuff of vena cava and the right renal vein being left with the inferior vena cava attached. By leaving the vena cava attached to the right vein, it is possible to fashion a venous conduit onto the renal vein, allowing for increased adaptability of the right kidney to any transplant situation. The separation is completed by dividing the anterior surface of the aorta, again being careful to avoid any vascular injury. At this point, the kidneys are placed separately into an iced euro-collins solution and packed in ice to await transplantation.

The actual techniques of multiple organ recovery and the resulting condition of the harvested organs have been well described by Starzl et al and Rosenthal et al from the University of Pittsburgh. There has been no detrimental effect on the eventual renal function or other organ function with multiple organ procurement techniques. Under most circumstances, the order of harvest has been heart, heart/lung, followed by liver, followed by kidneys. In all situations, at the time the heart or heart/lung has been removed, the liver and kidneys have been undergoing in situ cooling, and the time spent removing the organs at this point is only a matter of minutes with no warm ischemia.

Using these techniques, we have had minimal organ damage and waste due to procurement injury in more than 300 donor operations. The average time for the procurement of kidneys alone, using this technique, is approximately 1 to 1½ hours. The flexibility and adaptability of this technique allows for a multiorgan procurement without unduly prolonging the procedures or increasing the risk of damage to any of the organs involved.

SUGGESTED READING

Rosenthal JT, et al. Principles of multiple organ procurement from cadaver donors. Ann Surg 1983; 198:617.

Starzl TE, et al. Flexible procedure for multiple cadaveric organ procurement. Surg Gynecol Obstet 1984; 158:223.

Starzl TE, et al. An improved technique for multiple organ harvesting. Surg Gynecol Obstet 1987; 165:343.

Taylor RJ, Rosenthal JT. Kidney recovery from cadaver donors and kidney recovery from living related donors. AUA Update series 1990:50: vol. X.

RENOVASCULAR HYPERTENSION

HYPERTENSION SECONDARY TO RENAL ARTERIAL DISEASE

E. DARRACOTT VAUGHAN, Jr., M.D.
R. ERNEST SOSA, M.D.

It is estimated that 60 million adults in the United States have fixed hypertension, and of these 5 to 15 percent have hypertension secondary to renovascular disease. These patients tend to have severe hypertension which is difficult to control with antihypertensive medications. They have a higher incidence of malignant hypertension and cardiovascular complications than patients with essential hypertension, and their renal artery disease tends to progress, leading to further renal damage. Hypertensive patients should therefore be evaluated to identify the subset with renovascular hypertension (RVH). In addition, normotensive patients with renal impairment should be studied to identify underlying renal arterial disease. Once this is identified, treatment options include pharmacologic management, percutaneous transluminal angioplasty (PTA), and surgical correction of the renal artery lesion.

PATHOLOGY AND PATHOPHYSIOLOGY

There are two main types of renal artery disease, atherosclerotic (ASD) and fibromuscular (FMD) dysplasia (Table 1), and a number of less common causes of the disease. Both types of lesions progress, but ASD more commonly progresses to total occlusion, with renal loss and renal failure if bilateral. Moreover, ASD of the renal artery is part of diffuse vascular disease and the cerebral and coronary systems are often involved, whereas FMD is usually confined to the renal arteries.

After a renal arterial stenosis reaches a critical degree (about 70 percent), there is a decrease in renal blood flow, reduced perfusion pressure, reduced glomerular filtration rate (GFR), and reduced sodium and chloride delivery to the area of the macula densa in the distal tubule. In concert, these changes result in renin release, angiotensin II formation, and hypertension.

Table 1 Causes of Renovascular Hypertension

Common Causes
- Atherosclerosis (66%)
- Fibromuscular dysplasia (33%)
    - Intimal fibroplasia (about 5%)
    - Fibromuscular hyperplasia (about 2%)
    - Medial fibroplasia (about 80%)
    - Perimedial fibroplasia (about 15%)

Rare Causes
- Polyarteritis nodosa
- Takayasu's arteritis
- Arteriovenous fistula
- Aortic aneurysm
- Coarctation of aorta
- Middle aorta syndrome
- Radiation arteritis
- Cholesterol emboli
- Transplant renal artery stenosis
- Neurofibromatosis
- Renal artery aneurysm
- Renal artery emboli or thrombosis
- Extrinsic obstruction

Accordingly, appropriate studies of the renin-angiotensin system can identify about 80 percent of these patients (Fig. 1). If there is bilateral disease and azotemia, salt and water retention may occur, rendering renin measurements less reliable.

EVALUATION FOR RENOVASCULAR HYPERTENSION

There are no clear-cut characteristics of RVH, but there should be a high index of suspicion in children and young adults, patients with a documented short history (<5 years) of hypertension, cases of malignant hypertension, and patients with hypertension that has become difficult to control. On physical examination, the finding of a continuous systolic-diastolic abdominal bruit is helpful but by no means specific for RVH. Moreover, many patients with RVH have no features to distinguish them from patients with essential hypertension.

Further evaluation involves study of the renin-angiotensin system, as shown in Table 2. The peripheral plasma renin activity (PRA) is elevated in 80 percent of

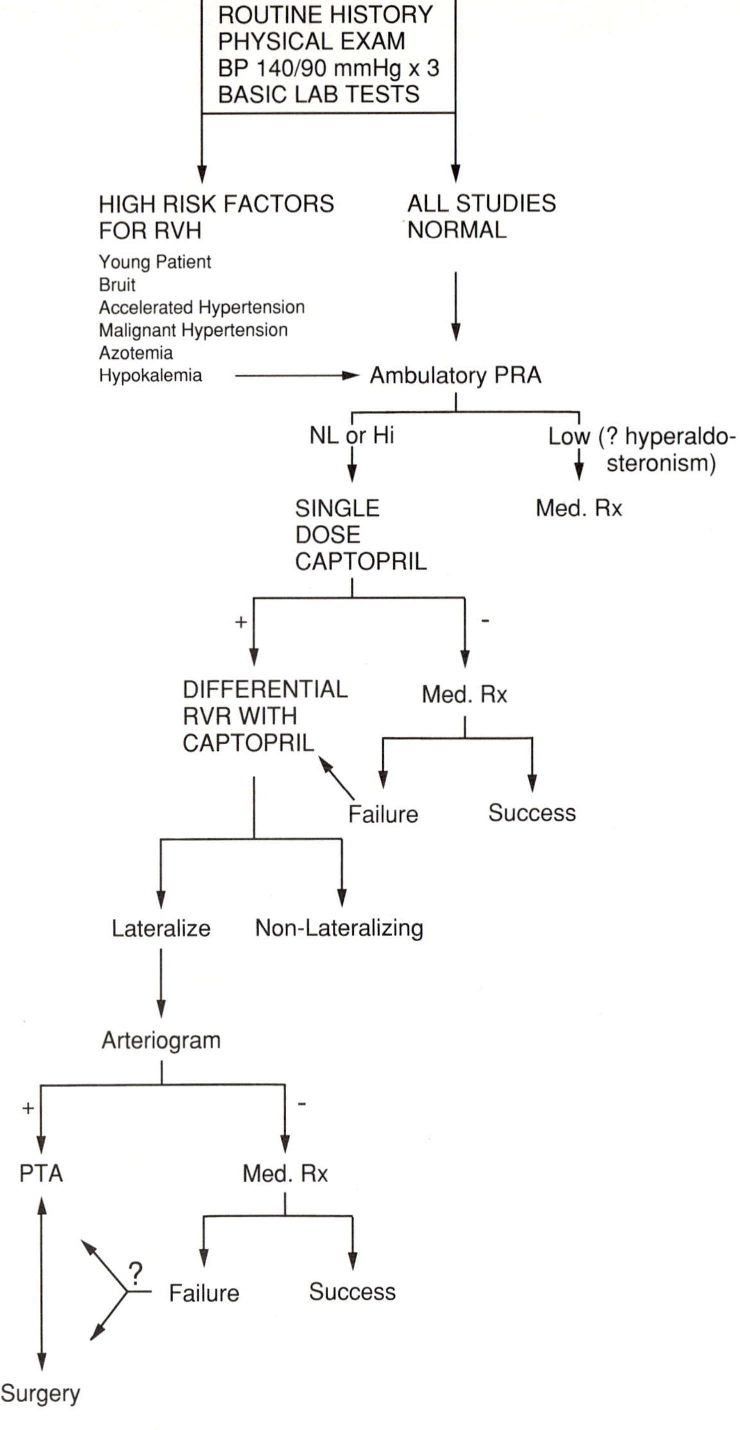

Figure 1   Evaluation plan to identify renovascular hypertension. (Modified from Sosa RE, Vaughan ED Jr. Evaluation of surgically curable hypertension. AUA Update Series 1983; (2)32.)

patients with RVH, and the captopril test specifically identifies almost all patients with the disease. Patients have to be off antihypertensive medications for accurate measurement of PRA, but beta blockers may be continued for the captopril test. If one or both of these tests are positive, we continue with renal vein renin sampling and a central digital subtraction angiogram (Fig. 1), often again using captopril to stimulate unilateral renin secretion. All these studies can be performed without hospitalization. An additional test currently under evaluation is the captopril DTPA scan. In patients with RVH, angiotensin converting enzyme inhibition

Table 2 Renin Values for Predicting Curability of Renovascular Hypertension

Peripheral Renin
Collection of samples (moderate sodium intake ± 100 mEq/day):
1. Ambulatory peripheral renin (PRA) and 24-h sodium excretion under ambulatory conditions (no antihypertensive medications)
2. PRA and blood pressure before and 30 and 60 min after 25-mg captopril (no medication or beta blockers alone)

Renal Vein Renins
Collection of supine:
1. With patient supine, collect blood samples for measurement of renin levels: sample from renal vein of kidney thought to be affected (V1), matching sample from inferior vena cava (A1), sample from renal vein of contralateral kidney (V2), and second matching sample from inferior vena cava (A2)
2. Enhance renin secretion by using converting enzyme inhibitor blockade

Criteria for Predicting Reversibility
1. High plasma renin level in relation to urinary sodium level; indicates hypersecretion of renin
2. Stimulated PRA >12 ng/ml/hr, change PRA >10, increase >150% rise in plasma renin level, and fall in blood pressure in response to converting enzyme inhibitor
3. In contralateral kidney, V2 − A2 = 0; indicates suppression of renin secretion in this kidney.
4. In affected kidney, V1 − A1 divided by A1 >0.5; indicates unilateral renin secretion and reduced renal blood flow
5. In patients with high plasma renin levels, low ratios of renal vein renin to aorta renin ([V1 − A1] divided by A1 + [V2 − A2] divided by A2 ≤0.5) indicate incorrect sampling or segmental disease; repeat measurements with segmental sampling.

reduces both perfusion pressure to the affected kidney and angiotensin II–mediated glomerular efferent arteriolar constriction, resulting in a dramatic fall in GFR filtration rate and thus DTPA uptake.

TREATMENT

It is our strong feeling that patients with RVH should have the lesion corrected by either renovascular surgery or angioplasty. However, there clearly are some patients, especially those who are elderly with diffuse ASD, who are not candidates for intervention. Thus, the role of medical management and the inherent dangers need to be reviewed.

The most widely quoted report of medical management was the randomized study of 214 patients by Hunt in 1973. The patients treated medically had a higher mortality rate, a higher incidence of cardiovascular events, and poorer blood pressure control than did their surgically treated counterparts. However, at the time these studies were performed, many of the effective drugs currently used in patients with RVH were not available. These studies therefore are useful for information on the natural history of RVH, but are inadequate to clearly determine blood pressure control with currently available drugs. In a more recent study, Greminger performed a retrospective multicenter analysis of 202 patients and concluded that the blood pressure control was similar in three groups treated with surgery, with angioplasty, or medically. However, again these were not clearly randomized, and the effects on differential renal function were not extensively studied.

With newer agents, effective medical management is available to maintain blood pressure control in patients who are subsequently undergoing surgery or angioplasty. Moreover, patients who refuse any type of intervention or who fail surgery or angioplasty can be treated.

A major guide in the selection of drugs for patients with RVH hypertension has been an understanding of the underlying physiology of the entity. It is now established in both animal models and humans that RVH is caused by abnormally high renin secretion from the ischemic kidney in most cases. Thus, the major breakthrough in the treatment of patients occurred with the development of beta-blocking agents that were effective in approximately 75 percent of patients with RVH. The recent introduction of angiotensin converting enzyme inhibitors has increased this figure to nearly 90 percent, and it is now apparent that these are the most potent antihypertensive drugs in the treatment of patients with RVH. In fact, the long-term effect of the blood pressure response to captopril has been found to be a good predictor of the response to successful surgical revascularization. Two studies have compared the result of the converting enzyme inhibitor enalapril with standard triple therapy (a diuretic, a beta-blocker, and a vasodilator), and both found that blood pressure was more effectively controlled with enalapril.

The major concern with medical management at the present time is not blood pressure control but maintenance of renal function. There have been numerous reports documenting the onset of reversible decrease in renal function associated with the use of converting enzyme inhibitors in patients with RVH. In patients with bilateral renal artery stenosis or renal artery stenosis in a solitary kidney, treatment with angiotensin converting enzyme inhibitors may sometimes cause dramatic decreases in renal function. Moreover, progression to total renal artery occlusion has been described, and in our experience occurs more commonly than has been reported in the literature. It is not uncommon to see a patient referred for percutaneous transluminal angioplasty (PTA) who on repeat study has a totally occluded renal artery and renal loss.

The theory to explain this phenomenon is that the effect of angiotensin II on the efferent glomerular arteriole that serves to maintain GFR in the presence of renal ischemia is lost with converting enzyme inhibition. This specific effect of converting enzyme inhibitors is additive to the simple effect of decreasing renal perfusion pressure across the stenosis. Texter has shown that nitroprusside infusion in patients with bilateral renal artery stenosis caused a marked reduction in GFR, and we have reproduced his findings in the two-kidney one-clip Goldblatt dog model. Clinically, nuclear renal scans have shown significant impairment of renal function in the ischemic kidney in patients with unilateral renal artery stenosis treated by captopril.

Therefore, in summary, it is our position that patients with documented RVH or those with bilateral renal artery stenosis and azotemia should be treated by PTA or surgery and not managed medically unless they represent an unacceptable surgical risk, refuse intervention, or have lesions that are thought to be technically uncorrectable. Whatever their situation, all patients with RVH who are treated pharmacologically must be carefully and routinely evaluated for changes in renal function and size.

Percutaneous Transluminal Renal Artery Angioplasty

PTA was first introduced by Dotter and Judkins in 1964 for the treatment of peripheral vascular stenoses. The difficulties associated with the technique were overcome by the introduction of a flexible, double-lumen balloon catheter by Gruntzig, permitting the development of percutaneous balloon angioplasty of renal artery stenoses. The fibromuscular dysplasias and unilateral, nonosteal, nonoccluded, atherosclerotic renal artery stenoses are the most suitable lesions for treatment with PTA. PTA has also been used in patients with inactive arteritis, those with recurrent stenosis after initially successful PTA, and those with anastomotic strictures of the renal artery after surgical correction.

The major group of patients who do not respond to PTA include those with diffuse ASD primarily involving the aorta that gives rise to a secondary occlusion of the renal artery ostium. Therefore, in ostial stenosis the success rate of PTA is poor, although in the occasional patient there is a long-term success. Second, patients with total occlusion of the renal artery are also poor candidates for the technique, although new laser technology may make the procedure more feasible. The management of patients with total renal artery occlusion is discussed later in this chapter. Finally, patients with multiple branch lesions, particularly at vessel bifurcations, are less likely to respond to angioplasty. This situation is only a relative contraindication to PTA and pertains primarily to patients with atherosclerotic disease.

The ideal patient for PTA is one with unilateral disease, positive renin indices, and FMD or nonosteal, nonoccluded atherosclerotic renal artery stenosis. A second indication to be discussed later is angioplasty for preservation of renal function.

One of the advantages of transluminal angioplasty is the ability to avoid general anesthesia, the relatively low morbidity of the procedure, and the short period of hospitalization. A team approach is important, to involve not only the radiologist but also medical and surgical teams who are familiar with the management of patients with hypotension and any potential surgical complication. Patients are often volume depleted owing to their angiotensin II–induced vasoconstriction prior to angioplasty, and often require vigorous hydration to avoid postangioplasty hypotension, electrolyte imbalances, and contrast medium–induced injury. Some of these complications can be avoided if patients who are on chronic converting enzyme inhibitors are allowed restoration of vascular volume before angioplasty. In contrast, the patients may also have an increase in blood pressure requiring medical management after angioplasty, or may simply maintain the pre-existing blood pressure for some time before resolution occurs. Accordingly, patients need to be in the hospital where they can receive careful blood pressure monitoring and fluid replacement.

There is conflict over the use of systemic anticoagulation during or after angioplasty. Some people use systemic heparinization, but most feel that aspirin administration is sufficient.

The results of renal angioplasty for both ASD and FMD have been excellent in properly selected patients. Reviewing the data from five recent series, the blood pressure benefit in FMD is about 88 percent and in ASD about 66 percent of all patients in whom PTA was attempted. Therefore, there is a general consensus at the present time that percutaneous angioplasty is the treatment of choice for patients with medial fibroplasia. The earlier prediction about restenosis has not proved accurate and more long-term successes are now in the literature. The results are also good in patients with ASD, particularly those with nonosteal lesions.

In summary, except for high-risk patients with diffuse ASD involving multiple arteries, including the aorta, it is generally agreed that PTA is the initial treatment of choice. Angioplasty is highly successful in the groups outlined above. In cases of failure, surgical intervention can be carried out. Patients who require complex aortic reconstruction or exhibit diffuse bilateral disease are best suited for surgery.

Surgical Management of Renovascular Hypertension

After the classic work of Goldblatt in 1934, it was only 3 years before Butler described the cure of hypertension in a patient with renal parenchymal disease by unilateral nephrectomy. Soon thereafter, Leadbetter and Burkland removed a kidney that pathologically was found to have a renal artery stenosis. Therefore, during the 1940s small kidneys were removed from hypertensive patients in the hope of controlling the blood pressure. However, in 1948 a careful review of the effect of nephrectomy on the treatment of hypertension revealed a dismal 19 percent success rate. However, one must remember that kidneys at that time were being removed primarily for parenchymal disease; angiography was not available and the concept of RVH had not been defined. As more cases were analyzed, it was realized that patients with unilateral renovascular disease fared somewhat better than those with unilateral parenchymal disease.

There obviously have been major advances in both patient selection and revascularization techniques since those early days. Nephrectomy is rarely used today and is reserved for totally nonfunctioning "endocrine" kid-

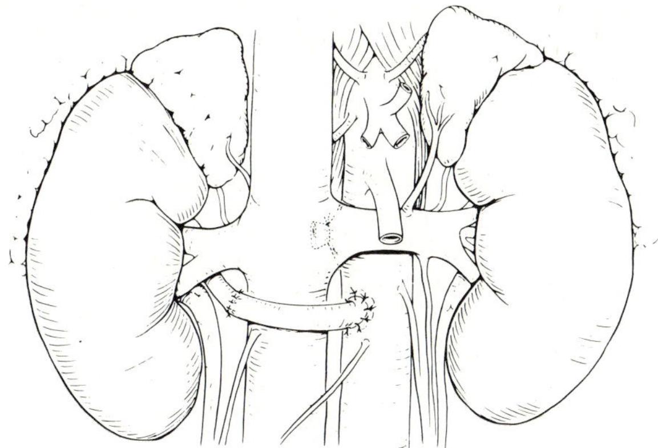

Figure 2 Aortic renal bypass graft with an autogenous vascular graft. (Courtesy of Dr. Andrew Novick.)

neys, after a failed revascularization procedure or in an extremely poor surgical risk patient with a normal contralateral kidney.

Thus, most patients are suitable for renal revascularization, and aortorenal bypass with an autogenous vascular graft is the preferred method (Fig. 2). However, in patients with diffuse ASD, the aorta is often involved, and the Cleveland Clinic group has made a major advance in championing the concept of avoiding the diseased aorta. In these cases techniques such as splenorenal bypass on the left (Fig. 3) or hepatorenal bypass on the right (Fig. 4), ileorenal bypass (Fig. 5), or renal autotransplantation (Fig. 6) are used.

The success rate following renal revascularization is excellent and fatalities low. The current results are markedly better than those described in the national cooperative study in 1975. A critical advance was made by Novick and colleagues, who evaluated patients with renovascular hypertension preoperatively and found the frequent coexistence of coronary and cerebrovascular disease. This study was stimulated by retrospective observations revealing that the major cause of morbidity and mortality following renal revascularization was not related to the kidneys themselves, but to coronary and cerebral events. Thus, at the present time, Novick and colleagues suggest that in addition to a careful history, physical examination, and electrocardiography, all operative candidates with ASD should undergo a cardiac stress test. If any of the latter assessments suggest the presence of coronary artery disease, these authors' policy is to perform coronary cineangiography and left ventriculography. Coronary artery bypass grafting is recommended before renal revascularization for patients with significant correctable coronary artery disease. In patients with severe uncorrectable coronary artery disease, major operative intervention for renovascular disease is associated with significant increased risk and is best deferred. In addition, the Cleveland Clinic group considers that there should also be a high index of suspicion for extracranial cerebrovascular disease. In such patients carotid arteriography is obtained preoperatively and again, if significant disease is found,

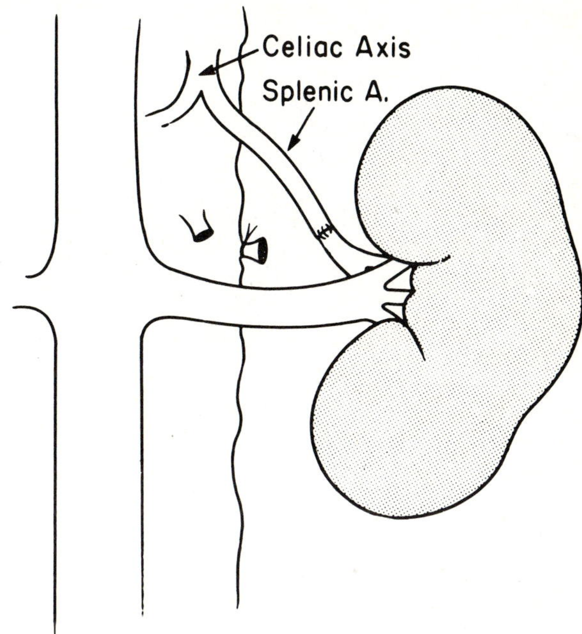

Figure 3 End-to-end splenorenal bypass to the left kidney. (Republished with permission by Sosa RE, Vaughan ED Jr. Renovascular hypertension. In: Gillenwater JY, Grayhack JT, Howards ST, Duckett JW, eds. Adult and pediatric urology. Chicago: Year Book, 1987:752.)

endarterectomy is recommended before revascularization is undertaken. Using these techniques, Novick and colleagues reported a 2 percent operative mortality rate while achieving a 91 percent improvement in blood pressure in 100 consecutive renal revascularizations for atherosclerotic RVH. However, most 60 percent of patients with ASD have improvement (showing reduction of diastolic blood pressure by over 15 mm Hg or being normotensive on treatment), while only 30 percent are cured (being normotensive without medication). These numbers are reversed in patients with FMH.

Techniques for renal revascularization have improved markedly over the last few years, and the success rate for surgeons who commonly perform these procedures is better than that achieved with renal angioplasty in patients with diffuse ASD. Moreover, there is now long-term follow-up information concerning these patients, and the delayed restenosis or occlusion rate is acceptably low. Comparable data are not yet available for PTA.

Renal Reconstruction or Angioplasty for Preservation of Renal Function

The risk of the progressive nature of renal artery lesions discussed earlier has called attention to the threat of atherosclerotic renal artery disease to overall renal function. This is now recognized as an important clinical issue separate from the problem of RVH. In addition, the Schreiber study from the Cleveland Clinic suggested that progression occurred primarily within the

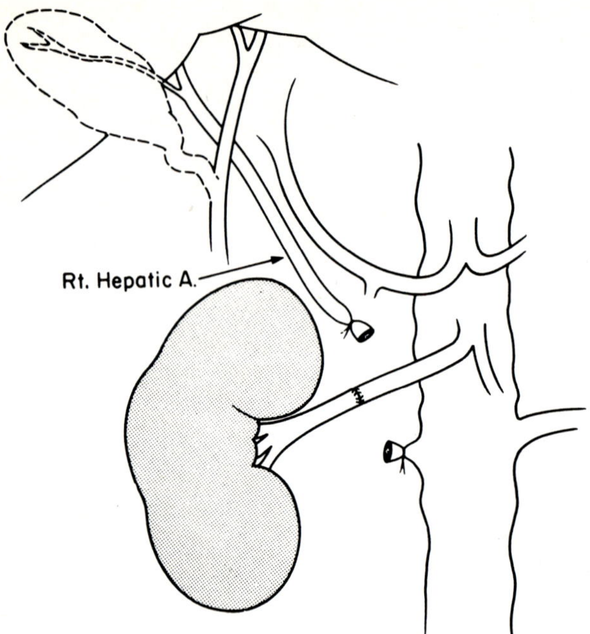

Figure 4 End-to-end hepatorenal bypass from the right hepatic artery to the right renal artery. An adjunctive cholecystectomy is necessary, because the gallbladder loses its nutrient artery. (Republished with permission by Sosa RE, Vaughan ED Jr. Renovascular hypertension. In: Gillenwater JY, Grayhack JT, Howards ST, Duckett JW, eds. Adult and pediatric urology. Chicago: Year Book, 1987:752.)

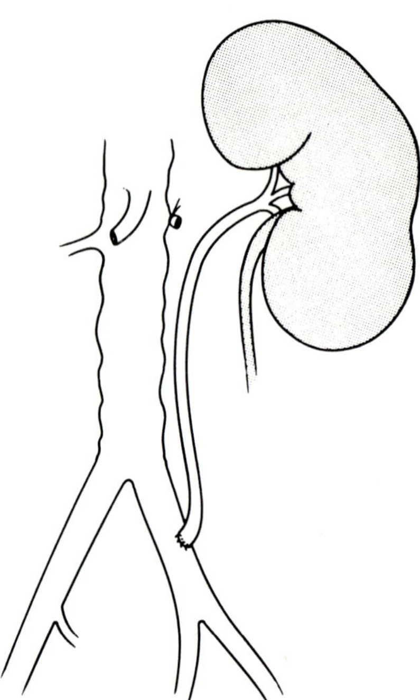

Figure 5 Renal revascularization by ileorenal bypass by means of a long saphenous vein graft. (Republished with permission by Sosa RE, Vaughan ED Jr. Renovascular hypertension. In: Gillenwater JY, Grayhack JT, Howards ST, Duckett JW, eds. Adult and pediatric urology. Chicago: Year Book, 1987:752.)

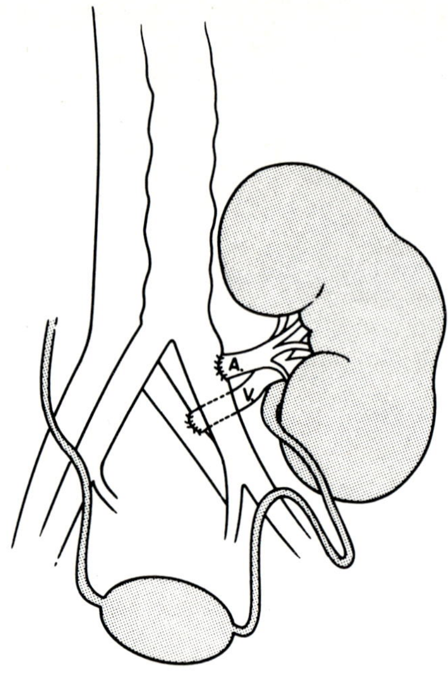

Figure 6 Renal revascularization by autotransplantation leaving the ureter intact. (Republished with permission by Sosa RE, Vaughan ED Jr. Renovascular hypertension. In: Gillenwater JY, Grayhack JT, Howards ST, Duckett JW, eds. Adult and pediatric urology. Chicago: Year Book, 1987:752.)

first 2 years of angiographic follow-up in patients with more than 50 percent stenosis on the initial angiogram. Moreover, blood pressure control was equal in the two groups, and loss of renal parenchyma could not be attributed to poor blood pressure control. In a separate study, Novick reviewed patients undergoing dialysis over a 10-year period and identified 25 patients with end-stage renal disease as a consequence of atherosclerotic renal artery disease.

Therefore, a second indication for intervention with angioplasty or revascularization is to preserve renal function, whether or not there is associated RVH.

Novick has established the following criteria for angiographic screening of atherosclerotic renal artery disease: (1) evidence of generalized atherosclerosis, (2) a unilateral small kidney, (3) mild to moderate azotemia (serum creatinine level greater than 1.5 mg per deciliter), and (4) hypertension. If the patient is subsequently found to have a high-grade arterial stenosis (greater than 75 percent) affecting the entire renal mass, i.e., when such a stenosis is present bilaterally or involves a solitary kidney, the author recommends intervention. One caveat is the level of renal function. The effect of baseline renal function on the outcome of surgical revascularization in elderly patients has been evaluated. For patients with preoperative serum creatinine levels of less than 3 mg per deciliter, postoperative renal function was stable and improved in 89 percent. Conversely, revascularization to preserve renal function in patients with serum creatinine levels of more than 4 mg per deciliter was not worthwhile because of advanced underlying renal parenchymal disease.

In a 10-year review of operative patients at the Cleveland Clinic, 161 of 241 patients with atherosclerotic disease were reported as undergoing surgical revascularization to achieve preservation of renal function. Within this group renal function improved in 93 patients (57.7 percent), was stable in 50 (31.3 percent), and deteriorated in 10 (6 percent).

On the basis of an earlier observation of Novick in 51 patients, Schwarten began in 1983 to perform transluminal angioplasty in a similar group of patients. He has reported on 32 patients with mild to moderate renal insufficiency. All patients had a serum creatinine level in the range of 2 to 3.1 mg per deciliter and kidneys over 9 cm in size. Fifteen patients had bilateral renal artery stenoses of more than 75 percent, and 17 had greater than 75 percent unilateral renal artery stenosis in a single functioning kidney. Angioplasty was performed using dilute contrast media and low volume, and in follow-up 23 patients were improved and seven exhibited no change; two patients were worse on a brief follow-up. Therefore, the early results of angioplasty appear to be similar to those reported for surgical intervention.

SUGGESTED READING

Butler AM. Chronic pyelonephritis and arterial hypertension. J Clin Invest 1937; 16:889–892.

Dotter CT, Judkins MP. Transluminal treatment of arteriosclerotic obstruction. Circulation 1964; 30:654–658.

Greminger P, Lüscher TF, Züber J, et al. Surgery, transluminal dilatation and medical therapy in the management of renovascular hypertension. Nephron 1986; 44 [Suppl 1]:36–39.

Hunt JC, Strong CS. Renovascular hypertension: mechanism, natural history and treatment. Am J Cardiol 1973; 32:562–570.

Leadbetter WF, Burkland CF. Hypertension in unilateral renal disease. J Urol 1938; 39:611–614.

Muller FB, Sealey JE, Case DB, et al. The captopril test for identifying renovascular disease in hypertensive patients. Am J Med 1986; 80:633–638.

Novick AC, Khauli RB, Vidt DG. Diminished operative risk and improved results following revascularization for atherosclerotic renovascular disease. Urol Clin North Am 1984; 11:435–449.

Novick AC, Textor SC, Bodie B, Khauli RB. Revascularization to preserve renal function in patients with atherosclerotic renovascular disease. Urol Clin North Am 1984; 11:477–490.

Schreiber MJ Jr, Novick AC, Pohl MA. The natural history of atherosclerotic and fibrous renal artery disease. World J Urol 1989; 7:59–63.

Schwarten DE. Percutaneous transluminal renal artery anigoplasty. In: NM Kaplan, BM Brunner, JH Laragh, eds, The kidney and hypertension. New York: Raven Press, 1987.

Sosa RE, Vaughan ED Jr. Renovascular hypertension: background, pathophysiology, pathology and clinical evaluation. AUA Update Series 1989; 8:138–144.

Sosa RE, Vaughan ED Jr. Hypertension of renal origin. World J Urol 1989; 7:64–71.

Textor SC, Novick AC, Tarazi RC, et al. Critical perfusion pressure for renal function in patients with bilateral atherosclerotic renovascular disease. Ann Intern Med 1985; 102:308–317.

Vaughan ED Jr, Buhler FR, Laragh JH, et al. Renovascular hypertension; renin measurements to indicate hypersecretion and contralateral suppression, estimate renal plasma flow and score for surgical curability. Am J Med 1973; 55:402.

Vaughan ED Jr, Sosa RE. Renovascular hypertension: treatment options. AUA Update Series 1989; 8:282–288.

HYPERTENSION IN UNILATERAL RENAL PARENCHYMAL DISEASE

DAVID A. GOLDFARB, M.D.
STEVAN B. STREEM, M.D.

Elevation of systemic arterial blood pressure can be associated with a wide range of diseases primarily affecting the parenchyma of a single renal unit. The hypertension associated with renal parenchymal disease is characterized by a decrease in the total number of functioning nephrons and, in some patients, abnormalities in sodium homeostasis and volume regulation that contribute to persistence of the pressor state. As in renovascular disease, the hypertension may result from local tissue destruction and ischemia with subsequent activation of the renin-angiotensin system.

Treatment of hypertension associated with unilateral renal parenchymal disease can be medical or surgical. In most patients, hypertension can be controlled with medication. By contrast, surgical cure rates for hypertension in renal parenchymal disease have been disappointing. In a classic review by Homer Smith in 1956, unilateral nephrectomy was reported to result in cure of hypertension in only 26 percent of patients. Since then, there have been many reports of surgical treatment of hypertension with nephrectomy or partial nephrectomy. Recent experience has shown that if the same criteria used to identify reversible, renin-mediated hypertension in patients with renovascular disease are strictly applied to patients with unilateral renal parenchymal disease, surgical results will be improved. The focus of this chapter is therefore to outline a diagnostic strategy that will permit appropriate selection of patients for either therapeutic option.

EVALUATION OF SURGICALLY CURABLE RENAL PARENCHYMAL HYPERTENSION

Criteria for the diagnosis of hypertension have been defined by the Joint National Committee on Detection, Evaluation and Treatment of High Blood Pressure (1988) as a sustained blood pressure of 140/90 mm Hg or more confirmed by at least three repeat measurements. Blood pressure should be measured while the patient is comfortably seated for several minutes, using a cuff of appropriate size. This definition has been established for patients older than 18 years of age; blood pressure in children is age related. In these cases, hypertension is defined as a sustained elevation in diastolic or systolic blood pressure more than two standard deviations above normal for any given age category.

Once the diagnosis of hypertension is established, further evaluation is required to determine whether there is a surgically reversible cause. A careful history and physical examination must be performed. Confirmation of a history of urinary infection, reflux, urolithiasis, trauma, flank pain, or hematuria suggests a possible renal cause. The mode of presentation may be helpful in identifying a secondary cause of hypertension. Abrupt onset of severe hypertension that is symptomatic (e.g., nausea, headache) or accompanied by evidence of end-organ damage should clearly warrant a search for a potentially reversible cause. Urinalysis may demonstrate pyuria, bacteriuria, or hematuria. Patients with significant proteinuria and casts may have glomerular disease, and this should be evaluated. Basic laboratory testing includes determination of blood urea nitrogen (BUN), serum creatinine, and electrolyte levels. A 24-hour urine collection should be evaluated for creatinine clearance, total protein, and sodium excretion.

A basic uroradiologic evaluation may next be made. The initial imaging study may be ultrasonography or intravenous urography (IVU), either of which may document abnormalities of the affected kidney and, equally important, exclude disease of the contralateral kidney. When indicated, voiding cystourethrography is performed to rule out vesicoureteral reflux. Radionuclide studies may also be indicated, because renal scarring may be more reliably detected with a dimercaptosuccinic acid (DMSA) scan than with IVU or ultrasonography. A Tc-99 diethylenetriaminepentaacetic acid (DTPA) scan is especially helpful in determining differential renal function when total or partial nephrectomy is being considered. Arteriography can be performed to exclude a renal artery lesion when surgical curability has been established, or for further investigation of possible neoplastic disease.

As an initial screening test, plasma renin activity (PRA) is indexed against a 24-hour urine sodium level. Patients with low PRA are unlikely to have surgically curable hypertension and should be treated with antihypertensive medication. Those with high PRA should be further evaluated with divided renal vein renin studies. Patients with normal PRA may also be evaluated with a captopril challenge test. This useful provocative test has identified surgically curable hypertension in 20 percent of renovascular patients who had normal PRA. When overall renal function is normal, captopril enhances renin secretion from the diseased kidney and lowers blood pressure. In patients who are not taking other antihypertensive medications, this is a highly sensitive, specific, and simple screening test. Divided renal vein studies are then performed in patients with high PRA or those with a positive captopril test to identify both increased renin secretion from the diseased kidney and suppression of renin secretion from the contralateral kidney.

Vaughn and colleagues at the Cornell Medical Center have developed criteria to predict surgically correctable hypertension. The renin increment from the diseased kidney should be 50 percent to maintain a steady-state renin level: $\frac{V_1-A}{A} \leq 0.5$ (V_1 = diseased kidney renal vein renin; A = infrarenal vena caval renin). As a physiologic response to hypersecretion of renin from the diseased kidney, renin secretion is suppressed in the normal contralateral kidney: $V_2 - A = 0$ (V_2 = normal kidney renal vein renin). At the Cleveland Clinic we have used a renal vein renin ratio of at least 1.5:1 (diseased: normal) as an indicator of surgical curability, provided that global renal function is normal and that renin secretion from the normal kidney is suppressed. Some patients have an elevated PRA or positive captopril test, yet on renal vein renin analysis the renin increment is less than 50 percent or the renal vein renin ratio is less than 1.5:1. In this setting, there may be a sampling error owing to malposition of the renal vein catheter, or unilateral parenchymal disease may be segmental. In the latter case, sampling from the main renal vein may be normal, since effluent blood from the diseased segment may be diluted with blood from the surrounding normal kidney. Selective sampling from the venous drainage of the affected segment may demonstrate a renin increment, and thus better guide appropriate treatment.

TREATMENT

Medical

Hypertension in unilateral renal parenchymal disease can be treated medically in most patients. Those with low PRA are likely to have volume-dependent hypertension and can be treated with diuretics. Patients with normal or high PRA usually respond to medications aimed at interruption of the renin-angiotensin system, such as beta blockers or converting enzyme inhibitors. Combined therapy may be required, including a diuretic and either a beta blocker or a converting enzyme inhibitor. Management of such patients in cooperation with an internist, a pediatrician, or a nephrologist is appropriate. Medical treatment is best suited for adult patients in whom mild hypertension can be controlled on a one- or two-drug regimen with minimal side effects. Children also are candidates for medical treatment, but every effort should be made to evaluate them for a potentially reversible cause to avoid life-long treatment with antihypertensive medications.

Surgical

Two groups of patients may benefit from surgery (Table 1). The first are those who have as an underlying

Table 1 Unilateral Renal Parenchymal Diseases Associated with Hypertension

Congenital/inflammatory disorders
  Reflux nephropathy
  Chronic pyelonephritis
  Ask-Upmark kidney
  Unilateral atrophic kidney
  Multicystic-dysplastic kidney
  Renal tuberculosis

Obstructive disorders
  Hydronephrosis (any cause)
  Ureteropelvic junction obstruction
  Simple renal cyst

Tumors
  Congenital mesoblastic nephroma
  Wilms' tumor
  Reninoma
  Renal cell carcinoma

Miscellaneous disorders
  Post-ESWL
  Post-traumatic
  Radiation nephritis

pathology those conditions that have been listed as inflammatory or congenital. Despite different mechanisms of initial injury, the final common end point is segmental or global renal scarring associated with a loss of nephrons and a variable amount of tissue ischemia. These patients must be completely evaluated and the indication for surgery clearly defined. A patient from this category who is ideally suited for surgical treatment will (1) strictly fulfill the described criteria for surgical curability, (2) have little or no renal function associated with the segment of kidney to be removed, and (3) have no detectable disease in the remaining renal tissue or contralateral kidney.

Hypersecretion of renin must be demonstrated from the affected renal segment or kidney. More important, however, is clear demonstration of contralateral renin suppression. Almost any renin elevation from the contralateral "normal" kidney may be taken as evidence of occult bilateral disease, and in such patients hypertension may persist after surgical intervention. In patients considered for surgery, a Tc-99 DTPA renal scan with differential renal function may be used to assess the diseased kidney's contribution to overall renal function. For nephrectomy to be considered, a kidney should contribute less than 10 to 15 percent of overall renal function. When kidney function is greater than this, a partial nephrectomy should be considered, at least when the disease is focal and segmental renal vein renins support the potential for cure. Finally, the remaining renal tissue after surgery must be normal. For example, compensatory hypertrophy suggests a completely normal contralateral kidney. In contrast, significant azotemia suggests bilateral disease with a decreased likelihood of surgical cure.

The second group of patients who may be cured surgically have pathologic conditions listed as obstruc-

tion or tumors. Acute unilateral renal obstruction is associated with activation of the renin-angiotensin system, although few patients with unilateral hydronephrosis have hypertension. There are many reported cases of renin-dependent hypertension accompanying a unilateral, chronically obstructed kidney. The association with hypertension notwithstanding, the primary indication for surgery in these patients is to relieve the obstruction and restore renal function. In kidneys with a substantial amount of remaining parenchyma, every effort should be made to re-establish unobstructed urinary drainage. The choice of procedure can be guided by the specific pathology. Occasionally, severe parenchymal loss from chronic obstruction is present, and nephrectomy rather than reconstruction is appropriate. This decision can be made on the basis of preoperative radiographic assessment (ultrasound and nuclear studies) or at the time of exploration. Surgical intervention for hydronephrosis can reasonably be expected to ameliorate the associated hypertension only when the criteria outlined for surgical curability have been satisfied.

In addition to the disease states outlined in Table 1, some conditions warrant further discussion. The association of hypertension with various tumors of the kidney has been well established. Up to 50 percent of patients with renal cell carcinoma or Wilms' tumor have been reported to be hypertensive. For both tumors, high renin content has been documented, and this may contribute to high blood pressure. Obviously, however, the primary indication for nephrectomy in these patients is removal of the tumor and not cure of hypertension.

The juxtaglomerular cell tumor (reninoma) is a rare cause of renal parenchymal hypertension that is usually found in young adults. These patients generally present with hypertension associated with hyperreninemia and secondary aldosteronism. The hyperaldosteronism can be severe and, like an aldosteronoma, is not suppressed with deoxycorticosterone. It is important to determine PRA, which when elevated in this clinical situation is pathognomonic of a renin-secreting tumor, thereby clearly distinguishing these patients from those with hyperaldosteronism, who will have low PRA. Lateralizing renal vein renin assays can identify which kidney contains the tumor. In these patients, angiography has usually been performed to exclude renovascular disease. It may, however, identify the tumor, which is generally small and often exhibits a hypovascular pattern visualized as a cortical lucency on the nephrogram phase. Ultrasound or computed tomography (CT) may also be useful for further investigation. In the future, magnetic resonance imaging (MRI) may prove to be a valuable adjunctive study. Reninomas are benign, so the primary indication for surgical intervention is relief of hypertension. Standard treatment is nephrectomy, which uniformly results in cure, although partial nephrectomy may also be successful.

Renal trauma is occasionally associated with persistent hypertension. Reports suggest that with appropriate initial management the incidence of post-traumatic hypertension is low. Ischemia from renal artery injury or a devitalized renal segment is one mechanism that can explain post-traumatic hypertension; a Page kidney, which results from a subcapsular hematoma or a perinephric collection (hematoma or urinoma), is another. Surgery is indicated when a causal relationship between the renal injury and hypertension can be documented. Again, nephrectomy or partial nephrectomy can be used to remove ischemic renal tissue and thus treat the hypertension.

Extracorporeal shock wave lithotripsy (ESWL) is one of the most common forms of renal traumatic injury today. Subcapsular or perinephric fluid accumulation can be observed in up to one third of patients undergoing ESWL. These fluid collections are usually small and reabsorbed within 6 weeks. Occasionally, serious bleeding may occur requiring transfusion, angiographic embolization, or even nephrectomy. Other acute renal changes that follow ESWL include the loss of corticomedullary demarcation, edema, and a decrease in renal plasma flow. Chronic renal changes from ESWL have been documented only in experimental animals and include interstitial fibrosis, with loss of tubules and glomeruli. The degree of injury has been correlated with the number of shock waves. The relationship between renal injury from ESWL and new-onset hypertension is a subject of concern and continued debate. Retrospective uncontrolled studies from the mid-1980s indicated that the annual incidence of hypertension was greater in ESWL patients than in the general population. Lingeman and colleagues from the Methodist Hospital of Indiana have reported blood pressure changes after ESWL and compared this large group with a similar cohort of stone-forming patients undergoing other forms of treatment for nephrolithiasis. After 2 years of follow-up, the annual incidence of new-onset hypertension in the ESWL group was no different from the non-ESWL group and was comparable with the annual incidence of hypertension in the general population. The annual increase in diastolic blood pressure, however, was significantly increased in ESWL patients (0.78 mm Hg) compared with non-ESWL patients (-0.88 mm Hg) and the general population (0.33 mm Hg). This difference does not seem to be clinically significant over a short period, but if the annual increase in blood pressure was to remain constant, many patients could be hypertensive in 10 to 15 years.

SUGGESTED READING

Javadpour N, Doppman JL, Scardino PT, Bartter FC. Segmental renal vein renin assay and segmental nephrectomy for correction of renal hypertension. J Urol 1976; 115:580–582.

Lingeman JE, Woods JR, Toth PD. Blood pressure changes following extracorporeal shock wave lithotripsy and other forms of treatment for nephrolithiasis. JAMA 1990; 263:1789–1794.

Smith HW. Unilateral nephrectomy in hypertensive disease. J Urol 1956; 76:686–701.

Vaughan ED, Buhler FR, Laragh JH, et al. Hypertension and unilateral parenchymal renal disease: evidence for abnormal vasoconstriction–volume interaction. JAMA 1975; 233:1177–1183.

RENAL ARTERY ANEURYSM

ANDREW C. NOVICK, M.D.

A renal artery aneurysm is a localized dilatation of the main renal artery or its branches, presumably due to weakening of the elastic tissue and media of the arterial wall. The incidence of renal artery aneurysms in the general population is not known. Estimates based on autopsy examinations or selected arteriographic studies are associated with an inherent bias. One postmortem angiographic study revealed saccular renal artery aneurysms in 9.7 percent of random autopsies. Renal artery aneurysms have been observed in 2.5 percent of patients undergoing renal arteriography for evaluation of hypertension, and in 1.5 percent of potential kidney donors undergoing arteriographic evaluation. The true incidence of renal artery aneurysms in the general population may be more accurately reflected in studies of patients undergoing abdominal aortography for nonrenal diseases. In two such series of 10,000 and 8,500 patients, the incidence of renal artery aneurysm was 0.3 and 0.09 percent, respectively.

ETIOLOGY AND CLASSIFICATION

Renal artery aneurysms may be caused by a variety of disorders, including atherosclerosis, fibrous dysplasia, arteritis, trauma, and neurofibromatosis. Alternatively, they may be present with no other apparent associated arterial disease. Some aneurysms in children may be congenital. The most useful classification recognizes four types of renal artery aneurysms, which are described below.

Saccular Aneurysm

The most common type of renal artery aneurysm is a saccular aneurysm, which is characterized by an outpouching from the renal artery, 1 to 5 cm in diameter, with a connecting channel of variable width. Saccular aneurysms usually occur at the bifurcation of the main renal artery or one of its branches, possibly because of a weakness in the arterial wall at this point (Fig. 1). They

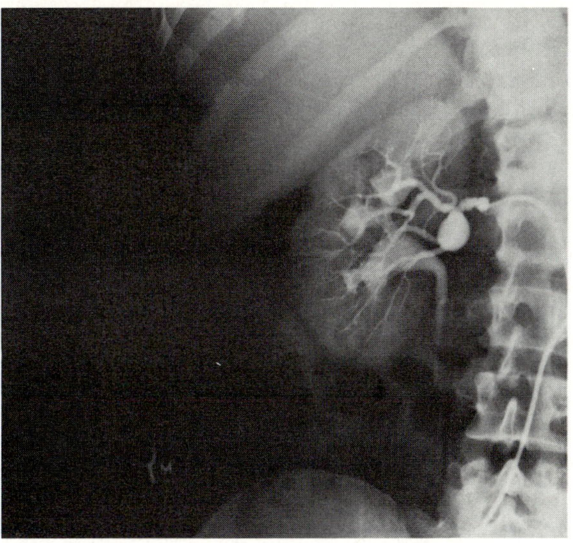

Figure 1 Right renal arteriogram shows a large saccular aneurysm at the bifurcation of the main renal artery.

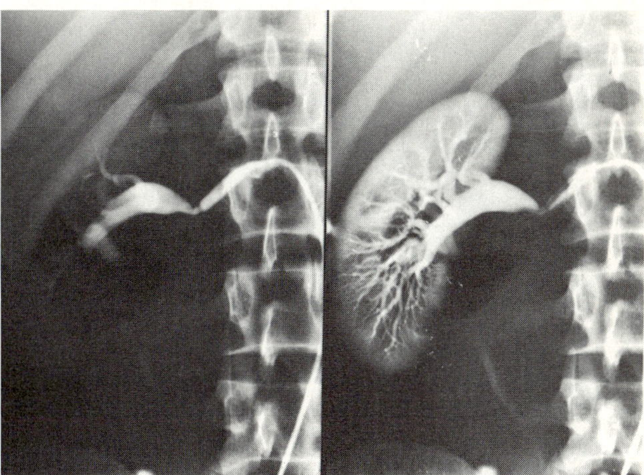

Figure 2 Right renal arteriogram shows a high-grade stenosis of the main renal artery from intimal fibroplasia with a post-stenotic fusiform aneurysm.

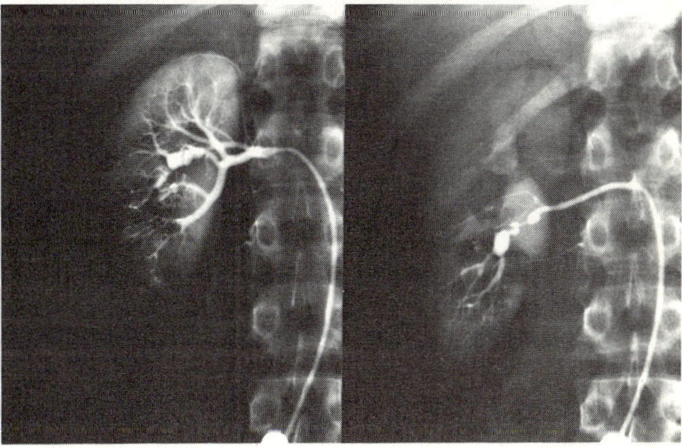

Figure 3 Selective right renal arteriography demonstrates two arteries supplying the right kidney with dissecting aneurysms (*arrows*).

may occur in association with medial fibroplasia of the renal artery, where intramural disruption of elastic tissue and loss of smooth muscle often leave the arterial wall composed of only a thin layer of connective tissue. Abnormalities of the media in neurofibromatosis may also predispose to aneurysmal development. Atherosclerotic aneurysmal involvement is generally a secondary process rather than a primary cause. When it occurs, the wall of the aneurysm may undergo calcification, and a mural thrombus may also develop within the aneurysmal lumen.

Fusiform Aneurysm

Fusiform aneurysms occur as a uniform dilatation of an entire segment of the renal artery to as much as three or four times its normal diameter. These aneurysms range in length from 1 to 3 cm and generally are not calcified. They are typically found in young hypertensive patients with stenosing fibrous dysplasia of the renal artery (Fig. 2). In such cases, the fusiform aneurysm is actually a post-stenotic dilatation and can involve either the main renal artery or its branches. The vast majority of patients with this type of aneurysm have significant associated renal ischemia and hypertension.

Dissecting Aneurysm

A dissecting aneurysm results from a tear in the internal elastic membrane of the renal artery; as blood flows through the opening, the intima is separated from the remainder of the arterial wall. This process may be contained to a localized dissection or may spread to involve one or more branches (Fig. 3). In some patients, the dissection may re-enter the lumen distally. Dissecting aneurysms are most often complications of renal arterial involvement with atherosclerosis, intimal fibro-

plasia, or perimedial fibroplasia. Less commonly, this type of aneurysm may occur as an extension of a dissecting aortic aneurysm.

Intrarenal Aneurysm

Intrarenal aneurysms make up approximately 15 to 20 percent of all renal artery aneurysms. They are usually saccular or fusiform and may be calcified (Fig. 4). These aneurysms can originate from atherosclerosis, fibrous dysplasia, trauma, congenital vascular malformations, polyarteritis nodosa, renal carcinoma, or closed needle biopsy of the kidney.

CLINICAL PRESENTATION

Renal artery aneurysms may occur at any age, but most are found in patients between 40 and 60 years of age. There is no predilection for either sex, and the right

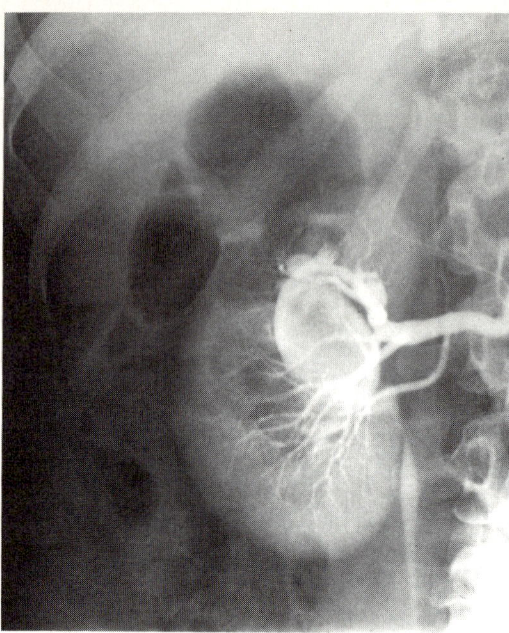

Figure 4 Right renal arteriogram shows an intrarenal arterial aneurysm.

and left renal arteries are involved equally. Of patients with renal artery aneurysms, approximately 30 percent have multiple lesions and 20 percent have bilateral lesions.

Most renal artery aneurysms are small and asymptomatic. The most common clinical manifestations are hypertension, subcostal or flank pain, hematuria, an abdominal bruit, and (rarely) a palpable pulsating mass. Renovascular hypertension occurs in 15 to 75 percent of patients and may be due to turbulent flow within an aneurysm, associated arterial stenosis, dissection, arteriovenous fistula formation, thromboembolism, or compression of adjacent arterial branches by a large aneurysm. Flank pain occurs in up to 30 percent of patients and may be due to aneurysmal expansion, acute dissection with infarction, or associated pyelocaliceal obstruction. An abdominal bruit may be auscultated in approximately 15 percent of patients with a renal artery aneurysm.

COMPLICATIONS

There are several potential complications of renal artery aneurysms. A saccular aneurysm may erode into the main renal vein or one of its branches, with formation of an arteriovenous fistula. Erosion into the renal pelvis may occur, with resultant hematuria. Mural thrombus formation may also occur within saccular aneurysms and may occasionally lead to peripheral renal embolization. Saccular aneurysms can enlarge over time to produce extrinsic compression either of renal artery branches or of the intrarenal collecting system. Throm-

bosis of the main renal artery or its branches with resultant infarction may occur as an acute event either in dissecting aneurysms or in aneurysms associated with stenosing vascular disease associated with an aneurysm.

Spontaneous rupture of a renal artery aneurysm is an important potential complication. Large, incompletely calcified saccular aneurysms may become soft, thin, and ulcerated between zones of calcification, thus predisposing to rupture. Poutasse recommended surgical repair of all noncalcified or incompletely calcified aneurysms larger than 1.5 cm in diameter to obviate this complication. Smith and Hinman reported ruptures occurring in 20 percent of patients with intrarenal aneurysms. Stanley and colleagues observed ruptures in four of 72 patients (5.6 percent) with renal artery aneurysms. Hageman and colleagues followed 25 patients with renal artery aneurysms larger than 2 cm for periods of 1 to 17 years, and no ruptures occurred.

Although there are scant data on the natural history of renal artery aneurysms, several factors predisposing to rupture have been identified. Harrow and Sloane reviewed the cases of 100 patients with noncalcified aneurysms and found a 24 percent incidence of rupture; in contrast, their review disclosed no rupture among 69 patients with calcified aneurysms. Hypertension is considered to be another important factor predisposing to rupture. Finally, several reports indicate an increased risk of aneurysmal rupture during pregnancy. It has been suggested that hormonal changes during pregnancy produce weakness of the arterial wall. This weakness, combined with an increase in cardiac output and blood volume and an increase in intra-abdominal pressure from the fetus, might result in aneurysmal rupture, which carries a high risk of mortality for both mother and fetus.

SELECTION FOR SURGERY

Surgical excision is indicated for a renal artery aneurysm, regardless of size, in the following situations:

1. Aneurysm causing renovascular hypertension.
2. Dissecting aneurysm.
3. Aneurysm associated with local symptoms such as flank pain or hematuria.
4. Aneurysm occurring in a woman of child-bearing age with a potential for pregnancy.
5. Aneurysm associated with functionally significant renal artery stenosis.
6. Aneurysm that has led to distal renal embolization.
7. Aneurysm with evidence of progressive expansion on serial radiographic studies.

In the absence of the above criteria, there is general agreement that renal artery aneurysms that are smaller than 2.0 cm and nonsymptomatic do not require operative intervention. These should be followed radiographically to detect any change in size. Aneurysms that

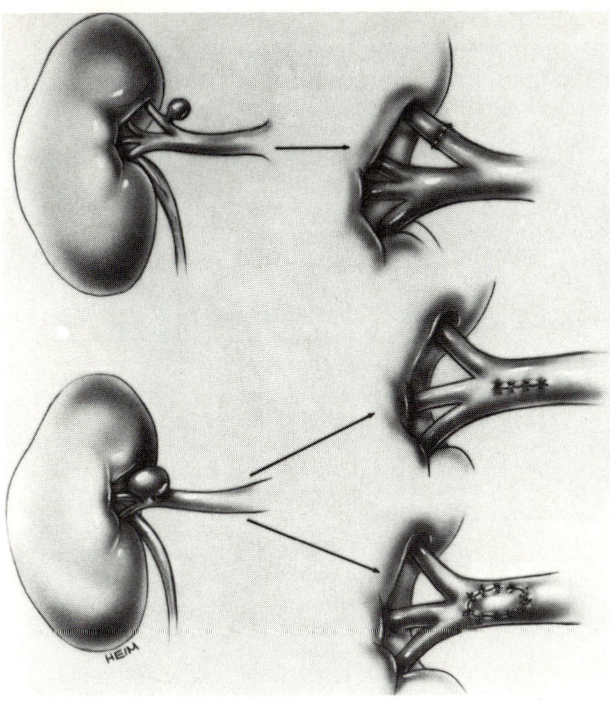

Figure 5 Methods of renal artery aneurysmectomy by segmental resection and reanastomosis (*above*) or aneurysmectomy with primary closure or patch angioplasty (*below*). (Republished with permission by Novick AC. Microvascular reconstruction of complex branch renal artery disease. Urol Clin North Am 1984; 11:465. © by Williams & Wilkins.)

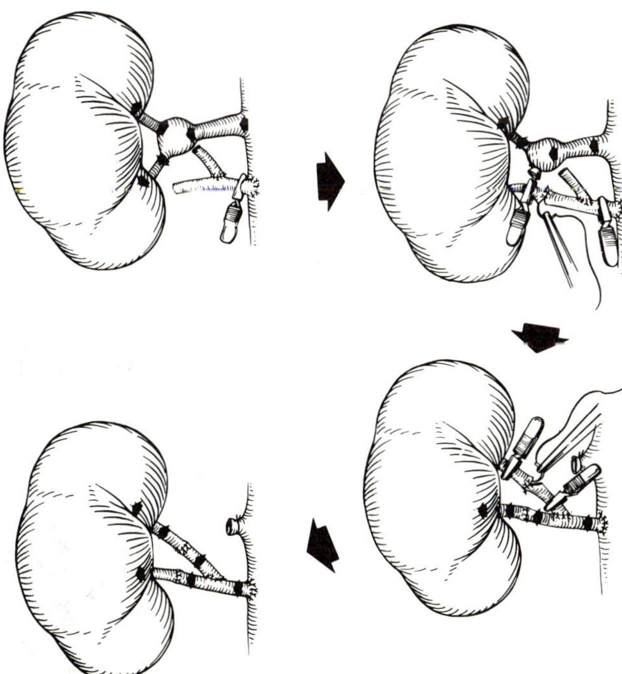

Figure 6 Technique of aortorenal bypass with a branched saphenous vein graft for repairs of two renal artery branches associated with an aneurysm. After anastomosis of the graft to the aorta (*top left*), end-to-end anastomosis to one of the renal artery branches is done while the remainder of the kidney is perfused (*top right*). After circulation is restored to the repaired branch, the remaining branch is anastomosed end to end to the other limb of the graft (*bottom right*) to complete the revascularization (*bottom left*).

are completely calcified may be followed with serial plain abdominal radiography at yearly intervals. For noncalcified or incompletely calcified aneurysms, I obtain serial arteriography at yearly or biyearly intervals to document stability in size and to monitor possible progression of associated stenosing arterial disease. Ultrasonography, computed tomography (CT), and magnetic resonance imaging (MRI) may be useful alternative noninvasive imaging tools, but their efficacy requires further elucidation. Radiographic evidence of serial aneurysmal enlargement warrants reconsideration of surgery to prevent rupture.

The management of asymptomatic patients with renal artery aneurysms greater than 2.0 cm in diameter is controversial. I believe there is an increased risk of rupture with aneurysms of this size when there is absent or incomplete calcification of the wall. My preference in such cases is therefore for surgical excision, which invariably reveals areas of the aneurysmal wall that are extremely thin.

SURGICAL TREATMENT

A variety of operations are available for patients with renal artery aneurysms who need surgical treatment. Total or partial nephrectomy is reserved for patients with renal infarction, severe ischemic renal atrophy, or particularly complex intrarenal aneurysms that cannot be repaired. Since the advent of microvascular and extracorporeal techniques, aneurysmectomy with preservation of the involved renal unit is currently possible in most cases.

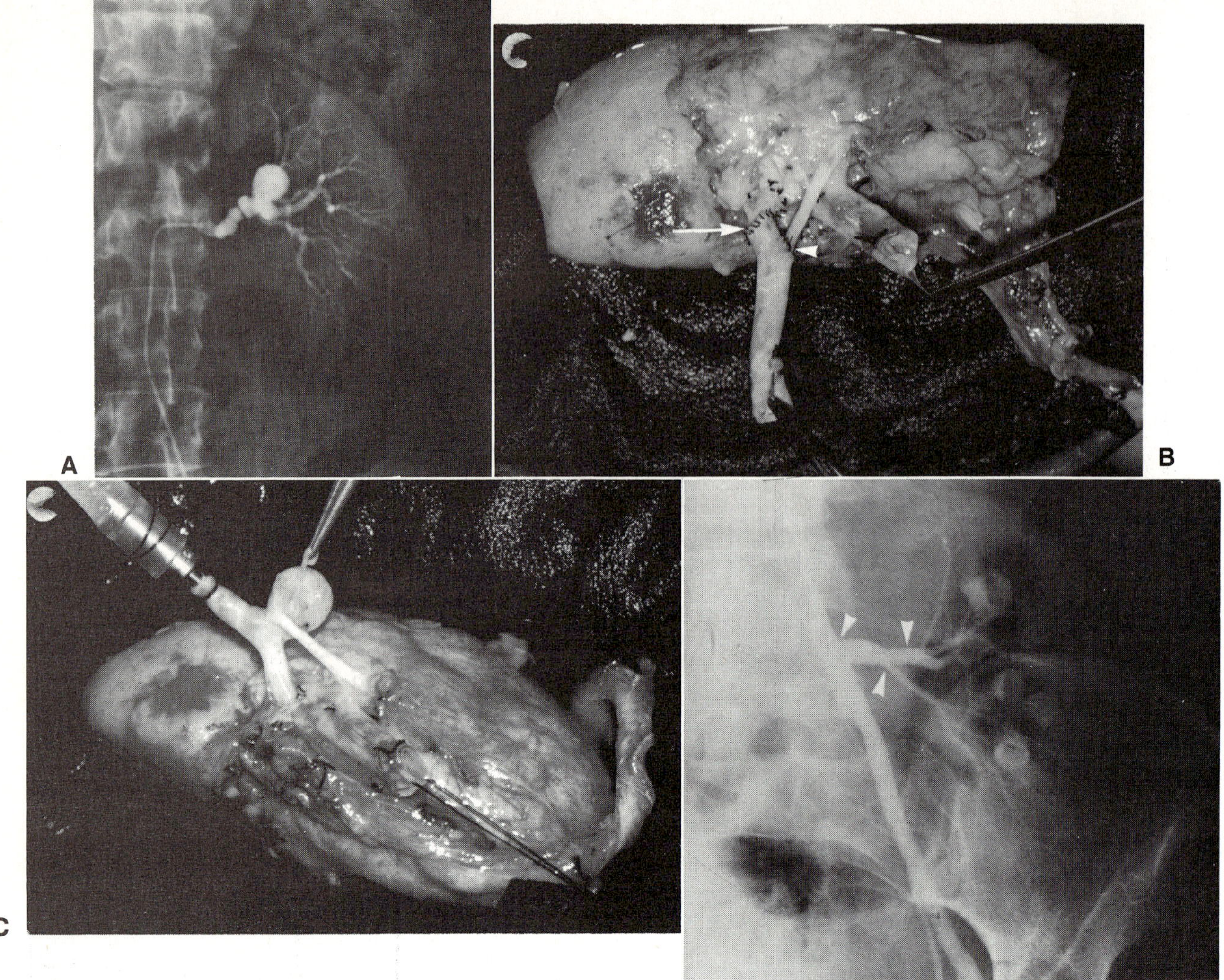

Figure 7 *A,* Left renal arteriogram shows fibrous dysplasia and aneurysm involving the main renal artery and primary branches. *B,* Operative photograph of removed flushed kidney after mobilization of the diseased main renal artery and two primary branches. *C,* Completed extracorporeal repair. After resection of diseased renal vessels, hypogastric arterial autograft was anastomosed end to end (*long arrow*) and side to end (*short arrow*) to primary branches. *D,* Autotransplantation was performed into the left iliac fossa with end-to-end anastomosis of the new renal artery to the common iliac artery. A postoperative arteriogram demonstrates patency of all arterial anastomoses (*arrowheads*). Republished with permission by Novick AC, et al. The role of renal autotransplantation in complex urological reconstruction. J Urol 1990; 143:452.

Renal artery aneurysms have a variable presentation, and vascular involvement may be focal or diffuse. For saccular aneurysms confined to the main renal artery, if the arterial wall at the base of the aneurysm is intact, in situ aneurysmectomy with either primary closure or patch angioplasty can be performed. Aneurysms with short focal involvement of the main renal artery or a proximal branch may also be simply resected with end-to-end arterial anastomosis (Fig. 5). When more extensive extrahilar vascular disease is present, aortorenal bypass with an autogenous graft is necessary.

Since most saccular aneurysms occur at the bifurcation of the renal artery, branch arterial revascularization is commonly required. With multiple branch involvement, segmental resection or complex arterioplastic re-

construction often necessitates prolonged renal ischemia and is best avoided. The best method of in situ revascularization in such cases is aortorenal bypass employing a branched vascular graft. Although the hypogastric artery may be removed intact with its branches, this type of graft is rarely long enough to reach from the aorta to the renal artery branches, especially on the right side where the vena cava is interposed. In these cases, a prefashioned branched saphenous vein graft is the best material for replacement of the diseased vessels. With this technique a multibranched graft may be created to allow revascularization of several renal artery branches. Vascular reconstruction is technically straightforward in that direct end-to-end anastomosis of each graft branch to a renal artery branch is performed. Finally, renal ischemia time is minimal, since each segmental arterial anastomosis is done separately, while perfusion to the remainder of the kidney continues (Fig. 6).

Extracorporeal aneurysmectomy with vascular reconstruction and autotransplantation is indicated for patients with intrarenal aneurysms involving multiple arterial branches. In patients with dissecting or partially calcified aneurysms, the diseased renal vessels may be difficult to mobilize in situ because of intense surrounding fibrotic reaction; some of these patients also are more safely and effectively managed with extracorporeal reconstruction. In this approach the kidney is removed and flushed with an intracellular electrolyte solution, and then submerged in ice slush saline to maintain hypothermia. I prefer to transect the ureter and place the removed kidney on a separate workbench for the extracorporeal repair. Alternatively, the ureter may be left intact and the repair made on the abdominal wall, although this may be more cumbersome.

The particular method of extracorporeal revascularization depends on the extent of renovascular involvement by the aneurysm and the presence of associated arterial stenosis. If the arterial wall at the base of the aneurysm is free of disease, aneurysmectomy with primary closure or patch angioplasty is possible. Aneurysms with short focal branch arterial involvement can also be resected with primary branch reanastomosis. With extensive intrarenal vascular disease, complete aneurysmal excision and revascularization with a branched autogenous graft is indicated. A hypogastric arterial graft is the preferred material for vascular reconstruction, since this vessel may be obtained intact with several of its branches (Fig. 7). Extracorporeal repair of the kidney is made to create a single main renal artery, so that autotransplantation may be performed with only one arterial anastomosis and no increase in revascularization time. The kidney is then autotransplanted to either iliac fossa, using the same technique as in renal allotransplantation, with ureteroneocystostomy as the method of restoring urinary continuity.

SUGGESTED READING

Hageman JH, et al. Aneurysms of the renal artery: problems of prognosis and surgical management. Surgery 1978; 84:563.

Harrow BR, Sloane JA. Aneurysm of renal artery: report of five cases. J Urol 1959; 81:35.

Novick AC. Renal artery aneurysms and arteriovenous fistulas. In: Novick AC, Straffon RA, eds. Vascular problems in urologic surgery. Philadelphia: WB Saunders, 1982.

Ortenberg J, Novick AC, Straffon RA, Stewart BH. Surgical treatment of renal artery aneurysms. Br J Urol 1983; 55:341.

Poutasse EF. Renal artery aneurysms. J Urol 1976; 113:443.

Smith JN, Hinman F. Intrarenal artery aneurysms. J Urol 1967; 97:990.

Stanley JC, et al. Renal artery aneurysms: significance of macroaneurysms exclusive of dissections and fibrodysplastic mural dilations. Arch Surg 1975; 110:1327.

RENAL ARTERY EMBOLISM AND THROMBOSIS

W. GRAHAM GUERRIERO, M.D.

The kidney is composed of five segments, each of which receives its own arterial blood supply. For this reason the kidney is known as an end-organ vascular system. Few collaterals are found, except for a few millimeters of cortex supplied by capsular arteries. Only small branches from the adrenal gland and aorta may feed the arterial tree. Acute interruption of renal arterial blood supply results in necrosis of the renal cortex and medulla. Experimentally, normothermic occlusion of the renal artery for 10 minutes will cause transient changes in renal function; these become permanent after 30 minutes and the whole kidney is lost after 180 minutes. For up to 180 minutes, some portion of the cortex will recover, but areas of persistent ischemia result in renovascular hypertension in most patients, and kidney function is markedly impaired the longer the renal artery is occluded.

If experimental occlusion of the renal artery results in complete death of the kidney after 180 minutes, why are there reports of successful revascularization of the kidney in patients with bilateral arterial thrombosis, with occlusion times of up to 24 hours? The only answer can be that the blockage was incomplete, that protection was afforded by hypothermia, or that collateral circulation was present. This is not the situation in most cases. Most authors writing on the subject today consider it unlikely that revascularization of the renal artery will be successful if occlusion has occurred more than 3 to 6 hours before the surgical procedure. In almost all reported cases of revascularization, impaired function or hypertension has been found after "successful" revascularization. Results reported have been so bad that some surgeons have taken the stance that an attempt to revascularize an acutely thrombosed kidney is never warranted. This simplistic approach has resulted in little effort to identify patients with early renal artery thrombosis, and may be denying successful repair to some of these patients.

An examination of the variables present in the patient population with renal arteries occluded by embolus or thrombosis may help surgeons select patients who may benefit from revascularization.

NATURE OF OCCLUSION OF RENAL ARTERY

Occlusion of the renal artery may occur as a result of embolus or thrombosis. Thrombosis may be secondary to dissecting aneurysm, intimal disruption secondary to blunt trauma (Fig. 1) or arteriosclerosis and associated thrombosis, or may be considered to be idiopathic. Embolus is statistically more common than thrombosis. An embolus to the renal artery usually arises from the heart, either (1) from a mural thrombus of the left ventricle secondary to a ventricular aneurysm, a myocardiopathy, or myocardial infarction; (2) from the left atrium as a result of an arrhythmia such as atrial fibrillation; or (3) from a cardiac valve as a result of a fibrin thrombus on a prosthetic valve or a mycotic thrombus on a valve leaflet. Embolus has been reported from valves damaged by rheumatic fever, but this is not common today. Diagnosis of a mural thrombus is best made by echocardiography, and once the embolus has been discovered, therapy is usually directed toward the cause of the thrombus and prevention of further embolization by anticoagulation. Other causes of emboli include vascular surgery of the thoracic aorta or the rare instance of a foreign body metastasizing to the renal

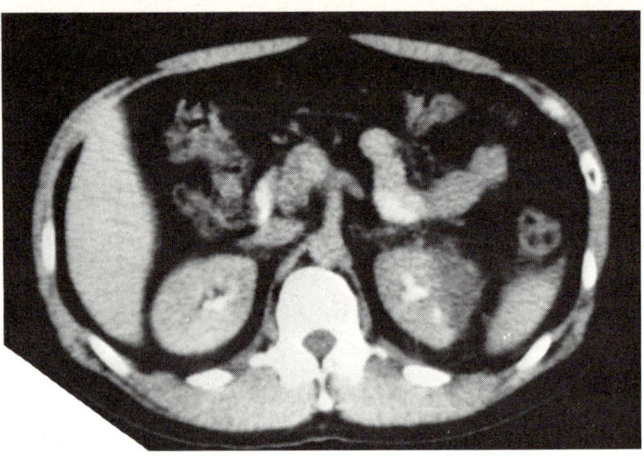

Figure 2 CT scan of the kidneys with contrast demonstrating poor renal perfusion and a wedge-shaped infarct.

artery, as, for example, after thrombosis of the contralateral artery with a wire coil.

When embolization or thrombosis of the renal artery occurs, there is intense, sudden flank pain similar to that seen with renal colic secondary to stone; the usual presumptive diagnosis in an ambulatory patient is that a stone has blocked the ureter. Patients with renal artery occlusion usually have microhematuria and minimal proteinuria, but significant degrees of leukocytosis and fever may be present.

The first study ordered is usually intravenous pyelography (IVP). This may show nothing if only a segmental infarction has occurred, or poor-to-absent excretion of dye may be noted on the side of the thrombosis. A "cortical rim sign" may be seen if collateral circulation to the peripheral renal cortex is present. The physician ordering the IVP should be suspicious of renal artery occlusion if no stone is seen and flank pain is severe and persistent. Computed tomography (CT) scan usually confirms the diagnosis by revealing areas of poor renal perfusion or wedge-shaped infarcts (Fig. 2). Arteriography will demonstrate a blocked branch or complete occlusion of the renal artery. Segmental occlusion is more common than total renal occlusion and is obviously a much less serious risk to the patient. Renal isotope scans may also suggest the diagnosis of renal artery thrombosis or embolism. Concomitant embolization of the extremities, particularly the toes, is frequently seen in patients who are showering emboli into the systemic circulation ("blue toe" sign).

TREATMENT OF RENAL ARTERY EMBOLIZATION

Surgical embolectomy has been performed infrequently for renal artery embolus, but reports in the literature suggest that successful relief of obstruction with surgery may be found in up to 82 percent of patients. Most patients selected for embolectomy are those with total renal artery occlusion. According to

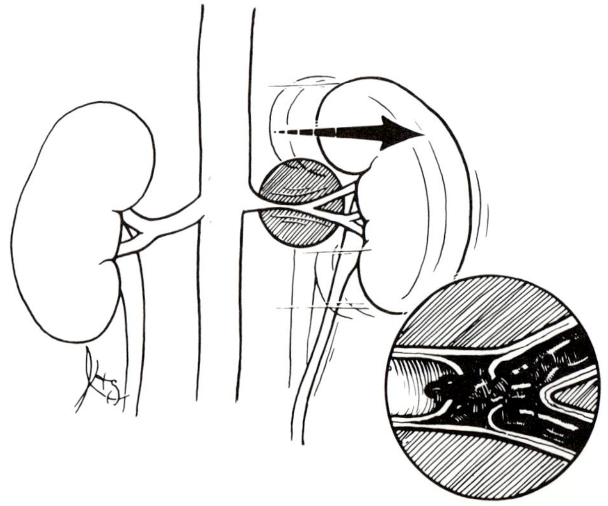

Figure 1 Intimal disruption of the renal artery. (Republished with permission from Guerriero WG, Kessler DL. Urologic injuries. East Norwalk, Appleton-Century-Crofts, 1984:14.)

Cass, surgical treatment of segmental infarction is not warranted unless an aneurysm is present.

Percutaneous transcatheter embolectomy has been reported by Buxton, but in most centers the choice of treatment is among surgical embolectomy, heparinization alone, or fibrinolytic therapy with streptokinase or urokinase. Although normalization of renal function has been reported by Campieri, most authors have been disappointed in the effectiveness of fibrinolytic therapy. There is a significant risk of bleeding when streptokinase is used, making it difficult to use the procedure in postoperative patients. There are few reports on fibrinolytic therapy with streptokinase. Further experience is necessary before it can be said that fibrinolytic therapy will produce results as good as early surgical re-establishment of renal artery blood flow.

Although surgery re-establishes flow in up to 80 percent of patients and hypertension may be ameliorated in patients with embolus, renal function is rarely improved, according to Ouriel and colleagues. Successful revascularization should mean a significant improvement in renal function, the absence of hypertension, and demonstration of renal arterial flow to a significant portion of the kidney by postoperative arteriography or renal scan. If these criteria are used, few reported cases have been successful.

Thrombosis

In children, thrombotic occlusion of the renal artery occurs spontaneously without known cause. In rare instances, it may occur in infants as a result of dehydration, but of course renal vein thrombosis is much more common in these small patients. Arterial occlusion of the renal artery may occur in infants as a result of embolus secondary to thrombosis of the ductus arteriosus, sepsis, or congenital heart disease. Thrombosis of the renal artery leads to hypertension and congestive heart failure. Woodard has suggested that immediate nephrectomy is required to save the life of these infants.

In adults, thrombosis is usually secondary to arteriosclerosis and ulceration of the renal artery and aorta, fibromuscular hyperplasia of the renal artery, a dissecting aneurysm of the aorta, renal artery aneurysm, complications of rejection after renal transplantation, or thrombocythemic states. Signs and symptoms of thrombosis are similar to those seen with embolism of the renal artery. In most cases of renal artery thrombosis, the artery is diseased and the clot is secondary to the disease process. Successful revascularization depends on correction of the disease process, the cause of thrombosis, and the presence of collateral circulation or incomplete occlusion to maintain renal viability. Segmental thrombosis is an indication for systemic anticoagulation but not an indication for surgery. As in the group with emboli, streptokinase therapy is promising, but return of function is not seen in most patients.

The results of therapy, both surgical and medical, for thrombosis and embolization of the renal artery have been disappointing. Only when the occlusion has been diagnosed in the first few hours or when collateral circulation has been present have good results been obtained. Correction of the condition leading to the thrombosis, e.g., dehydration, hypercoagulable state, aneurysm, or arterial sclerosis, is mandatory: just aspirating the clot or passing a Fogarty balloon is almost never successful.

Preoperative signs that a revascularization surgical procedure may be successful include demonstration of a partial occlusion, the presence of collateral circulation as demonstrated by a cortical rim sign on IVP or CT, a disease process that has led to slow occlusion of the renal artery with only a thrombosis to complete the process, early diagnosis, visualization of the renal artery distal to the occlusion, and preservation of renal size. Some authors have suggested preoperative biopsy to determine renal viability. At the time of surgery, good back flow from the kidney is accepted as a favorable prognostic sign, and the intraoperative Doppler may be useful for demonstrating good blood flow.

RENAL ARTERY THROMBOSIS SECONDARY TO BLUNT TRAUMA

Thrombosis of the renal artery secondary to blunt trauma occurs as a result of stretching and rupture of the intima of the artery, as when the patient is thrown from a car or suddenly decelerates for any other reason, such as falling from a height (Fig. 1). These injuries frequently go unrecognized because of other injuries that are more obvious and often immediately life-threatening. Although the patient may have microhematuria, gross hematuria is unlikely unless there is other urologic injury such as a deep cortical laceration, a fractured kidney, or rupture of the bladder. Nonvisualization of the kidney is discovered when IVP or CT scan is obtained for hematuria or other suspected abdominal injuries. Discovery on the operating table is unlikely unless these studies have been performed or unless another renal injury is present that mandates surgical correction.

In most cases of renal artery thrombosis, recognition does not occur within the first few hours after injury. It is often 24 or more hours before microhematuria alerts the surgical team to the possibility of renal injury. The classic test for this injury is arteriography, but CT usually provides enough information for surgical exploration if time is a problem, because most arteriograms show only occlusion near the aorta with a nub of artery visible. In some instances the tear is only partial, and some dye is seen beyond the injury. As in spontaneous thrombosis, this is a favorable sign that should lead to a surgical attempt at correction of the occlusion. Segmental arterial injuries are not usually repaired, because the amount of parenchymal loss is generally insignificant. Infarction of the kidney caused by complete arterial occlusion causes pain, leukocytosis, fever, and microhematuria. These symptoms are self-limiting, and only when hypertension is persistent is nephrectomy necessary in most cases. The less than satisfactory long-term results of revascularization procedures for traumatic thrombosis of the renal artery have led some authors to recommend no surgery for unilateral thrombosis unless impaired renal function is found or bilateral thrombosis is present. In a review by Spirnak and Resnick in 1987, only 17 cases of bilateral renal artery thrombosis were found to be documented in the literature. Ten patients underwent attempted revascularization, but only four were successful. In another study in 1981, Clark and associates found 34 patients who had undergone revascularization procedures for unilateral thrombosis; in only five was some degree of renal function salvaged, and in only one case was a patient normotensive with normal renal function. Time to revascularization in Clark's series ranged from 4 to 12 hours; the best result was seen in the patient who had occlusion for only 4 hours. Of the 34 patients reported by Clark and associates, 12 eventually required nephrectomy for hypertension. Spirnak and Resnick, on the basis of their own experience and that of Clark and associates, recommended that revascularization be attempted only when bilateral thrombosis is present. Cosby and Peterson have suggested that the course of unrepaired thrombosis is not always predictable. Recannulization does occur and function has been reported to return in some cases. Thus, performance of bilateral, immediate nephrectomy when thrombosis of both renal arteries is discovered is not the best course. Only after observation can one be sure that nephrectomy is necessary. According to Cosby and Peterson, one patient in their experience had significant improvement in function after exploration without repair. Thus, if surgical correction is not carried out, one should perform nephrectomy only as a secondary procedure when bilateral thrombosis is present. Review of the literature reveals that the most effective method of revascularization appear to be venous bypass using saphenous vein or inferior mesenteric vein after extraction of the thrombus and autotransplantation. Embolectomy and thrombectomy alone do not appear to be effective.

Few authors have much experience with renal artery thrombosis, and published reports are anecdotal at best. Attempts to summarize the literature also appear to be unrewarding, since many factors have led to failures in these patients. Conflicting opinions exist over whether surgery or fibrinolytic therapy is best in cases of spontaneous thrombosis and thromboembolism, and the value of surgery for unilateral, traumatic thrombosis is not revealed by a careful review of the literature. Some conclusions, however, can be made in regard to the management of these patients: (1) unilateral renal artery thrombosis secondary to blunt trauma should be aggressively treated if the time from injury to repair is less than 6 hours, or later, if the injury can be shown to have resulted only in partial occlusion; (2) unilateral traumatic thrombosis should not be explored after 24 hours unless nephrectomy is necessary for hypertension; (3) nephrectomy is indicated for uncontrollable hypertension, or pain and toxic symptoms, but should be deferred if possible when bilateral thrombosis is present until one can be sure that significant recovery of function will not occur; (4) treatment of embolism or spontaneous thrombosis of the renal artery should be aggressive and may be either surgical or medical, using streptokinase or urokinase; and (5) surgical treatment of thrombosis of the renal artery associated with arteriosclerotic disease or dissecting aneurysm produces the best results when there is preservation of renal size, demonstration of partial occlusion, slow development of the occlusive process, minimal signs of occlusion (such as leukocytosis, pain, and fever), and the presence of collateral circulation. Treatment should be directed at correction of the condition that led to the thrombosis, and treatment is surgical in all instances.

A nihilistic approach to the treatment of thromboembolism of the renal artery will lead to maximal loss of renal units. No progress can be made in the treatment of this disease unless an attempt is made to find those patients who will benefit from surgery or fibrinolytic therapy, through early diagnosis and recognition of the signs of preservation of renal viability.

SUGGESTED READING

Clark DE, et al. Renal arterial injuries caused by blunt trauma. Surgery 1981; 90:87–96.

Cosby RL, et al. Traumatic renal artery thrombosis. Am J Med 1986; 81:890–894.

Ouriel K, et al. Acute renal artery occlusion: when is revascularization justified? J Vasc Surg 1987; 5:348–355.

Peterson NE, et al. Traumatic renal infarction (review article). J Trauma 1989; 29:158–167.

Spirnak JP, et al. Revascularization of traumatic thrombosis of the renal artery. Surg Gynecol Obstet 1987; 164:22–26.

RENAL VEIN DISORDERS

STEVEN W. SIEGEL, M.D.

Renal vein thrombosis and left renal vein hypertension are venous abnormalities associated with renovascular hypertension. Renal vein thrombosis occurs in diverse clinical settings, and the diagnosis and management of this disorder depends on the age of the patient.

RENAL VEIN THROMBOSIS

In neonates, renal vein thrombosis is typically associated with dehydration, which may be secondary to vomiting, diarrhea, or sepsis. It is also more common in children of diabetic mothers, or after traumatic delivery. In this setting, a generalized thrombosis begins in the intrarenal venous system and extends outward to the renal vein. The etiology may be similar in adults owing to states of dehydration or hypercoagulability but may also include neoplasia, nephrotic syndrome, and systemic disorders, such as amyloidosis.

A low threshold of suspicion is required to make a diagnosis in both groups. The clinical presentation in infants may include the presence of flank mass, hematuria, and thrombocytopenia secondary to platelet aggregation in the thrombus. Adults who develop acute thrombosis may complain of flank pain, and there may also be associated signs of flank tenderness, hypertension, gross or microscopic hematuria, and proteinuria. Chronic renal vein thrombosis in adults may present more subtly and include additional findings of lower extremity edema and venous collateralization, such as a noncollapsing, left-sided varicocele.

Radiographic diagnosis in both groups includes renal ultrasonography or computed tomography (CT), which may reveal increased renal size in the absence of hydronephrosis or mass. Intravenous pyelography may show nonfunction. Renal angiography can disclose nonspecific findings of stretched interlobar arteries and nonvisualization of the renal vein. A definitive diagnosis can usually be established with venography, which can often be accomplished through the umbilical vein in neonates.

Treatment is centered around management of precipitating factors such as dehydration and sepsis. In adults with acute thrombosis, anticoagulation should be instituted with systemic heparinization followed by warfarin administration. Thrombolysis may not occur rapidly with systemic anticoagulation therapy and can be associated with significant hemorrhagic complications in children. Fibrinolytic therapy with streptokinase or urokinase may result in more prompt recovery of renal function, and the role of these therapies continues to be evaluated. It appears that direct thrombolytic therapy is likely to be more effective among neonates and in adults with nontraumatic acute renal vein thrombosis. This may emerge as the treatment of choice in anuric patients with bilateral renal vein thrombosis in a solitary kidney. The roles of selective venous infusion versus systemic therapy need to be further evaluated.

Surgery may be considered in patients who do not respond to medical management. Nephrectomy is the treatment of choice among patients with renal venous infarction who develop uncontrollable sepsis or hypertension. Thrombectomy is rarely effective, owing to the centripetal propagation of the thrombus, but may be considered in patients with acute bilateral thrombosis or renal vein thrombosis in a solitary kidney who do not respond to conservative treatment. Surgery may also be the treatment of choice in patients with chronic thrombosis secondary to an underlying malignancy, when therapy for both disorders can be combined. In such cases a transabdominal approach is necessary in order to gain full control of the vena cava above and below the level of the thrombus. Rarely, a combined thoracoabdominal approach may be needed to allow cardiac bypass for complete thrombectomy.

RENAL VEIN HYPERTENSION

Abnormal pressure gradients between the left renal vein and vena cava, often referred to as renal vein entrapment or the "nutcracker syndrome," can result in a state of relative venous hypertension. Patients may present with flank pain and/or hematuria, which results from renal pelvic and ureteral varices or from submucosal renal caliceal or forniceal veins under increased pressure owing to the state of venous hypertension.

Diagnosis is made when patients with unexplained and persistent hematuria have undergone a negative routine evaluation, including renal angiography. Renal venography with measurement of renal vein to vena cava pressure gradients are necessary to establish the diagnosis. Appropriate treatment may initially include bed rest, hydration, and transfusion as indicated. If bleeding persists, more aggressive measures may be performed, including caudal relocation and reimplantation of the left renal vein into the vena cava. Occasionally, ligation of renal pelvic or ureteral varices may be sufficient to resolve hematuria. Rarely, partial or simple nephrectomy may be required for refractory cases.

SUGGESTED READING

Kay R. Renal vein thrombosis. In: Novick, AC, Straffon RA, eds. Vascular problems in urologic surgery. Philadelphia: WB Saunders, 1982:205.

Stewart BH, Reiman G. Left renal venous hypertension "nutcracker" syndrome managed by direct renocaval re-implantation. Urology 1982; 20:265.

VOIDING DISORDERS

OBSTRUCTION TO VOIDING

FRANK HINMAN, Jr., M.D.

Obstruction to voiding is evidenced clinically by difficulty (or inability) to begin urinating, poor flow, and incomplete emptying, with resultant middle and upper tract damage. The cause differs among infants (posterior urethral valves), girls and boys (dysfunctional voiding on a training-psychological basis), women (habit and hysteria), and older men (prostatic obstruction).

OBSTRUCTION IN INFANTS

Bladder neck obstruction, if it occurs at all in infants or children, is secondary to valves or dyssynergia and should be treated as such. Avoid surgery of the vesical neck without detailed urodynamic evaluation.

Obstruction by congenital posterior urethral valves is damaging. Three types are recognized, of which two have clinical significance: type I (sails or exaggerated plicae colliculi extending distally from either side of the verumontanum to attach to the anterolateral walls of the urethra) and type III (diaphragms with small central perforations distal or proximal to the verumontanum but separate from it). Either type forces the detrusor to higher pressures, resulting in dilatation of the posterior urethra, thickening of the bladder wall, and severe upper tract obstructive changes and renal failure. A voiding cystogram establishes the diagnosis. These babies should be referred to the intensive care unit of a pediatric tertiary care facility.

In severe cases, treatment begins by inserting a feeding tube in the bladder. Determine serum and molality to find if the dehydration is hypotonic or hypertonic. If hypotonic, treat dehydration and shock with colloidal volume expanders (20 ml per kilogram of body weight given rapidly) and maintenance fluids (100 ml per kilogram of body weight per day of 0.2 percent normal saline with 5 percent dextrose). Correct electrolyte imbalance; watch out for hyperkalemia by electrocardiogram (ECG) monitoring.

If the urethral catheter cannot be maintained, place a suprapubic tube percutaneously to tide the infant over the difficult days. Consider percutaneous nephrostomies or, better, cutaneous pyelostomies or loop ureterostomy if the response to bladder drainage is poor.

Ablation of the valve may be done at once in an infant in good balance or later after control of sepsis and shock. Endoscopic removal is best, but requires great care not to injure the delicate urethra by overdilatation. First, calibrate the urethra and perform a meatotomy. If the urethra still will not accommodate the instrument, perform a perineal urethrostomy. Use a straight-ahead lens to visualize the valve and confirm the presence of trabeculation. Pressing on the filled bladder will elevate the cusp and allow the electrode to hold it away from the wall during division with the cutting current. Type I valves may be divided near the verumontanum; type III valves are cut in three places. Leave a catheter in place if infection or bleeding is present. Postoperatively, observe the child for electrolyte imbalance and infection. Perform a repeat cystogram if there are complications, and as a routine in 2 to 3 months. Carry out elective reconstruction of the upper urinary tract later.

OBSTRUCTION IN BOYS AND GIRLS

Children with day and night wetting may have vesicourethral dysfunction on a behavioral basis. When severe, this constitutes the non-neurogenic–neurogenic bladder syndrome. Attempts by the child at sphincteric urinary control are futile in the face of uncontrollable bladder contractions. These contractions produce not only symptoms of the syndrome, but also anatomic and functional changes: vesical trabeculation, distortion of the ureterovesical orifices, and dilatation of the upper tracts along with residual urine and consequent bacteriuria. These changes are indistinguishable from obstructive or, particularly, neurogenic factors; these causes must therefore be ruled out.

Urodynamic investigations are seldom needed in these children, but show incoordination between detrusor contraction and the expected but not forthcoming urethral sphincter relaxation.

Since these children are usually toilet trained initially, the incoordination appears to be a learned behavior or habit, perhaps as a response to under-appreciated detrusor contractions.

The four approaches to treatment are suggestion, including hypnosis; retraining and bladder drill; biofeedback; and drug administration. Usually a combination is needed.

The first method to be applied systematically was suggestion with hypnotherapy. It was used in conjunction with other modalities, including anticholinergic drugs such as imipramine (Tofranil) in doses of 25 mg three times a day, often with a fourth dose at bedtime, which was continued until suggestion therapy was well under way. Antibacterial medication was given for infection. Fecal retention was managed by digitally breaking up the fecal mass and by use of an enema of sodium biphosphate-sodium phosphate. This was followed by nightly administration of a stool softener and laxative. Milk was withdrawn from the diet. Parents were instructed to ensure the use of mutually understandable terminology, to be sure they had confidence in the child's ability to overcome the handicap, and to dwell on every success by praise and awards. Finally, the suggestion therapy from the family was supplemented by that from the physician, to plant the ideas in the child that would lead to success in urinary control. Hypnosis is a state of markedly increased suggestibility, and ideas so placed, may last a lifetime. The psychological disturbances may also be the result rather than the cause of the voiding disturbance. Although some patients with voiding disorders initially had abnormally high psychopathology scores, these returned to normal in those patients who were urologically cured.

Biofeedback therapy was introduced for women with detrusor instability. It is a more formalized approach than suggestion and retraining, but achieves its results through similar routes.

Urodynamic biofeedback may be useful in children. After surface electrodes are applied to the perianal skin to record perineal electromyography (EMG), the child is placed on a commode containing a urinary flowmeter where he or she can see a tracing of both signals. The child learns to recognize the relationship between sphincter relaxation and urinary flow so that he or she may suppress the sphincter dyssynergia during each voiding. Proponents emphasize the need to establish close rapport with the family and with the child, who in turn is selected because of motivation to learn and a willingness to participate. Children over 10 years old are the best candidates. Reportedly, it is better if only one member of the urodynamic team works with the child, to provide continuity of rapport and learning. Success, urodynamically and clinically, has been reported in a high proportion of patients within 24 to 48 hours of in-hospital training, an improvement that lasted through the follow-up period. Since each of these children had been instructed to double void, to relax during voiding, and to spend more time during the synchronous voiding, the improvement may have stemmed as much from the obviously intense educational process focusing on the child's voiding habits as from the bladder drill regimen itself.

Formal psychotherapy is not valuable. Experience in treating psychogenic impotency has shown that suggestion and retraining are more direct and practical.

Pharmacologic manipulation is incorporated in almost all programs of therapy. Agents used have included anticholinergics to reduce the effect on the uninhibited detrusor contractions, diazepam to affect the striated muscle reaction, and phenoxybenzamine to block the alpha-adrenergic contraction of the vesical neck.

In summary, many poorly understood factors may be involved and many agents needed in the treatment of an individual child. Detailed urodynamic assessment is probably not needed for most children. Rather, retraining based on history and clinical evaluation alone can be effective.

OBSTRUCTION IN WOMEN

Acute obstruction to urination in women is a manifestation of hysteria and is treated accordingly.

Chronic incomplete emptying in women is rarely (if ever) due to vesical neck obstruction or strictures. Rather, it is an acquired pattern probably secondary to habitual deferral of urination. These women are unable to perform the normal sequence of voiding: relaxation of the perineum with concomitant contraction of the detrusor and opening of the bladder neck. They regularly strain to void, to push the urine out by abdominal pressure, which in turn reflexively contracts the perineal musculature, cutting off flow.

The treatment is re-education. Decreasing urethral irritation or psychogenic urethral contraction will help.

OBSTRUCTION IN MEN

Benign prostatic hypertrophy (BPH) is the most common cause of obstruction in men, although prostatitis and urethral stricture are not rare.

Treatment of patients with BPH may be conservative or surgical. A patient can be managed conservatively if he does not feel that his daily life is disturbed and he is not suffering renal damage. Re-examination every 6 months is advised to detect incipient damage (and to pick up incidental carcinoma). Alpha-blocking agents may be used to carry a patient through an obstructive crisis. An alternative for a few men may be intermittent self-catheterization. It is simple and safe, but operation is usually preferable.

Operation will be needed in 15 to 20 percent of patients. Overflow incontinence and persistent total obstruction are mandatory indications. Recurrent infection, vesical calculi, and severe bleeding are also strong indications for surgery. Optional indications are more flexible. Surgery may be worthwhile if the irritative symptom of frequency interferes with daytime activities and nocturia disturbs sleep. If the obstructive symptoms of a slow stream (less than 10 ml per second) and dribbling are present, operation is worthwhile. Residual urine volumes over 60 ml probably warrant correction. It is advisable to counsel patients that impotence occurs in up to 30 percent of cases. The expected retrograde ejaculation may be psychologically upsetting. Incontinence is a rare complication. The objective of surgery is to remove all the adenoma and leave the true prostate (surgical capsule) behind. The method of choice is transurethral resection (TUR), except for glands so large that they would be technically difficult to remove with this technique. Spinal anesthesia is preferred. Water is satisfactory for irrigation, since the syndrome following extravasation from the capsule results from hypervolemia and hyponatremia, not from hemolysis. It is treated by diuretics and an intravenous infusion of sodium to restore the serum level to normal. The operative mortality for TUR is less than 0.4 percent, and hospitalization is for less than 4 days. Suprapubic or retropubic prostatectomy is limited to large glands that cannot be removed transurethrally in the safe period of 1 hour. Good results can be expected from surgery.

Urethral strictures occur in 6 percent, a result of urethral manipulation by the resectoscope. The obstructive symptoms resolve if the operation has been done adequately, and the irritative ones generally clear. BPH is a common disease that may disable the patient and damage his urinary tract. Since operation carries a low incidence of morbidity and mortality, it is the current treatment of choice for men who have sufficient functional impairment to warrant it.

Alternative methods to TUR are pharmacologic or incisional intervention. An alpha-blocking agent (phenoxybenzamine, 10 mg at bedtime) will relax the vesical neck and capsule and often improve voiding. Instead of the adenoma being removed by TUR, the capsule can be induced to relax its grip on the adenoma and, through it, on the urethra by a deep incision through the entire thickness of the vesical neck and prostate.

Obstruction is harmful because it causes stasis, with consequent retention of bacteria, and back pressure, resulting in renal damage. Selection of a remedy based on its cause will allow the physician to reverse the process.

NEUROGENIC URINARY RETENTION

EDWARD J. McGUIRE, M.D.

ETIOLOGY

The causes of neurogenic urinary retention vary from the common to the distinctly rare. The most common causes are nonspecific and are associated with spinal or general anesthesia; complex operative procedures on the intervertebral discs or the vertebral column; operative procedures involving dural manipulation; those involving the pelvic floor or external anal sphincter; and, in children, procedures on or near the urethra. Extensive intracranial procedures can also be associated with temporary urinary retention. The precise mechanisms whereby these procedures, in common with traumatic injury to the vertebral column (e.g., a compression fracture), result in loss of reflex voiding is unknown. Procedures on or near the dura mater, on or near the sacral roots, and on the intervertebral discs can result in a spinal shock–like state involving bowel and bladder function, but not somatic motor or sensory activity.

Reflex vesical contractility and reflex and volitional control of the bladder are highly complex processes that involve neural activity at all levels of the central nervous system. Supraspinal influences are both facilitatory and inhibitory to lower urinary tract function, but in most circumstances inhibitory influences appear to predominate. For example, deep general or spinal anesthesia is almost never associated with involuntary voiding. Experimentally, cats, despite gross bladder overfilling, do not show reflex vesical contractility under anesthesia at various depths, including very light or very deep anesthesia. Grossman and colleagues showed that normal children did not develop reflex bladder contractile activity under light general anesthesia, but children with day- and nighttime incontinence did. A variety of influences may result in loss of reflex voiding, which appears to be a more vulnerable process than that which normally operates to modulate and inhibit vesical contractility. In the aggregate, those processes that modulate or inhibit vesical contractility constitute the storage mode of lower urinary tract function, and appear to be dominant.

Given that a number of noxious stimuli may result in transient loss of reflex vesical contractility (or a paradoxical preponderance of inhibitory factors on the lower urinary tract), and that these noxious stimuli produce their effect by unknown mechanisms, the problem is not so much how to deal with these directly but rather how to plan effective management of transient urinary retention. Prolonged vesical overdistention related to lack of reflex voiding can produce a permanent bladder muscular or neuromuscular injury. Thus, prospective management of patients at risk for transient loss of reflex activity is an important aspect of care. Chronic Foley catheter drainage carries with it a risk of infection, induction of bladder compliance abnormalities, and urethral damage. It further prevents monitoring of the patient's ability to void until the catheter is removed. For these reasons and because loss of reflex vesical contractility related to nonspecific events is associated with normal, very low bladder pressures, patients with these conditions are ideally suited for intermittent catheterization as a temporary method of management. This technique requires 4- to 6-hour catheterization with measurement of recovered volumes. Volumes greater than 500 to 600 ml should be avoided and intermittent catheterization schedules adjusted to prevent accumulation of larger bladder volumes.

ANCILLARY METHODS

Pharmacologic stimulation of reflex contractility, with or without a reduction of outlet resistance, to improve voiding function has not been demonstrated to be effective or to hasten recovery of reflex vesical contractility. The data available are largely anecdotal and have not been derived from rigidly controlled double-blind studies. Nevertheless, various agents and combinations of agents *may* have some role in the management of transient urinary retention in specific circumstances. This usually occurs when some underlying vesical or urethral abnormality, e.g., prostatic hypertrophy or diabetes, is pre-existent to an episode of retention. Bethanechol chloride (Urecholine) may facilitate existing reflex vesical contractility but should be avoided in patients with total denervation injuries and those with urethral obstruction. Combined use of bethanechol chloride and alpha-blocking agents has some theoretical basis, but there are no real data on whether this actually works. Reflex vesical contractility involves both contraction of the bladder and opening of the proximal urethral sphincter. If some process such as benign prostatic hypertrophy interferes with urethral opening, an alpha-blocking agent may be effective in facilitating voiding. In that specific circumstance, the agent should be used alone and not in conjunction with bethanechol chloride.

URODYNAMIC TESTING IN CASES OF NONSPECIFIC NEUROGENIC URINARY RETENTION

Urodynamic testing is often advocated when retention persists for more than 1 or 2 days. Neurosurgeons may ask for consultation and urodynamic testing to determine whether a true neural praxis exists. Cystometry generally reveals a low-pressure bladder with no detrusor reflex response. Although this is often interpreted as a "hypotonic" bladder, it is in fact often normal, since the normal bladder pressure response to filling is minimal. A lack of electromyographic activity recorded from the anal or external urethral sphincter during bladder filling is abnormal, indicating the lack of a normal guarding reflex response, but the finding is relatively subtle. Bulbocavernosus reflex testing, manual or electrical, measures a somatic afferent, somatic efferent response involving the pudendal nerve, and is not very useful in terms of *bladder function,* although it may provide information about sacral cord function or the degree of generalized reflex depression in spinal shock. Sensation reported by the patient during cystometrography is subjective, but it seems likely that the pathway subserving cortical recognition of bladder filling is not the same as the pathway subserving reflex contractility. Thus, the presence or absence of reported sensation is not useful in most cases as a prognostic or diagnostic clue.

SPECIFIC CAUSES OF NEUROGENIC RETENTION

Supraspinal Disease

A cardiovascular accident (CVA), a stroke, elevated intracranial pressure, or a frontal lobe lesion can produce total detrusor areflexia. Particularly in the acute stages after a CVA, a profound depression in reflex bladder activity is common. Although this is usually followed later by the development of uninhibited bladder contractility and incontinence, the initial problem is urinary retention. Most neurologic or neurosurgical patients who develop urinary retention are treated by Foley catheter drainage. This may be necessary for hourly urinary output monitoring, but after 48 to 72 hours it becomes more a matter of convenience. Chronic Foley catheter drainage results over time in loss of bladder capacity, loss of low-pressure bladder compliance, urinary tract infection, and urethral inflammation, all of which may be prejudicial to later efforts to control reflex vesical contractility. It is clear from a longitudinal functional study of patients with neurogenic retention related to spinal cord injury or peripheral neural lesions that intermittent catheterization for prolonged periods (up to 3 to 5 years) is not associated with the functional and morphologic changes associated with Foley or suprapubic catheter drainage. This is particularly true of disorders of compliance that have the most direct effect on ureteral and renal function. Disorders of compliance can be almost totally prevented by prompt initiation of intermittent catheterization; this should be employed as soon as practicable in patients who develop neurogenic retention related to intracranial processes. Intermittent catheterization, when used for temporary or permanent management of bladder dysfunction related to a neural injury or disease, should be monitored by pressure volume curves (cystometrography) rather than simple volume determinations. Pressure volume curves provide precise information on bladder responses to filling. Bladder pressure at those volumes obtained by intermittent catheterization should be kept below 10 to 12 cm H_2O to prevent infection, as well as to prevent the interaction of intravesical pressure and outlet resistance, which appears to be the mechanism for permanent loss of compliance in neurogenic vesical dysfunction. Loss of compliance is the single most important factor in the deterioration of upper tract function in these conditions.

Peripheral and Low Central Neural Lesions

Peripheral neural injuries related to pelvic extirpative operative procedures, pelvic trauma, radiation, or violent trauma below T-12 induce true detrusor areflexia related to a loss of pelvic nerve integrity or, if the injury occurs within the vertebral canal, to the components of the pelvic nerve. In general, trauma, whether surgical, radiotherapeutic, or violent, produces both sensory and motor decentralization. Specific disease processes such as tabes dorsalis or diabetes mellitus result in isolated sensory decentralization, while poliomyelitis induces isolated motor decentralization.

Injury to the *preganglionic* motor nerve supply to the bladder can occur to the motor nerve cell bodies in the sacral spinal cord, to the axon between the motor nerve cell body and to the peripheral ganglion located in the bladder wall. Complete preganglionic injury results in preservation of the postganglionic nerve cell and axon and the neuromuscular junction. Although this situation has been traditionally associated with "flaccid" bladder dysfunction, this is not the case, and motor decentralization carries a risk of development of a hypertonic bladder with a loss of compliance and loss of normal urine storage. This ultimately endangers ureteral and renal function. This process appears to be accelerated by chronic Foley or suprapubic tube drainage. Since adverse compliance changes can occur in any case of decentralization of the bladder, chronic catheter drainage should be avoided in favor of intermittent catheterization. Injuries that result in pelvic nerve damage are often temporary and incomplete, and recovery can be expected in a substantial percentage of patients. Therefore, preservation of normal bladder storage behavior is important for patients who later recover normal function, and also for those with permanent injury. At present the best way to achieve this is by intermittent catheterization. In a series of patients followed here at the University of Michigan with lower motor neuron injuries, resultant from bladder decentralization after radical hysterectomy, none developed abnormalities of bladder compliance when managed entirely by intermittent catheterization. A decentralized bladder will not be improved by bethanechol chloride administration, nor will recovery of reflex vesical contractility be hastened by alpha-blocking agents or cholinergic agents, which may serve only to impair continence. Patients with areflex vesical function, who can void by straining to completion, are almost always also incontinent with cough or exercise; thus, efforts to encourage voiding by the Valsalva or Credé technique are not helpful and can be dangerous. Intermittent catheterization is the preferred method of management. Patients with permanent vesical decentralization managed continually by intermittent catheterization never develop loss of compliance, bladder trabeculation, and leakage related to a hypertonic detrusor response to filling, which commonly occurs in patients managed by catheter drainage or various maneuvers to induce voiding by increased abdominal pressure. It is now clear that the deleterious effects on bladder storage seen after decentralization of the bladder are related to the interaction of the bladder and a fixed sphincter mechanism that maintains sufficient pressure to require bladder pressures in excess of 40 cm H_2O to drive urine across the sphincter. Once such changes in bladder storage function become well established, they are difficult to reverse, and achievement of low-pressure reservoir capability may then require augmentation cystoplasty.

Urinary Retention Associated with Suprasacral Spinal Cord Injury or Disease

Spinal cord injury results in a period of spinal shock during which all reflex activity is markedly depressed or absent below the level of the injury. While external urethral sphincter activity is minimal or absent, internal sphincter closure is maintained in spinal shock, and Credé voiding is thus impossible (except in patients with a nonfunctional internal sphincter that antedates the spinal cord injury). The ideal method of management of bladder dysfunction in the spinal shock state is intermittent catheterization. Over time, patients with upper motor neuron lesions or lesions between C1 and T12 often redevelop reflex vesical contractility with detrusor sphincter dyssynergia. Untreated, this discoordinate bladder and sphincter relationship leads to progressive increases in intravesical pressure, and if sustained over long periods a loss of bladder compliance, back pressure effect on the ureters, symptomatic febrile urinary tract infection, epididymitis and orchitis, pyelonephritis, upper tract struvite stone formation, hypertension, and death.

Patients with spinal cord injury treated continuously from shortly after injury by intermittent catheterization do not develop high-pressure vesical dysfunction, and can be managed by intermittent catheterization indefinitely or until normal reflex contractility is re-established in those with incomplete injuries. Surprisingly, some 25 percent of patients with upper motor neuron lesions never again redevelop reflex vesical contractility and can be managed permanently without drugs by intermittent catheterization (either self-administered or provided by an attendant). About 70 percent of patients do require anticholinergic agents to prevent urinary leakage, but these are effective at fairly low dosages, and the typical trabeculated, thick-walled, neurogenic bladder never develops. These findings strongly suggest that typical high-pressure neurogenic vesical dysfunction results from the interaction of areflex bladder with a discoordinate sphincter over time, a process that can be circumvented by early employment of intermittent catheterization.

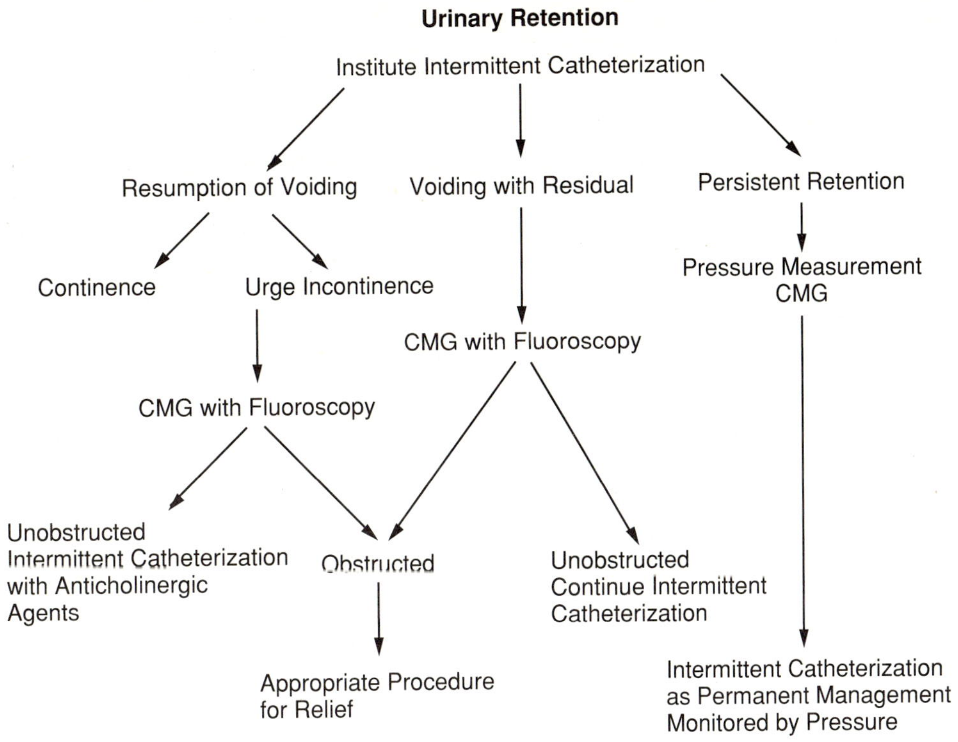

Urinary Retention

Figure 1 Flow chart for management of patients with urinary retention.

Multiple Sclerosis

Demyelinating diseases result in neurogenic vesical dysfunction similar in expression to that encountered after spinal cord injury, but not identical. The diseases are progressive, unlike spinal cord injury, and deterioration in function usually occurs with time despite treatment. Some 60 to 70 percent of multiple sclerosis patients presenting with uncomfortable bladder symptoms (which include urgency, frequency, and incontinence) show large to very large residual urine volumes. In most this is the result of detrusor external sphincter dyssynergia, which can be treated in males by sphincterotomy, or in both sexes by intermittent self-catheterization and anticholinergic agents. About 10 to 15 percent of these patients have residual urine volumes in excess of 500 ml and on urodynamic evaluation show detrusor areflexia. These individuals do not initially require anticholinergic agents when begun on intermittent catheterization, but about 50 percent, when so treated, ultimately redevelop reflex detrusor dysfunction and leakage and require these agents.

Urodynamics and Intermittent Catheterization in Neurogenic Disease

Of all the factors that determine outcome in patients treated for bladder dysfunction by intermittent catheterization, none is more important than adequate control of vesical pressure to those volumes obtained at the time of such catheterization (Fig. 1). Periodic urodynamic testing to ensure that pressures are low is an essential element in management by this or any other technique.

SUGGESTED READING

Grossman HB, Koff SA, Diokno AC. Cystometry in children. J Urol 1977; 117:646.

POSTPROSTATECTOMY URINARY INCONTINENCE

STEVEN P. PETROU, M.D.
DAVID M. BARRETT, M.D.

The patient's opinion as to whether his prostatectomy was successful depends largely on his postoperative continence. Postprostatectomy continence depends on the efficacy of urethral closure from the verumontanum to the proximal bulbous urethra. The urethral sphincter in this area consists of an inner layer of mucosal lining accompanied by vascular tissue, a middle layer of elastic tissue and smooth muscle, and an outer layer of intrinsic and extrinsic skeletal muscle. The inner layer of mucosal lining provides an all-important sealing effect. The intrinsic skeletal muscle is slow twitch and slow fatiguing, providing a resting tonus, while the extrinsic skeletal muscle is able to provide a rapid but fast-tiring volitional contraction. The extrinsic striated muscle is innervated by the pudendal nerve. The smooth muscles of this distal urethral sphincter mechanism contain alpha-adrenergic receptors and are innervated by the pelvic nerve.

The complication of urinary incontinence after both simple and radical prostatectomy is not uncommon. Rates of incontinence range from 0.5 to 40 percent. With improving optics for transurethral surgery, as well as refined nerve-sparing techniques for radical prostatectomy, the incidence of postprostatectomy incontinence may decrease. The key to successful therapy for postprostatectomy incontinence lies in a clear elucidation of its precise cause.

ETIOLOGY

Postprostatectomy incontinence is not due to sphincteric damage alone. Other etiologies include detrusor instability, decreased bladder wall compliance, and a combination of these. Not to be forgotten is overflow incontinence secondary to outlet obstruction due to a urethral stricture or bladder neck contracture.

Radiotherapy may alter both bladder and sphincter mechanism. Radiation sequelae such as decreased tissue viability and fibrosis decrease bladder compliance and predispose patients with sphincter malfunction to urinary incontinence.

Detrusor instability may develop secondary to urinary tract infection (UTI). Dysuria should not be automatically attributed to postinstrumentation urethritis or cystitis. Appropriate antibiotic therapy guided by culture and sensitivity tests is warranted.

DIAGNOSIS

Evaluation of the postoperative incontinent patient should include a careful history and physical examination, urinalysis and urine culture, urodynamics, cystourethroscopy, and renal function studies. The physician's discretion should govern the use of these tests within the appropriate postoperative time frame. During the first 6 months after surgery, we concentrate on the physical examination to rule out bladder distention and obstructive phenomena such as phimosis or metal stenosis. If available, ultrasound postvoid residual measurements are an excellent method to assess bladder emptying. The physical examination should include an efficient neurologic examination, including assessment of the anal sphincter tone, perianal sensation, presence of a bulbocavernosal reflux, and presence of the appropriate sensorium. No urologic physical examination is complete without a rectal examination, which should be done to rule out any local neoplastic recurrences. Evaluation of the perigenital skin will allow the physician to determine the severity of urinary leakage. Urinalysis and urine culture should be obtained to rule out UTI.

If bladder emptying cannot be ascertained, a No. 20 Fr catheter is passed to ensure absence of obstruction and also to check any postvoid residual. If the patient has an elevated bladder volume (more than 150 ml) and no evidence of obstruction, a water cystometrogram is obtained. Clean intermittent catheterization may be needed. If a catheter cannot be passed, cystoscopy is performed with suitable anesthesia to evaluate and treat a possible urethral stricture or bladder neck contracture.

Proper performance of the Janet exercises helps optimize the chances of rapid attainment of continence (Table 1). These exercises should be performed once a day as specified to avoid chronic fatigue of the pelvic floor musculature. Clinical observations suggest that the once-a-day routine provides the best results.

During the 6- to 12-month postoperative period, therapy and diagnosis should be tailored to the severity of the symptoms. Patients who are improving, or who have minimal to mild stress incontinence and wear two or fewer absorbent pads per day, may simply be observed during this period.

In patients with severe incontinence (using more than two pads per day) a formal incontinence work-up

Table 1 Janet Exercises for Bladder Control

1. If possible, perform exercise upon rising

2. With both rectal and bladder muscles, try to hold back urine

3. Walk around the room concentrating on holding back urine, then cough

4. Bend over and pick up something from the floor; sit on a chair and then stand up

5. Relax rectal and bladder muscles and start to void; when the stream has started, tighten muscles again to stop the stream

6. Repeat 3, 4, and 5 above twice, then empty the bladder completely

7. Perform the exercise only once each day

may be instituted at this time. This should include history taking, neurourologic physical examination, and urinary bacteriologic studies. We also include cystourethroscopy and urodynamics studies. The cystourethroscopy helps to classify the appearance of the distal sphincter mechanism, bladder neck, and bladder. The urodynamics study categorizes bladder wall compliance and detrusor activity. If the urodynamics do not correlate with the history, provocative measures such as coughing, standing, and a Valsalva maneuver should be instituted at the time of the urodynamics studies. Electromyographic studies help to assess external sphincter activity, but are not integral to the urodynamics study at this time. A uroflometric study should be obtained. Video studies, although an extremely helpful adjunct to urodynamics, are not obtained at our institution in this clinical setting.

PHARMACOLOGIC THERAPY

If the clinical evaluation of the incontinent patient leads to a diagnosis that includes detrusor instability or low bladder compliance, pharmacologic therapy is indicated. An unstable detrusor or decreased bladder compliance may respond to several types of agents, including anticholinergics (propantheline bromide), musculotropic relaxants (oxybutynin chloride, dicyclomine), and tricyclic antidepressants (imipramine). The emphasis of the therapy is upon optimization of detrusor stability and bladder compliance before surgery is contemplated. Therapy is usually started about 3 to 6 months postoperatively. The usual starting doses are oxybutynin chloride, 5 mg orally three to four times a day; dicyclomine, 20 mg orally four times a day; propantheline bromide, 15 to 30 mg orally every 4 to 6 hours; and imipramine, 25 mg orally four times a day. Side effects of propantheline and oxybutynin include dry mouth, pupillary dilatation, drowsiness, tachycardia, and decreased intestinal motility. Side effects of the imipramine include abnormal liver function, rash, obstruction jaundice, weakness, fatigue, sedation, tremor, and agranulocytosis. Imipramine works very well with anticholinergic medications, because their effects are additive. Thus, if optimal results are not obtainable with one agent, combination therapy may be used. Treatment is continued for 2 to 3 months, at which time the patient is clinically reassessed. If compliance or detrusor instability has not been optimized, the pharmacologic regimen is readjusted. If the symptoms have abated, the pharmacologic therapy is not altered until the 12-month postoperative check, at which time a pharmacologic wean may be instituted. If the patient has continued incontinence but optimized detrusor stability or bladder compliance, he is a surgical candidate.

The key to assessment of the efficacy of the pharmacologic therapy is to remember that the incontinence may be a mixed variety, i.e., of both sphincteric and vesical dysfunction. If the patient is still incontinent, it does not mean that the medical therapy has failed. Urodynamic testing will help indicate whether medical therapy is working.

SURGICAL APPROACH

After the appropriate time has elapsed and detrusor instability or bladder compliance has been optimally addressed, the patient may be considered an appropriate surgical candidate. He usually has mixed emotions about another possible procedure; he wants to be socially continent, but feels that he has just recovered from an operation.

There are many continence-restoring procedures, ranging from endoscopy to open surgery. Bladder neck reconstruction may be considered, but the postoperative changes in the tissues from the previous prostatectomy often make this a technically difficult procedure. Procedures that increase urethral resistance by compression of the bulbar urethra with intrinsic tissues have been described but not generally used. These include urethral compression by ischial and bulbocavernosal muscle plication, crural cross and approximation, and embedding the urethra between the corpora cavernosum.

Periurethral injection techniques have been developed using both polytetrafluoroethylene (polytef) paste and crosslinked collagen. These are viable concepts currently under clinical investigation. Prosthetic devices include both passive and active devices. Kaufman described a passive device that applied continuous compression on the bulbar urethra; although modified, the device is not currently used. In 1976 Rosen developed an active device consisting of an occluding balloon that, when inflated, compressed the urethra against two contra-member arms. This is a good concept, but clinical results have not led to its widespread use.

The cornerstone of our treatment of postprostatectomy incontinence is the artificial genitourinary sphincter (AGUS), which consists of three basic components: the balloon reservoir, the inflatable cuff, and the control assembly. The balloon reservoir is constructed to provide a preset specific pressure within the hydraulic system. The pressure produced is dependent on the elasticity in the wall of the balloon and the amount of fluid in the system. Although the cuff is manufactured in several sizes and is for either bladder neck or bulbous urethral placement with post–radical prostatectomy incontinence patients as well as post-transurethral prostatectomy patients, we place the cuff only around the bulbous urethra. This is technically much easier than addressing the postoperative bladder neck. The control assembly of the sphincter is approximately 1.2 cm wide and 3.3 cm long. The upper part of the control assembly contains the resistor and valves needed to transfer fluid to and from the cuff. The bottom half of the control assembly is a bulb that the patient squeezes to transfer fluid within the device. The deactivation button is on the control assembly. This activates the valves that, when seated, block the fluid pathway so that fluid in the pressure reservoir cannot get to the cuff, and vice versa. When the patient wishes to void, the control assembly is squeezed two to three times. This forces fluid from the cuff into the reservoir, which opens the cuff and allows urine to pass through the urethra. The balloon reservoir then repressurizes the cuff through the control assembly resistors, and within 3 to 4 minutes the urethra is closed.

Before surgical placement of the artificial sphincter, a careful physical examination must be made to rule out any cutaneous infections. If needed, a Foley catheter should be anchored for 1 to 2 weeks to promote skin healing. Sterility of the urine must be ascertained preoperatively. Hair is removed just before surgery to reduce the bacterial colonization in the small cuts that accompany shaving. The patient is positioned in an exaggerated bent-leg dorsolithotomy position for bulbourethral placement. A No. 12 French urethral catheter is anchored after appropriate prepping and draping, and the bladder is drained and then irrigated with 100 ml of antibiotic solution.

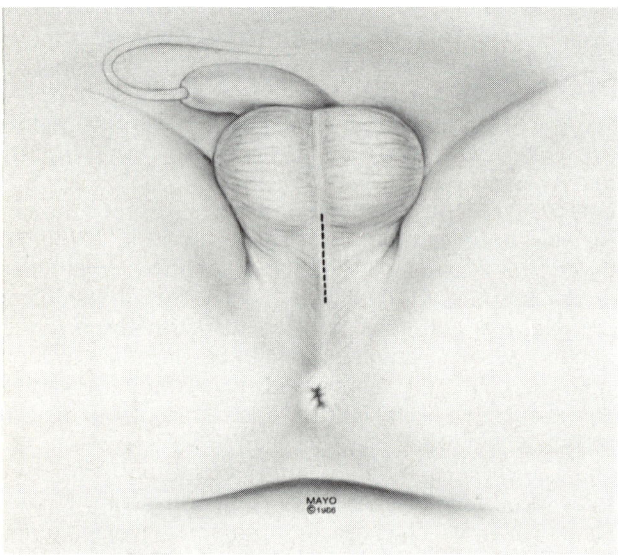

Figure 1 Incision in the perineum for bulbous urethra cuff placement.

For bulbous urethral cuff placement, a small midline perineal incision is made over the bulbous urethra (Fig. 1). The urethra is adequately mobilized to accept a 2-cm wide cuff (Fig. 2). When the urethral plane is established, we routinely place a 4.5-cm cuff around this mobilized urethra (Fig. 3). We consider that measurement is not mandatory, and uniformly use the 4.5-cm cuff. The pressure reservoir is placed in a developed pocket beneath the rectus muscle and anterior rectus fascia. Its tubing is brought through a separate stab incision in the anterior rectus fascia and brought down the appropriate plane to connect with the pump tubing. We routinely fill the reservoir with 22 ml of an iso-osmotic contrast medium to ensure appropriate fluid volume in the system. For most patients with uncomplicated bulbous urethral cuffs, we place a 61- to 70-cm pressure balloon reservoir. If the patient is at high risk, i.e., status postradiotherapy, the 51- to 60-cm pressure reservoir is used to minimize tissue pressure ischemia. The control assembly is placed in the scrotum in a lateral dependent position. The quick-connect tubing connections can be used, but we make all tubing connections with 2-0 Prolene. Upon completion of the sphincter placement and after the skin has been closed, we deactivate the mechanism. The Foley catheter is left in place overnight and removed on the first postoperative morning.

POSTOPERATIVE MANAGEMENT

Postoperative discomfort is moderate. Ice packs to the scrotum help reduce the symptoms. The patient may enjoy a transient continence postoperatively, but this usually resolves after the postoperative edema resolves. If the patient has difficulty voiding, the postvoid residual is checked. If the recorded volume is greater than 100 ml, he is placed on a clean intermittent catheterization program using a No. 12 French catheter. Activation is performed 6 to 8 weeks postoperatively. Indwelling

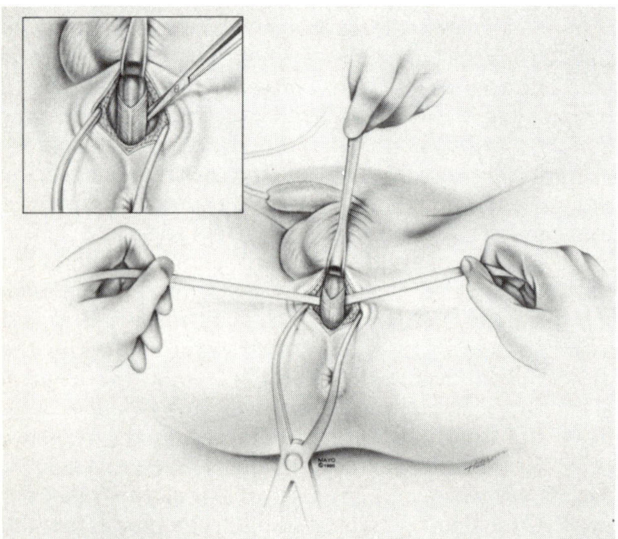

Figure 2 Mobilization of the urethra for cuff placement.

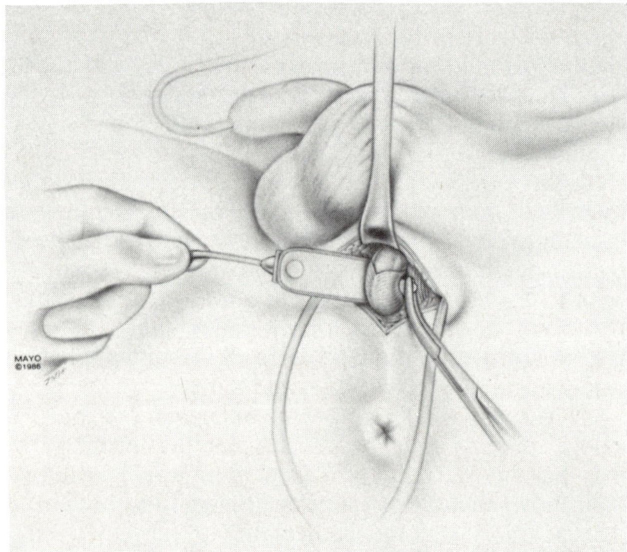

Figure 3 Placement of a cuff around the mobilized urethra.

catheters or external occlusion clamps should not be used or should be deactivated. Upon the patient's return for activation, an inflate-deflate radiograph is obtained to confirm an appropriate volume of contrast material in the system. Before activation, the patient is re-educated about the sphincter operation. Concepts of nighttime sphincter activation should be reinforced as well as that of the second pumping at the time of voiding to ensure maximum bladder drainage if necessary. Patient education should also include his recognition that prophylactic antibiotics should be given before any instrumentation procedure (e.g., dental work).

COMPLICATIONS AND SEQUELAE

The ability of the cuff to provide external urethral compression to ensure satisfactory coaptation of the urethral mucosa is the key to achieving continence. Unfortunately, this pressure may lead to ischemia of underlying tissues and possible erosion of the cuff. Erosion may manifest itself as a recurrence of incontinence as well as a periprostatic infection. Nighttime deactivation in theory provides a period of decreased compression, thus lessening possible vascular ischemia. This should be emphasized to patients who are dry when recumbent. Erosion most often presents 3 to 4 months after implantation. If it occurs in the immediate postoperative period, it is usually due to an unrecognized iatrogenic urethral entry. Cardinal symptoms of erosion or impending erosion include perineal or scrotal pain, recurrent incontinence, UTI, and bloody urethral discharge. Diagnostic steps should include cystourethroscopy and retrograde urethrography. If the diagnosis of erosion is confirmed, the cuff should be removed and a course of intravenous antibiotics given. A silicone catheter may be placed in the bladder for optimal bladder drainage for approximately 2 weeks. A retrograde urethrogram should be obtained to rule out any extravasation before removal of the urethral catheter.

There may be erosion without the presence of an infectious process. If so, the cuff should be removed and a stainless steel plug used to occlude the tubing. A course of antibiotics should be instituted. After 3 months and a negative preoperative evaluation, a new cuff may be placed at a site different from that of the original sphincter cuff. If an infectious process is diagnosed, the entire device should be removed and a reimplantation performed at a later operative setting (approximately 3 to 6 months later).

As with any other approach to the treatment of incontinence, the potential for recurrent incontinence does exist with the artificial genitourinary sphincter. Potential causes include UTI with associated detrusor instability, cuff erosion, fluid loss from the sphincter system, occlusion of the control assembly secondary to debris, and improper operation of the device by the patient. Upon his initial presentation with recurrent incontinence, it is wise to begin with an inflate-deflate film to rule out system leaks or tubing kinks of the sphincter system. Physical examination should include

an examination of the cuff assembly to ensure that it has not been inactivated accidentally by the patient. If the inflate-deflate film is normal, cystourethroscopy is needed to rule out a urethral erosion, and urodynamics studies should be performed to evaluate detrusor instability. A urinalysis and urine culture should be obtained to rule out UTI. If these tests are negative, a urethral pressure profile should be performed in the appropriate setting. If the urethral pressure profile appears low, the patient may benefit by an increase in balloon reservoir pressure or by downsizing to a 4.5-cm cuff if this is not already the cuff size in place.

If no contrast material appears on the inflate-deflate film, a leak is diagnosed and surgical exploration is needed. At the time of surgery, it is advisable to check the reservoir and cuff assembly first, since these are easier to isolate. Electrical continuity testing may be used to check for leaks. Unfortunately, the cuff is the most common site of leakage, and also the most technically difficult to replace. If no leak can be demonstrated intraoperatively, the entire sphincter system should be replaced.

Control assembly function can usually be assessed by examination and pumping of the control assembly. Inability to compress the plunger may signify a mechanical malfunction as well as a tubing kink or occlusion with particulate matter.

A patient with an artificial sphincter needs to be alert to several possible situations. As mentioned before, any invasive procedure, including dental work, should be performed with antibiotic prophylaxis. The patient and his family should also realize that in an emergency the health care team must be made aware of the sphincter's presence. The sphincter must be deactivated before catheter placement. If long-term catheterization is needed, a urologist should be consulted for a suprapubic tube placement under fluoroscopic guidance.

For patients with postprostatectomy incontinence, the artificial genitourinary sphincter offers a well-established therapy choice. With the appropriate surgical techniques and antibiotic prophylaxis, infection rates can be maintained at 2 percent. In the Mayo Clinic experience, socially acceptable continence rates have been achieved in more than 90 percent of patients. It is hoped that, with increasing interest in the field of incontinence, further improvements in incontinence therapy will be developed.

SUGGESTED READING

Barrett DM, Goldwasser B. The artificial urinary sphincter: current management philosophy. AUA Update Series, Lesson 32, Volume V, 1986.

Gundian JC, Barrett DM, Parulker BG. Mayo Clinic experience with the use of the AMS 800 artificial urinary sphincter for urinary incontinence following radical prostastectomy. J Urol 1989; 142: 1459–1461.

Igel TC, Barrett DM, Segura JW, et al. Perioperative and postoperative complications from bilateral pelvic lymphadenectomy and radical retropubic prostatectomy. J Urol 1987; 137:1189.

Wein AJ, Barrett DM. Voiding function and dysfunction: a logical and practical approach. Chicago: Year Book, 1988.

NEUROGENIC URINARY INCONTINENCE

EMIL A. TANAGHO, M.D.

Neurogenic incontinence is a difficult problem to manage successfully; to achieve this, a proper understanding of its basic mechanism is essential. In one sense it is totally different from other types of incontinence, yet it can overlap and needs proper evaluation to be distinguished from other symptomatically similar forms. Neurogenic incontinence can simulate overflow and urge incontinence, and occasionally stress incontinence, although the mechanism is completely different.

ANATOMIC CONSIDERATIONS

Urinary continence is dependent on the functional integrity of the lower urinary tract and its two main components, the urinary bladder (as a reservoir) and the bladder outlet (as a sphincteric mechanism). Although some cases of neurogenic incontinence are due primarily to the failure of one component or the other, the cause often is a combination of the two.

Urinary Bladder

The urinary bladder, which is innervated by the autonomic nervous system (primarily its parasympathetic division originating from the sacral segment S2-S4) is a mesh of muscle bundles capable of expanding to accommodate volumes up to a normal range of 400 to 500 ml while sustaining a constant, relatively low intravesical pressure of about 10 cm H_2O. The normal bladder can perceive the sensation of fullness; when it is ready for emptying, active contraction of the detrusor will lead to an increase in intravesical pressure and a synchronous opening of the sphincteric mechanism, resulting in voiding and complete emptying. Although the bladder is an involuntary muscular organ, it is under voluntary control, permitting the individual either to initiate contractions or to inhibit them under complete volition.

Sphincteric Mechanism

This is composed of two distinct elements, both intrinsic to the bladder outlet: the smooth muscle component, which constitutes what is commonly called the internal sphincter, and the striated muscular component, commonly known as the external sphincter. Both are innervated by the sacral segment of the spinal cord, and function in coordination with the detrusor muscle at the initiation of voiding. The internal sphincteric mechanism, although not an anatomic entity as a sphincteric muscle, represents a direct continuation of the detrusor muscle. With progressive bladder filling, it tightens progressively to maintain continence. When the capacity is exceeded, active opening of the internal meatus will lead to a drop in the sphincteric closure pressure. The striated external sphincter is innervated via the pudendal nerve by somatic fibers that likewise are under voluntary control and permit relaxation in coordination with detrusor activity; this allows lowering of the pelvic floor as well as a further decrease in the urethral closure pressure in the anatomic segment it surrounds.

CLASSIFICATION

Urinary incontinence as a result of neurogenic dysfunction can be classified as active or passive. The former is noted primarily in patients with a spastic lesion, in whom the sphincteric mechanism is active. Although the mechanism is not under voluntary control, it still exerts adequate closure pressure, if not higher than normal. However, these patients also have a hyperreflexive detrusor with uninhibited contractions, and this hyperactivity will increase the intravesical pressure in excess of the sphincteric pressure, leading to leakage of urine. In passive incontinence the sphincteric mechanism is weakened or completely lacking. Although the intravesical pressure is not abnormally high, any increase in intra-abdominal pressure will cause it to exceed the already low outlet resistance, resulting in urinary leakage.

Generally speaking, active incontinence is encountered most commonly with suprasegmental lesions (upper motor neuron lesions), and passive incontinence with lesions involving the micturition center or more distal to that level. Urinary incontinence can also be classified as due to the detrusor or the sphincter. The former corresponds to active urinary incontinence and the latter to passive incontinence.

A more common classification is based on the functions of the lower urinary tract: urinary incontinence due to failure of the reservoir or of retention.

Failure of Reservoir Function

In addition to the hyperreflexiveness with uninhibited contractions commonly encountered in suprasegmental lesions, poor compliance in the detrusor muscle can cause loss of reservoir function. Bladders so affected can be contractile or contracted. As a result of poor compliance, the intravesical pressure rises progressively with minimal bladder filling to exceed the outlet resistance and cause urinary leakage. Thus, since no specific activity is the cause, it might be considered separately from the initial classification of active incontinence. Not uncommonly, this is encountered in meningomyelocele patients who essentially have a lower motor neuron lesion, but, their bladders having lost compliance early, subsequently exhibit progressively increasing intravesical pressure with minimal bladder filling. These patients often have partial lesions, and to some extent still significant striated sphincteric activity capable of offering a certain degree of outlet resistance, although not enough to overcome the increased intravesical pressure. This particular group of patients is important because they often have a significant back pressure effect in the upper urinary tract leading to early deterioration and possible vesicoureteral reflux or lower ureteral obstruction. Indeed, once this group is recognized, it should be managed aggressively because of the potential damage to the upper urinary tract.

Failure of Retention Function

As discussed above, the sphincteric mechanism has two components: the internal sphincter, which receives its innervation primarily from the autonomic nervous system, with a major contribution from the pelvic parasympathetic fibers and the lower thoracic/upper lumbar sympathetic fibers; and the external sphincter, which receives its main innervation from the somatic nerve fibers carried along the pudendal nerve.

Lesions involving the sacral segment of the cauda equina, if complete, will result in a total loss of activity of both the smooth and striated muscular components. The bladder neck usually is widely funneled, and the external sphincter loses its spontaneous activity and offers minimal resistance. These patients are prone to incontinence, although not uncommonly the level of the lesion renders the bladder musculature itself atonic and lax and the intravesical pressure low. As a result, they can retain certain volumes, but they experience leakage with any increase in intravesical pressure and can never use their full bladder capacity. Thus, although incontinence is severe, the upper urinary tract is protected because these patients cannot build up sufficient intravesical pressure to interfere with its integrity. Most often, however, the clinical picture is not as complete as described, and one component retains some activity: e.g., with some activity in the internal sphincter and a complete loss in the striated sphincter, the entire pelvic floor would be flaccid and atonic.

DIAGNOSIS

Urinary incontinence in the presence of a significant neuropathy poses no diagnostic dilemma; the purpose of evaluation is to define the exact mechanism, i.e., one originating from detrusor or sphincteric dysfunction or from a combination. The difficulty arises when the neuropathy is not clear, such as in patients with multiple sclerosis as well as spinal stenosis, or those with disc problems in addition to partial traumatic damage to the spinal cord.

One caveat: even when the neuropathy is clear, one must establish that this is not another form of incontinence: a male patient may also have overflow incontinence from a mechanical obstruction, or a female may also have severe urinary incontinence from anatomic stress. After a complete urologic and neurologic history has been taken, radiographic evaluation is important to demonstrate the integrity of the upper urinary tract, the status of the reservoir, and the state of the sphincteric mechanism. Intravenous pyelography, cystourethrography, and if possible cinefluoroscopy are helpful.

An essential element in the evaluation is a urodynamic study, to demonstrate whether detrusor or sphincteric dysfunction is the underlying cause. The following are valuable: bladder responses to progressive filling; the sphincteric pressure profile and its response to progressive filling and the initiation of voiding; detrusor hyperreflexia and uninhibited activity (in patients with hyperreflexia); electromyelographic studies of the striated urinary sphincter; and, in selected patients, the response to neurostimulation of sacral roots and pudendal nerve, with or without blocking and measurement of latencies.

Incontinence arising from uninhibited detrusor contractions or detrusor hyperreflexia or poor compliance can be easily delineated. Cases arising from sphincteric weakness, precipitous sphincteric relaxation and decrease in pressure, or a lack of electromyographic activity of the pelvic floor musculature and external sphincter are all significant. Establishing the integrity of the sacral root reflex arc by neurostimulation of the sacral roots, with simultaneous recording of intravesical and intraurethral pressures at the levels of the internal and the external sphincter, can be valuable to achieve the proper diagnosis. Responses of the external sphincter and pelvic floor musculature to active contraction, to progressive bladder filling, and to sacral root stimulation are informative when multiple causes overlap.

It is important to determine the relative extent of each factor (sphincteric weakness or detrusor hyperreflexia) to direct management toward the predominating cause.

TREATMENT

Management is generally difficult. The approach should be guided by the need to rehabilitate the neuropathic condition and to alleviate the potentially damaging sequelae. The choice of treatment varies with the severity of the lesion, its potential progression, and the integrity of the system at the time of initiation of therapy. Especially in spinal cord injury and meningomyelocele patients, the earlier the treatment is instituted, the greater is the chance of preserving the integrity of the entire urinary system.

Conservative Management

Failure of Reservoir Function

A proper understanding of the function and capacity of the bladder and the role of detrusor hyperreflexia is essential in the management of reservoir dysfunction. Fortunately, this lends itself to pharmacologic manipulation to suppress the detrusor hyperreflexia; if this is successful, the patient may regain adequate reservoir function to maintain dryness for a reasonable time: 2 to 4 hours. Drug response depends on the initial functional bladder capacity, the extent of spasticity and hyperreflexia, and the presence of any significant lack of compliance due to collagen deposition and mural changes in the bladder wall.

Anticholinergic Drugs. These are used primarily to treat detrusor hyperreflexia and uninhibited contractions. Although many anticholinergic drugs are of significant clinical value, the one most commonly used is oxybutynin (Ditropan), a tertiary amine anticholinergic drug with antispasmodic action. The usual dosage is 5 mg two to four times a day, depending on the patient's tolerance and responses. Side effects are dry mouth, some drowsiness, palpitations, and occasional nausea. Patients should be careful to stay below their threshold of tolerance; this agent is contraindicated in those with high intraocular pressure.

Propantheline bromide (Pro-Banthine) is usually less effective than oxybutynin, but occasionally a combination of the two is effective. The usual dosage is 15 mg two to three times a day, with perhaps a larger dose at bedtime. Side effects are dry mouth, visual disturbances, and increased intraocular pressure. Some patients tolerate propantheline better than oxybutynin.

Imipramine hydrochloride (Tofranil) is a tricyclic antidepressant with a strong anticholinergic, antimuscarinic action and a significant effect on detrusor hyperreflexia. The usual dosage is 25 mg two to four times daily by mouth. Side effects are dry mouth, constipation, blurred vision, and drowsiness.

Antihistaminic Drugs. These produce an anticholinergic effect by antagonizing the histamine-mediated release of acetylcholine. Chlorpheniramine maleate can be taken alone in the long-acting 8.0-mg capsules/tablets orally twice a day or in combination with 75 mg of phenylpropanolamine hydrochloride (Ornade Spansules). The latter produces an anticholinergic effect on the detrusor as well as alpha-receptor stimulation to improve outlet resistance.

Musculotropic Relaxant Drugs. These exert an effect by direct depression of smooth muscle activity. The most common is flavoxate hydrochloride (Urispas), 200 mg three to four times daily by mouth.

Failure of Retention Mechanism

The first line of conservative management in this group of patients is intermittent catheterization. Although these individuals have very low outlet resistance, they also have an atonic bladder and can retain various volumes before they start to leak. Regular intermittent catheterization every 4 to 6 hours, depending on the total functional capacity, will eliminate leakage most of the time. Patients who are not able to empty the bladder before it reaches the leaking point (i.e., when the increase in intravesical pressure becomes excessive) can wear minimal protection.

Pharmacologic manipulation is less successful in this group, but alpha-receptor stimulants may be of some value. Ephedrine sulfate has a stimulating effect on both alpha and beta receptors and is usually given in 30- to 60-mg dosages three to four times daily orally. Phentermine resin (Ionamin) is a sympathomimetic drug with a stimulating effect on both alpha and beta receptors, which increases urethral sphincteric smooth muscle activity and partially relaxes the detrusor muscle. It is usually given in a 15-mg dose two to three times daily orally.

Surgical Management

The goal again is rehabilitation of the system to restore its normal function. However, this is not always feasible, and other principles may be applicable.

Sphincterotomy. This is an attempt to eliminate all outlet resistance and is commonly used in spastic hyperreflexive situations so that the bladder will remain completely empty with the use of an external appliance or condom catheter. This is applicable in male patients only. Many people consider this the easiest way to preserve the upper urinary tract, but it clearly is not a rehabilitative approach and may actually interfere with other more helpful modes of treatment.

Bladder Augmentation. This is a valuable means of improving reservoir function, especially in patients with very poor compliance owing to actual mural changes and chronic hypertrophy. When the bladder cannot expand even under anesthesia, but the sphincteric mechanism is adequate, the capacity can be augmented by detubularized bowel segments. Most of the time these patients have to rely on intermittent catheterization postoperatively, but they will have regained continence and preserved the upper urinary tract.

Artificial Sphincter Implant. This is useful in patients with a severe degree of sphincteric damage in association with low-pressure, large-capacity bladders; in males it is applied around the bulbous urethra. When the device is deflated, the patient can void either by detrusor contraction (if some capability is preserved) or by straining and the Valsalva maneuver. A complete sphincterotomy can precede the implant operation. Intermittent catheterization is rarely necessary; in fact, it is hazardous in the presence of a urethral cuff and can lead to significant urethral damage.

Urinary Diversion to Continent Reservoirs. I view this as a defeatist approach that should be reserved for cases of progressively deteriorating upper urinary tract function. Even then, because free drainage is essential, a simple conduit is preferable.

Other Approaches. These are to be condemned: denervation of the bladder through cystolysis or transvesical transection and resuturing, and denervation of the bladder base through phenol or alcohol injection. Although early results from these measures were encouraging, the long-term result has always been complete failure.

Neurosurgical Approach: Neurostimulation. In selected cases of detrusor hyperreflexia, neurostimulation of the sacral roots has been effective in suppressing the hyperactivity, relying on the known reflex response of the detrusor muscle to stimulation of the somatic component of the sacral plexus (which aborts and inhibits detrusor contractility). If patients with detrusor hyperreflexia and spinal cord injury, meningomyelocele, multiple sclerosis, and other neuropathies show significant improvement in symptoms after temporary testing, a permanent sacral root electrode is placed over the most responsive root, usually S3.

Dorsal Rhizotomy. Complete dorsal rhizotomy of S2-S4 extra- or intradurally is very effective in eliminating detrusor hyperreflexia and vastly increasing bladder capacity. I have seen increases from a 150- or 200-ml capacity to 600 to 800 ml. Dorsal rhizotomy alone definitely improves reservoir function. However, in patients with suprasegmental lesions and spastic upper motor neuron lesions, it is beneficial to add electrode

implantation on the sacral roots to induce detrusor contraction and bladder evacuation (the so-called bladder pacemaker). This combination has achieved complete rehabilitation of properly selected patients.

SUGGESTED READING

Beck RP. Neuropharmacology of the lower urinary tract in women. Obstet Gynecol Clin North Am 1989; 16:753–771.

Goldwasser B, Barrett DM, Wein AJ. Surgery of the neuropathic bladder. In: Libertino JA, ed: Pediatric and adult reconstructive urologic surgery. 2nd ed. Baltimore: Williams & Wilkins, 1987:419.

McGuire EJ. The innervation and function of the lower urinary tract. J Neurosurg 1986; 65:278–285.

O'Donnell WF. Urological management in the patient with acute spinal cord injury. Crit Care Clin 1987; 3:599–617.

Tanagho EA, Schmidt RA, Orvis BR. Neural stimulation for control of voiding dysfunction: a preliminary report in 22 patients with serious neuropathic voiding disorders. J Urol 1989; 142:340–345.

URINARY INCONTINENCE IN CHILDREN

WILLIAM C. HULBERT, Jr., M.D., F.A.A.P.
RONALD RABINOWITZ, M.D., F.A.A.P., F.A.C.S.

Urinary incontinence in children is a common complaint and often functional in origin. The history and physical examination can be extremely helpful in distinguishing between a functional and a structural cause of incontinence, and also is important in differentiating congenital from acquired structural abnormalities. By 3 to 4 years of age, most children have achieved daytime urinary control, but one in eight still has nocturnal enuresis. Bladder capacity progressively increases during childhood and can be calculated by adding 2 to the age (in years) and converting to ounces. That is, the average 2-year-old has a 4-oz capacity bladder, the average 4-year-old has a 6-oz capacity bladder, and so on. Approximately 85 percent of children are dry at night by age 5. By age 10, approximately 5 percent still have nocturnal enuresis. The incidence decreases to approximately 1 percent by the midteens.

Our obligation to patients who present with incontinence is to make certain that there is no underlying anatomic, infectious, or neurologic basis for the problem. The majority benefit most from a thorough office evaluation and supportive reassurance that includes options for symptomatic relief. Adjunctive radiologic or urodynamic studies are sometimes indicated.

HISTORY

As in many areas of pediatric urology, the history may be of utmost importance (Table 1). Initially, one needs to determine whether the incontinence is daytime, nighttime, or both. Nighttime wetting may be only functional, whereas both daytime and nighttime wetting may suggest an underlying structural abnormality. The volume wet may also be important. A large volume at discrete intervals suggests an infrequent voider who is simply "too busy" to take the time to void until it is too late, whereas a child who has damp pants may be suspected of having uninhibited bladder spasms. Frequency of voiding can be a clue to the underlying etiology. Frequent voiding is more suggestive of an irritable bladder secondary to spasms, infection, or neurogenic incontinence. A history of urinary urgency is important as evidence of bladder contractility. Some families provide a vivid verbal picture of squatting, cramping, and posturing that occurs frequently and represents attempts by the child to control uninhibited bladder contractions. It is important to take a dietary

Table 1 Historical Factors in Urinary Incontinence

Timing: day/night
Timing: wetting/voiding
Volume
Frequency
Urgency
Diet
Trauma
Infection
Associated symptoms

history, because caffeine intake may contribute to urinary incontinence. Incontinence may also be secondary to infection, either bacterial or viral. In some children the bladder irritability causing incontinence may significantly outlast the duration of active infection. It is important to take a history of both the voiding and wetting patterns. In girls, wetting that occurs shortly after voiding is suggestive of vaginal voiding. In boys, similar symptoms suggest zipper compression of the urethra or a urethral diverticulum. In girls, a normal voiding pattern with persistent urinary drainage is suggestive of an ectopic ureter. A history of persistent urinary drainage observed while changing the diaper of a female infant is likewise suggestive of ectopic ureter.

It is important to be certain that there is no history of trauma that could impact on urinary continence. Straddle injury, including bicycle seat trauma, is a common cause of urethral stricture in males. A previous endoscopy, or urethral intubation for some other type of procedure (e.g., cardiac, orthopedic, or neurosurgical), may result in traumatic stricture. Previous surgery of the spine, pelvis, or rectal area for such conditions as imperforate anus are important historical aspects. Other historical factors that may be important include associated orthopedic, neurologic, or gastrointestinal symptoms. Gait disturbances, developmental delay, severe constipation, and rectal incontinence may all suggest urinary incontinence secondary to an underlying structural or multisystem etiology.

PHYSICAL EXAMINATION

The physical examination is extremely important in evaluating children with urinary incontinence. Simple observations about their gait and activity in the examining room and their ability to climb onto the examining table are helpful in gross motor evaluation. The abdomen should be observed and examined for such findings as a distended bladder or other mass. The spine should be checked for signs of spinal dysraphism, including skin depressions, dimples, and hairy patches. Defects on observation or palpation of the spine may indicate the need for further radiographic investigation of this area. Deep tendon reflexes, superficial sensory reflexes, and the bulbocavernosus reflex can be checked, in addition to the anal wink and anal sphincter tone. The female perineum should be examined for persistent urinary drainage. In males, observation is made for an accessory

urethra or any other penile deformity such as megalourethra. In an uncircumcised male, a very tight phimotic foreskin may act as a storage container for urine, resulting in postvoid wetting. The urine should also be examined for infection, glucose, red blood cells, and specific gravity. Important aspects of the physical examination are listed in Table 2.

EVALUATION

In some children with urinary incontinence in whom an underlying structural abnormality is suspected, radiographic evaluation may be indicated. Ultrasonography is the least invasive screening study and is often completely adequate. However, as it is very observer dependent, it is important that the ultrasonographer be familiar with the various pediatric congenital anomalies. A complete evaluation of the urinary tract should include a search for orthotopic and ectopic kidneys, possible duplication anomalies, dilated ureters, and urine in the vagina. Ultrasonography over a spinal dimple can determine its depth and attachment to the spine. More detailed anatomic studies include voiding cystourethrography (VCUG) and intravenous urography. A view of the spine is also obtained in these studies and, if indicated, more detailed spinal studies may include magnetic resonance imaging (MRI).

In some children, urodynamic testing may help to define voiding dynamics more accurately. The two most helpful studies are cystometry and leak point pressure.

In some children, endoscopy is necessary to further define the cause of urinary incontinence. Both cystourethroscopy and vaginoscopy may be valuable in searching for an ectopic ureter or other problem.

TREATMENT

The management of children with urinary incontinence depends on the underlying etiology (Table 3). Often this is a functional disturbance, the diagnosis of which is made from a detailed history. These disturbances may be managed by changes in mechanical acts

Table 2 Physical Evaluation in Urinary Incontinence

Abdomen
Spine
Rectum
Urethra
Perineum
Gross motor function
Neurologic function
Urine

Table 3 Etiologies of Urinary Incontinence

Functional
  Mechanical
  Infrequent voiding
  Nocturnal
  Diurnal
  Urinary tract infections
  Uninhibited bladder spasms
  Dysfunctional urinary frequency urgency syndrome
Structural
  Ureteral ectopy
  Obstruction
  Trauma
  Foreign body
  Tumor
  Neurogenic

of voiding, changes in voiding habits, changes in bowel evacuation habits, changes in diet, or pharmacologic manipulation. Other aspects of urinary incontinence in children may be secondary to structural abnormalities that may require more invasive or surgical therapy.

Mechanical disturbances of urination that cause postvoid wetting can be seen in boys and girls. In girls, voiding with the legs together commonly causes urine to back up into the vagina and remain stored there until the girl is ambulatory, at which time it gradually leaks out. This usually occurs 10 to 15 minutes after completion of voiding and is seen in both young girls and adolescents. It is most commonly noted in girls who wear slacks as opposed to skirts. If they pull the slacks down only to the midthigh or knee level, they cannot separate their legs sufficiently during urination to prevent this vaginal voiding. The diagnosis is made by history, no diagnostic studies being necessary, and management involves voiding in a straddling position on the toilet. Slacks must be pulled down to the ankles. In some instances, it may be necessary to have the girl sit backward on the toilet and face the tank to enable her to sufficiently separate the thighs during voiding.

In boys, postvoid wetting may also be a functional mechanical problem caused by zipper constriction of the penile urethra. In these boys, some urine is stored in the urethra distal to the external sphincter because of compression against the distal urethra by the zipper, or by the elastic waistband of the underwear, if the penis is exposed by lowering the pants. This is usually seen in preadolescent or adolescent males. Before any studies are obtained to look for a structural abnormality such as a urethral diverticulum, observation of the voiding technique or having the boy void without anything compressing the urethra will determine the etiology.

A dietary history may be important in children with urinary incontinence, especially that associated with urinary frequency and urgency. In many children, significant urinary symptoms can occur with dietary intake of caffeine, as in soft drinks, tea, or chocolate. In many instances, simply discontinuing caffeine from the diet may resolve the urinary symptoms.

Frequency of voiding is an important aspect of the history of a child with urinary incontinence. If the child is a very infrequent voider on a chronic basis, the wetting may be secondary to waiting too long to urinate. These are usually children who become extremely absorbed in play and repress the urge to void until the bladder has become too distended. They then either completely empty their bladder or leak a small amount of urine on the way to the toilet. A change in their voiding routine will solve this problem without the need for any type of diagnostic study. The child is placed on a timed voiding routine with behavioral modification: he or she is encouraged to urinate before each meal and snack as well as before bedtime. A chart is constructed with spaces for breakfast, lunch, snack, dinner, and bedtime with a space for the child to place a star, sticker, or whatever with each void. In this fashion, the child participates in changing the voiding habit. Through a

positive reinforcement technique, rather than coercion or punishment, there is a better chance of achieving a long-lasting beneficial change.

Nocturnal enuresis is an extremely common problem, usually managed by pediatricians but often referred for urologic evaluation. In the vast majority of children with isolated nocturnal enuresis, there is no urologic structural abnormality; the condition is self-limited and spontaneous resolution is the norm. However, in some children this may not occur until adolescence, especially when there is a family history of late resolution. Conditioning therapy with an enuresis alarm has a high success rate in children who awaken to the sound of the alarm. However, some children who are profoundly deep sleepers may not be aroused by the alarm. In these, a low dose of imipramine for a few months in conjunction with the enuresis alarm may be sufficient. Additional success in pharmacologic management of nocturnal enuresis has been reported with anticholinergic medications and 1-deamino-(8-D-arginine)-vasopressin (DDAVP), a synthetic vasopressin analog. The relapse rates with these medications are higher than with the conditioning device, and pharmacologic therapy is generally reserved for patients resistant to other interventions. Because anticholinergic medications seem to be more successful for children with both day and night symptoms, the specifics of use is discussed in that section of the chapter. DDAVP has been approved for use in nocturnal enuresis since 1990. Nasal spray application of the medication is convenient and precise, successful dosing occurring with 20 to 40 μg at bedtime. Side effects are minimal, and 30 to 50 percent of patients achieve a meaningful improvement in enuresis. Relapse is frequent, however, and the medication is expensive. DDAVP may be most useful for episodic control of wetting in difficult social situations (e.g., overnight visits, camping) for children who are found to respond during trials.

When there is both daytime and nighttime wetting, the initial management is aimed at the daytime symptoms. Obviously, one must be certain that there is no urinary infection. Infection can cause both daytime and nighttime wetting without other symptoms and indicates the need for uroradiographic investigation: VCUG and either renal ultrasonography or intravenous urography. The wetting secondary to infection usually resolves with antibiotic sterilization of the urine. In the absence of a structural urologic abnormality, frequent recurrent urinary infections manifested by urinary incontinence are managed by long-term antibacterial prophylaxis, usually with sulfamethoxazole-trimethoprim or nitrofurantoin. In the absence of infection, some children have incontinence secondary to uninhibited bladder spasms. These patients have urinary frequency and urgency and may or may not have nighttime wetting. Children with the dysfunctional urinary frequency urgency syndrome usually wet only small volumes (damp pants) and often have significant posturing maneuvers such as squatting or sitting on a fist. If no other etiology is identified (e.g., diet, infection), these children are best managed with oxybutynin. Low dosages are given initially, with gradual increase to a maintenance level. The maximal dose is 1 mg per year of age twice a day up to age 5, and 5 mg one to three times a day thereafter. Side effects, seen in approximately half the patients, can include dry mouth, flushing, and blurred vision, as well as behavioral changes and sleep disturbances. Children may be significantly symptomatic from the temperature-regulating side effects in warm climates. If the wetting resolves, the medication is gradually and progressively tapered over a few weeks. Some children whose symptoms do not respond to oxybutynin do respond to propantheline or imipramine with the same type of management.

Most children with urinary incontinence do not have a structural abnormality, but it is important to distinguish those who do, because resolution may be easily attained with correction of the structural abnormality. Again, the history and physical examination are of utmost importance.

A girl who has a normal voiding pattern in conjunction with persistent wetting should be suspected of having an ectopic ureter distal to the sphincter (distal urethra, urethrovaginal septum, vagina). Sometimes the ectopic orifice can be visualized on external examination. There may be a history of persistent wetting and a constantly fluid-filled vagina during the time of diapering. Evaluation includes VCUG to evaluate for reflux, intravenous urography (IVU) to outline ureteral anatomy, a renal scan if there is a doubt about the function of the system associated with the ectopic ureter, and possible ultrasonography to visualize parenchymal thickness and the degree of ureteral dilatation if the system does not function. The involved ureter is usually the upper pole of a duplex system. If the system does not function, an upper pole heminephroureterectomy is indicated; if it does function, an ipsilateral ureteroureterostomy to the intravesical ureter is our preferred method of management.

Urinary incontinence in males can occur secondary to urethral obstruction, associated with straining to void and occasionally with hematuria. A congenital etiology may include posterior urethral valves or an anterior urethral diverticulum with an obstructing distal lip. An acquired etiology is urethral stricture. In both of these conditions, in addition to straining, there commonly is prolonged voiding. Diagnosis is made by VCUG and, in the case of severe stricture, retrograde urethrography. Urinary incontinence can also occur in uncircumcised males with severe phimosis who develop ballooning of the foreskin secondary to entrapped urine. The urine gradually leaks from the ballooned foreskin after completion of voiding. Circumcision or dilatation of the foreskin meatus may be necessary. Another urethral cause of urinary incontinence in boys is an anterior urethral diverticulum that stores urine during voiding, and later drains. Management of all these urethral obstructions is endoscopic. For some large diverticuli, open resection and urethroplasty is necessary.

In the face of urinary infection or hematuria, along with urinary incontinence, radiographic investigation is indicated: VCUG and an intravenous urogram. Stones and occasionally a foreign body may be found, representing the nidus for the underlying infection.

An uncommon cause of urinary incontinence is tumor. Sarcomas of the bladder neck, prostate, and vagina can present with urinary incontinence due to involvement of the sphincter, obstruction, or external irritative symptoms. Likewise, tumors of the spinal cord can cause urinary incontinence on a neurogenic basis. Evaluation of these tumors includes radiographic staging and either biopsy or excision, usually with concomitant chemotherapy with or without radiation therapy. It should be noted that, even in the presence of extensive tumor involvement of the lower urinary tract, combined chemotherapy and radiation with limited extirpative surgery can salvage a functional lower urinary tract.

The most common structural abnormality associated with urinary incontinence in children is myelodysplasia. This represents a wide range of spinal defects with a similarly wide range of physical and neurologic findings. Many conditions, such as myelomeningocele, are obvious at birth. Some, such as sacral agenesis and tethered spinal cord, may only be suggested by subtle abnormalities such as a dermal sinus or fat pad over the sacrum. Although about 10 to 20 percent of patients with myelomeningocele are found to have congenital renal abnormalities, the remainder usually start with normal kidneys. It is the detrusor and the function of the bladder outlet that determines continence, and which, over time, can cause problems with the upper tracts.

Therapy is determined by first evaluating bladder function; this does not necessarily correspond to the level of the spinal lesion, and patchy deficits are often seen. In addition to investigation with ultrasonography and VCUG, urodynamics may be helpful. The bladder capacity is estimated and a leak point pressure as well as detrusor contractility is determined on urodynamic investigation. The measured intravesical pressure at the point of urethral urinary leakage (the leak point) is important for estimating the risk of upper tract deterioration over time. A leak point of greater than 40 cm of water signifies detrusor-sphincter dyscoordination that can lead to hydronephrosis or reflux in time. Bladder storage and sphincteric function are also the important factors in obtaining continence. Bladder storage can be improved and bladder contractions inhibited by pharmacologic implementation, including oral and/or intravesical oxybutynin. If there is sufficient sphincteric competence, clean, intermittent self-catheterization may allow emptying and significantly increase the functional storage capacity, converting an incontinent neurogenic bladder to a continent one.

Further outlet resistance can sometimes be obtained pharmacologically with imipramine or alpha-adrenergic medications. In the presence of markedly increased intravesical pressures with a small functional bladder capacity that is unresponsive to medication, intestinal augmentation or some other storage-increasing technique can be used to increase bladder capacity and decrease intravesical pressure. This, in combination with intermittent catheterization, can convert the patient to urinary continence in addition to decreasing the risk of upper tract damage, without resort to urinary diversion.

SUGGESTED READING

Koff SA. Estimating bladder capacity in children. Urology 1983; 21:248.

Koff SA. Enuresis. In: Walsh PC, Gittes RF, Perlmutter AD, Stamey TA, eds. Campbell's urology. 5th ed. Philadelphia: WB Saunders, 1985:2179.

McLorie GA, Husmann DA. Incontinence and enuresis. Pediatr Clin North Am 1987; 34:1159–1174.

Rockney R, Caldamone AA. The management of persistent primary enuresis. Prob Urol 1990; 4:9.

STRESS INCONTINENCE IN FEMALES

SHLOMO RAZ, M.D.
DEBORAH R. ERICKSON, M.D.
ERNEST M. SUSSMAN, M.D.

Normal continence in females results from a balance of forces that include anatomic position of the bladder neck and urethra, urethral length, intrinsic urethral closure pressures (seal), and urethral responses to changes in abdominal pressures. Deficiency of a single factor does not usually result in urinary incontinence, since it can be counteracted by other compensatory mechanisms. For example, many women have altered anatomic position of the bladder and urethra, but not all these women are incontinent. Incontinence is more likely to occur when compensatory factors, such as the ability of the urethra to seal or the urethral responses to stress, also are impaired. The anatomic defect is most commonly caused by childbirth, but the presentation of stress incontinence is often near the time of menopause. This delay in presentation suggests that estrogens have a role in maintaining the compensatory factors.

The condition of genuine stress incontinence is present when urine is lost through the urethra during periods of increased intra-abdominal pressure, in the absence of a detrusor contraction. In spite of the complexity and multifactorial etiology of stress incontinence in women, for clinical purposes it can be divided into two types. The first type, anatomic incontinence, is associated with a change in position of the bladder neck relative to the pubic symphysis. The sphincteric unit is displaced to a low, dependent position. As previously mentioned, this anatomic change per se is not the only reason for incontinence; more complex functions also are impaired. However, it is known that most women who have this type of incontinence experience resolution if the bladder neck and proximal urethra are restored to a high retropubic position.

The second type of stress incontinence is due to intrinsic deficiency of the urethral sphincter mechanism

(ISD). In this type, the sphincteric unit itself is poorly functioning. The most common conditions responsible for damaging the delicate urethral closure mechanism include radiation, multiple surgeries, or neurologic disease such as myelomeningocele or sacral arc lesions. The goal of surgery in these cases is to provide coaptation, support, and compression to the open urethra. Anatomic malposition and ISD may coexist. If they do, a surgical procedure designed primarily to reposition the bladder neck, without providing additional coaptation, is less likely to be successful.

The three main choices for treatment of stress incontinence are pharmacologic, behavioral, and surgical. For mild degrees of stress incontinence, behavioral treatment (Kegel exercises) may offer relief. Some women may also experience improvement from alpha-adrenergic medications, but there is a concern that the long-term safety of vasoconstrictive drugs has not been established. Estrogen supplementation can improve incontinence in selected elderly women with atrophic changes. Usually a surgical approach for stress incontinence is preferable.

PREOPERATIVE EVALUATION

A complete history taking and physical examination should be performed to determine the type of incontinence present, identify concomitant pathology, and ascertain that the patient is medically fit for surgery. Urinary infection should be sought and eradicated if present. Laboratory, radiologic, or other preoperative testing should be done as needed according to the patient's medical condition. The extent of urologic evaluation required is related to the complexity of the presentation. Urodynamic, endoscopic, radiologic, or videourodynamic evaluation is indicated in patients who have obstructive symptoms, neurologic disease, previous anti-incontinence surgery, previous radiation therapy or trauma, or other complex histories.

The goals of the preoperative urologic evaluation include the following: (1) making the subjective and objective clinical diagnosis of stress incontinence; (2) determining whether the incontinence is due to anatomic position of the bladder neck, intrinsic urethral sphincter damage, or both; (3) evaluating the degree of prolapse of the anterior vaginal wall; (4) identifying other concomitant pathology that requires surgical treatment at the same time as the anti-incontinence procedure; (5) evaluating for bladder instability; and (6) ensuring adequate bladder emptying.

Subjective and Objective Clinical Diagnosis

The subjective diagnosis is made from the patient's history. It is important to distinguish between stress incontinence and incontinence due to stress-induced detrusor instability. Genuine stress incontinence usually causes urine loss that coincides exactly with the period of increased intra-abdominal pressure. Stress-induced instability usually causes urine loss that occurs a few seconds after the stress maneuver begins and continues even after the maneuver is finished.

The objective diagnosis is made by direct observation of leakage through the urethra during stress maneuvers (Marshall test). It should be corroborated by either cystoscopy, Valsalva leak point pressure, or lateral cystography with resting and straining. I prefer the lateral cystogram because it gives valuable anatomic information (the "physical examination in the standing position") and provides a hard copy for documentation. One caveat about the lateral cystogram is that intravesical pressure is not monitored, so incontinence due to stress-induced detrusor instability may be misdiagnosed as stress incontinence.

Determining Whether the Incontinence is Due to Anatomic Position of the Bladder Neck, Intrinsic Urethral Sphincter Damage, or Both

It is essential to make this diagnosis because the goals of surgery are different for each type of incontinence. This can be a difficult determination, and it is seldom possible to make a definitive decision based on any single test. In the history, patients with pure bladder neck hypermobility usually describe a mild to moderate degree of incontinence, with leakage occurring mainly during vigorous activity. Patients with ISD tend to have a severe degree of incontinence and leakage with minimal activity. This history is not specific, however, because patients with severe hypermobility also complain of leakage with minimal activity. On physical examination, patients with hypermobility have visible descent of the bladder neck and proximal urethra with leakage of urine during stress maneuvers, and the leakage stops after unobstructed elevation of the bladder neck (Marshall test). On the other hand, demonstration of stress incontinence through a correctly positioned urethra is diagnostic of ISD.

If a urethroscope is held at the midurethra and the patient is asked to cough or strain, hypermobility can be visualized. Urethral coaptation also can be assessed endoscopically. Good coaptation suggests a normal sphincter unit, while a persistently open, fixed urethra suggests ISD. Lateral cystography during resting and straining is also helpful. Most patients with only hypermobility have a closed urethra at rest, and urethral

descent with leakage of contrast while straining. Most patients with ISD have an open bladder neck at rest, and they may leak while standing still. One caveat about the lateral cystogram is that detrusor instability also can cause opening of the bladder neck at rest and leakage of contrast while the patient is standing still. Consideration of the entire clinical picture should enable the surgeon to decide whether the stress incontinence is due to anatomic position, ISD, or both.

Some clinicians believe that very high urethral pressures make the diagnosis of stress incontinence unlikely and that very low pressures (less than 15 to 20 cm water) suggest intrinsic sphincter dysfunction. However, a reliable correlation between urethral pressures and the presence or type of incontinence has not been established.

Evaluating the Degree of Prolapse of the Anterior Vaginal Wall

It is important to recognize a cystocele. Bladder neck suspension without concurrent cystocele repair can result in obstruction due to kinking as the cystocele hangs down below the supported bladder neck. The type of repair is chosen according to the degree of cystocele. A minimal cystocele can be corrected by a bladder neck suspension procedure. For moderate cystocele without a central fascial defect, the four-corner suspension provides effective repair. Severe cystocele requires repair of the central hernia by approximating the pubocervical fascia and cardinal ligaments in the midline, and bladder suspension if a lateral defect also is present.

Identifying Other Concomitant Pathology

Examples of such abnormalities include rectocele, enterocele, uterine mass, and prolapse.

Evaluating for Bladder Instability

Stress incontinence in women is often accompanied by urgency or urge incontinence. If a woman complains of urgency, urge incontinence, or precipitant micturition, this is believed to be detrusor instability even if not demonstrated on cystometry. Some women do not initiate detrusor contractions in the unfamiliar testing situation, and other patients' uninhibited contractions are hidden because, with a low outlet resistance, the contraction does not create a detectable rise in pressure. Also, although this diagnosis is not made solely on the basis of history, the most common cause of voiding without awareness is detrusor instability. I do perform cystometry for women with these complaints, to look for abnormalities in bladder capacity or compliance that may suggest an underlying neurologic or inflammatory disorder.

Patients who complain of both stress and urge incontinence require careful evaluation. If (1) the history is definite for stress incontinence, (2) the physical examination demonstrates bladder neck hypermobility and a positive Marshall test, (3) cystoscopy confirms hypermobility and excludes bladder pathology, and (4) videourodynamic study confirms that leakage does occur in the absence of a detrusor contraction, I perform anti-incontinence surgery. Often the urgency resolves after the stress incontinence is corrected.

The use of cystometry to diagnose asymptomatic detrusor instability in women with pure stress incontinence is controversial. I do not believe it to be necessary, because the finding of asymptomatic instability would not alter the plans for surgery.

Ensuring Adequate Bladder Emptying

The postvoid residual should be checked before performing anti-incontinence surgery. Patients with a high residual, or those complaining of obstructive symptoms, require further investigation to rule out obstruction or poor bladder contractility.

SURGICAL PROCEDURES TO CORRECT ANATOMIC INCONTINENCE

For incontinence due only to anatomic malposition of the sphincteric unit, three types of procedure may be used: anterior repair, retropubic suspension, and vaginal (needle) bladder neck suspension.

The anterior repair operations are modifications of the Kelly plication. These may repair cystoceles but do not reposition the bladder neck to a high retropubic position. I do not recommend the anterior repair as a treatment for stress incontinence: it has a greater long-term failure rate than the suspension procedures.

The choice between a vaginal and retropubic approach should be based on the surgeon's experience and expertise and on the presence of concomitant pathology that would require treatment through a vaginal or abdominal incision.

The three most commonly used retropubic operations are the Marshall-Marchetti-Krantz (MMK) procedure, the paravaginal repair, and the Burch colposuspension. For the MMK procedure, interrupted sutures are used to anchor the upper vaginal wall and lateral urethra (extraluminally) to the pubic periosteum. Additional sutures can be used to anchor the bladder wall to the rectus muscle. For the paravaginal repair, the vaginal wall and overlying fascia, lateral to the bladder neck and urethra, are approximated to the obturator fascia. For the Burch colposuspension, the lateral vaginal wall is suspended from Cooper's ligament bilaterally. When a retropubic operation is chosen, I generally use the Burch suspension. It is a straightforward procedure, the risk of osteitis pubis is negligible because the periosteum is not entered, and postoperative obstruction is rare because the sutures are placed far lateral to the urethra. If the vaginal wall will not reach Cooper's ligament, or if concomitant cystocele repair is required, I use the paravaginal repair.

The Burch procedure is well described. Briefly, the retropubic space is exposed through a midline or Pfannenstiel incision. The proximal urethra, bladder, and lateral vagina are mobilized, care being taken not to dissect directly upon the urethra or urethrovesical junction. Cooper's ligaments are identified, and care is taken to dissect the fat away from the pelvic side wall, since fat interferes with the formation of adhesions. The assistant's fingers are placed into the vagina to elevate it toward Cooper's ligaments, and absorbable interrupted sutures are used for fixation. It is not necessary (in fact, some surgeons think it is not desirable) for the vaginal wall to be completely apposed to Cooper's ligament. Suspension from the ligament is sufficient provided that the bladder neck and urethra are brought into a high retropubic position. The formation of adhesions between the lateral vagina and pelvic side wall will maintain the proper position. Burch's continence rate for 143 women was 93 percent. A combined series from a literature review (15 articles) showed a continence rate of 85 percent.

If the patient does not require abdominal surgery to treat concomitant pathology, I prefer a vaginal (needle) bladder neck suspension because the recovery time is quicker, pain is less, and the hospital stay is shorter. Several variations of the original Pereyra needle suspension have been described, including modifications by Pereyra himself. The most commonly used variations are the Stamey, the Cobb-Ragde, the Raz, and the Gittes.

In the Stamey procedure, long needles are passed through small, bilateral, transverse suprapubic incisions to the periurethral fascia, which is exposed through a T-shaped vaginal incision. Cystoscopy is performed to visualize the indentation, which indicates that the needle is placed at the desired location adjacent to the bladder neck. A nonabsorbable suture with a dacron buttress is used for suspension. The long needle brings one end of the suture to the suprapubic incision, and a second needle pass is made, lateral to the first, to transfer the other end. The ends are tied over the bridge of abdominal fascia between them.

The Cobb-Ragde procedure differs from the Stamey in two ways. First, a barrel knot is used as a buttress instead of a dacron sleeve. Second, a double-pronged needle is used, which reduces by half the number of passes required and provides a consistent 1-cm bridge of abdominal fascia between the ends of the suture. Cystoscopy is performed to exclude urethral or bladder injury.

The Gittes procedure is similar except that no incisions, vaginal or abdominal, are used. The nonabsorbable suspending sutures incorporate the whole vaginal wall at the level of the bladder neck. Through a small puncture in the suprapubic area, a needle is passed to the vaginal area. The ends of the sutures are passed through the eye of the needle and transferred to the suprapubic area. The sutures are tied independently over the fascia. After a short period the vaginal sutures are re-epithelialized. The advantage of this procedure is that it can be performed under local anesthesia.

The Raz modification of the Pereyra procedure

differs from these three because it includes mobilization of the urethropelvic ligament. This ligament is a condensation of the periurethral fascia and endopelvic (superior levator) fascia, which suspends the urethra to the tendinous arc of the obturator fascia. This mobilization provides several advantages. First, it allows tension-free suspension, which is especially important in secondary procedures. Second, entry into the retropubic space allows the needle passage to be accomplished by fingertip guidance, reducing the risk of bladder or urethral injury. Third, helical sutures are applied under vision into the desired structures: the strong fascia of the urethropelvic ligament and the anterior vaginal wall excluding the epithelium. Fourth, the strength of the anchor can be tested by a steady pull on the sutures. Fifth, placement of the sutures is lateral to the urethra, minimizing the risk of injury or obstruction.

My technique will be reviewed in detail. With the patient in the lithotomy position, a suprapubic tube and urethral Foley catheter are placed. An Allis clamp grasps the anterior vaginal wall midway between the external meatus and the bladder neck. Two oblique incisions are made lateral to the urethra and bladder neck. Spreading dissection is performed from the lateral edges of these incisions, with the scissors above the glistening periurethral fascia and under (from the vaginal surgeon's viewpoint) the vaginal wall and levator muscle. Dissection continues to the junction of the urethropelvic ligament with the tendinous arc. At this point the retropubic space is entered with closed scissors, aiming toward the ipsilateral shoulder. Blunt finger dissection frees the lateral edge of the urethropelvic ligament from the tendinous arc and pubic bone. This freed edge provides the strong anchoring tissue for bladder neck suspension.

Bilateral helical No. 1 polypropylene sutures are then placed in two steps. For the first step, the needle is passed through the anterior vaginal wall, parallel to and excluding the epithelium. By extending these passes posteriorly and medially, a small cystocele can be corrected. For the second step, opened Russian forceps are placed into the retropubic space and pushed medially, to expose the freed edge of the urethropelvic ligament. Two or three passes are made through this strong anchoring tissue. After this, the strength of the fascia is tested with a steady pull on the polypropylene sutures. It is important to place these sutures at the level of the bladder neck, because distal placement can cause urethral kinking and obstruction. It also is important to place the sutures at the lateral edge of the freed urethropelvic ligament, because placement too close to the urethra can result in urethral obstruction, injury, or intrinsic sphincter deficiency.

A small, transverse suprapubic incision is deepened to expose the fascia. A double-pronged needle is passed close to the midline. The initial needle penetration should be made just superior to the pubic bone, in a relatively fixed area of the abdominal fascia. Passing sutures through the mobile part of the abdominal wall can result in prolonged postoperative pain, especially

with movement. After the needle points have penetrated the rectus fascia and muscle, the rest of the passage to the vaginal incision is made with direct fingertip guidance, avoiding injury to the bladder or urethra.

The ends of the polypropylene sutures are transferred to the suprapubic incision. Cystoscopy is performed to ensure that no bladder or urethral injury has occurred and to confirm that good elevation of the bladder neck can be produced by gently pulling upward on the polypropylene sutures. The vaginal incision is closed before the suspension sutures are tied over the rectus fascia. It is not necessary to tie the suspension sutures under tension.

The results of bladder neck suspension were reviewed in 17 articles; all patients had at least 6 months' follow-up. When all the procedures were considered together, the continence rate was 84 percent (range 61 to 94 percent). When the various modifications were considered separately, continence rates were as follows: Stamey, 632/779 (81 percent); Pereyra-Raz, 90/108 (83 percent); Cobb-Ragde, 56/62 (90 percent); Gittes 32/38 (84 percent).

SURGICAL PROCEDURES FOR INTRINSIC SPHINCTER DEFICIENCY

If the preoperative evaluation demonstrates that the patient has ISD, procedures to increase urethral coaptation and support should be considered. The three options currently available are the suburethral sling, artificial sphincter, and periurethral bulking injection of polytetrafluoroethylene (PTFE) or collagen.

Periurethral PTFE injections can be performed in the office under local anesthesia and repeated if necessary. PTFE is especially useful in patients who have a high risk for surgery. I offer periurethral PTFE injection as an option to women who have stress incontinence in spite of good urethral support, in the understanding that a PTFE injection carries a lower probability of success than a sling procedure. Five series of PTFE injections from the literature were combined, and the overall results were 59 percent cured, 16 percent improved, and 25 percent failed. Initial reports on the use of collagen for patients with ISD are encouraging. At this time, the FDA is considering its approval for periurethral injection.

Reports concerning the artificial urinary sphincter in female patients have shown variable results. I seldom use the artificial sphincter in women. Many of my patients with ISD have severe damage to the urethrovaginal septum, which leads to a greater incidence of long-term complications such as tissue atrophy, erosion, or infection. Another concern is the possibility of pump malfunction, fluid leak, tubing kink, or other mechanical problems. I believe that incontinence can be resolved just as effectively with a sling procedure as with an artificial sphincter. I therefore prefer to use sling procedures for women with ISD who are medically fit for surgery.

Slings can be made from autologous or synthetic material. Synthetic slings have a much higher rate of local complications such as erosion, infection, and fistula. The most commonly used autologous slings are made from fascia (placed through a vaginal, abdominal, or combined approach) or vaginal wall. The latter involves less extensive surgery and less pain than the fascial sling. For patients with an excessively short or scarred vagina, I use the abdominal fascia sling.

Different procedures for placement of the abdominal fascia sling have been described. Briefly, a transverse suprapubic incision is made to harvest a 1×12 cm strip of rectus fascia. A helical suture is placed at each end of the sling before excising it from the fascia. Some surgeons also use the suprapubic incision to enter the retropubic space and mobilize the anterior bladder wall and urethra from the superior aspect of the vagina, but I do not believe that this mobilization is necessary. A midline or U-shaped vaginal incision is made. Lateral dissection with entry into the retropubic space, similar to that for a bladder neck suspension, is performed. Tunnels are created on each side of the urethra to connect the vaginal and suprapubic incisions. One end of the sling is passed down from the suprapubic incision, around the bladder neck, and up through the tunnel on the other side. Interrupted sutures maintain the correct position of the sling at the bladder neck. The vaginal incision is closed before the ends of the sling are sutured to the anterior abdominal fascia, just above the pubic bone. Although some surgeons recommend cystoscopy or intraoperative urethral pressure profilometry to determine the correct tension while the ends of the sling are tied, I believe the sling should be tied with minimal tension.

A review of the literature on fascial slings for recurrent stress incontinence or other etiologies for ISD (six articles) gave a continence rate of 86 percent. Complications for the combined series included superficial wound infection (4 percent), vesicovaginal fistula (0.8 percent), and necrosis of the fascial strips causing recurrent incontinence (0.5 percent). Although transient obstructive voiding difficulty was common, the incidence of permanent retention in this review was 3 percent.

The vaginal wall sling is my preferred approach, and the important points are emphasized here. An inverted U-shaped incision is made on the anterior vaginal wall with the apex of the U just below the external meatus. A transverse incision connects the legs of the U at the level of the bladder neck. This creates an island of vaginal wall under the urethra. The vaginal wall posterior to the island is mobilized to make a flap sufficient to cover the island. Lateral dissection and entry into the retropubic space are performed as described for the bladder neck suspension. Four helical polypropylene sutures are placed, one at each corner of the island. All four sutures include the periurethral fascia, and the anterior vaginal wall except for the epithelium. The proximal sutures also include the freed edge of the urethropelvic ligaments. All four sutures are transferred to the suprapubic area in the same manner as described for the bladder neck suspension. The posterior vaginal wall flap is advanced to cover the island. Care is taken to tie the suspension sutures without tension. A minimal amount of tension is needed to improve urethral coaptation and support; excessive tension serves only to increase the risk of postoperative urinary retention. The continence rate in our first report on the vaginal wall sling for women with various causes of ISD was 81 percent.

SUGGESTED READING

Blaivas JG, Chancellor M. Complicated stress urinary incontinence. Semin Urol 1989; 7:103.

Burch JC. Cooper's ligament urethrovesical suspension for stress incontinence. Am J Obstet Gynecol 1968; 100:764.

Karram MM, Bhatia NN. Transvaginal needle bladder neck suspension procedures for stress urinary incontinence: a comprehensive review. Obstet Gynecol 1989; 73:906.

Leach GE, Zimmern P, Staskin D, et al. Surgery for pelvic prolapse. Semin Urol 1986; 4:43.

Little NA, Juma S, Raz S. Surgical treatment of stress urinary incontinence. Semin Urol 1989; 7:86.

Little NA, Juma S, Raz S. Bladder neck suspension and formal cystocele repair for severe anterior vaginal wall prolapse. J Urol (in press).

McGuire EJ. Pubovaginal sling. In: Hinman F, ed. Atlas of urologic surgery. Philadelphia: WB Saunders, 1989:455.

Nichols DH, Randall CL. Vaginal surgery. Baltimore: Williams & Wilkins, 1976.

Raz S, Klutke CG, Golomb J. Four-corner bladder and urethral suspension for moderate cystocele. J Urol 1989; 142:712.

Raz S, Siegel AL, Short JL, Snyder JA. Vaginal wall sling. J Urol 1989; 141:43

Richardson AC, Edmonds PB, Williams NL. Treatment of stress urinary incontinence due to paravaginal fascial defect. Obstet Gynecol 1981; 57:357.

Tanagho EA. Colpocystourethropexy: the way we do it. J Urol 1976; 116:751.

Turner-Warwick R. Turner-Warwick vagino-obturator shelf urethral repositioning procedure. In: Gingell C, Abrams P, eds. Controversies and innovations in urological surgery. New York: Springer-Verlag, 1988:195.

Webster GD. Female urinary incontinence. In: Glenn JF, ed. Urologic surgery. Philadelphia: JB Lippincott, 1983:665.

IMPOTENCE

ARTERIAL ETIOLOGY OF IMPOTENCE

TOM F. LUE, M.D.

Within the past decade, innovative studies have effected a better understanding of the physiology of penile erection. Consequently, new functional tests and new therapies for the penile arterial and venous systems are being developed and interest in penile surgery has been revived. This chapter will summarize the advances in our understanding of arteriogenic impotence and present a treatment strategy based on these advances.

PATHOGENESIS

Increased flow in the penile artery and its three branches is essential for erection. In a recent study, Watanabe showed that penile blood flow increases from an average of 1.95 to 10.71 ml per 100 grams per minute during visual sexual stimulation and from 2 to 6.28 ml per 100 grams per minute after intracavernous injection of 20 µg of prostaglandin E_1 (PGE_1). Therefore, stenosis or occlusion of the terminal aorta or hypogastric, pudendal, or penile arteries can result in erectile failure. In addition, the cavernous artery, the helicine arterioles, and the inter- and intracellular architecture and function of the penile erectile tissue can be affected by diminished inflow. Our recent ultrastructural studies revealed atrophy of intracavernous smooth muscle, fibrous replacement, and neural degeneration in patients with poor penile arterial flow. Michal and associates found the incidence and age at onset of coronary disease and impotence to be parallel. Although arterial insufficiency can result from trauma or a congenital anomaly, arteriogenic impotence in most cases is a component of a generalized atherosclerotic process. The associated risk factors include hypercholesterolemia, cigarette smoking, diabetes mellitus, radiation, hypertension, and perineal trauma.

With moderate arterial stenosis, the initial symptoms are delay in initiating erection, necessity for increased stimulation, and early detumescence. With severe luminal compromise, partial to complete erectile failure ensues. The degree can vary among patients owing to the great variation in penile size and adequacy of the venous occlusion mechanism. Other factors such as obesity, cigarette smoking, and psychologic overlay can also aggravate erectile failure.

DIAGNOSIS OF ARTERIOGENIC IMPOTENCE

Except in traumatic cases, the typical history is one of gradual onset: progression from symptoms of delayed initiation of erection, necessity of greater stimulation, occasional premature ejaculation, and lessened rigidity to complete erectile failure. Some patients may present with an inability to maintain erection once the sexual act begins, suggestive of the pelvic steal syndrome in which blood flow is diverted to the skeletal muscle during intercourse. A history of intermittent claudication, myocardial infarction, hypercholesterolemia, diabetes mellitus, hypertension, or cigarette smoking also strongly suggests an arterial cause. Physical examination should be directed at signs of vascular disease such as poor peripheral pulse, skin changes, and bruit. Laboratory testing should include fasting blood glucose and lipid profile.

Diagnostic Tests

If arterial flow is measured in the flaccid state, results will not reflect the functional capacity of the penile arteries and could be misleading. Ideally, a test should be performed before and after the patient attains erection. The commonly used functional tests for vasculogenic impotence are briefly discussed below.

Office Screening Tests

Penile Brachial Pressure Index. Penile blood pressure is measured by a Doppler stethoscope with a pediatric blood pressure cuff placed at the root of the penis. When compared with brachial pressure, an index of less than 0.6 suggests penile arterial disease. However, the fact that this measurement is obtained in the flaccid state makes it unreliable.

CIS Test (Combined Intracavernous Injection and Stimulation). In my clinical observation of 100 patients after intracavernous vasodilator injection, 68 developed a much better erection after manual stimulation. On the basis of this, we added manual genital stimulation (with the option of sexually explicit magazines) to intracavernous injection to test for penile hemodynamics. Results can also give some indication of whether the patient has an adequate reflexogenic erection (spinal reflex arc) and whether he is under major psychological inhibition at the time of the test. For example, if the patient has a partial erection 15 minutes after injection of vasodilators, and if the addition of manual genital stimulation results in a sustained rigid erection, his reflexogenic erection is relatively intact and he has not been inhibited during the test. The details of our CIS test are summarized in Table 1. In my practice this test is used as a screening procedure.

Prevention of Priapism. The patient is routinely observed for 1 hour in the office. If full erection persists after 45 minutes, a diluted alpha-adrenergic agent is injected into the corpus cavernosum until detumescence occurs (epinephrine, 10 to 20 µg, or phenylephrine, 200 µg, every 5 minutes until detumescence). The patient is also told not to engage in masturbation or sexual intercourse on the day of the test (this is included in the written consent form).

Additional Tests

Duplex Ultrasound or Color Ultrasound Scanning. Real-time ultrasonography and pulsed Doppler scanning, or color Doppler, can be used to examine the penile structures and cavernous arteries before and after intracavernous injection of a vasodilator. Because the arterial diameter and flow rate change during different phases of erection, they are measured within 5 minutes of injection and, if necessary, after self-stimulation. The normal values (obtained in potent patients studied for reasons other than impotence) are: (1) postinjection diameter of more than 0.08 cm, (2) peak flow velocity of over 30 cm per second, and (3) strong pulsation of the thin-walled cavernous arteries. The advantages of this test are its noninvasiveness and sensitivity; the disadvantages are the expense of the equipment and the operator dependency of the results.

Cavernous Arterial Occlusion Pressure. Padma-Nathan and associates introduced this test to measure the cavernous arterial pressure. After intracavernous injection of papaverine and phentolamine, normal saline solution is infused to raise the intracavernous pressure to more than 150 mm Hg. When the infusion is stopped, the intracavernous pressure begins to decrease. The pressure at which the arterial pulse becomes audible is the cavernous artery occlusion pressure. The normal value is a gradient of less than 20 mm Hg between the cavernous and brachial arteries. Results correlate well with those of arteriography. The advantage is the less costly equipment (compared with the duplex ultrasound scanner); the disadvantage is its moderate invasiveness.

Pharmacologic Arteriography. Because of the low flow rate in a flaccid penis, visualization of the cavernous

Table 1 Combined Injection and Stimulation (CIS) Test

1. Complete explanation of procedure (including possible complications and necessity of a second injection if erection lasts >1 hr); consent obtained

2. Intracavernous injection of 10 µg prostaglandin E_1 (PGE_1); observation for 15 min

3. Good erection lasting >45 min: phenylephrine* injection to prevent priapism

   Partial erection: add manual genital stimulation
      Good erection >30 min: phenylephrine* injection
      Partial erection: add vacuum constriction device

4. Adequate erection: advise injection plus constriction device
   Inadequate erection: increase PGE_1 up to 25–40 µg in next few visits

5. Additional vascular work-up if patient wishes

*Phenylephrine solution: 200-µg intracavernous injection every 5 min until detumescence.

arteries has been universally poor if penile arteriography is performed under local anesthesia. With the introduction of intracavernous vasodilator injection, various authors have shown excellent visualization with this technique. Because of potential complications and high cost, I recommend this test only if penile arterial surgery is contemplated.

For the investigation of arteriogenic impotence, I begin with the CIS test in the office. If the patient achieves a prompt and sustained erection, no further vascular test is performed. If he does not, duplex ultrasonography before and after intracavernous injection of PGE_1 is performed to assess arterial function. I believe that duplex ultrasound scanning gives a better assessment of cavernous arterial function than arteriography, although the latter provides information of the proximal large arteries. Duplex ultrasonography is far less expensive and virtually risk free.

PREFERRED TREATMENT

I believe that treatment should begin with the least invasive therapy such as oral medication (e.g., yohimbine or a vasodilator) or a vacuum constriction device. If these are not effective or are unacceptable to the patient, more invasive therapies such as intracavernous injection should be advised. In my opinion, only when these alternatives fail should surgery be recommended. Of course, there are exceptions. For example, in a young man with traumatic injury to a penile vessel, revascularization may be a better alternative than life-long injection therapy or a vacuum constriction device.

Nonsurgical Therapies

Nonsurgical therapies include yohimbine, oral vasodilators, a vacuum constriction device, intracavernous injection, a combination of the constriction device with injection, and transluminal angioplasty. The first four choices are discussed elsewhere in this volume.

Combined Vacuum Constriction Device and Intracavernous Injection

In patients who cannot achieve adequate erection with either intracavernous injection or a vacuum constriction device alone, the combination may be helpful. This is especially true in patients with severe vascular disease and those with fibrosis of the erectile tissue secondary to priapism or failed prosthesis insertion.

Transluminal Angioplasty

Balloon dilatation of the stenotic area of the aortic bifurcation and iliac artery has restored potency in some patients. With improved instruments and refined technique, balloon angioplasty of the distal arteries (internal pudendal, common penile, or proximal cavernous) is technically feasible. However, the success rate is limited by the high rate of recurrence of stenosis.

Surgical Therapies

Arterial Surgery

Because the distal and proximal penile arteries differ notably in size and hemodynamics, the distal internal pudendal, common penile, and cavernous arteries will be discussed separately from the aortic bifurcation, hypogastric, and proximal internal pudendal arteries.

Distal Arterial Disease. In our recent series of 657 impotent patients who underwent duplex ultrasonography, 80 percent were found to have some degree of cavernous arterial insufficiency. Theoretically, arterial reconstruction or bypass would be the ideal therapy (Table 2). However, the cavernous artery, with a diameter of 1 mm, delivers only several milliliters per minute of flow in the flaccid state, a feature that has severely hindered the success of distal penile arterial surgery. On the basis of our clinical experience and animal studies, the following procedures are believed to have the best chance of success from a hemodynamic point of view:

1. Anastomosis of a donor artery (usually epigastric) to the dorsal artery of the penis in patients with large communicating branches between the dorsal and cavernous arteries. Theoretically, this procedure will carry enough flow to the corpora cavernosa, but large collaterals between the dorsal and cavernous arteries are seen in less than 20 percent of cases.
2. Retrograde anastomosis of a donor artery to the proximal stump of a dorsal artery (if the occlusion occurs at the common penile artery proximal to its trifurcation). The patent cavernous artery will

Table 2 Penile Vascular Reconstructive Techniques

Common penile-dorsal-cavernous arteries
  Balloon dilatation (Bookstein)
  Arteriocorporeal bypass
    Epigastric-corporeal (Michal)
    Femoral-saphenous vein-corporeal (LeVeen)
  Arterioarterial bypass
    Epigastric-dorsal (end-to-side; Michal)
    Epigastric-dorsal (retrograde; Goldstein, Sharlip)
    Epigastric-cavernous (Crespo)
  Arteriovenous bypass
    Femoral-saphenous–deep dorsal vein (LeVeen)
    Epigastric–deep dorsal vein–corporeal (Virag)
    Epigastric-dorsal artery and vein (Hauri)

Aortohypogastric-pudendal arteries
  Balloon dilatation
  Endarterectomy
  Bypass

Combined arterial and venous surgery
  Epigastric-dorsal artery (or epigastric artery–dorsal vein)
    + plication of crura (Goldstein)
    + suture ligation of cavernous and crural veins (Lue)

then be able to draw blood from the new source during erection.

3. Variations of arteriovenous or arterioarteriovenous anastomoses to increase the distal run-off and provide retrograde flow to the corpora cavernosa (see Table 2). Early results have been encouraging, because these types of anastomoses have a better likelihood of remaining patent owing to the large distal run-off. In animal experiments, we found that a high pressure in the deep dorsal vein after the arteriovenous anastomosis is essential to divert blood to the corpora cavernosa and prevent venous leakage. Therefore, ligating both proximal and distal portions of the deep dorsal vein may improve the surgical outcome if the anastomosis can remain patent. However, several questions remain. How much retrograde flow from the deep dorsal vein to the corpora cavernosa is actually delivered when, during tumescence, the venous channels are compressed and flow is restricted? Do the emissary veins enlarge under the constant high pressure from the arteriovenous anastomosis? If so, do they eventually become the source of venous leakage? What is the long-term effect of subjecting the erectile tissue to a retrograde high-pressure system with highly oxygenated blood?

One major concern of arterial surgery is the recent finding of altered penile erectile tissue in elderly patients and in those with diabetes mellitus or generalized vascular disease, and the frequent association of arterial insufficiency and venous leakage. This end-organ disease may prevent cure of potency even if the arterial anastomosis is patent and enough flow is delivered to the erectile tissue. Further research on the incidence, detection, and reversibility of end-organ changes is urgently needed.

Proximal Arterial Disease.   Because of the size and greater flow rate of these vessels, balloon dilatation or reconstructive surgery of an isolated lesion has a reasonably high success rate. In patients with generalized atherosclerosis, however, impotence usually recurs with progression of the arterial disease. To achieve a higher success rate, the distal penile arteries should be assessed by techniques in addition to the traditional pudendal arteriography. Duplex ultrasonography, before and after intracavernous injection of a vasodilator or measurement of the cavernous artery occlusion pressure, would give the best assessment of the cavernous arteries. Pharmacologic cavernosometry and cavernosography are also required to evaluate the venous occlusion mechanism. In selected patients in whom the integrity of the cavernous erectile tissue is in doubt, electron microscopic examination of a biopsy sample may be indicated.

Patient Selection.   The best candidates are young men with a history of perineal injury but no venous leakage. Patients with generalized atherosclerosis, diabetes, or chronic hypertension; those who smoke heavily; and those who are older than 65 years usually do not have a favorable response.

Preoperative Preparation.   It is essential that diagnostic tests be performed by experienced personnel. These should include duplex sonography or cavernous artery occlusion pressure, cavernosometry, cavernosography, and pharmacologic arteriography.

Choice of Procedure.   Retrograde epigastric-dorsal artery bypass is the procedure of choice for patients with isolated internal pudendal or common penile arterial disease. If the cavernous artery is stenotic or occluded, epigastric artery–dorsal vein anastomosis is appropriate.

Postoperative Course.   To prevent excessive hematoma formation and ecchymosis, a 7-mm Jackson-Pratt suction drain is placed at the end of surgery and removed the next day. The patient is instructed to abstain from sexual intercourse for 4 weeks. Anticoagulant therapy is initiated on the first postoperative day (5 gr aspirin every day or dipyridamole, 25 mg three times daily) and continued for at least 12 months.

Complications.   Bleeding, anastomosis disruption, penile shortening, numbness, thrombosis of the anastomosis, and glans hypervascularization (in patients with epigastric artery–dorsal vein anastomosis) have all been reported. Once glans hypervascularization is detected, surgical ligation of the remaining tributaries of the deep dorsal vein will be needed to prevent glanular sloughing.

Combined Arterial and Venous Surgery

Several investigators suggested procedures to increase both the arterial flow and venous resistance. Among these are Virag's deep dorsal vein arterialization, Hauri's epigastric–dorsal artery–dorsal vein anastomosis, and Goldstein's epigastric–dorsal artery–dorsal vein ligation. Theoretically, these procedures should achieve a higher success rate because they simultaneously correct problems of supply and drainage.

In patients with combined arterial insufficiency and venous leakage, I prefer an inguinoscrotal incision to approach the penis and a paramedian incision to harvest the epigastric artery. I first perform suture ligation of the cavernous and crural veins after resection of the most proximal segment of the deep dorsal vein from the hilum of the penis to about 2 cm distal to the periprostatic plexus. This is followed by epigastric artery–proximal dorsal vein end-to-end anastomosis. In addition, the distal dorsal vein is ligated about 1 to 2 cm from the glans after valvotomy to prevent glans hypervascularization. This technique results in high intraluminal pressure in the deep dorsal vein, and theoretically higher venous resistance and retrograde flow into the corpus cavernosum. If the postoperative results in these patients prove to be superior over the long term, we can look forward to a new and exciting era of penile vascular surgery.

The preoperative preparation, postoperative course, and complications are similar to those of epigastric artery–dorsal vein anastomosis. However, in selecting patients, only those with combined arterial insufficiency and venous leakage who do not have clinical evidence of corporeal fibrosis and a neurologic deficit would be recommended for this procedure.

Prosthetic Surgery

The Small-Carrion prosthesis, introduced in 1975, was the first satisfactory semirigid prosthesis. It came in different sizes and lengths, had greater flexibility than previous devices, and fit the entire length of the corpora cavernosa. To improve concealment, many new devices subsequently emerged: the Finney hinged silicon rod (Surgitech), the Jonas prosthesis, the AMS malleable and Mentor malleable, and the Omniphase and Duraphase from Dacomed.

Aiming for a better cosmetic appearance, Scott developed the ingenious inflatable prosthesis. Over the years, numerous modifications have been made to improve its durability and reduce the complication rate, which was reported to be as high as 54 percent at first. To decrease the incidence of wear, dilatation, and leakage, the Mentor inflatable made of Bioflex was introduced in 1983. Recently, single- and two-component modifications of the inflatable prosthesis aimed at simplifying the implantation process have become available (e.g., Hydroflex [AMS], Flexi-Flate [Surgitech], and Resipump [Mentor]). Many recent studies have shown improved device reliability and patient-partner satisfaction. The major complications include device malfunction, device protrusion, infection, and persistent pain.

Preoperative Preparation.   Pre-, intra-, and postoperative antibiotic coverage is essential in any prosthetic surgery. The patient is shaved in the operating room and scrubbed with povidone-iodine (Betadine) solution for 10 minutes. Preoperative urine cultures must be negative. If these are positive, the operation is postponed until the source is identified and adequately treated.

Table 3 Author's Indications for Penile
Prosthesis Implantation

Patients with poor response to intracavernous injection and vacuum
constriction devices
  Those who are inappropriate candidates for vascular surgery for
    following reasons
    Generalized arterial disease
    Advanced age
    Heavy smoking, drug abuse
    Chronic systemic disease: e.g., diabetes, renal failure
  Those who decline other treatment options

Patients with good response to intracavernous injection and vacuum
constriction devices
  Those who decline other treatment options
  Those with systemic diseases that contraindicate other options:
    e.g., coagulopathy, sickle cell disease

Skin Incision. I prefer a penoscrotal incision for a
semirigid and an infrapubic incision for an inflatable
prosthesis. Others prefer a penoscrotal incision for both.
Because of the relative stiffness of the Dacomed Duraphase and Omniphase prostheses, a circumcision incision is recommended for these. I found a small (7-mm)
Jackson-Pratt drain placed in the scrotal sac overnight to
be helpful in minimizing scrotal hematoma so that the
patient can begin to activate the inflatable device several
days after surgery.

Postoperative Course. I routinely continue antibiotic therapy for 1 week and advise the patient to activate
the inflatable prosthesis 3 to 5 days after surgery when
the pain becomes tolerable.

Indications for Penile Prosthesis Implantation.
Before the introduction of intracavernous vasodilator
injection therapy and vacuum constriction devices, a
penile prosthesis was the only effective treatment for
erectile dysfunction besides psychological counseling.
Tens of thousands were implanted, with indications that
were somewhat loose. Any patient with a poor erection
on nocturnal penile tumescence testing was a candidate,
as were patients with good nocturnal tumescence who
failed to improve with psychotherapy.

The high success rate of the newer, less invasive
therapies has clouded the indications for prosthetic surgery. Although the goal of the patient and his partner is
still the primary consideration of the treating urologist,
the fact that successful alternative treatments are currently available should be fully explained. Table 3 lists
the indications for prosthetic surgery in my practice.

PATIENT'S GOAL-DIRECTED APPROACH TO DIAGNOSIS AND TREATMENT OF IMPOTENCE

At my institution, after detailed history taking, physical examination, and routine laboratory testing, the pa-

Table 4 Treatment Options versus Tests

1. Oral medication or vacuum erection device
     No further testing
2. Intracavernous injection therapy
     CIS test*
3. Penile prosthesis
     CIS or NPT† test
4. Venous surgery
     CIS test
     Duplex scanning or measurement of cavernous artery occlusion
       pressure
     Cavernosometry and cavernosography
5. Arterial surgery (or mixed arterial and venous surgery)
     CIS test
     Duplex scanning or cavernous artery occlusion pressure
     Cavernosometry and cavernosography
     Pharmacologic arteriography

*CIS, Combined injection and stimulation (see Table 1).
†NPT, Nocturnal penile tumescence.

tient is given a pamphlet containing various treatment
options currently available. Because impotence is a functional disease, I believe that the patient's medical and
psychological conditions and his desired treatment can
be used to direct further diagnosis and treatment (Table
4). For example, if the patient is interested only in a
vacuum constriction device, no further testing is performed. However, if the patient is interested in vascular
surgery and is a good candidate, several vascular tests are
advised. The different tests for the different treatments
desired are listed in Table 4.

SUGGESTED READING

Goldstein I. Arterial revascularization procedures. Semin Urol 1986;
  4:252–258.
Hauri D. A new operative technique in vasculogenic erectile impo-
  tence. World J Urol 1986; 4:237–249.
Lue TF, Mueller SC, Jow YR, Hwang TI-S. Functional evaluation of
  penile arteries with duplex ultrasound in vasodilator-induced
  erection. Urol Clin North Am 1989; 16:799–807.
Lue TF. Penile venous surgery. Urol Clin North Am 1989; 16:607–611.
Padma-Nathan H. Evaluation of the corporal veno-occlusive
  mechanism: dynamic infusion cavernosometry and cavernosography.
  Semin Intervent Radiol 1989; 6:205.
Persson C, Diederichs W, Lue TF, Yen TSB, Fishman IJ, McLin PH,
  Tanagho EA: Correlation of altered penile ultrastructure with
  clinical arterial evaluation. J Urol 1989; 142:1462–1468.
Valji K, Bookstein JJ. Transluminal angioplasty in the treatment of
  arteriogenic impotence. Cardiovasc Intervent Radiol 1988; 11:
  245–252.
Virag R. Revascularization of the penis. In: Bennett AH, ed.
  Management of male impotence. Baltimore: Williams & Wilkins,
  1982:219.

NEUROGENIC ETIOLOGY OF IMPOTENCE

JERZY B. GAJEWSKI, M.D., FRCSC
R. BREWER AULD, M.D., FRCSC
SAID A. AWAD, M.B., FRCSC

Erection is controlled by the central (spinal and supraspinal centers) and peripheral nervous systems. The hypothalamus plays an integrating role for different afferent sexual stimuli and efferent pathways. Afferent impulses are provided from the peripheral erogenous regions and from thalamic (visual), limbic (emotion and memory), and rhinencephalic (olfactory) areas. These afferents also connect to the cerebral cortex. The regulation of ascending and descending erectile impulses in the spine is localized in two centers: one that modulates sympathetic control is at the T10-T12 level, and the other parasympathetic innervation is at S2-S4. The parasympathetic efferents, via the pelvic nerves, produce erection by relaxing cavernous and arteriolar smooth muscle. The sympathetic efferents, via the hypogastric nerves, cause detumescence by contracting these smooth muscles. Somatic innervation from the dorsal penile and internal pudendal nerves provides afferent stimuli from the penis.

Three different types of erections have been described: reflexogenic, psychogenic, and nocturnal. Reflexogenic erections result from tactile stimuli (afferents) from the penis and groin area traveling via the pudendal nerve to the spine and triggering an efferent response at the spinal level. Stimuli from the brain (audiovisual or fantasy) cause psychogenic erections. Nocturnal erections are not well understood. Disruption of the nervous system at any level can cause erectile dysfunction. Disruption of neurogenic control may occur centrally at the supraspinal or spinal levels or in the peripheral nervous system. Examples of each are listed in Table 1.

PATIENT POPULATION

In about 10 percent of impotent men seen in our Sexual Dysfunction Clinic the impotence has a neurogenic cause (excluding patients with diabetes mellitus). The mean age of these patients is 42 years. Half of them have spinal cord lesions (paraplegics and quadriplegics). The second largest group consists of individuals with multiple sclerosis. Most patients present with early loss of erection or have semierections of insufficient rigidity to achieve penetration. Sixty percent of our patients decide to have treatment after their initial evaluation and information session.

EVALUATION

All patients are evaluated according to a standardized clinic protocol. We begin the history taking by asking specific questions about their sexual dysfunction relating to penile tumescence, rigidity, deformity, and pain and the duration of the problem. The patient's libido should be determined. It is important to ask about the status of erections before the event that led to neurologic injury. Current or previous medical problems are established, especially possible neurogenic lesions. In patients with spinal cord injury, a detailed description of the injury and treatment should be documented. Bladder function and management must be established. Medications are recorded and their potential role in the erectile problem clarified. Smoking habits and alcohol intake should be documented. It is important to evaluate patients' personal and social support systems. This is integrated with the basic psychological assessment.

Physical examination includes routine physical and detailed urologic and neurologic investigation. Examination of the external genitals provides evidence of diseases (e.g., Peyronie's) or malformations (congenital or traumatic). Sensory and reflex testing provides information about the spinal and peripheral status of the neurologic system. Laboratory studies include tests of serum testosterone and serum glucose levels, and of liver function.

Response to intracorporeal injection of pharmacologic agents (papaverine, phentolamine, or prostaglandin E_1 [PGE_1]) is most useful in supporting a neurogenic cause and illustrating a practical mode of treatment.

Studies reserved for particular individuals or for research include evaluation of the vascular supply by a duplex Doppler ultrasonography, nocturnal penile tumescence (NPT), electromyography (EMG) of the cavernosal smooth muscles, sacral and cortical evoked potentials, dorsal nerve conduction velocity studies,

Table 1 Etiology of Neurogenic Dysfunction

Supraspinal	Spinal	Peripheral
Cerebrovascular accident (CVA)	Injury (trauma or surgery)	Diabetes mellitus
Parkinsonism	Multiple sclerosis	Alcoholism
Epilepsy	Tumor	Injury (trauma or surgery)
Tumor	Syringomyelia	Vitamin deficiency
Alzheimer's disease	Discopathy	Metals and chemicals
	Spina bifida	Drugs
	Tabes dorsalis	

sweating tests, skin ultratremor, biothesiometry, and cystometrography (CMG).

TREATMENT

Information

We inform patients of all options available: intracorporeal injection of pharmacologic agents, vacuum constriction devices, and penile prostheses. Success with oral pharmacologic agents such as yohimbine for patients with neurogenic dysfunction is infrequent and no longer recommended. The efficacy of oral dopa-agonists is currently being assessed. Electrostimulation for erectile dysfunction also shows therapeutic possibilities as a treatment option.

Consideration is given to associated medical problems such as autonomic dysreflexia, spasticity, skin erosion, and decubiti. Selection also depends on manual dexterity, comprehension, communication, and mobility. In some instances the participation of a patient's sexual partner is advantageous. The partner may assume an active role in treatment, assist in different sexual techniques, and help with handling of other devices the patient may have (e.g., Foley catheter, condom, stoma).

Intracorporeal Injection

Intracorporeal injection of a pharmacologic agent is the preferred treatment for impotence of neurogenic cause when response is good on test injection and the patient is agreeable.

All our patients receive an intracorporeal injection test during initial evaluation. Owing to the corporeal supersensitivity of neurogenic patients to pharmacologic agents, the initial dosage should be one tenth of the usual one. Table 2 shows appropriate initial dosages of different pharmacologic agents. A mixture of papaverine and phentolamine is more potent than either drug alone, and the dosage of an individual drug should be reduced even more. PGE_1 is the most potent of the three. Papaverine is a smooth muscle relaxant that affects penile arteries and smooth muscles of the corporeal body. Subsequently, arterial flow increases, cavernous tissues expand, and venous outflow decreases. Phentolamine, an alpha blocker, acts on the vasculature only. The vascular smooth muscle relaxing effect of PGE_1 is not well understood.

Table 2 Dosages of Pharmacologic Agents for Intracorporeal Injection

Drug	Normal Dosage	Reduced Dosage†
Papaverine	40–65 mg	4–6 mg
Phentolamine*	0.5–2.5 mg	0.1–0.5 mg
Prostaglandin E_1	15–30 μg	1–3 μg

*In combination with papaverine.
†For testing of neurogenic impotence.

Teaching sessions are arranged if good penile tumescence and rigidity results from the test dose. If the patient is unable to inject himself, a willing partner may be taught the technique. Usually, one or two teaching sessions are given by the clinic nurse. Autoinjection is given in the midshaft of the penis at 10 or 2 o'clock positions, avoiding visible veins and using an insulin syringe with 28G1/2" needle. The needle should be positioned perpendicular to the skin and the medication injected slowly. Erection usually develops in 10 to 15 minutes and lasts 30 to 60 minutes, depending on dosage. It is advisable to alternate injection sites side to side. We suggest waiting 48 hours or more between successive injections.

Complications from the initial injection test are rare, but hematoma, ecchymosis, or malinjection (1 percent) may occur. Hypotensive reactions have been described. Occasionally, patients with preserved sensation may briefly experience mild burning in the corpora. This is less frequently seen with mixed injections and is usually well tolerated. PGE_1 causes penile burning or prolonged painful sensation in 30 percent of patients 10 minutes after injection, and this occasionally interferes with sexual enjoyment.

The most significant unwanted reaction is priapism, which occurs most commonly in men with impotence of neurogenic and psychogenic etiology. We define priapism as a continuous, painful, erection lasting longer than 6 hours. This occurs in 3 to 5 percent of patients after injections of papaverine or a mixture of papaverine and phentolamine. Once individual dosage has been determined, prolonged erections are rare. PGE_1 is less often associated with priapism because it is rapidly inactivated. Priapism is reversed by irrigation of the corpora with normal saline using sterile precautions through a No. G18 butterfly needle, especially if the priapism has been prolonged. Approximately 10 to 15 ml of blood is aspirated from the corpora and the same amount of saline is infused. If tumescence persists, irrigation is continued with an epinephrine solution (1 mg in 1 L of 0.9 percent sodium chloride). Close monitoring of blood pressure is recommended. In all cases we have been able to achieve detumescence. Other clinics use a single injection of metaraminol (2 to 4 mg), epinephrine (15 μg), or phenylephrine (200 to 500 μg). Metaraminol is considered an unsafe and unpredictable compound. In patients with severe ischemic heart disease or a recent myocardial infarction, treatment with alpha-mimetic agents should be undertaken with extreme caution. Oral vasoconstrictive agents such as pseudoephedrine (120 mg), phenylpropanolamine (30 mg), or phenylephrine (10 mg) may also be used to prevent prolonged erections.

The long-term effects of injection on the corporeal tissue are unknown. Painless fibrotic lesions occur in 5 to 10 percent of patients within 1 year of treatment with monoinjection of papaverine. Mixed injection or PGE_1 induces fibrosis less frequently. Some of these lesions spontaneously resolve when injections are stopped.

Papaverine is considered a hepatotoxic agent. However, abnormal liver function tests are rare in these patients and occur predominantly in those with an alcoholic background.

Treatment with papaverine or phentolamine is relatively inexpensive; PGE_1 can be 10 to 15 times more expensive. In our experience, successful results are achieved in 88 percent of patients at 1-year follow-up. Lack of a partner is the main cause for discontinuance of the treatment.

Vacuum Constriction Devices

A conservative alternative to self-injection is the use of vacuum constriction devices (ErecAid, Osbon; VED, Mission; Catalyst, Dacomed; Response or Touch, Mentor; Pos-T-Vac, Pos-T-Vac Inc). These consist of a cylinder, a pump, and a constriction ring. The constrictor is stretched over the base of the cylinder, and the lubricated cylinder is placed over the penis to attain a closed system. The pump removes air from the system, creating negative pressure around the erectile tissue, and an erection occurs within 1 to 5 minutes. The constriction ring is slipped onto the base of the penis to sustain the erection, and the cylinder and pump are set aside. In patients who are able to achieve an erection but have difficulty sustaining it, the use of a constriction device for venous entrapment may be adequate treatment. The achieved erection is distal to the constriction ring, and the penis pivots at the base. Manual assistance to achieve penetration may be required. This should be discussed with the patient and his partner and they must be prepared to make adjustments in sexual techniques. Because of decreased blood flow through the penile tissue, there may be edema, increase in penile circumference, coldness, and cyanosis. It is recommended not to exceed 30 minutes of constriction time. One must be careful to select patients who do not have problems with skin erosion due to condom drainage, or those with indwelling Foley catheters. These patients are more susceptible to cutaneous excoriation, and a lubricant applied to the ring will reduce the incidence of skin trauma. The device is relatively contraindicated in patients taking anticoagulants or those with blood dyscrasias. Patients with preserved peripheral sensation may experience some discomfort if the negative pressure is too high. It is important, especially in patients with no sensation, that devices have a safety mechanism to vent excessive negative pressure (220 mm Hg). The constriction ring may impair ejaculation in 30 to 50 percent of patients. Some rings are of a special design to minimize urethral obstruction. The most common technical problem is difficulty with creating an air-tight seal when the cylinder is placed over the flaccid penis. Results are improved by the use of lubricants and different-size cylinder inserts, shaving of pubic hair, and appropriate instruction. Careful selection of the size and type of constriction ring is important. Insufficient tightness may allow detumescence. Treatment is inexpensive except for the initial investment to purchase the device. We have observed good results (60 percent success) from

this technique in patients with both neurogenic and non-neurogenic erectile dysfunction. The major objection is that it is too mechanical, intruding into the intimacy of sexual activity.

Penile Prostheses

Implantation of a penile prosthesis is also an effective treatment. It may be the primary modality selected, but it is particularly useful in those who fail to respond to other forms of therapy: e.g., those with impaired manual dexterity or poor vision or without a consistent partner. Patients who have difficulty maintaining condom drainage may find that the implant makes condom application easier.

Extensive consultation with the patient and his partner regarding the type of prosthesis to be implanted is mandatory. Samples of prostheses should be shown to the patient and the costs of each discussed; obviously, mechanical or inflatable prostheses are more expensive.

The different types of penile prosthesis are presented in Table 3. Rod prostheses are easy to implant, have long-term mechanical stability, and are associated with low malfunction rates. These prosthesis, however, do not change girth or length and tend to erode more often than the inflatable devices, especially in patients with poor sensation. This is particularly true in patients with indwelling Foley catheters or on intermittent catheterization. The erosion rate may reach 50 percent. This may be improved by creating a perineal urethrostomy for catheterization. Rod prostheses result in transurethral instrumentation being more difficult. In the absence of perineal urethrostomy, longer instruments may be necessary. These are not readily available in most urologic centers.

Inflatable prostheses are more of a surgical challenge, carry a greater risk of malfunction, and are more expensive. However, the advantage in patients with decreased sensation is that there is less likelihood of erosion. A routine endoscopic instrument can be used if necessary. The three-piece inflatable prosthesis produces the most natural erection, and when deflated causes no embarrassment.

All patients should be free of infection before the planned surgery. In particular, the urine culture should be negative. A providone-iodine (Betadine) bath is advisable the night before surgery. Perioperative cover-

Table 3 Penile Prostheses

Rods	Mechanical	Inflatable
Rigid	OmniPhase	One-piece — self-contain
Small-Carrion	DuraPhase	Flexi-Flate II
Semirigid		Hydroflex
Flexi-rod II		Two-piece
Malleable		GFS Mark II
Jonas		Uni-Flate 1000
AMS 600		Three-piece
		IPP Mentor
		AMS 700 CX

age with broad-spectrum antibiotics is mandatory. We usually give oral antibiotics for 10 days after surgery.

Implantation of the prosthesis is a simple procedure. We usually use a penoscrotal incision for both semirigid and inflatable devices, even when implanting a three-piece device. Careful measurement of the corporeal length is important. If corporeal rods or cylinders are too long, pain may result and erosion is more likely to occur. If the length is inadequate, penile deformity may be associated with penetration problems. Intraoperative antibiotic irrigation of the prosthesis and the corpora prevents infection. In patients who require an indwelling urinary catheter or condom drainage, suprapubic drainage is indicated until the incision is healed. Implantation of prostheses may be performed as a 1-day surgical procedure, but hospitalization may be required for other medical or logistic factors.

Complications from penile prosthesis surgery are now infrequent. A satisfactory result is observed in 80 to 90 percent. Pain observed immediately after the opera-

tion in some patients usually disappears and rarely requires removal of the device. Infection is rare, but when present, with or without erosion, usually necessitates implant removal. Removal of a single rod or portion of the inflatable device may be adequate. Restoration of device function is best delayed to allow eradication of infection, but immediately successful replacement of infected devices is reported.

SUGGESTED READING

Junemann KP, Alken P. Pharmacotherapy of erectile dysfunction: a review. Int J Impotence Res 1989; 1:71–93.
Malloy TR, Wein AJ. Current status of penile prostheses. Int J Impotence Res 1989; 1:153–165.
Nadig PW. Six years' experience with the vacuum constriction device. Int J Impotence Res 1989; 1:55–58.
Steidle CP, Mulcahy JJ. Erosion of penile prosthesis: a complication of urethral catheterization. J Urol 1989; 142:736–739.
Witherington R. Vacuum constriction device for management of erectile impotence. J Urol 1989; 141:320–322.

IMPOTENCE SECONDARY TO SURGERY

ALAN H. BENNETT, M.D.

Several factors must be considered before ascribing the development of sexual dysfunction to a specific surgical procedure. Many reports in the literature that indicate impotence as a complication of a procedure or treatment offer few control studies to substantiate the cause-and-effect relationship being noted. The pretreatment status of sexual performance is rarely known, and the change in sexual function is based on subjective and historical data and not objective testing such as the use of intracavernous vasoactive drugs, nocturnal penile tumescence testing, and dynamic cavernometrics. Most recent studies on the causes of sexual dysfunction indicate multiple factors in nearly 50 percent of patients. Psychogenic factors are the primary component in one third of patients, and vascular causes in almost one half. Obviously, there is a direct relationship between a surgical event and impotence in many patients, but the above-mentioned issues must be considered before incriminating the surgical procedure or treatment as the sole cause of the resultant sexual dysfunction. Sexual dysfunction after surgery may present as erectile dysfunction, ejaculatory dysfunction, or elements of both.

Three general classifications can be developed in which impotence may be a result of surgery: procedures completely extrinsic to the genitourinary tract, urologic procedures, and nonurologic procedures.

An example of a common operation that may result in sexual dysfunction is a cardiac procedure. Psychogenic factors obviously play a role in this situation and, when combined with a partial arteriogenic factor from generalized atherosclerosis, may account for erectile dysfunction. This is true for any major surgical procedure in older males. Fear of causing bodily harm by coitus may be a prominent factor in cardiac, transplant, and ostomy patients.

Many urologic procedures may directly affect the erectile and ejaculatory mechanisms. Scar tissue or a poor surgical outcome from hypospadias and epispadias repairs or circumcision may result in penile curvature or pain during the erectile state. This is also true of urethral stricture repair and the various procedures (especially patch graft) performed for the curvature associated with Peyronie's disease. Any reparative procedure for lack of testicular descent or hernia repair in infancy or childhood can result in testicular atrophy, which if bilateral may result in lack of sufficient testosterone to stimulate libido. Obviously, bilateral orchiectomy produces the same result. Patients undergoing partial penectomy for carcinoma should be advised that sensation and corporal filling may be impaired postoperatively. The impotence associated with transurethral resection of the prostate should be categorized into disturbances of ejaculation (common) and of erectile dysfunction (rare and poorly documented). Transurethral resection or Y-V–plasty of the bladder neck, once regularly performed in young males, often produced retrograde ejaculation. Radical cystoprostatectomy for bladder carcinoma, and total prostatectomy for carcinoma of the prostate, commonly resulted in erectile dysfunction, but since the advent of nerve-sparing procedures, potency after these operations is often possible.

Nongenitourinary surgery that often is associated with impotence can be divided into neural-ablative procedures (retroperitoneal lymphadenectomy, abdominal perineal resection or total colectomy for carcinoma, abdominal aneurysm surgery, and various spinal cord operations) and procedures in which the penile blood supply may be reduced or interrupted (aneurysm repair, lower extremity arterial bypass procedures, and renal transplantation). Pure nerve injury of the sympathetic chain usually results in ejaculatory disturbances (lack of seminal fluid or anejaculation), but disturbances of erectile function are also possible.

The evaluation and treatment of sexual dysfunction secondary to surgical procedures have changed dramatically in the last decade. Penile prosthesis placement was the only option for these men 10 years ago, but today it should be considered only as a last resort. The discovery by Virag that intracorporal papaverine could produce an erectile response and his seminal work on vasoactive drugs, have resulted in accurate methods of diagnosing and treating all forms of erectile dysfunction. The only patients who do not respond to intracorporal vasoactive drugs are those who have severe arterial or corporovenous occlusive disease. Patients with psychogenic or purely neurogenic causes for erectile dysfunction generally respond to low doses of vasoactive drugs. Recently, combinations of these agents, especially papaverine, phentolamine, and prostaglandin E_1 (PGE_1) have reduced the volume and concentrations of these drugs, thereby increasing the safety of their use.

Before proceeding with intracorporal vasoactive drug testing, a careful history taking and physical examination is important. An artificial erection by saline infusion with a tourniquet or by intracorporal vasoactive drugs should outline the curvature or adhesive bands that may have resulted from an earlier penile procedure. A variety of reparative procedures, ranging from a simple release of fibrous bands to a Nesbitt procedure, are in the armamentarium of every urologist. Before any corrective penile procedure is begun, however, an assessment of corporal filling and retention by means of vasoactive drug testing and dynamic cavernosometry is essential. Repair of a curvature in a man who has a flaccid erection will not result in a happy patient!

An important consideration in patients with sexual dysfunction caused by a neural disruption is the natural reparative process. Many patients gradually recover erectile function with time. No invasive procedure should be undertaken until a reasonable period (up to 2 years) has elapsed. As mentioned, these patients, who often have a normal vascular supply, respond to small doses of self-administered intracorporal vasoactive drugs (pharmacologic erection programs [PEP]).

Obviously, a total loss of testicular tissue will result in the need for supplementation to stimulate libido. However, up to 15 percent of patients with sexual dysfunction have some degree of endocrine dysfunction. Thus, a measurement of the serum testosterone level is important. Other hormonal measurements such as prolactin, follicle stimulating hormone (FSH), and luteinizing hormone (LH) are not necessary unless there is an abnormality in the testosterone level. Simple correction of the testosterone deficiency may be rewarding in men with documented low levels, but PEP may also be indicated in older males with multiple etiologic factors.

Retrograde ejaculation after surgical procedures to the bladder neck may respond to oral administration of sympathomimetic drugs or alpha-adrenergic agonists such as ephedrine. However, postorgasm urinary alkalinization and urethral catheterization is usually the means necessary to capture seminal fluid. Lack of emission from nerve damage will not respond to pharmacotherapy.

For patients who do not respond to PEP or are unwilling to accept it as treatment, options include vacuum pump devices, vascular/surgical procedures, or penile prostheses. Most patients with vasculogenic impotence, including many with corporovenous occlusive disease, respond to PEP. Vascular corrective procedures should be reserved for nonsmoking men under 55 years of age without other concurrent disease such as diabetes. No vascular procedure should be performed until the patient has had an adequate trial of PEP. Results of penile vascular repair for impotence indicate a wide variation in success rates (20 to 90 percent). Many of the "successes" still require PEP to produce adequate rigidity for penetration.

For total loss of the phallus, a variety of plastic reconstructive procedures have been developed employing penile implants. However, these appendages provide only coital function.

Thus, treatment is available for all men rendered impotent by a surgical procedure. PEP provides the safest, least expensive form of therapy for most patients. Time will heal some. For the rest, vascular reconstruction, vacuum constriction devices, and penile implants are available.

SUGGESTED READING

Bennett AH. Management of male impotence. Int Perspect Urol 1982; 5.

Virag R. Vasoactive drugs: papaverine and impotence. Editions du Ceri, 1987.

Whitehead ED. Surgical treatment of erectile impotence. Curr Op Urol 1989; 227–313.

PENILE PROSTHESES

DROGO K. MONTAGUE, M.D.

Men suffering from sexual dysfunction today have a better opportunity of finding more effective relief than was ever available in the past. We have a better understanding of normal sexual anatomy and physiology, and more useful knowledge concerning the pathophysiology of various disorders of sexual function. The means currently available to evaluate complaints of sexual dysfunction include history, physical examination, psychological assessment, endocrine evaluation, nocturnal penile tumescence testing, infusion pharmacocavernosometry, duplex ultrasonography, pharmacocavernosography, penile arteriography, and neurodiagnostic testing. After diagnostic evaluation, men with sexual dysfunction can usually be placed into one of three broad diagnostic categories: psychogenic dysfunction; endocrine dysfunction; or organic, nonendocrine dysfunction. Men with psychogenic dysfunction should initially be treated by a sex therapist. Men with endocrine abnormalities, who in my experience constitute approximately 3 to 5 percent of men with sexual dysfunction, can usually be effectively treated with systemic medication. The largest number of these patients have organic, nonendocrine dysfunction. In the past, penile prosthesis implantation was, for the most part, the only treatment available to men in this category. Today, other treatment alternatives are available, but penile prostheses still remain a prime treatment option for these men.

THERAPEUTIC ALTERNATIVES

Treatment alternatives for men with organic, nonendocrine erectile dysfunction include vacuum constriction devices, intracavernous injection therapy, penile vascular surgery, and penile prosthesis implantation.

Vacuum Constriction Devices

Except for men who have limited use of their hands, men with certain hematologic disorders such as sickle cell disease, and men who are on anticoagulants, vacuum constrictive devices can be used by almost all men with organic, nonendocrine erectile dysfunction. The effect produced by these devices resembles a normal erection in that the glans penis and corpus spongiosum are erect; however, in the corpora cavernosa the erection is confined to the penile portion of these erectile bodies, and coupling of the penis to body movement is not ideal. Compared with other methods of treatment, vacuum constrictive devices are relatively inexpensive, and this therapy is reversible. The rubber band or constricting ring used with these devices impedes ejaculation, and leaving the band or ring in place for more than 30 minutes is not recommended. I have found that many men regard a vacuum constrictive device as interfering considerably with the aesthetics of coitus.

Intracavernous Injection Therapy

The direct injection of vasoactive medication into the corpora cavernosa can produce an erection, and intracorporeal drugs have been used widely for both diagnostic and therapeutic purposes. A patient on intracavernous injection therapy must give himself an injection each time he has coitus; however, the erection that results can usually be sustained for an hour or more without a band or ring, and thus there is only moderate interference with coitus. Men who use this method of treatment should be seen for regular follow-up, and the costs of these visits plus the costs of medication, syringes, and needles make this method relatively expensive in the long run. Complications include prolonged erections, penile fibrosis, and hepatotoxicity. Should complications occur or if the patient loses interest, this method of treatment is reversible.

Penile Vascular Surgery

Penile vascular surgery consists of various penile arterial revascularization procedures for arterial insufficiency and penile venous ligation procedures for correction of corporeal-venous occlusive dysfunction. These procedures have the advantage, when they are successful, of restoring normal erections. However, strict diagnostic criteria are used to select candidates for these operations, which can be offered only to a relatively small subset of men with organic, nonendocrine erectile dysfunction. Furthermore, short-term results, in terms of the percentage of men who have restoration of erections that are usable for coitus, are relatively low compared with those of other treatment methods. Long-term results at this time are unknown.

Penile Prosthesis Implantation

Penile prosthesis implantation is a form of treatment that is applicable to nearly every man with organic, nonendocrine erectile dysfunction. Success, in terms of the restoration of the ability to have coitus, should be achieved in more than 95 percent of cases. Penile prostheses interfere little, if at all, with coitus, and periodic follow-up visits are not necessary. The primary disadvantage of penile prosthesis implantation is that it should be considered irreversible.

PREFERRED APPROACH

Patient Selection

Patients who are candidates for penile prosthesis implantation should be offered other treatment options such as a vacuum constrictive device or intracavernous injection therapy. Patients who are candidates for penile vascular surgery should be told of the existence of these procedures.

Success with penile prosthesis implantation in terms of primary healing without infection, erosion, sizing and positioning errors, or early mechanical failure is greater than 95 percent, but patient and partner satisfaction is less. Patients and partners who are not satisfied after a successful procedure clearly did not have their expectations met. While no amount of preoperative counseling will ensure realistic expectations in every case, the urologist should make every effort to counsel the patient adequately, and whenever possible his partner, before implantation. Both should understand that a prosthesis produces an artificial erection that is different from a normal one. The flaccid appearance of the penis is also changed. The amount of difference between a normal state and the postimplant state varies according to variations in anatomy and the type of prosthesis chosen. However, regardless of the type of prosthesis, almost every man with a penile implant reports that his erection is not as long as his normal erection used to be.

Penile sensation is usually not changed after prosthesis implantation, and orgasm and ejaculation, if intact preoperatively, should be preserved. The patient should be warned about the possibility of infection, which usually requires complete removal of the prosthetic device. Mechanical failure and the need for possible future revision should also be discussed with potential implant recipients.

Timing of Surgery

Penile prosthesis implantation should not be offered to a patient with recent-onset erectile dysfunction until it is reasonably certain that the dysfunction is permanent. Patients who experience erectile dysfunction after an injury or a surgical procedure sometimes regain normal erections as healing takes place. A waiting period of 6 to 12 months is reasonable in most cases.

Device Selection

A dozen or more penile prostheses are currently available in the United States (Table 1). In most instances, it is appropriate to provide the potential implant recipient with a choice of at least two and possibly three devices. Nonhydraulic prostheses offer the advantages of simplicity and, in most cases, low costs. A permanent erection is produced, and the positionability between the downward (noncoital) and upward (coital) states varies according to the prosthesis selected.

Hydraulic implants can be grouped into one-, two-, and three-piece devices. One-piece devices are paired implants confined to the corpora cavernosa. The two-piece varieties are paired corporeal cylinders connected to a scrotal pump-reservoir. Three-piece hydraulic prostheses consist of paired corporeal cylinders attached to a scrotal pump, which in turn is connected to an abdominal fluid reservoir.

One-piece hydraulic implants become rigid when

Table 1 Types of Penile Prosthesis

Nonhydraulic devices	Hydraulic devices
Semirigid	One-piece
Small-Carrion	AMS Dynaflex
	Flexi-Flate
Hinged	
Flexi-Rod II	Two-piece
	Mentor GFS
Malleable	Uniflate 1000
AMS Malleable 600	
Jonas Silicon-Silver	Three-piece
Mentor Malleable	AMS Ultrex
	Mentor Inflatable
Positionable	
DuraPhase	
Mechanically activated	
OmniPhase	

inflated; when deflated, they lose part of this rigidity. There is no change in the size of a one-piece device between the deflated and inflated states. When palpated within the penis, these implants feel more natural than most semirigid rod prostheses.

Two-piece hydraulic implants do increase both in size and rigidity when inflated. However, the combined pump-reservoir often produces a detectable bulge in the scrotum. Also, because the volume of fluid in the pump-reservoir is limited, there is often some compromise in either the amount of erection or the degree of flaccidity.

Three-piece hydraulic devices employ a small pump that is readily accommodated within the scrotum and a large abdominal fluid reservoir, which is not detectable. Because a large volume of fluid is available for transfer to and from the cylinders, these devices produce, on average, the best flaccid and erect appearances.

These considerations should be made known to the patient so that he can select an implant type to best meet his needs. Also, if the potential implant recipient appears interested in any of the inflatable devices, the urologist should judge his ability to operate the device. In this regard, intelligence, motivation, manual dexterity, and strength are all important factors.

Finally, certain anatomic factors may make one implant type more desirable than another. In patients who are at high risk for erosion (e.g., spinal cord injury patients), hydraulic devices offer a lower risk of erosion. In patients with erectile dysfunction due to Peyronie's disease, a malleable or positionable nonhydraulic implant will usually both straighten the penis and provide adequate rigidity. If a hydraulic device is implanted in a patient with chordee due to Peyronie's disease, a simultaneous straightening procedure (corporoplasty) may also be needed.

Preoperative Preparation

At the time of prosthesis implantation, the urine should be sterile and there should be no dermatitis or potentially infected skin lesions in the operative field.

The patient is given intravenous antibiotics 1 hour before the procedure; these should be bactericidal and should provide coverage against both gram-positive and gram-negative organisms. I currently use gentamicin and a cephalosporin; if the patient is allergic to penicillin, I substitute vancomycin for the cephalosporin. Shaving to remove hair from the operative field should be done immediately before the procedure. The operative field is then scrubbed with povidone-iodine (Betadine) or other suitable surgical preparation solutions. Paper drapes are used because cloth drapes become permeable to bacteria when wet.

Surgical Approach

Penile prostheses have been implanted through a variety of incisions (Table 2), many of which are no longer in common use. Those still frequently used include infrapubic, dorsal subcoronal, ventral penile midline, penoscrotal, and transverse upper scrotal incisions. I prefer the transverse upper scrotal incision for implantation of the three-piece AMS Ultrex prosthesis, and the ventral midline penile incision for the one-piece AMS Dynaflex prosthesis. I also favor the ventral penile midline incision for implantation of both the AMS Malleable 600 and the DuraPhase prostheses. I have found the lateral inguinoscrotal incision, popularized by Lue for penile venous ligation, useful for access to the entire length of both corpora cavernosa for penile prosthesis implantation in patients with extensive intracorporeal fibrosis.

Postoperative Course

All my implants are inserted under either general or spinal/epidural anesthesia. I insert a urethral catheter and remove it on the first postoperative day. Most patients are discharged from the hospital on the second day after surgery. All prostheses are kept up on the lower abdomen for the first 4 postoperative weeks.

The body reacts to silicone by forming a fibrous pseudocapsule around it. If a patient with an inflatable device keeps the penis in a dependent position while this pseudocapsule is forming, a permanent ventral chordee may result. If the implant recipient with a two- or three-piece hydraulic device keeps the device fully or partially inflated during the healing process, the reservoir will be only partially full, and the pseudocapsule that forms around this reservoir will prevent complete deflation of the prosthesis. For this reason, all two- and three-piece devices should be kept fully deflated while healing is taking place. A pseudocapsule will form around the deflated cylinders; however, when the device is first inflated at the 4-week postoperative visit, the pressure generated by the pumping process will stretch the pseudocapsule, and the quality of the erection will not be impaired in any way.

Complications

Complications of penile prosthesis implantation are shown in Table 3. Infection is inherent in all surgical procedures, but infection in the space around a prosthetic device poses certain special considerations. Bacteria adhere to the surface of prosthetic devices, and antibiotic treatment alone is rarely sufficient to clear these infections. Periprosthetic infections almost always require removal of the entire prosthesis. Reimplantation of a penile prosthesis at a later date is often difficult because of the resultant intracorporeal fibrosis. Salvage procedures for infected prostheses represent an attempt to avoid this fibrosis. In a salvage procedure, the infected device is completely removed and the operative field copiously irrigated with antibiotic solution. A new prosthesis is implanted and antibiotic treatment (according to intraoperative cultures and sensitivities) is continued for up to 6 weeks postoperatively. These salvage procedures are successful in approximately 80 percent of patients.

In the early to middle 1970s, device-related mechanical complications occurred in as many as 50 percent of recipients of inflatable penile prostheses. Improvements in both prosthesis design and implantation techniques have resulted in a dramatic reduction in these types of complications. The AMS Ultrex prosthesis, and its predecessor, the AMS 700CX prosthesis have controlled expansion cylinders that to date have eliminated cylinder aneurysms and have resulted in a dramatic decline in cylinder leaks. Kinkproof tubing with these devices has eliminated tubing kinks, and a special connector system has significantly lowered connector-related leaks. In the

Table 2 Surgical Approaches to Penile Prosthesis Implantation

Above penis	Penile
Suprapubic	Dorsal subcoronal
Transverse	Degloving
Midline	Dorsal midline
	Ventral midline
Infrapubic	Penoscrotal
Transverse	
Midline	Below penis
	Transverse upper scrotal
Lateral to penis	Perineal
Inguinoscrotal	

Table 3 Complications of Penile Prosthesis Implantation

Surgical	Device related (mechanical)
Infection (superficial)	Semirigid rod breakage
Hematoma	Hydraulic leaks
Phimosis	Cylinders
Paraphimosis	Tubing
Urinary retention	Connectors
	Pump
Device related (nonmechanical)	Reservoir
Sizing errors	Cylinder aneurysms
Malposition	Tubing kinks
Erosion	Spontaneous deflation
Infection (periprosthetic)	Spontaneous inflation
Tissue loss	
Fibrosis	

past 5½ years, I have implanted the AMS 700CX device in 113 men, with only two mechanical complications: a tubing leak, and a cylinder leak.

PROS AND CONS

In spite of the recent development of alternative forms of treatment for men with organic, nonendocrine erectile dysfunction, penile prosthesis implantation still continues to be a prime treatment. It is appropriate for almost every man with an erectile disorder of this nature, and its success rate is better than 95 percent in experienced hands. A man can use a penile prosthesis with little or no interference in the love-making process. Long-term follow-up visits are not needed, and mechanical complication rates, which were high in the past, are acceptable with current prostheses and implantation techniques.

However, penile prosthesis implantation should be considered essentially irreversible. If a man is dissatisfied with a penile implant, it can be removed, and vacuum constriction devices and intracavernous injection therapy have both been successfully used in former implant recipients. However, it is far better for patients who are uncertain regarding their choice of treatment to try either or both of the nonsurgical options before proceeding with penile prosthesis implantation.

SUGGESTED READING

Carson CC, Robertson CN. Late hematogenous infection of penile prostheses. J Urol 1988; 139:50–52.
Furlow WL, Motley RC. The inflatable penile prosthesis: clinical experience with a new controlled expansion cylinder. J Urol 1988; 139:945–946.
Montague DK. Periprosthetic infections. J Urol 1987; 138:68–69.
Montague DK. Penile prostheses. In: Montague DK, ed. Disorders of male sexual function. Chicago: Year Book, 1988.
Mulcahy JJ. Use of CX cylinders in association with AMS 700 penile prosthesis. J Urol 1988; 140:1420–1421.

PHARMACOLOGIC ERECTION PROGRAMS

ADRIAN W. ZORGNIOTTI, M.D.

Pharmacologic erection has become an accepted alternative to penile implantation. Tens of thousands of injections have been administered or, more often, self-administered throughout the world. There have been very few reports of serious complication and the procedure appears to be safe and well tolerated, considering that actual use by patients is out of physicians' hands but not deprived of their overall supervision.

Informed consent should include a statement of risks and benefits and a discussion of alternative methods currently available for impotence: penile implantation, pharmacologic erection, microsurgical revascularization and veno-occlusive disorder "leak" surgery where appropriate, and vacuum erection devices. Of these choices, only pharmacologic erection programs (PEP) and microsurgery alter flow within the penis to produce erection. Advocates of implant and vacuum devices say that erection is achieved, but this is untrue.

Intracavernous injection, since it is less invasive, is preferable to implantation in patients who have intercourse infrequently. Many choose this in preference to the treatment alternatives if they have had a chance to try it and understand that it produces erection on demand. Penile injection is nearly painless and produces penetration in more than 75 percent of patients who become sexually aroused. In some centers, the patient is given an injection and then observed for erectile response in the clinical setting. It is important to insist on actual coitus, because some men obtain a pharmacologic erection by vigorous self-stimulation but not with sexual intercourse. These patients are then taught self-injection, only to be disappointed by the results.

PLAN FOR INTRACAVERNOUS SELF-INJECTION OF VASOACTIVE MATERIALS

Correct diagnosis through evaluation of the patient involves history taking, physical examination, tests of serum testosterone and prolactin levels, penile blood pressure determinations, and plethysmography (Table 1). Dynamic duplex ultrasonography, psychological testing, and snap gauge or nocturnal penile tumescence testing can be used when appropriate. Invasive arteriography and cavernosography are not suitable for patients in whom injection or implantation is planned.

Intercourse after injection precedes the teaching of self-injection. The patient is given the intracavernous agent and observed for 3 to 5 minutes. He receives a written reminder to call the practitioner after 4 hours, and if he manifests no untoward effects, he may leave the office at once to rejoin his partner, who must be available not more than a 30- to 40-minute journey from the office. Allowing about 3 hours for intercourse, the patient must report his results, and if erection persists make plans to return to the office for de-erection. About 6 percent of patients develop prolonged erection, which can become priapism if allowed to go untreated. Because of this, trial injections are best made in the early afternoon so that

Table 1 Evaluation for PEP

History and physical examination
Laboratory studies: serum testosterone and prolactin (specimen taken before 9:00 AM), fasting blood sugar, cholesterol, and triglycerides
Penile blood pressure determinations
Penile plethysmography
Penile ultrasonography with Doppler velocimetry
Intercourse trial

Other examinations:
  Psychological testing
  Nocturnal penile tumescence testing

Not indicated for PEP
  Selective penile arteriography
  Cavernosometry and cavernosography (with certain exceptions)

---

the practitioner can avoid emergency treatment at 2 AM.

If the patient obtained a full erection and was successful, he can be told it is reasonably certain that the problem is vascular and can be overcome by PEP, and that the venous outflow restriction mechanism appears to be intact. On the basis of his own observation, the patient can decide whether he wishes to learn self-injection.

If the practitioner has access to duplex Doppler ultrasonography, it is desirable to combine the trial injection with a dynamic study. This allows the practitioner to have hard documentation of the vascular status of the penis in the patient's chart for future reference. The study consists of measurement of corporeal arterial diameter before and after the intracavernous administration of papaverine. Blood flow velocities are also determined. As soon as the study is completed, the patient rejoins his partner as described above.

A certain amount of art is required to select the correct agent and dosage in patients with differing etiologies and degrees of vascular impairment. In general, 30 mg of papaverine hydrochloride with 0.5 mg of phentolamine mesylate or 5 to 10 μg of alprostadil (prostaglandin E_1 [PGE_1]) represent safe initial doses for most trials. There are exceptions: patients with impotence secondary to neurologic disease should receive much lower doses (5 to 10 mg of papaverine) followed by close supervision. This is true also for cases of psychogenic impotence or of acute anxiety in a newlywed who has failed to consummate his marriage.

If the trial is unsuccessful, it may be repeated, increasing the dosage or changing pharmacologic agents. An occasional problem arises when one dose fails to produce erection and a slightly higher one results in a prolonged erection. In such cases, it may be better to experiment with PGE_1, which appears to be more benign in the presence of prolonged erection, since this agent is metabolized by the corporeal tissues.

If several trials at intercourse are unsuccessful and if corporo-occlusive dysfunction leakage can be demonstrated, this may be corrected relatively easily by surgery. It may not restore potency, but it may make

it possible for the patient to then enter the pharmacologic program.

When there has been successful intercourse, the patient may wish to learn self-injection. Alternative treatments should be explained and an informed consent signed.

The patient receives formal instruction in all phases of the self-injection technique, including preparation of a sterile injection and injection at the base of the penis, avoiding the urethra, neurovascular bundle, and superficial veins. Injection into the corpus cavernosum is different from subcutaneous injection in several particulars: (1) it is not necessary to aspirate blood from the corpus before injecting; (2) to ensure that the corpus cavernosum is entered, the patient must be aware of the change in resistance as the needle passes through the tunica albuginea, and should inject only if this characteristic "give" is felt; and (3) the complication of fibrosis can be diminished by avoiding extravasation into the corporeal tissues. The injection should be into the corporeal spaces. If undue resistance is felt on the syringe plunger, the needle can be withdrawn for 1 mm, thus eliminating the resistance; free injection into the corporeal spaces then takes place.

A 10-ml multiple-dose vial is dispensed containing enough material for ten injections per month, or about two per week. These should be relabeled with an expiration date of 1 month. When the supply is exhausted or goes beyond the expiration date, a new supply is given. All solutions, except unmixed papaverine, require storage under refrigeration.

The patient receives ten single-use syringes, alcohol wipes, and printed instructions to supplement actual training in the penile injection technique. The following syringes are preferred:

1. 1-ml disposable allergist syringes with attached 27-gauge 3/8-inch needle (Becton and Dickinson No. 5541). With this shorter ultrasharp needle, the patient can insert it to the hub with less concern about injecting outside a small corpus.
2. 3-ml syringes (Becton and Dickinson No. 9585), which do not come with a needle. A 27-gauge 1/2-inch and a 30-gauge 1/2-inch needle are available. Both give satisfactory results, but the 30-gauge needle is delicate and should not be given to patients who are just learning the technique.

In the interests of safety, restriction to ten times a month is acceptable to most men. It may also be advantageous to experiment with the dosage to arrive at a minimum consistent with penetration. This may be difficult to explain to certain patients who equate success with the degree of stiffness, rather than successful penetration. If they are told that, by using the lowest dose possible, they will be prolonging the effective time that they will be able to do this, there is usually acceptance.

The patient reports monthly to obtain a new supply and to have his penis palpated for fibrous changes. At this time, modifications in medication can be made. Once or twice during the year, a blood sample for liver function testing is suggested. Minor changes in liver function can be detected with papaverine administration and do not appear to be significant.

COMPLICATIONS

Fibrosis

At this writing, complications are rare and usually consist of transitory pains in the penis or ecchymosis due to perforation of a superficial skin vein. After several months of injections, 4 percent of patients are found to have areas of induration of the penis that can be circumscribed, nodular, and nontender. These indurations do not always correspond to the site of injection. They usually do not interfere with continuation of injections, and some subside spontaneously. Subsidence is noted after discontinuation of injection. This has been identified as fibrosis and can interfere with penile prosthesis insertion. Treatment is not necessary, although the presence of fibrosis may be associated with the development of tolerance to the pharmacologic agent. There is evidence that these changes are inflammatory in nature, and the use of non-steroidal anti-inflammatory agents is recommended.

Prolonged Erection

This condition is not priapism and is usually seen with the first trial injection. It is rare to note this complication once the patient is established in a self-injection program. A patient who develops a rigid erection that does not subside should be treated on an emergency basis and seen within 4 to 6 hours of injection. This precaution should be followed unless the practitioner believes that spontaneous subsidence will take place. It is always better to err on the side of prudence.

The patient can be given 60 mg of pseudoephedrine to be taken orally to terminate an erection. If this fails, he should return to the office for de-erection, which involves irrigation of the corpora with 3 to 5 ml of phenylephrine solution (0.1 mg per milliliter in saline). This is followed by aspiration of both corpora, and can be repeated as necessary. The erection is converted into a tumescence, which will subside over the next few hours. Phenylephrine is preferred because it produces only minor cardiogenic effects, although systolic hypertension is a possibility. Dopamine, 1:3,000 in saline, is also effective. Metaraminol should be avoided for this purpose. Sometimes considerable patience is needed to de-erect a patient, but I have not found surgical intervention necessary in anyone.

How to Proceed with Prolonged Erection

First, place the patient supine and check vital signs. Note that the penis is probably pulsatile, indicating high flow. Prepare the penis and drape.

Second, take a 10- or 20-ml syringe with a "slip tip" (this is preferable to a Luer-Lok) and attach a 1 1/2-inch 21-gauge needle (a larger one is not required). Pull up 4 to 6 ml of phenylephrine solution (0.1 mg per milliliter of saline) and, with a quick jab, insert the needle into the base of the penis on the most lateral surface. Skin anesthesia is not necessary. Placement of the needle in this location will allow free passage from one corpus to the other through the septum that separates these.

Inject 3 to 5 ml of phenylephrine into the corpora, noting that the erection will be considerably stiffened. After 2 to 3 minutes the erection may detumesce by itself, and the needle may be withdrawn and pressure applied. It is more likely that this will not occur, and aspiration of the corpora should be begun one at a time. When the syringe becomes filled with unclotted blood, it can be detached and emptied without withdrawing the needle from the corpus, so that injection with phenyl-ephrine and aspiration may be repeated. Usually less than 30 ml of blood needs to be aspirated for the penis to de-erect but remain tumescent. At this point the needle may be removed and pressure applied for a few minutes. The use of 18- and 19-gauge needles is not necessary for aspiration of this unclotted blood; these also produce a hematoma, which the 21-gauge needle does not. A Coban dressing can be applied, but this is usually unnecessary and the penis returns to the flaccid state in a few hours.

The patient should be advised to avoid sexual activity, including further intracavernous injection, for several days. When prolonged erection occurs, a retrial can be performed with a lower dose. Sometimes a correct dose is elusive and, in spite of dose titration, an all-or-nothing result is obtained, so that either no erection or a prolonged erection is produced. This makes an implant a preferred solution.

IMPORTANCE OF SUPERVISION

The key to success lies in careful selection of patients, avoiding those who have normal function or are unreliable or psychologically unstable. Alcoholics with cirrhosis should also be avoided. The clinician must insist on continuing supervision with regular follow-up visits. Around-the-clock emergency response is important to confront the infrequent problems that may arise. The best-qualified practitioner to deal with the possible complications is the urologist who is willing to provide such ongoing supervision.

LIABILITY

Questions of liability should be carefully considered before embarking on a PEP. A frequent question concerns the use of FDA-approved drugs for unapproved purposes. The FDA does not come between the patient and physician, who is free to prescribe any drug whose safety and efficacy has been demonstrated and

Table 2 Formulary

Drug	Formulation	Recommended dosage
Papaverine hydrochloride*	30 mg/ml	0.5–2.0 ml
Papaverine hydrochloride	30 mg/ml	0.5–2.0 ml
+ Phentolamine mesylate†	0.5–1.0 mg/ml	
Alprostadil (PGE$_1$)	10 µg/ml	0.5–1.0 ml
Super mixture†		
Papaverine hydrochloride	10 ml	
30 mg/ml		
Phentolamine	10 mg	
Alprostadil	100 µg	0.3–1.5 ml
De-erection drugs		
Pseudoephedrine	60-mg tablet	PO
Phenylephrine (saline)	0.1 mg/ml	4.0 ml‡

*Does not need refrigeration; all others do.
†Stock solution.
‡Intracavernous.

has FDA approval. The corner drug store does not carry products for impending gangrene (papaverine), for pheochromocytoma (phentolamine), or for emergency treatment of a major cardiac anomaly in a neonate (alprostadil). For most practitioners, dispensing is the only way to supply these drugs to the patient, but the physician assumes responsibility for the outcome of treatment.

I believe that intracavernous injections for erectile failure are safe, provided that the patient is trained and supervised and does not abuse these. At the initial interview, many patients say they do not want a prosthesis, a fact that the prudent clinician should note in the chart for future reference.

FINANCIAL CONSIDERATIONS

A service has been rendered by teaching the patient how to self-inject. In addition, acquisition and preparation of the drugs needed and maintenance of a 24-hour response to emergency needs must be factored in. The practitioner will do well to consider what a penile implant or penile revascularization costs in arriving at a just fee for this service, which has quality of life as well as medical implications.

THE FUTURE OF INTRACAVERNOUS INJECTION THERAPY

The pharmacology of injected substances is undergoing change. Single- or two-agent formulations may well be supplanted by mixtures of multiple agents (Table 2). These produce erection in patients in whom the current injections have failed. At present, mixtures of papaverine, phentolamine, and PGE$_1$ are being tested. Multiple agents may activate smooth muscle relaxation more readily than single agents and provide a better erection.

SUGGESTED READING

Lue TF. Intracavernous drug administration: its role in diagnosis and treatment of impotence. Semin Urol 1990; 8:100–106.
Zorgniotti A, Lizza EF. Diagnosis and usuagement of impotence. Philadelphia: BC Decker, 1991.

ENDOCRINE DISORDERS AND IMPOTENCE

DONALD R. BODNER, M.D.

Impotence is defined as the inability to obtain and sustain a satisfactory erection to permit penetration and successful completion of the sexual act. It has been estimated that 10 million American men are impotent. In the past it was thought that the etiology of impotence was psychogenic in as many as 90 percent of cases. With a better understanding of the mechanism of erection and with newer diagnostic tests to assess erectile dysfunction, an organic cause can be found in at least 50 percent of cases. Since most cases of impotence are neither purely organic nor psychogenic but mixed in etiology, it is important to evaluate the patient with complaints of sexual dysfunction in a comprehensive and multidisciplinary approach to establish the diagnosis and determine the most effective therapy.

Along with vascular and neurologic disease, endocrine disorders are a major cause of impotence. In general urologic practices, endocrinopathies account for impotence in approximately 15 percent of patients being evaluated for erectile dysfunction. In endocrine specialty clinics, the incidence is higher, about 35 percent. Diabetes mellitus, a frequently treated endocrine disease, is a common cause of organic impotence. It is estimated that 15 percent of diabetic men between the ages of 30 and 40 years and 55 percent of diabetic men by age 55 complain of erectile dysfunction. Approximately 75 percent of men with diabetes for more than 10 years also complain of impotence. Impotence is a more common complication of diabetes than either eye or kidney disease, and impotence in diabetes mellitus can be secondary to a multitude of factors, including hyperglycemia and acidosis, small vessel disease, neurologic involvement, endocrine abnormality, medication, and psychogenic factors.

The causes of erectile dysfunction include general medical illness, drugs, alcohol, gross obesity, aging, endocrine abnormalities, neurologic disorders, vasculogenic disease, surgery, and psychologic factors. Endocrine etiologies can be found in patients with systemic illness, those taking medications or alcohol, obese or aging individuals, and those with defined endocrinopathic disorders.

Evaluation of patients with impotence that is thought to be secondary to an endocrine etiology should include a careful history and physical examination. The history should include the nature of the onset of the erectile problem. Was it gradual or sudden in onset? Can the patient obtain good erections with one partner or at certain times and not at others? A detailed list of medications and alcohol consumption is central in the evaluation. The age of onset of puberty should be elicited along with previous surgeries involving the testicles or hernia repairs, or any history of testicular infection. Change in vision should be noted. Physical examination should include examination of the size and consistency of the testicles, hair distribution, the size of the prostate, and the presence of perineal sensation and rectal tone. The abdomen should be examined for the previous surgical scars, the breast for gynecomastica, and the extremities for the quality of pulses. Visual fields should be tested when hypogonadotropic hypogonadism is suspected.

To evaluate the hypothalamic-pituitary-gonadal axis, in theory, serum testosterone, follicle-stimulating hormone (FSH), luteinizing hormone (LH), and prolactin levels are obtained. Studies have shown, however, that if the serum testosterone level is normal it is unusual to find an abnormality in this axis. Therefore, to minimize cost, serum testosterone test is made to screen for organic impotence. If the testosterone value is low, serum prolactin, FSH, and LH tests are made.

HYPERPROLACTINEMIA

Hyperprolactinemia is found in approximately 5 percent of patients presenting with impotence. Most of these are taking medications known to increase the serum prolactin, such as alpha-methyldopa, estrogens, phenothiazines, and reserpine. Treatment includes changing the medication when possible. A few patients with hyperprolactinemia have a pituitary adenoma as the source of the elevated prolactin. Diagnosis can be confirmed by magnetic resonance imaging (MRI) or computed tomography (CT) of the sella turcica. Treatment includes the judicious use of bromocryptine; only a minority require surgical ablation. The daily dosage of bromocryptine is gradually increased to a total of 5 to 7.5 mg. Gastric intolerance is the most frequent side effect of this medication. It is a rare patient in this group who needs exogenous testosterone.

HYPERGONADOTROPIC HYPOGONADISM

Hypergonadotropic hypogonadism, although rare, is perhaps the most common endocrine abnormality causing erectile dysfunction. A low serum testosterone level in the presence of elevated serum gonadotropins is diagnostic. End-organ testicular failure is responsible for this condition. Genetic abnormalities affecting sex development, such as Kleinfelter's syndrome (XXY), previous testicular surgery, trauma, torsion, or infection (e.g., mumps orchitis), can lead to this condition. Physical examination reveals atrophic or absent testicles. Treatment consists of testosterone replacement, which is best given intramuscularly because oral absorption is erratic. Replacement is best accomplished with testosterone enanthate, 300 mg intramuscularly every 2 to 3 weeks.

HYPOGONADOTROPIC HYPOGONADISM

Hypogonadotropic hypogonadism is a rare cause of impotence and may be associated with prolactinomas. Serum values of testosterone, LH, and FSH are low, while serum prolactin levels are elevated. Kallmann's syndrome of congenital olfactory-genital dysplasia can produce hypogonadotropic hypogonadism and has been associated with erectile dysfunction. Imaging the pituitary gland with either MRI or CT is central in the evaluation. Treatment consists of eliminating the causative factor when possible. If this is not possible or not desired by the patient, exogenous testosterone replacement should be instituted with testosterone enanthate as described above.

It is thought that thyroid dysfunction does not lead to impotence, but both hyper- and hypothyroidism have been associated with erectile dysfunction. An elevated serum testosterone level secondary to an elevated sex hormone binding globulin may be associated with hyperthyroidism. Decreased libido in the presence of elevated serum testosterone should lead one to suspect hyperthyroidism and check thyroid functions. When thyroid function studies are abnormal, endocrine referral should be made.

YOHIMBINE

Yohimbine, an alpha$_2$ adrenoreceptor blocker derived from the bark of the yohimbehe tree, has been considered an aphrodisiac in the Western world for many years, but only in recent decades have clinical trials of this agent been made. Double-blind, placebo-controlled trials with yohimbine have been limited. Giving one tablet three times daily to patients with psychogenic impotence does appear to be beneficial. Yohimbine's effectiveness in restoring potency in patients with documented organic impotence is less convincing and unproved. Further studies are warranted.

DISCUSSION

In summary, patients with erectile dysfunction should be evaluated by a multidisciplinary approach, because in those with endocrine and other organic causes there may be concurrent psychogenic issues related to the erectile dysfunction that must be addressed. Hormonal replacement should be instituted only when decreased levels of serum testosterone are documented and the patient has been adequately evaluated. Empiric hormone administration for the treatment of erectile dysfunction in the presence of normal serum testosterone and normal endocrine evaluation is not warranted. Hormonal manipulation is required in a minority of patients and should be reserved for those in whom a definite endocrine abnormality has been documented.

It must be remembered that in many patients with impotence, the etiology is mixed, and correcting the organic factor alone may be insufficient to restore satisfactory erectile function. These patients should be evaluated and treated in a multidisciplinary setting. When erections are not sufficiently restored by appropriate hormonal replacement, other organic therapies can be combined once psychogenic factors have been eliminated. These organic treatments include intracorporeal injection of vasoactive medications, the use of external suction devices, and the implantation of penile prostheses. Each of these treatment options is discussed in detail in a separate chapter.

SUGGESTED READING

McClure RD. Endocrine evaluation and therapy of erectile dysfunction. Urol Clin North Am 1988; 15:000–000.

Morales A, Condra M, Owen JA, et al. Is yohimbine effective in the treatment of organic impotence? Results of a controlled trial. J Urol 1987; 137:1168–1171.

Susset JG, Tessier CD, Wincze J, et al. Effect of yohimbine hydrochloride on erectile impotence: a double-blind study. J Urol 1989; 141:1360–1363.

VACUUM DEVICE FOR THE TREATMENT OF IMPOTENCE

ELROY D. KURSH, M.D.

The concept of using a vacuum to establish an erection is not new. In 1917 the United States Patent Office issued a patent to Otto Lederer for a device that allowed "persons considered to be completely impotent to perform sexual intercourse in a normal manner." The patent stated that "by creating a vacuum, the blood is compelled to enter the cavernosum, whereby the erection is produced. By means of the ring remaining on the root of the penis, an erection is maintained for a considerable time after the sleeve has been removed." Modifications of the vacuum pump have been patented since this original invention. Despite the fact that a vacuum pump has been available for more than 15 years, there was little if any acceptance for the device by the medical community until the last few years. I also doubted whether the pump could induce a satisfactory erection.

The vacuum pump (ErecAid System by Osbon) has been used as one alternative treatment for impotence in the Male Sexual Health Center for the last 18 months. After undergoing a thorough evaluation by a multidisciplinary team of physicians including psychiatrists, psychologists, and urologists, patients are classified as having organic, psychogenic, or mixed impotence. The comments made below regarding the vacuum pump are based on experience in over 40 patients in a study performed in a prospective manner (supported by a grant from Osbon) and the reported experience in the literature.

USE OF THE VACUUM PUMP

A number of vacuum pumps are currently available. My only experience is with the ErecAid System, a patented, FDA-approved device marketed by Osbon Medical Systems and commercially available by prescription. Like other similar vacuum systems, the device consists of a cylinder connected by a plastic tube to a hand-held vacuum pump. An elastic constriction band is stretched around the open end of the cylinder before it is used. A water-soluble lubricant is liberally applied to the lower abdomen, the base of the penis, and the cylinder opening to help create a tight seal between the vacuum pump and the patient. The cylinder is placed over the flaccid penis and firmly pressed against the body to create an air-tight seal. Air is removed from the cylinder by using the pump to create the vacuum, which draws blood into the corpora cavernosa of the penis. An erection-like state is produced in the penis in 30 seconds to 7 minutes, after which the constriction band is slipped from the cylinder to the base of the penis to help maintain the erection. It has been shown that penile blood flow continues, albeit at a reduced rate, while the constriction band is left in place. Upon removal of the band, the penis becomes flaccid again and penile blood pressure immediately returns to preusage levels. Because of concerns regarding complications related to ischemia, maintenance of the erectile state has been limited to 30 minutes. If more than 30 minutes of tumescence is desired by the patient, the constriction band should be removed for several minutes before the device is used again.

Reports indicate that 77 percent of patients achieved a penile longitudinal rigidity of more than 454 g buckling force, the minimum considered adequate by sleep laboratories. The amount of vacuum applied ranged from 175 to 380 mm Hg.

The erection produced by the external vacuum device differs from a normal erection in several ways. Men who have severe impotence with little or no spontaneous erectile capacity maintain tumescence only distal to the constricting bands. Therefore, the proximal fixed part of the penis remains flaccid, causing penile pivoting, which may make penetration and sexual intercourse difficult. The skin temperature of the penis falls an average of 0.96°C over 30 minutes owing to reduced arterial inflow. The vacuum and constricting bands cause congestion of the extracorporeal penile tissues, indicated by distention of the superficial veins, which establishes a larger circumference than that of normal erections. Although it has also been reported that the device makes antegrade ejaculation impossible owing to urethral occlusion, the sensation of climax is unaffected.

Although no corporeal fibrosis, penile gangrene, penile skin necrosis, or urethral strictures have been reported, use of the vacuum has been relatively contraindicated in patients with blood dyscrasias such as sickle cell disease. Because of concern over possible bleeding complications, it has also been relatively contraindicated in men on anticoagulants. Patients with impaired manual dexterity may also have difficulty using the device, but in these cases the pump can be employed by the partner.

EXPERIENCE WITH THE VACUUM PUMP

Experience has shown that the external vacuum pump produces an erection sufficient for intercourse in approximately 90 percent of men with impotence of a variety of causes. My experience and that of others has shown that there is a definite learning curve in gaining proficiency with the pump. Most men require at least four practice sessions and up to 1 month of use to get the device to work properly. Patients should be told not to be discouraged when they begin to use the pump.

Patients use the vacuum pump approximately four times a month, and 80 percent of attempts result in successful erection. There is a statistically significant improvement in the quality of erections produced by the vacuum pump during foreplay and intercourse over baseline levels. Not all the men use the pump for intercourse, and others do not use the device until after engaging in foreplay. The frequency of intercourse attempts is significantly increased in the early months of evaluation, but by 1 year it is not increased over baseline data. Significant gains are also noted in the frequency with which men are able to reach orgasm during intercourse and in sexual satisfaction, although the assessment criteria do not show a change in sexual desire. In general, results reveal an improvement in self-esteem but no change in levels of depression or anxiety.

Twenty-five patients engaged in various forms of sexual activity without the vacuum pump: masturbation (18 men), foreplay (23), and intercourse (19). Interestingly, the quality of erections of the 19 men who had occasional intercourse without the vacuum pump is noted as being improved even without the device, but the difference is not statistically significant.

Partners also report enhanced satisfaction with lovemaking. Women are able to achieve orgasm more frequently during intercourse, but like their spouses, their sexual desire remains unchanged.

The pump appears to have a relatively high degree of patient acceptance, my drop-out rate being only 21 percent. Most patients left the program after 1 to 3 months. This is in marked contrast to patients on a self-injection program (using varying amounts of papaverine and phentolamine) in whom a drop-out rate of 59 percent was noted. Reasons for dropping out include failure of the system, with complaints of insufficient rigidity or duration of erection to sustain intercourse (four men), or insufficient fixation of the base of the penis, resulting in pivoting (one man). One patient dropped out because of complaints of penile numbness despite the fact that the pump produced a reasonable erection. Some men also leave the program for reasons unrelated to the device, such as a relationship conflict or the recovery of spontaneous erectile capacity. The data indicate that the pump produced adequate erections in 47 of 52 men, or 90 percent of the sample.

ADVERSE EFFECTS

There are relatively few adverse effects associated with use of external vacuum devices. Ecchymosis of the penis, probably due to excess vacuum, has been reported to develop in 12 percent of users, and minor petechiae of the penile skin has been noted in up to 25 percent. Both of the latter problems were noted to be painless and to disappear without intervention.

It has been reported that urethral occlusion by the constricting band prevents normal emission of semen, with concomitant distention of the bulbous urethra. This has been considered to be the cause of painful ejaculation in a few patients. Contrary to previous studies, my own experience with the vacuum pump reveals that only 40 percent of patients variably experienced blocked ejaculation. Therefore, the data suggest that vacuum devices need not be prematurely rejected as a treatment alternative for couples who are trying to conceive. When blocked ejaculation occurred, none of my patients reported this as a particular problem for them.

Discomfort appears to be a problem primarily at the beginning of treatment: many report initial discomfort most often at the site of the constriction band. This usually subsides with continued use and experimentation. Discomfort due to too rapid pumping or too much vacuum can be easily reduced by slowing the process and stopping earlier.

A few patients complain of pain due to the suctioning of scrotal tissue or extraneous tissue from around the base of the penis; this tissue is drawn into the cylinder and trapped distal to the rubber constriction bands. It is therefore important that the inside diameter of the opened end of the vacuum cylinder should correctly fit the patient. When this problem occurs, it can generally be alleviated by placement of a plastic insert into the cylinder neck, thus reducing the inside diameter of the opening.

Although varying degrees of penile pivoting or inadequate fixation of the penis occur, only a few patients feel that this interferes with satisfactory sexual functioning. In men with mild or moderate impotence, penile pivoting can often be alleviated by engaging in foreplay before using the vacuum pump, in order to obtain a partial erection and fixation of the penis proximal to the constriction band.

Another drawback is that the device is cumbersome. The equipment may be somewhat difficult to transport. Use of the device and application of the constriction band may interfere with the naturalness and spontaneity of shared intimacy.

DISCUSSION

As life expectancy continues to increase, more couples express an interest in maintaining an excellent quality of life. There is increasing awareness and openness in discussing sexual dysfunction, which increases significantly with age. More and more men are requesting that something be done to alleviate their impotence and restore normal sexual functioning.

In recent years, much has been learned about the physiology of erection, and treatment options continue to expand. Medical therapy such as alteration of hypertensive medication or appropriate hormone replacement is possible in some individuals. Self-injection of the penis with vasoactive drugs has increased in popularity, and new agents are becoming available to reduce some of the potential side effects, making this a more desirable form of therapy. Some highly selected patients may be candidates for venous ligation or arterial revascularization.

The vacuum pump is a useful addition to the current arsenal of treatment alternatives for dealing with impotence. In planning any intervention to restore potency, a number of factors must be considered: patients' demands, partners' acceptance of the treatment, ease and versatility of use, and the effectiveness of intervention, which includes the incidence and severity of adverse effects and overall costs. Applying these criteria, the external vacuum device measures up extremely well, making it the least invasive, least expensive, and safest of the current medical interventions for impotence.

Patients should be given the opportunity to make an informed decision regarding the various treatment options. This is particularly applicable to the treatment of impotence as the therapeutic options continue to expand. It has been my experience that if patients are told the therapeutic alternatives in an unbiased manner, they generally choose to start therapy with the vacuum pump. The vacuum pump appears to be a logical alternative with which to begin therapy in most men whose impotence is due to irreversible organic factors.

SUGGESTED READING

Nading PJ, Ware JC, Blumoff R. Noninvasive device to produce and maintain an erection-like state. Urology 1986; 26:126.

Nelson RP. Nonoperative management of impotence. J Urol 1988; 139:2.

Witherington R. Suction device therapy in the management of erectile impotence. Urol Clin North Am 1988; 15:123.

Witherington R. Vacuum constriction device for management of erectile impotence. J Urol 1989; 141:320.

PSYCHOLOGICAL FACTORS OF IMPOTENCE

STEPHEN B. LEVINE, M.D.

The act of intercourse is a psychosomatic drama that involves a man's sense of self, his personal and his partner's requirements for arousal, and his physiologic capacity to sequester blood in his corpora cavernosa. Impotent men who consult with a urologist usually appear eager to be "fixed"; they do not want to be told about the complex interactions between body and mind, let alone about the psychological nuances involved in partner communications. Unfortunately, events that occur in the sexual arena are complex. The act of intercourse is psychosomatic. Many cases of organic impotence have important psychological contributants; many cases of psychogenic impotence involve subtle organic background factors. Instead of identifying and dealing with all the factors that contribute to the man's problem, physicians often behave as though the etiology of erectile dysfunction is simply organic or psychogenic. An evaluation based on such a belief is fraught with danger. The patient's wish for a simple solution, and the physician's need to deal with a busy office efficiently, can create a clinical process that yields a high level of misdiagnosis and ineffective treatment.

THERAPEUTIC ALTERNATIVES FOR PSYCHOGENIC IMPOTENCE

1. Provision of the diagnosis and a follow-up appointment.
2. Referral for psychiatric evaluation:
   a. as a consultant in case management.
   b. for subsequent care.
   c. for advice about use of organic intervention.
3. Referral for individual psychotherapy.
4. Referral for relationship therapy.
5. Suggested reading about the nature of psychogenic impotence.
6. Prescription of medication with a follow-up visit:
   a. yohimbine.
   b. trinitroglycerin paste.
7. Vacuum pump.
8. Intracavernosal injections.
9. Prosthesis.

KNOWING WHAT IT IS LIKE TO BE IMPOTENT: PERFORMANCE ANXIETY

My first step in treating an impotent man is to facilitate his trust in me. One of the ways this happens derives from my understanding of what the patient is experiencing as a result of his erectile dysfunction. I originally learned this from Masters and Johnson's 1970 description of performance anxiety and have had it confirmed hundreds of times. I now understand that most men who lose their erections experience performance anxiety no matter what the cause of their impairment may be. Performance anxiety is a vigilant preoccupation with the state of erection that keeps the average man from sensually experiencing lovemaking. Rather than giving himself over to the pleasures of touching and being touched, he thinks about the adequacy of his erection. The anticipation or dread of the loss of erection is highly destructive; it precludes arousal by substituting anxiety and inattention to sensation. The man with performance anxiety goes through the motions of lovemaking, instead of participating in a relaxed, sensual manner.

The adequate performance of intercourse is so highly valued as a male behavior that almost all men readily worry about the quality of their erections with a partner. The fact that an impotent man seems excessively worried about his performance is not, therefore, evidence that the etiology is psychogenic; diabetics with severe autonomic neuropathy can have just as much performance anxiety.

PREFERRED APPROACH: THERAPY AS DIAGNOSTIC ASSESSMENT

At the conclusion of an initial diagnostic assessment, I hope to be able to classify every case into one of four categories: psychogenic, organic, mixed psychogenic-organic, or idiopathic. I am typically alerted to the psychogenic diagnosis by one of two aspects of the history: a selective pattern of adequate erection formation and maintenance; a change in the man's social, vocational, or family life before the onset of the problem. However, sometimes I am required to see a man or a man and his wife for therapy before I can be certain to which of the four categories his case belongs.

Selective Pattern. The report of adequate erections during the night or early mornings, during kissing or petting behaviors, during masturbation, with certain partners, in response to magazines or videos, or spontaneously suggests a strong psychogenic component. When normal erections are periodically present, I look for an organic factor that might explain their inconstancy. Such factors include periodic substance abuse, medication use, or exacerbations of chronic medical diseases such as congestive heart failure or multiple sclerosis. When these are lacking, I consider the patient's age in relationship to his sexual drive manifestations.

Middle age has a dramatic influence on the psychogenically impaired man's ability to obtain normal erections. The diagnosis is easiest to make in young men because their drive, ease of arousal, and degree of responsiveness to erotic stimuli are great. Sexual neurophysiology slows as men become middle-aged. Their marital problems, vocational disappointments, and concerns over children compete more powerfully with the slower, less intense arousal, thereby making the typical selective psychogenic pattern of erections more difficult to discern. Particularly after the age of 55 years, a man's self-report of his erectile pattern is less reliable as an indicator of the cause of his erectile dysfunction.

Significant Social Changes. I have seen many psychogenically impotent men with initial histories of no adequate erections under any circumstances for many months. In making this diagnosis in men older than 55 years of age, I am therefore more heavily influenced by what has changed in the man's life since the onset of the erectile dysfunction than by his patterns of erection. If little has changed and adequate erections are rarely in evidence, I strongly suspect organic impotence. If much has changed before the onset of the erectile problem (e.g., job loss, divorce, wife's death, marital deterioration) and if there have been no adequate erections for months, I presume psychogenic impotence.

Dealing with the Uncertainty of the Initial Evaluation. The outcome of therapy is heavily dependent upon correct diagnosis. Organic and mixed psychogenic-organic impotence do not completely respond to psychotherapies, and organic treatments for psychogenic cases do not produce good results in most cases. When the diagnosis is uncertain, the process may be aided by a review of the history with the partner, a trial of psychotherapy, a sleep laboratory evaluation of nocturnal tumescence and rigidity, and home monitoring of these parameters. Invasive testing may not be helpful, since normal, age-adjusted data are not available, and reduced blood pressure or flow does not mean that other organic and psychogenic factors are absent. In the long run, I believe it is better for the patient for me to be uncertain than to be wrong.

THERAPY IMPLICATIONS OF THE TWO TYPES OF PSYCHOGENIC IMPOTENCE

My decision about the management of psychogenic impotence greatly depends upon whether the patient has primary or secondary psychogenic impotence. Men with primary psychogenic impotence have been consistently unable to have intercourse throughout their lives. They are a distinct minority in clinical settings that specialize in this problem.

The most prevalent form of psychogenic impotence develops after a sustained period of secure erectile functioning. Such secondary psychogenic impotence outnumbers primary cases by approximately 10:1. Psychogenic impotence is separated into these two broad categories because the pathogeneses, therapeutic tasks, and prognoses are very different.

Primary impotence requires long-term individual psychotherapy, has a poorer prognosis, and is usually associated with a major variation of sexual identity, such as paraphilia, gender identity disorder, or homosexual preferences. Occasionally, men whose histories suggest an entirely conventional sexual identity have primary impotence; like those men with gender identity problems, they have a limited motivation to have intercourse.

Mental health clinicians classify secondary impotence according to the psychological factors that have triggered the erectile dysfunction. Treatment recommendations and prognosis depend upon these factors. The following is a list of the five most frequent psychological triggers for psychogenic impotence:

1. *Deterioration of the Nonsexual Relationship.* The usual clinical recommendation is marital therapy, and the prognosis depends upon the interest of both partners.
2. *Divorce.* The clinical recommendation is usually for a brief, supportive therapeutic relationship to help deal with the continuing emotional pain arising from the separation and divorce, and the fears of emotional injury with the next partner.
3. *Death of Spouse.* A widower's impotence is usually treated with brief supportive therapy and generally carries an excellent prognosis.
4. *Vocational Failure.* This type of impotence often is self-limited and responds quickly when the work crisis is past. If the man has lost his job because of continued substance abuse or vocational incompetence, the prognosis for prompt recovery without psychotherapeutic intervention may be poor.
5. *Loss of Personal or Spousal Health.* Many physical illnesses may lead to erectile impairment through psychological responses to the alterations in life style and sense of attractiveness. Although a middle-aged wife's mastectomy may lead to temporary impotence, the fate of the couple's future sexual function depends heavily upon the reactions of both husband and wife. Brief couples therapy can be useful when impotence is precipitated by serious physical illness.

Two assumptions partially explain why some men become impotent and others do not under these five circumstances: (1) the impotent man expects that he should be able to perform sexually regardless of social circumstances; (2) he is unable to quickly label and understand his feelings, and his uncooperative penis expresses his feelings for him.

TOWARD AN UNDERSTANDING OF PSYCHOTHERAPY

Psychotherapies for psychogenic impotence are conducted outside the urologist's realm. However, the urologist is often the first to see the patient and make the referral to a psychotherapist. He may eventually offer an organic treatment if the psychotherapist fails to reverse the problem after a year or more of regular therapy. After consultation with the therapist, it is reasonable to treat men with chronic psychogenic impotence who have been refractory to psychotherapy with a vacuum pump, intracavernosal injections, or a prosthesis. However, the urologist should be alert for the man with chronic psychogenic impotence who requests an organic treatment as a means of avoiding psychotherapy. Such interventions have a high risk of not being helpful, and occasionally can be psychologically disastrous.

It is fortunate for many psychogenically impotent men that a complete understanding of the causes of the problem through psychotherapy is not necessary. Some men spontaneously recover from their problem within a short time without insight or therapy. Others respond to therapeutic suggestions that decrease performance anxiety. Some seem to improve in response to conversations that help them work through the social changes that triggered the symptom; others need to work through the earlier life events that set up the meanings of the recent life changes. There are also men for whom no therapy is sufficient to restore potency with a partner.

The adequacy of psychotherapy for psychogenic factors in impotence depends upon the psychotherapist's ability to perceive the emotional forces within the patient's life. The process of therapy strengthens or rejects the causal hypotheses generated during the evaluation; it continues until the patient is better or the clinician and patient agree that progress does not currently seem possible.

Therapy works by helping the man answer the question, "What caused my impotence?" To the patient initially presenting to the urologist, the diagnosis of psychogenic impotence means that he cannot have intercourse because of some problem in living. To the psychotherapist, it means the man does not feel safe in emotionally attaching to another person. At the end of therapy, both patient and therapist have a fairly good understanding of why the patient did not feel safe having intercourse.

It is important for the urologist to understand that secondary psychogenic impotence is the patient's way of resolving a hidden, unarticulated drama precipitated by events in his life. The inability of the penis to attain rigidity is a useful protective device created by a knowing part of the patient's psyche. This part is far more powerful than the man's social expectations for intercourse. The psychotherapist tries to help the patient to recognize the original drama, deal with it emotionally, and appreciate the dangers from which his mind is protecting him. Therapy removes the mystery from the situation and provides dignity by helping the man make sense of the problem at a deeper level.

PSYCHOGENIC IMPOTENCE FREQUENTLY HAS AN INCOMPLETE RESOLUTION

Although physicians love to see psychogenically impotent men who can be quickly helped, these cases do not represent the majority; there are many more men with secondary impotence who do not attain fast or complete symptomatic relief. Like all psychogenic symptoms, impotence can be difficult to resolve completely and permanently. Many men never entirely get over their problem. Many factors, such as the patient's fear of talking, the therapist's inability to conceptualize the cause, spousal lack of cooperativeness, and poor insurance coverage, can interfere with resolution. Even when conditions are ideal, the results may not be attained efficiently because resistance to conceptualizing the original drama must be worked through with patience, tact, and creativity.

This same general notion also applies to organic interventions for psychogenic impotence that mechanically restore penile rigidity: vacuum pumps, intracavernosal injections, and prostheses. At best, the intervention restores the mechanical capacity to achieve intercourse. However, the psychosomatic drama of sex occurs between two individuals and involves both their minds and their bodies. Mechanical therapy can be very useful when the other factors involved in the drama are lined up correctly.

Yohimbine or a small amount of vasodilator paste is currently replacing testosterone pills or injections as something the doctor can give the patient. This is face-saving for some men and functions as a placebo-like assist while they spontaneously get over their problem, but the urologist needs to consider that it may actually delay the patient's seeking therapy that might lead to a more efficient resolution. Referral from a urologist to a mental health professional or "sex therapist" is most readily accomplished if the urologist works regularly with the mental health professional and lets the patient know that it is standard office practice to ensure the best care possible for this problem. After working for 5 years with urologists, I am convinced that we do far more good for patients working together than in isolation.

SUGGESTED READING

Levine SB. Sex is not simple. Columbus, OH: Psychology Publishing Company, 1989.

Lieblum S, Rosen R. Erectile failure: assessment and treatment. New York: Guilford Press, 1991.

Schiavi RC, Schreiner-Engel P, Mandeli J, et al. Healthy aging and male sexual function. Am J Psychiatry 1990; 147:766–771.

INFERTILITY

AZOOSPERMIA

ROBERT D. OATES, M.D.
LARRY I. LIPSHULTZ, M.D.

Azoospermia, or absence of sperm in the ejaculate, can result from many diverse etiologic conditions, ranging from reparable obstructive disorders to uncorrectable intrinsic testicular failure. It is helpful to subclassify azoospermia as either "low"-volume ejaculate (<1 ml) or "normal"-volume ejaculate (>1 ml). This categorization defines and clarifies the primary causes for the azoospermia. Table 1, which is a compilation of the potential causes, shows clearly how important this breakdown can be. Further evaluation and the treatment strategies eventually employed depend on an accurate diagnosis based on clinical information provided by the history, physical examination, and laboratory data. This chapter concentrates on the surgical options available for the treatment of azoospermia.

LOW-SEMEN-VOLUME AZOOSPERMIA

Neurologic Etiologies

If the ejaculate volume of a properly collected semen specimen is repeatedly less than 1 ml, both anatomic and neurologic causes should be sought to explain the low volume (see Table 1). The patient profile may reveal an obvious "neurologic" etiology such as spinal cord injury, previous retroperitoneal lymph node dissection, multiple sclerosis, or diabetes mellitus. All of these disorders may result in an inability to ejaculate secondary to consequent neurologic impairment of the ejaculatory sequence. If such an easily recognized condition is present, it is important to obtain a postejaculate urine specimen to identify retrograde ejaculation. In this pathologic state, the seminal fluid travels from the prostatic urethra, where it is delivered and deposited by the ejaculatory ducts, backward into the bladder (retrograde) and not forward out of the urethral meatus (antegrade). Table 2 lists the steps necessary to perform an adequate analysis of this specimen. As can be

seen, there is no reason to catheterize the patient unless he also has a voiding disorder that precludes routine collection of the postejaculate urine. If it is diagnosed, retrograde ejaculation occasionally can be converted to normal antegrade ejaculation by pharmacologic therapy (Table 3). If this fails, the postejaculate urine–semen mixture is processed appropriately for intracervical or intrauterine insemination (Table 2). Surgical therapy is not indicated for retrograde ejaculation because it necessarily would involve major reconstructive surgery of the bladder neck region. Both anatomic (e.g., previous Y-V-plasty, previous transurethral resection of the prostate [TURP]) and neurologic (diabetes mellitus, pharmacologic sympathectomy) causes exist for retrograde semen flow.

When retrograde ejaculation is not present in

Table 1 Etiology of Azoospermia

Low-Volume Ejaculate (< 1 ml)

Neurologic	*Anatomic*
Failure of emission	Absence/aplasia of
Spinal cord injury	seminal vesicles
Retroperitoneal lymph	± congenital vasal
node dissection	agenesis
Diabetes mellitus	Ejaculatory duct
	obstruction
Retrograde ejaculation	Urethral stricture
As above "failure of	Retrograde ejaculation
emission"	Previous Y-V-plasty
Idiopathic	bladder neck
Pharmacologic	Previous TURP
Multiple sclerosis	Previous TURBN
Ejaculatory incompetence	

Normal-Volume Ejaculate (> 1 ml)

Nonanatomic (nonobstructive)	*Anatomic/Obstructive*
Primary testicular failure	Vasal
(High FSH)	Vasal occlusion, e.g.,
Germinal cell aplasia	vasectomy
Complete maturation	Vasal agenesis
arrest	
	Epididymal
Secondary testicular failure	Congenital malunions
(Low FSH)	Epididymitis
Hypothalamic disease,	Young's syndrome
e.g., Kallman's	
Pituitary disease	

Table 2 Detection of Retrograde Ejaculation: Postejaculate Urinalysis

1. Patient voids to completion
2. Patient ejaculates (masturbation or intercourse)
3. Patient voids again into sterile container as soon as possible
4. Unspun specimen is checked for presence of sperm; if present, steps 5–8 may be carried out
5. Specimen is immediately centrifuged at 300–600 g × 10 min
6. Pellet is resuspended in 1 ml of appropriate buffer
7. Mixture is analyzed for sperm density (per ml) and motility
8. If appropriate, insemination is performed. If insemination is planned, patient ingests $NaHCO_3$ tabs (650 mg × 4) qid × 2 days (to alkalinize urine component) and drinks 500 ml of water ½ hr before collection (to dilute urine component)

Table 3 Pharmacologic Therapy of Retrograde Ejaculation

1. Pseudoephedrine HCl 60 mg PO q.i.d. × 10–14 days prior to ejaculation
2. Ephedrine sulfate 25–50 mg PO q.i.d. × 10–14 days prior to ejaculation
3. Phenylpropanolamine HCl 75 mg b.i.d.–t.i.d. × 10–14 days prior to ejaculation
4. Imipramine hydrochloride 25–50 mg t.i.d. × 10–14 days prior to ejaculation

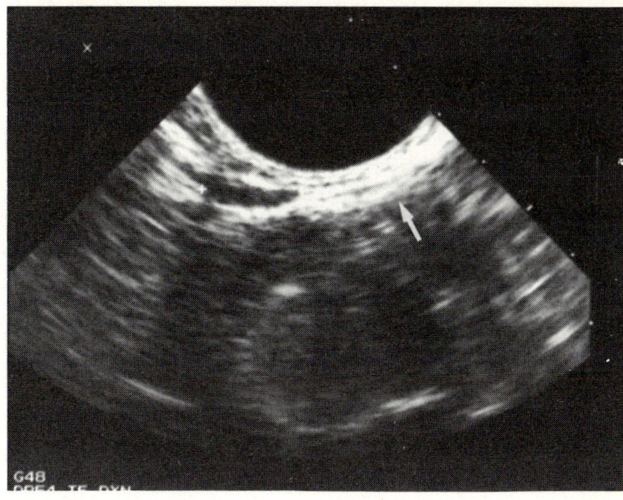

Figure 1 Transrectal ultrasonography (TRUS) (transverse image) demonstrating a thin, atrophic right seminal vesicle (cursors) and absence of the left seminal vesicle (the arrow points to the anticipated location) in a patient with CAV who presented with low-semen-volume azoospermia.

disorders such as spinal cord injury or retroperitoneal lymph node dissection, a failure of the entire ejaculatory sequence is likely. Emission, or the deposition of both seminal vesicle secretions and sperm-rich fluid from the vasal ampulla into the prostatic urethra, is under sympathetic neural control. When this innervation is disrupted, emission will not occur. Electrical stimulation of these structures by a transrectal probe has recently been shown to result in successful semen retrieval in 80 to 90 percent of patients so treated. Electroejaculation has therefore made possible the collection of sperm in the neurologically impaired, anejaculatory population, and numerous pregnancies have now been reported. Proper semen processing and spousal management are important to the successful attainment of pregnancy.

Anatomic/Obstructive Etiologies

If retrograde ejaculation is not present in the low-volume azoospermia patient, and if there is no reason to suspect a complete neuropathic failure of emission (e.g., no history of retroperitoneal surgery), an anatomic abnormality or distal ductal obstruction is a highly likely possibility. Transrectal ultrasonography (TRUS) most accurately defines these potential etiologies by precisely visualizing and characterizing the seminal vesicles, terminal vasa, and ejaculatory ducts.

Congenital Absence of the Vasa

Bilateral seminal vesicle aplasia or hypoplasia is often associated with bilateral congenital absence of the vasa (CAV), as both are manifestations of the same embryologic mishap that hinders the proper development of the mesonephric duct and its derivatives (ureter, seminal vesicle, vas deferens, ejaculatory duct, and distal two thirds of the epididymis). The combination of low semen volume, azoospermia, normal testicular size and consistency, and *nonpalpable vasa* on careful physical examination is diagnostic of this condition, and routine scrotal exploration is unwarranted. CAV is detected in 1 percent of the infertile male population. TRUS detects the distal ductal abnormalities in 80 percent and renal ultrasonography defines any upper tract anomalies in 20 percent of patients with CAV (Fig. 1). Epididymal anatomic malformations can be determined on physical examination if strict attention is paid to palpation of all regions. The caput is invariably present but the corpus and cauda epididymidis may also exist, either unilaterally or bilaterally. This helps in choosing the side to be explored at the time of microscopic epididymal sperm aspiration (MESA). Recent trials of MESA combined with in vitro fertilization (IVF), gamete intrafallopian transfer (GIFT), or zygote intrafallopian transfer (ZIFT) have clearly shown that sperm directly aspirated from the epididymal remnant are capable of fertilization and that pregnancy can now be achieved despite the presence of this hitherto untreatable disorder. Although not yet clearly defined, the probability of achieving pregnancy depends on a host of factors, including male and female baseline fertility potential, the length of epididymal remnant available, and the quality and quantity of sperm obtained. Early results indicate a 10 to 30 percent chance of conception per cycle. Obviously, there must be continual coordination and communication between the urologist and the reproductive endocrinologist/gynecologist, since the aspiration of the sperm must be performed coincident with oocyte harvest.

TECHNIQUE OF MICROSCOPIC EPIDIDYMAL SPERM ASPIRATION

On the basis of the physical examination or previous surgical findings, the side with the longest epididymal remnant is selected for exploration and MESA. The spermatic cord is anesthetized at the level of the pubic tubercle with instillation of 10 ml of 0.5 percent bupivacaine. The skin over the proposed incision site is similarly blocked. Coupled with small amounts of intravenous sedation, this generally offers sufficient anesthesia. The scrotum is opened in standard fashion and the testicle and cord structures are delivered into the wound. The epididymis is inspected to confirm the preoperative assessment. Usually, the dilated tubules in the most distal region of the epididymal remnant contain a thick, creamy fluid that is either slightly yellow or light brown. This material constitutes nothing more than debris and represents the degenerated sperm and epididymal secretions that are pushed to this region by the constant low-level flow emanating from the testicle and proximal epididymis. Proximal to these areas, there usually are dilated tubules that appear white or clear. With the epididymis pinched between index finger and thumb, epididymal tubules can be "pushed" upward, tight against the undersurface of the overlying epididymal tunics. This tunical tissue is carefully incised 1 cm with microscissors so that an individual tubule can be brought to the surface and isolated. A micro-bipolar forceps on low power is used to gently coagulate all bleeding points. In addition, the mesentery of the epididymis, which harbors many of the incoming blood vessels, can be squeezed to occlude blood flow and thus aid in the necessary hemostasis.

The selected tubule is incised longitudinally on its presenting surface for approximately 3 mm with a fine ophthalmology (Beaver) blade. Released, rapidly flowing fluid must be immediately and continuously aspirated into a 3-ml syringe with an attached 22- or 24-gauge angiocath plastic tip (Fig. 2). When the "squeezing pressure" on the epididymis is slightly reduced, the opened tubule will fall back and the margins of the incised tunics will form a crater from which the extravasating fluid can more easily be aspirated. When the plunger is at its limit, the tiny amount of fluid collected in the syringe is forcibly expelled into a sterile conical tube containing 0.5 ml of appropriate media, e.g., Human Tubal Fluid (HTF). The tube is kept warm (37°C) at all times on a formal warming tray or submersed in a temperature-controlled water bath. This first aspirate is also microscopically surveyed on a clean glass slide. If motile sperm are present, this tubule is repeatedly aspirated with the original syringe until it produces no more fluid (even with both proximal and distal milking), or until enough motile sperm have been extracted for whatever advanced reproductive technique has been chosen.

If no motile sperm are detected, a tubule 1 cm more proximal is selected and the procedure repeated. If the epididymal remnant is small (composed only of efferent ducts), squeezing the testicle itself may result in fluid flow from the *intra*testicular rete testis, which is in direct continuity with the *extra*testicular efferent duct tubules. This sperm may indeed be capable of both motility and oocyte fertilization and is therefore worth retrieving. Once collection is complete, all tubular incisions are approximated delicately with 10-0 nylon suture, while the overlying tunics are coated with 9-0 nylon. This

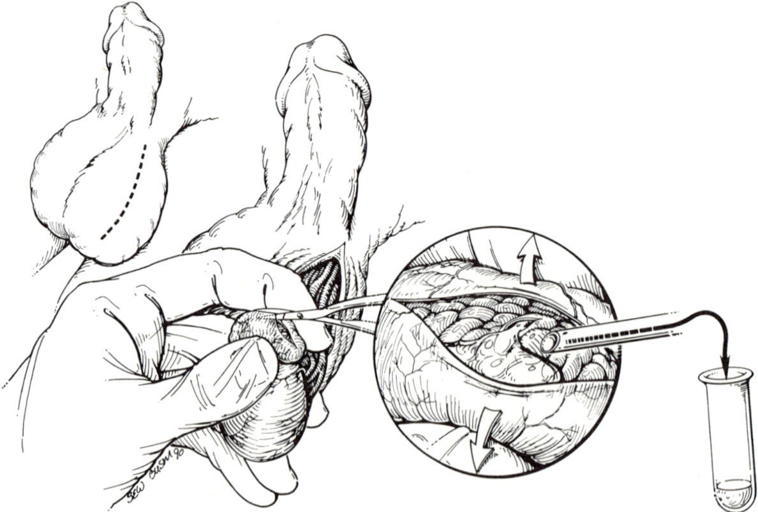

Figure 2 Technique of microscopic epididymal sperm aspiration. After isolation and incising of an individual, dilated epididymal tubule (*inset*), the streaming fluid is gently aspirated and placed into an appropriate warmed medium, such as modified Human Tubal Fluid (HTF) medium (Irvine Scientific), for later processing.

allows for possible re-exploration and reaspiration of this side if the couple do not achieve conception. The technical aspects of sperm recovery are important, but most crucial to the success of the entire concept is proper spousal management and proper sperm processing once motile spermatozoa have been obtained. This can be accomplished only in conjunction with an advanced reproductive program whose participants are well versed in manipulating substandard sperm specimens.

Ejaculatory Duct Obstruction

TRUS is also extremely useful in detecting the various anatomic abnormalities associated with complete and partial ejaculatory duct obstruction or stenosis. Since the ejaculatory duct (ED) is formed by the confluence of the duct of the seminal vesicle and the terminal ampullary region of the vas, an occlusion of the ED will result in diminished semen volume (70 percent of which is derived from the seminal vesicles) and also a blockage of sperm flow into the ejaculate. The regional anatomy, as defined by TRUS, can dictate the precise operative approach for correction: transurethral resection of the ejaculatory ducts (TURED).

TECHNIQUE OF TRANSURETHRAL RESECTION OF THE EJACULATORY DUCTS

TURED should be performed only when the diagnosis of ejaculatory duct obstruction is confirmed or highly probable. Ejaculate volume *must* be low, and either azoospermia or severe oligospermia may exist as well. TRUS may have identified a midline prostatic cyst, variably referred to as an "ejaculatory duct cyst," "müllerian duct cyst," or "urogenital sinus cyst." This cyst is immediately below the verumontanum (Fig. 3*A*). If such a cyst is identified, the operative approach is that of simple TUR of the verumontanum. With the standard resectoscope loop, only the verumontanum is resected. The cut into the prostatic substance, however, must be of sufficient depth for entering into and unroofing the cyst, approximately 0.5 to 1 cm (Fig. 4). The resection must not be carried distal to the most distal aspect of the veru for fear of inadvertent damage to the external sphincter. Once the cyst is entered, entrapped whitish fluid may flow instantly from the cyst cavity. Often a calculus can be visualized in the cyst, but removal is not mandatory. There is absolutely no need for routinely "scoping" the cyst. The ejaculatory ducts enter into the

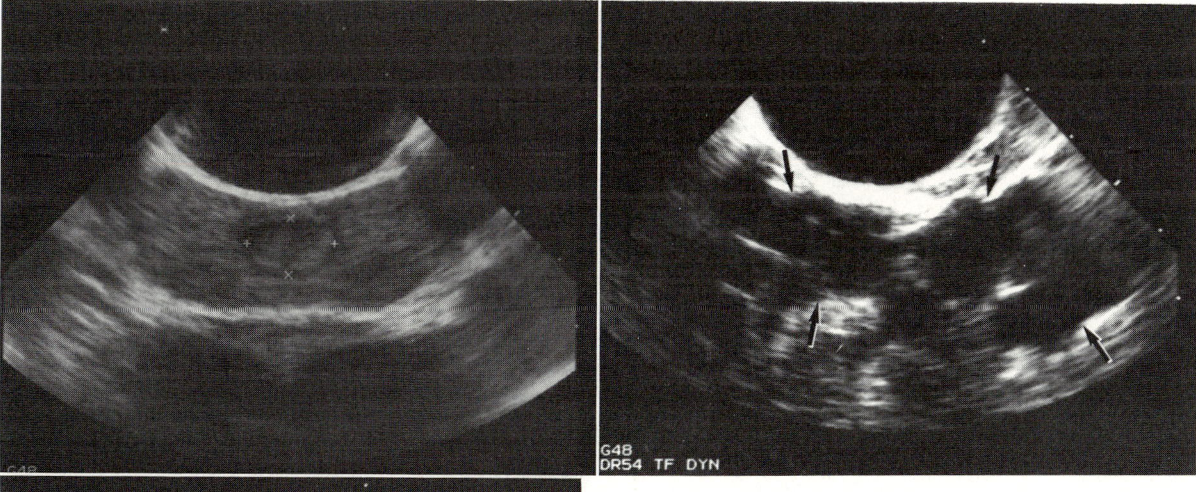

Figure 3 *A,* TRUS (transverse image at the level of the midprostate) demonstrating an enlarged midline cyst (cursors) filled with seminal fluid (seen churning within on real-time examination). This cyst resided immediately below the verumontanum, had each ejaculatory duct opening into it laterally, and was easily opened with transurethral resection (TUR) of the verumontanum. *B,* TRUS (transverse image at the level of the seminal vesicles) revealing massive distention of both seminal vesicles secondary to ejaculatory duct obstruction (outlined by arrows). No distinct borders of seminal vesicles could be established (contrast with Fig. 1). *C,* TRUS (transverse image at the level of the midprostate) displaying a dilated right ejaculatory duct secondary to distal stenosis.

cyst walls laterally, and if flow of seminal fluid is noted, the purpose of the surgery has been realized. However, the procedure to remove obstruction may be successful even though efflux of seminal fluid is not seen immediately. Only the subsequent semen analysis is confirmatory. The edges of the resected margin are lightly electrocoagulated and the resectoscope is removed. A urethral catheter is placed and removed on the second postoperative day. A semen analysis is performed 2 weeks later.

If TRUS has not defined a clear-cut midline structure but shows only suggestive evidence of ejaculatory duct obstruction with distended or enlarged seminal vesicles and/or dilated ejaculatory ducts (Fig. 3B, C), the operative approach is different. Depending on the level of confidence engendered by the history, physical examination, laboratory results, and TRUS, vasography may be helpful before TUR. Vasography is not used routinely, however, because any surgical transgression into the delicate vas deferens may lead to scarring and occlusion.

If vasography is in fact needed to help define the ejaculatory duct, operative magnification (microscope or optical loupes) is recommended. The scrotal vas may be isolated and a hemitransection of the vasal wall performed to expose the lumen; a fine ophthalmologic blade is helpful. This incision is carried only through the *anterior* seromuscular and mucosal layers. With a 22-gauge plastic angiocath tip placed in the opened lumen, 5 to 10 ml of a 50:50 combination of contrast agent and indigo carmine as the instillate is slowly injected distally (abdominally, as in Fig. 5). Vasography should *never* be performed in a "retrograde" direction to define the epididymis, as this may result in rupture of the thin-walled epididymal tubule and thus unnecessarily create an additional obstruction. After vasography, closure of the vas is performed with interrupted 10-0 sutures (mucosal layer) and 9-0 sutures (seromuscular layer). Alternatively, a thin angiographic catheter can be introduced through the vas and into the vasal lumen, but the potential for submucosal instillation and extravasation of fluid is much higher.

If the ejaculatory ducts are unobstructed, the blue fluid will pass easily into the prostatic urethra and bladder, indicating patency; no radiographs are necessary. However, if fluid flow is impeded, a formal pelvic x-ray examination will provide visualization of the distal ductal anatomy, often imaging a dilated ED as well as an absence of flow of the radiodense instillate into the prostatic urethra and bladder—classic vasographic findings indicative of ejaculatory duct obstruction (Fig. 6). With a cold knife, incisions in the prostatic floor from just distal to the bladder neck to just proximal to the verumontanum and just lateral to the midline are accomplished. These cuts should enter into the ejaculatory ducts as they course through the prostatic substance from their origin posterolaterally to their termination anteromedially in the prostatic urethra (see Fig. 4). Blue-tinged seminal fluid should be released if the obstructed ducts are successfully incised. Rarely, the vas will be seen to terminate well short of its predicted transformation into the ejaculatory duct, and no entrance into the ejaculatory ducts can be transurethrally achieved. This anatomic occurrence is most likely secondary to complete obliteration of, or maldevelopment of, the terminal ductal system. Again, light coagulation of all incised areas is accomplished and an indwelling urethral catheter left in place. A secondary

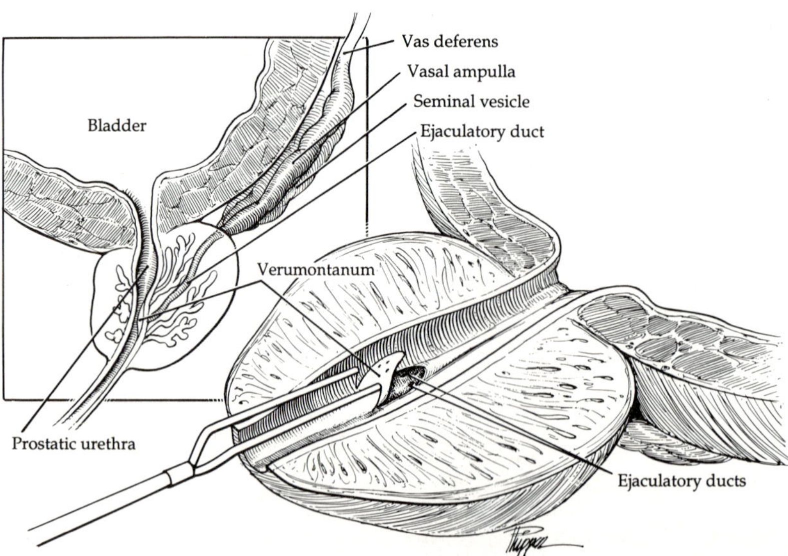

Figure 4 Technique of TUR of the ejaculatory duct in cases of obstruction in association with a midline cyst. The upper left inset demonstrates the course of a normal ejaculatory duct through prostatic substance.

epididymal obstruction may coexist and must be identified if the patient has return of adequate semen volume but remains azoospermic. In these instances, a routine microscopic epididymovasostomy will also be necessary.

NORMAL-VOLUME AZOOSPERMIA

Nonanatomic (nonobstructive) azoospermia is not a surgically correctable disorder and will not be considered further here. However, to confirm the diagnosis of primary testicular failure, a testicular biopsy is often required. "Normal-volume" anatomic (obstructive) azoospermia is obviously best treated with surgical therapy. Vasectomy, congenital malunions of the epididymis and vas, and occlusive sequelae secondary to epididymitis are managed with vasal-vasal or vasal-epididymal anastomoses, and the surgical technique is covered in detail in the chapters *Vasovasostomy* and *Vasoepididymostomy.* Azoospermia as a result of bilateral congenital absence of the vasa may be associated with embryologic defects in seminal vesicle development and therefore may be accompanied by low semen volume. However, the disorder can also be present in patients with normal semen volume if seminal vesicle anatomy is normal on at least one side. Surgical therapy is reviewed above.

TECHNIQUE OF OPEN TESTICULAR BIOPSY

Spermatic cord block is accomplished with 5 to 10 ml of 0.5 percent bupivacaine instilled at the level of the pubic tubercle. A small amount is injected into the skin of the scrotum and a 2-cm transverse incision made. The assistant holds the testicle and pushes it anteriorly so that it is tight against the undersurface of the scrotal wall. Most important, the epididymis must be palpated and kept in a posterior position to avoid inadvertent surgical entry into this structure. The incision is deepened through the dartos muscle, and finally the tunica vaginalis is encountered and opened the full width of the incision. Hemostats are appropriately placed on the edge of the tunica to help in retraction. With a No. 11 blade, a 1-cm incision is made into the tunica albuginea of the testicle. The seminiferous tubules that extrude are sharply excised and gently dragged across, or multiply touched to, a sterile glass slide, which is immediately cytofixed. The specimen is then placed into Bouin's or Zenker's solution for permanent section. Formalin should *not* be used, because the fixation is suboptimal for testicular biopsy. The edges of the opened tunica are lightly coagulated and closed with 4-0 chromic suture. A fluff gauze scrotal support and ice pack are placed. Good

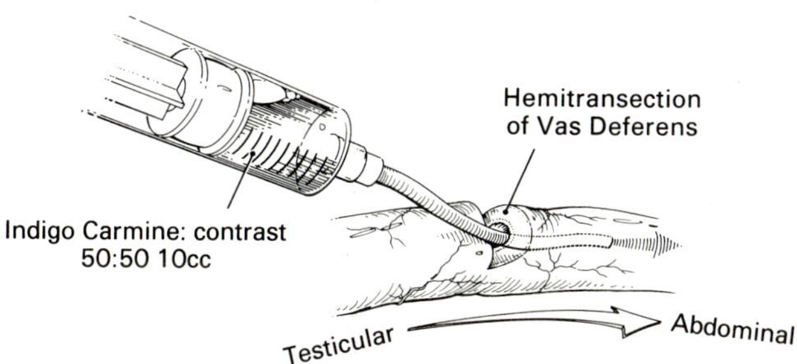

Figure 5 Technique of vasography. A 50:50 mixture of indigo carmine (to impart the blue tinge) and contrast agent is instilled into the vas after a transverse hemivasotomy. Injection is only in the "abdominal" and never in the "testicular" direction. Pelvic radiography is immediately performed.

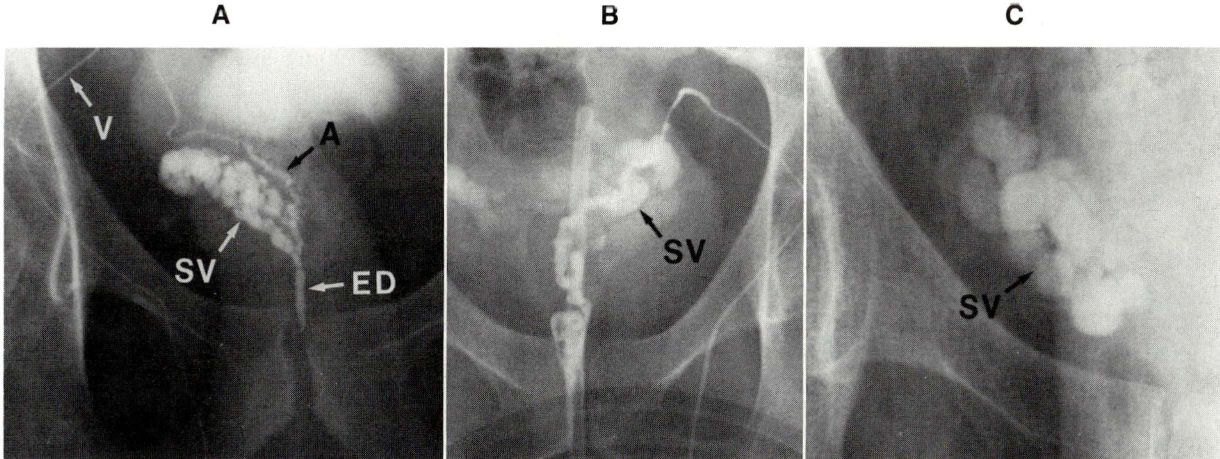

Figure 6 *A,* Normal vasogram. Clearly seen are the delicate vas deferens (V), the slightly corkscrew distal vasal ampulla (A), the normal internal contour of the seminal vesicle (SV), and the ejaculatory duct (ED). Contrast material is collecting in the bladder, indicating patency of the system. *B, C,* Abnormal vasograms. The seminal vesicles are seen to be enlarged (moderately in *B* and massively in *C*) and no contrast material is flowing into the bladder. Both *B* and *C* therefore exhibit classic vasographic findings of ejaculatory duct obstruction.

compression for 24 hours is crucial in preventing scrotal hematomas. If the ejaculate volume is normal, there is *absolutely no need* to carry out vasography at this time. If the biopsy is normal, vasography at the time of biopsy may seriously hamper any reconstructive surgery planned for the future.

SUGGESTED READING

Carson CC. Transurethral resection of the verumontanum for ejaculatory duct stenosis and oligospermia. In: Thompson W, Harrison RF, Bonnar J, eds. The male factor in human infertility diagnosis and treatment. Lancaster: MTP Press, 1984:191.

Goldstein M, Schlossberg S. Men with congenital absence of the vas deferens often have seminal vesicles. J Urol 1988; 140:85–86.

Jequier AM, Cummins JM, Gearon C, et al. A pregnancy achieved using sperm from the epididymal caput in idiopathic obstructive azoospermia. Fertil Steril 1990; 53:1104–1105.

Ohl DA, Bennet CJ, McCabe M, et al. Predictors of success in electroejaculation of spinal cord injured men. J Urol 1989; 142: 1483–1485.

Shangold GA, Cantor B, Schreiber JR. Treatment of infertility due to retrograde ejaculation: a simple, cost-effective method. Fertil Steril 1990; 54:175–177.

Silber SJ, Balmaceda J, Borrero C, et al. Pregnancy with sperm aspiration from the proximal head of the epididymis: a new treatment for congenital absence of the vas deferens. Fertil Steril 1988; 50:525–529.

ABNORMAL SPERM MORPHOLOGY AND MOTILITY

PETER N. SCHLEGEL, M.D.
MARC GOLDSTEIN, M.D.

Evaluation of the infertile man should include a carefully performed history taking and physical examination, laboratory evaluation of endocrine function, and a complete semen analysis. History and physical examination alone produce a presumptive diagnosis of the cause of infertility in over 90 percent of men in our practice. Endocrine function tests (serum LH, FSH, testosterone, and 17β-estradiol levels) are used to quantify the performance of the hypothalamic-pituitary-gonadal axis in men. Semen analysis results provide the best individual parameter to predict the likelihood of a man fathering a child.

The semen analysis should be repeated with separate specimens over a period of at least 2 months. We agree with many andrologists that a single normal semen analysis is adequate to evaluate fertility potential in most men. However, fertility is defined by the presence or absence of children in a relationship, not the likelihood of fathering a child in the future. So, despite having a low fertility potential, a man may still be considered "fertile." Similarly, a man considered to have normal fertility potential may not father a child by chance or other confounding (including female) factors. Therefore, a semen analysis evaluation does not automatically categorize an individual as infertile, despite abnormal semen parameters. Rather, an abnormal semen analysis provides the urologist with the indication that it may be necessary to intervene for an individual patient to improve his chances to contribute to a pregnancy.

Many additional laboratory methods for evaluating sperm function have been proposed, including hamster zona-free oocyte penetration assay, computerized sperm motion analysis, biochemical evaluations (ATP and acrosin content), hypo-osmotic swelling test, flow cytometry, and the human hemizona attachment assay. However, these additional and sometimes expensive tests have not yet proved of value in guiding the urologist in the management of infertility. The evaluation of men with a suspected immunologic cause of infertility may be aided by assays for antisperm antibodies. Our experience is that a carefully performed history and physical examination with endocrine testing and semen analysis provides adequate information to allow delineation of the likely cause of male factor infertility and to direct initial therapy.

SPERM MORPHOLOGY

The importance of sperm morphology in semen analysis is controversial. Several methods for determining the percentage of normal morphologic forms have been proposed, and many different criteria of normal semen values for morphology are used. Since the morphologic evaluation is subjective, great variability is seen between different technicians, even within the same laboratory. Some variables that may decrease errors in interpretation of semen morphology include the use of clean slides, preparation of very thin smears, and standardized fixation and staining techniques.

Standard criteria for evaluation of sperm morphology, as proposed by the World Health Organization (WHO), include only the presence of an oval sperm head, with no examination of sperm acrosome, neck, midpiece or tail defects, or cytoplasmic droplets. Not surprisingly, great intraobserver variation occurs with these criteria. Most laboratories in the United States use the standard WHO semen analysis criteria for evaluation.

Strict criteria for evaluation of sperm morphology has been predominantly used by research and in vitro fertilization (IVF) groups in the past. With these criteria, sperm are considered normal only if the sperm head has a smooth oval configuration with a well-defined acrosome covering 40 to 70 percent of the head, and an absence of neck, midpiece, or tail defects. No cytoplasmic droplets greater than half the size of the sperm head may be present. The normal sperm head measures 5 to 6 μm in length and 2.5 to 3.5 μm in width. Using these strict criteria, sperm morphology is the best predictive index of semen analysis for the likelihood of fertilization and subsequent pregnancy rates during IVF. If less than 4 percent of normal forms are present, fertilization is highly unlikely; if more than 14 percent of normal forms are present by these criteria, normal fertilization rates are expected.

Extremely rare, isolated disorders of men with uniform sperm morphologic abnormalities have been reported. These sperm may range from having no motility to having moderately normal motility, but the morphologic abnormality tends to be relatively uniform throughout the entire population of sperm. We have noted no pregnancies with these patients but recommend referring them for consideration in an IVF program. It is possible that fertilization could be induced with insertion of these morphologically abnormal sperm under the zona pellucida.

Unfortunately, there is no specific successful treatment for the typical patient with abnormal sperm morphology. As previously discussed, a careful search for correctable factors (such as varicocele, environmental toxins) should be performed in infertile men with abnormal sperm morphology to improve their fertility potential.

SPERM MOTILITY

Sperm motility is defined both by the percentage of sperm that are motile and by the quality of forward progression of that motility. Criteria for normal motility have ranged from 30 to 85 percent of sperm in the ejaculate. We have used a total of 50 percent of motile sperm in the ejaculate as our lower value for a normal semen analysis with forward progression of 2 on a scale of 1 to 4 (Table 1). Although sperm motility is not as good a predictive criterion of fertility potential as sperm concentration or strict criteria morphology, impaired sperm motility in a semen analysis may provide a sensitive clue to the presence of varicocele, immunologic factors, infection, toxic agents, or epididymal dysfunction that may impair fertility.

Table 1 Grading of Motility (Forward Progression)

Forward Progression	Description
1	Poor motility
2	Fair motility
3	Good forward progression
4	Excellent forward progression

Table 2 Potential Technical Factors That May Impair Apparent Sperm Motility During Semen Analysis

Excessive delay between production and delivery of specimen to semen analysis laboratory

Excessive heating or cooling of specimen during transport to laboratory

Contamination of specimen with K-Y jelly or soap during masturbation

Use of condoms containing contraceptive agents

Use of a container toxic to sperm (or containing traces of toxic agents, i.e., drug containers)

Excessive delay at laboratory in examining specimens

Collection and Processing of Semen Specimens

Unfortunately, sperm motility is also easily affected by a number of factors related to the collection and analysis of a semen specimen (Table 2). Semen specimens for analysis should be collected after 2 to 3 days of abstinence in a sterile container that has been previously evaluated and found not to affect the motility of normal sperm. The importance of complete specimen collection should be stressed to the patient, avoiding contamination with soap, K-Y jelly, or other agents used during masturbation. The specimen should preferably be procured in a room reserved for that purpose at the laboratory. If necessary, the specimen may be transported to the laboratory within 1 hour of ejaculation, with the specimen maintained as close to body temperature as possible (e.g., in the inner pocket of a coat). Some plasticizers may affect sperm motility, so the patient should be encouraged to use the standard container tested by the laboratory.

Some men are unable to produce a semen specimen by masturbation for psychological or religious reasons. These men should use a Silastic condom specially designed for collection of semen during intercourse without adversely affecting sperm quality. After analysis of a first specimen, the importance of following the specific guidelines needed for semen collection should be re-emphasized to the patient.

Oligoasthenoteratozoospermia

After potentially confounding causes of falsely decreased sperm motility in a semen specimen have been eliminated, the finding of decreased motility should be evaluated in light of the other semen parameters (Fig. 1). This allows for an important distinction between isolated impairment of sperm motility and a finding of impaired motility in conjunction with low sperm concentration and abnormal sperm morphology, the oligoasthenoteratozoospermia syndrome. Most commonly, impaired sperm motility is seen in conjunction with other semen

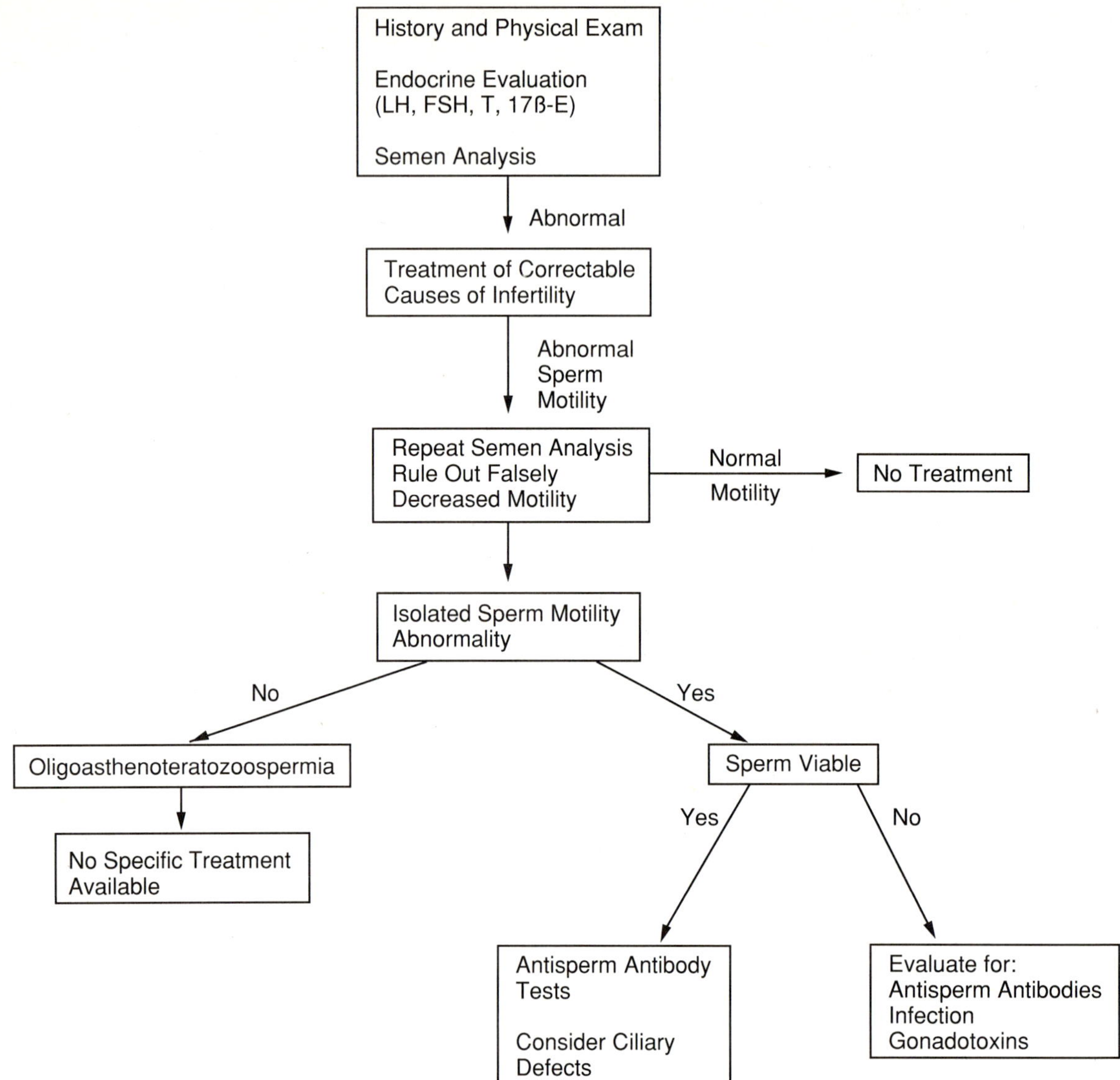

Figure 1 Algorithm for management of men with abnormal sperm motility.

abnormalities. As previously discussed, treatable causes of testicular dysfunction should be addressed. The prognosis for recoverability of function may be further assessed in these patients on the basis of serum levels of FSH, as well as the size and consistency of the testes. Other potential therapies for these patients are reviewed in the chapter on Oligospermia.

Impaired Motility and Necrospermia

Patients found to have isolated defects in sperm motility should also be evaluated to determine whether the sperm are viable, or if they are predominantly dead (necrospermic). Necrospermic specimens may result if the semen is contaminated with urine, if overwhelming infection is present, and in some patients affected by toxins. The presence of infection is evaluated by determining the number of white blood cells (WBC)

present. If these are elevated (>3 WBC per sperm or $>10^6$ WBC per milliliter), semen culture should be performed and specific therapy given for any pathogens isolated. In the absence of specific therapeutic indications, "shotgun" antibiotic therapy for men is discouraged because of the potentially detrimental effects of some antibiotics on fertility.

Contamination of semen with urine is uncommon and may be difficult to diagnose. It is occasionally found in some patients with diabetes. For these patients, neurologic dysfunction may cause poor bladder neck closure during ejaculation, resulting in an ejaculate partially containing urine or in retrograde ejaculation. This condition may be associated with increased semen volume and decreased semen pH, with otherwise unexplained poor sperm motility. These patients may be treated by alkalinizing the urine with Polycitra, 20 ml four times a day starting the night before the specimen is produced. They should empty the bladder just before masturbation, and catheterization may be necessary if significant retrograde ejaculation occurs.

Most gonadotoxins decrease spermatogenesis and decrease sperm counts as well as affecting sperm motility. However, some agents such as gossypol, the agent derived from cottonseed oil and used as an antifertility agent in China, may affect epididymal function without preventing sperm production, resulting in poor sperm motility.

Impaired Motility and Live Sperm

Impaired sperm motility with live sperm may be associated with antisperm antibodies, infection, caused by defects in the sperm tail, or by abnormalities in sperm biochemistry. The presence of sperm clumping in the semen specimen may be associated with immobilizing antisperm antibodies, or even infection. Most commonly, patients with impaired sperm motility and clumping have elevated semen levels of antisperm antibodies, suggesting an immunologic cause for their infertility. These patients often have an improvement in sperm function that parallels a decrease in semen antisperm antibodies. Isolated total lack of sperm motility, with viable sperm, strongly suggests the presence of sperm tail function abnormalities, the immotile cilia syndrome.

Antisperm Antibodies

We use the immunobead test to evaluate for antisperm antibodies. Some sperm motility must be present in order to evaluate whether the beads are attached to sperm or merely overlying sperm in the immunobead test. Binding to greater than 10 percent of sperm by beads is considered a positive result, and if associated with infertility, is an indication for treatment. The advantages of the immunobead test include the ability to differentiate immunoglobulin subtypes (IgM, IgG, IgA) present in sperm and to determine the location of antisperm antibodies on the sperm.

Optimal treatment for antisperm antibodies in men is controversial, because of the potentially adverse effects of treatment with high-dose corticosteroids. Case reports of aseptic necrosis of the hip, as well as the known adverse effects of prednisone on ulcer disease, have persuaded some clinicians to avoid corticosteroid treatment for infertile men. Alternative therapy involves referral of men with infertility associated with antisperm antibodies for IVF. We have encountered no significant adverse effects from corticosteroid treatment in infertile men on low-dose intermittent therapy. Previous reports of adverse effects are associated with long-term, high-dose corticosteroid treatment. Men who are candidates for treatment are given 20 mg of prednisone daily for 1 week beginning on the 21st day after the start of his partner's menstrual cycle. The maximal benefit of treatment is then achieved at the time of ovulation.

Patients are followed with repeat semen analyses and immunobead tests every 3 months and the prednisone dose is titrated upward to a maximum of 60 mg per day for 7 days a month, until pregnancy, improvement in semen analysis, or reduction in antisperm antibody levels is noted. Although some investigators have suggested that corticosteroid therapy is indicated only under investigational review board approval, we consider it appropriate to treat men with low-dose intermittent corticosteroids after providing them detailed informed consent.

Infertile men with varicocele have a higher prevalence of antisperm antibodies than infertile men without varicocele. In our experience, microsurgical varicocelectomy is highly effective in eliminating these antibodies. Unilateral vasal, epididymal, or ejaculatory duct obstruction is also associated with high levels of antibodies against sperm surface antigens. When feasible, repair of obstruction may be indicated, since it should result in decreased antibody levels.

Sperm Tail Defects

A defect in ciliary function may be suspected if there is a history of bronchitis or sinusitis with impaired sperm motility. The best recognized disorder involving these defects is Kartagener's syndrome, which consists of situs inversus, chronic sinusitis, and bronchiectasis. These abnormalities are attributed to an absence in the dynein arms from the nine microtubular filament couplets in the axoneme complex of the sperm tail. The lack of dynein arms leads to the nonmotile condition of the sperm and appears to be associated with the immotility of cilia in the bronchial tree, as well as the rotational abnormalities that result in situs inversus. Patients may have only minor defects of spokes of dynein arms, absence of central microtubules, or complete absence of the dynein arms, as occurs in Kartagener's syndrome. Therefore, the range of abnormalities in ciliary defects and associated clinical syndromes may be wide. The association between chronic sinus or bronchial disease and nonmotile sperm should lead the urologist to suspect a ciliary defect. The diagnosis is made by electron microscopic ultrastructural studies of sperm. Until recently, no treatment has been available to allow these patients to have children except artificial insemination or adoption. Recent advances in micromanipulation of eggs as part of IVF have allowed subzonal insertion of nonmotile sperm next to the egg and subsequent fertilization of those eggs with implantation, pregnancies, and live births.

Young's syndrome (epididymal obstruction associated with chronic sinopulmonary infections) usually presents with azoospermia. The epididymal obstruction is associated with sludging of viscous fluid in the epididymal tubules. These patients may be treated with vasoepididymostomy, usually to the caput region of the epididymis. Micropuncture aspiration of sperm from the epididymis in conjunction with IVF may also be effective for these men.

Sperm Biochemical Defects

Another purported rare defect in sperm motility has been attributed to a defect in protein-carboxylmethylase activity, an enzyme associated with changes in chemotaxis in bacteria. When no specific diagnosis can be reached and there is an isolated lack of sperm motility, a specific defect in sperm biochemistry may be postulated. IVF is a possible therapeutic intervention for these patients.

Empirical Treatment for Poor Sperm Motility

Several medical treatments have been proposed for the management of impaired sperm motility as well as oligospermia. These include systemic administration of agents known to be associated with increased sperm motility in vitro, such as kallikrein and caffeine, as well as the phosphodiesterase inhibitor, pentoxifylline. These agents, as well as drugs with endocrinologic action such as clomiphene citrate, have not been demonstrated to increase semen parameters or pregnancy rates significantly. Therefore, we do not currently advocate the nonspecific medical treatment of patients with impaired sperm motility.

Topically administered caffeine, pentoxifylline, theophylline, carnitine and acetylcarnitine, arginine, cyclic AMP, and kallikrein have all been shown to increase sperm motility in some patients. However, it is not well documented that the increase in motility is then translated into increased fertilization rates with these sperm. It is possible that some of these agents merely simulate the capacitation process rather than actually change the fertilizing potential of sperm. One of the agents, pentoxyfylline, is a fueradical scavenger and may therefore decrease the potential adverse effects of impaired or dying sperm on the potentially functional sperm. Other authors have cautioned against the topical use of methylxanthines on sperm because these have a known teratogenic action in animals. This teratogenicity has not been demonstrated in humans. We do not advocate topical treatment of sperm to artificially enhance sperm motility until this intervention is shown to translate into improved fertilization and pregnancy rates.

SUGGESTED READING

Amelar RD, Dubin L, Schoenfeld C. Sperm motility. Fertil Steril 1980; 34:197–215.

Gagnon C, ed. Controls of sperm motility: biological and clinical aspects. Boca Raton, FL: CRC Press, 1990.

Kruger TF, Acosta AA, Simmons KF, et al. Predictive value of abnormal sperm morphology in *in vitro* fertilization. Fertil Steril 1988; 49:112–117.

Schlegel PN, Chang TSK, Marshall FF. Antibiotics: potential hazards to male fertility. Fertil Steril 1991; 55(2):235–242.

Sigman M, Vance ML. Medical treatment of idiopathic infertility. Urol Clin North Am 1987; 14:459–469.

Note: page numbers followed by (*t*) indicate tables; page numbers followed by (*f*) indicate figures.

N